DIC	disseminated intravascular coagulation
DMSO	dimethylsulfoxide
DNA	deoxyribonucleic acid
DOT	(US) Department of Transportation
2,3-DPG	2,3-diphosphoglycerate
DRG	diagnosis-related group
DSTR	delayed serologic transfusion reaction
DTT	dithiothreitol
EACA	epsilon aminocaproic acid
EBAA	Eye Bank Association of America
ECMO	extracorporeal membrane oxygenation
ECV	extracorporeal volume
EDTA	ethylenediaminetetraacetic acid
EIA	enzym
ELBW	extre
ELISA	enzyı
EMAs	emer
EPO	eryth
FACT	Foun Cellu
FcR	Fc ga
FDA	Food
FFP	Fresl
FMH	fetor
FNAIT	fetal/ thror
FNHTR	febri react
FTA-ABS	fluor abso
G-CSF	gran
GalNAc	N-ac
GM-CSF	gran stim
GMP	gooc
GPIa	glyc
GPA	glyc
GPB	glyc
GPC	glyc
GPD	glyc
GTP	goc
GVHD	gra
Gy	Gra
HAV	hep
HAZMAT	haz
Hb	hen
HBc	hep
HBsAg	hepatitis B surface antigen
HBV	hepatitis B virus
Hct	hematocrit
HCT/Ps	human cells, tissues, and cellular and tissue-based products
HCV	hepatitis C virus
HDFN	hemolytic disease of the fetus and newborn
HES	hydroxyethyl starch
HHS	(US) Department of Health and Human Services
HIT	heparin-induced thrombocytopenia
HIV	human immunodeficiency virus
HNA	human neutrophil antigen
	antigen
	rogenitor cell
	resis (HPC, Apheresis)
	blood (HPC, Cord
	row (HPC, Marrow)
	tem cell
	tem cell transplantation
	nphotropic virus, type I
	fusion reaction
	ic syndrome
	ulin test
	Transport Association
	nesion molecule-1
	r individual donation
	n
	pha
	ta
	new drug
	malized ratio
	ogy reference
	ciety of Blood
	ganization for
	ocytopenia
	it
	nune globulin
	genase

LDL	low-density lipoprotein
LISS	low-ionic-strength saline
LN_2	liquid nitrogen
LR	leukocyte-reduced
MAC	membrane attack complex
2-ME	2-mercaptoethanol
MF	mixed field
MHC	major histocompatibility complex
MNC	mononuclear cell
MoAb	monoclonal antibody
MPHA	mixed passive hemagglutination assay
mRNA	messenger ribonucleic acid
MSDS	material safety data sheet
MSM	males who have sex with other males
NAIT	neonatal alloimmune thrombocytopenia
NAN	neonatal alloimmune neutropenia
NAT	nucleic acid testing
NHLBI	National Heart, Lung, and Blood Institute
NIH	National Institutes of Health
NIPA	nonimmunologic protein adsorption
NK	natural killer
NMDP	National Marrow Donor Program
NRC	Nuclear Regulatory Commission
NRF	National Response Framework
OSHA	Occupational Safety and Health Administration
p	probability
PAD	preoperative autologous (blood) donation
PBS	phosphate-buffered saline
PCH	paroxysmal cold hemoglobinuria
PCR	polymerase chain reaction
PEG	polyethylene glycol
PF24	Plasma Frozen Within 24 Hours After Phlebotomy
PPE	personal protective equipment
PRA	panel-reactive antibody
PRCA	pure red cell aplasia
PRP	platelet-rich plasma
PRT	pathogen reduction technology
PT	prothrombin time or proficiency testing
PTP	posttransfusion purpura
PTT	partial thromboplastin time
PVC	polyvinyl chloride
QA	quality assessment or quality assurance
QC	quality control
QSE	Quality System Essential
RBCs	Red Blood Cells (blood donor unit)
RFLP	restriction fragment length polymorphism
rFVIIa	recombinant Factor VIIa
Rh	Rhesus factor
RHAG	Rh-associated glycoprotein
RhIG	Rh Immune Globulin
RIBA	recombinant immunoblot assay
RIPA	radioimmunoprecipitation assay
RNA	ribonucleic acid
RPR	rapid plasma reagin (serologic test for syphilis)
RT	room temperature or reverse transcriptase
SCF	stem cell factor
SD	standard deviation or solvent/detergent
SNP	single nucleotide polymorphism
SOP	standard operating procedure
SPRCA	solid-phase red cell adherence
TA	transfusion-associated
TACO	transfusion-associated circulatory overload
TCR	T-cell receptor
TMA	transcription-mediated amplification
TNCs	total nucleated cells
TNF-α	tumor necrosis factor alpha
TPE	therapeutic plasma exchange
TPO	thrombopoietin
TRALI	transfusion-related acute lung injury
TSE	transmissible spongiform encephalopathy
TTP	thrombotic thrombocytopenic purpura
UCB	umbilical cord blood
UDP	uridine diphosphate
UNOS	United Network for Organ Sharing
USC	United States Code
vCJD	variant Creutzfeldt-Jakob disease
VLBW	very low birthweight
vWD	von Willebrand disease
vWF	von Willebrand factor
WAIHA	warm autoimmune hemolytic anemia
WB	whole blood or Western blot
WBC	white blood cell
WHO	World Health Organization
WNV	West Nile virus

Technical Manual

17TH EDITION

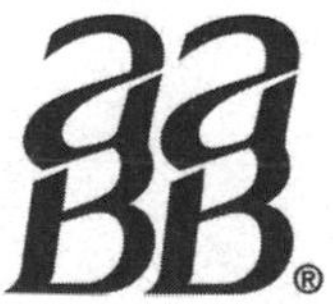

Other related publications available from the AABB:

Technical Manual and Standards for Blood Banks and Transfusion Services on CD-ROM

Transfusion Therapy: Clinical Principles and Practice, 3rd Edition
Edited by Paul D. Mintz, MD

Transfusion Medicine Self-Assessment and Review, 2nd Edition
By Douglas P. Blackall, MD; Priscilla I. Figueroa, MD; and Jeffrey L. Winters, MD

Blood Transfusion Therapy: A Physician's Handbook, 10th Edition
Edited by Karen King, MD

Practical Guide to Transfusion Medicine, 2nd Edition
By Marian Petrides, MD; Laura Cooling, MD; Gary Stack, MD, PhD; and Lanne Maes, MD

Transfusion Medicine Interactive: A Case Study Approach CD-ROM
By Marian Petrides, MD; Roby Rogers, MD; and Nora Ratcliffe, MD

To purchase books or to inquire about other book services, including digital downloads and large-quantity sales, please contact our sales department:

- 866.222.2498 (within the United States)
- +1 301.215.6499 (outside the United States)
- +1 301.951.7150 (fax)
- www.aabb.org>Resources>Marketplace

AABB customer service representatives are available by telephone from 8:30 am to 5:00 pm ET, Monday through Friday, excluding holidays.

Technical Manual

17TH EDITION

Edited by

John D. Roback, MD, PhD
Emory University Hospital
Atlanta, GA

Brenda J. Grossman, MD, MPH
Washington University School of Medicine
St. Louis, MO

Teresa Harris, MT(ASCP)SBB, CM, CQIA, CQA(ASQ)
American Red Cross
Washington, DC

Christopher D. Hillyer, MD
New York Blood Center
New York, NY

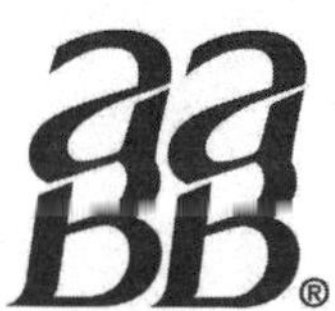

Mention of specific products or equipment by contributors to this AABB publication does not represent an endorsement of such products by the AABB nor does it necessarily indicate a preference for those products over other similar competitive products. Any forms and/or procedures in this book are examples. AABB does not imply or guarantee that the materials meet federal, state, or other applicable requirements. It is incumbent on the reader who intends to use any information, forms, policies, or procedures contained in this publication to evaluate such materials for use in light of particular circumstances associated with his or her institution.

AABB authors are requested to comply with a conflict of interest policy that includes disclosure of relationships with commercial firms. A copy of the policy is located at http://www.aabb.org.

Efforts are made to have publications of the AABB consistent in regard to acceptable practices. However, for several reasons, they may not be. First, as new developments in the practice of blood banking occur, changes may be recommended to the *Standards for Blood Banks and Transfusion Services*. It is not possible, however, to revise each publication at the time such a change is adopted. Thus, it is essential that the most recent edition of the *Standards* be consulted as a reference in regard to current acceptable practices. Second, the views expressed in this publication represent the opinions of authors. The publication of this book does not constitute an endorsement by the AABB of any view expressed herein, and the AABB expressly disclaims any liability arising from any inaccuracy or misstatement.

AABB
8101 Glenbrook Road
Bethesda, Maryland 20814-2749

ISBN No. 978-1-56395-315-6
Printed in the United States

Cataloging-in-Publication Data

Technical manual / editor, John D. Roback—17th ed.
p. ; cm.
Including bibliographic references and index.
ISBN 978-1-56395-315-6
1. Blood Banks—Handbooks, manuals, etc. I. Roback, John D. II. AABB.
[DNLM: 1. Blood Banks-laboratory manuals. 2. Blood Transfusion-laboratory manuals. WH 25 T2548 2011]
RM172.T43 2011
615'.39—dc23
DNLM/DLC

Technical Manual Authors

Colleen A. Aronson, MT(ASCP)SBB
James P. AuBuchon, MD
Jamie Blietz, MBA, CAE
Robert A. Bray, PhD
Stella T. Chou, MD
Laura Cooling, MD, MS
Geoff Daniels, PhD, FRCPath
Robertson D. Davenport, MD
Janice Davis-Sproul, MAS, MT(ASCP)SBB
Katharine A. Downes, MD
Anne F. Eder, MD, PhD
William P. FitzGerald, LTC USA (Ret)
Susan A. Galel, MD
Howard M. Gebel, PhD
N. Rebecca Haley, MD
Betsy W. Jett, MT(ASCP), CQA(ASQ)CQM/OE
Cassandra D. Josephson, MD
Jana Julleis, MBA, MT(ASCP)SBB
Diane M. Kadidlo, MT(ASCP)SBB
Ram Kakaiya, MD, MBBS
Melanie S. Kennedy, MD
Patricia M. Kopko, MD
Thomas A. Lane, MD
Regina M. Leger, MSQA, MT(ASCP)SBB, CMQ/OE(ASQ)
Jill Leonard, MT(AMT)
Sandy L. Liles, MT(ASCP)SBB
William B. Lockwood, PhD, MD
Christine Lomas-Francis, MSc, FIBMS
Catherine A. Mazzei, MD
Jeffrey McCullough, MD
Janice G. McFarland, MD
David H. McKenna, MD
John D. McMannis, PhD
Tania L. Motschman, MS, MT(ASCP)SBB, CQA(ASQ)
Theresa Nester, MD
Marilyn S. Pollack, PhD
Mark A. Popovsky, MD
Glenn Ramsey, MD
Donna M. Regan, MT(ASCP)SBB
Rita A. Reik, MD
Ira A. Shulman, MD
Bonnie L. S. Sink, BSN, RN, HP(ASCP)
James W. Smith, MD, PhD
Steven L. Spitalnik, MD
Simon Stanworth, MD, DPhil
Ruth D. Sylvester, Lt Col, USAF (Ret), MS, MT(ASCP)SBB
Alan Tinmouth, MD, FRCPC, MSc
Christopher A. Tormey, MD
Lance D. Trainor, MD
Phyllis S. Walker, MS, MT(ASCP)SBB
Jonathan H. Waters, MD
Connie M. Westhoff, PhD, MT(ASCP)SBB
Susan L. Wilkinson, EdD, MS, MT(ASCP)SBB, CQA(ASQ)
James C. Zimring, MD, PhD

Acknowledgments

THE 17TH EDITION OF the *Technical Manual* was the work of many dedicated individuals. In addition to the chapter authors, I would like to thank my three associate editors: Brenda Grossman, Teresa Harris, and Chris Hillyer. Their efforts and long hours in revising and rewriting chapters during the review process made my job immeasurably easier. Teresa, in particular, took the lead in revising the methods sections, a job she is eminently more qualified to undertake than I. If you enjoy the content of the 17th edition, all credit should go to the associate editors and the authors. Laurie Munk, Jennifer Boyer, Jay Pennington, and their colleagues are an unmatched publication resource. Their knowledge of transfusion medicine is encyclopedic, matched only by their grammatical acumen. If the text reads well, it is due to their efforts. Should you find problems with the 17th edition, however, the blame resides with me.

We would also like to acknowledge the members of the following committees and program units for their expert review of chapters, methods, and appendices for the 17th edition of the *Technical Manual.*

REVIEWING COMMITTEES

AABB Cellular Therapies Section
AABB Interorganizational Task Force on Domestic Disasters and Acts of Terrorism
Cellular Therapies Standards Program Unit
Cellular Therapies Accreditation Program Unit
Clinical Transfusion Medicine Committee
Circular of Information Task Force
Donor Center Accreditation Program Unit
Donor History Task Force
Immunohematology Reference Laboratories Standards Program Unit
Immunohematology Reference Laboratories Accreditation Program Unit
Information Systems Committee
Molecular Testing Accreditation Program Unit
Perioperative Accreditation Program Unit
Perioperative Standards Program Unit
Quality Management Standards Subcommittee
Quality Systems Accreditation Subcommittee
Relationship Testing Standards Program Unit
Tissue Committee
Transfusion Services Accreditation Program Unit
Transfusion Transmitted Diseases Committee

Finally, we would like to thank the editors, authors, and program unit members of the 16th and earlier editions of the *Technical Manual* for selected tables, figures, methods, and written sections of the chapters that could not be improved upon, and thus were used again in the 17th edition.

John D. Roback, MD, PhD
Chief Editor

Preface

THE EDITORS ARE pleased to present the 17th edition of the *Technical Manual.* This is the second edition to use the revised format, which includes listing authorship for each chapter. In preparing the 17th edition, we carefully considered the comments received after publication of the 16th edition, both from readers and from authors. Many believed that the new format was successful in bringing the necessary levels of expertise to the preparation of each chapter. However, they also suggested a number of changes that have now been incorporated into the present edition. For example, Chapter 10 was expanded through the addition of several pages of basic and applied immunology as a primer for later immunohematology chapters. A section on hemovigilance was added to Chapter 27 in keeping with AABB's expanding commitment to this important quality and safety activity. Another significant change was the inclusion of several "Key Points" at the end of each chapter, which should be useful for both students and experienced readers alike.

We believe that with the revised format a modest amount of author rotation is beneficial. Thus, for the 17th edition we recruited new authors for three chapters; additional authorship changes were also made for five other chapters. These changes should help to keep the text of the 17th edition fresh while also maintaining continuity with earlier editions.

One aspect of the *Technical Manual* that has not changed is the commitment of the AABB and the editors to extensive, multi-layered technical review. Each chapter was reviewed and revised at least twice by an editor. The chapters were also submitted to subject matter-appropriate committees for detailed content review (see list in Acknowledgments). All chapters were then subjected to additional regulatory, AABB standards, legal, and editorial review prior to publication. Finally, as noted above, many highly knowledgeable readers functioned as an ad hoc "post-publication" review committee for the 16th edition by bringing errors and omissions to the editors' notice. We have carefully considered each of the issues that was raised and where appropriate included revised text in the 17th edition. Because the field of blood banking, transfusion medicine, and cellular therapy is complex, detail-oriented, and continues to evolve, we once again invite all readers to contact us if they should find omissions, errors, and inconsistencies in the 17th edition, or if they would like to suggest ways to improve the next edition of the *Technical Manual.* We value your opinions and look to the readership for assistance in keeping this valuable resource up to date with our dynamically evolving field.

It is important for readers to realize that, in the opinions of the chapter authors and the editors, the methods chosen for inclusion in the 17th edition represent best technical practices. However, these methods are not the only approaches that fulfill the requirements of AABB *Standards*; readers may choose to use other approaches. Furthermore, should you find that any method or statement in the *Technical Manual* is in conflict with the *Standards*, the authority of the *Standards* supersedes that of the *Technical Manual.*

John D. Roback, MD, PhD
Chief Editor

Contents

BLOOD GROUPS

CLINICAL CONSIDERATIONS IN TRANSFUSION PRACTICE

TRANSPLANTATION

METHODS

Chapter 1

Quality Management Systems: Theory and Practice

◆

Tania L. Motschman, MS, MT(ASCP)SBB, CQA(ASQ);

Betsy W. Jett, MT(ASCP), CQA(ASQ)CQM/OE; and

Susan L. Wilkinson, EdD, MS, MT(ASCP)SBB, CQA(ASQ)

A PRIMARY GOAL of transfusion medicine, cellular therapies, and clinical diagnostics is to promote high standards of quality in all aspects of patient care and related products and services. This commitment to quality is reflected in standards of practice set forth by the AABB. AABB standards use a "quality management system" as the framework for quality. A quality management system includes the organizational structure, responsibilities, policies, processes, procedures, and resources established by executive management to achieve and maintain quality. (A glossary of quality terms used in this chapter is included in Appendix 1-1.)

The establishment of a formal quality assurance program is required under the Centers for Medicare and Medicaid Services (CMS) Clinical Laboratory Improvement Amendments (CLIA)[1] and the Food and Drug Administration (FDA) current good manufacturing practice (cGMP) and current good tissue practice (cGTP) regulations.[2-5] The FDA regulations in the *Code of Federal Regulations* (CFR) Title 21, Part 211.22 require an independent quality control or quality assurance unit that has responsibility for the overall quality of the facility's finished product and authority to control the processes that may affect this product[3] (see frequently used CFR quality-related citations in Appendix 1-2). Professional and accrediting organizations, such as the AABB,[6,7] College of American Pathologists (CAP),[8] The Joint Commission,[9,10] Clinical and Laboratory Standards Institute (CLSI),[11] and the Foundation for the Accreditation of Cellular Therapy (FACT)[12] have also established requirements and guidelines to address quality

Tania L. Motschman, MS, MT(ASCP)SBB, CQA(ASQ), Regulatory and Accreditation Manager, Department of Laboratory Medicine and Pathology, Mayo Clinic, Rochester, Minnesota; Betsy W. Jett, MT(ASCP), CQA(ASQ)CQM/OE, Chief Operations Officer, Department of Transfusion Medicine, National Institutes of Health, Bethesda, Maryland; and Susan L. Wilkinson, EdD, MS, MT(ASCP)SBB, CQA(ASQ), Associate Director and Associate Professor, Hoxworth Blood Center, University of Cincinnati, Cincinnati, Ohio

The authors have disclosed no conflicts of interest.

issues. The International Organization for Standardization (ISO) quality management standards (ISO 9001) are generic to any industry and describe the important minimum elements of a quality management system.[13] In addition, the *Health Care Criteria for Performance Excellence*[14] published by the Baldrige National Quality Program provides an excellent framework for implementing quality on an organizational level.

The AABB has defined the minimum elements that must be addressed in its Quality System Essentials (QSEs).[15] The AABB QSEs were developed to be compatible with ISO 9001 standards, the FDA *Guideline for Quality Assurance in Blood Establishments*,[5] and other FDA quality system approaches.[16,17]

QUALITY CONCEPTS

Quality Control, Quality Assurance, and Quality Management

The purpose of *quality control* (QC) is to provide feedback to operational staff about the state of a process that is in progress. It tells staff whether to continue (everything is acceptable) or whether to stop until a problem has been resolved (something is found to be out of control). Product QC is performed to determine whether the product or service meets specifications. Historically, transfusion services and donor centers have used many QC measures as standard practice in their operations. Examples include reagent QC, clerical checks, visual inspections, and measurements such as temperature readings on refrigerators and volume or cell counts performed on finished blood components.

Quality assurance activities are not tied to the actual performance of a process. Rather, they include activities such as the development of documents like standard operating procedures (SOPs) to ensure that processes are performed consistently and correctly, training of personnel, and qualification of materials and equipment. They also include retrospective review and analysis of operational performance data to determine if the overall process is in a state of control and to detect shifts or trends that require attention. Quality assurance provides information to process managers regarding levels of performance that can be used in setting priorities for process improvement. Examples of quality assurance activities in transfusion medicine and cellular therapies include record reviews, monitoring of quality indicators, and internal assessments.

Quality management considers interrelated processes in the context of the organization and its relations with customers and suppliers. It addresses the leadership role of executive management in creating a commitment to quality throughout the organization, the understanding of suppliers and customers as partners in quality, the management of human and other resources, and quality planning. The quality systems approach described in this chapter encompasses all of these activities. It ensures application of quality principles throughout the organization, and it reflects the changing focus of quality efforts from detection to prevention.

Juran's Quality Trilogy

Juran's Quality Trilogy is one example of a quality management approach. This model centers around three fundamental processes for managing quality in any organization: planning, control, and improvement.[18(p2.5)]

The *planning* process for a new product or service includes activities to identify requirements, to develop product and process specifications that meet those requirements, and to design the process. During the planning phase, the facility must perform the following steps:

1. Establish quality goals for the project.
2. Identify the customers.
3. Determine customer needs and expectations.
4. Develop product and service specifications to meet customer, operational, regulatory, and accreditation requirements.

5. Develop operational processes for production and delivery, including written procedures and resources requirements.
6. Develop process controls and validate the process in the operational setting.

The results of the planning process are referred to as design output.[13]

Once the plan is implemented, the *control* process provides a feedback loop for operations that includes the following:

1. Evaluation of performance.
2. Comparison of performance to goals.
3. Action to correct any discrepancy between the two.

It addresses control of inputs, production, and delivery of products and services to meet specifications. Process controls should allow staff to recognize when things are going wrong and to either make appropriate adjustments to ensure the quality of the product or stop the process. An important goal in quality management is to establish a set of controls that ensure process and product quality but that are not excessive. Controls that do not add value should be eliminated in order to conserve limited resources and to allow staff to focus attention on those controls that are critical to the operation. Statistical tools, such as process capability measurement and control charts, allow the facility to evaluate process performance during the planning stage and in operations. These tools help determine if a process is stable (ie, in statistical control) and if it is capable of meeting product and service specifications.[18(pp22.19)]

Quality *improvement* is intended to attain higher levels of performance for an organization either by creating new or better features that add value or by removing existing deficiencies in the process, product, or service. Opportunities to improve may be related to deficiencies in the initial planning process; unforeseen factors that are discovered on implementation; shifts in customer needs; or changes in starting materials, environmental factors, and other variables that affect the process. Improvements must be based on data-driven analysis; an ongoing program of measurement and assessment is fundamental to that process.

Process Approach

In its most generic form, a process includes all of the resources and activities that transform an input into an output. An understanding of how to manage and control processes in transfusion medicine, cellular therapies, and clinical diagnostic activities is based on this simple equation:

INPUT → PROCESS → OUTPUT

For example, a key process for donor centers is donor selection. The "input" includes the individual who presents for donation and all of the resources required for the donor health screening. Through a series of activities (a process) including verification of eligibility (based on the results of prior donations, a mini-physical, and a health history questionnaire), an individual is deemed an "eligible donor." The "output" is either an eligible donor who can continue to the next process (blood collection) or an ineligible donor who is deferred. When the selection process results in a deferred donor, the resources (inputs) associated with that process do not continue through the process but contribute to the cost of quality. One way that donor centers attempt to minimize this cost is to educate potential donors before screening so that those who are not eligible do not enter the selection process.

Strategies for managing a process should address all of its components, including its interrelated activities, inputs, outputs, and resources. Supplier qualification, formal agreements, supply verification, and inventory control are strategies for ensuring that the inputs to a process meet specifications. Personnel training and competence assessment, equipment maintenance and control, management of documents and records, and implementation of appropriate in-process controls provide assurance that the process will operate as intended. End-product testing and inspection, customer feedback, and outcome measurement provide data to help evaluate the quality of the product and to improve the process as a whole. These output measurements and quality indicators are used to evaluate the effectiveness of the process and process controls.

To manage a system of processes effectively, the facility must understand how its processes interact and what cause-and-effect relationships exist between them. In the donor selection scenario, the consequences of accepting a donor who is not eligible reach into almost every other process in the facility. For example, if a donor with a history of high-risk behavior is not identified as such during the selection process, the donated unit(s) may return positive test results for one of the viral marker assays, triggering follow-up testing, look-back investigations, and donor deferral and notification procedures. Components must be quarantined and their discard documented. Personnel involved in collecting and processing the unit(s) are at risk of exposure to infectious agents. Part of quality planning is to identify these relationships so that quick and appropriate corrective action can be taken when process controls fail. It is important to remember that operational processes include not only product manufacture or service creation, but also the delivery of a product or service. Delivery generally involves interaction with the customer. The quality of that transaction is critical to customer satisfaction and should not be overlooked in the design and ongoing assessment of the quality management system.

Service vs Production

Quality management principles apply equally to a broad spectrum of activities, from those related to processing and production to those involving the interactions between individuals in the delivery of a service. However, different strategies may be appropriate when there are differing expectations related to customer satisfaction. Although the emphasis in a production process is to minimize variation in order to create a product that consistently meets specifications, service processes require a certain degree of flexibility to address customer needs and circumstances at the time of the transaction. In production, personnel need to know how to maintain uniformity in the day-to-day operation. In service, personnel need to be able to adapt the service in a way that meets customer expectations but does not compromise quality. To do this, personnel must have sufficient knowledge and understanding of interrelated processes to use independent judgment appropriately, or they must have ready access to higher-level decision-makers. When one designs quality management systems for production processes, it is useful to think of the process as the driver, with people providing the oversight and support needed to keep it running smoothly and effectively. In service, people are the focus; the underlying process provides a foundation that enables staff to deliver safe and effective services that meet the needs of the customers in almost any situation.

Quality Management as an Evolving Science

The principles and tools that are used in quality management today will change as research provides new knowledge of organizational behavior, as technology provides new solutions, and as the field of transfusion medicine and cellular therapies presents new challenges. Periodic assessments of the quality management system will help identify practices that are no longer effective or that could be improved through the use of new technology or new tools.

PRACTICAL APPLICATION OF QUALITY MANAGEMENT PRINCIPLES

The remainder of this chapter discusses the elements of a quality management system and practical application of quality management principles to the transfusion medicine, cellular therapies, or clinical diagnostics environments. These basic elements include the following:

- Organization and leadership.
- Customer focus.
- Facilities, work environment, and safety.
- Human resources.
- Suppliers and materials management.
- Equipment management.
- Process management.
- Documents and records.
- Information management.
- Management of nonconforming events.
- Monitoring and assessment.
- Process improvement.

Organization and Leadership

The facility should be organized in a manner that promotes effective implementation and management of its operational and quality management system. The structure of the organization must be documented, and the roles and responsibilities for the provision of tests, products, and services must be clearly defined. These provisions should include a description of the relationships and avenues of communication between organizational units and those responsible for key quality functions. Each facility may define its structure in any format that suits its operations. Organizational trees or charts that show the structure and relationships are helpful.

The facility should define in writing the authority and responsibilities of executive management to establish and maintain the quality management system. These responsibilities include the following:

- Establishing a quality policy and associated quality goals and quality objectives.
- Providing adequate facilities as well as human, equipment, and material resources to carry out the operations of the facility and the quality management system.
- Ensuring design and effective implementation of new or modified processes and procedures.
- Participating in the review and approval of quality and technical policies, processes, and procedures.
- Enforcing adherence to operational and quality policies, processes, and procedures.
- Overseeing operations and regulatory and accreditation compliance.
- Periodically providing review and assessment of quality management system effectiveness.

Executive management support for the quality management system goals, objectives, and policies is critical to the success of the program. Executive management needs to communicate its commitment to quality and create an organizational culture in which quality principles can grow and flourish.

The individual designated to oversee the facility's quality functions should report directly to management. In addition to having the responsibility to coordinate, monitor, and facilitate quality system activities, this person has the authority to recommend and initiate corrective action when appropriate.[5] The designated individual need not perform all of the quality functions personally. Ideally, this person should be independent of the facility's operational functions. In small facilities, this independence may not always be possible and may require some creativity. Depending on the size and scope of the organization, the designated oversight person may work in the transfusion service, may have laboratory-wide responsibilities, may have a staff of workers (eg, a quality unit), or may be part of an organization-wide quality unit (eg, hospital quality or risk management). Individuals with dual quality and operational responsibilities should not provide quality oversight for operational work they have performed (see 21 CFR 211.194).[3]

Quality oversight functions may include the following[5]:

- Review and approval of SOPs and training plans.
- Review and approval of validation plans and results.
- Review and approval of document control and record-keeping systems.
- Audit of operational functions.
- Development of criteria for evaluating systems.
- Review and approval of suppliers.

- Review and approval of product and service specifications (eg, the requirements to be met in the manufacture, distribution, or administration of blood components, cellular therapy products, tissue, and derivatives).
- Review of reports of adverse reactions, of deviations in the manufacturing process, of nonconforming products and services, and of customer complaints.
- Participation in decisions to determine if blood components, cellular therapy products, tissue, derivatives, and services are suitable for use, distribution, or recall.
- Review and approval of corrective action plans.
- Surveillance of problems (eg, event or incident reports, Form FDA 483 observations, or customer complaints) and the effectiveness of corrective actions implemented to solve those problems.
- Use of data resources to identify trends and potential problems before a situation worsens and patients and/or products are affected.
- Preparation of periodic (as specified by the organization) reports of quality issues, trends, findings, and corrective and preventive actions.

Quality oversight functions may be shared among existing staff, departments, and facilities or, in some instances, may be contracted to an outside firm. The goal is to provide as much of an independent evaluation of the facility's quality activities as possible. Policies, processes, and procedures should exist to define the roles and responsibilities of all individuals in the development and maintenance of these quality goals. Quality management system policies and processes should be applicable across the entire facility. A blood bank, tissue bank, transfusion service, or cellular therapy product service need not develop its own quality policies if it is part of a larger entity whose quality management system addresses all of the minimum requirements. The quality management system should address all matters related to compliance with federal, state, and local regulations and accreditation standards that are applicable to the organization.

Customer Focus

A primary focus for any organization interested in quality is serving the needs of its customers. Customers have a variety of needs and expectations. The most appropriate way to ensure that these needs and expectations are met is for the facility and its customer to define them in an agreement, a contract, or another documented format. Additional information on agreements can be found in the "Suppliers and Materials Management" section.

When planning for new or changed products or services, the customer's needs and expectations should be taken into account. If these changes are determined to be critical to the quality or effectiveness of the products and services provided by the facility, they should be incorporated into the product or service specifications as customer requirements. The facility must have a process to manage the needs and expectations that are not met. For example, for a facility that has agreed to provide daily delivery of leukocyte-reduced components to one of its customers, processing components in a manner that ensures adequate leukocyte removal is critical to the quality of this product. Such an expectation should be incorporated into the product specifications. However, daily delivery of products is a customer need and expectation, but it is not critical to the quality of the manufactured product. The facility should have a process to manage this agreed-upon expectation and to ensure that the product delivery mechanism meets this customer need. If this need cannot be met, the facility should have a process to address this failure.

Once agreements have been made between the facility and its customers, there should be a means to obtain feedback from the customer to ensure that the facility is meeting the customer's expectations. Mechanisms for obtaining such feedback proactively include satisfaction surveys and periodic review of agreements. Reactive feedback is obtained through customer complaints. A review of event data may also indicate failures to meet customer needs and expectations. Data obtained through these mechanisms should be evaluated, and appropriate follow-up action must be taken. One such action could be to change the agreement. Inadequately addressing customer concerns or failing to meet expectations may result in loss of the customer.

Facilities, Work Environment, and Safety

The facility should provide a safe workplace with adequate environmental controls and emergency procedures for the safety of the patients, donors, staff, and visitors. Space allocation, building utilities, and the communication infrastructure should adequately support the activities of the facility. The facility should be kept clean and well maintained so that the products and services provided are not compromised. Procedures should be in place to address the following:

- General safety.
- Disaster preparedness, response, and recovery.
- Biological safety (blood-borne pathogens).
- Chemical safety.
- Fire safety.
- Radiation safety, if applicable.
- Discard of biologic and other hazardous substances.

cGMP regulations require quality planning and control of the physical work environment, including the following:

- Adequate space and ventilation.
- Sanitation and trash disposal.
- Equipment for controlling air quality and pressure, humidity, and temperature.
- Water systems.
- Toilet and hand-washing facilities.

An evaluation of the infrastructure and its limitations before implementation of procedures or installation of equipment will help to ensure maximum efficiency and safety. A more thorough discussion of facilities and safety can be found in Chapter 2.

Human Resources

This element of the quality management system is aimed at management of personnel, including selection, orientation, training, competence assessment, and staffing.

Selection

Each facility should have a process to provide adequate numbers of qualified personnel to perform, verify, and manage all activities in the facility. Qualification requirements are determined on the basis of job responsibilities. The selection process should consider the applicant's qualifications for a particular position as determined by education, training, experience, certifications, licensure, or a combination of them. For laboratory testing staff, the standards for personnel qualifications should be compatible with the regulatory requirements established under CLIA.[1] Job descriptions are required for all personnel involved in processes and procedures that affect the quality of tests, products, and services. Effective job descriptions clearly define the qualifications and responsibilities of the positions as well as the reporting relationships they involve.

Orientation, Training, and Competence Assessment

Once hired, employees should be oriented to their position and to the organization's policies and procedures. The orientation program should include facility-specific requirements and an introduction to policies that address issues such as safety, quality, computers, security, and confidentiality. The job-related portion of the orientation program covers the operational issues specific to the work area. Training should be provided for each procedure for which employees have responsibility. The ultimate result of the orientation and training program is to deem new employees competent to work independently in performing the duties and responsibilities defined in their job descriptions. Time frames should be established to accomplish this goal. Before the introduction of a new test or service, existing personnel should be trained to perform their newly assigned duties and must be deemed competent. During orientation and training, the employee should be given the opportunity to ask questions and to seek additional help or clarification. All aspects of the training should be documented, and the facility trainer or designated facility management representative and the employee should mutually agree about the determination of competence.

FDA cGMP training is required for staff involved in the manufacture of blood and blood components.[3] Likewise, cGTP training is required for personnel involved in activities for human cells, tissue, and cellular and tissue-based products (HCT/Ps).[4] Such training should provide staff with an understanding of the regulatory basis for the facility's policies and procedures as well as the specific application of the cGMP and cGTP requirements as described in the facility's own written operating procedures. This training should be provided at periodic intervals to ensure that personnel remain familiar with regulatory requirements.

To ensure that skills are maintained, the facility should have regularly scheduled competence evaluations of all staff members whose activities affect the quality of laboratory testing, manufacture of products, or provision of products or services.[1,5-10] Depending on the nature of the job duties, such assessments may include written evaluations; direct observation of activities; review of work records or reports, computer records, and QC records; testing of unknown samples; and evaluation of the employee's problem-solving skills.[5] For testing personnel, CMS requires that the following methods be used, when applicable, for each test system annually:

- Direct observations of
  - Routine patient test performance (including patient preparation, if applicable), specimen handling, processing, and testing.
  - Performance of instrument maintenance and function checks.
- Monitoring the recording and reporting of test results.
- Review of intermediate test results or worksheets, quality control records, proficiency testing results, and preventive maintenance records.
- Assessment of
  - Test performance through testing previously analyzed specimens, internal blind testing samples, or external proficiency testing samples.
  - Problem-solving skills.

A formal competency plan that includes a schedule of assessments, a defined minimum for acceptable performance, and remedial measures is one way to ensure appropriate and consistent competence assessments. Assessments need not be targeted at each individual test or procedure performed by the employee; instead, they can be grouped together to assess similar techniques or methods. Written tests can be used effectively to evaluate problem-solving skills and to cover many topics by asking one or more questions for each area to be assessed. CMS requires that employees who perform testing be assessed semiannually during the first year that patient specimens are tested and annually thereafter.[1] Initial training verification activities may serve as the first of these competence assessments.

The quality oversight personnel should assist in the development, review, and approval of training programs, including the criteria for retraining.[5] Quality oversight personnel also monitor the effectiveness of the training program and competence evaluations, and they make recommendations for changes as needed. In addition, The Joint Commission requires analysis of aggregate competence assessment data for the purpose of identifying staff learning needs.[9]

Staffing

Management should have a staffing plan that describes the number and qualifications of personnel needed to perform the functions of the facility safely and effectively. There should be an adequate number of staff to perform the

operational activities and to support the activities of the quality management system. Organizations should assess staffing effectiveness by evaluating human resource indicators (eg, overtime, staff injuries, staff satisfaction) in conjunction with operational performance indicators (eg, adverse events, patient complaints). The results of this evaluation should feed into the facility's human resource planning process, along with projections based on new or changing operational needs.

Suppliers and Materials Management

Materials, supplies, and services used as inputs to a process are considered "critical" if they affect the quality of products and services being produced. Examples of critical supplies are blood components, blood bags, test kits, and reagents. Examples of critical services are infectious disease testing, blood component irradiation, transportation, equipment calibration, and preventive maintenance services. The suppliers of these materials and services may be internal (eg, other departments within the same organization) or external (outside vendors). Supplies and services used in the collection, testing, processing, preservation, storage, distribution, transport, and administration of blood components, cellular therapy products, tissue, and derivatives that have the potential to affect quality should be qualified before use and obtained from suppliers who can meet the facility's requirements. The quality management system should include a process to evaluate the suppliers' abilities to meet qualification requirements. Three important elements are 1) supplier qualification; 2) agreements; and 3) receipt, inspection, and testing of incoming supplies.

Supplier Qualification

Critical supplies and services must be qualified on the basis of defined requirements. Similarly, the supplier should be qualified to ensure a reliable source of materials. The facility should clearly define requirements or expectations for the suppliers and should share this information with staff and the supplier. The ability of suppliers to consistently meet specifications for a supply or service should be evaluated along with performance relative to availability, delivery, and support. The following are examples of factors that could be considered to qualify suppliers:

- Licensure, certification, or accreditation.
- Supply or product requirements.
- Review of supplier-relevant quality documents.
- Results of audits or inspections.
- Review of quality summary reports.
- Review of customer complaints.
- Review of experience with the supplier.
- Cost of materials or services.
- Delivery arrangements.
- Financial security, market position, and customer satisfaction.
- Support after the sale.

A list of approved suppliers should be maintained, including both primary suppliers and suitable alternatives for contingency planning. Critical supplies and services should be purchased only from those suppliers who have been qualified. Once suppliers are qualified, periodic evaluation of supplier performance helps to ensure the supplier's continued ability to meet requirements. Tracking the supplier's ability to meet expectations gives the facility valuable information about the stability of the supplier's processes and commitment to quality. Documented failures of supplies or suppliers to meet defined requirements should result in immediate action by the facility, including notification of the supplier, quality oversight personnel, and management with contracting authority, if applicable. Supplies may need to be replaced or quarantined until all quality issues are resolved.

Agreements

Contracts and agreements define expectations and reflect concurrence of the parties involved. Periodic review of agreements ensures that expectations of all parties continue to be met. Changes should be mutually agreed upon and incorporated as needed.

Transfusion and cellular therapy services should maintain written contracts or agreements with outside suppliers of critical materials and services such as blood components, irradiation, compatibility testing, or infectious disease marker testing. The outside supplier may be another department within the same facility that is managed independently, or it may be another facility (eg, contract manufacturer). The contracting facility assumes responsibility for the manufacture of the product; for ensuring the safety, purity, and potency of the product; and for ensuring that the contract manufacturer complies with all applicable product standards and regulations. Both the contracting facility and the contractor are legally responsible for the work performed by the contractor.

It is important for the transfusion or cellular therapy service to participate in the evaluation and selection of suppliers. The service should review contracts and agreements to ensure that all important aspects for their critical materials and services are addressed. Examples of issues that could be addressed in an agreement or contract include the responsibility for a product or blood sample during shipment; the responsibility of the supplier to promptly notify the facility when changes have been made that could affect the safety of blood components, cellular therapy products, tissue, derivatives, or services for patients; and the responsibility of the supplier to notify the facility when information is discovered indicating that a product may not be considered safe, such as during look-back procedures.

Receipt, Inspection, and Testing of Incoming Supplies

Before acceptance and use, critical materials, such as reagents, blood components, cellular therapy products, tissue, and derivatives should be inspected and tested (if necessary) to ensure that they meet specifications for their intended use. It is essential that supplies used in the collection, processing, preservation, testing, storage, distribution, transport, and administration of blood, components, tissue, and cellular therapy products also meet FDA requirements.

The facility must define acceptance criteria for critical supplies (see 21 CFR 210.3)[3] and must develop procedures to control and prevent inadvertent use of materials that do not meet specifications. Corrective action may include returning the material to the vendor or destroying it. Receipt and inspection records provide the facility with means to trace materials that have been used in a particular process and also provide information for ongoing supplier qualification.

Equipment Management

Equipment that must operate within defined specifications to ensure the quality of blood components, cellular therapy products, tissue, derivatives, and services is referred to as "critical" equipment in the quality management system. Critical equipment may include instruments, measuring devices, and computer systems (hardware and software). Activities designed to ensure that equipment performs as intended include qualification, calibration, maintenance, and monitoring. Calibration, functional and safety checks, and preventive maintenance should be scheduled and performed according to the manufacturer's recommendations and regulatory requirements of the FDA[2,4] and CMS.[1] Written procedures for the use and control of equipment should comply with the manufacturer's recommendations unless an alternative method has been validated by the facility and, in some instances, approved by the appropriate regulatory and accrediting agencies.

When one selects new equipment, it is important to consider not only the performance of equipment as it will be used in the facility, but also any supplier issues regarding ongoing service and support. There should be a written plan for installation, operational, and performance qualifications. The plan should provide for 1) installation according to the manufacturer's specifications, 2) verification of the equipment's functionality before use by ensuring that the criteria established by the

manufacturer for its intended use are met, and 3) assurance that the equipment performs as expected in the facility's processes. After installation, there should be documentation of any problems and the follow-up actions taken. Recalibration and requalification may be necessary if repairs are made that affect the critical operating functions of the equipment. Recalibration and requalification should also be considered when existing equipment is relocated.

The facility must develop a mechanism to uniquely identify and track all critical equipment, including equipment software versions, if applicable. The unique identifier may be the manufacturer's serial number or a unique identification applied by the transfusion or cellular therapy service or assigned through a laboratory-wide or organization-wide identification system. Maintaining a list of all critical equipment helps in the control function of scheduling and performing functional and safety checks, calibrations, preventive maintenance, and repair. The equipment list can be used to ensure that all appropriate actions have been performed and recorded. Evaluation and trending of equipment calibration, maintenance, and repair data will assist the facility in assessing the functionality of the equipment, managing defective equipment, and identifying equipment that may need replacement. When equipment is found to be operating outside acceptable parameters, the potential effects on the quality of products or test results must be evaluated and documented.

Process Management

Written and approved policies, processes, and procedures must exist for all critical functions performed in the facility, and these functions must be carried out under controlled conditions. Each facility should have a systematic approach for identifying, planning, and implementing new (and making changes to existing) policies, processes, and procedures that affect the quality of the facility's tests, products, or services. Such activities should include a review of at least the following:

- Customer needs and expectations.
- Accreditation and regulatory requirements.
- Specifications to be met.
- Risk assessment.
- Performance measures.
- Nonconformance analyses.
- Current available knowledge (eg, other successful practices).
- Resource needs (eg, financial, facility, human, materials, and equipment).
- Interrelationships of the new or changed process(es) with other processes.
- Documents needed for the new or changed process(es).

The documents developed should be reviewed by management personnel with direct authority over the process and by quality oversight personnel before implementation. Changes should be documented, validated, reviewed, and approved. Additional information on policies, processes, and procedures can be found in the "Documents and Records" section later in this chapter.

Once a process has been implemented, the facility should have a mechanism to ensure that procedures are performed as defined and that critical equipment, reagents, and supplies are used in conformance with manufacturers' written instructions and facility requirements. Table 1-1 lists elements that constitute sound process control (among other elements of a quality management system). A facility using critical equipment, reagents, or supplies in a manner that is different from the manufacturer's directions should have validated such use. If the activity is covered under regulations for blood and blood components or HCT/Ps, the facility may be required to request FDA approval to operate at variance to requirements (see 21 CFR 640.120[2] or 21 CFR 1271.155[4]). If a facility believes that changes to the manufacturer's directions would be appropriate, it should encourage the manufacturer to make such changes in the labeling (ie, the package insert or user manual).

TABLE 1-1. Components of a Quality Management System

Quality System Component	Quality Functions
Organization and leadership	♦ Organization structure and function ♦ Leadership roles and responsibilities, authority, and relationships ♦ Establishment of a quality management system ♦ Customer needs ♦ Planned products and services ♦ Documented, followed, and improved policies, processes, and procedures ♦ Quality representative ♦ Management reviews ♦ Provision of adequate resources ♦ Adequate design and effective implementation ♦ Conformance to requirements ♦ Effective communication ♦ Effective process improvement
Customer focus	♦ Customer requirements ♦ Agreements ♦ Customer feedback
Facilities, work environment, and safety	♦ Minimal health and safety risks ♦ Design and space allocations ♦ Clean work environment ♦ Controlled environment ♦ Communication and information management systems ♦ Storage facilities ♦ Health and safety programs ♦ Hazard discards ♦ Emergency preparedness
Human resources	♦ Adequate and qualified staff ♦ Job descriptions and qualifications ♦ Defined roles and responsibilities for all staff and their reporting relationships ♦ Staff selection ♦ New hire orientation ♦ Training on quality systems, job-related activities, and safety ♦ Staff competence ♦ Continuing education ♦ Staff identifying information ♦ End-of-employment activities
Suppliers and materials management	♦ Supplier qualification ♦ Agreement reviews ♦ Qualifying incoming materials ♦ Inventory management ♦ Adequate storage conditions ♦ Receipt, inspection, and testing of incoming materials and products ♦ Acceptance and rejection of materials and products ♦ Tracing critical supplies

TABLE 1-1. Components of a Quality Management System (Continued)

Quality System Component	Quality Functions
Equipment management	♦ Selection and acquisition ♦ Unique identification ♦ Verification of performance ♦ Installation, operation, and performance qualification ♦ Calibration ♦ Preventive maintenance and repairs ♦ Retirement
Process management	♦ Process development ♦ Change control ♦ Process validation ♦ Process implementation ♦ Adherence to policies, processes, and procedures ♦ Quality control program ♦ Inspection of products and services ♦ Concurrent creation of records ♦ Requirements for critical activities ♦ Traceability
Documents and records	♦ Standardized formats ♦ Document creation ♦ Unique identification ♦ Review and approval process ♦ Use and maintenance ♦ Change control ♦ Archiving and storage ♦ Retention and destruction
Information management	♦ Confidentiality ♦ Prevention of unauthorized access ♦ Data integrity ♦ Backup data ♦ Alternative system
Management of nonconforming events	♦ Detection of deviations and nonconformances ♦ Complaint file ♦ Adverse event reporting ♦ Investigations ♦ Immediate actions
Monitoring and assessment	♦ Monitoring and assessment of specified requirements ♦ Quality indicators ♦ Internal and external assessments ♦ Laboratory proficiency testing ♦ Data analyses
Process improvement	♦ Identifying opportunities for improvement ♦ Systems approach to continual improvement ♦ Root cause evaluation ♦ Corrective and preventive action plans ♦ Monitoring for effectiveness

Process Validation

Validation is used to demonstrate that a process is capable of achieving planned results.[13] It is critical to validate processes in situations where it is not feasible to measure or inspect each finished product or service in order to fully verify conformance with specifications. However, even when effective end-product testing can be achieved, it is advisable to validate important processes to generate information that can be used to optimize performance. Prospective validation is used for new or revised processes. Retrospective validation may be used for processes that are already in operation but were not adequately validated before implementation. Concurrent validation is used when required data cannot be obtained without performance of a "live" process. If concurrent validation is used, data are reviewed at predefined periodic intervals before final approval for full implementation occurs. Modifications to a validated process may warrant revalidation, depending on the nature and extent of the change. It is up to the facility to determine the need for revalidation on the basis of its understanding of how the proposed changes may affect the process.

Test Method Validation

When the laboratory wishes to implement a non-waived test using an FDA-approved or -cleared test system, CLIA requires that the performance specifications, which were established by the manufacturer, be verified by the laboratory before reporting patient results.[1] At a minimum, the laboratory must demonstrate that it can obtain performance specifications comparable to the manufacturer for accuracy, precision, reportable range, and reference intervals (normal values).

If the laboratory develops its own methodology, introduces a test system not subject to FDA approval or clearance, or makes modifications to an FDA-approved or -cleared test system, or if the manufacturer does not provide performance specifications, then the laboratory must establish the test system performance specifications before reporting patient results. At a minimum, the following must be established for the test system:

- Accuracy.
- Precision.
- Reportable range of test results for the test system.
- Reference intervals (normal values).
- Analytical sensitivity.
- Analytical specificity, including interfering substances.
- Any other performance characteristic required for test performance (eg, specimen or reagent stability).

Based on performance specifications, the laboratory must also establish calibration and control procedures and document all activities for test method validation (see 42 CFR 493.1253).[1]

Validation Plan

Validation should be planned if it is to be effective. Development of a validation plan is best accomplished after one obtains an adequate understanding of the system, or framework, within which the process will occur. The plan should include conducting the process as designed. Additionally, a significant amount of effort should be targeted at attempts to "break" the process in order to identify process weaknesses and limitations. Many facilities develop a template for the written validation plan to ensure that all aspects are adequately addressed. Although no single format for a validation plan is required, most plans include the following common elements:

- System description.
- Purpose or objectives.
- Risk assessment.
- Responsibilities.
- Validation procedures.
- Acceptance criteria.
- Approval signatures.
- Supporting documentation.

The validation plan should be reviewed and approved by quality oversight personnel.

Staff responsible for carrying out the validation activities should be trained in the process before the plan is executed. The results and conclusions of these activities may be appended to the approved validation plan or may be recorded in a separate document. This documentation typically contains the following elements:

- Expected and observed results.
- Interpretation of results as acceptable or unacceptable.
- Corrective action for and resolution of unexpected results.
- Explanation of and rationale for any deviations from the validation plan.
- Conclusions and limitations.
- Approval signatures.
- Supporting documentation.
- Implementation time line.

When a validation process does not produce the expected outcome, its data and corrective actions must be documented as well. The responsible quality oversight personnel should provide final review and approval of the validation plan, results, and corrective actions and determine whether new or modified processes and equipment may be implemented or implemented with specified limitations.

Equipment Validation

Validation of new equipment used in a process should include installation qualification, operational qualification, and performance qualification, as follows[19]:

- Installation qualification demonstrates that the instrument is properly installed in environmental conditions that meet the manufacturer's specifications.
- Operational qualification demonstrates that the installed equipment operates as intended. It focuses on the capability of the equipment to operate within the established limits and specifications supplied by the manufacturer.
- Performance qualification demonstrates that the equipment performs as expected for its intended use in the processes established by the facility and that the output meets the facility's specifications. It evaluates the adequacy of equipment for use in a specific process that uses the facility's own personnel, procedures, and supplies in a normal working environment.

Computer System Validation

The FDA considers computerized systems to include "hardware, software, peripheral devices, personnel, and documentation."[20] End-user validation of computer systems and the interfaces between systems should be conducted in the environment where they will be used. Testing performed by the vendor or supplier of computer software is not a substitute for computer validation at the facility. End-user acceptance testing may repeat some of the validation performed by the developer, such as load or stress testing and verification of security, safety, and control features, in order to evaluate performance under actual operating conditions. In addition, the end-user should evaluate the ability of personnel to use the computer system as intended within the context of actual work processes. The hardware and software interface should be designed so that staff can navigate successfully and respond appropriately to messages, warnings, and other functions. Depending on the nature of the computer functionality, changes to the computer system may result in changes to the way a process is performed. If this occurs, process revalidation should also be performed. As with process validation, quality oversight personnel should review and approve validation plans, results, and corrective actions and should determine whether implementation may proceed with or without limitations. Facilities that develop their own software should refer to FDA guidance regarding general principles of software validation for additional information.[21]

Quality Control

QC testing is performed to ensure the proper functioning of materials, equipment, and methods during operations. QC performance expectations and acceptable ranges should be defined and readily available to staff so that they will recognize unacceptable results and trends in order to respond appropriately. The frequency for QC testing is determined by the facility in accordance with the applicable CMS, FDA, AABB, state, and manufacturer requirements. QC results should be documented concurrently with performance.[2] Records of QC testing should include the following:

- Identification of personnel performing test.
- Identification of reagents (including lot numbers, expiration dates, etc).
- Identification of equipment.
- Testing date and, when applicable, time.
- Results.
- Interpretation (eg, meets or fails to meet established criteria).
- Reviews.

Unacceptable QC results must be investigated and corrective action must be implemented, if indicated, before repeating the QC procedure or continuing the operational process. If products or services were provided since the last acceptable QC results were obtained, it may be necessary to evaluate the conformance of these products or services. Specific examples of the application of validation and quality controls are included in Appendices 1-3 and 1-4.

Documents and Records

Documentation provides a framework for understanding and communication throughout the organization. Documents describe how processes are intended to work, how they interact, where they must be controlled, what their requirements are, and how to implement them. Records provide evidence that the process was performed as intended and provide information needed to assess the quality of products and services. Together, documents and records are used by quality oversight personnel to evaluate the effectiveness of a facility's policies, processes, and procedures. An example of quality system documentation is provided in ISO 9001 and includes the following items[13]:

- The quality policy and objectives.
- A description of the interactions between processes.
- Documented procedures for the control of documents, records, and nonconforming products and for corrective action, preventive action, and internal quality audits.
- Records related to the quality management system, operational performance, and product or service conformance.
- All other "documents needed by the organization to ensure the effective planning, operation, and control of its processes."

Written policies, process descriptions, procedures, work instructions, labels, forms, and records are all part of the facility's documentation system. They may be paper-based or electronic. Documents provide a description or instructions regarding what is *supposed* to happen; records provide evidence of what *did* happen. A document management system provides assurance that documents are comprehensive, current, and available and that records are accurate and complete. A well-structured document management system links policies, process descriptions, procedures, forms, and records together in an organized and workable system.

Documents

Documents should be developed in a format that conveys information clearly and that provides staff with the necessary instructions and templates for recording data. The CLSI offers guidance regarding general levels of documentation[11] as well as detailed instructions on how to write procedures.[22] General types of documentation are described below.

POLICIES. Policies communicate the highest-level goals, objectives, and intent of the organization. The rest of the organization's documentation will interpret and provide instruction regarding implementation of these policies.

PROCESSES. Process documents describe a sequence of actions and identify responsibilities, decision points, requirements, and acceptance criteria. Process diagrams or flow charts are often used for this level of documentation. It is helpful to show process control points on the diagram as well as flow of information and handoffs between departments or work groups.

PROCEDURES AND WORK INSTRUCTIONS. These documents provide step-by-step directions on how to perform job tasks and procedures. Procedures and work instructions should include enough detail to perform the task correctly but not so much as to make them difficult to read. The use of standardized formats will help staff know where to find specific elements and will facilitate implementation and control. External documents may also be incorporated into the facility's procedures manual by reference; for example, those from a manufacturer's manual or package insert. Relevant procedures should be available to the staff in each area where the corresponding job tasks are performed.[2,5,8]

FORMS. Forms provide a template for capturing data either on paper or electronically. These documents specify the data requirements called for in SOPs and processes. Forms should be carefully designed for ease of use, to minimize the likelihood of errors, and to facilitate the retrieval of data and information. The forms should be designed to effectively capture outcomes and support process traceability. When it is not immediately evident what data should be recorded or how to record them, forms should include instructions about usage. For quantitative data, the form should indicate units of measure. Computer data entry and review screens are a type of form.

LABELS. Product labels, such as blood component or HCT/P labels, are critical materials that are subject to many of the requirements in a document management system. Many facilities maintain a master set of labels that can be used as a reference to verify that only currently approved stock is in use. New label stock should be verified as accurate before it is put into inventory; comparison against a master label provides a mechanism for accomplishing this verification. Change control procedures should be established for the use of on-demand label printers, to prevent nonconforming modification of label format or content.

Each facility should have a defined process for developing and maintaining documents. It should include basic elements required for documents; procedures for review and approval of new or revised documents; a method for keeping documents current; control of document distribution; and a process for archiving, protecting, and retrieving obsolete documents. Training should be provided to the staff responsible for the content of new or revised documents. Document management systems include these established processes:

- Verifying the adequacy of the document before approval and issuance.
- Periodically reviewing, modifying, and reapproving documents as needed to keep them current.
- Identifying changes and revision status.
- Ensuring that documents are legible, identifiable, and readily available in the locations where they will be used.
- Retaining and retrieving previous versions for the required retention period.
- Preventing unintended use of outdated or obsolete documents.
- Protecting documents from alteration, damage, or unintended destruction.

External documents that are incorporated by reference become a part of the document management system and should be identified and controlled. The facility should have a mechanism to detect changes to external documents in its system, such as manufacturers' package inserts or user manuals, so that corresponding changes to procedures and forms can be made.

When new or revised policies, process descriptions, procedures, or forms are added to or replaced in the facility's manual, the documents should be marked with the date that they have been put into use (ie, effective date).

One copy of retired documents should be retained as defined by existing and applicable standards and regulations.

A master list of all current policies, process descriptions, procedures, forms, and labels is useful for maintaining document control. It should include the document title, the individual or work group responsible for maintaining it, the revision date, the unique document identifier, and the areas where it is used. It should also identify the number and location of controlled copies in circulation. Copies of documents that will be used in the workplace should be identified and controlled to ensure that none is overlooked when changes are implemented.

Records

Records provide evidence that critical steps in a procedure have been performed appropriately and that products and services conform to specified requirements. Review of records is an important tool to help evaluate the effectiveness of the quality management system. Records should be created concurrently with the performance of each significant step and should clearly indicate the identity of the individuals who performed each step and when it occurred.[2,6,7] The process for managing records should address the following items:

- Creation and identification of records.
- Protection from accidental or unauthorized modification or destruction.
- Verification of completeness, accuracy, and legibility.
- Storage and retrieval.
- Creation of copies or backups.
- Retention periods.
- Confidentiality.

Record-keeping systems should allow for ready retrieval within time frames established by the facility and should permit traceability of blood, components, cellular therapy products, tissue, and derivatives as required by federal regulations.[2,4] Specific requirements for records to be maintained by AABB-accredited facilities are included in the relevant set of AABB standards.

When forms are used for capturing or recording data, steps, or test results, the forms become records. Data should be recorded in a format that is clear and consistent. The facility should define a process and time frames for record review to ensure accuracy, completeness, and appropriate follow-up. It should determine how reports and records are to be archived and how to define their retention period. When copies of records are retained, the facility should verify that each copy contains the complete, legible, and accessible content of the original record before the original is destroyed.

If records are maintained electronically, adequate backups should exist in case of system failure. Electronic records should be readable for the entire length of their retention period. Obsolete computer software that is necessary to reconstruct or trace records should also be archived appropriately. If the equipment or software used to access archived data cannot be maintained, the records should be converted to another format or copied to another medium to permit continued access. Converted data should be verified against the original to ensure completeness and accuracy. Electronic media such as magnetic tapes, optical disks, or online computer data storage are widely used for archiving documents. Records kept in this manner must meet FDA requirements for electronic record-keeping.[23] Microfilm or microfiche may also be used to archive records. The medium selected should be appropriate for the retention requirements.

Each facility should have a policy for altering or correcting records. A common practice is to record the change along with the date, the identity of the person making the change, and the evidence of review by a responsible person. In some instances, it may also be important to include the reason for the change. The original recording must not be obliterated in written records; the original may be crossed out with a single line, but it should remain legible. Write-overs and scratch-outs are not permissible. Electronic records must permit tracking of both original and corrected data and must include the date and user identification of the person making the change. There should be a process for controlling changes. A method for referencing changes to records, one that is linked to the original records, and a system for reviewing changes for completeness and accuracy are essential. Audit trails for changed data in computerized systems are required by the FDA.[23]

The following are issues that might be considered when planning record storage:

- Storage of records in a manner that protects them from damage and from accidental or unauthorized destruction or modification.
- Degree of accessibility of records in proportion to frequency of their use.
- Method and location of record storage related to the volume of records and the amount of available storage space.
- Availability of properly functioning equipment, computer hardware, and software to view archived records.
- Documentation that all records copied, microfiched, or converted to electronic images legitimately replace originals that may be stored elsewhere or destroyed.
- Retention of original color-coded records when only black-and-white reproductions are available.

Considerations for electronic records include the following:

- A method of verifying the accuracy of data entry.
- Prevention of unintended deletion of data or access by unauthorized persons.
- Adequate protection against inadvertent data loss (eg, when a storage device is full).
- Validated safeguards to ensure that a record can be edited by only one person at a time.
- Security of and access to confidential data.

To link relevant personnel to recorded data, the facility should maintain a record of names; of inclusive dates of employment; and of corresponding signatures, identifying initials, or identification codes of personnel authorized to create, sign, initial, or review reports and records. Magnetically coded employee badges and other computer-related identifying methods are generally accepted in lieu of written signatures, provided the badges or other methods meet electronic record-keeping requirements.

Information Management

The quality management system should ensure the confidentiality and appropriate use of data and information. Oral and written communication of information should be included. Privacy of patient and donor records should be addressed to maintain the security and confidentiality of such records.

The system must prevent unauthorized access, modification, or destruction of the data and information. Individuals who are authorized to make changes to data should be defined by name, code, or job responsibility. Computer systems should be designed with security features to prevent unauthorized access and use. Systems may include levels of security defined by job responsibility and administered by the use of security codes and passwords.

The integrity of data should be maintained so that data are retrievable and usable. Periodic checks of data integrity should be conducted for critical data to ensure that they have not been inadvertently modified or lost or have become inaccessible. When data are sent manually or electronically from one point to another, a process should be in place to ensure that the data accurately and reliably reached their final destination in a timely manner.

A backup disk or tape should be maintained for critical data in the event of an unexpected loss from the storage medium. It is advisable to store backup or archived computer records and databases off-site at a sufficient distance to ensure that disasters will not affect both the originals and the backups. The storage facility should be secure. Environmental conditions should be maintained in a way that protects and preserves the equipment and media for the duration of their storage. Temperature and humidity should be monitored and controlled. An archival copy of the computer operating system and applications software should be stored in the same manner.

The facility should develop and maintain alternative systems to ensure access to critical data and information in the event that computerized data or the primary sources of information are not available. The backup and recovery procedures for computer downtime should be defined, with validation documentation to show that the backup system works properly. The associated processes should be tested periodically to ensure that the backup system remains effective. Special consideration should be given to staff competence and readiness to use the backup system.

Management of Nonconforming Events

The quality management system should include a process for detecting, investigating, and responding to events that result in deviations from accepted policies, processes, and procedures or in failures to meet requirements, as defined by the facility, AABB standards, or applicable regulations.[2,4] This process includes the discovery of nonconforming products and services as well as adverse reactions to donation, blood components, cellular therapy products, tissues, or derivatives. The facility should define how to perform the following:

- Document and classify occurrences.
- Determine the effect, if any, on the quality of products or services.
- Evaluate the effect on interrelated activities.
- Analyze the event to understand root causes.
- Implement corrective action as appropriate, including notification and recall, on the basis of investigation and root cause analysis.
- Implement preventive actions as appropriate on the basis of analysis of aggregate data about events and their causes.
- Report to external agencies when required.
- Evaluate effectiveness of the corrective actions and preventive actions taken.

The CLSI has published a consensus standard on occurrence management that explores event management in more detail.[24]

Facility personnel should be trained to recognize and report such occurrences. Depending on the severity of the event and risk to patients, donors, and products, as well as the likelihood of recurrence, investigation into contributing factors and underlying causes may be warranted. The cGMP regulations require an investigation and documentation of the results if a specific event could adversely affect patient safety or the safety, purity, or potency of blood or components.[2,3] The cGTP regulations require similar activities for deviations and for possible product contamination or communicable disease transmission.[4] Tools and approaches for performing root cause analysis and implementing corrective action are discussed in the section on process improvement. A summary of the event, investigation, and any follow-up must be documented. Table 1-2 outlines suggested components of an internal event report.

Fatalities related to blood collection or transfusion or HCT/Ps must be reported as soon as possible to the FDA Center for Biologics Evaluation and Research (CBER) [see 21 CFR 606.170(b) and 1271.350(a)(i), respectfully]. Instructions for reporting to CBER are available in published guidance[26] and on the FDA website.[27] A written follow-up report must be submitted within 7 days of the fatality and should include a description of any new procedures implemented, to avoid recurrence. AABB *Association Bulletin #04-06* provides additional information, including a form to be used for reporting donor fatalities.[28]

Regardless of their licensure and registration status with the FDA, all donor centers, blood banks, and transfusion services must promptly report biological product deviations—and information relevant to these events—to the FDA[2,29] using Form FDA-3486 when the event 1) is associated with manufacturing (ie, collecting, testing, processing, packing, labeling, storing, holding, or distributing); 2) represents a deviation from cGMP, from established specifications, or from applicable regulations or standards, or a deviation that is

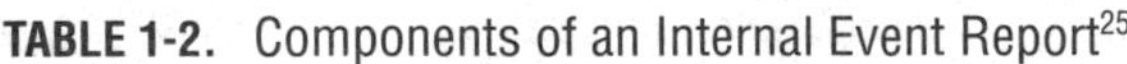

TABLE 1-2. Components of an Internal Event Report[25]

Who	◆ Identity of reporting individual(s) ◆ Identity of individual(s) involved (by job title) in committing, compounding, discovering, investigating, and initiating any immediate action ◆ Patient or donor identification ◆ Reviewer(s) of report
What	◆ Brief description of event ◆ Effects on and outcome to patient, donor, blood component, or tissue ◆ Name of component and unit identification number ◆ Manufacturer, lot number, and expiration of applicable reagents and supplies ◆ Immediate action taken
When	◆ Date of report ◆ Date and time event occurred ◆ Date and time of discovery ◆ Collection and shipping dates of blood component(s) ◆ Date (and time, if applicable) that immediate action was taken
Where	◆ Physical location of event ◆ Where in process event was detected ◆ Where in process event was initiated
Why and How	◆ Explanation of how event occurred ◆ Contributing factors to event ◆ Root cause(s)
Follow-up	◆ External reports or notifications (eg, FDA,* manufacturer, or patient's physician) ◆ Corrective actions ◆ Implementation dates ◆ Effectiveness of actions taken ◆ Linkage to preventive action if appropriate

*All blood establishments (including licensed, registered but unlicensed, and unregistered transfusion services)[2] (21 CFR 606.121) are required to notify the FDA in cases of deviations from cGMP, applicable standards, or established specifications that may affect the safety, purity, or potency of biological products or otherwise cause the biological products to be in violation of the Food, Drug, and Cosmetic Act or the Public Health Service Act (21 CFR 600.14).[2] The FDA has identified the following examples as reportable events if components or products are released for distribution:

- ◆ Arm preparation not performed or performed incorrectly.
- ◆ Units released from donors who are (or should have been) either temporarily or permanently deferred because of their medical history or a history of repeatedly reactive viral marker tests.
- ◆ Shipment of a unit with repeatedly reactive viral markers.
- ◆ ABO/Rh or infectious disease testing not performed according to the manufacturer's package insert.
- ◆ Units released from donors for whom test results were improperly interpreted because of testing errors related to improper use of equipment.
- ◆ Units released before completion of all tests (except as an emergency release).
- ◆ Sample used for compatibility testing that contains incorrect identification.
- ◆ Testing error that results in the release of an incorrect unit.
- ◆ Incorrectly labeled blood components (eg, ABO, expiration date).
- ◆ Incorrect crossmatch label or tag.
- ◆ Storage of biological products at the incorrect temperature.
- ◆ Microbial contamination of blood components when the contamination is attributed to an error in manufacturing.

Deviations involving a distributed HCT/P and relating to core cGTP requirements must also be reported to the FDA if the deviation occurred in the facility or in a facility that performed a manufacturing step for it under contract, agreement, or other arrangement.[4] Each report must contain a description of the HCT/P deviation, information relevant to the event and the manufacture of the HCT/P involved, and information on all follow-up actions that have been or will be taken in response to the deviation.

FDA = Food and Drug Administration; cGMP = current good manufacturing practice; cGTP = current good tissue practice; CFR = *Code of Federal Regulations.*

unexpected or unforeseen; 3) may affect the safety, purity, or potency of the product; 4) occurs while the facility had control of, or was responsible for, the product; and 5) involves a product that has left the control of the facility (ie, has been distributed).

Using the same form, facilities must also promptly report biological product deviations associated with a distributed HCT/P if the event represents a deviation from applicable regulations, standards, or established specifications that relate to the prevention of communicable disease transmission or HCT/P contamination. This includes events that currently may be unexpected or unforeseeable but may relate to the transmission or potential transmission of a communicable disease or may lead to HCT/P contamination.[4]

More information concerning biological product deviation reporting can be found on the FDA website.[30]

There must also be a mechanism to report medical device adverse events to the FDA and to the device manufacturer.[8,31] The Joint Commission encourages reporting of sentinel events, including hemolytic transfusion reactions involving the administration of blood or components having major blood group incompatibilities.[9,10]

Hemovigilance systems also provide an opportunity to detect, investigate, and respond to events that result in deviations from safe blood transfusion and collection practices. Two such systems have been implemented in the United States. The Centers for Disease Control and Prevention (CDC) National Healthcare Safety Network Hemovigilance Module, developed with expert input from AABB, is being used by hospitals to track and reduce adverse events associated with blood transfusion. The Donor Hemovigilance System—developed through the efforts of the US Department of Health and Human Services Office of Public Health and Science, AABB, and AABB's member blood donor programs—is being used by blood collection centers to track and reduce adverse events associated with blood donation. The ultimate goal of these hemovigilance systems is to improve patient safety and donor health.[32]

Each facility should track reported events and look for trends. The use of classification schemes may facilitate trend analysis and typically involves one or more of the following categories: the nature of the event, the process (or procedure) in which the event occurred, the outcome and severity of the event, and the contributing factors and underlying causes. If several events within a relatively short period involve a particular process or procedure, that process or procedure should be further investigated. The most useful schemes involve use of multiple categories for each event, which allow data to be sorted in a variety of ways so that patterns, previously not obvious, can emerge (see example in Table 1-3). Such sorting or stratification can result in identification of situations that require closer monitoring or of problems needing corrective or preventive action. For smaller facilities that may not have sufficient data to note trends, pooling data with a larger entity (eg, the laboratory or all transfusion services in a health-care system) or following national trends from data provided by organizations such as the AABB, CAP, or The Joint Commission, may also prove helpful. The extent of monitoring and the length of time to monitor processes will depend on the frequency of the occurrence and the critical aspects of the occurrences. Reporting and monitoring of events are essential problem identification methods for process improvement activities in a quality management system.

Occasionally, there may be a need for a facility to deviate from approved procedures in order to meet the unique medical needs of a particular patient. When this situation arises, a medically indicated exception is planned and approved in advance by the facility's medical director. The rationale and nature of the planned exception should be documented. Careful consideration should be given to maintaining a controlled process and to verifying the safety and quality of the resulting product or service. Any additional risk to the patient must be disclosed.

TABLE 1-3. Example of an Event Classification

Event: A unit of Red Blood Cells from a directed donor was issued to the wrong oncology patient. The unit was not transfused.
Event Classification ♦ Type of event: patient ♦ Procedure involved: issuing products ♦ Process involved: blood administration ♦ Product involved: Red Blood Cells ♦ Location: Transfusion Service ♦ Other factors: directed donor ♦ Other factors: oncology patient
Underlying Causes ♦ Proximate cause: two patients with similar names had crossmatched blood available ♦ Root cause: inadequate procedure for verification of patient identification during issue
Outcome ♦ Severity: serious, FDA reportable ♦ Patient: no harm, correct product was obtained and transfused ♦ Product: no harm, product returned to inventory ♦ Donor: not applicable
Successful Barriers ♦ Problem detected during the patient identification verification step of blood administration

FDA = Food and Drug Administration.

Monitoring and Assessment

The quality management system should describe how the facility monitors and evaluates its processes. Assessments are systematic examinations to determine whether actual activities comply with planned activities, are implemented effectively, and achieve objectives. Depending on the focus, assessments can include 1) evaluation of process outputs (ie, results), 2) the activities that make up a process as well as its outputs, or 3) a group of related processes and outputs (ie, the system). Assessments can be internal or external and can include quality assessments, peer review, self-assessments, and proficiency testing. Evaluations typically include comparison of actual results to expected results.

Internal Assessments

Internal assessments may include evaluation of quality indicator data, targeted audits of a single process, or system audits that are broader in scope and may cover a set of interrelated processes. These assessments should be planned and scheduled. The details of who performs the assessments and how they are performed should be addressed. Assessments should cover the quality system and the major operating systems found in the donor center and in the transfusion or cellular therapy service.

In addition, there should be a process for responding to the issues raised as a result of the assessment, including review processes and time frames. The results should be documented and submitted to management personnel who have authority over the process assessed as well as to executive management. Management should develop corrective action plans with input from the operational staff and quality oversight personnel for any deficiencies noted in the assessment. Quality oversight personnel should track progress toward implementation of corrective actions and monitor them for effectiveness.

For one to make the best use of these assessments, there should be a process to track, trend, and analyze the problems identified so that opportunities for improvement can be recognized. Early detection of trends makes it possible to develop preventive actions before patient safety, blood, components, tissues, or derivatives are adversely affected. Evaluation summaries provide information useful for addressing individual or group performance problems and for ensuring adequacy of test methods and equipment. In addition to review of assessment results and summaries, any associated corrective or preventive action should be reviewed by executive management.

Quality Indicators

Quality indicators are specific performance measurements designed to monitor one or more processes during a defined time and are useful for evaluating service demands, production, adequacy of personnel, inventory control, and process stability. These indicators can be process-based or outcome-based. Process-based indicators measure the degree to which a process can be consistently performed. An example of a process-based indicator is measurement of turnaround time from blood product ordering until transfusion. Outcome-based indicators are often used to measure what does or does not happen after a process is or is not performed. Counting incorrect test result reports is an example of such an indicator. For each indicator, thresholds are set that represent warning limits, action limits, or both. These thresholds can be determined from regulatory or accreditation requirements, from benchmarking, or from internal facility data.

Tools frequently used for displaying quality indicator data are run charts and control charts. In a run chart, time is plotted on the x axis and values on the y axis. In control charts, the mean of the data and the upper and lower control limits, which have been calculated from the data, are added to the chart. Single points outside the upper and lower control limits result from special causes. Statistical rules for interpreting consecutive points outside 1 standard deviation (SD), 2 SD, and 3 SD should be used to recognize a process that is out of control. The root cause should be determined, and corrective action should be initiated, if indicated.

Blood Utilization Assessment

The activities of blood usage review committees in the transfusion setting are an example of internal assessment. Guidelines are available from the AABB for both adult and pediatric utilization review.[33-35] Peer review of transfusion practices, required by the AABB, is also required by The Joint Commission[9] for hospital accreditation, by CMS[1] for hospitals to qualify for Medicare reimbursement, and by some states for Medicaid reimbursement.

Transfusion audits provide a review of policies and practices to ensure safe and appropriate transfusions and are based on measurable, predetermined performance criteria (see Chapter 28). Transfusion services should investigate an adequate sampling of cases (eg, 5% of the number of cases occurring within a defined time frame, or 30 cases—whichever is larger). Audits assess the facility's performance and effectiveness in the following[6]:

- Ordering practices.
- Patient identification.
- Sample collection and labeling.
- Infectious and noninfectious adverse events.
- Near-miss events.
- Usage and discard.
- Appropriateness of use.
- Blood administration policies.
- The ability of services to meet patient needs.
- Compliance with peer-review recommendations.

One method of assessing the blood administration process is to observe a predetermined number of transfusions by following the unit of blood as it is issued for transfusion and as it is transfused.[34]

Assessments of transfusion safety policy and practice may include a review of transfusion reactions and transfusion-transmitted diseases. The review committee may monitor policies and practices for notifying recipients or recipients' physicians of recalled products and for notifying donors of abnormal test results. Other assessments important in transfusion practice include the review of policies for informed consent, indications for transfusion, release of directed donor units, and outpatient or home transfusion. Additional assessments should include, where appropriate, 1) therapeutic apheresis, 2) the use of blood recovery devices, 3) procurement and storage of hematopoietic progenitor cells, 4) perioperative autologous blood collection, 5) procurement and storage of tissue, and 6) evaluation of evolving technologies and products such as growth factors and cytokines.

External Assessments

External assessments include inspections, surveys, audits, and assessments performed by those not affiliated with the organization, such as the AABB, CAP, CMS, Commission on Office Laboratory Accreditation, FACT, the FDA, The Joint Commission, or state and regional departments of health. Participation in an external assessment program provides an independent objective view of the facility's performance. External assessors often bring broad-based experience and knowledge of best practices that can be shared. Such assessments are increasingly being performed unannounced or with minimal notification. In the preparation phase, there is typically some data gathering and information to submit to the organization performing the assessment. To be practiced and ready, facilities can also prepare by performing internal audits and by conducting drills to ensure that the staff can answer questions. For most external assessments, there is an increased emphasis on observations of the processes and dialogue with non-management staff, so preparation is key. During the assessment phase, it is important to know who is responsible for the assessors or inspectors during the time they are in the facility. Clear descriptions of what information can be given to these individuals—and in what form—will help the facility through the assessment or inspection process. After the assessment, identified issues should be addressed. Usually, a written response is submitted.

Proficiency Testing for Laboratories

Proficiency testing (PT) is one means for determining that test systems (including methods, supplies, and equipment) are performing as expected. As a condition for certification, CMS requires laboratories to participate successfully in an approved PT program for CLIA-regulated testing performed routinely. When no approved PT program exists for a particular analyte, the laboratory must have another means to verify the accuracy of the test procedure at least twice annually.[1] Some accrediting agencies may require more frequent verification of accuracy.

PT must be performed using routine work processes and conditions if it is to provide meaningful information. Handling and testing of PT samples should be the same as with patient or donor specimens, except that a CLIA-certified laboratory is prohibited from discussing the PT or sending the samples to a laboratory with a different CLIA number during the active survey period, even if the two laboratories are within the same organization and even if that would be the routine manner for handling patient or donor specimens. Supervisory review of the summary evaluation report should be documented along with investigation and corrective action for results that are unacceptable. Quality oversight personnel should monitor the PT program and verify that test systems are maintained in a state of control and that appropriate corrective action is taken when indicated.

Process Improvement

Continuous improvement is a fundamental goal in any quality management system. In transfusion and cellular therapies and clinical diagnostics, this goal is tied to patient safety goals and expectations for the highest quality health care. The importance of identifying, in-

TABLE 1-4. Applicable Joint Commission Performance Improvement Standards[9,10]

◆ The organization collects data to monitor its performance, including the following: – Blood and blood component use. – All confirmed transfusion reactions.
◆ The organization compiles and analyzes data.
◆ The organization improves performance on an ongoing basis.

vestigating, correcting, and preventing problems cannot be overstated. The process of developing corrective and preventive action plans involves identification of problems and their causes as well as the identification and evaluation of solutions to prevent future problems. This process should also include evaluation of near-miss events and a mechanism for data collection and analysis, as well as follow-up to evaluate the effectiveness of the actions taken. Statistical tools and their applications may be found in publications from the AABB and the American Society for Quality.[36-38] The Joint Commission standards for performance improvement are outlined in Table 1-4.[9,10]

Corrective action is defined as the action taken to address the root causes of an *existing* nonconformance or other undesirable situation in order to reduce or eliminate recurrence. Preventive action is defined as the action taken to reduce or eliminate the *potential* for a nonconformance or other undesirable situation in order to prevent occurrence. Corrective action can be thought of as a *reactive* approach to address the root causes of actual nonconformances, deviations, complaints, and process failures, whereas preventive action can be thought of as a *proactive* approach to address the underlying causes of anticipated problems identified through the analysis of data and information.[39] In contrast, remedial action is defined as the action taken to alleviate the *symptoms* of existing nonconformances or any other undesirable situation.[40] Remedial action addresses only the visible indicator of a problem, not the actual cause (see comparisons in Table 1-5). Effective corrective and preventive action cannot be implemented until the underlying cause is determined and the process is evaluated in relationship to other processes. Pending such evaluation, it may be desirable to implement interim remedial action.

Identification of Problems and Their Causes

Sources of information for process improvement activities include process deviations, nonconforming products and services, customer complaints, QC records, PT, internal audits, quality indicators, and external assessments. Active monitoring programs may be set up to help identify problem areas. These programs should be representative of the facility processes, should be consistent with organizational goals, and should reflect customer needs. Preparation of a facility quality report, at least annually, in which data from all these sources are aggregated and analyzed, can be a

TABLE 1-5. Comparison of Remedial, Corrective, and Preventive Actions[39]

Action	Problem	Approach	Outcome
Remedial	Existent	Reactive	Alleviates symptoms
Corrective	Existent	Reactive	Prevents recurrence
Preventive	Nonexistent	Proactive	Prevents occurrence

valuable tool to identify issues for performance improvement.

Once identified, problems should be analyzed to determine their scope, their potential effects on the quality management and operational systems, their relative frequency, and the extent of their variation. Such an analysis is important to avoid tampering with processes that are merely showing normal variation or problems with little effect.

Identifying underlying causes for an undesirable condition or problem can be accomplished by an individual or group. The more complex the problem and the more involved the process, the greater the need to enlist a team of individuals and to formalize the analysis. Three commonly used tools for identifying underlying causes in an objective manner are process flowcharting, use of the "repetitive why," and the cause-and-effect diagram.

A process flow chart gives a detailed picture of the multiple activities and important decision points within that process. By examining this picture, one may identify problem-prone areas.

The "repetitive why" is used to work backward through the process. One repeatedly asks the question, "Why did this happen?" until 1) no new information can be gleaned; 2) the causal path cannot be followed because of missing information; or 3) further investigation is impractical, impossible, or outside the boundaries of the organization. Use of the "repetitive why" prevents the mistake of interpreting an effect as a cause.

The cause-and-effect diagram, also known as the Ishikawa or fish-bone diagram, uses a specialized form of brainstorming that breaks down problems into "bite-sized" pieces. (An example of a cause-and-effect diagram is shown in Fig 1-1.) The method used in the diagram is designed to focus ideas around the component parts of a process as well as to give a pictorial representation of the ideas that are generated and their interactions. When using the cause-and-effect diagram, one looks at equipment, materials, methods, environment, and human factors.

These tools identify both active and latent failures. Active failures are those that have an immediate adverse effect. Latent failures are those more global actions and decisions with potential for damage that may lie dormant and may become evident only when triggered by the presence of localized factors. The key to successfully determining root cause is to avoid stopping too soon or getting caught in the trap of placing blame on an individual.

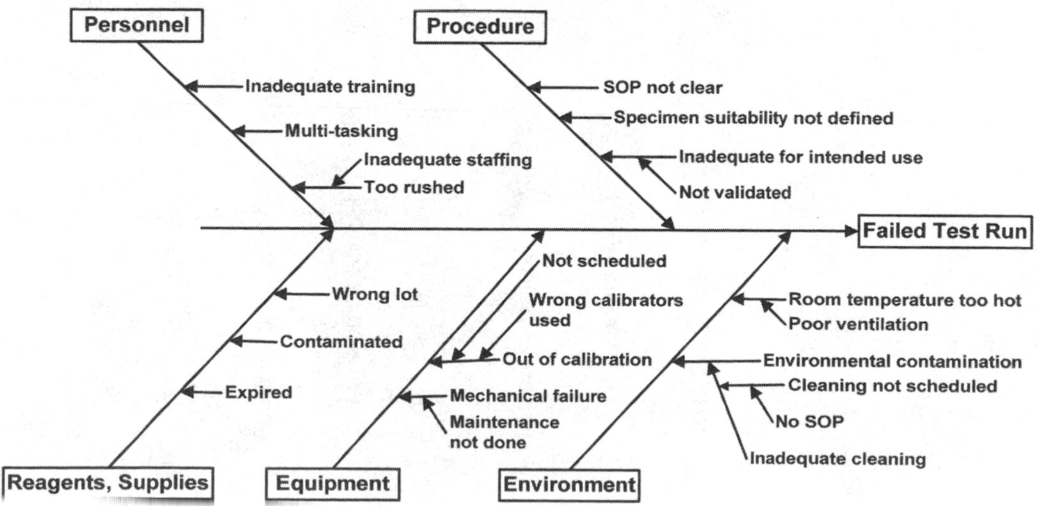

FIGURE 1-1. Example of a cause-and-effect diagram. SOP = standard operating procedure.

Most problems, particularly those that are complex, have several root causes. A method that can be of use when such problems occur is the Pareto analysis. A chart of causes, laid out in order of decreasing frequency, is prepared. Those that occur most frequently are considered the "vital few"; the rest are considered the "trivial many." This method offers direction about where to dedicate resources for maximal effect. An example of a Pareto chart is shown in Fig 1-2.

Identification and Evaluation of Solutions

Potential solutions to problems are identified during the creative phase of process improvement. Brainstorming and process flow charting can be particularly helpful in this phase. Benchmarking with other organizations can also be helpful. Possible solutions should be evaluated relative to organizational constraints and should be narrowed down to those most reasonable. Individuals who perform the process are usually the most knowledgeable about what will work. They should be included when possible solutions are being considered. Individuals with knowledge of the interrelationships of processes and the more "global" view of the organization should also be included. Solutions may fail if representatives with those perspectives are not involved.

Potential solutions should be tested before full implementation, with a clear plan relative to methods, objectives, timelines, deci-

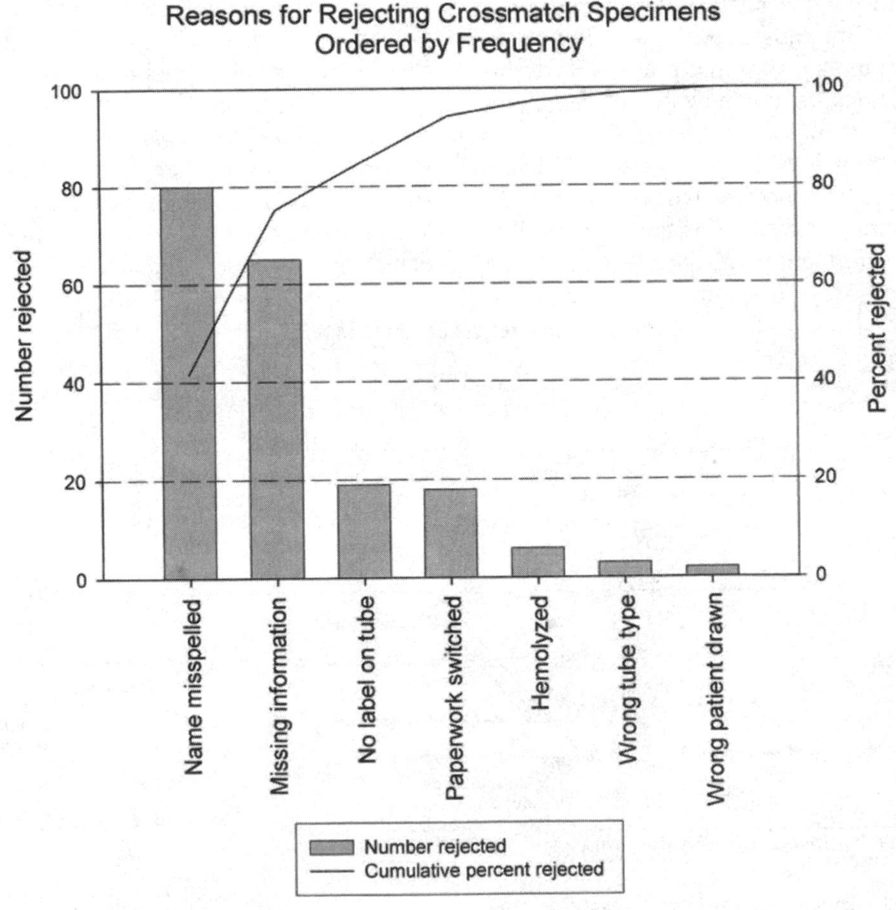

FIGURE 1-2. Example of a Pareto chart.

sion points, and algorithms for all possible results of the trial. Large-scale solutions can be tried on a limited basis and can be expanded if successful; small-scale solutions can be implemented pending an effectiveness evaluation. Data should be collected to evaluate the effectiveness of the proposed change. Data can be collected by the methods used initially to identify the problems or by methods specially designed for the trial. Once solutions have been successfully tested, full implementation can occur. After implementation, data should be collected—on at least a periodic basis—to ensure the continuing effectiveness and control of the changed process.

Other Process Improvement Methods

Failure Modes and Effects Analysis is a systematic step-wise approach for identifying all possible failures within a process, product, or service; for studying and prioritizing the consequences, or effects, of those failures; and for eliminating or reducing the failures, starting with those of highest priority. Despite their relative complexity, LEAN and Six Sigma process improvement methods from the manufacturing industry are finding increasing use in the health-care setting. LEAN emphasizes speed and efficiency. Six Sigma emphasizes precision and accuracy. Six Sigma uses the DMAIC data-driven approach to problem solving: define, measure, analyze, improve, and control. Application of those principles and techniques can improve performance, reduce costs and waste, cut time, and eliminate non-value-added actions. Additional information about both methods can be found on the website of the American Society for Quality.[41]

KEY POINTS

1. **Organization and Leadership.** A defined organizational structure as well as top management's support and commitment to the quality policy, goals, and objectives are key to ensuring the success of the program.
2. **Customer Focus.** Quality organizations should understand and meet or exceed customer needs and expectations. These needs and expectations should be defined in a contract, agreement, or other documented format, with opportunities to obtain feedback from the customer.
3. **Facilities, Work Environment, and Safety.** Procedures related to general safety; biological, chemical, and radiation safety; fire safety; and disaster preparedness are required. Space allocation, building utilities, ventilation, sanitation, trash, and hazardous substance disposal must support the operations of the organization.
4. **Human Resources.** Quality management of all personnel addresses adequate staffing levels and staff selection, orientation, training, and competence assessment, as well as specific regulatory requirements.
5. **Suppliers and Materials Management.** Suppliers of critical materials and services (ie, those affecting quality) should be qualified, and requirements should be defined in contracts or agreements. All critical materials should be inspected and tested upon receipt to ensure specifications are met.
6. **Equipment Management.** Critical equipment may include instruments, measuring devices, and computer hardware and software. This equipment must be uniquely identified and operate within defined specifications, as ensured by qualification, calibration, maintenance, and monitoring.
7. **Process Management.** A systematic approach to develop new and control changes to policies, processes, and procedures includes process validation, test method validation, computer system validation, equipment validation, and quality control. Validation must be planned, and results reviewed and accepted.

8. **Documents and Records.** Documents include policies, processes, procedures, work instructions, forms, and labels. Records provide evidence that the process was performed as intended and allow assessment of the quality of products and services.
9. **Information Management.** Unauthorized access, modification, or destruction of information must be prevented, and confidentiality of patient and donor records maintained. Data integrity should be assessed periodically, and backup devices, alternative systems, and archived documents maintained.
10. **Management of Nonconforming Events.** Deviations from facility-defined requirements, standards, and regulations must be addressed by documenting and classifying occurrences, assessing the effect on quality, implementing remedial action, and reporting to external agencies as required.
11. **Monitoring and Assessment.** Evaluation of facility processes includes internal and external assessments, monitoring of quality indicators, blood utilization assessment, proficiency testing, and analysis of data.
12. **Process Improvement.** Opportunities for improvement may be identified from deviation reports, nonconforming products and services, customer complaints, quality control records, proficiency testing results, internal audits, quality indicator monitoring, and external assessments. Process improvement includes determination of root causes, implementation of corrective actions and preventive actions, and evaluation of the effectiveness of these actions.

REFERENCES

1. Code of federal regulations. Title 42, CFR Part 493. Washington, DC: US Government Printing Office, 2010 (revised annually).
2. Code of federal regulations. Title 21, CFR Parts 606, 610, 630, and 640. Washington, DC: US Government Printing Office, 2010 (revised annually).
3. Code of federal regulations. Title 21, CFR Parts 210 and 211. Washington, DC: US Government Printing Office, 2010 (revised annually).
4. Code of federal regulations. Title 21, CFR Parts 1270 and 1271. Washington, DC: US Government Printing Office, 2010 (revised annually).
5. Food and Drug Administration. Guideline for quality assurance in blood establishments. (July 11, 1995) Rockville, MD: CBER Office of Communication, Outreach, and Development, 1995.
6. Carson TH, ed. Standards for blood banks and transfusion services. 27th ed. Bethesda, MD: AABB, 2011.
7. Fontaine M, ed. Standards for cellular therapy product services. 5th ed. Bethesda, MD: AABB, 2011 (in press).
8. Laboratory Accreditation Program checklists. Chicago: College of American Pathologists, 2010.
9. Hospital accreditation standards. Oakbrook Terrace, IL: Joint Commission Resources, 2011.
10. Laboratory accreditation standards. Oakbrook Terrace, IL: Joint Commission Resources, 2011.
11. Quality management system: A model for laboratory services; approved guideline (GP26-A4), 4th ed. Wayne, PA: Clinical and Laboratory Standards Institute, 2011.
12. FACT-JACIE international standards for cellular therapy product collection, processing, and administration. 4th ed. Omaha, NE: Foundation for the Accreditation of Cellular Therapy and the Joint Accreditation Committee of ISCT and EBMT, 2008.
13. ANSI/ISO/ASQ Q9001-2008 series—quality management standards. Milwaukee, WI: ASQ Quality Press, 2008.
14. Baldrige National Quality Program. Health care criteria for performance excellence. Gaithersburg, MD: National Institute of Standards and Technology, 2010 (revised annually).
15. Quality program implementation. Association bulletin #97-4. Bethesda, MD: AABB, 1997.
16. Food and Drug Administration. Guidance for industry: Quality systems approach to pharmaceutical cGMP regulations. (September 2006) Rockville, MD: CBER Office of Communication, Outreach, and Development, 2006.

17. Code of federal regulations. Title 21, CFR Part 820. Washington, DC: US Government Printing Office, 2010 (revised annually).
18. Juran JM, Godfrey AB. Juran's quality handbook. 5th ed. New York: McGraw-Hill, 1999.
19. Food and Drug Administration. Guidance for industry: Process validations: General principles and practices. (January, 2011) Rockville, MD: CBER Office of Communication, Outreach, and Development, 2011.
20. Food and Drug Administration. Glossary of computerized system and software development terminology. (August 1995) Rockville, MD: Division of Field Investigations, Office of Regional Operations, Office of Regulatory Affairs, 1995.
21. Food and Drug Administration. Guidance for industry: General principles of software validation: Final guidance for industry and FDA staff. (January 11, 2002) Rockville, MD: CBER Office of Communication, Outreach, and Development, 2002.
22. Laboratory documents: Development and control; approved guideline. 5th ed (GP2-A5). Wayne, PA: Clinical and Laboratory Standards Institute, 2006.
23. Code of federal regulations. Title 21, CFR Part 11. Washington, DC: US Government Printing Office, 2010 (revised annually).
24. Management of nonconforming laboratory events; approved guideline. 1st ed (GP32-P). Wayne, PA: Clinical and Laboratory Standards Institute, 2007.
25. Motschman TL, Santrach PJ, Moore SB. Error/incident management and its practical application. In: Duckett JB, Woods LL, Santrach PJ, eds. Quality in action. Bethesda, MD: AABB, 1996:37-67.
26. Food and Drug Administration. Guidance for industry: Notifying FDA of fatalities related to blood collection or transfusion. (September 22, 2003) Rockville, MD: CBER Office of Communication, Outreach, and Development, 2003.
27. Food and Drug Administration. Transfusion/donation fatalities: Notification process for transfusion related fatalities and donation related deaths. Rockville, MD: Center for Biologics Evaluation and Research, 2007. [Available at http://www.fda.gov/BiologicsBloodVaccines/SafetyAvailability/ReportaProblem/TransfusionDonationFatalities/default.htm (accessed September 19, 2010).]
28. Reporting donor fatalities. Association bulletin #04-06. Bethesda, MD: AABB, 2004.
29. Food and Drug Administration. Guidance for industry: Biological product deviation reporting for blood and plasma establishments. (October 18, 2006) Rockville, MD: CBER Office of Communication, Outreach, and Development, 2006.
30. Food and Drug Administration. Biological product deviations: Includes human tissue and cellular and tissue-based product (HCT/P) reporting (BPDR). Rockville, MD: Center for Biologics Evaluation and Research, 2010. [Available at http://www.fda.gov/BiologicsBloodVaccines/SafetyAvailability/ReportaProblem/BiologicalProductDeviations/default.htm (accessed September 19, 2010).]
31. Code of federal regulations. Title 21, CFR Part 803. Washington, DC: US Government Printing Office, 2010 (revised annually).
32. Strong DM, AuBuchon J, Whitaker B, Kuehnert MJ. Biovigilance initiatives. ISBT Science Series 2008;3:77-84.
33. Shulman IA, Lohr K, Derdiarian AK, et al. Monitoring transfusionist practices: A strategy for improving transfusion safety. Transfusion 1994;34:11-15.
34. Becker J, Blackall D, Evans C, et al, for the Scientific Section Coordinating Committee. Guidelines for blood utilization review. Bethesda, MD: AABB, 2001.
35. Strauss RG, Blanchette VS, Hume H. National acceptability of American Association of Blood Banks Hemotherapy Committee guidelines for auditing pediatric transfusion practices. Transfusion 1993;33:168-71.
36. Vaichekauskas L. You need the tools to do the job. In: Walters L, ed. Introducing the big Q: A practical quality primer. Bethesda, MD: AABB Press, 2004:181-206.
37. Walters L. So many tools, so little understanding. In: Walters L, Carpenter-Badley J, eds. S[3]: Simple Six Sigma for blood banking, transfusion, and cellular therapy. Bethesda, MD: AABB Press, 2007:9-24.
38. Tague NR. The quality toolbox. 2nd ed. Milwaukee, WI: ASQ Quality Press, 2005.
39. Motschman TL. Corrective versus preventive action. AABB News 1999;21(8):5,33.
40. Russell JP, Regel T. After the quality audit: Closing the loop on the audit process. 2nd ed. Milwaukee, WI: ASQ Quality Press, 2000.
41. Learn about quality. Milwaukee, WI: American Society for Quality, 2010. [Available at http://www.asq.org/learn-about-quality/ (accessed September 19, 2010).]

◆ APPENDIX 1-1
Glossary of Commonly Used Quality Terms

Biovigilance	The collection and analysis of adverse event data for the purpose of improving outcomes in the use of blood products, organs, tissues and cellular therapies.
Calibration	Comparison of measurements performed by an instrument to those made by a more accurate instrument or standard for the purpose of detecting, reporting, and eliminating errors in measurement.
Change control	Established procedures for planning, documenting, communicating, and executing changes to infrastructure, processes, products, or services. Such procedures include the submission, analysis, decision-making, approval, implementation, and postimplementation review of the change. Formal change control provides a measure of stability and safety and avoids arbitrary changes that might affect quality.
Control chart	A graphic tool used to determine whether the distribution of data values generated by a process is stable over time. A control chart plots a statistic vs time and helps to determine whether a process is in control or out of control according to defined criteria (eg, a shift from a central line or a trend toward upper or lower acceptance limits).
Design output	Documents, records, and evidence in any other format used to verify that design goals have been met. Design output should identify characteristics of a product or service that are crucial to safety and function and to meeting regulatory requirements. It should contain or make reference to acceptance criteria. Examples of design output include standard operating procedures; specifications for supplies, reagents, and equipment; identification of quality control requirements; and results of verification and validation activities.
End-product test and inspection	Verification through observation, examination, or testing (or a combination) that the finished product or service conforms to specified requirements.
Near-miss event	An unexpected occurrence that did not adversely affect the outcome but could have resulted in a serious adverse event.
Process capability	Ability of a controlled process to produce a service or product that fulfills requirements. Also, a statistical measure of the inherent process variability for a given characteristic relative to design specifications. The most widely accepted formula for process capability is Six Sigma.
Process control	Activities intended to minimize variation within a process in order to produce a predictable output that meets specifications.
Qualification	Demonstration that an entity is capable of fulfilling specified requirements. Verification of attributes that must be met or complied with in order for a person or thing to be considered fit to perform a particular function. For example, equipment may be qualified for an intended use by verifying performance characteristics such as linearity, sensitivity, or ease of use. An employee may be qualified on the basis of technical, academic, and practical knowledge and skills developed through training, education, and on-the-job performance.

◆ APPENDIX 1-1

Glossary of Commonly Used Quality Terms (Continued)

Quality assurance	Activities involving quality planning, control, assessment, reporting, and improvement necessary to ensure that a product or service meets defined quality standards and requirements.
Quality control (QC)	Operational techniques and activities used to monitor and eliminate causes of unsatisfactory performance at any stage of a process.
Quality indicators	Measurable aspects of processes or outcomes that provide an indication of the condition or direction of performance over time. Quality indicators are used to monitor progress toward stated quality goals and objectives.
Quality management	The organizational structure, processes, and procedures necessary to ensure that the overall intentions and direction of an organization's quality program are met and that the quality of the product or service is ensured. Quality management includes strategic planning, allocation of resources, and other systematic activities such as quality planning, implementation, and evaluation.
Requirement	A stated or obligatory need or expectation that can be measured or observed and that is necessary to ensure quality, safety, effectiveness, or customer satisfaction. Requirements can include things that the system or product must do, characteristics it must have, and levels of performance it must attain.
Specification	Description of a set of requirements to be satisfied by a product, material, or process indicating, if appropriate, the procedures to be used to determine whether the requirements are satisfied. Specifications are often in the form of written descriptions, drawings, professional standards, and other descriptive references.
Validation	Demonstration through objective evidence that the requirements for a particular application or intended use have been met. Validation provides assurance that new or changed processes and procedures are capable of consistently meeting specified requirements before implementation.
Verification	Confirmation, by examination of objective evidence, that specified requirements have been met.

♦ APPENDIX 1-2
Code of Federal Regulations Quality-Related References

Topic	Code of Federal Regulations, Title 21		
	Biologics, Blood	Drugs	Tissue, HCT/Ps
Personnel	600.10, 606.20	211.25, 211.28	1271.170
Facilities	600.11, 606.40	211.42-58	1271.190
Environmental control and monitoring			1271.195
Equipment	606.60	211.63-72, 211.105	1271.200
Supplies and reagents	606.65	211.80	1271.210
Standard operating procedures	606.100	211.100-101	1270.31, 1271.180
Process changes and validation		211.100-101	1271.225, 1271.230
Quality assurance/quality control unit		211.22	
Label controls	610.60-64, 606.120-122	211.122-130	1271.250, 1271.370
Laboratory controls	606.140	211.160	
Records and record reviews	600.12, 606.160	211.192, 211.194, 211.196	1270.33, 1271.270
Receipt, predistribution, distribution	606.165	211.142, 211.150	1271.265
Adverse reactions	606.170	211.198	1271.350
Tracking		211.188	1271.290
Complaints		211.198	1271.320
Reporting deviations	600.14, 606.171		1271.350
Storage	640.2, 640.11, 640.25, 640.34, 640.54, 640.69		1271.260

HCT/Ps = human cells, tissues, and cellular and tissue-based products.

◆ APPENDIX 1-3

Statistical Tables for Binomial Distribution* Used to Determine Adequate Sample Size and Level of Confidence for Validation of Pass/Fail Data

A. Confidence Levels (%) for Percent Conforming

		Requirement for % Conforming				Requirement for % Conforming	
		90%	95%			90%	95%
Sample Size	No. of Failures	% Confidence		Sample Size	No. of Failures	% Confidence	
10	0	65.1	–	50	0	99.5	92.3
	1	26.4	–		1	96.6	72.1
20	0	87.8	64.2		2	88.8	45.9
	1	60.8	26.4		3	75.0	–
	2	32.3	–		4	56.9	–
30	0	95.8	78.5		5	38.4	–
	1	81.6	44.6	60	0	99.8	95.4
	2	58.9	–		1	98.6	80.8
	3	35.3	–		2	94.7	58.3
40	0	98.5	87.1		3	86.3	35.3
	1	91.9	60.1		4	72.9	–
	2	77.7	32.3		5	56.3	–
	3	57.7	–		6	39.4	–
	4	37.1	–				

This table answers the question, *How confident am I that [90 or 95]% of all products manufactured will meet specifications if I have tested __ number of samples and found __ number to be nonconforming (failures)?*

*Data from Alion System Reliability Center. [See calculator at http://src.alionscience.com (accessed September 19, 2010).]

(Continued)

◆ APPENDIX 1-3

Statistical Tables for Binomial Distribution* Used to Determine Adequate Sample Size and Level of Confidence for Validation of Pass/Fail Data (Continued)

B. Minimum Sample Size for Percent Conforming

	Requirement for Percent Conforming								
	90% Confidence Level			95% Confidence Level			99% Confidence Level		
	90%	95%	99%	90%	95%	99%	90%	95%	99%
No. of Failures	Sample Size			Sample Size			Sample Size		
0	22	29	45	46	59	90	230	299	459
1	39	47	65	77	94	130	388	467	662
2	53	63	83	106	125	166	526	625	838
3	66	76	98	133	180	198	664	773	1002
4	78	90	113	159	208	228	789	913	1157
5	91	103	128	184	235	258	926	1049	1307
6	104	116	142	209	260	288	1051	1186	1453
7	116	129	158	234	286	317	1175	1312	
8	128	143	170	258	310	344	1297	1441	
9	140	154	184	282	336	370	1418		
10	152	167	197	306	361	397			

This table answers the question, *How many samples do I need to test with ___ number of failures if I want to have [90, 95, or 99]% confidence that [90, 95, or 99]% of all products will meet specifications?*

*Data from Alion System Reliability Center. [See calculator at http://src.alionscience.com (accessed September 19, 2010).]

◆ APPENDIX 1-4

Suggested Quality Control Performance Intervals for Equipment and Reagents*

Equipment and Reagent	Frequency of Quality Control
Refrigerators/freezers/platelet storage	
Refrigerators	
◆ Recorder	Daily
◆ Manual temperature	Daily
◆ Alarm system board (if applicable)	Daily
◆ Temperature charts (review daily)	Weekly
◆ Alarm activation	Quarterly
Freezers	
◆ Recorder	Daily
◆ Manual temperature	Daily
◆ Alarm system board (if applicable)	Daily
◆ Temperature charts (review daily)	Weekly
◆ Alarm activation	Quarterly
Platelet incubators	
◆ Recorder	Daily
◆ Manual temperature	Daily
◆ Temperature charts (review daily)	Weekly
◆ Alarm activation	Quarterly
Ambient platelet storage	Every 4 hours
Laboratory equipment	
Centrifuges/cell washers	
◆ Speed	Quarterly
◆ Timer	Quarterly
◆ Function	Yearly
◆ Tube fill level (serologic)	Day of use
◆ Saline fill volume (serologic)	Weekly
◆ Volume of antihuman globulin dispensed (if applicable)	Monthly
◆ Temperature check (refrigerated centrifuge)	Day of use
◆ Temperature verification (refrigerated centrifuge)	Monthly

(Continued)

◆ APPENDIX 1-4

Suggested Quality Control Performance Intervals for Equipment and Reagents* (Continued)

Equipment and Reagents	Frequency of Quality Control
Heating blocks/waterbaths/view boxes	
◆ Temperature	Day of use
◆ Quadrant/area checks	Periodically
Component thawing devices	Day of use
pH meters	Day of use
Blood irradiators	
◆ Calibration	Yearly
◆ Turntable (visual check each time of use)	Yearly
◆ Timer	Monthly/quarterly
◆ Source decay	Dependent on source type
◆ Leak test	Twice yearly
◆ Dose delivery check (with indicator)	Each irradiator use
◆ Dose delivery verification	
– Cesium-137	Yearly
– Cobalt-60	Twice yearly
– Other source	As specified by manufacturer
Thermometers (vs NIST-certified or traceable)	
◆ Liquid-in-glass	Yearly
◆ Electronic	As specified by manufacturer
Timers/clocks	Twice yearly
Pipette recalibration	Quarterly
Sterile connecting device	
◆ Weld check	Each use
◆ Function	Yearly
Blood warmers	
◆ Effluent temperature	Quarterly
◆ Heater temperature	Quarterly
◆ Alarm activation	Quarterly

◆ APPENDIX 1-4
Suggested Quality Control Performance Intervals for Equipment and Reagents* (Continued)

Equipment and Reagents	Frequency of Quality Control
Blood collection equipment	
Whole blood equipment	
◆ Agitators	Day of use
◆ Balances/scales	Day of use
◆ Gram weight (vs NIST-certified)	Yearly
Microhematocrit centrifuge	
◆ Timer check	Quarterly
◆ Calibration	Quarterly
◆ Packed cell volume	Yearly
Cell counters/hemoglobinometers	Day of use
Blood pressure cuffs	Twice yearly
Apheresis equipment	
◆ Checklist requirements	As specified by manufacturer
Reagents	
Red cells	Day of use
Antisera	Day of use
Antiglobulin serum	Day of use
Transfusion-transmissible disease marker testing	Each test run
Miscellaneous	
Copper sulfate	Day of use
Shipping containers for blood and component transport (usually at temperature extremes)	Twice yearly

*Note: The frequencies listed above are suggested intervals, not requirements. For any new piece of equipment, installation, operational, and performance qualifications must be performed. After the equipment has been suitably qualified for use, ongoing quality control (QC) testing should be performed. Depending on the operational and performance qualification methodology, the ongoing QC may initially be performed at a greater frequency than one ultimately wishes to use. Once a track record of appropriate in-range QC results has been established (during either equipment qualification or the ongoing QC), the frequency of testing can be reduced. At a minimum, the frequency must comply with the manufacturer's suggested intervals; if no such guidance is provided by the manufacturer, the intervals given in this table would be appropriate to use.
NIST = National Institute of Standards and Technology.

Chapter 2

Facilities, Work Environment, and Safety

◆

Betsy W. Jett, MT(ASCP), CQA(ASQ)CQM/OE; Susan L. Wilkinson, EdD, MS, MT(ASCP)SBB, CQA(ASQ); and Tania L. Motschman, MS, MT(ASCP)SBB, CQA(ASQ)

THE PHYSICAL WORK environment can have a significant impact on the safety, efficiency, and effectiveness of work processes and on the quality of work process outcomes. It should be designed and managed in a way that meets operational needs and provides for the safety of staff and visitors. The layout of the physical space; management of utilities such as water and air ventilation; flow of personnel, materials, and waste; and ergonomic factors should all be considered in the facility management plan.

In addition to providing adequate facilities, the organization must develop and implement a safety program that defines policies and procedures for safe work practices and emergency response. Such a program also includes requirements for training, hazard communication, use of engineering controls, and protective equipment. All employees are responsible for protecting their own safety and the safety of others by adhering to policies and procedures set forth in the facility safety program.

The AABB requires accredited transfusion medicine, cellular therapy, and clinical diagnostic services to plan, implement, and maintain a program to minimize risks to the health and safety of donors, patients, volunteers, and employees from biological, chemical, and radiological hazards.[1,2] Other professional and accrediting organizations, including the College of American Pathologists (CAP), the Clinical and Laboratory Standards Institute (CLSI), and The Joint Commission, have similar or more detailed safety program requirements.[3-6]

US federal regulations and recommendations intended to protect the safety of workers and the public in health-care settings are listed

Betsy W. Jett, MT(ASCP), CQA(ASQ)CQM/OE, Chief Operations Officer, Department of Transfusion Medicine, National Institutes of Health, Bethesda, Maryland; Susan L. Wilkinson, EdD, MS, MT(ASCP)SBB, CQA(ASQ), Associate Director and Associate Professor, Hoxworth Blood Center, University of Cincinnati, Cincinnati, Ohio; and Tania L. Motschman, MS, MT(ASCP)SBB, CQA(ASQ), Regulatory and Accreditation Manager, Department of Laboratory Medicine and Pathology, Mayo Clinic, Rochester, Minnesota
The authors have disclosed no conflicts of interest.

in Appendix 2-1. The contents of these regulations and guidelines are discussed in more detail in each section of this chapter. US state and local government regulations should be reviewed as well to identify any additional safety requirements. State and local building codes address architectural and construction safety requirements. Trade and professional organizations such as those listed in Appendix 2-1 also provide relevant safety recommendations.

FACILITIES

Facility Design and Workflow

Effective design and maintenance of facilities, along with the physical organization of work activities, can help to reduce or eliminate many potential hazards. Facility design, workflow, and maintenance also affect process efficiency, productivity, error rates, employee and customer satisfaction, and the quality of products and services.

During the design phase for a new or renovated space, the location and flow of personnel, materials, and equipment should be considered in the context of the processes to be performed. Adequate space must be allotted for personnel movement, for location of supplies and large equipment, and for private or distraction-free zones for certain manufacturing tasks (eg, donor interviewing, record review, and blood component labeling). The facility must be able to accommodate designated "clean" and "dirty" spaces and to provide for controlled movement of materials and waste in and out of these areas so as to avoid contamination. Chemical fume hoods and biological safety cabinets (BSCs) should be located away from drafts and high-traffic areas. The number and location of eyewash stations and emergency showers must also be considered. Water sources for reagent preparation must be provided. Staff handling hazardous materials must have ready access to handwashing sinks. For certain pieces of heavy equipment, such as irradiators, load-bearing capacity must be taken into account.

Laboratories must be designed with adequate illumination, electrical power, and conveniently located electrical outlets. Emergency backup power sources, such as uninterruptible power supplies and backup generators, should be considered to ensure that blood components, cellular therapy products, and critical reagents are not compromised during power failures. The National Electrical Code[7] is routinely used as a national guideline for the design of essential electrical distribution systems, with modifications approved by the local building authority having jurisdiction.

Heating, ventilation, and air conditioning must be adequate for the needs of the facility. Environmental monitoring systems should be considered for laboratories that require positive or negative air pressure differentials, or where air filtration systems are used to control particle levels. The nationally accepted specifications for ventilation are published by the American Society of Heating, Refrigerating, and Air-Conditioning Engineers.[8]

Housekeeping

The workplace should be kept clean and free of clutter. Work surfaces and equipment should be regularly cleaned and disinfected. Items that may accumulate dust and debris should not be stored above clean supplies or work surfaces. Exits and fire safety equipment must not be blocked or obstructed in any way. Receptacles and disposal guidelines for nonhazardous solid waste and biohazardous, chemical, and radiation waste should be clearly delineated. Housekeeping responsibilities, methods, and schedules should be defined for every work area. Written procedures, initial training, continuing education of personnel, and ongoing monitoring of housekeeping effectiveness are essential to safe operations.

Clean Rooms

Clean room facilities should be considered for open processing activities that cannot be accommodated in a BSC. Laboratories that process cellular therapy products may choose to adopt clean room specifications and maintenance practices to meet the requirements of the Food and Drug Administration (FDA) current good tissue practice (cGTP) regulations.[9] International standards for clean rooms are published by the International Organization for Standardization (ISO) and provide specifications for general manufacturing applications to limit airborne particulates, contaminants, and pollutants.[10] They also provide specific guidance for pharmaceutical and biotechnology applications that include methods to assess, monitor, and control biocontamination.[11] Aspects of a biocontamination control system include 1) developing air sampling plans using validated equipment, 2) assessing biocontamination of surfaces, textiles, and liquids, 3) evaluating laundering processes, and 4) maintaining personnel training and work practices.

Restricted Areas

Hazardous areas should be clearly and uniformly identified with warning signs in accordance with federal Occupational Safety and Health Administration (OSHA) and Nuclear Regulatory Commission (NRC) standards so that personnel entering or working around them are aware of existing biological, chemical, or radiation dangers.[12-15] Staff members not normally assigned to these areas should receive adequate training to avoid endangering themselves. Risk areas can be stratified. For example, "high-risk" areas might include those that contain chemical fume hoods, BSCs, and storage areas for volatile chemicals or radioisotopes. Technical work areas might be considered "moderate risk" and restricted to laboratory personnel. Administrative and clerical areas are generally considered "low risk" and not restricted. Guidelines for restricted access based on biosafety levels are published by the US Department of Health and Human Services (DHHS).[16] When possible, functions not requiring special precautions should be separated from those performed in restricted areas.

Casual visitors should not be allowed in restricted areas. Children should not be allowed in areas where they could be exposed to hazards and should be closely supervised in those areas where their presence is permitted. Organizations should consider establishing specific safety guidelines for visitors with business in restricted areas and verifying that safety guidelines were received and understood before the visitors access the area.

Mobile Sites

Mobile blood collection operations can present special challenges. Responsibility for site safety is generally assigned to an individual with adequate knowledge to recognize safety concerns and with the authority to address them in a timely manner. An advance safety survey of the proposed collection site will help to ensure that hazards are minimized. All mobile personnel should be trained to recognize unsafe conditions and understand how to effectively implement infection control policies and procedures in a variety of settings.

Hand-washing access is essential at collection sites. Carpeted or difficult-to-clean surfaces may be covered using an absorbent overlay with waterproof backing to protect them from possible blood spills. Portable screens and crowd control stations and ropes are helpful in directing traffic flow to maintain safe work areas. Food service areas should be physically separated from areas for blood collection and storage. Blood-contaminated waste must be either returned to a central location for disposal or packaged and decontaminated in accordance with local regulations for medical wastes. Trained staff must perform this decontamination with particular attention paid to cleanup of mobile sites after blood collection.

Ergonomics

Consideration in physical design should be given to ergonomics and to accommodations for individuals covered under the Americans with Disabilities Act (42 USC §§2101-12213, 1990). Several factors may contribute to employee fatigue, musculoskeletal disorder syndromes, or injury, including the following[17]:

- Awkward postures—positions that place stress on the body such as reaching over-

head, twisting, bending, kneeling, or squatting.
- Repetition—performing the same motions continuously or frequently.
- Force—the amount of physical effort used to perform work.
- Pressure points—pressing the body against hard or sharp surfaces.
- Vibration—continuous or high-intensity hand/arm or whole-body vibration.
- Other environmental factors—extreme high or low temperatures; lighting too dark or too bright.

Both the total time per work shift and the length of uninterrupted periods of work can be significant in contributing to physical problems. Actions to correct problems associated with ergonomics may include the following:

- Engineering improvements to reduce or eliminate the underlying cause, such as making changes to equipment, workstations, or materials.
- Administrative improvements, such as providing variety in tasks; adjusting work schedules and work pace; providing recovery or relaxation time; modifying work practices; ensuring regular housekeeping and maintenance of work spaces, tools, and equipment; and encouraging exercise.
- Provision of personal protective equipment (PPE) such as gloves, knee and elbow pads, footwear, and other items that employees should wear to protect themselves against injury.

SAFETY PROGRAM

An effective safety program starts with a well-thought-out safety plan. This plan identifies the applicable regulatory requirements and describes how they will be met. In general, institutions are required to do the following:

- Provide a workplace free of recognized hazards.
- Evaluate all procedures for potential exposure risks.
- Evaluate each employment position for potential exposure risks.
- Identify hazardous areas or materials with appropriate labels and signs.
- Educate staff, document training, and monitor compliance.
- Apply Standard Precautions (including Universal and Blood and Body Fluid Precautions) to the handling of blood, body fluids, and tissues.
- Dispose of hazardous waste appropriately.
- Report incidents and accidents, and provide treatment and follow-up.
- Provide ongoing review of safety policies, procedures, operations, and equipment.
- Develop facility policies for disaster preparedness and response.

Safety programs should consider the needs of all persons affected by the work environment. Most obvious is the safety of technical staff members, but potential risks for blood donors, ancillary personnel, volunteers, visitors, housekeeping staff, and maintenance and repair workers must also be evaluated. Appropriate provisions must be applied if these individuals cannot be excluded from risk areas.

Laboratories should appoint a safety officer who can provide general guidance and expertise.[4] A safety officer might develop the safety program, oversee orientation and training, perform safety audits, survey work sites, recommend changes, and serve on or direct the activities of safety committees. Facilities using hazardous chemicals and radioactive materials often assign specially trained individuals to oversee chemical and radiation protection programs as needed.[12,15] Five basic elements must be addressed for each type of hazard covered in the safety program:

- Training.
- Hazard identification and communication.
- Engineering controls and PPE.
- Safe work practices, including waste disposal.
- Emergency response plan.

Management controls should be established to ensure that these elements are implemented, maintained, and effective. Management is responsible for the following:

- Developing and communicating the written plan.
- Ensuring implementation and providing adequate resources.
- Providing access to employee health services related to prevention strategies and treatment of exposures.
- Monitoring compliance and effectiveness.
- Evaluating and improving the safety plan.

Basic Elements of a Safety Program

Training

Employees must be trained to recognize the hazards in their workplace and the appropriate precautions to take in order to manage hazards safely. Supervisors are responsible for assessing and documenting each employee's understanding of and ability to apply safety precautions before independent work is permitted. Safety training must precede even temporary work assignments if significant potential for exposure exists. Staff members who do not demonstrate the requisite understanding and skills must undergo retraining. These requirements apply not only to laboratory staff but also to housekeeping and other personnel who may come into contact with hazardous substances or waste. Table 2-1 lists topics to cover in work safety training programs.

Hazard Identification and Communication

Employees must know when they are working with hazardous substances and must know where the substances are located in the workplace. Organizations are required to provide information about workplace hazards to their employees to help reduce the risk of occupational illnesses and injuries. This communication is achieved by means of signage, labels on containers, written information, and training programs.

Engineering Controls and Personal Protective Equipment

Whenever possible, the physical workspace should be designed to eliminate any potential for exposure. When elimination is not possible, protective gear must be provided to protect the employee. Engineering controls are physical plant controls or equipment such as sprinkler systems, chemical fume hoods, and needleless systems that isolate or remove the hazard from the workplace. PPE is specialized clothing or equipment, such as gloves, masks, and laboratory coats, worn by an employee for protection against a hazard. Employees should remove their PPE such as gloves and laboratory coats and should wash their hands with soap and water when leaving a laboratory area. General guidance on the use of engineering controls and PPE is included in Appendix 2-2.

Safe Work Practices

Employees must be trained to know how to work with hazardous materials in ways that protect themselves, their coworkers, and the environment. Safe work practices are defined as tasks performed in a manner that reduces the likelihood of exposure to workplace hazards. General recommendations for safe work practices are included in Appendix 2-2.

Emergency Response Plan

When engineering and work practice controls fail, employees must know how to respond promptly and appropriately. The purpose of advance planning is to control the hazardous situation as quickly and safely as possible. Regular testing of the emergency response plan will identify areas for improvement and will also build confidence in the staff to respond effectively in a real situation. OSHA requires a written plan for facilities with more than 10 employees. Verbal communication of the plan is acceptable for facilities with 10 or fewer employees.[18]

Management Controls

Supervisory personnel must monitor safety practices in their areas of responsibility. Continuing attention to safety issues should be addressed in routine staff meetings and training sessions. Periodic audits performed by a safety professional help to increase safety awareness. Management should seek staff input for the design and improvement of the facility's safety plan.

The safety program, with its policies, guidelines, and supporting references to regulatory documents, should be detailed in a safety manual and made available to all personnel at risk. That manual, along with operational procedure manuals, should be reviewed on a regular basis and updated as technology evolves and new information becomes available. Work sites and safety equipment should be inspected regularly to ensure compliance and response readiness. Checklists may be helpful in documenting safety inspections and assessing safety preparedness.[3,4,19]

Employee Health Services

Hepatitis Prophylaxis

All employees routinely exposed to blood must be offered hepatitis B virus (HBV) vaccine if

TABLE 2-1. Topics to Cover in a Work Safety Training Program

Work safety training programs should ensure that all personnel:
◆ Have access to a copy of pertinent regulatory texts and an explanation of the contents.
◆ Understand the employer's exposure control plan and how to obtain a copy of the written plan.
◆ Understand how hepatitis and human immunodeficiency virus (HIV) are transmitted and how often; be familiar with the symptoms and consequences of hepatitis B virus (HBV), hepatitis C virus, and HIV infection.
◆ Know that they are offered vaccination against HBV.
◆ Recognize tasks that pose infectious risks, and distinguish them from other duties.
◆ Know what protective clothing and equipment are appropriate for the procedures they will perform and how to use them.
◆ Know and understand the limitations of protective clothing and equipment (eg, different types of gloves are recommended according to the permeability of the hazardous material to be used).
◆ Know where protective clothing and equipment are kept.
◆ Become familiar with and understand all requirements for work practices specified in standard operating procedures for the tasks they perform, including the meaning of signs and labels.
◆ Know how to remove, handle, decontaminate, and dispose of contaminated material.
◆ Know the appropriate actions to take and the personnel to contact if exposed to blood or other biologic, chemical, or radiologic hazards.
◆ Know the corrective actions to take in the event of spills or personal exposure to fluids, tissues, and contaminated sharp objects; the appropriate reporting procedures; and the medical monitoring recommended when parenteral exposure may have occurred.
◆ Know their right for access to medical treatment and medical records.
◆ Know fire safety procedures and evacuation plans.

they do not already have HBV-protective antibodies (ie, anti-HBs). OSHA requires that the vaccine be offered at no cost to all employees and, if any employee refuses the vaccine, that the refusal be documented.[14]

Monitoring Programs

The employer must provide a system for monitoring exposure to certain substances as defined in the OSHA standard if there is reason to believe that exposure levels routinely exceed the recommended action level.[20]

Medical First Aid and Follow-up

When requested by a worker who has sustained known or suspected blood exposure, monitoring for HBV, hepatitis C virus (HCV), and human immunodeficiency virus (HIV) infection should be provided, with appropriate counseling. In some states, consent is required for this voluntary testing; rejection of offered testing must be documented. The usual schedule would include immediate tests on the worker and on the source of the potentially infectious material, with follow-up testing of the worker at intervals after exposure.[13,14] All aspects of accident follow-up should be appropriately documented.

The Centers for Disease Control and Prevention (CDC) has published recommendations for both pre-exposure and post-exposure prophylaxis if the contaminating material is HBV-positive or if this information is unknown.[21] Hepatitis B Immune Globulin is usually given concurrently with hepatitis B vaccine in cases of penetrating injuries. When administered in accordance with the manufacturer's directions, both products are very safe and carry no documented risk for infection with HBV, HCV, or HIV. Post-exposure prophylaxis for HIV is continually evolving; policies are generally based on Public Health Service recommendations[21] and on current standards of practice.

Reporting Accidents and Injuries

When an injury occurs, as much relevant information as possible should be documented (see Table 2-2). The supervisor should complete any accident reports and investigation forms required by the institution's insurer and by worker's compensation agencies. Medical records for individual employees should be preserved for the duration of employment plus 30 years, with few exceptions.[21]

OSHA requires health service employers with 11 or more workers to maintain records of occupational injuries and illnesses requiring a level of care that exceeds the capabilities of a person trained in first aid.[22] Records of first aid provided by a nonphysician for minor injuries such as cuts or burns do not have to be retained. Initial documentation must be completed within 6 days of the incident. All logs, summaries, and supplemental records must be preserved for at least 5 years beyond the calendar year of occurrence. Employers must report fatalities and injuries resulting in the hospitalization of three or more employees to OSHA within 8 hours of the accident.[22]

Latex Allergies

With the increased use of gloves, there has been a rise in the number of health care workers with latex allergies. Adverse reactions associated with latex, powdered gloves, or both include contact dermatitis, allergic dermatitis, urticaria, and anaphylaxis. Medical devices that contain latex must bear a caution label. The National Institute for Occupational Safety and Health (NIOSH) offers the following recommendations[23]:

- Make latex-free gloves available as an alternative to latex. Encourage use of latex-free gloves for activities and work environments where there is minimal risk of exposure to infectious materials.
- If latex gloves are used, provide reduced-protein, powder-free gloves. (Note: This is not a requirement, but a recommendation to reduce exposure.)
- Use good housekeeping practices to remove latex-containing dust from the workplace.

TABLE 2-2. Information for Possible Inclusion in Injury Reports

♦ Name and address of the injured person
♦ Time of the injury (hour, day, month, year)
♦ Specified place where the injury occurred
♦ Details of the injured person's activities at the time of injury
♦ Nature of the injury (eg, bruise, laceration, burn, etc)
♦ Part of the body injured (eg, head, arm, leg, etc)
♦ Nature of the known or potential agent, in cases of exposure to pathologic organisms or other hazardous materials
♦ Nature of medical attention or first aid applied in the workplace
♦ Date the injured person stopped work
♦ Date the injured person returned to work
♦ Injured person's statement of the events leading to the injury
♦ Statements from witnesses, if applicable
♦ Cause of the injury
♦ Corrective action taken or recommendations for corrective action
♦ Supervisor notification and signature
♦ Signature of employee

- Use work practices that reduce the chance of reaction, such as hand washing and avoiding oil-based hand lotions.
- Provide workers with education programs and training materials about latex allergy.
- Periodically screen high-risk workers for latex allergy symptoms.
- Evaluate current prevention strategies.
- If symptoms of latex allergy develop, have workers avoid direct contact with latex and consult a physician about allergy precautions.

FIRE PREVENTION

Fire prevention relies on a combination of facility design that is based on the National Fire Protection Association (NFPA) Life Safety Code,[24] defined processes to maintain fire protection systems in good working order, and fire safe work practices. The Life Safety Code includes both active and passive fire protection systems (eg, alarms, smoke detectors, sprinklers, exit lights in corridors, and fire-rated barriers).

Training

Fire safety training is recommended at the start of employment and at least annually thereafter. Training should emphasize prevention and an employee's awareness of the work environment, including how to recognize and report unsafe conditions, how to report fires, where the nearest alarm and fire containment equipment are located and their use, and what the evacuation policies and routes are.

All staff members in facilities accredited by CAP or The Joint Commission are required to participate in fire drills at least annually.[3,5] In areas where patients are housed or treated, The Joint Commission requires quarterly drills on each shift. Staff participation and understanding should be documented.

Hazard Identification and Communication

Emergency exits must be clearly marked with an "EXIT" sign. Additional signage must be posted along the exit route to show the direction of travel if it is not immediately apparent. All flammable materials should be labeled with appropriate hazard warnings, and flammable storage cabinets should be clearly marked.

Engineering Controls and Personal Protective Equipment

Laboratories storing large volumes of flammable chemicals are usually built with 2-hour fire separation walls, or with 1-hour separation if there is an automatic fire extinguishing system.[4] Permanent exit routes must be designed to provide free and unobstructed exit from all parts of the facility to an area of safety. Secondary exits may be required for areas larger than 1000 square feet; consult local safety authorities having jurisdiction, such as the local fire marshal and the NFPA. Fire detection and alarm systems should be provided in accordance with federal, state, and local regulations.

Safe Work Practices

All fire equipment should be inspected on a regular basis to ensure good working order. Fire extinguishers should be made readily available, and the staff should be trained to use them properly. Emergency exit routes must be clear of anything that would obstruct evacuation efforts. Exit doors must not be locked in such a way that egress is impeded. Housekeeping and inventory management plans should be designed to control the accumulations of flammable and combustible materials stored in the facility. In areas where sprinkler systems are installed, all items should be stored at least 18 inches below the sprinkler head. Local fire codes may require greater clearance.

Emergency Response Plan

The fire emergency response plan should encompass both facility-wide and area-specific situations. It should describe reporting and alarm systems; location and use of emergency equipment; roles and responsibilities for the staff during the response; "defend in place" strategies; and conditions for evacuation, evacuation procedures, and exit routes.[5,18] When a fire occurs, the general sequence for immediate response should be to 1) rescue anyone in immediate danger; 2) activate the fire alarm system and alert others in the area; 3) confine the fire by closing doors and shutting off fans or other oxygen sources if possible; and 4) extinguish the fire with a portable extinguisher if the fire is small, or evacuate if it is too large to manage.

ELECTRICAL SAFETY

Electrical hazards, including fire and shock, may arise from use of faulty electrical equipment; damaged receptacles, connectors, or cords; or unsafe work practices. Proper use of electrical equipment, periodic inspection and maintenance, and hazard recognition training are essential to help prevent accidents that may result in electric shock or electrocution. The severity of shock depends on the path that the electrical current takes through the body, the amount of current flowing through the body, and the length of time that current is flowing through the body. Even low-voltage exposures can lead to serious injury.[25]

Training

Safety training should be designed to make employees aware of electrical hazards associated with receptacles and connectors and to help them recognize potential problems such as broken receptacles and connectors, improper electrical connections, damaged cords, and inadequate grounding.

Hazard Identification and Communication

The safety plan should address the proper use of receptacles and connectors. Equipment that does not meet safety standards should be marked to prevent accidental use.

Engineering Controls and Personal Protective Equipment

OSHA requires that electrical systems and equipment be constructed and installed in a way that minimizes the potential for workplace hazards. When purchasing equipment, the facility should verify that it bears the mark of an OSHA-approved independent testing laboratory such as Underwriters Laboratories (UL).[26] Adequate working space should be provided around equipment to allow easy access for safe operation and maintenance. Ground-fault circuit interrupters should be installed in damp or wet areas.

Safe Work Practices

Electrical safety practices are focused around two factors: 1) proper use of electrical equipment and 2) proper maintenance and repair. Staff should not plug or unplug equipment from an electrical source with wet hands. Overloading circuits with too many devices may cause the current to heat the wires to a very high temperature and may generate a fire. Damaged receptacles and faulty electrical equipment must be tagged and removed from service until they have been repaired and checked for safety. Flexible cords should be secured to prevent tripping and should be protected from damage from heavy or sharp objects. Flexible cords should be kept slackened to prevent tension on electrical terminals, and cords should be checked regularly for cut, broken, or cracked insulation. Extension cords should not be used in lieu of permanent wiring.

Emergency Response Plan

In case of an emergency, when it is not possible to decrease the power or disconnect equipment, the power supply should be shut off from the circuit breaker. If it is not possible to interrupt the power supply, a nonconductive material such as dry wood should be used to pry a victim from the source of current.[25] Victims must not be touched directly. Emergency first aid for victims of electrical shock must be sought. Water-based fire extinguishers should not be used on electrical fires.

BIOSAFETY

The facility must define and enforce measures to minimize the risk of exposure to biohazardous materials in the workplace. Requirements published by OSHA (Bloodborne Pathogens Standard)[14] and recommendations published by the US DHHS[13,16] provide the basis for an effective biosafety plan.

Bloodborne Pathogens Standard

The OSHA Bloodborne Pathogens Standard is intended to protect employees in all occupations where there is a risk of exposure to blood and other potentially infectious materials. It requires that the facility develop an Exposure Control Plan and describes appropriate engineering controls, PPE, and work practice controls to minimize the risk of exposure. It also requires employers to provide hepatitis B vaccination for any staff members with occupational exposure, to provide medical follow-up in case of accidental exposure, and to keep records related to accidents and exposures.

Standard Precautions

Standard Precautions represent the most current recommendations by the CDC to reduce the risk of transmission of blood-borne pathogens and other pathogens in hospitals. Originally published in 1996 in the *Guidelines for Isolation Precautions in Hospitals,*[13] Standard Precautions build on earlier recommendations, including Body Substance Isolation (1987), Universal Precautions (1986), and Blood and Body Fluid Precautions (1983). The Bloodborne Pathogens Standard refers to the use of Universal Precautions. However, OSHA recognizes the more recent guidelines from the CDC and, in Directive CPL 02-02-069, allows hospitals to use acceptable alternatives, including Standard Precautions, as long as all other requirements in the standard are met.[27]

Standard Precautions apply to all patient care activities regardless of diagnosis where there is a risk of exposure to 1) blood; 2) all body fluids, secretions, and excretions, except sweat; 3) nonintact skin; and 4) mucous membranes.

Biosafety Levels

Recommendations for biosafety in laboratories are based on the potential hazards for specific infectious agents and the activities performed.[16] Biosafety recommendations include guidance on both engineering controls and safe work practices. The four biosafety levels are designated in ascending order, with increasing protection for the personnel, the environment, and the community.

Biosafety Level 1 (BSL-1) involves work with agents of no known or of minimal potential hazard to laboratory personnel and the environment. Activities are usually conducted on open surfaces, and no containment equipment is needed.

Biosafety Level 2 (BSL-2) work involves agents of moderate potential hazard to personnel and the environment, usually from contact-associated exposure. Most blood bank laboratory activities are considered BSL-2. Precautions described in this section will focus on BSL-2 requirements. Laboratories should consult the CDC or the National Institutes of Health (NIH) guidelines for precautions appropriate for higher levels of containment.

Biosafety Level 3 (BSL-3) includes work with indigenous or exotic agents that may cause serious or potentially lethal disease as a result of exposure to aerosols (eg, *Mycobacterium tuberculosis*) or by other routes that would result in grave consequences to the infected host (eg, HIV). Recommendations for work at BSL-3 are designed to contain biohazardous aerosols and to minimize the risk of surface contamination.

Biosafety Level 4 (BSL-4) applies to work with dangerous or exotic agents that pose high individual risk of life-threatening disease from aerosols (eg, agents of hemorrhagic fevers, filoviruses). BSL-4 is not applicable to routine blood-bank-related activities.

Training

OSHA requires annual training for all employees whose tasks carry risk of infectious exposure.[14,27] Training programs must be tailored to the target group, both in level and content. General background knowledge of biohazards, understanding of control procedures, or work experience cannot meet the requirement for specific training, although assessment of such knowledge is a first step in planning program content. Workplace volunteers require at least as much safety training as do paid staff members who are performing similar functions.

Hazard Identification and Communication

The facility's Exposure Control Plan communicates the risks present in the workplace and describes controls to minimize exposure. BSL-2 through BSL-4 facilities must have a biohazard sign posted at the entrance when infectious agents are in use. The sign serves to notify personnel and visitors about the presence of infectious agents, provides a point of contact for the area, and indicates any special protective equipment or work practices required.

Biohazard warning labels must be placed on containers of regulated waste; on refrigerators and freezers containing blood or other potentially infectious material; and on other containers used to store, transport, or ship blood or other potentially infectious materials. Blood components that are labeled to identify their contents and that have been released for transfusion or other clinical use are exempted.

Engineering Controls and Personal Protective Equipment

OSHA requires that hazards be controlled by engineering or work practices whenever possible. Engineering controls for BSL-2 laboratories include limited access to the laboratory when work is in progress and BSCs or other containment equipment for work that may involve infectious aerosols or splashes. Handwashing sinks and eyewash stations must be available. The work space should be designed so that it can be easily cleaned, and benchtops should be impervious to water and resistant to chemicals and solvents. To help prevent exposure or cross-contamination, work area telephones can be equipped with speakers to eliminate the need to pick up the receiver. Computer keyboards and telephones can be covered with plastic. Such equipment should be cleaned on a regular basis and when visibly soiled.

BSCs are primary containment devices for handling moderate-risk and high-risk organisms. There are three types—Classes I, II, and III—with Class III providing the highest protection to the worker. In addition to protecting personnel during the handling of biohazardous materials, a BSC may be used to prevent contamination of blood and cellular therapy products during open processing steps. A comparison of the features and applications for the three classes of cabinets is provided in Table 2-3.[28] BSCs are not required by Standard Precautions, but centrifugation of open blood samples or manipulation of units known to be positive for hepatitis B surface antigen (HBsAg) or HIV are examples of blood bank procedures for which a BSC could be useful. The effectiveness of the BSC is a function of directional airflow inward and downward, through a high-efficiency filter. Efficacy is reduced by anything that disrupts the airflow pattern (eg, arms moving rapidly in and out of the BSC, rapid movements behind an employee using the BSC, downdrafts from ventilation systems, or open laboratory doors). Care should be taken not to block the front intake and rear exhaust grills. Performance of the BSC should be certified annually.[29]

Injuries from contaminated needles and other sharp objects (sometimes called sharps) continued to be a major concern in health-care settings even after the Bloodborne Pathogens Standard went into effect. In 2001, OSHA revised the standard to include reference to engineered sharps injury protections and to needleless systems.[30] It requires that employers implement appropriate new control technologies and safer medical devices in Exposure Control Plans and that employers solicit input from their employees to identify, evaluate, and select engineering and work practice controls. Examples of safer devices are needleless systems and self-sheathing needles in which the sheath is an integral part of the device.

Decontamination

Reusable equipment and work surfaces that may be contaminated with blood require daily cleaning and decontamination. Obvious spills on equipment or work surfaces should be cleaned up immediately; routine wipe-downs with disinfectant should occur at the end of each shift or on a regular basis that provides equivalent safety. Equipment that is exposed to blood or other potentially infectious material must be decontaminated before servicing or shipping. When decontamination of all or a portion of the equipment is not feasible, a biohazard label stating which portions remain contaminated should be attached before servicing or shipping the equipment.

Choice of Disinfectants

The Environmental Protection Agency (EPA) maintains a list of chemical products that have been shown to be effective hospital antimicrobial disinfectants.[31] The Association for Professionals in Infection Control and Epidemiology also publishes a guideline to assist health-care professionals in decisions involving judicious selection and proper use of specific disinfectants.[32] For facilities covered under the Bloodborne Pathogens Standard, OSHA allows the use of EPA-registered tuberculocidal disinfectants, EPA-registered disinfectants that are effective against both HIV and HBV, a diluted bleach solution to decontaminate work surfaces, or a combination of them.[27]

Before selecting a product, workers should consider several factors. Among them are the type of material or surface to be treated, the hazardous properties of the chemical

TABLE 2-3. Comparison of Classes I, II, and III Biological Safety Cabinets*

Category	Main Features	Intended Use	Common Applications
Class	Unfiltered room air is drawn into the cabinet. Inward airflow protects personnel from exposure to materials inside the cabinet. Exhaust is high-efficiency particulate air (HEPA) filtered to protect the environment. It maintains airflow at a minimum velocity of 75 linear feet per minute (lfpm) across the front opening (face velocity).	Personal and environmental protection	To enclose equipment (eg, centrifuges) or procedures that may generate aerosols
Class I (General—applies to all types of Class I cabinets)	Laminar flow (air moving at a constant velocity in one direction along parallel lines) is used. Room air is drawn into the front grille. HEPA-filtered air is forced downward in a laminar flow to minimize cross-contamination of materials in the cabinet. Exhaust is HEPA filtered.	Personal, environmental, and product protection	Work with microorganisms assigned to Biosafety Levels 1, 2, or 3 Handling of products where prevention of contamination is critical, such as cell culture propagation or manipulation of blood components in an open system
Class I, A	Around 75% of air is recirculated after passing through a HEPA filter. Face velocity = 75 lfpm.	See Class II, general	See Class II, general

(Continued)

TABLE 2-3. Comparison of Classes I, II, and III Biological Safety Cabinets* (Continued)

Category	Main Features	Intended Use	Common Applications
Class II, B1	Around 70% of air exits through the rear grille, is HEPA filtered, and is then discharged from the building. The other 30% is drawn into the front grille, is HEPA filtered, and is recirculated. Face velocity = 100 lfpm.	See Class II, general	Allows for safe manipulation of small quantities of hazardous chemicals and biologics
Class II, B2	All 100% of air is exhausted; none is recirculated. A supply blower draws air from the room or outside and passes it through a HEPA filter to provide the downward laminar flow. Face velocity = 100 lfpm.	See Class II, general	Provides both chemical and biological containment; is more expensive to operate because of the volume of conditioned room air being exhausted
Class II, B3	Although similar in design to Type A, the system is ducted and includes a negative pressure system to keep any possible contamination within the cabinet. Face velocity = 100 lfpm.	See Class II, general	Allows for safe manipulation of small quantities of hazardous chemicals and biologics
Class III	Cabinet is airtight. Materials are handled with rubber gloves attached to the front of the cabinet. Supply air is HEPA filtered. Exhaust air is double HEPA filtered or may have one filter and an air incinerator. Materials are brought in and out of the cabinet either through a dunk tank or a double-door pass-through box that can be decontaminated. Cabinet is kept under negative pressure.	Maximum protection to personnel and environment	Work with Biosafety Level 4 microorganisms

*Data from the US Department of Health and Human Services.[28]

such as corrosiveness, and the level of disinfection required. After a product has been selected, procedures need to be written to ensure effective and consistent cleaning and treatment of work surfaces. Some factors to consider for effective decontamination include the contact time, the type of microorganisms, the presence of organic matter, and the concentration of the chemical agent. Workers should review the basic information on decontamination and should follow the manufacturer's instructions.

Storage

Hazardous materials must be segregated, and areas for different types of storage must be clearly demarcated. Blood must be protected from unnecessary exposure to other materials, and vice versa. If transfusion products cannot be stored in a separate refrigerator from reagents, specimens, and unrelated materials, areas within the refrigerator must be clearly labeled, and extra care must be taken to reduce the likelihood of spills and other accidents. Storage areas must be kept clean and orderly; food or drink is never allowed where biohazardous materials are stored.

Personal Protective Equipment

Where hazards cannot be eliminated, OSHA requires employers to provide appropriate PPE and clothing and to clean, launder, or dispose of PPE at no cost to their employees.[14] Standard PPE and clothing include uniforms, laboratory coats, gloves, face shields, masks, and safety goggles. Indications and guidelines for their use are discussed in Appendix 2-2.

Safe Work Practices

Safe work practices appropriate for Standard Precautions include the following:

- Wash hands after touching blood, body fluids, secretions, excretions, and contaminated items, whether or not gloves are worn.
- Wear gloves when touching blood, body fluids, secretions, excretions, and contaminated items, and change gloves between tasks.
- Wear a mask and eye protection or a face shield during activities that are likely to generate splashes or sprays of blood, body fluids, secretions, and excretions.
- Wear a gown during activities that are likely to generate splashes or sprays of blood, body fluids, secretions, or excretions.
- Handle soiled patient-care equipment in a manner that prevents exposure; ensure that reusable equipment is not used for another patient until it has been cleaned and reprocessed appropriately; and ensure that single-use items are discarded properly.
- Ensure that adequate procedures are defined and followed for the routine care, cleaning, and disinfection of environmental surfaces and equipment.
- Handle soiled linen in a manner that prevents exposure.
- Handle needles, scalpels, and other sharp instruments or devices in a manner that minimizes the risk of exposure.
- Use mouthpieces, resuscitation bags, or other ventilation devices as an alternative to mouth-to-mouth resuscitation methods.
- Place in a private room those patients who are at risk of contaminating the environment or who are not able to maintain appropriate hygiene (eg, patients with tuberculosis).

Laboratory Biosafety Precautions

Several factors need to be considered when assessing the risk of blood exposures among laboratory personnel. Some factors include the number of specimens processed, personnel behaviors, laboratory techniques, and type of equipment.[33] The laboratory director may wish to institute BSL-3 practices for procedures that are considered to be higher risk than BSL-2. When there is doubt whether an activity is BSL-2 or BSL-3, the safety precautions for BSL-3 should be followed. BSL-2 precautions that are applicable to the laboratory setting are summarized in Appendix 2-3.

Considerations for the Donor Room

The Bloodborne Pathogens Standard acknowledges a difference between hospital patients and healthy donors, in whom the prevalence of infectious disease markers is significantly lower. The employer in a volunteer blood donation facility may determine that routine use of gloves is not required for phlebotomy as long as the following conditions exist[14]:

- The policy is periodically reevaluated.
- Gloves are made available to those who want to use them, and their use is not discouraged.
- Gloves are required when an employee has cuts, scratches, or breaks in skin; when there is a likelihood that contamination will occur; while an employee is drawing autologous units; while an employee is performing therapeutic procedures; and during training in phlebotomy.

Procedures should be assessed for risks of biohazardous exposures and risks inherent in working with a donor or patient during the screening and donation processes. Some techniques or procedures are more likely to cause injury than others, such as using lancets for finger puncture, handling capillary tubes, crushing vials for arm cleaning, handling any unsheathed needles, cleaning scissors, and giving cardiopulmonary resuscitation.

In some instances, it may be necessary to collect blood from donors known to pose a high risk of infectivity (eg, collection of autologous blood or Source Plasma for the production of other products such as vaccines). The FDA provides guidance for collecting blood from such "high-risk" donors.[34] The most recent regulations and guidelines should be consulted for changes or additions.

Emergency Response Plan

Table 2-4 lists steps to take when a spill occurs. Facilities should be prepared to handle both small and large blood spills. Good preparation for spill cleanup includes several elements.

TABLE 2-4. Blood Spill Cleanup

◆ Evaluate the spill.
◆ Wear appropriate protective clothing and gloves. If sharp objects are involved, gloves must be puncture-resistant, and a broom or other instrument should be used during cleanup to avoid injury.
◆ Remove clothing if it is contaminated.
◆ Post warnings to keep the area clear.
◆ Evacuate the area for 30 minutes if an aerosol has been created.
◆ Contain the spill if possible.
◆ If the spill occurs in the centrifuge, turn the power off immediately and leave the cover closed for 30 minutes. The use of overwraps helps prevent aerosolization and helps contain the spill.
◆ Use absorbent material to mop up most of the liquid contents.
◆ Clean the spill area with detergent.
◆ Flood the area with disinfectant and use it as described in the manufacturer's instructions. Allow adequate contact time with the disinfectant.
◆ Wipe up residual disinfectant if necessary.
◆ Dispose of all materials safely in accordance with biohazard guidelines. All blood-contaminated items must be autoclaved or incinerated.

- Work areas designed so that cleanup is relatively simple.
- A spill kit or cart prepared to contain all necessary supplies and equipment with instructions for their use. It should be placed near areas where spills are anticipated.
- Responsibility assigned for kit or cart maintenance, spill handling, record-keeping, and review of significant incidents.
- Personnel trained in cleanup procedures and procedures for reporting significant incidents.

Biohazardous Waste

Medical waste is defined as any waste (solid, semisolid, or liquid) generated in the diagnosis, treatment, or immunization of human beings or animals in related research, production, or testing of biologics. Infectious waste includes disposable equipment, articles, or substances that may harbor or transmit pathogenic organisms or their toxins. In general, infectious waste should be either incinerated or decontaminated before disposal in a sanitary landfill.

If state law allows, blood and components, suctioned fluids, excretions, and secretions may be carefully poured down a drain connected to a sanitary sewer. Sanitary sewers may also be used to dispose of other potentially infectious wastes that can be ground and flushed into the sewer. State and local health departments should be consulted about laws and regulations on disposal of biologic waste into the sewer.

Laboratories should clearly define what will be considered hazardous waste. For example, in the blood bank all items contaminated with liquid or semiliquid blood are biohazardous. Items contaminated with dried blood are considered hazardous if there is potential for the dried material to flake off during handling. Contaminated sharp objects are always considered hazardous because of the risk for percutaneous injury. However, items such as used gloves, swabs, plastic pipettes with excess liquid removed, or gauze contaminated with small droplets of blood may be considered nonhazardous if the material is dried and will not be released into the environment during handling.

Guidelines for Biohazardous Waste Disposal

Employees must be trained before handling or disposing of biohazardous waste, even if it is packaged. The following disposal guidelines are recommended[35]:

- Identify biohazardous waste consistently; red seamless plastic bags (at least 2 mm thick) or containers carrying the biohazard symbol are recommended.
- Place bags in a protective container with closure upward to avoid breakage and leakage during storage or transport.
- When transported over public roads, the waste must be prepared and shipped according to US Department of Transportation (DOT) regulations.
- Discard sharps (eg, needles, broken glass, glass slides, and wafers from sterile connecting devices) in rigid, puncture-proof, leakproof containers.
- Put liquids in leakproof, unbreakable containers only.
- Do not compact waste materials.

Storage areas for infectious material must be secured to reduce accident risk. Infectious waste must never be placed in the public trash collection system. Most facilities hire private carriers to decontaminate and dispose of infectious or hazardous waste. The facility should disclose all risks associated with the waste in their contracts with private companies. The carrier is responsible for complying with all federal, state, and local laws for biohazardous (medical) waste transport, treatment, and disposal.

Treating Infectious or Medical Waste

Facilities that incinerate hazardous waste must comply with EPA standards of performance for new stationary sources and emission guidelines for existing sources.[36] In this regulation, a hospital/medical/infectious waste incinerator (HMIWI) is any device that combusts any amount of hospital waste or medical/infectious waste.

Decontamination of biohazardous waste by autoclaving is another common method for decontamination or inactivation of blood samples and blood components. The following elements are considered in determining processing time for autoclaving:

- Size of load being autoclaved.
- Type of packaging of item(s) being autoclaved.
- Density of items being autoclaved.
- Number of items in single autoclave load.
- Placement of items in the autoclave, to allow for steam penetration.

It is useful to place a biologic indicator in the center of loads that vary in size and contents to evaluate optimal steam penetration times. The EPA provides detailed information about choosing and operating such equipment.[35]

For decontamination, material should be autoclaved for a minimum of 1 hour. For sterilization, longer treatment times are needed. A general rule for decontamination is to process 1 hour for every 10 pounds of waste being processed. Usually, decontaminated laboratory wastes can be disposed of as nonhazardous solid wastes. The staff should check with the local solid waste authority to ensure that the facility is in compliance with regulations for the area. Waste containing broken glass or other sharp items should be disposed of in a method consistent with policies for the disposal of other sharp or potentially dangerous materials.

CHEMICAL SAFETY

One of the most effective preventive measures that a facility can take to reduce hazardous chemical exposure is to choose alternative nonhazardous chemicals whenever possible. When the use of hazardous chemicals is required, purchasing in small quantities reduces the risks associated with storing excess chemicals and later dealing with their disposal.

OSHA requires that facilities using hazardous chemicals develop a written Chemical Hygiene Plan (CHP) and that the plan be accessible to all employees. The CHP should outline procedures, equipment, PPE, and work practices that are capable of protecting employees from hazardous chemicals used in the facility.[15,20] The CHP must also provide assurance that equipment and protective devices are functioning properly and that criteria to determine implementation and maintenance of all aspects of the plan are in place. Employees must be informed of all chemical hazards in the workplace and must be trained to recognize chemical hazards, to protect themselves when working with these chemicals, and to know where to find information about particular hazardous chemicals. Safety audits and annual reviews of the CHP are important control steps to help ensure that safety practices comply with the policies set forth in the CHP and that the CHP is up to date.

Establishing a clear definition of what constitutes hazardous chemicals is sometimes difficult. Generally, hazardous chemicals are those chemicals that pose a significant health risk if an employee is exposed to them or that pose a significant physical risk, such as fire or explosion, if handled or stored improperly. Categories of health and physical hazards are listed in Tables 2-5 and 2-6. Appendix 2-4 lists examples of hazardous chemicals that may be found in the blood bank. The *NIOSH Pocket Guide to Chemical Hazards* provides a quick reference for many common chemicals.[37]

The facility should identify a qualified chemical hygiene officer to be responsible for determining guidelines for hazardous materials.[20] The chemical hygiene officer is also accountable for monitoring and documenting accidents and for initiating process change as needed.

Training

Employees who may be exposed to hazardous chemicals must be trained before they begin work in an area where hazards exist. If a new employee has received prior training, it may

TABLE 2-5. Categories of Health Hazards

Hazard	Definition
Carcinogens	Cancer-producing substances
Irritants	Agents causing irritations (edema, burning, etc) to skin or mucous membranes upon contact
Corrosives	Agents causing destruction of human tissue at the site of contact
Toxic or highly toxic agents	Substances causing serious biologic effects following inhalation, ingestion, or skin contact with relatively small amounts
Reproductive toxins	Chemicals that affect reproductive capabilities, including chromosomal damages and effects on fetuses
Other toxins	Hepatotoxins, nephrotoxins, neurotoxins, agents that act on the hematopoietic systems, and agents that damage the lungs, skin, eyes, or mucous membranes

not be necessary to retrain the individual, depending on the employer's evaluation of the new employee's level of knowledge. New employee training is likely to be necessary regarding such specifics as the location of the relevant material safety data sheets (MSDSs), details of chemical labeling, the PPE to be used, and site-specific emergency procedures.

Training must be provided for each new physical or health hazard when it is introduced into the workplace, but not for each new chemical that falls within a particular hazard class.[15] For example, if a new solvent is brought into the workplace and the solvent has hazards similar to existing chemicals for which training has already been conducted, then the employer need only make employees aware of the new solvent's hazard category (eg, corrosive, irritant). However, if the newly introduced solvent is a suspected carcinogen and carcinogenic hazard training has not been provided before, then new training must be conducted for employees with potential exposure. Retraining is advisable as often as necessary to ensure that employees understand the hazards linked to the materials with which

TABLE 2-6. Categories of Physical Hazards

Hazard	Definition
Combustible or flammable chemicals	Chemicals that can burn (includes combustible and flammable liquids, solids, aerosols, and gases)
Compressed gases	A gas or mixture of gases in a container under pressure
Explosives	Unstable or reactive chemicals that undergo violent chemical change at normal temperatures and pressure
Unstable (reactive) chemicals	Chemicals that could be self-reactive under conditions of shocks, pressure, or temperature
Water-reactive chemicals	Chemicals that react with water to release a gas that is either flammable or presents a health hazard

they work, particularly any chronic and specific target-organ health hazards.

Hazard Identification and Communication

Hazard Communication

Employers must prepare a comprehensive hazard communication program for all areas using hazardous chemicals to complement the CHP and to "ensure that the hazards of all chemicals produced or imported are evaluated, and that information concerning their hazards is transmitted to employers and employees."[15] The program should include the labeling of hazardous chemicals, instructions on when and how to post warning labels for chemicals, directions for managing MSDS reports for hazardous chemicals in the facilities, and employee training.

Safety materials made available to employees should include the following:

- The facility's written CHP.
- The facility's written program for hazard communication.
- Identification of work areas where hazardous chemicals are located.
- Required list of hazardous chemicals and their MSDSs. (It is the responsibility of the facility to determine which chemicals may present a hazard to employees. This determination should be based on the quantity of chemical used; the physical properties, potency, and toxicity of the chemical; the manner in which the chemical is used; and the means available to control the release of, or exposure to, the chemical.)

Hazardous Chemical Labeling and Signs

The Hazard Communication Standard requires manufacturers of chemicals and hazardous materials to provide the user with basic information about the hazards of these materials through product labeling and MSDSs.[15] Employers are required to provide the following to employees who are expected to work with these hazardous materials: information about what the hazards of the materials are, how to read the labeling, how to interpret symbols and signs on the labels, and how to read and use the MSDSs. MSDS forms typically include the following:

- Identification.
- Hazard(s) identification.
- Composition/information on ingredients.
- First-aid measures.
- Fire-fighting measures.
- Accidental release measures.
- Handling and storage.
- Exposure controls/personal protection information.
- Physical and chemical properties.
- Stability and reactivity.
- Toxicologic information.
- Ecologic information.
- Disposal considerations.
- Transport information.
- Regulatory information.
- Other information.

At a minimum, hazardous chemical container labels must include the name of the chemical, name and address of the manufacturer, hazard warnings, labels, signs, placards, and other forms of warning to provide visual reminders of specific hazards. The label may refer to any MSDS for additional information. Labels applied by the manufacturer must remain on containers. The user may add storage requirements and dates of receipt, opening, and expiration. If chemicals are aliquotted into secondary containers, the secondary container must be labeled with the name of the chemical and appropriate hazard warnings. Additional information such as precautionary measures, concentration if applicable, and date of preparation are helpful but not mandatory. It is a safe practice to label all containers with their content, even water. Transfer containers used for temporary storage need not be labeled if the person performing the transfer retains control and intends the containers for immediate use. Information regarding acceptable standards for hazard communication labeling is provided by the NFPA[38] and the National Paint and Coatings Association.[39]

Signs meeting OSHA requirements must be posted in areas where hazardous chemicals are used. Decisions on where to post warning signs are based on the manufacturer's recommendations on the chemical hazards, the quantity of the chemical in the room or laboratory, and the potency and toxicity of the chemical.

Material Safety Data Sheets

The MSDS identifies the physical and chemical properties of a hazardous chemical (eg, flash point, vapor pressure), its physical and health hazards (eg, potential for fire, explosion, signs and symptoms of exposure), and precautions for safe handling and use. Specific instructions in an individual MSDS take precedence over generic information in the Hazardous Materials (HAZMAT) program.

Employers must maintain copies of the required MSDSs in the workplace for each hazardous chemical and must ensure that MSDS copies are readily accessible during each work shift to employees when they are in their work areas. When household consumer products are used in the workplace in the same manner that a consumer would use them [ie, where the duration and frequency of use (and therefore exposure) are not greater than those the typical consumer would experience], OSHA does not require that an MSDS be provided to purchasers. However, if exposure to such products exceeds that normally found in consumer applications, employees have a right to know about the properties of such hazardous chemicals. OSHA does not require or encourage employers to maintain an MSDS for nonhazardous chemicals.

Engineering Controls and Personal Protective Equipment

Guidelines for laboratory areas in which hazardous chemicals are used or stored must be established. Physical facilities, and especially ventilation, must be adequate for the nature and volume of work conducted. Chemicals must be stored according to chemical compatibility (eg, corrosives, flammables, oxidizers) and in minimal volumes. Bulk chemicals should be kept outside work areas. NFPA standards and others provide guidelines for proper storage.[4,38,40]

Chemical fume hoods are recommended for use with organic solvents, volatile liquids, and dry chemicals with a significant inhalation hazard.[4] Although constructed with safety glass, most fume hood sashes are not designed as safety shields. Hoods should be positioned in an area where there is minimal foot traffic to avoid disrupting the airflow and compromising the containment field.

PPE that may be provided, depending on the hazardous chemicals used, includes chemical-resistant gloves and aprons, shatterproof safety goggles, and respirators.

Emergency showers should be available to areas where caustic, corrosive, toxic, flammable, or combustible chemicals are used.[4,41] There should be unobstructed access, within 10 seconds, to the showers from the areas where hazardous chemicals are used. Safety showers should be periodically flushed and tested for function, and associated floor drains should be checked to ensure that drain traps remain filled with water.

Safe Work Practices

Hazardous material should not be stored or transported in open containers. Containers and their lids or seals should be designed to prevent spills or leakage in all reasonably anticipated conditions. Containers should be able to safely store the maximum anticipated volume and should be easy to clean. Surfaces should be kept clean and dry at all times. When an employee is working with a chemical fume hood, all materials should be kept at a distance of at least 6 inches behind the face opening. The vertical sliding sash should be positioned at the height specified on the certification sticker. The airfoil, baffles, and rear ventilation slot must not be blocked. Appendix 2-5 lists specific chemicals and suggestions on how to work with them safely.

Emergency Response Plan

The time to prepare for a chemical spill is before a spill occurs. A comprehensive employee training program should provide each employee with all tools necessary to act responsibly at the time of a chemical spill. The employee should know response procedures, should be able to assess the severity of a chemical spill, should know or be able to quickly look up the basic physical characteristics of the chemicals, and should know where to find emergency response phone numbers. The employee should be able to assess, stop, and confine the spill; either clean up the spill or call for a spill cleanup team; and follow up on the report of the spill. The employee must know when to ask for assistance, when to isolate the area, and where to find cleanup materials.

Chemical spills in the workplace can be categorized as follows[42]:

- *Incidental releases* are spills that are limited in quantity and toxicity and that pose no significant safety or health hazard to the employee. They may be safely cleaned up by the employees familiar with the hazards of the chemical involved in the spill. Waste from the cleanup may be classified as hazardous and must be disposed of in the proper fashion. Appendix 2-6 describes appropriate responses to incidental spills.
- *Releases that may be incidental or may require an emergency response* are spills that may pose an exposure risk to the employees depending on the circumstances. Considerations such as the hazardous substance properties, the circumstances of release, and mitigating factors play a role in determining the appropriate response. The facility's emergency response plan should provide guidance about how to determine whether the spill is incidental or requires an emergency response.
- *Emergency response releases* are spills that pose a threat to health and safety regardless of the circumstances surrounding their release. The spill may require evacuation of the immediate area. The response typically comes from outside the immediate release area by personnel trained as emergency responders. These spills include, but are not limited to, spills that involve immediate danger to life or health, serious threat of fire or explosion, and high levels of toxic substances.

Appendix 2-7 addresses the management of hazardous chemical spills. Spill cleanup kits or carts tailored to the specific hazards present should be available in each area. The kits or carts may contain the following: rubber gloves and aprons, shoe covers, goggles, suitable aspirators, general absorbents, neutralizing agents, broom, dust pan, appropriate trash bags or cans for waste disposal, and cleanup directions. Chemical absorbents such as clay absorbents or spill blankets can be used for cleaning up a number of chemicals and thus may be easier for the employee to use in spill situations.

With any spill of a hazardous chemical, but especially with a carcinogenic agent, it is essential to refer to the MSDS and to contact a designated supervisor or designee trained to handle these spills and hazardous waste disposal.[4] Facility environmental health and safety personnel can also offer assistance. The employer must assess the extent of the employee's exposure. After an exposure, the employee must be given an opportunity for medical consultation to determine the need for a medical examination.

Another source of a workplace hazard is the unexpected release of hazardous vapors into the environment. OSHA has set limits for exposure to hazardous vapors from toxic and hazardous substances.[43] The potential risk associated with a chemical is determined by the manufacturer and is listed on the MSDS. See Table 2-7 for a listing of the limits of exposure.

Chemical Waste Disposal

Most laboratory chemical waste is considered hazardous and is regulated by the EPA through the Resource Conservation and Recovery Act (42 USC §6901 et seq, 1976). This regulation specifies that hazardous waste can be legally disposed of only at an EPA-approved disposal

TABLE 2-7. Regulatory Limits for Exposure to Toxic and Hazardous Vapors[36]

Limit	Definition
Permissible exposure limit	The maximum concentration of vapors in parts per million (ppm) that an employee may be exposed to in an 8-hour day/40-hour work week.
Short-term exposure limit	The maximum allowable concentration of vapors that an employee may be exposed to in a 15-minute period, with a maximum of four exposures per day allowed with at least 1 hour between each.
Ceiling limit	The maximum concentration of vapors that may not be exceeded instantaneously at any time.

facility. Disposal of chemical waste into a sanitary sewer is regulated by the Clean Water Act (33 USC §1251 et seq, 1977), and most US states have strict regulations concerning disposal of chemicals in the water system. Federal and applicable state regulations should be consulted when a facility is setting up and reviewing facility waste disposal policies.

RADIATION SAFETY

Radiation can be defined as energy in the form of waves or particles emitted and propagated through space or a material medium. Gamma rays are electromagnetic radiation, whereas alpha and beta emitters are examples of particulate radiation. The presence of radiation in the blood bank, either from radioisotopes used in laboratory testing or from self-contained blood irradiators, requires additional precautions and training.[4,44]

Radiation Measurement Units

The measurement unit quantifying the amount of energy absorbed per unit mass of tissue is the Gray (Gy) or rad (radiation absorbed dose); 1 Gy equals 100 rads.

Dose equivalency measurements are more useful than simple energy measurements because dose equivalency measurements take into account the effectiveness of the different types of radiation to cause biologic effects. The ability of radiation to cause damage is assigned a number called a quality factor (QF). For example, exposure to a given amount of alpha particles (QF = 20) is far more damaging than exposure to an equivalent amount of gamma rays (QF = 1). The common unit of measurement for dose equivalency is the rem (roentgen or rad equivalent man). Rem is the dose from any type of radiation that produces biologic effects in man equivalent to one rad of x-rays, gamma rays, or beta rays. To obtain dose from a particular type of radiation in rem, the number of rad should be multiplied by the QF (rad × QF = rem). Because the QF for gamma rays, x-rays, and most beta particles is 1, the dose in rad is equal to the dose in rem for these types of radiation.

Biologic Effects of Radiation

Any harm to tissue begins with the absorption of radiation energy and subsequent disruption of chemical bonds. Molecules and atoms become ionized or excited (or both) by absorbing this energy. The direct action path leads to radiolysis or formation of free radicals that in turn alter the structure and function of molecules in the cell.

Molecular alterations can cause cellular or chromosomal changes, depending on the amount and type of radiation energy absorbed. Cellular changes can manifest as a visible somatic effect (eg, erythema). Changes at the chromosome level may manifest as leukemia or other cancers, or possibly as germ cell defects that are transmitted to future generations.

Several factors influence the level of biologic damage from exposure, including the type of radiation, the part of the body exposed, the total absorbed dose, and the dose rate. The total absorbed dose is the cumulative amount of radiation absorbed in the tissue. The greater the dose, the greater the potential for biologic damage. Exposure can be acute or chronic. The low levels of ionizing radiation likely to occur in blood banks should not pose any detrimental risk.[45-48]

Regulations

The NRC controls use of radioactive materials by establishing licensure requirements. States and municipalities may also have requirements for inspection, licensure, or both. The type of license for using radioisotopes or irradiators will depend on the scope and magnitude of the use of radioactivity. US facilities should contact the NRC and the appropriate state agencies for license requirements and applications as soon as such activities are proposed.

Each NRC-licensed establishment must have a qualified radiation safety officer who is responsible for establishing personnel protection requirements and for proper disposal and handling of radioactive materials. Specific radiation safety policies and procedures should address dose limits, employee training, warning signs and labels, shipping and handling guidelines, radiation monitoring, and exposure management. Emergency procedures must be clearly defined and readily available to the staff.

In 2005, the NRC imposed additional security requirements for high-risk radioactive sources, including those used in blood irradiators. The purpose of the increased controls is to reduce the risk of unauthorized use of radioactive materials that may pose a threat to public health and safety. Those 2005 measures include controlled access, approval in writing of individuals deemed trustworthy and reliable to have unescorted access, a system of monitoring to immediately detect and respond to unauthorized access, and documentation of authorized personnel and monitoring activities.[49] In 2007, a requirement for fingerprinting was added.[50]

Exposure Limits

The NRC sets standards for protection against radiation hazards arising from licensed activities, including dose limits.[12] Such limits, or maximal permissible dose equivalents, are a measure of the radiation risk over time and serve as standards for exposure. The occupational total effective-dose-equivalent limit is 5 rem/year. The shallow dose equivalent limit (skin) is 50 rem/year, the extremity dose equivalent limit is 50 rem/year, and the eye dose equivalent limit is 15 rem/year.[12,45] Dose limits for an embryo or fetus must not exceed 0.5 rem during the pregnancy.[12,45,50,51] Employers are expected not only to maintain radiation exposure below allowable limits, but also to keep exposure levels as far below these limits as can reasonably be achieved.

Radiation Monitoring

Monitoring is essential for early detection and prevention of problems resulting from radiation exposure. Monitoring is used to evaluate the facility's environment, work practices, and procedures, and to comply with regulations and NRC licensing requirements. Monitoring is accomplished with the use of dosimeters, bioassays, survey meters, and wipe tests.[4]

Dosimeters, such as film or thermoluminescent badges, rings, or both, measure personnel radiation doses. The need for dosimeters depends on the amount and type of radioactive materials in use; the facility radiation safety officer will determine individual dosimeter needs. Film badges must be changed at least quarterly and in some instances monthly, must be protected from high temperature and humidity, and must be stored at work away from sources of radiation.

Bioassays, such as thyroid and whole body counting or urinalysis, may be used to determine if there is radioactivity inside the body and, if so, how much. If necessary, bioassays are usually performed quarterly and after an incident where accidental intake may have occurred.

Survey meters are sensitive to low levels of gamma or particulate radiation and provide a quantitative assessment of radiation hazard. Survey meters can be used to monitor storage areas for radioactive materials or wastes, testing areas during or after completion of a procedure, and packages or containers of radioactive materials. Survey meters must be calibrated annually by an authorized NRC licensee. Selection of appropriate meters should be discussed with the radiation safety officer.

In areas where radioactive materials are handled, all work surfaces, equipment, and floors that may be contaminated should be checked regularly with a wipe test. In the wipe test, a moistened absorbent material (the wipe) is passed over the surface and then counted for radiation.

Training

Personnel who handle radioactive materials or who work with blood irradiators must receive radiation safety training before beginning work. This training should cover an explanation of the presence and potential hazards of radioactive materials found in the employee's specific work area, general health protection issues, emergency procedures, and radiation warning signs and labels in use. Instruction in the following areas is also suggested:

- NRC regulations and license conditions.
- The importance of observing license conditions and regulations and of reporting violations or conditions of unnecessary exposure.
- Precautions to minimize exposure.
- Interpretation of results of monitoring devices.
- Requirements for pregnant workers.
- Employees' rights.
- Documentation and record-keeping requirements.

The need for refresher training is determined by the license agreement between the NRC and the facility.

Engineering Controls and Personal Protective Equipment

Although self-contained blood irradiators present little risk to the laboratory staff and film badges are not required for routine operation, blood establishments with irradiation programs must be licensed by the NRC.[46]

The manufacturer of the blood irradiator usually accepts responsibility for radiation safety requirements during transportation, installation, and validation of the unit as part of the purchase contract. The radiation safety officer can help oversee the installation and validation processes and should confirm that appropriate training, monitoring systems, procedures, and maintenance protocols are in place before use and that they reflect the manufacturer's recommendations. Suspected malfunctions must be reported immediately so that appropriate actions can be initiated.

Blood irradiators should be located in secure areas so that only trained individuals have access. Fire protection for the unit must also be considered. Automatic fire detection and control systems should be readily available in the immediate area. Blood components that have been irradiated are not radioactive and pose no threat to the staff or the general public.

Safe Work Practices

Each laboratory should establish policies and procedures for the safe use of radioactive materials. They should include requirements for following general laboratory safety principles, appropriate storage of radioactive solutions, and proper disposal of radioactive wastes. Radiation safety can be improved with the following procedures:

- Minimizing the time of exposure by working as efficiently as possible.

- Maximizing the distance from the source of the radiation by staying as far from the source as possible.
- Maximizing shielding (eg, by using a self-shielded irradiator or by wearing lead aprons) when working with certain radioactive materials. These requirements are usually stipulated in the license conditions.
- Using good housekeeping practices to minimize the spread of radioactivity to uncontrolled areas.

Emergency Response Plan

Radioactive contamination is the dispersal of radioactive material into or onto areas where it is not intended—for example, the floor, work areas, equipment, personnel clothing, or personnel skin. The NRC regulations state that gamma or beta radioactive contamination cannot exceed 2200 dpm (disintegrations per minute) per 100 cm^2 in the posted (restricted) area, or 220 dpm/100 cm^2 in an unrestricted area such as corridors; for alpha emitters, these values are 220 dpm/100 cm^2 and 22 dpm/100 cm^2, respectively.[52]

If a spill occurs, employees' contaminated skin surfaces must be washed several times, and the radiation safety officer must be notified immediately for further guidance. Others must not be allowed to enter the area until emergency response personnel arrive.

Radioactive Waste Management

Policies for the disposal of radioactive waste, whether liquid or solid, should be established with input from the radiation safety officer.

Liquid radioactive waste may be collected into large sturdy bottles labeled with an appropriate radiation waste tag. The rules for separation by chemical compatibility apply. Bottles must be carefully stored to protect against spillage or breakage. Dry or solid waste may be sealed in a plastic bag and tagged as radiation waste. The isotope, the activity of the isotope, and the date that the activity was measured should be placed on the bag. Radiation waste must never be discharged into the facility's drain system without prior approval by the radiation safety officer.

SHIPPING HAZARDOUS MATERIALS

The US DOT regulations[53] for transportation of hazardous materials are harmonized with the international standards published annually by the International Air Transport Association (IATA).[54] These regulations provide specific instructions about identifying, classifying, packaging, marking, labeling, and documenting hazardous materials to be offered for shipment on public roadways or by air. Hazardous materials commonly shipped by transfusion medicine, cellular therapy, and clinical diagnostic services include infectious substances, biologic substances, liquid nitrogen, and dry ice. Specimens are classified as Category A if they are known or likely to contain infectious substances in a form that is capable of causing permanent disability or life-threatening or fatal disease in otherwise healthy humans or animals when an exposure occurs. The proper shipping name is "infectious substances, affecting humans" (UN2814) or "infectious substances, affecting animals only" (UN2900).

Specimens that may contain infectious substances but that do not have the level of risk described above are classified as Category B and the proper shipping name is "biological substance, category B" (UN3373). HIV in culture or HBV in culture is classified as a Category A infectious substance, but those same viruses present in a patient blood specimen are classified as Category B. Patient specimens with minimal likelihood that pathogens are present are exempt from hazardous materials regulations if the specimens are properly packaged and marked. Blood components, cell therapy products, and tissue for transfusion or transplantation are not subject to hazardous material regulations. Method 1-1 provides additional shipping instructions for safe transport of these materials. However, the most recent revision of the IATA or DOT regulations should be consulted for the most current classification, packaging, and labeling requirements, as well as for limitations in the volumes of hazardous materials that can be packaged together in one container.

GENERAL WASTE MANAGEMENT

Those responsible for safety at a facility must be concerned with protecting the environment as well as all staff members. Every effort should be made to establish facility-wide programs to reduce solid wastes, including nonhazardous and, especially, hazardous wastes (ie, biohazardous, chemical, and radiation wastes). A hazardous waste reduction program instituted at the point of use of the material achieves several goals. It reduces the institutional risk for occupational exposures to hazardous agents, reduces "cradle to grave" liability for disposal, and enhances compliance with environmental requirements to reduce pollution generated from daily operations of the laboratory.[35,55,56] Facilities can minimize pollution of the environment by practicing the "three R's": reduce, reuse, and recycle. Seeking suitable alternatives to the use of materials that create hazardous waste and separating hazardous waste from nonhazardous waste can reduce the volume of hazardous waste and can decrease costs for its disposal.

A goal of waste management should be to reduce to a minimum the volume of hazardous material. Noninfectious waste should always be separated from infectious waste. Changes in techniques or materials to reduce the volume of infectious waste or render it less hazardous should be carefully considered, and employees should be encouraged to identify safer alternatives wherever possible.

Facilities should check with state and local health and environmental authorities for current requirements for storage and disposal of a particular multihazardous waste before creating that waste. If creating the multihazardous waste cannot be avoided, the volume of waste generated should be minimized. In some states, copper sulfate contaminated with blood is considered a multihazardous waste. The disposal of this waste poses several problems with transportation from draw sites to a central facility for disposal of the final containers. State and local health departments must be involved in the review of transportation and disposal practices where this is an issue, and procedures must be developed in accordance with state and local regulations as well as those of the US DOT.

KEY POINTS

1. Facilities should be designed and maintained in a way that supports the work being done in the physical space. Designing the space to accommodate planned work flow, the need to restrict certain areas, the movement of materials and waste, the location of equipment, special air-handling requirements, and other critical aspects of the operation will help ensure safety for staff and visitors as well as the quality of products and services.
2. The facilities safety program should 1) strive to reduce hazards in the workplace, 2) ensure that staff are trained to handle known hazards and potential risks, 3) ensure that known hazards are clearly identified and marked, and 4) describe policies and procedures for workplace safety and emergency response.
3. Safety programs should address fire, electrical, biological, chemical, and radioactive hazards that may be found in the facility.
4. For each type of hazard, five basic elements that must be covered are 1) training, 2) hazard identification and communication, 3) engineering controls and personal protective equipment, 4) safe work practices including waste disposal, and 5) an emergency response plan.
5. Management controls ensure that the safety program is implemented, maintained, and effective. Management is responsible for 1) developing and communicating the written plan, 2) ensuring implementation and providing adequate resources, 3) providing access to employee health services related to prevention strategies and treatment of exposures, 4) monitoring compliance and effectiveness, and 5) evaluating and improving the safety plan.

REFERENCES

1. Carson TH, ed. Standards for blood banks and transfusion services. 27th ed. Bethesda, MD: AABB, 2011.
2. Fontaine M, ed. Standards for cellular therapy product services. 5th ed. Bethesda, MD: AABB, 2011 (in press).
3. Laboratory Accreditation Program laboratory general checklist. Chicago: College of American Pathologists Commission on Laboratory Accreditation, 2010.
4. Clinical laboratory safety; approved guideline. 2nd ed. NCCLS Document GP17-A2. Wayne, PA: Clinical and Laboratory Standards Institute, 2004.
5. Hospital accreditation standards. Oakbrook Terrace, IL: The Joint Commission, 2011.
6. Laboratory accreditation standards. Oakbrook Terrace, IL: The Joint Commission, 2011.
7. NFPA 70—National electrical code. Quincy, MA: National Fire Protection Association, 2008.
8. ANSI/ASHRAE Standard 62.1-2007. Ventilation for acceptable indoor air quality. Atlanta, GA: American Society of Heating, Refrigerating, and Air-Conditioning Engineers, Inc., 2007.
9. Code of federal regulations. Human cells, tissues, and cellular and tissue-based products. Title 21, CFR Part 1271.190. Washington, DC: US Government Printing Office, 2010 (revised annually).
10. International Organization for Standardization. ISO-14644: Cleanrooms and associated controlled environments, Parts 1-8. ISO/TC 209. Geneva, Switzerland: ISO, 1999-2007.
11. International Organization for Standardization. ISO-14698: Cleanrooms and associated controlled environments—bio-contamination control, Part 1: General principles and methods. ISO/TC 209. Geneva, Switzerland: ISO, 2003.
12. Code of federal regulations. Standards for protection against radiation. Title 10, CFR Part 20. Washington, DC: US Government Printing Office, 2010 (revised annually).
13. Siegel JD, Rhinehart E, Jackson M, et al. 2007 Guideline for isolation precautions: Preventing transmission of infectious agents in healthcare settings. Atlanta, GA: Centers for Disease Control and Prevention (Healthcare Infection Control Practices Advisory Committee), 2007. [Available at http://www.cdc.gov/hicpac/pdf/isolation/Isolation2007.pdf (accessed September 21, 2010).]
14. Code of federal regulations. Occupational exposure to bloodborne pathogens; final rule. Title 29, CFR Part 1910.1030. Washington, DC: US Government Printing Office, 2010 (revised annually).
15. Code of federal regulations. Hazard communication standard. Title 29, CFR Part 1910.1200. Washington, DC: US Government Printing Office, 2010 (revised annually).
16. US Department of Health and Human Services, Centers for Disease Control and Prevention, and National Institutes of Health. Biosafety in microbiological and biomedical laboratories. 5th ed. Washington, DC: US Government Printing Office, 2007.
17. Bernard B, ed. Musculoskeletal disorders and workplace factors: A critical review of epidemiologic evidence for work-related musculoskeletal disorders of the neck, upper extremity, and low back. NIOSH publication no. 97-141. Washington, DC: National Institute for Occupational Safety and Health, 1997.
18. Code of federal regulations. Emergency action plans. Title 29, CFR Part 1910.38. Washington, DC: US Government Printing Office, 2010 (revised annually).
19. Wagner KD, ed. Environmental management in healthcare facilities. Philadelphia: WB Saunders, 1998.
20. Code of federal regulations. Occupational exposure to hazardous chemicals in laboratories. Title 29, CFR Part 1910.1450. Washington, DC: US Government Printing Office, 2010 (revised annually).
21. Centers for Disease Control and Prevention. Public Health Service guidelines for the management of occupational exposures to HBV, HCV, and HIV and recommendations for postexposure prophylaxis. MMWR Morb Mortal Wkly Rep 2001; 50:1-52.
22. Code of federal regulations. Access to employee exposure and medical records. Title 29, CFR Part 1910.1020. Washington, DC: US Government Printing Office, 2010 (revised annually).
23. National Institute for Occupational Safety and Health. NIOSH Alert: Preventing allergic reactions to natural rubber latex in the workplace. (June 1997) NIOSH publication no. 97-135. Washington, DC: NIOSH, 1997. [Available at

http://www.cdc.gov/niosh/latexalt.html (accessed September 21, 2010).]
24. NFPA 101: Code for safety to life from fire in buildings and structures. Quincy, MA: National Fire Protection Association, 2009.
25. Fowler TW, Miles KK. Electrical safety: Safety and health for electrical trades student manual. (January 2002) NIOSH publication no. 2002-123. Washington, DC: National Institute for Occupational Safety and Health, 2002.
26. Occupational Safety and Health Administration. OSHA technical manual: TED 1-0.15A. Washington, DC: US Department of Labor, 1999.
27. Occupational Safety and Health Administration. Enforcement procedures for the occupational exposure to bloodborne pathogens. Directive CPL 02-02-069. Washington, DC: US Department of Labor, 2001.
28. US Department of Health and Human Services, Centers for Disease Control and Prevention, and National Institutes of Health. Primary containment for biohazards: Selection, installation, and use of biological safety cabinets. Appendix A in: Biosafety in microbiological and medical laboratories. 5th ed. Washington, DC: US Government Printing Office, 2009. [Available separately at http://www.cdc.gov/biosafety/publications (accessed September 21, 2010).]
29. Richmond JY. Safe practices and procedures for working with human specimens in biomedical research laboratories. J Clin Immunoassay 1988;11:115-19.
30. Code of federal regulations. Occupational exposure to bloodborne pathogens; needlesticks and other sharps injuries; final rule. Title 29, CFR Part 1910.1030. Fed Regist 2001;66:5317-25.
31. US Environmental Protection Agency. ATP—tested actively registered hospital disinfectant products. (March 2010) Washington, DC: EPA Office of Pesticide Programs, 2010. [Available at http://www.epa.gov/oppad001/chemreg index.htm (accessed October 12, 2010).]
32. Rutala WA. APIC guideline for selection and use of disinfectants. Am J Infect Control 1996; 24:313-42.
33. Evans MR, Henderson DK, Bennett JE. Potential for laboratory exposures to biohazardous agents found in blood. Am J Public Health 1990;80:423-7.
34. Food and Drug Administration. Memorandum: Guideline for collection of blood products from donors with positive tests for infectious disease markers ("high risk" donors). (October 26, 1989) Rockville, MD: CBER Office of Communication, Outreach, and Development, 1989.
35. US Environmental Protection Agency. EPA guide for infectious waste management. EPA/530-SW-86-014. NTIS #PB86-199130. Washington, DC: National Technical Information Service, 1986.
36. Code of federal regulations. Occupational safety and health standards, Subpart Z—toxic and hazardous substances; air contaminants. Title 29, CFR Part 1910.1000. Washington, DC: US Government Printing Office, 2010 (revised annually).
37. NIOSH pocket guide to chemical hazards. Washington, DC: National Institute for Occupational Safety and Health, 2005. [Available at http://www.cdc.gov/niosh/npg (accessed November 8, 2010).]
38. NFPA 704—Standard for the identification of the hazards of materials for emergency response. Quincy, MA: National Fire Protection Association, 2001.
39. HMIS implementation manual. 3rd ed. Neenah, WI: JJ Keller and Associates, Inc., 2001.
40. Lisella FS, Thomasston SW. Chemical safety in the microbiology laboratory. In: Fleming DO, Richardson JH, Tulis JJ, Vesley D, eds. Laboratory safety, principles, and practices. 2nd ed. Washington, DC: American Society for Microbiology Press, 1995:247-54.
41. American National Standards Institute. American national standards for emergency eyewash and shower equipment. ANSI Z358.1-1998. New York: ANSI, 1998.
42. Occupational Safety and Health Administration. Inspection procedures for 29 CFR 1910.120 and 1926.65, paragraph (q): Emergency response to hazardous substance releases. OSHA directive CPL 02-02-073. Washington, DC: OSHA Office of Health Enforcement, 2007.
43. Code of federal regulations. Air contaminants: Toxic and hazardous substances. Title 29, CFR Part 1910.1000. Washington, DC: US Government Printing Office, 2010 (revised annually).
44. Cook SS. Selection and installation of self-contained irradiators. In: Butch S, Tiehen A, eds. Blood irradiation: A user's guide. Bethesda, MD: AABB Press, 1996:19-40.

45. Beir V. Health effects of exposure to low levels of ionizing radiation. Washington, DC: National Academy Press, 1990:1-8.
46. Regulatory guide 8.29: Instruction concerning risks from occupational radiation exposure. Washington, DC: Nuclear Regulatory Commission, 1996.
47. NCRP report no. 115: Risk estimates for radiation protection: Recommendations of the National Council on Radiation Protection and Measurements. Bethesda, MD: National Council on Radiation Protection and Measurements, 1993.
48. NCRP report no. 105: Radiation protection for medical and allied health personnel: Recommendations of the National Council on Radiation Protection and Measurements. Bethesda, MD: National Council on Radiation Protection and Measurements, 1989.
49. US Nuclear Regulatory Commission. EA-05-090. Enforcement action: Order imposing increased controls (licensees authorized to possess radioactive material quantities of concern). (November 14, 2005) Rockville, MD: NRC, 2005.
50. US Nuclear Regulatory Commission. RIS 2007-14. Fingerprinting requirements for licensees implementing the increased control order. (June 5, 2007) Rockville, MD: NRC, 2007.
51. US Nuclear Regulatory Commission regulatory guide 8.13: Instruction concerning prenatal radiation exposure. Washington, DC: NRC, 1999.
52. Nuclear Regulatory Commission regulatory guide 8.23: Radiation surveys at medical institutions. Washington, DC: NRC, 1981.
53. Code of federal regulations. Hazardous materials regulations. Title 49, CFR Parts 171-180. Washington, DC: US Government Printing Office, 2010 (revised annually).
54. International Air Transport Association. Dangerous goods regulations manual. 48th ed. Montreal, PQ, Canada: IATA, 2010 (revised annually).
55. United States Code. Pollution prevention act. 42 U.S.C. §§13101 and 13102 et seq. Washington, DC: US Government Printing Office, 2009.
56. Clinical laboratory waste management. Approved guideline—second edition GP5-A2. Wayne, PA: Clinical and Laboratory Standards Institute, 2002.

◆ APPENDIX 2-1
Safety Regulations and Recommendations Applicable to Health-Care Settings

Agency/Organization	Reference	Title
Federal Regulations and Recommendations		
Nuclear Regulatory Commission (NRC)	10 CFR 20	Standards for Protection Against Radiation
	10 CFR 36	Licenses and Radiation Safety Requirements for Irradiators
	Guide 8.29	Instruction Concerning Risks from Occupational Radiation Exposure
Occupational Safety and Health Administration (OSHA)	29 CFR 1910.1030	Occupational Exposure to Blood-borne Pathogens
	29 CFR 1910.1020	Access to Employee Exposure and Medical Records
	29 CFR 1910.1096	Ionizing Radiation
	29 CFR 1910.1200	Hazard Communication Standard
	29 CFR 1910.1450	Occupational Exposure to Hazardous Chemicals in Laboratories
Department of Transportation (DOT)	49 CFR 171-180	Hazardous Materials Regulations
Environmental Protection Agency (EPA)		EPA Guide for Infectious Waste Management
Centers for Disease Control and Prevention (CDC)		Guideline for Isolation Precautions in Hospitals
Food and Drug Administration (FDA)	21 CFR 606.3-606.171	Current Good Manufacturing Practice for Blood and Blood Components
	21 CFR 630.6	General Requirements for Blood, Blood Components, and Blood Derivatives
	21 CFR 640.1-640.120	Additional Standards for Human Blood and Blood Products
	21 CFR 211.1-211.208	Current Good Manufacturing Practice for Finished Pharmaceuticals
	21 CFR 1270	Human Tissue Intended for Transplantation
	21 CFR 1271	Human Cells, Tissues, and Cellular and Tissue-Based Products

(Continued)

◆ APPENDIX 2-1

Safety Regulations and Recommendations Applicable to Health-Care Settings (Continued)

Agency/Organization	Reference	Title
Trade and Professional Organizations		
National Fire Protection Association (NFPA)	NFPA 70	National Electrical Code
	NFPA 70E	Electrical Safety Requirements for Employee Workplaces
	NFPA 101	Life Safety Code
	NFPA 99	Standards for Health Care Facilities
	NFPA 704	Standard for the Identification of the Hazards of Materials for Emergency Response
National Paint and Coatings Association		Hazardous Materials Identification System (HMIS) Implementation Manual
International Air Transport Association (IATA)		Dangerous Goods Regulations

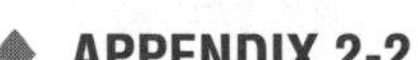

APPENDIX 2-2
General Guidelines for Safe Work Practices, Personal Protective Equipment, and Engineering Controls

UNIFORMS AND LABORATORY COATS

Closed laboratory coats or full aprons over long-sleeved uniforms or gowns should be worn when personnel are exposed to blood, corrosive chemicals, or carcinogens. The material of required coverings should be appropriate for the type and amount of hazard exposure. Plastic disposable aprons may be worn over cotton coats when there is a high probability of large spills or splashing of blood and body fluids; nitrile rubber aprons may be preferred when pouring caustic chemicals.

Protective coverings should be removed before leaving the work area and should be discarded or stored away from heat sources and clean clothing. Contaminated clothing should be removed promptly, placed in a suitable container, and laundered or discarded as potentially infectious. Home laundering of garments worn in Biosafety Level 2 areas is not permitted because unpredictable methods of transportation and handling can spread contamination, and because home laundering techniques may not be effective.[1]

GLOVES

Gloves or equivalent barriers should be used whenever tasks are likely to involve exposure to hazardous materials.

TYPES OF GLOVES

Glove type varies with the task:

- Sterile gloves: for procedures involving contact with normally sterile areas of the body.
- Examination gloves: for procedures involving contact with mucous membranes, unless otherwise indicated, and for other patient care or diagnostic procedures that do not require the use of sterile gloves.
- Rubber utility gloves: for housekeeping chores involving potential blood contact, for instrument cleaning and decontamination procedures, and for handling concentrated acids and organic solvents. Utility gloves may be decontaminated and reused but should be discarded if they show signs of deterioration (peeling, cracks, discoloration) or if they develop punctures or tears.
- Insulated gloves: for handling hot or frozen material.

INDICATIONS FOR USE

The following guidelines should be used to determine when gloves are necessary[1]:

- For donor phlebotomy when the health-care worker has cuts, scratches, or other breaks in his or her skin.
- For phlebotomy of autologous donors or patients (eg, therapeutic apheresis procedures, intraoperative red cell collection).
- For persons who are receiving training in phlebotomy.
- When handling "open" blood containers or specimens.
- When collecting or handling blood or specimens from patients or from donors known to be infected with a blood-borne pathogen.
- When examining mucous membranes or open skin lesions.
- When handling corrosive chemicals and radioactive materials.
- When cleaning up spills or handling waste materials.

(Continued)

◆ APPENDIX 2-2
General Guidelines for Safe Work Practices, Personal Protective Equipment, and Engineering Controls (Continued)

- When the likelihood of exposure cannot be assessed because of lack of experience with a procedure or situation.

The Occupational Safety and Health Administration (OSHA) does not require the routine use of gloves by phlebotomists working with healthy prescreened donors or the changing of unsoiled gloves between donors if gloves are worn.[1,2] Experience has shown that the phlebotomy process is low risk because donors typically have low rates of infectious disease markers. Also, exposure to blood is rare during routine phlebotomy, and other alternatives can be used to provide barrier protection, such as using a folded gauze pad to control any blood flow when the needle is removed from the donor's arm.

The employer whose policies and procedures do not require routine gloving should periodically reevaluate the potential need for gloves. Employees should never be discouraged from using gloves, and gloves should always be available.

GUIDELINES ON USE

Guidelines for the safe use of gloves by employees include the following[3,4]:

- Securely bandage or cover open skin lesions on hands and arms before putting on gloves.
- Change gloves immediately if they are torn, punctured, or contaminated; after handling high-risk samples; or after performing a physical examination (eg, on an apheresis donor).
- Remove gloves by keeping their outside surfaces in contact only with outside and by turning the glove inside out while taking it off.
- Use gloves only where needed, and avoid touching clean surfaces such as telephones, door knobs, or computer terminals with gloves.
- Change gloves between patient contacts. Unsoiled gloves need not be changed between donors.
- Wash hands with soap or other suitable disinfectant after removing gloves.
- Do not wash or disinfect surgical or examination gloves for reuse. Washing with surfactants may cause "wicking" (ie, the enhanced penetration of liquids through undetected holes in the glove). Disinfecting agents may cause deterioration of gloves.
- Use only water-based hand lotions with gloves, if needed; oil-based products cause minute cracks in latex.

FACE SHIELDS, MASKS, AND SAFETY GOGGLES

Where there is a risk of blood or chemical splashes, the eyes and the mucous membranes of the mouth and nose should be protected.[5] Permanent shields, fixed as a part of equipment or bench design, are preferred (eg, splash barriers attached to tubing sealers or centrifuge cabinets). All barriers should be cleaned and disinfected on a regular schedule.

Safety glasses alone provide impact protection from projectiles but do not adequately protect eyes from biohazardous or chemical splashes. Full-face shields or masks and safety goggles are recommended when permanent shields cannot be used. Many designs are commercially available; eliciting staff input on comfort and selection can improve compliance on use.

Masks should be worn whenever there is danger from inhalation. Simple, disposable dust masks are adequate for handling dry chemicals, but respirators with organic vapor filters are preferred for areas where noxious fumes are produced (eg, for cleaning up spills of noxious materials). Respirators should be fitted to their specific wearers and checked annually.

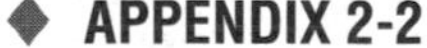

◆ APPENDIX 2-2
General Guidelines for Safe Work Practices, Personal Protective Equipment, and Engineering Controls (Continued)

HAND WASHING

Frequent thorough hand washing is the first line of defense in infection control. Blood-borne pathogens generally do not penetrate intact skin, so immediate removal reduces the likelihood of transfer to a mucous membrane or broken skin area or of transmission to others. Thorough washing of hands (and arms) also reduces the risks from exposure to hazardous chemicals and radioactive materials.

Hands should always be washed before leaving a restricted work area, before using a biosafety cabinet, between medical examinations, immediately after becoming soiled with blood or hazardous materials, after removing gloves, and after using the toilet. Washing hands thoroughly before touching contact lenses or applying cosmetics is essential.

OSHA allows the use of waterless antiseptic solutions for hand washing as an interim method.[2] These solutions are useful for mobile donor collections or in areas where water is not readily available for cleanup purposes. If such methods are used, however, hands must be washed with soap and running water as soon as feasible thereafter. Because there is no listing or registration of acceptable hand-wipe products similar to the one that the Environmental Protection Agency maintains for surface disinfectants, consumers should request data from the manufacturer to support advertising claims.

EYEWASHES

Laboratory areas that contain hazardous chemicals must be equipped with eyewash stations.[3,6] Unobstructed access, within 10 seconds from the location of chemical use, must be provided for these stations. Eyewashes must operate so that both of the user's hands are free to hold open the eyes. Procedures and indications for use must be posted, and routine function checks must be performed. Testing eyewash fountains weekly helps ensure proper function and flushes out the stagnant water. Portable eyewash systems are allowed only if they can deliver flushing fluid to the eyes at a rate of at least 1.5 liters per minute for 15 minutes. They should be monitored routinely to ensure the purity of their contents.

Employees should be trained in the proper use of eyewash devices, although prevention—through consistent and appropriate use of safety glasses or shields—is preferred. If a splash occurs, the employee should be directed to keep his or her eyelids open and to use the eyewash according to procedures, or the employee should go to the nearest sink and direct a steady, tepid stream of water into his or her eyes. Solutions other than water should be used only upon a physician's direction.

After adequate flushing (many facilities recommend 15 minutes), follow-up medical care should be sought, especially if pain or redness develops. Whether washing the eyes is effective in preventing infection has not been demonstrated, but it is considered desirable when accidents occur.

1. Code of federal regulations. Occupational exposure to bloodborne pathogens; final rule. Title 29, CFR Part 1910.1030. Fed Regist 1991; 56:64175-82.
2. Occupational Safety and Health Administration. Enforcement procedures for the occupational exposure to bloodborne pathogens. OSHA instruction CPL 02-02-069. Washington, DC: US Government Printing Office, 2001.
3. Clinical laboratory safety; approved guideline. 2nd ed (GP17-A2). Wayne, PA: Clinical and Laboratory Standards Institute, 2004.
4. Food and Drug Administration. Medical glove powder report. (September 1997) Rockville, MD: Center for Devices and Radiological Health, 2009. [Available at http://www.fda.gov/MedicalDevices/DeviceRegulationandGuidance/GuidanceDocuments/ucm113316.htm (accessed September 21, 2010).]

5. Inspection checklist: General laboratory. Chicago: College of American Pathologists, 2010.
6. American National Standards Institute. American national standards for emergency eyewash and shower equipment. ANSI Z358.1-1998. New York: ANSI, 1998.

♦ APPENDIX 2-3
Biosafety Level 2 Precautions

Biosafety Level 2 precautions as applied in the blood establishment setting include at least the following[1,2]:

- ♦ High-risk activities are appropriately segregated from lower risk activities, and the boundaries are clearly defined.
- ♦ Bench tops are easily cleaned and are decontaminated daily with a hospital disinfectant approved by the Environmental Protection Agency.
- ♦ Laboratory rooms have closable doors and sinks. An air system with no recirculation is preferred, but not required.
- ♦ Workers are required to perform procedures that create aerosols (eg, opening evacuated tubes, centrifuging, mixing, or sonicating) in a biological safety cabinet or equivalent, or to wear masks and goggles in addition to gloves and gowns during such procedures. (Note: Open tubes of blood should not be centrifuged. If whole units of blood or plasma are centrifuged, overwrapping is recommended to contain leaks.)
- ♦ Gowns and gloves are used routinely and in accordance with general safety guidelines. Face shields or their equivalents are used where there is a risk from splashing.
- ♦ Mouth pipetting is prohibited.
- ♦ No eating, drinking, smoking, applying cosmetics, or manipulating contact lenses occurs in the work area. All food and drink are stored outside the restricted area, and laboratory glassware is never used for food or drink. Personnel are instructed to avoid touching their face, ears, mouth, eyes, or nose with their hands or other objects, such as pencils and telephones.
- ♦ Needles and syringes are used and disposed of in a safe manner. Needles must never be bent, broken, sheared, replaced in sheath, or detached from syringe before being placed in puncture-proof, leakproof containers for controlled disposal. Procedures are designed to minimize exposure to sharp objects.
- ♦ All blood specimens are placed in well-constructed containers with secure lids to prevent leaking during transport. Blood is packaged for shipment in accordance with regulatory agency requirements for etiologic agents or clinical specimens, as appropriate.
- ♦ Infectious waste is not compacted and is decontaminated before its disposal in leakproof containers. Proper packaging includes double, seamless, tear-resistant, orange or red bags that are enclosed in protective cartons. Both the carton and the bag inside display the biohazard symbol. Throughout delivery to an incinerator or autoclave, waste is handled only by suitably trained persons. If a waste management contractor is used, the agreement should clearly define the respective responsibilities of the staff and the contractor.
- ♦ Equipment to be repaired or submitted for preventive maintenance, if potentially contaminated with blood, must be decontaminated before its release to a repair technician.
- ♦ Accidental exposure to suspected or actual hazardous material is reported to the laboratory director or responsible person immediately.

1. Clinical laboratory safety; approved guideline. 2nd ed (GP17-A2). Wayne, PA: Clinical and Laboratory Standards Institute, 2004.
2. Fleming DO. Laboratory biosafety practices. In: Fleming DO, Richardson JH, Tulis JJ, Vesley D, eds. Laboratory safety, principles, and practices. 2nd ed. Washington, DC: American Society for Microbiology Press, 1995:203-18.

◆ APPENDIX 2-4
Sample List of Hazardous Chemicals that May Be Encountered in the Blood Bank

Chemical	Hazard
Ammonium chloride	Irritant
Bromelin	Irritant, sensitizer
Calcium chloride	Irritant
Carbon dioxide, frozen (dry ice)	Corrosive
Carbonyl iron powder	Oxidizer
Chloroform	Toxic, suspected carcinogen
Chloroquine	Irritant, corrosive
Chromium-111 chloride hexahydrate	Toxic, irritant, sensitizer
Citric acid	Irritant
Copper sulfate (cupric sulfate)	Toxic, irritant
Dichloromethane	Toxic, irritant
Digitonin	Toxic
Dimethyl sulfoxide (DMSO)	Irritant
Dry ice (carbon dioxide, frozen)	Corrosive
Ethidium bromide	Carcinogen, irritant
Ethylenediaminetetraacetic acid (EDTA)	Irritant
Ethyl ether	Highly flammable and explosive, toxic, irritant
Ficin (powder)	Irritant, sensitizer
Formaldehyde solution (34.9%)	Suspected carcinogen, combustible, toxic
Glycerol	Irritant
Hydrochloric acid	Highly toxic, corrosive
Imidazole	Irritant
Isopropyl (rubbing) alcohol	Flammable, irritant
Liquid nitrogen	Corrosive
Lyphogel	Corrosive
2-Mercaptoethanol	Toxic, stench
Mercury	Toxic
Mineral oil	Irritant, carcinogen, combustible
Papain	Irritant, sensitizer
Polybrene	Toxic
Sodium azide	Toxic, irritant, explosive when heated

♦ APPENDIX 2-4
Sample List of Hazardous Chemicals that May Be Encountered in the Blood Bank (Continued)

Chemical	Hazard
Sodium ethylmercurithiosalicylate (thimerosal)	Highly toxic, irritant
Sodium hydrosulfite	Toxic, irritant
Sodium hydroxide	Corrosive, toxic
Sodium hypochlorite (bleach)	Corrosive
Sodium phosphate	Irritant, hygroscopic
Sulfosalicylic acid	Toxic, corrosive
Trichloroacetic acid (TCA)	Corrosive, toxic
Trypsin	Irritant, sensitizer
Xylene	Highly flammable, toxic, irritant

◆ APPENDIX 2-5
Specific Chemical Categories and How to Work Safely with Them

Chemical Category	Hazard	Precautions	Special Treatment
Acids, alkalis, and corrosive compounds	Irritation Severe burns Tissue damage	During transport, protect large containers with plastic or rubber bucket carriers. During pouring, wear eye protection and chemical-resistant-rated gloves and gowns as recommended. Always ADD ACID TO WATER, never water to acid. When working with large jugs, have one hand on the neck and the other hand at the base, and position them away from the face.	Store concentrated acids in acid safety cabinets. Limit volumes of concentrated acids to 1 liter per container. Post cautions for materials in the area. Report changes in appearance (perchloric acid may be explosive if it becomes yellowish or brown) to chemical safety officer.
Acrylamide	Neurotoxic Carcinogenic Absorbed through the skin	Wear chemically rated gloves. Wash hands immediately after exposure.	Store in a chemical cabinet.
Compressed gases	Explosive	Label contents. Leave valve safety covers on until use. Open valves slowly for use. Label empty tanks.	Transport using hand trucks or dollies. Place cylinders in a stand or secure them to prevent falling. Store in well-ventilated separate rooms. Do not store oxygen close to combustible gas or solvents. Check connections for leaks with soapy water.

◆ APPENDIX 2-5
Specific Chemical Categories and How to Work Safely with Them (Continued)

Chemical Category	Hazard	Precautions	Special Treatment
Flammable solvents	Classified according to flash point—see material safety data sheet Classified according to volatility	Use extreme caution when handling. Post "NO SMOKING" signs in working area. Have a fire extinguisher and solvent cleanup kit in the room. Pour volatile solvents under suitable hood. Use eye protection when pouring and chemical-resistant neoprene gloves. No flame or other source of possible ignition should be in or near areas where flammable solvents are being poured. Label as "FLAMMABLE."	Make every attempt to replace hazardous materials with less hazardous materials. Store containers larger than 1 gallon in a flammable solvent storage room or in a fire safety cabinet. Ground metal containers by connecting the can to a water pipe or ground connection; if recipient container is also metal, it should be electrically connected to the delivery container while pouring.
Liquid nitrogen	Freeze injury Severe burns to skin or eyes	Use heavy insulated gloves and goggles when working with liquid nitrogen.	The tanks should be securely supported to avoid being tipped over. The final container of liquid nitrogen (freezing unit) must be securely supported to avoid tipping over.

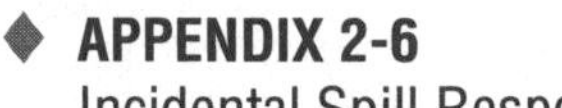

APPENDIX 2-6
Incidental Spill Response*

Chemicals	Hazards	PPE	Control Materials
Acids Acetic Hydrochloric Nitric Perchloric Sulfuric Photographic chemicals (acid)	If inhaled, causes severe irritation. Contact causes burns to skin and eyes. Spills are corrosive. Fire or contact with metal may produce irritating or poisonous gas. Nitric, perchloric, and sulfuric acids are water-reactive oxidizers.	Acid-resistant gloves Apron and coveralls Goggles and face shield Acid-resistant foot covers	Acid neutralizers or absorbent Absorbent boom Leakproof containers Absorbent pillow Mat (cover drain) Shovel or paddle
Bases and caustics Potassium hydroxide Sodium hydroxide Photographic chemicals (basic)	Spills are corrosive. Fire may produce irritating or poisonous gas.	Gloves; impervious apron or coveralls Goggles or face shield; impervious foot covers	Base control/neutralizer Absorbent pillow Absorbent boom Drain mat Leakproof container Shovel or paddle
Chlorine Bleach Sodium hypochlorite	Inhalation can cause respiratory irritation. Liquid contact can produce irritation of the eyes or skin. Toxicity is caused by alkalinity, possible chlorine gas generation, and oxidant properties.	Gloves (double set of 4H undergloves and butyl or nitrile overgloves); impervious apron or coveralls Goggles or face shield Impervious foot covers (neoprene boots for emergency response releases) Self-contained breathing apparatus (emergency response releases)	Chlorine control powder Absorbent pillow Absorbent Absorbent boom Drain mat Vapor barrier Leakproof container Shovel or paddle
Cryogenic gases Carbon dioxide Nitrous oxide Liquid nitrogen	Contact with liquid nitrogen can produce frostbite. Asphyxiation (displaces oxygen). Anesthetic effects (nitrous oxide).	Full face shield or goggles; neoprene boots; gloves (insulated to protect from the cold)	Hand truck (to transport cylinder outdoors if necessary) Soap solution (to check for leaks) Putty (to stop minor pipe and line leaks)

◆ APPENDIX 2-6
Incidental Spill Response* (Continued)

Chemicals	Hazards	PPE	Control Materials
Flammable gases Acetylene Oxygen gases Butane Propane	Simple asphyxiate (displaces air). Anesthetic potential. Extreme fire and explosion hazard. Release can create an oxygen-deficient atmosphere.	Face shield and goggles; neoprene boots; double set of gloves; coveralls with hood and feet	Hand truck (to transport cylinder outdoors if needed) Soap solution (to check for leaks)
Flammable liquids Acetone Xylene Methyl alcohol toluene Ethyl alcohol Other alcohols	Vapors harmful if inhaled (central nervous system depressants). Harmful through skin absorption. Extreme flammability. Liquid evaporates to form flammable vapors.	Gloves (double set of 4H undergloves and butyl or nitrile overgloves); impervious apron or coveralls; goggles or face shield; impervious foot covers	Absorbent Absorbent boom Absorbent pillow Shovel or paddle (nonmetal, nonsparking) Drain mat Leakproof containers
Formaldehyde and glutaraldehyde 4% formaldehyde 37% formaldehyde 10% formalin 2% glutaraldehyde	Harmful if inhaled or absorbed through skin. Irritant to skin, eyes, and respiratory tract. Formaldelyde is a suspected human carcinogen. Keep away from heat, sparks, and flame (37% formaldehyde).	Gloves (double set of 4H undergloves and butyl or nitrile overgloves); impervious apron or coveralls; goggles; impervious foot covers	Aldehyde neutralizer or absorbent Absorbent boom Absorbent pillow Shovel or pallet (nonsparking) Drain mat Leakproof container
Mercury Cantor tubes Thermometers Barometers Sphygmomanometers Mercuric chloride	Mercury and mercury vapors are rapidly absorbed in respiratory tract, GI tract, or skin. Short-term exposure may cause erosion of respiratory or GI tracts, nausea, vomiting, bloody diarrhea, shock, headache, or metallic taste.	Gloves (double set 4H undergloves and butyl or nitrile overgloves); impervious apron or coveralls; goggles; impervious foot covers	Mercury vacuum or spill kit Scoop Aspirator Hazardous waste containers Mercury indicator powder Absorbent Spatula Disposable towels

(Continued)

◆ APPENDIX 2-6
Incidental Spill Response* (Continued)

Chemicals	Hazards	PPE	Control Materials
Mercury (Continued)	Inhalation of high concentrations can cause pneumonitis, chest pain, dyspnea, coughing, stomatitis, gingivitis, and salivation. Avoid evaporation of mercury from tiny globules by quick and thorough cleaning.		Sponge with amalgam Vapor suppressor

*This list of physical and health hazards is not intended as a substitute for the specific MSDS information. In the case of a spill or if any questions arise, always refer to the chemical-specific MSDS for more complete information.
PPE = personal protective equipment; GI = gastrointestinal; MSDS = material safety data sheet.

◆ APPENDIX 2-7
Managing Hazardous Chemical Spills

Actions	Instructions for Hazardous Liquids, Gases, and Mercury
Deenergize.	Liquids: For 37% formaldehyde, deenergize and remove all sources of ignition within 10 feet of spilled hazardous material. For flammable liquids, remove all sources of ignition. Gases: Remove all sources of heat and ignition within 50 feet for flammable gases. Remove all sources of heat and ignition for nitrous oxide release.
Isolate, evacuate, and secure the area.	Isolate the spill area and evacuate everyone from the area surrounding the spill except those responsible for cleaning up the spill. (For mercury, evacuate within 10 feet for small spills or 20 feet for large spills.) Secure the area.
Have the appropriate personal protective equipment (PPE).	See Appendix 2-2 for recommended PPE.
Contain the spill.	Liquids or mercury: Stop the source of spill if possible. Gases: Assess the scene; consider the circumstances of the release (quantity, location, ventilation). If circumstances indicate it is an emergency response release, make appropriate notifications; if release is determined to be incidental, contact supplier for assistance.
Confine the spill.	Liquids: Confine spill to initial spill area using appropriate control equipment and material. For flammable liquids, dike off all drains. Gases: Follow supplier's suggestions or request outside assistance. Mercury: Use appropriate materials to confine the spill (see Appendix 2-6). Expel mercury from aspirator bulb into leakproof container, if applicable.
Neutralize the spill.	Liquids: Apply appropriate control materials to neutralize the chemical (see Appendix 2-6). Mercury: Use mercury spill kit if needed.
Spill area cleanup.	Liquids: Scoop up solidified material, booms, pillows, and any other materials. Put used materials into a leakproof container. Label container with name of hazardous material. Wipe up residual material. Wipe spill area surface three times with detergent solution. Rinse areas with clean water. Collect supplies used (goggles, shovels, etc) and remove gross contamination; place into separate container for equipment to be washed and decontaminated. Gases: Follow supplier's suggestions or request outside assistance. Mercury: Vacuum the spill using a mercury vacuum, or scoop up mercury paste after neutralization and collect the paste in designated container. Use sponge and detergent to wipe and clean spill surface three times to remove absorbent. Collect all contaminated disposal equipment and put into hazardous waste container. Collect supplies and remove gross contamination; place them into a separate container for equipment that will be thoroughly washed and decontaminated.

(Continued)

♦ APPENDIX 2-7
Managing Hazardous Chemical Spills (Continued)

Actions	Instructions for Hazardous Liquids, Gases, and Mercury
Dispose.	Liquids: For material that was neutralized, dispose of it as solid waste. Follow facility's procedures for disposal. For flammable liquids, check with facility safety officer for appropriate waste determination. Gases: The manufacturer or supplier will instruct the facility about disposal if applicable. Mercury: Label with appropriate hazardous waste label and Department of Transportation diamond label.
Report.	Follow appropriate spill documentation and reporting procedures. Investigate the spill; perform root cause analysis if needed. Act on opportunities for improving safety.

Chapter 3

Regulatory Issues in Blood Banking

◆

Glenn Ramsey, MD

◆3

EVERY YEAR, MORE than 5.5 million people in America depend on the safety and efficacy of blood components and other blood products as an essential part of their medical care.[1] To protect the public health, the federal government regulates the manufacture of blood products under the laws for pharmaceutical agents and biologics. From this perspective, blood products are especially complicated biological drugs that are collected from individual donors, then manufactured (often one dose, or blood component, at a time), stored under specific conditions, and administered to patients using specialized testing procedures and medical devices. Blood banks and transfusion services are medical laboratories that are regulated under public health laws for health-care facilities. Government-approved accreditation programs, although voluntary, can demonstrate compliance with regulations for the purpose of mandatory laboratory certification.

FEDERAL LAWS AND REGULATIONS FOR DRUGS

In the United States, when federal laws are enacted, they are published chronologically as statutes and placed into the appropriate one of 50 subject areas (titles) of the United States Code (USC).[2] The government agency responsible for the law [in the case of blood, the Food and Drug Administration (FDA)] then writes regulations (rules) to enforce the law. Proposed rules for public comment and final rules, along with background and interpretive information, are published chronologically in the daily *Federal Register*.[3] The current edition of all rules is collated annually in the appropriate subject area (title) of the *Code of Federal Regulations* (CFR), and an unofficial online edition of the CFR is updated daily.[4] In the CFR, Title 21 is for food and drugs, and Title 42 includes health care.

Some rules have associated guidance documents, which are published online by the agency to provide current thinking about regulatory topics. Guidances are recommendations, not requirements, but they are usually followed by industry. Memoranda to blood establishments were issued before 1998, but some are still active references. Each type of these publications can be accessed from the FDA Blood and Blood Products web page, which provides links to lists of documents in reverse chronological order.[5]

Glenn Ramsey, MD, Medical Director, Blood Banks, Northwestern Memorial Hospital and Children's Memorial Hospital, Department of Pathology, Feinberg School of Medicine, Northwestern University, Chicago, Illinois
The author has disclosed no conflicts of interest.

The FDA regulates drugs and medical devices under the Food, Drug, and Cosmetic Act. Sections 1 through 910 of that act are the same as Sections 301 through 399a of USC Title 21.[6] Blood products are included in the definition of drugs because they are intended to cure, mitigate, treat, or prevent disease (21 USC 321).[7,8] The law requires manufacturers to register with the FDA, obtain biologics license approvals, and follow current good manufacturing practice (cGMP). It also prohibits adulteration and misbranding, authorizes inspections, and defines civil and criminal penalties for violations. The act controls the use of unapproved drugs and devices during their investigational phases and during public health emergencies.

Medical devices include instruments, in-vitro reagents, and their parts and accessories for the diagnosis and treatment of disease. The FDA classifies devices as Class I, II, or III, in ascending order of associated risk [21 USC 360(c)].[9,10] Class I devices have no potential unreasonable risk. Class II devices must meet performance standards beyond basic FDA regulations. Some Class I devices and most Class II devices must be cleared by the FDA based on substantial equivalence with another device already marketed. This process is called 510(k) clearance, referring to the applicable section of the act describing the submission of applications to the FDA for such devices (21 USC 360).[9] Class III devices pose potential unreasonable risk and require specific premarket approval from the FDA, as do unprecedented new devices before their class is determined.

BIOLOGICAL PRODUCTS

Biological products come from living sources and include blood, blood components, derivatives, therapeutic serum, and vaccines applicable to the prevention or treatment of disease. They are regulated by Section 351 (42 USC 262) of the Public Health Service Act, which includes licensure, labeling, inspections, recalls, and penalties for violations in producing biological drugs. This set of regulations provides the core of federal law most specific to blood products.[11] Section 361, "Regulations to Control Communicable Diseases" (42 USC 264), grants the Surgeon General inspection and quarantine powers to prevent the spread of infectious diseases and is invoked in the regulation of tissues (see below).[12]

The FDA's key regulations enforcing the Food and Drug Act and the Public Health Service Act are in Title 21 of the CFR, "Food and Drugs," and in particular, Parts 200 through 299 for drugs, 600 through 680 for biologicals, 800 through 898 for devices, and 1270 through 1271 for tissues.[13] Table 3-1 lists selected parts relevant for manufacturing biologicals. The FDA home page (www.fda.gov) has links to pertinent laws in the USC and regulations in the CFR.

Within the FDA, the Center for Biologics Evaluation and Research (CBER) (www.fda.gov/BiologicsBloodVaccines) regulates blood products and most other biological therapies. The Center for Devices and Radiological Health (CDRH) (www.fda.gov/MedicalDevices) regulates most medical devices, but CBER retains primary jurisdiction over medical devices used with blood and cellular products. The FDA's Office of Regulatory Affairs (ORA) has responsibility for all field operations, which includes inspections and investigations.

As part of the development process for FDA regulations and guidances, several forums are offered for input from the public and from regulated groups.[14] Proposed rules and draft guidances are published to invite written comments, and these comment files, or dockets, are accessible online (www.regulations.gov). When final rules are published in the *Federal Register*, the accompanying commentaries respond to key questions raised. The FDA also receives petitions, which are written requests to write or change regulations. Expert opinions on current issues are sought from several advisory committees, including the FDA's committees on blood products and on cellular, tissue, and gene therapies, and the Department of Health and Human Services (HHS) committee on blood safety and availability. The FDA also hosts public meetings and hearings on selected topics.

Facilities may apply to CBER for approval of exceptions or alternative procedures to the

TABLE 3-1. Regulations of Interest in Title 21 of the CFR (Food and Drugs)

Topic	Section	Topic	Section
FDA general		Donor notification	630.6
Enforcement	1-19	Blood product standards	640
Research and development	50-58	Donor suitability	640.3
Labeling	201	Blood collection	640.4
cGMP for drugs	210-211	Blood testing	640.5
Biological products	600-680	Red Blood Cells	640.10-.17
General	600	Platelets	640.20-.27
Licensing	601	Plasma	640.30-.34
cGMP for blood components	606	Cryoprecipitated AHF	640.50-.56
Personnel, resources	606.20-.65	Exceptions, alternatives	640.120
Standard operating procedures	606.100	Medical devices	800-898
Labeling	606.120-.122	Adverse events	803
Compatibility testing	606.151	Hematology and pathology	864
Records	606.160-.165	Tissues	
Adverse reactions	606.170	Tissues for transplantation	1270
Product deviations	606.171	Cellular and tissue-based products	1271*
Establishment registration	607	General provisions	1271.1-.20
General standards	610	Registration and products	1271.21-.37
Donor testing	610.40	Donor eligibility	1271.45-.90
Donor deferral	610.41	cGTP	1271.145-.320
Look-back	610.46-.48	Section 361 provisions†	1271.330-.440
Dating periods	610.53		

*The following citations represent Subparts A, B, C, D, and E-F, respectively.
†Autologous and related donors (see text).
cGMP = current good manufacturing practice; cGTP = current good tissue practice.

regulations for blood products under 21 CFR 640.120(a). Those that are granted are periodically published, although individual circumstances may not apply to other facilities.[15]

LICENSURE AND REGISTRATION

Blood establishments are classified in three general categories of regulation by the FDA: 1) licensure and registration for interstate commerce, 2) registration for manufacturers not involved in interstate commerce, and 3) exemption from registration for transfusion services as described in the regulations.[16-17] Licensed and/or registered facilities are inspected by the FDA. For transfusion services that perform minimal manufacturing and are certified for reimbursement by the Centers for Medicare and Medicaid Services (CMS), the

FDA accepts CMS-sanctioned laboratory inspections and CMS approval, according to terms of a memorandum of understanding (MOU) with CMS.[18] However, the FDA still has jurisdiction and may inspect if warranted. All military blood facilities, including transfusion services, register with and are inspected by the FDA under another MOU with the Department of Defense.[19]

Facilities seeking licensure use the Biologics License Application (BLA, Form 356h)[20] to apply for both their establishment license and for the products they wish to have licensed for interstate commerce. Subsequent license amendments are handled according to the potential for adverse effects of the changes.[21] Unlicensed blood products, whether from a licensed or an unlicensed facility, may be shipped across state lines for a medical emergency if necessary, but this should be unscheduled and infrequent.[22] The shipping facility must retain documentation of the emergency for FDA review.

Facilities must register annually with the FDA if they collect, manufacture, prepare, or process blood products (Form FDA 2830).[20,23] Transfusion services are exempt from this requirement if they are approved for reimbursement by CMS and their preparation activities are basic, such as preparing Red Blood Cells from whole blood, converting unused plasma to Recovered Plasma, pooling components, reducing leukocytes with bedside filters, or collecting blood only in emergencies. However, facilities that routinely collect blood (including autologous units) or perform such procedures as irradiation, washing, laboratory leukocyte reduction, freezing, deglycerolization, and rejuvenation must register as community or hospital blood banks. Transfusion services that act as depots for forwarding a blood bank's products to other hospitals must register as distribution centers. Clinical laboratories performing infectious disease testing required for blood donors must register unless they are CMS approved. If blood irradiation is performed outside the blood bank or transfusion service, such as in a nuclear medicine department, that facility must register as well.

FDA INSPECTIONS

New facilities are generally inspected within 1 year by a team from CBER and ORA. Subsequent routine inspections are generally performed by ORA every 2 years or earlier depending on the compliance history of the facility.

ORA publishes online manuals and instructions for FDA investigators for inspections in general and for inspections of licensed and unlicensed blood banks in particular.[24,25] The blueprints for blood bank inspections are the general regulations for cGMP and drugs (21 CFR 210-211) and the specific requirements for blood components (21 CFR 606).[26] Routine inspections address the FDA's five required layers of blood safety—donor screening, donor testing, product testing, quarantining, and monitoring and investigating problems. Investigators review the following operational systems that create these safety layers: quality assurance, donor eligibility, product testing, quarantine/inventory management, and production and processing. Full inspections of all systems are designated Level I. After a favorable inspection profile, facilities with four or five systems sometimes may have streamlined Level II inspections of three systems. (Focused inspections for problems or fatalities need not follow these formats.) Within each system, the investigators review standard operating procedures, personnel and training, facilities, equipment calibration and maintenance, and records. Specific requirements for individual systems and processes are discussed in detail in their respective chapters of this book.

If the investigator judges that significant objectionable practices, violations, or conditions are present under which a drug or device is or could be adulterated or injurious to health, these observations are written and presented to the facility (Form 483). Investigators are instructed to seek and record the management's intentions for corrections.[24] However, most facilities also respond in writing immediately with questions or corrective actions. Final determination of violation is made after ORA review.

The agency can take a number of steps in response, including no action at all. For significant violations, the FDA may choose to issue a warning letter, an advisory action to provide the facility with the opportunity for voluntary compliance. Enforcement actions are categorized as administrative, judicial, or recall. Administrative actions include formal citations of violation and—for licensed facilities—suspension or revocation of license. Judicial actions range from seizure of products to court injunctions, civil monetary penalties, and criminal prosecution. The FDA may also conduct recalls if necessary. ORA's *Regulatory Procedures Manual* provides details of available sanctions.[27]

BLOOD-RELATED DEVICES

CBER has lead responsibility in collaboration with CDRH for equipment marketed for the transfusion service and for the collection and processing of blood products, hematopoietic stem cells, and autotransfusions.[28,29] This includes diagnostic tests for infectious disease in blood donors and pretransfusion testing in patients. Blood bank computer software programs are CBER-approved devices. Most blood-related devices are in Class II and cleared by 510(k) equivalence. Examples of Class I devices are copper sulfate solutions for hemoglobin screening, blood grouping view boxes, and heat sealers. Human immunodeficiency virus (HIV) and hepatitis B and C virus (HBV, HCV) donor tests are regulated as Class II or III devices. Screening tests for blood donations are regulated under BLAs. BLAs and Class III devices require specific premarket approval. Each category of device is assigned a code, and all cleared or approved vendors and products for that code are searchable in the Establishment Registration and Device Listing database on the FDA CDRH website.[30]

Serious adverse events related to medical devices must be reported (21 CFR 803).[31] User facilities must report death or serious injuries in which a device was or may have been a factor. Serious injury is defined as being life-threatening, causing permanent impairment or damage, or needing medical or surgical intervention. These reports are sent to the device maker on FDA Medwatch Form 3500A[20] within 10 working days, and deaths must also be reported to the FDA. In years when a Form 3500A report is submitted, an annual summary must be sent to the FDA by January 1 of the following year (Form 3419).[20] Users may voluntarily report other device-related adverse events to the FDA (Form 3500).[20] All possible adverse events, whether reported or not, must be investigated and kept on file for 2 years.

HEMATOPOIETIC PROGENITOR CELLS AS TISSUES

Unmanipulated marrow cell transplants are regulated by the Health Research and Services Administration of HHS, which also oversees marrow and cord blood donations and transplants coordinated by the National Marrow Donor Program. Other hematopoietic progenitor cells (HPCs) collected before May 25, 2005 are regulated by FDA rules for tissue transplants in 21 CFR 1270.[13] The FDA's 2005 regulations in 21 CFR 1271 for human cells, tissues, and cellular and tissue-based products (HCT/Ps) have applied to HPCs collected on or after May 25, 2005.[13,32,33]

HCT/P manufacturers must comply with rules for 1) facility registration and product listing; 2) donor eligibility, including testing for communicable diseases; and 3) production according to current good tissue practice (cGTP). (See Table 3-1.) Registrants using FDA Form 3356[20] report each type of their HPCs in three categories: 1) HCT/Ps as described in 21 CFR 1271.10(a), 2) biologics, or 3) drugs. Table 3-2 outlines how the FDA defines, regulates, and (when applicable) approves each type of HPC. Basic peripheral blood stem cells (PBSCs) from autologous or first- or second-degree related donors are in the first category, which is regulated mainly with regard to preventing transmission of communicable diseases or contamination (Public Health Service Act, Section 361, 42 USC 264).[12] Typical PBSCs from unrelated donors are biologics, and the FDA is considering licensure requirements for them. Beginning in 2011, most unrelated umbilical cord cells must be licensed (see Chapter

TABLE 3-2. US Regulations for Manufacturers of Hematopoietic Progenitor Cells[34]

Type of HPC Product	Jurisdiction Category	Key Regulations (21 CFR except as noted)	FDA Premarket Licensure, Approval, or Clearance?	FDA Compliance Program Manual[35,36]
Unmanipulated marrow	HHS Health Resources and Services Administration	42 US Code 274(k)	No	Not applicable
HPCs collected before May 25, 2005	Tissues, 21 CFR 1270 (before May 25, 2005)	1270 1271 Subparts A-B (see Table 3-1)	No	7341.002A[37]
Autologous or allogeneic related-donor* HPCs	PHS Act Section 361: HCT/Ps	1271.10(a)[†] (must meet all criteria) 1271 A-F	No	7341.002[35] 7342.007 Addendum[38] (imported products)
Unrelated-donor peripheral blood HPCs	PHS Act Section 351: Biologics	1271 A-D	Planned	7341.002[35]
Unrelated-donor umbilical cord cells	Section 351: Biologics	1271 A-D FDA Guidance[39] FDA Draft Guidance[40]	Yes (after October 20, 2011): licensure or IND application for nonqualifying products	7341.002[35]
HPCs with altered characteristics or different function (including somatic cell therapy), or HPCs combined with drug	Cellular and Gene Therapy, CBER	1271 A-D	Yes: IND and BLA	7345.848[41]
HPCs combined with medical device	CBER and CDRH, as determined	1271 A-D	Yes: investigational device exemption and BLA	7382.845[42]

*First- or second-degree relative.

†21 CFR 1271.10(a) as applied to Section 361 (see full rule for details) requires that HPCs be 1) minimally manipulated (biological characteristics unaltered), 2) for homologous use only (similar function as original tissue), 3) not combined with another article (except water; crystalloids; or sterilizing, preserving, or storage agents with no new safety concerns), and 4) used in autologous transfusion or in allogeneic transfusion of donations from a first- or second-degree relative.

HPCs = hematopoietic progenitor cells from manipulated marrow, peripheral blood, and umbilical cord blood (includes donor lymphocyte infusions); CFR = Code of Federal Regulations; FDA = Food and Drug Administration; HHS = Department of Health and Human Services; PHS = Public Health Service; HCT/Ps = Human cells, tissues, and cellular and tissue-based products, as defined by 2005 tissue regulations [21 CFR 1271.3(d)]; IND = investigational new drug; CBER = Center for Biologics Evaluation and Research, FDA; BLA = biologics license application; CDRH = Center for Devices and Radiological Health, FDA.

31). Any HPC that is more than minimally manipulated (eg, by expansion, property alteration, gene therapy) or is used for a different function (eg, tissue engineering) is categorized as a drug and must have premarket approval.

The FDA specifies required donor infectious disease tests for tissue donors and posts lists of tests licensed or cleared for this indication.[43] The elements of cGTP are analogous to cGMP for blood products. A circular of information, *Circular of Information for the Use of Cellular Therapy Products,* is jointly written by the AABB and other organizations for users of these products.[44] The AABB and the Foundation for Accreditation of Cellular Therapy set voluntary standards and accredit facilities for collection and processing of HPCs. (See Chapters 29 and 30.)

The FDA tissue regulations do not apply to facilities that receive, store, and administer tissues but do not perform any manufacturing steps. However, The Joint Commission has hospital standards for handling and tracing tissues and investigating adverse events (TS.03.01.01 to 03.03.01).[45] (See Chapter 32.)

MANAGING RECALLS AND WITHDRAWALS

The FDA's requirements for monitoring and investigating problems with drugs extend to the time after a product's release. When blood banks discover after distribution that a blood product was in violation of rules, standards, specifications, or cGMP, they must report the problem to the FDA and to their consignee. These problems compose a subset of biological product deviations (BPDs)—events in which the safety, purity, or potency of a distributed blood product may be affected—which, again, must be reported to the FDA.[46]

A recall is defined as removal or correction of a marketed product that is in violation of the law (21 CFR 7.3).[47] The FDA classifies recalls by severity. Most blood component recalls are in Class III, not likely to cause adverse health consequences. Class II recalls are for products that may cause temporary adverse effects or remotely possible serious problems. Class I recalls involve a reasonable probability of serious or fatal adverse effects. All recalls are published by the FDA and involve about 1 in 2000 blood components issued in the United States.[48-50]

Market withdrawals are required for products found to be in minor violation. Problems beyond the control of the manufacturer, such as postdonation donor information, are often in this category. Withdrawals are much more common than recalls but are not published.

Transfusion services need to have procedures and training for rapid responses as advised when recalls and withdrawals are received, along with records of actions, reviews, and follow-up, as indicated. Accreditation requirements of the AABB (Standard 7.1) and the College of American Pathologists (CAP: TRM.42120 and TRM.42170) address aspects of this topic.[51,52]

Most of these blood components are transfused before notice is received of their nonconformance. In some recent blood guidances on infectious diseases, the FDA has included recommendations on whether or not to notify the recipient's physician about transfused units. In cases of possible recent infectious-disease exposure in donors or transfusion recipients, the seroconversion window periods for tests should be kept in mind. This can be helpful either for scheduling prospective testing or for reviewing retrospective results, such as a donor who has been retested since an exposure. A general set of recommendations about managing common BPDs has been published for consideration.[53]

The most common reasons for BPDs and blood component recalls are given in Table 3-3. Look-backs on units from donors found after donation to have HIV or HCV are discussed elsewhere (Chapter 8).

MEDICAL LABORATORY LAWS AND REGULATIONS

CMS regulates all US medical laboratories under Section 353 of the Public Health Service Act, as amended by the Clinical Laboratory Improvement Amendments [CLIA; 42 USC 263(a)].[55] Regulations for CLIA are found at 42

TABLE 3-3. Most Common Reasons for Biological Product Deviations and Blood Component Recalls

Biological Product Deviations (Ranked by number of events)	Blood Component Recalls (Ranked by number of units)
Malaria travel/residence	Collection sterility and arm preparation
Variant Creutzfeldt-Jakob disease travel/residence	Storage temperature
Postdonation illness	Production according to current good manufacturing practice
Tattoo	Donor suitability
Donor deferral missed via incorrect donor identification	Product quality control

Biological product deviations shown are from licensed establishments.[54] Blood component recalls are compiled from Food and Drug Administration Enforcement Reports.[50] Market withdrawals are not included in public recalls data.

CFR 493.[56] The law and regulations establish the requirements and procedures for laboratories to be certified under CLIA, both a general requirement and a prerequisite for receiving Medicare and Medicaid payments.

In broad terms, all laboratories must have adequate facilities and equipment, supervisory and technical personnel with training and experience appropriate to the complexity of testing, a quality system (see Chapter 1), and successful ongoing performance in CMS-approved proficiency testing (PT).[57] All laboratories must register with CMS, are subject to inspection by CMS or its designees, and must be recertified every 2 years.

Laboratory requirements start by addressing the complexity of tests performed. All laboratory tests are rated for complexity by the FDA for CMS as waived, moderate complexity, and high complexity. Waived tests are simple and easily performed with limited technical training. Examples include over-the-counter tests, urinalysis dipsticks, copper sulfate specific-gravity hemoglobin screens, spun microhematocrits, and some simple devices for measuring hemoglobin. Laboratories that perform only waived tests register with CMS for a certificate of waiver. The Centers for Disease Control and Prevention provides technical and advisory support to CMS for laboratory regulation and has published practice recommendations for waived testing sites.[58]

Nonwaived tests are classified as moderate or high complexity based on a scoring system of needs for training, preparation, interpretive judgment, and other factors (42 CFR 493.17). The FDA CDRH website provides a searchable database ("CLIA Database") for the complexity of specific tests.[30] For example, manual reagents for compatibility testing are of moderate complexity, automated systems for immunohematology and hematology testing are moderate or high complexity, and viral tests for blood donors are high-complexity tests.

Blood banks and transfusion services have three pathways for CMS approval[59]: 1) certificate of compliance: approval via state health department inspections using CMS requirements; 2) certificate of accreditation: approval via a CMS-approved accrediting organization; and 3) CMS-exempt status: licensure programs for nonwaived laboratories in New York and Washington States are accepted by CMS.

The CLIA regulations delineate general requirements for facilities; quality systems, including quality assurance and quality control; and management and technical personnel qualifications. High-complexity tests require more stringent personnel qualifications. Im-

TABLE 3-4. Hospital Regulations and Accreditation Issues for Transfusion Therapy and Safety

		Reference	
Category	**Subject**	**CMS**	**The Joint Commission**[45]
Transfusion practices	Medical staff: measuring, assessing, and improving blood component use		MS.05.01.01
	Blood management performance standards (as a selectable option on list of hospital performance measures)		In development[64]
Transfusion reaction prevention	Administering transfusions in accordance with state law and medical staff policies and with special training for nonphysicians	482.23(c)(3)[65(p180)]	HR.01.02.01
	Using two patient identifiers for laboratory specimens and blood administration, and labeling samples in presence of patient		NPSG.01.01.01
	Eliminating transfusion errors related to patient misidentification: two-person or automated bedside verification before transfusion		NPSG.01.03.01
Transfusion reaction evaluation	Reporting and monitoring all transfusion reactions	482.23(c)(4)[65(p181)]	PI.01.01.01
ABO hemolytic transfusion reactions	"Never event": No CMS payment for hospital-acquired condition ICD-9-CM[66] code 999.6, ABO incompatibility reaction	Medicare fee-for-service payments: Hospital-acquired conditions[67] Fed Regist 2007;72:47207[3]	
	Reviewable sentinel event: hemolytic transfusion reaction involving "major blood group incompatibilities"		Sentinel Event program[68]

CMS = Centers for Medicare and Medicaid Services.

munohematology laboratories have standards for blood supply agreements, compatibility testing, blood storage and alarms, sample retention, positive identification of blood product recipients, investigation of transfusion reactions, and documentation (42 CFR 493.1103 and 493.1271). Viral and syphilis serologic tests are part of the immunology requirements. CMS has published guidelines for conducting surveys (inspections).[60]

CMS has approved six laboratory accreditation organizations with requirements meeting CMS regulations[61]: the AABB, American Osteopathic Association, American Society for Histocompatibility and Immunogenetics (ASHI), CAP, COLA (formerly the Commission on Office Laboratory Accreditation), and The Joint Commission. The Joint Commission has cooperative agreements with CAP and COLA to accept their laboratory accreditations in facility surveys by The Joint Commission.[62]

AABB and CAP can coordinate joint surveys if desired by facilities seeking both accreditations. CMS may perform their own follow-up surveys to validate the accreditation organizations.

CMS requires successful PT for ongoing laboratory certification of nonwaived testing. Within each laboratory section, CMS regulations specify tests and procedures (regulated analytes) that must pass approved PT if the laboratory performs them. The CMS website has a list of approved PT providers.[63] PT is discussed in Chapter 1.

HOSPITAL REGULATIONS AND ACCREDITATION

In addition to laboratory testing requirements, CMS has regulations for blood administration and the evaluation of transfusion reactions. The Joint Commission incorporates these CMS regulations and has more detailed requirements for monitoring transfusion practices and preventing transfusion errors. The Joint Commission also requires hospitals to select and adopt approved performance measures for focused quality improvement, and it is developing performance measures in blood management for its list of options. Table 3-4 lists key provisions from CMS and The Joint Commission for hospital transfusion services.

STATE AND LOCAL REGULATIONS

All state and local laws and regulations for laboratories and blood banks apply, and must be adhered to. Each state has its own professional licensure requirements for medical and laboratory personnel. CLIA supplanted general laboratory regulations in many states. However, facilities should be familiar with their local requirements, which may extend beyond federal rules in areas such as donor age limits, directed donations, personnel qualifications, adverse event reports, inspection practices, laboratory certification, and transfusion consent. In some situations, facilities providing interstate products or services must comply with local regulations in the customer's location. Some states accept approved accreditation programs for their laboratory requirements.

CONCLUSION

Blood components and other blood products are regulated as pharmaceutical agents, and blood banks and transfusion services are also regulated as medical laboratories. These many requirements make compliance complex. However, close regulation underscores the recognized importance to public health of safe, effective blood products provided via good laboratory practices, using the quality systems described in Chapter 1 and the procedures discussed throughout this manual.

KEY POINTS

1. The US Food and Drug Administration (FDA) regulates the manufacture and use of drugs and medical devices. This includes blood components, blood-derived biological products,

and their ancillary testing and transfusion equipment. The FDA website (www.fda.gov) provides links to blood-related regulations in Title 21 of the *Code of Federal Regulations* (CFR) and to explanatory guidances.

2. The FDA requires licensure and registration for blood manufacturers engaged in interstate commerce, and registration alone for manufacturing activities such as irradiation or washing. Transfusion services performing only basic component preparation need not register but must have laboratory approval from the US Centers for Medicare and Medicaid Services (CMS).
3. Licensed and registered blood facilities are inspected by the FDA every 2 years, with focus on current good manufacturing practice (cGMP; 21 CFR 210-211) and blood component requirements (21 CFR 606). Observations of significant noncompliance or hazards are provided to the facility for its response and correction and may result in a spectrum of sanctions ranging up to license revocation and criminal prosecution.
4. Hematopoietic progenitor cells (HPCs) for transplantation are regulated as tissues by the FDA, with emphasis on preventing transmission of infections and contamination in autologous or closely related allogeneic transplants. The FDA plans to introduce licensure requirements for unrelated allogeneic HPCs, beginning with umbilical cord transplants in 2011.
5. The FDA requires drug (and blood) manufacturers to conduct recalls or market withdrawals when noncompliance is found after products are issued, such as for donor malaria risk or potentially compromised component sterility. Transfusion services should have procedures for evaluating and managing these notices for their potential impact on patients transfused with such products.
6. All US medical laboratories must be approved by CMS every 2 years. Laboratory regulations emphasize adequate facilities and qualified personnel commensurate with the complexity of testing, and they require ongoing successful performance in proficiency testing from CMS-approved vendors. Laboratory approval by CMS is granted via inspections performed by CMS-approved accrediting agencies or by state health departments.
7. Health-care facilities also have CMS regulations for their activities, and The Joint Commission and other organizations accredit many hospitals for CMS compliance. CMS and The Joint Commission have requirements for monitoring transfusion practices, evaluating adverse transfusion reactions, and preventing mistransfusions.

REFERENCES

1. US Department of Health and Human Services. 2009 National blood collection and utilization survey report. Washington, DC: Department of Health and Human Services, 2011 (in press). (Available at http://www. aabb.org/programs/biovigilance/nbcus/Pages/default.aspx.)
2. United States code. Washington, DC: US Government Printing Office, 2010. [Available at http://www.gpoaccess.gov/uscode/index.html (accessed November 15, 2010).]
3. Federal register. Washington, DC: National Archives and Records Administration (daily). [Available at http://www.gpoaccess.gov/fr/index.html (accessed November 15, 2010).]
4. Electronic code of federal regulations (e-CFR). Washington, DC: Office of the Federal Register, National Archives and Records Administration, 2010. [Available at http://ecfr.gpoaccess.gov (accessed November 15, 2010).]
5. Food and Drug Administration. Blood and blood products. Rockville, MD: CBER Office of Communication, Outreach, and Development, 2010. [Available at http://www.fda.gov/BiologicsBloodVaccines/BloodBloodProducts/default.htm (accessed November 15, 2010).]
6. Food and Drug Administration. Section number reference: Federal Food, Drug, and Cosmetic Act. Rockville, MD: FDA, 2009. [Available at http://www.fda.gov/RegulatoryInformation/Legislation/FederalFoodDrugandCosmetic

ActFDCAct/ucm086299.htm (accessed November 15, 2010).]
7. United States code. Title 21, USC Part 321. Washington, DC: US Government Printing Office, 2006.
8. Food and Drug Administration. Compliance policy guides. CPG 230.120—Human blood and blood products as drugs. Rockville, MD: FDA Office of Regulatory Affairs, 2009. [Available at http://www.fda.gov/ICECI/Compliance Manuals/CompliancePolicyGuidanceManual/ucm073863.htm (accessed November 15, 2010).]
9. Food and Drug Administration. FD&C Act Chapter V: Drugs and devices. Rockville, MD: FDA, 2009. [Available at http://www.fda.gov/RegulatoryInformation/Legislation/Federal FoodDrugandCosmeticActFDCAct/FDCAct ChapterVDrugsandDevices/default.htm (accessed November 15, 2010).]
10. Food and Drug Administration. General and special controls. Rockville, MD: FDA Center for Devices and Radiological Health, 2009. [Available at http://www.fda.gov/MedicalDe vices/DeviceRegulationandGuidance/Over view/GeneralandSpecialControls/default.htm (accessed November 15, 2010).]
11. United States code. Title 42, USC Part 262. Washington, DC: US Government Printing Office, 2006.
12. United States code. Title 42, USC Part 264. Washington, DC: US Government Printing Office, 2006.
13. Code of federal regulations. Title 21, CFR Parts 200-299, 600-680, 800-898, and 1270-1271. Washington, DC: US Government Printing Office, 2010 (revised annually).
14. Food and Drug Administration. Comment on regulations. Rockville, MD: FDA, 2008. [Available at http://www.fda.gov/AboutFDA/Con tactFDA/CommentonRegulations/default.htm (accessed November 15, 2010).]
15. Food and Drug Administration. Exceptions and alternative procedures approved under 21 CFR 640.120(b) (revised periodically). Rockville, MD: CBER Office of Communication, Outreach, and Development, 2010. [Available at http://www.fda.gov/BiologicsBloodVac cines/BloodBloodProducts/Regulationofthe BloodSupply/ExceptionsandAlternativeProce dures/default.htm (accessed November 15, 2010).]
16. Food and Drug Administration. Compliance policy guides. CPG Sec. 230.110—Registration of blood banks, other firms collecting, manufacturing, preparing or processing human blood or blood products. Rockville, MD: FDA Office of Regulatory Affairs, 2000. [Available at http://www.fda.gov/ICECI/ComplianceMan uals/CompliancePolicyGuidanceManual/ucm073862.htm (accessed November 15, 2010).]
17. Code of federal regulations. Title 21, CFR Part 607.65(f). Washington, DC: US Government Printing Office, 2010 (revised annually).
18. Food and Drug Administration. MOU 225-80-4000. Memorandum of understanding between the Health Care Financing Administration and the Food and Drug Administration. (June 6, 1983) Rockville, MD: FDA, 1983. [Available at http://www.fda.gov/AboutFDA/PartnershipsCollaborations/Memorandaof UnderstandingMOUs/DomesticMOUs/ucm 116313.htm (accessed November 15, 2010).]
19. Food and Drug Administration. MOU 225-74-7017. Memorandum of understanding between the Department of Defense and the Food and Drug Administration. (June 19, 1974) Rockville, MD: FDA, 1974. [Available at http://www.fda.gov/AboutFDA/PartnershipsCollab orations/MemorandaofUnderstandingMOUs/DomesticMOUs/ucm115877.htm (accessed November 15, 2010).]
20. Food and Drug Administration. FDA forms. Rockville, MD: FDA, 2010. [Available at http://www.fda.gov/AboutFDA/ReportsManuals Forms/Forms/default.htm (accessed November 15, 2010).]
21. Food and Drug Administration. Guidance for industry. Changes to an approved application: Biological products: Human blood and blood components intended for transfusion or for further manufacture. (July 2001) Rockville, MD: CBER Office of Communication, Outreach, and Development, 2001. [Available at http://www.fda.gov/BiologicsBloodVaccines/GuidanceComplianceRegulatoryInformation/Guidances/Blood/ucm076729.htm (accessed November 15, 2010).]
22. Food and Drug Administration. Compliance policy guides. CPG Sec. 220.100. IS shipment of biological products for use in medical emergencies. Rockville, MD: FDA Office of Regulatory Affairs, 2000. [Available at http://www.fda.gov/ICECI/ComplianceManuals/Compli ancePolicyGuidanceManual/ucm073860.htm (accessed November 15, 2010).]

23. Code of federal regulations. Title 21 CFR Part 607.21. Washington, DC: US Government Printing Office, 2010 (revised annually).
24. Food and Drug Administration. Investigators operations manual 2009. Rockville, MD: FDA Office of Regulatory Affairs, 2010. [Available at http://www.fda.gov/ICECI/Inspections/IOM/default.htm# Content (accessed November 15, 2010).]
25. Food and Drug Administration. 7342.001. Inspection of licensed and unlicensed blood banks, brokers, reference laboratories, and contractors. (updated December 2010) Rockville, MD: FDA Office of Regulatory Affairs, 2006. [Available at http://www.fda.gov/BiologicsBloodVaccines/GuidanceComplianceRegulatoryInformation/ComplianceActivities/Enforcement/CompliancePrograms/ucm095226.htm (accessed November 15, 2010).]
26. Code of federal regulations. Title 21, CFR Parts 210, 211, and 606. Washington, DC: US Government Printing Office, 2010 (revised annually).
27. Food and Drug Administration. Regulatory procedures manual (March 2010). Rockville, MD: FDA Office of Regulatory Affairs, 2010. [Available at http://www.fda.gov/ICECI/ComplianceManuals/RegulatoryProceduresManual/default.htm (accessed November 15, 2010).]
28. Food and Drug Administration. Intercenter agreement between the Center for Biologics Evaluation and Research and the Center for Devices and Radiological Health. (October 31, 1991) Rockville, MD: CBER Office of Communication, Outreach, and Development, 1991. [Available at http://www.fda.gov/CombinationProducts/JurisdictionalInformation/ucm121175. htm (accessed November 15, 2010).]
29. Food and Drug Administration. Devices regulated by the Center for Biologics Evaluation and Research. Rockville, MD: CBER Office of Communication, Outreach, and Development, 2010. [Available at http://www.fda.gov/BiologicsBloodVaccines/DevelopmentApprovalProcess/510kProcess/ucm133429.htm (accessed November 15, 2010).]
30. Food and Drug Administration. Medical device databases. Rockville, MD: FDA Center for Devices and Radiological Health, 2010 (revised monthly). [Available at http://www.fda.gov/MedicalDevices/DeviceRegulationandGuidance/Databases/default.htm (accessed November 15, 2010).]
31. Code of federal regulations. Title 21, CFR Part 803. Washington, DC: US Government Printing Office, 2010 (revised annually).
32. Food and Drug Administration. Tissues and tissue products. Rockville, MD: CBER Office of Communication, Outreach, and Development, 2009. [Available at http://www.fda.gov/BiologicsBloodVaccines/TissueTissueProducts/default.htm (accessed November 15, 2010).]
33. Halme DG, Kessler DA. Regulation of stem-cell-based therapies. N Engl J Med 2006;355:1730-5.
34. Food and Drug Administration. Guidance for industry: Regulation of human cells, tissues, and cellular and tissue-based products (HCT/Ps)—small entity compliance guide. (August 2007) Rockville, MD: CBER Office of Communication, Outreach, and Development, 2007. [Available at http://www.fda.gov/BiologicsBloodVaccines/GuidanceComplianceRegulatoryInformation/Guidances/Tissue/ucm073366.htm (accessed November 15, 2010).]
35. Food and Drug Administration. 7341.002—Inspection of human cells, tissues, and cellular and tissue-based products (HCT/Ps). (updated January 4, 2011) Rockville, MD: CBER Office of Communication, Outreach, and Development, 2005. [Available at http://www.fda.gov/BiologicsBloodVaccines/GuidanceComplianceRegulatoryInformation/Compliance Activities/Enforcement/CompliancePrograms/ucm095207.htm (accessed November 15, 2010).]
36. Food and Drug Administration. Compliance programs (CBER). Rockville, MD: CBER Office of Communication, Outreach, and Development, 2009. [Available at http://www.fda.gov/BiologicsBloodVaccines/GuidanceComplianceRegulatoryInformation/ComplianceActivities/Enforcement/CompliancePrograms/default.htm (accessed November 15, 2010).]
37. Food and Drug Administration. 7341. 002A—Inspection of tissue establishments. (updated January 4, 2011) Rockville, MD: CBER Office of Communication, Outreach, and Development, 2007. [Available at http://www.fda.gov/BiologicsBloodVaccines/GuidanceComplianceRegulatoryInformation/ComplianceActivities/Enforcement/CompliancePrograms/ucm095218.htm (accessed November 15, 2010).]
38. Food and Drug Administration. 7342.007 Addendum—Imported human cells, tissues, and

cellular and tissue-based products (HCT/Ps). (January 1, 2010) Rockville, MD: CBER Office of Communication, Outreach, and Development, 2010. [Available at http://www.fda.gov/BiologicsBloodVaccines/GuidanceCompliance RegulatoryInformation/ComplianceActivities/Enforcement/CompliancePrograms/ucm 095250.htm (accessed November 15, 2010).]

39. Food and Drug Administration. Guidance for industry: Minimally manipulated, unrelated allogeneic placental/umbilical cord blood intended for hematopoietic reconstitution for specified indications. (October 2009) Rockville, MD: CBER Office of Communication, Outreach, and Development, 2009. [Available at http://www.fda.gov/downloads/BiologicsBloodVaccines/GuidanceComplianceRegulatoryInformation/Guidances/Blood/UCM 187144.pdf (accessed November 15, 2010).]
40. Food and Drug Administration. Guidance for industry and FDA staff: Investigational new drug applications (INDs) for minimally manipulated, unrelated allogeneic placental/umbilical cord blood intended for hematopoietic reconstitution for specified indications. Draft guidance. (October 2009) Rockville, MD: CBER Office of Communication, Outreach, and Development, 2009. [Available at http://www.fda.gov/downloads/BiologicsBloodVaccines/GuidanceComplianceRegulatoryInformation/Guidances/Blood/UCM187146.pdf (accessed November 15, 2010).]
41. Food and Drug Administration. 7345. 848—Inspection of biological drug products. (October 1, 2010) Rockville, MD: CBER Office of Communication, Outreach, and Development, 2010. [Available at http://www.fda.gov/BiologicsBloodVaccines/GuidanceCompliance RegulatoryInformation/ComplianceActivities/Enforcement/CompliancePrograms/ucm095393.htm (accessed November 15, 2010).]
42. Food and Drug Administration. Inspection of medical device manufacturers. Program 7382.845. (June 15, 2006) Rockville, MD: FDA Center for Devices and Radiological Health, 2006. [Available at http://www.fda.gov/MedicalDevices/DeviceRegulationandGuidance/GuidanceDocuments/ucm072753.htm (accessed November 15, 2010).]
43. Food and Drug Administration. Testing HCT/P donors for relevant communicable disease agents and diseases. Rockville, MD: CBER Office of Communication, Outreach, and Development, 2010. [Available at http://www.fda.gov/BiologicsBloodVaccines/SafetyAvailability/TissueSafety/ucm 095440.htm (accessed November 15, 2010).]
44. AABB, America's Blood Centers, American Association of Tissue Banks, American Red Cross, American Society for Apheresis, American Society for Blood and Marrow Transplantation, College of American Pathologists, Foundation for the Accreditation of Cellular Therapy, ICCBBA, International Society for Cellular Therapy, Joint Accreditation Committee, National Marrow Donor Program, and Netcord. Circular of information for the use of cellular therapy products. Bethesda, MD: AABB, 2009. [Available at http://www.aabb.org/resources/bct/Documents//coi_ct1109.pdf (accessed November 15, 2010).]
45. The Joint Commission. 2010 Comprehensive accreditation manual for hospitals: The official handbook (CAMH). Oakbrook Terrace, IL: The Joint Commission, 2010.
46. Food and Drug Administration. Biological product deviations. Rockville, MD: CBER Office of Communication, Outreach, and Development, 2010. [Available at http://www.fda.gov/BiologicsBloodVaccines/SafetyAvailability/ReportaProblem/BiologicalProduct Deviations/default.htm (accessed November 15, 2010).]
47. Code of federal regulations. Title 21, CFR Part 7.3. Washington, DC: US Government Printing Office, 2010 (revised annually).
48. Ramsey G, Sherman LA. Blood component recalls in the United States. Transfusion 1999;39:473-8.
49. Ramsey G, Sherman LA. Blood component recalls in the United States, 1998 (letter). Transfusion 2000;40:253-4.
50. Ramsey G. Blood component recalls in the United States, 2006 (abstract). Transfusion 2007;47(Suppl 3S):34A.
51. Carson TH, ed. Standards for blood banks and transfusion services. 27th ed. Bethesda, MD: AABB, 2011.
52. College of American Pathologists Laboratory Accreditation Program checklists. Northfield, IL: College of American Pathologists, 2010 (revised annually).
53. Ramsey G. Managing recalls and withdrawals of blood components. Transfus Med Rev 2004;18:36-45.
54. Food and Drug Administration. Biological product and HCT/P deviation reports. Annual summary for fiscal year 2009. Rockville, MD:

CBER Office of Communication, Outreach, and Development, 2010. [Available at http://www.fda.gov/BiologicsBloodVaccines/SafetyAvailability/ReportaProblem/BiologicalProductDeviations/ucm129757.htm (accessed November 15, 2010).]

55. United States code. Title 42, USC Part 263a. Washington, DC: US Government Printing Office, 2006.
56. Code of federal regulations. Title 42, CFR Part 493. Washington, DC: US Government Printing Office, 2010 (revised annually).
57. Rauch CA, Nichols JH. Laboratory accreditation and inspection. Clin Lab Med 2007;27: 845-58.
58. Howerton D, Anderson N, Bosse D, et al. Good laboratory practices for waived testing sites: Survey findings from testing sites holding a certificate of waiver under the Clinical Laboratory Improvement Amendments of 1988 and recommendations for promoting quality testing. MMWR Re-comm Rep 2005;54(RR-13):1-32.
59. Department of Health and Human Services. Clinical Laboratory Improvement Amendments (CLIA): How to obtain a CLIA certificate. (March 2006) Baltimore, MD: HHS Centers for Medicare and Medicaid Services, 2006. [Available at http://www.cms.hhs.gov/CLIA/downloads/HowObtainCLIACertificate.pdf (accessed November 15, 2010).]
60. Department of Health and Human Services. Interpretive guidelines for laboratories. Appendix C. Survey procedures and interpretive guidelines for laboratories and laboratory services. Baltimore, MD: HHS Centers for Medicare and Medicaid Services, 2010. [Available at http://www.cms.hhs.gov/CLIA/03_Interpretive_Guidelines_for_Laboratories.asp (accessed November 15, 2010).]
61. Department of Health and Human Services. List of approved accreditation organizations under CLIA. Baltimore, MD: HHS Centers for Medicare and Medicaid Services (undated). [Available at http://www.cms.hhs.gov/CLIA/downloads/AO. List.pdf (accessed November 15, 2010).]
62. The Joint Commission. Laboratory services. Facts about the cooperative accreditation initiative. (April 2010) Oakbrook Terrace, IL: The Joint Commission, 2010. [Available at http://www.jointcommission.org/AccreditationPrograms/Laboratory Services/coop_accreditation.htm (accessed November 15, 2010).]
63. Department of Health and Human Services. CLIA-approved proficiency testing programs—2010. Baltimore, MD: HHS Centers for Medicare and Medicaid Services, 2010. [Available at http://www.cms.hhs.gov/CLIA/downloads/ptlist.pdf (accessed November 15, 2010).]
64. The Joint Commission. Performance measurement initiatives. Oakbrook Terrace, IL: The Joint Commission, 2010. [Available at http://www.jointcommission.org/PerformanceMeasurement/PerformanceMeasurement (accessed November 15, 2010).]
65. Department of Health and Human Services. State operations manual. Appendix A—Survey protocol, regulations and interpretive guidelines for hospitals (rev. 47, June 5, 2009). Baltimore, MD: HHS Centers for Medicare and Medicaid Services, 2009. [Available at http://cms.hhs.gov/manuals/Downloads/som107ap_a_hospitals.pdf (accessed November 15, 2010).]
66. National Center for Health Statistics and Centers for Medicare and Medicaid Services. ICD-9-CM: International classification of diseases, 9th revision; clinical modification, CD-ROM 2010. Los Angeles: Practice Management Information Corporation, 2010.
67. Department of Health and Human Services. Hospital-acquired conditions (HAC) in acute inpatient prospective payment system (IPPS) hospitals. (May 2010) Baltimore, MD: HHS Centers for Medicare and Medicaid Services, 2010. [Available at http://www.cms.hhs.gov/HospitalAcqCond/Downloads/HACFactsheet.pdf (accessed November 15, 2010).]
68. The Joint Commission. Sentinel event. Oakbrook Terrace, IL: The Joint Commission, 2010. [Available at http://www.jointcommission.org/SentinelEvents (accessed November 15, 2010).]

Chapter 4

Disaster Management

Jamie Blietz, MBA, CAE; William P. FitzGerald, LTC USA (Ret); and Ruth D. Sylvester, Lt Col, USAF (Ret), MS, MT(ASCP)SBB

◆4

MUCH HAS BEEN learned over the past decade about preparing for and responding to disasters. Whether the disaster is from natural forces (eg, hurricane, earthquake, flood, or pandemic influenza) or is the result of a human event (eg, terrorism, human accidents), organizations around the world have put forth tremendous resources to counteract and to mitigate the threats related to such events.

The goal of this chapter is to provide an overview of disaster management and to discuss the various functional areas and issues that blood collection and hospital facilities should consider in their planning and response strategies. This chapter is more strategic than procedural in nature. Many of the specific and tactical procedures can be found in the AABB *Disaster Operations Handbook*, which should be considered as a complementary text to this chapter.[1]

It is important to point out that the chapter title "Disaster Management" encompasses much more than just preparing for a disaster. It addresses the entire cycle of disaster management, including elements often overlooked in traditional disaster plans. Even though this chapter focuses primarily on emergency management strategies used in the United States, many of the methods can also be adapted for use in other countries. Hospital-based blood banks and transfusion services should note that many of the items contained in this chapter are intended for stand-alone organizations (eg, blood collection centers) and may already be addressed in the hospital's overall disaster plan. However, hospital staff members should review both their hospital and departmental disaster plans to ensure that blood-related issues (including cellular and related biologic therapies) are sufficiently covered.

BACKGROUND

Cycle of Disaster Management

The cycle of disaster management shown in Fig 4-1 includes four functional areas: mitiga-

Jamie Blietz, MBA, CAE, Director, National Blood Exchange, AABB, Bethesda, Maryland; William P. FitzGerald, LTC USA (Ret), Senior Advisor, Biomedical Preparedness, American Red Cross, Washington, District of Columbia; Ruth D. Sylvester, Lt Col, USAF (Ret), MS, MT(ASCP)SBB, Director, Regulatory Services, America's Blood Centers, Washington, District of Columbia

The authors have disclosed no conflicts of interest.

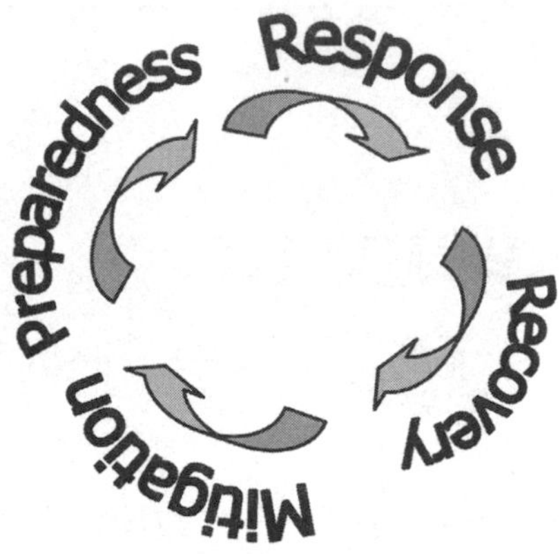

FIGURE 4-1. The cycle of disaster management.

tion, preparedness, response, and recovery.[2] Organizations should consider each of these areas when creating an effective disaster management program.

- *Mitigation* efforts are focused on making permanent changes to plant and property in order to reduce the overall exposure to various known hazards. Mitigation strategies typically involve the "where" and "how" of building physical structures and protecting employees and assets (eg, building code requirements, flood plain analysis, storm shelters). Mitigation techniques also involve taking relatively minor steps to reduce loss or injury (eg, fastening bookshelves or file cabinets to a wall).
- *Preparedness* focuses on areas of risk that cannot be addressed through mitigation efforts alone. Emergencies are dynamic and complex events, and careful preparation efforts are needed to reduce the loss of life and property while sustaining business operations. Preparation efforts begin with a thorough risk analysis of all known hazards (both natural and human) that could potentially affect an organization (eg, fire, severe storm, earthquake, terrorism). Based on the risk assessment, planning efforts should focus on the people and organizational systems that are most likely to be affected. Effective preparation involves a continual improvement process whereby the disaster plan is routinely tested by a series of real or simulated events (drills) through which gaps are identified and remedied.
- *Response* takes place during an emergency and typically involves time-sensitive action steps taken by the staff to protect life and property and to stabilize the organization (eg, communication with staff, evacuation procedures, response to customers and the media). Effective response strategies are centered on clearly outlined processes or procedures and on well-defined lines of authority that can be practiced during drills and can be implemented during any time of the day or night (eg, night and weekend shifts).
- *Recovery* efforts begin once the initial response actions have taken place. Efforts focus on restoring critical lifeline systems in order to resume and maintain business operations (eg, communications, water, power, sewage). Recovery efforts complete the cycle of disaster management by providing insight into additional mitigation strategies that can be deployed for future emergencies.

Risk Assessment

The cornerstone of an effective disaster management program is a thorough risk assessment of the known hazards that can affect the organization. Risk can be defined as the potential losses (physical, economic, social) associated with a hazard and can be defined in terms of expected probability and frequency, causative factors, and locations or areas affected.[3] The goal of risk assessment is to identify and reduce the number of potential risks associated with a hazard, given its probability of occurrence and scope. Potential hazards that are generated *externally* include natural events such as earthquakes, floods, wildfires, pandemics, and hurricanes, as well as human events such as terrorism or industrial accidents, including chemical, hazardous material, and nuclear power plant emergencies.[4]

Another class of potential hazards to consider involves events that may occur *internal-*

ly at the respective organization. Examples of internal hazards include internal flooding caused by a burst water pipe or fire sprinkler malfunction, fires, natural gas leaks, workplace violence, and hazardous spills. Each of those hazards may involve the disruption of services and the evacuation of staff, donors, and patients. For instance, what is the potential risk to stored blood components and patients if the hospital's blood bank should become flooded or must be relocated because of smoke damage from a fire?

There are many approaches to conducting an effective risk assessment. Even though this text does not provide guidance on a specific risk assessment process, a sample risk assessment chart is provided in Table 4-1, which highlights the major functional areas and hazards to consider. For instance, a facility located in an area of seismic activity would list earthquakes as a potential external hazard and would need to determine the immediate effect on its operational status (human, property, business) and the resources needed to recover and restore operations. Conversely, the same organization may be located far away from hurricane and flood zones and would accordingly reflect that situation on its risk assessment chart. The AABB *Disaster Operations Handbook* contains a section listing common hazards, including impact factors as well as preparedness and response strategies.

Emergency Management in the United States

Emergency management as an organized function or profession has evolved over the past two centuries in the United States, beginning with the passage of the Congressional Fire Disaster Relief Act of 1803 in response to an extensive fire that swept through Portsmouth, NH, overwhelming local and state resources. World wars, catastrophic disasters, and nuclear threats have further shaped emergency management concepts and have created an academic discipline with standard procedures and processes. It is important for staff members to understand the basics of emergency management when creating a disaster management program so that an organization can communicate effectively when working with emergency management professionals during an event or a drill.

- **Emergency Management Agencies (EMAs).** EMAs are local, tribal, state, and federal agencies tasked with helping individuals and organizations deal with all cycles of disaster management. These agencies are staffed by both full-time and volunteer per-

TABLE 4-1. Risk Assessment Chart with Sample Data[4]

	Probability of Occurrence	Human Effect	Property Effect	Business Effect	Recovery Resources Needed	Total
Type of Disaster	High Low 5 ↔ 1	High Low 5 ↔ 1	High Low 5 ↔ 1	High Low 5 ↔ 1	High Low 5 ↔ 1	
External Hazards						
Earthquake	5	3	4	5	4	21
Hurricane	1	1	1	2	2	7
Internal Hazards						
Flooding	4	1	4	3	2	14
Workplace Violence	2	5	2	4	1	14

sonnel (emergency managers) and use standard methods when responding to a disaster (eg, Incident Command System or ICS).[5] A listing of state EMA websites can be found at http://www.emergencymanagement.org.

- **Levels of Disaster Support.** Emergencies are inherently local events requiring citizens, local organizations, and "first responders" to be prepared for identified hazards (eg, earthquake, hurricane). State and national support systems are in place to assist if a local municipality is overwhelmed by a disaster.
- **National Response Framework (NRF).** The NRF (formerly the National Response Plan) is a federally operated "all hazards" response plan that is activated in response to a presidentially declared disaster under the Robert T. Stafford Disaster Relief and Emergency Assistance Act (amended June 2006).[6,7] Under this act, the federal government's action, coordinated by the Department of Homeland Security (DHS), provides support (personnel, assets, financial support) to state and local governments that are overwhelmed during a major disaster. The need for blood is covered under the medical and public health section of the NRF (Emergency Support Function No. 8).[6] Blood collection and hospital facilities should be familiar with the language contained in the NRF in order to request and receive assistance during major emergencies.
- **AABB Interorganizational Task Force on Domestic Disasters and Acts of Terrorism (AABB Disaster Task Force).** The AABB Disaster Task Force was formed in January 2002 and provides support to blood collection and transfusion facilities during major emergencies and when the NRF is activated under the Stafford Act. Facilities should review the AABB Disaster Task Force response plan and integrate the specific response processes into organizational disaster plans.[1]
- **Homeland Security Advisory System (HSAS).** At the federal level, the DHS assesses critical infrastructure vulnerabilities and communicates protective measures that individuals and organizations can take when information about a potential threat has been received (eg, changes in airline security screening). The DHS currently uses three communication vehicles to convey threat and protective measure information: 1) Homeland Security Threat Advisories, 2) Homeland Security Information Bulletins, and 3) the Color-Coded Threat Level System.[8]
- **National Incident Management System (NIMS).** The NIMS is a nationally accepted system for helping responders from various jurisdictions to communicate and coordinate their response efforts.[9] The NIMS uses a unified approach for incident management with standard command and management structures and emphasizes preparedness, mutual aid, and resource management. Organizations should be familiar with NIMS protocols so that they are prepared to communicate effectively with responding organizations (eg, police, fire, and the Federal Emergency Management Agency, or FEMA). Online training courses are located at http://training.fema.gov/IS/crslist.asp (accessed October 12, 2010).
- **National Disaster Medical System (NDMS).** The NDMS is a cooperative asset-sharing program directed by the Department of Health and Human Services (DHHS) that augments local medical care when an emergency exceeds the scope of a community's health-care system. The NDMS comprises more than 9000 medical and support personnel from federal, state, and local governments; from the private sector; and from civilian volunteers.[10]

Major Disaster Management Factors for Blood and Transfusion

In conjunction with comprehensive disaster planning strategies, blood collection and hospital facilities should consider the following factors that have been identified as key issues for blood and blood components from collection to transfusion.[11-14]

Most of the blood and blood components in the United States are collected, processed, tested, and stored at regional blood centers and must be delivered to hospitals before transfusion. During an emergency, this "just-in-time" delivery system results in the need for close coordination between blood centers and the hospitals they serve, which involves robust communication and information systems, transportation and logistics support, and critical utilities such as fuel and power to ensure that blood can be transported and stored at required temperatures.

Emergency management personnel are often unaware of issues related to the collection, processing, storage, and distribution of blood and blood components and may assume that blood is collected and stored directly in hospitals. As a result of this misconception, blood-related issues are often overlooked during real and simulated disasters (eg, the need for transportation and logistics support). A continuing process of education for emergency managers at both the local and national levels is needed to increase their awareness of issues related to blood.

Historically, most disasters required relatively few units of blood for transfusions related to the event; however, the public response to disasters has traditionally resulted in an increase in blood donations regardless of the true medical need for transfusions. A sudden increase in unexpected blood donations can disrupt both local and national blood supplies. Efforts should be made to establish the true medical need for blood during a disaster and to communicate this need to organizations within the blood community, to blood donors, and to the public through a clear and consistent messaging strategy.[11-14]

In disasters resulting in injuries that do require blood transfusions to treat victims, the local blood inventory is the primary source for the initial treatments. Because blood collected in response to the disaster takes from 24 to 48 hours to process, it is critical for the local blood supply to remain at ample levels to treat victims of potential hazards as defined in the organizational risk assessment. The AABB Disaster Task Force recommends maintaining a 5- to 7-day supply [combined inventory at the blood collector and hospital(s) it serves] to address potential disasters.[1] Efforts will be made to resupply the affected facilities from neighboring blood collection centers or through national support by the AABB Disaster Task Force. However, it should be estimated that blood being transported from outside the immediate vicinity would take from 12 to 24 hours to be delivered to the affected hospital.

Disasters created by humans and resulting from the use of biologic, chemical, radiologic, or nuclear agents may result in widespread donor deferrals and in the potential quarantine of blood components already in the manufacturing process or storage until the nature and effect of the agent can be determined. In addition, in the event of an influenza pandemic, blood supplies may be severely strained for weeks as a result of extremely high staff absenteeism and donor shortages as individuals become ill, need to stay home to take care of loved ones, or fear exposure to influenza in public places. An influenza pandemic could also severely affect the availability of needed supplies as manufacturers face similar absenteeism problems and transportation difficulties.[15] Hospitals and transfusion services should develop blood shortage management plans to maximize the probability of optimal blood distribution and use during a severe shortage. Such plans can achieve the consistency and collaboration crucial to the equitable allocation of scarce blood resources in times of severe shortage.

Finally, certain disasters may affect a blood collector's ability to collect and process blood throughout the duration of an event, thus straining the local blood supply for days or weeks. For instance, as a hurricane approaches, a blood collector may suspend collections for a few days before and after the storm has passed, resulting in a significant loss of expected collections. Elective surgeries are typically postponed during the same period, thereby helping to alleviate the strain on supply. However, lessons learned from previous disasters indicate that blood collection and transfusion facilities should prepare for the potential acute shortage of blood components in the days following a hurricane-type event, with special attention given to the supply of platelets. Facilities should work to augment supplies before a predictable hazard (eg, hurricane or severe winter storm) and should contact the AABB Disaster Task Force for support if routine supply channels are inadequate to bolster supplies before or after the event has occurred.

BUSINESS OPERATIONS PLANNING

Business operations planning is generally approached as a three-step process: assembling a planning team; analyzing the current situation, including hazards and capabilities; and developing a plan to continue operations in the event of an emergency. Once planning has been completed, implementation of the plan (which includes training and testing as well as evaluating and revising the plan[16,17]) can proceed.

Disaster Planning Team

The first step in disaster planning is to identify the person or team of people in an organization who are responsible for emergency operations planning. The number of people involved will depend on the size and complexity of an operation. Assistance will be needed from key people such as an organization's accountant, attorney, human resources staff, and insurance agent. Additionally, establishing an early liaison with local EMAs can be vital to the success of a disaster plan in an actual emergency.

Once the team has been formed, a project plan should be developed to identify the key steps and a timeline for completion. Business continuity planning has proliferated over the past 5 years as organizations have seen human and natural disasters wreak havoc in the United States and abroad. References, training materials, and tool kits with step-by-step instructions and templates are widely available on the Internet and should be acquired and used.[16-19]

Analysis of Current Situation

The success of disaster planning depends on a risk analysis of the current situation (see section on risk assessment, earlier). This assessment includes the process of determining the hazards to which an organization is vulnerable, the probability of each hazard occurring, and the anticipated effect of each event on human and physical resources as well as on business operations.[4,16] For example, a potential event may have catastrophic consequences for infrastructure and human resources, but the likelihood of its occurring may be minuscule.

The best option to ensure uninterrupted business operations is to prevent disasters before they occur.[19,20] Effective prevention strategies can be used for risks such as fire, power interruption, facility security, and workplace violence. What cannot be prevented should be mitigated. For example, locating essential operations away from flood plains, having multiple sources (not necessarily multiple suppliers) of critical supplies, and relocating vital records to upper floors in flood-prone areas are all mitigation strategies.

For those risks that cannot be prevented or adequately mitigated, plans must be made to continue essential operations. Plans should be developed for events that have a high likelihood of occurring as well as low probability events with potentially catastrophic consequences (eg, Category 5 hurricane or pandemic influenza).

Continuity of Operations Plan

A Continuity of Operations Plan (COOP) is a plan to ensure continued operation of essential functions in the event of an emergency or a disaster.[16] A COOP should be developed so that the plan is independent of the event and covers the range of emergencies determined to be the most likely or with such a significant effect that their inclusion is merited. The areas identified in Table 4-2 are the minimum needed in a COOP. Hospital-based blood banks and transfusion services may be part of the overall hospital or laboratory COOP; however, the various planning documents should be reviewed to ensure that issues specific to blood and transfusion are sufficiently covered. Such plans are required by the AABB in *Standards for Blood Banks and Transfusion Services*[21] as well as by The Joint Commission.[22] The elements in the table are discussed below.

Essential Functions

Essential functions are those that must be carried out to ensure business continuity, such as the storage of blood and blood components and their transportation and delivery to hospitals. Even though collections, component preparation, and testing may be interrupted, the continued viability of a blood center depends on its ability to provide hospital customers with blood. Blood can be imported from outside the affected area to ensure an adequate inventory until collections can be resumed. Likewise, hospitals must be certain that they can receive, store, and transfuse blood to patients in need.

COOP Decision Trees

COOP operations and decisions are best thought out in advance, during normal operations. Flow charts and decision trees that list options can be developed to guide leaders during emergency operations. Such charts and trees can be developed in group sessions and refined using lessons learned from. exercises and real-world events. An example of a decision tree developed to support blood bank operations is available on the Internet.[23]

TABLE 4-2. Essential Elements of a Continuity of Operations Plan (COOP)[16,17]

1. Identify essential processes and functions required for continued operations.
2. Develop decision trees for implementation of the COOP.
3. Consider alternate facility options.
4. Establish safety and security plans for staff facilities and fleet vehicles.
5. Identify and ensure protection and survivability of vital records and databases.
6. Review insurance coverage and ensure adequacy for potential risks.
7. Establish minimum cash reserves necessary to continue operations for 90 days.
8. Develop an emergency communications plan.
9. Establish a chain of command and an order of succession for decision-making authority.
10. Develop a plan for dealing with the news media.
11. Identify designated spokespersons, and train them to handle risk and emergency communications.
12. Plan to maintain supplies and logistical support for operations.
13. Evaluate utility needs and develop contracts or memoranda of agreement (MOA) to ensure replenishment and restoration of essential utilities.
14. Review information technology (IT) systems and develop redundancies to ensure that vital systems and their supporting subsystems remain operational during an emergency.
15. Identify staffing issues including essential personnel and key contacts necessary to carry out essential functions as well as human resource considerations of employee compensation and benefits during and after the disaster.
16. Develop procedures for transitioning back to normal operations.

Alternate Facilities

Alternate facilities that can be used to continue operations should be identified during the planning phase of a COOP. Thought should be given to the need for equipment, supplies, information technology (IT) support, and other items at the alternate location. Consideration should also be given to practical locations for alternate facilities. For example, an alternate facility across the street will most likely be similarly affected by an external disaster. If funding is not available to pay for an alternate facility, the organization should consider establishing documented agreements with other organizations in the area to provide alternate existing space if one facility is incapacitated.

Security and Safety

In the event of a disaster, security can become a major issue, from security of the facility and fleet to security of the staff and information systems.[24] For example, crowd control may become an issue if large numbers of donors gather at collection locations, or in the event of special screening requirements during a pandemic influenza outbreak. In natural disasters where fuel shortages occur, the security of fuel supplies can become a major challenge. A COOP should include the measures that will be necessary to ensure the security of all critical resources.

Planners should review their organizational security plan and should determine if the plan adequately addresses changes in the threats and hazards to the local area. Coordination with EMA officials can provide information on threat or risk assessments. Planners should consider the implementation of measures to increase the security of their facilities and for their staff, volunteers, and donors during changes in the HSAS.[8] Measures should include at least the following:

- Appropriate personnel background checks for staff, volunteers, and contractors who require access to irradiators in accordance with federal and state guidelines.
- Appropriate security for irradiators in accordance with federal and state guidelines.
- Use of security cameras to monitor entrances, parking lots, fuel points, and storage areas.
- Positive identification checks at entrances to buildings, parking lots, and loading docks.
- Use of contractor-provided security personnel.
- Increased police patrols in the immediate area.
- Coordination with sponsors at mobile drive sites.
- Distribution of brochures that discuss a facility's security and safety measures for staff, volunteers, and donors.

Planners should ensure that the facility is in compliance with all local building codes and applicable Occupational Safety and Health Administration (OSHA) regulations. The actions that have been implemented should be discussed with the local EMA and the insurance company, and any suggestions that they may provide should be put into effect.[17]

Vital Records

The protection of vital records is especially critical in an industry that depends on records to document the safety and availability of blood. In addition to donor records, the organizational human resource files, legal records, payroll records, and financial records such as accounts receivable and accounts payable are also critical to the survivability of a business.[25] Records of insurance policies, bank account numbers, and supplies of blank checks must be available during emergency operations to ensure continuity of operations. Corporation records, strategic plans, and records of research must also be maintained. Redundancy of computerized records should be established through periodic creation of copies or real-time backup on a duplicate server. Geographic considerations must be taken into account in identifying off-site storage locations. Not all records are maintained electronically, so provisions to safely keep paper copies of records must be considered, especially if alternate facility operations are implemented.

Insurance

Adequate insurance is essential to the survivability of any business. The two major types of insurance coverage are property and liability. Key provisions of policies include valuation of property; perils covered, such as flooding, wind, and power interruptions; deductibles; and how to file claims. Another key consideration is business interruption insurance to cover loss of income. Additional background information is available from a variety of resources, including the Small Business Administration and insurance companies.[24,26]

Cash Reserves

The single most crucial element in determining the survivability of a business is access to cash that will support a business until normal operations can be resumed.[20,27] Cash reserves, equal to several months' worth of operational expenses, should be accrued during normal operations. Other options for obtaining cash after a disaster include Small Business Administration loans, conventional bank loans, and lines of credit.

Emergency Communications Plan

Communication systems are often the first assets to be strained during an emergency. Telecommunication systems can quickly become overloaded or jammed, computer systems may be disrupted because of a loss of power, and the staff may become separated, resulting in general confusion and an organization's inability to make fast-paced decisions during and after a disaster. Clear, quick, and effective communication is vital in protecting life and property during a disaster. Organizations should invest heavily in ensuring that the staff can communicate both internally and externally and should develop an Emergency Communications Plan (ECP). No single definition or all-encompassing set of procedures exists for an ECP, but organizations should consider the following areas when designing a plan.

IDENTIFYING INTERNAL AND EXTERNAL AUDIENCES FOR THE ECP. Blood collection and hospital facilities should work to identify and map the essential internal departments and personnel that need to communicate both during a disaster (response) and after a disaster (recovery). It may be helpful to classify these individuals and groups by their relative importance toward ensuring continuity of operations (ie, essential employees). At some level, all employees need to be included in the ECP, because all employees will need to receive information regarding the evacuation or response procedures and the operational status of the facility (ie, when to report back to work).

External audiences need to be identified and assessed on their ability to communicate with an organization (eg, vendors must have an ECP for communications with an organization). For instance, a hospital blood bank or transfusion service should identify all essential departments or personnel, or both, at their related blood supplier(s). Conversely, blood centers should identify the key departments and personnel at hospitals or the testing providers that need to be contacted during and after an emergency.

KEY CONTACTS. A key contact list should be periodically updated and maintained for all of the critical internal and external personnel, departments, and organizations that require communication during an emergency. Internal contact lists should include essential personnel and key leadership. External contact lists should include customers, suppliers, and vendors of critical supplies, as well as other key business resources such as insurance agents, utility services, legal representatives, and banking personnel.

The contact list should be readily available both electronically (eg, on a personal digital assistant) and in printed form (eg, on a laminated card) for emergency response personnel to use during a disaster. In addition to main contact telephone numbers, facilities should consider collecting redundant contact information for each individual contact (ie, telephone, cellular telephone, home telephone, e-mail, text messaging address). For organizational contacts (eg, blood bag supplier, delivery services, electrical utility provider), facilities should obtain alternate direct ("back door") contact information in order to bypass standard voice answering systems during an emergency. Consideration should also be given to collecting key contact information for individuals during nonbusiness hours (eg, night or weekend shift contacts).

Human resources staff and legal counsel should be consulted to ensure that they support the collection of staff contact information. In some cases, the staff may resist providing such personal contact information.

CHAIN OF COMMAND. Leadership is critical for maintaining control and direction during a disaster. Organizations should clearly define and communicate to all personnel and external partners who will be (or who are) in charge of a given event.[4(pp27-28)] In addition to a primary authority, clearly defined lines of decision-making authority, delegation, and communication should be established among the leadership team and employees. First-responder organizations (eg, fire) use a process known as the ICS to provide for a coordinated response with a clear chain of command. Facilities should review their respective ICS plans periodically to ensure they are up to date.[28]

STRATEGIES FOR COMMUNICATION REDUNDANCY AND COMPATIBILITY. Perhaps the most critical challenge that organizations face during real or simulated disasters is the ability (or inability) to communicate using routine methods. These methods quickly become overloaded or jammed, requiring organizations to use alternate communication channels. It is vital to identify and test these redundant communication channels before a disaster because significant delays can occur in switching to alternate methods during an event, resulting in the potential loss of life and property.

No single method is used by organizations to design communications redundancy. Local and state jurisdictions vary greatly in their use of emergency communications equipment (eg, radios used by fire and police) as well as the local telecommunications infrastructure and capacity (eg, cell sites). Organizations should acquire multiple redundancies and should list them in order of importance and use during an emergency.[4(pp31-32)] The following are common communication redundancy options to consider:

- **Land-Line Telephones.** Traditional land-based telephones, typically the first option in an ECP, are vulnerable to becoming jammed or inoperable during an emergency. To bypass congestion on the telephone lines, critical health entities such as blood centers and hospitals should consider participating in the Government Emergency Telecommunications Service (GETS). This federally funded program provides emergency access and priority processing in local and long distance networks during an emergency.[29]
- **Wireless Telephones.** Experience during major disasters has shown that cellular networks have a limited capacity for calls and quickly become overloaded during an emergency. Facilities should consider participating in the Wireless Priority Service (WPS) program. Similar to GETS, this federally funded program provides priority access to cellular network calling queues.[29]
- **Satellite Telephones.** Satellite telephones do not rely on land-based or wireless networks. Typically they connect directly to a satellite network. The major drawback of satellite communication is that the handset antenna must have a clear "view" of the sky and cannot be used in buildings (although externally mounted antennas can circumvent this issue).
- **VOIP Telephones.** Voice-over-Internet protocol (VOIP) technologies have replaced many analog or "traditional telephone" systems used by organizations and households. VOIP technology transmits voice as data (packet files) over the Internet or a local area network (LAN) and offers users a greater flexibility in services (eg, forwarding calls to a VOIP handset). However, there are disadvantages in using VOIP systems during an emergency because they rely on ac-

cess to a computer network (eg, Internet) and electrical power at the user's location. Organizations should carefully trace and test their VOIP networks to ensure that adequate redundancies are in place for the equipment to function during an emergency (eg, sufficient battery backup).

- **Facsimile.** Fax machines are still widely used in laboratory settings and provide a quick way to disseminate information to large groups of people (assuming that both the sender and receiver have electrical power and access to telecommunications). One hidden benefit of fax machines that rely on traditional analog signals (ie, not digital or VOIP) is that analog-based fax machines can often be used as an alternate method for voice communications if the machines are not connected to the main telephone system. If the main system loses power, the analog function on the fax machine may still be accessible.
- **E-mail.** E-mail can be an effective way to communicate with large groups of people provided there is electrical power and Internet access. As an additional method of redundancy, organizations should consider having essential personnel maintain e-mail addresses on nationally hosted services (eg, Yahoo, Google, and so forth). Alternate e-mail addresses can be used if an organization's main e-mail system becomes inoperable (eg, personnel can still gain access to e-mail if they have a computer and access to the Internet).
- **Text Messaging.** Short messaging service is a standard feature on most cell phones and has been used during major emergencies when land-based and wireless telecommunications are overloaded or inoperable. Because text messages are relatively small and contain only a few bytes of data, such messages can often be delivered even if networks are busy or overwhelmed.[30]
- **Social Media.** Social media networks such as Facebook and Twitter have grown significantly in the past few years and many hospitals and blood centers use these platforms to regularly communicate with donors and the public. Although these networks would not necessarily be useful as a primary emergency communication channel, they should be considered by the public relations departments of facilities as a way to keep the public and donors informed about an event (eg, to prevent donor surge or inform about facilities reopening after a hurricane).
- **Amateur Radio.** Amateur, or "ham," radio systems and protocols have been used to support emergency communication during major disasters and emergencies. Many possible configurations can be considered when using amateur radio systems (eg, working with local ham clubs or having trained personnel on site). Facilities should contact local amateur radio operators and discuss the structure for emergency communication.[31-34]
- **Two-Way Radio.** Two-way radios are typically used by first-responder organizations (eg, fire and police) when responding to emergencies. Blood centers and hospitals should contact their local EMAs and request access to these networks during an emergency (eg, obtain handsets and receive training on system and emergency communication protocols).
- **Websites.** Websites can be used to convey or collect information from both internal and external groups (assuming users have electrical power and Internet access). In addition to the organization's main website, facilities should consider having a private website that is hosted in another city or state and that can be accessed by personnel when the main site is down. This site can be used by staff to "check in" and receive information if the main facility has been damaged or destroyed.
- **Word of Mouth.** When technology-based communication systems fail, organizations should have a procedure for relaying information by word of mouth both internally and externally. For instance, if a blood supplier is unable to contact hospital customers during or after an event, the supplier should have a set process for sending personnel to establish and maintain contact with the affected facilities (eg, sending

blood delivery drivers to check with each facility for blood needs).

- **Local Media Outlets.** Local media outlets (eg, radio and television) can be used to convey general messages on the status of a facility or to relay specific instructions to staff, donors, and the public. For instance, a local radio station can broadcast a message indicating that a blood center or hospital is closed but that "essential personnel" should report for work.

COMMUNICATION WITH LOCAL, STATE, AND NATIONAL EMERGENCY RESPONSE AGENCIES. In addition to communicating with routine suppliers and vendors, facilities should establish and maintain relationships with local, tribal, state, and national emergency response organizations as shown in Fig 4-2 (see also section on working with EMAs, later, and Appendix 4-1). In particular, blood collection and transfusion facilities should identify those agencies that can assist with obtaining 1) transportation support for components and staff, 2) power restoration, 3) fuel for backup generators (diesel), 4) fuel for fleet and essential staff vehicles, 5) communication support, 6) security if staff or property is threatened, and 7) other utilities support (telecommunications, Internet). Facilities should educate these agencies on how the blood supply operates both locally and nationally (eg, "just-in-time" delivery methods and the need to deliver blood from regional blood centers to hospitals) and should request that the facility be deemed a "critical health entity" or "critical infrastructure entity" in the emergency response structure.[35]

In most cases, the transfusion service obtains access to these organizations through the main hospital disaster response administration and may not need to contact them directly. In such cases, the transfusion service should establish and maintain relationships with the proper internal disaster preparedness and response personnel and should educate them about how the local blood supply functions (eg, blood supplies must be delivered from a blood center; the blood supplies need local storage and blood crossmatching).

National assistance during disasters (eg, coordination of national media messages and resupply of blood components to the affected facilities) is provided through the AABB Disaster Task Force in coordination with other national and federal organizations. Along with

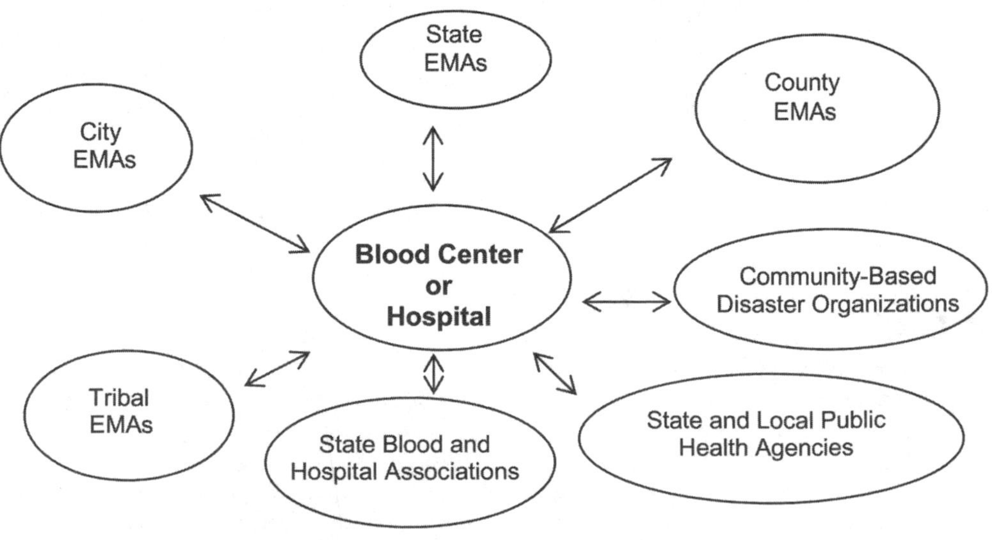

FIGURE 4-2. Communication with external agencies. EMAs = emergency management agencies.

local planning efforts, blood collection and transfusion facilities are encouraged to integrate the task force response system into their disaster plans. The response system is described in the AABB *Disaster Operations Handbook* on the AABB website.[1]

WORKING WITH PUBLIC MEDIA. Creating and disseminating a clear and consistent message about the status of the local and national blood supply is a critical component of an ECP. Historically, most events require relatively few units of blood for transfusions related to the disaster; however, the public's response to disasters has traditionally resulted in an increase in blood donations regardless of the true medical need for transfusions.[11-14] An unexpected surge in blood donations can negatively impact the local blood supply by straining resources needed to collect, test, manufacture, and store blood, as well as by creating a temporary oversupply of blood that tends to be followed by a decline in donations in subsequent months.

Preventing the effect of unnecessary donor surge or requesting specific individuals to donate (eg, group O red cell or platelet donors) can be accomplished by working with public media outlets to effectively convey messages about the status of the blood supply following a disaster. The AABB Disaster Task Force has developed media-related resources for facilities to use, including boilerplate press releases that are contained in the AABB *Disaster Operations Handbook*.[1] The following issues should be considered when working with public media organizations:

- **Trained Media Spokesperson(s).** Speaking with reporters or giving interviews can be tricky and may result in a "crisis within a crisis" if not handled properly. Only individuals who have received prior media training in risk and emergency communication should be allowed to speak with the members of the media. Specific steps should be taken before, during, and after an interview.[36] For instance, written background information should be provided to a reporter before the interview, and a spokesperson should focus the most salient points of the message into "sound bites" that can be quoted in a story. Another technique that can be used successfully when communicating with the media is message mapping.[37] Message maps assist communicators in the development and synthesis of complex information by focusing on three key messages delivered in three short sentences with a total of 27 words. This process accommodates both broadcast and print media. Most important, a spokesperson should never speak "off the record" with a reporter. Many other tips and techniques can be used to ensure that the correct messages are conveyed. One resource for such tips is the Northwest Center for Public Health Practice in collaboration with Public Health—Seattle and King County.[38]
- **Maintenance of Relationships with Media Contacts.** If one is to reduce the chance of miscommunication, it is critical to develop and maintain ongoing relationships with media contacts. Further, it is important to educate these contacts about blood and blood components, especially as they relate to emergencies.
- **Preprepared Press Materials.** The organization should consider drafting as many template press materials as possible ahead of time. These materials should include brief biographical sketches, fact sheets, and potential scenarios (eg, no need for blood to support the disaster, specific blood component/type donations needed, etc).
- **Local News vs National Headlines.** It is important to remember that most of the local news stations are connected to national news outlets and that local messages may affect other organizations across the country. For instance, a tragic disaster (with little or no blood-related needs) may be "picked up" on national news networks or services, thereby prompting an outpouring of support from individuals in other states, including blood donors. To prevent unnecessary donor surge (or to recruit donors), the AABB Disaster Task Force urges facilities to coordinate their local messages with the task force (see *Disaster Operations Hand-*

book[1] for contact information), which should ensure that the blood community, donors, and the public receive clear and consistent messages regarding the status of the blood supply.

Logistics

During the formulation of a COOP, facility planners must place heavy emphasis on the management of daily operations that includes making available the supplies and equipment required to perform essential functions related to 1) the recruitment of donors, 2) collecting the donated blood, 3) manufacturing and testing blood components, and 4) delivering the components to the hospital for transfusion to the patient. During a disaster or terrorist incident the normal logistical systems may not be present or capable of providing the necessary support. Key areas for consideration are transportation, "just-in-time" systems, storage, contracts, and biohazard issues.

TRANSPORTATION. Past disaster and terrorist events, as well as experience with National Special Security Events such as the presidential inauguration and international political summits, have clearly demonstrated the vulnerability of transportation systems. Blood centers should coordinate with their local EMAs to ensure that vehicles engaged in collecting or distributing blood are duly authorized as emergency support vehicles and are granted the appropriate clearances to operate on the roads. Additionally, memoranda of understanding, agreements or statements of understanding, or agreements should be established with the appropriate EMAs regarding access to the roads and use of law enforcement, National Guard and state militia personnel, or vehicles to deliver blood. Under the provisions of the NRF, the DHHS can request the Department of Transportation (DOT) to assist with the movement of blood by air, rail, water, and motor vehicle.[6] Such requests should be directed to the AABB Disaster Task Force.[1]

"JUST-IN-TIME" SYSTEMS. Many blood centers and hospitals have adopted just-in-time supply systems in an effort to minimize expenses associated with the storage of large quantities of supplies, materials, the maintenance of storage facilities, and staff. Blood centers and hospitals should determine the critical items required for their business operations, the associated resupply capability of the vendor (including manufacturing schedule and transport timelines), the shelf life of the supply item, and any storage requirements (special environmental factors).

STORAGE. Planners should consider the storage capacity of their customers and any local storage companies that may be suitable for an emergency storage site. Contingency contracts or contingency clauses to existing contracts with customers and ice and dry-ice suppliers should be considered. Temporary storage space may be provided by the use of commercial containers, including validated refrigerated containers, that could be placed at the blood center, depending on space and electric power. Additionally, some commercial containers have their own generators. The local EMA may permit storage of consumables at municipal disaster supply facilities at no cost.

CONTRACTS. All vendor contracts should include wording that identifies the process for emergency delivery of supplies, equipment, and services. Vendors and suppliers should provide their key disaster or emergency contacts, including phone numbers (office, cell, and home), e-mail addresses, and fax numbers. The vendor or supplier should have a disaster plan that demonstrates the ability to meet a facility's supply requirement in the event of a disaster, terrorist incident, or pandemic influenza outbreak. It is advisable to include a disaster plan requirement in all vendor contracts. Another consideration is the development of contracts containing noncompete agreements with local competitor organizations in the event of disasters.

BIOHAZARDS. In the aftermath of a disaster or terrorist incident, the disposal of biohazardous material may become a serious problem for a blood center or hospital. Planners should incorporate appropriate language in their biohazard material disposal contracts that will ensure that the vendor establishes a contingency plan to meet the facility's requirements. The blood center and hospital should coordinate with the EMA and the fire or safety agencies and should provide information on the types of biohazardous wastes that are generated by the facility. Organizations that have irradiators should provide local fire or safety agencies with a detailed building plan that includes photographs of the ingress routes to the device, photographs of the device, and the manufacturer's specifications and contact information. Affected facilities should contact the AABB Disaster Task Force[1] if the local and state EMA authorities cannot provide assistance.

Utilities

Blood centers and hospitals rely on the provision of utility services (electricity, water, fuel, sewage disposal, telecommunications, and access to the Internet) from a variety of sources, such as municipalities or public or privately owned companies. The lack of one or more of these services can severely affect the business operations of a facility. Planners should establish contingency support plans with their service providers. These plans should include emergency points of contact at the utility service provider, with their telephone numbers and e-mail addresses. Most utility services have priority lists for service restoration during emergencies. Planners should solicit the support of the local EMA and hospitals to ensure that their organization will receive designation for priority restoration of services. This should be done during the planning process and not during or after an emergency. The following actions may mitigate the effect of lost service.[1]

ELECTRICITY. It is important to install and conduct tests of an auxiliary generator for the blood center or hospital. Each generator should be able to provide power to heating, ventilation, and air conditioning (HVAC) systems and other critical equipment. Consideration should be given to the use of uninterruptable power sources for critical systems (computers). Facilities should have OSHA-approved emergency lighting systems, flashlights, and batteries for staff use. In September 2006, The Joint Commission recommended in a *Sentinel Event Alert* that health-care institutions routinely review their emergency power systems. The alert also established steps that should be taken by institutions to ensure that they have adequate power for patients and critical systems.[39]

WATER AND HYGIENE. Water is essential for staff health and may be required for refrigeration equipment, manufacturing, and testing procedures. Planners should establish an emergency supply of drinking water and water for hand washing on the basis of the number of staff members, volunteers, and donors that a facility may have. A stock rotation plan should be based on the expiration date of all bottled water. Use of alcohol-based sanitizers will reduce the amount of water required to support personal hygiene. Loss of access to municipal water may have a negative impact on the facility's HVAC and on the use of restrooms. Plans should be established for movement of blood components and test tubes to alternate manufacturing and testing sites in the event that the municipal water supply is not available.

FUEL (ALL TYPES). All fixed-site facilities should have an adequate on-site fuel storage capacity for all auxiliary generators, fuel-based heating plants, and vehicles on the basis of consumption rates, vendor resupply capabilities, and their COOP. The blood center or hospital should take appropriate action to ensure that all storage tanks are full (only approved gasoline and diesel fuel containers and heating fuel tanks should be used) when advance warning of an impending natural disaster or an increase in the HSAS threat level occurs. Additionally, planners should ensure that the blood center or hospital is placed on the vendor's priority service list, that an automatic emergency resupply delivery of the fuel is established according to the facility's on-site storage capacity, and that the vendor's emergency contact data are provided. Planners should coordinate with the EMA to gain access to the necessary fuels if shortage prevents the supplier from delivering necessary fuel products in support of the essential staff and fleet vehicles.

SEWAGE. Loss of the sewage disposal system can produce major health issues for the staff, volunteers, and donors. The use of portable or temporary restrooms may provide an immediate solution to the lack of service but may not be available if the facility does not have a contingency contract with a vendor. Organizations can use small waste disposal systems that are available at sporting goods, camping, and recreational vehicle supply stores and marine supply stores. Use of portable or temporary restrooms or camping disposal systems requires the provision of hand sanitation systems, considerations for privacy, and a waste removal system or contractor.

TELECOMMUNICATIONS. Loss of an organization's telephone system will severely affect its ability to conduct business operations. The ability to contact staff, volunteers, donors, vendors, local EMAs, and hospitals is a critical function to which planners must devote extensive planning. Blood centers and hospitals should review the federal Telecommunications Priority Service (TPS) program and the capability it provides. TPS offers priority provisioning and restoration of national security and emergency preparedness (NS/EP) telecommunications services. NS/EP telecommunications services are those services critical to the maintenance of a state of readiness or the response to and management of an event or crisis that causes or could cause harm to the population, damage property, or threaten the security of the United States.[29] (See the "Emergency Communications Plan" section for more information.)

INFORMATION TECHNOLOGY SYSTEMS. Facilities use a vast array of computer-based IT systems to conduct their daily business operations. Many of these systems rely on complex communications networks and often route data and voice communications through the Internet. Planners should analyze these systems and determine the effect on business applications during periods when the networks are interrupted or destroyed. Contingency planning for IT systems is especially critical for blood collection and transfusion facilities because many of these systems are regulated and contain critical information about the donors, the components they have donated, and where the components have been stored and distributed.

Alternative data centers, file backups, offsite storage procedures, and possible outsourcing options should be established. If the blood center or hospital outsources the storage of vital records and files (eg, emergency operating records, legal and financial records), consideration should be given to the proximity of the outsourced records to the facility and ease of access to the records and files. Facilities should be familiar with the outsourcing vendor's contingency plans (whether the vendor has more than one site, 24/7 access, and emergency power). If a facility's staff maintains files locally on computers, steps should be initiated to move files to shared drives and portable hard drives to maintain backup copies of vital records and files on the servers. In some situations, the organization may have to revert to manual procedures until normal operations are reestablished. FEMA's *Continuity Guidance Circular 1* provides a template for ensuring access to critical information and systems.[18] Further, organizations should continually review and amend their IT department policies and procedures to protect critical IT systems and to reduce cyber-attacks.[40]

Staffing

Blood centers and hospitals depend on their highly trained, competent, and motivated staff and volunteers to be successful in their mission of recruiting blood donors and collecting, manufacturing, testing, and distributing blood components. Management should involve staff and volunteers in all aspects of the emergency planning process. Management should promote preparedness to staff and volunteers and should encourage them to complete family preparedness plans.[4,17,35]

ESSENTIAL PERSONNEL. During the emergency planning process, the management team should identify those staff members and volunteers (if applicable) who are responsible for essential functions that provide the vital services required to maintain business operations. Each department should develop a "smart book" that details its essential functions, its essential personnel who accomplish them, its vital information and records, its contract information, and its customer information. Employees who are deemed essential because of their assigned responsibilities should receive extensive training in the facility's emergency plans and should participate in disaster training exercises in order to refine operational procedures under emergency conditions. Consideration should be given to establishing alternate work sites and/or implementing telework programs to mitigate the effects that the loss of the blood center or hospital may have on operations. The human resources department should work with management to ensure that employee-training plans provide for the succession of personnel into those positions held by designated essential personnel should the incumbent become unavailable. Management should also plan for housing, feeding, and providing fuel to essential personnel to help them get to and from work when the local infrastructure is not operational.[18]

FAMILY SUPPORT PLANS. Management should help staff and volunteers develop family support plans.[35] These plans should include the building of a home disaster kit, establishment of a safe room for the family to gather during an emergency, an evacuation plan and assembly point outside the home, an out-of-area contact person (family member or friend) to whom family members can provide their personal status, and assurance that children's schools have an emergency plan for sheltering the children and procedures for releasing children to a designated representative.[41] The plans should ensure that all pets are included.[42-44]

CROSS-FUNCTIONAL TRAINING. Planners, in close coordination with the human resources department and, if applicable, any collective bargaining units, should develop a cross-functional training program that identifies personnel whose duties are not in support of the facility's essential functions during a response to a disaster. These duties should then be reassigned to staff members whose duties are within the essential functions. These reassigned personnel may perform as drivers, public affairs representatives, recruiters, and other nonregulatory staff. Human resources and management should develop the necessary modifications to the affected employee or volunteer job descriptions, develop training plans, and conduct initial and refresher training as required. Management may need to negotiate with labor unions to modify any existing contracts.

HUMAN RESOURCES ISSUES. Of importance to employees—beyond the safety of loved ones and provisions of food and shelter—will be issues such as salary continuation, flexible work schedules, implementation of telework procedures, and benefits.[4,18] For many organizations, decisions on such issues became paramount following Hurricane Katrina, when thousands of people were displaced or relocated from the affected area. Because these issues are influenced by many factors, having a predeveloped decision matrix can be particularly helpful during times of crisis.

SHELTER-IN-PLACE ORDERS. During a disaster, industrial accident, or terrorist-related event, the local EMA may issue a shelter-in-place order to mitigate the effect of an event on people. Management should establish areas within their facilities where staff, volunteers, and donors can congregate for the duration of the event. Planners can consult with the local EMA to determine what supplies may be needed (such as water, food, first aid kits, blankets, cots, flashlights, plastic sheeting, duct tape, crank- or battery-powered radios, and spare batteries). Guidelines for supplies for emergency shelter operations can also be found on the FEMA website.[45] Quantities of shelter-in-place supplies will depend on the risk assessment findings. Management should ensure that all staff and volunteers are cognizant of their roles and responsibilities if a shelter-in-place order is issued.[18,46,47]

EMPLOYEE ASSISTANCE (MENTAL HEALTH). It is not unusual during times of heightened threat or in the aftermath of a disaster or terrorist-related incident for staff and volunteers to exhibit physical manifestations or other signs of stress, or loss of work productivity. Management should establish procedures for monitoring the workplace environment in an effort to identify such situations early and to initiate programs such as employee counseling and similar actions. Some organizations have an employee assistance program that provides services at no expense to the staff and volunteers. Management should review all health-care programs to determine if the employees are covered for external professional assistance. Facilities may contact the local EMA and public health officials to gain access to local or state-sponsored programs. Additional assistance may be available through professional associations.[48-50]

Key to minimizing tensions is the development of crisis communications that are directed solely to the staff, volunteers, and their family members and that provide information on actions to be taken in response to the threat or the event. In addition, people who have experienced a disaster may have special recovery needs.[17]

WORKING WITH EMERGENCY MANAGEMENT AGENCIES

Most incidents are managed locally.[9] The blood center or hospital management team should establish a good working relationship with the EMA that is responsible for disaster and terrorist response operations in its city or town.[5] In many instances, the blood center or hospital will have a working relationship with the local public health department and the hospital association, and this can be used to introduce the blood center or hospital management team to the EMA management team. Management should provide informational briefings to members of the EMA and the public health department about the mission of the organization, the scope of its operations, and the effect on local health-care facilities if the blood center or hospital is not operational.

Management should also become familiar with the NIMS and NRF documents and should consider enrolling in FEMA online educational courses[28] or disaster training courses provided by the state and local community. Management should request that the EMA provide informational briefings to key staff of the blood center or hospital. During the exchange with the EMA, management should discuss resource issues (transportation assistance, fuel support, storage, security, inclusion in EMA notification systems, and assignment of a blood center or hospital liaison in the EMA). Management should invite the EMA to participate in its organization's disaster exercises and should actively encourage the EMA to include the blood center or hospital in its exercise programs.

Communications Links with EMAs

Blood centers and hospitals should coordinate with the local EMA for inclusion in local emergency communications systems. These systems may include established video teleconference or conference calls, blast facsimile networks, EMA mailgroups, and 800-MHz radio networks. Further, blood centers should seek admission to any priority networks established by the local hospitals to improve communications during an incident.

EMA Command Center

The EMA will normally establish an emergency command center that may be referred to as an emergency operations center (EOC) or similar title. The EOC will be structured along the five major functional areas as found in the ICS: command, operations, planning, logistics, and finance and accounting. The EOC staff will include representatives from the jurisdiction's police, fire, utilities, public affairs, public health, education, and ambulance departments and the office of the senior elected official; liaisons from the county and state may be present as well as local nongovernmental agencies that support disaster response. The EOC will operate on a 24/7 basis and will monitor its jurisdiction for potential disasters or terrorist-related incidents. The EOC will conduct training exercises to ensure that disaster response agencies are trained, that standard operating procedures are effective, that interoperability of communications is verified, and that contingency plans can be executed.[9]

Incident Command System

The ICS resulted from the obvious need for a new approach to the problem of managing rapidly moving wildfires in the early 1970s. At that time, emergency managers faced a number of problems, such as the following:

- Too many people reporting to one supervisor.
- Different emergency response organizational structures.
- Lack of reliable incident information.
- Inadequate and incompatible communications.
- Lack of a structure for coordinated planning between agencies.
- Unclear lines of authority.
- Terminology differences between agencies.
- Unclear or unspecified incident objectives.

Designing a standardized emergency management system to remedy such problems took several years and extensive field testing. The ICS was developed by an interagency task force working in a cooperative local, state, and federal interagency effort called FIRESCOPE (Firefighting Resources of California Organized for Potential Emergencies). Early in the development process, four essential requirements became clear, as follows:

1. The system must be organizationally flexible to meet the needs of incidents of any kind and size.
2. Agencies must be able to use the system on a day-to-day basis for routine situations as well as for major emergencies.
3. The system must be sufficiently standard to allow personnel from a variety of agencies and diverse geographic locations to rapidly meld into a common management structure.
4. The system must be cost effective.

Initial ICS applications were designed for responding to disastrous wildfires. It is interesting to note that characteristics of these wildfire incidents are similar to those seen in many other kinds of situations involving law enforcement and hazardous materials (see http://www.nimsonline.com). For example, wildfires have the following characteristics:

- They can occur with no advance notice.
- They develop rapidly.
- Unchecked, they may grow in size or complexity.
- Personal risk for response personnel can be high.
- Several agencies often have some on-scene responsibility.
- They can very easily become multijurisdictional.
- They often have high public and media visibility.
- Risk of life and property loss can be high.
- Cost of response is always a major consideration.

The NIMS mandated the adoption of the ICS to facilitate the domestic incident command and management operations by the federal agencies. The NIMS also required that field command and management functions be performed in accordance with a standard set of ICS organizations, doctrine, and procedures.[9]

In October 2005, the US Secretary of Homeland Security informed the nation's governors that Homeland Security Presidential Directive No. 5 (HSPD-5), titled "Management of Domestic Incidents," required that "all federal preparedness assistance funding for states, territories, local jurisdictions, and tribal entities be dependent on NIMS compliance."[51] The Secretary's letter placed added emphasis on the importance of the ability of the United States to manage domestic incidents through a single NIMS.[9,52]

Participating with EMAs in Disaster Drills

The National Strategy for Homeland Security directed the establishment of a national exercise strategy. HSPD-8 directed the DHS to establish a "National Exercise Program" (NEP).[52] DHS charged the Grants and Training Division to develop a program that identifies and integrates national-level exercise activities and that will ensure those activities serve the broadest community of learning.

In addition to full-scale, integrated, national-level exercises, the NEP provides for tailored exercise activities that serve as the primary DHS vehicle for training national leaders and staff. The NEP enhances the collaboration among partners at all levels of government for assigned homeland security missions. National-level exercises provide the means to conduct "full-scale, full-system tests" of collective preparedness, inter-operability, and collaboration across all levels of government and the private sector.[52] The program also incorporates elements to allow identification of implications of changes to homeland security strategies, plans, technologies, policies, and procedures.[52]

Blood centers and hospitals should seek inclusion in disaster drills or exercises by contacting their local EMAs. Participation in local, state, and federal exercises will increase a facility's preparedness and will increase awareness by the emergency preparedness officials at all levels about the critical role that the blood community plays in providing the blood components required by victims of a disaster or terrorist-related incident and about the resources that are required to do so.

REGULATORY CONSIDERATIONS IN EMERGENCIES

The blood community is highly regulated, and even slight changes to processes and procedures can have far-reaching effects for facilities and patients, especially during an emergency. Blood collection and transfusion facilities should carefully consider the regulatory issues within their disaster management plans.

Federal Agencies Involved

The blood community is regulated by numerous agencies. The Center for Biologics Evaluation and Research (CBER) of the Food and Drug Administration (FDA) has the primary responsibility to ensure the safety and efficacy of all biologic products, which includes blood and blood components. The Center for Devices and Radiological Health (CDRH), another arm of the FDA, regulates medical devices and radiation-emitting devices. Although the FDA is responsible for the safety of blood components and medical devices, the DOT regulates the movement of cargo, including blood, blood components, and progenitor cells through the transportation network. OSHA ensures the safety of the US workforce. Likewise, the mission of the Environmental Protection Agency (EPA) is to protect human health and the environment. The Centers for Medicare and Medicaid Services (CMS) under the Clinical Laboratory Improvement Amendments (CLIA '88) have oversight of patient testing that occurs at blood centers, hospital blood banks, and transfusion services. Consideration must be given to the regulations and requirements of each of these agencies when developing emergency response plans. Such regulatory considerations generally fall into three categories: effect on available blood components, effect on donors, and potential consequences on operations.

Effects on Components in Available Inventory

All blood centers and hospitals must have written procedures to follow in the event of an emergency. These procedures should address the provisions for emergency power and continuous temperature monitoring during storage and should document the temperature at least every 4 hours. Should the allowable storage conditions be exceeded, temperature extremes (either high or low) should be identified as well as any other effects, such as exposure to smoke or water.[53] Consideration should also be given to nontraditional emergencies that may affect blood, such as a radiologic event or exposure to a biologic or chemical agent.[54,55] Components potentially exposed in an event should be quarantined, and a determination of component suitability should be made. When the quality, safety, purity, or potency of a component is in question, CBER should be consulted. An exception or variance may be needed to use components in certain situations. Additionally, the AABB Disaster Task Force is available to assist facilities with questions about a component's safety, purity, or potency during a disaster.

All blood released for use during a disaster should be fully tested, including testing for infectious diseases. An exception to full testing would be made in the event that all blood supplies are exhausted, that resupply is not possible, and that blood is needed immediately to save lives. Blood testing samples should be retained for retrospective testing after a disaster. Thorough documentation of the circumstances is essential, and physicians should be notified as to what tests have been completed on the blood.[21]

In very extreme circumstances, the FDA may issue emergency guidance to help ensure an adequate blood supply. For example, on September 11, 2001, the FDA issued "Policy Statement on Urgent Collection, Shipment, and Use of Whole Blood and Blood Components Intended for Transfusion to Address Blood Supply Needs in the Current Disaster Situation."[57] Blood collection facilities should closely follow all developments regarding donor deferrals and all emergency FDA guidance during times of disaster.

Effects on Donors

Disasters can affect donor eligibility, particularly emergencies involving any potential infectious diseases or hazardous chemicals. Agents should be evaluated for 1) transmissibility through blood transfusion, 2) potential to harm recipients, and 3) potential for any asymptomatic period after exposure and before or after the actual disease period when the donor may be infectious. If an agent is determined to be transmissible, a deferral period that ensures an adequate period of safety from infectivity or adverse effect must be identified, and donors must be deferred appropriately. As with component suitability, CBER and national blood organizations should be consulted for potential donor deferral issues.

Potential Consequences on Operations

Emergencies involving power outages, floods, or structural damage to facilities will disrupt normal operations. Disasters that do not directly affect the blood center or hospital physical infrastructure can still disrupt operations. For example, a pandemic influenza outbreak may cause severe staffing shortages with up to 40% absenteeism.[15] Collections should be performed only by facilities that routinely collect blood. Facilities that collect only autologous blood should not attempt to collect allogeneic blood during a disaster.

Adequate staffing can be an issue immediately before and after an emergency while staff members tend to their families and personal needs. Only staff trained in regulated functions should be used. Volunteers can be used to perform nonregulated functions such as predonation education and maintenance of the canteen. Likewise, appropriate licensure is required to safely operate fleet vehicles. Emergency plans can include maintaining a list of staff trained in multiple functions. For example, staff members who have transferred from one area to another (who have maintained competency in the prior area) could be used in the previous function with appropriate certification and any necessary commercial vehicle licenses.[58] Key to any and all decisions made during disasters should be the safety and well-being of facility staff.

Equipment and supplies should also be assessed for exposure to water, humidity, and temperature extremes. CDRH has published an information guide about the effect of disasters on medical devices; it can be useful in planning as well as responding to disasters.[59]

Records Management

Vital records must be secured and maintained. These documents include records of donors, donations, manufacturing, testing, quality assurance, and disposition. If these records are damaged or lost during a disaster, blood in inventory at that time may require quarantine and recall. Efforts should be made to retrieve and preserve any damaged records. CBER should be consulted to determine disposition of inventory when records are lost.

TESTING THE DISASTER PLAN

Continual improvement of a disaster plan is critical for maintaining a high state of readiness for future emergencies, and participation in disaster drills is one way to achieve this goal. By simulating the conditions of a real disaster, a facility can identify and correct deficiencies and gaps in the disaster plan.

Internal vs External Disaster Drills

Drills can be conducted internally (eg, fire drill, hazardous spill cleanup) or in conjunction with other organizations. Multiple-organization disaster drills are typically conducted by local or state emergency management agencies. Unfortunately, blood-related issues are often overlooked in the exercise scenarios that are developed by these agencies because many of the planners are unaware of how blood is collected, stored, and distributed to hospitals. Blood collection and transfusion facilities must educate these emergency managers about how the blood system operates specifically as it relates to the just-in-time delivery methods that are used to transport units from a regional blood center to a hospital. Further, facilities should consider becoming routinely involved with emergency management agencies by participating in regular meetings and events.

Types of Disaster Drills and Training

Disaster drills range from informal discussions about improving response methods, to full-scale, real-time exercises that involve hundreds of organizations. Each method can be used by a single organization or in conjunction with multiple organizations. When an organization participates in drills with other organizations (ie, full-scale exercise), it is important for blood collection and transfusion facilities to "inject" blood-related scenarios into the drill during the planning stages. For example, drills should include 1) the need to transport blood from a blood center to a hospital (or hospitals) to treat victims when local roads have been damaged or destroyed or 2) the effect of an unknown biologic agent release on the local blood supply, the donors (ie, deferral of donors), or both. The basic types of drills are categorized below.[28,60]

- **Orientation and Education Sessions.** Orientation and education sessions are regularly scheduled meetings to discuss the roles and responsibilities of personnel as well as the policies and procedures to be used during an emergency. Such sessions are generally focused on training, on identifying needs and concerns related to the existing disaster plan, or both.
- **Tabletop Exercises.** Participants typically meet in a conference room setting and discuss their organizational responsibilities in responding to a given scenario (eg, HAZMAT spill, earthquake). Tabletop exercises are a cost-effective way to quickly identify areas of overlap or confusion and to resolve issues of coordination and responsibility.
- **Walk-Through Drills.** Participants should actually perform their emergency duties for a given disaster scenario in order to identify specific issues that need to be addressed in the disaster plan. For instance, the disaster response plan may call for essential personnel to set up a command post in a conference room; upon conducting a walk-through drill, staff members might discover that there are not enough electrical outlets or network ports for computers and phones.

- **Functional Drills.** Functional drills test a specific functional area (eg, communication procedures and equipment) and take place in real time in order to put stress on the system being tested. Participants then evaluate, identify, and resolve problem areas.
- **Evacuation Drills.** Participants perform evacuation procedures and trace evacuation routes in order to identify hazards (eg, cluttered stairways, blocked exits) that may prevent personnel from quickly exiting and meeting in a designated area where all personnel can be fully accounted for. Participants note areas for improvement, and modifications are made to the evacuation plan.
- **Full-Scale Exercises.** A potential emergency (eg, fire, earthquake, terrorism) is simulated in real time to test multiple systems and their related organizations for a coordinated response. Full-scale exercises are typically sponsored by local, state, or national emergency management agencies and may range in length from hours to days. Significant preplanning and postevaluation efforts are conducted to derive significant learning points and corrective actions.

After-Action Review

Perhaps the most significant aspect of a well-executed drill or real disaster is the after-action review process. During this process, participants evaluate "what worked well" and "what did not work well," with the aim of identifying lessons learned and then implementing corrective actions after the drill or incident to improve future responses.

Continual Quality Improvement

Disaster planning and response are not static processes, and organizations should strive for continuous quality improvement in order to maintain a high state of readiness for the next emergency. This state can be accomplished by regular participation in drills, followed by a well-designed after-action review process. In addition, facilities are encouraged to share the significant learning points from drills or real disasters with AABB so that they can benefit the entire blood community.

SUMMARY OF LESSONS LEARNED FROM RECENT DISASTERS

Blood collection facilities and hospitals around the world have dealt with significant disasters in recent years. Hurricanes, tsunamis, earthquakes, fires, industrial accidents, and terrorism have tested emergency response systems, and organizations have used the learning points from these events to further sharpen their disaster plans. Many of these lessons are integrated within this chapter and can be found in the AABB *Disaster Operations Handbook.*[1] Table 4-3 summarizes learning points from events in the past few years.

Blood collection and transfusion facilities are encouraged to share the major learning points from real or simulated disasters that they have experienced. AABB has taken on the task of collecting such lessons and sharing them with facilities around the world through articles, education sessions, and the AABB *Disaster Operations Handbook.*[1] Facilities with information to share should contact the AABB through the AABB National Blood Exchange at 1.800.458.9388 or send an e-mail to nbe@aabb.org.

CONCLUSION

In the wake of disasters such as 1) the September 11, 2001 attacks on the World Trade Center and the Pentagon, 2) the rail transit bombings in Great Britain and Spain, and 3) the devastating natural disasters that occur every year, organizations around the world have focused significant attention and resources in strengthening their disaster plans. Given the heightened awareness of the need for organizations to be prepared, both the public and members of the press are holding organizations to the highest standards of excellence for ensuring that all necessary planning efforts have been made to protect both life and property from known threats. As was witnessed in

TABLE 4-3. Summary of Lessons Learned from Recent Disasters and Events

Event	Lessons Learned
NIH Multiple Events[61] 5/2001 - 11/2004 The NIH Clinical Center Department of Transfusion Medicine experienced several events, including a credible bomb threat, a broken steam pipe, and a partial building collapse. All events required the rapid evacuation and relocation of the facility to an alternate work site.	◆ Develop a full-scale evacuation plan including contingencies for moving staff, patients, components, equipment, and services to predetermined alternate work locations. ◆ Develop a procedure to notify critical partners (nurses, doctors, suppliers) of the alternate work site location. ◆ Keep a doctor and administrative staff nearby for support. ◆ Practice transferring phone lines to alternate locations, and develop redundancies for computer access. ◆ Determine methods to postpone nonurgent transfusions until alternate sites are operational. ◆ Consider irradiating components, when such products are necessary, before evacuation (ie, cannot move irradiators). ◆ Develop communication contingencies for notifying night and weekend staff of the facility status. ◆ Develop a list of critical supplies to relocate to the new work site during the evacuation.
Tropical Storm Allison (Houston)[62] 6/2001 Widespread flooding prompted the complete evacuation of Hermann Memorial Hospital. The blood bank, located in the basement, was completely destroyed along with the entire laboratory. Hundreds of blood components were lost.	◆ Emergency generators were located on the roof, but the mechanical switches for the generators were in the basement and malfunctioned when the basement flooded. ◆ Abrupt loss of emergency power prohibited removing blood and blood storage equipment. ◆ Upon reconstruction of the hospital, the blood bank was moved to the 8th floor (above the potential flooding zone). ◆ Rebuilding the blood bank took 5 weeks.
US World Trade Center and Pentagon Attacks 9/11/2001 In a series of coordinated suicide terrorist attacks, hijackers flew two commercial passenger planes into the World Trade Center and a third plane into the Pentagon; passengers crashed a fourth plane into a field near Shanksville, PA.	◆ Blood centers and hospitals need to quickly determine the true medical need for blood related to the event. ◆ Facilities should not collect blood components in excess of the true medical need. ◆ Only trained personnel who have maintained competency in functional areas (eg, phlebotomy) should be allowed to perform tasks in those areas. ◆ Unnecessary donor surges need to be prevented through clear and consistent messages to the blood community, donors, and the public.
US Northeast Power Outage 8/14/2003 - 8/15/2003 A massive power outage occurred and shut down 21 power plants across several Northeast states.	◆ Establish redundant water sources for critical functions (eg, testing, air conditioning, restrooms). ◆ Establish alternate testing sites and procedures to redirect samples if the main primary testing center has no power. ◆ Establish alternate fuel sources that rely on redundant power sources to pump fuel. ◆ Ensure that the facility is a on the priority list for power and water restoration. ◆ Obtain "back door" numbers for the local power company to determine where service is being restored.

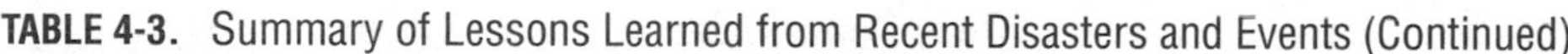

TABLE 4-3. Summary of Lessons Learned from Recent Disasters and Events (Continued)

Event	Lessons Learned
Multiple US Hurricanes Multiple years (2002 - 2007) Several major hurricanes struck the United States and affected blood collection and distribution of components to hospitals.	◆ Blood centers should consider dispersing components to hospitals before a hurricane. ◆ Blood centers should disperse fleet vehicles to prevent damage to all in one location. ◆ Focus on the "cone of uncertainty" rather than the projected path of the hurricane, in case of unexpected turns before landfall. ◆ Have an emergency communications plan for contacting the staff, donors, and the public about the status of the facility. ◆ If the facility is closed, make sure security systems are programmed correctly (ie, doors may be programmed to automatically unlock at preset times). ◆ Test generators regularly, and ensure that the generator is protected from the elements (high wind and horizontal rain). ◆ Ensure that mobile generators and the building have compatible connectors.
London Subway Bombings[63] 7/5/2005 The London transportation network was subjected to a series of terrorist attacks. Many hospitals activated their major incident (MI) plans.	◆ The pathology MI plan must be an integral part of the hospital's MI plan. ◆ The plan should consider: – Early alert of the hospital transfusion laboratory. – Ongoing communication with all key personnel, including communication about stand-down procedures. – Alternative modes (eg, walkie-talkies and runners) if the switchboard, mobile phones, or e-mails fail. ◆ The hospital transfusion laboratory must have dedicated external phone and fax lines to NHSBT offices. ◆ MI policies should include the following: – When and how to place emergency blood orders. – Early communication to the British NBS of the potential need for blood, components, and tissue. – Handling of potential donor inquiries. ◆ Guidance for the management of massive hemorrhage should be incorporated into MI policies; policies should cover surgical and medical control of bleeding. ◆ Blood samples should be taken as early as possible, and care must be taken to label samples correctly; gender must be included, with default to female if unidentified. ◆ Patient MI identification must be compatible with other IT systems, including the blood bank. ◆ Group-specific blood should be issued once the blood group is known and identification is confirmed. ◆ Systems must maintain blood traceability and temperature control in the MI setting. ◆ Policies should cover the organization of the transfusion laboratory staff; staff must have identification to enter restricted areas where needed. ◆ Key personnel must be aware of the NBS antidote service. ◆ Plans must include maintaining essential services and restarting normal services as soon as possible.

(Continued)

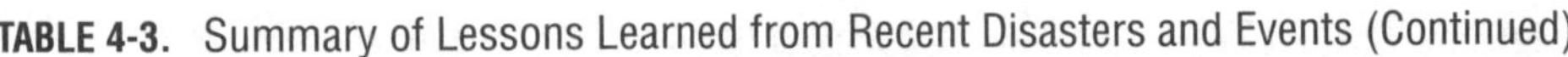

TABLE 4-3. Summary of Lessons Learned from Recent Disasters and Events (Continued)

Event	Lessons Learned
Tsunami (Indian Ocean) 12/26/2004 An earthquake measuring 9.0 on the Richter scale struck off the western coast of northern Sumatra, triggering massive tidal waves from Indonesia to Somalia.	◆ Establish a national disaster plan with routine disaster drills at all levels. ◆ Establish an alternative communication system when regular telephone and mobile phone services are disrupted or inoperable. ◆ Establish a system to contact donors with rare blood types. ◆ Clearly designate the top manager of the blood center to communicate with communities and media about how they can help during and after a crisis. ◆ Include suppliers (especially blood bag and infectious-marker reagent suppliers) as stakeholders for the emergency plan and exercise. ◆ If actual blood needs have been met, ask additional donors to register or schedule a future blood donation. ◆ Establish routine training and disaster drills for a group of volunteers who can come and assist regular staff during an emergency. ◆ Routinely update contact information for all means of transportation for component delivery. ◆ Train administrative staff to perform noncritical technical work and mobilize them to assist technical staff during a disaster. ◆ Establish relationships with transfusion services abroad so that support of specialized components can be sent as quickly as possible.
Fire at Gulf Coast Regional Blood Center[61,64] 2/12/2005 A four-alarm fire at Gulf Coast Regional Blood Center in Houston, TX, destroyed the primary warehouse and caused significant damage in several surrounding departments, including blood collection and distribution. Critical supplies were destroyed as well as several hundred units of blood and platelet components.	◆ Develop a contingency plan for the rapid movement of blood components to alternate storage facilities; consider the need to ice, pack, transport, and track components (eg, sequentially number containers). ◆ Conduct routine fire drills to ensure that staff know what to do and where to safely exit the building. ◆ Senior leadership should emphasize employee and donor safety during and after an event. ◆ Notify quality assurance personnel immediately after a fire to assess systems and procedures needed to restore operations. ◆ Have a procedure to notify appropriate authorities (ie, FDA, FBI) after a fire. ◆ Chronologically document recovery efforts for the FDA. ◆ Consider establishing an off-site communications command center. ◆ Have contingency agreements to replace supplies and to import needed blood components. ◆ Assign a primary spokesperson to work with the news media. ◆ Review insurance coverage and consider the following: ◆ True replacement value of property contents (machinery and equipment). ◆ True value of the building. ◆ Real potential of business interruption. ◆ Value of a good relationship with insurer and validation of disaster plan with insurer.

TABLE 4-3. Summary of Lessons Learned from Recent Disasters and Events (Continued)

Event	Lessons Learned
Fire at Gulf Coast Regional Blood Center[61,64] (Continued)	◆ Have a process to monitor air quality in buildings that have received fire damage. ◆ Review building plans and systems to ensure adequate fire and smoke detection systems are in place; install cameras in critical areas to monitor remotely. ◆ Develop restoration contingency plans; determine the order in which critical functions are to be restored (eg, hospital services, consultation or reference laboratory, donor testing).
Hurricane Katrina (US)[65] 8/25/2005 and 8/29/2005 Hurricane Katrina made landfall in southeast Florida, causing minimal disruption to blood collection and transfusion facilities. Then it struck Louisiana and the Gulf Coast region, causing catastrophic damage and forcing the temporary or permanent closure of several hospitals and of the primary blood collection center in New Orleans.	◆ Relocate critical operations to areas exposed to less risk. ◆ Create redundant facilities for critical operations. ◆ Relocate critical functions to higher floors in a building (eg, electrical room, records). ◆ Include communicating with board of directors in the disaster plan to identify specific administrative rendezvous locations. ◆ Accumulate a 75-day strategic cash reserve. ◆ Use text messaging to communicate with staff and provide necessary devices and training. ◆ Develop and maintain a crisis website where staff and the board of directors can read and post information related to the facility's status and the whereabouts of the staff. ◆ Include hospital line staff in critical communications between the blood center and the hospital. ◆ Convert critical documents into an electronic format, and back up on a secure server outside the immediate area. ◆ Secure mainframe host provider for the computer system outside the immediate service area. ◆ Provide a wallet-sized emergency contact list for easy reference by staff and board members. ◆ Use an 800-MHz (or equivalent) telephone system for constant communication with clients; have hospitals include the blood center in disaster plans. ◆ Meet periodically with hospital management and other clients to acquire and exchange recent modifications to disaster plans.
Operation Enduring Freedom 10/2001 through present Operation Enduring Freedom is a full-scale military action in support of the global war on terrorism; it requires blood support for medical interventions.	◆ Maintain the ability to rapidly expand collection capabilities on short notice to meet military contingencies. ◆ Ensure contracts are in place to purchase blood components and supplies at all times for contingencies. ◆ Consider potential donor deferrals for countries involved as soon as possible in contingency. ◆ Make transportation systems for delivery of blood to theater of operations both flexible and adaptable.

(Continued)

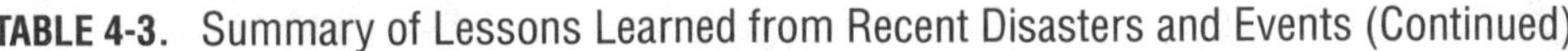

TABLE 4-3. Summary of Lessons Learned from Recent Disasters and Events (Continued)

Event	Lessons Learned
Operation Iraqi Freedom 3/2003 - 9/2010 Operation Iraqi Freedom was a full-scale military action in support of the global war on terrorism; it required blood support for medical interventions.	♦ Be able to sustain increased collections for extended periods. ♦ Be able to target specific ABO blood types for specialized components. ♦ Be flexible to adapt to changes in component requirements as the delivery of health care on the battlefield changes (consider apheresis platelets in theater). ♦ Use training to sustain personnel, especially in specialty areas such as apheresis.
Top Official Exercises (Topoff) Topoff 2—5/12/2003 - 5/16/2003 Topoff 3—4/4/2005 - 4/8/2005 Full-scale federal exercises involving hundreds of governmental and private organizations simulate various scenarios, including terrorist bombings (radiologic and chemical) and the release of biologic agents.	♦ Maintain a list of emergency points of contact and update the list regularly. ♦ Ensure that the staff is trained in emergency contact procedures, especially during off-duty hours. ♦ Develop a robust and up-to-date information distribution system. ♦ Develop and use an after-action reporting process to capture lessons learned. ♦ Establish contact and lines of communication with local and state departments of public health. ♦ Identify alternative transportation services for blood and supplies.
Novel H1N1 Influenza A Outbreak and Pandemic 4/2009 - 8/2010 Outbreak of an influenza that rapidly spread throughout the world and was declared a pandemic by the World Health Organization (WHO).	♦ Early command and control is important to facilitate communication. ♦ Planning is more important than the plan *(flexibility is critical)*. ♦ Messaging needs to be clear to explain the nature of the threat. ♦ Over- and under-reactions should be avoided among staff, donors, public, etc. ♦ Such events should be primarily a public health issue, but blood facilities may need to take action. ♦ Public health messages may present potential for blood donor confusion. ♦ Facility plan must discuss pandemic phases in terms of severity in order to avoid confusion with WHO pandemic phases. ♦ Donor deferrals are variable around the world. ♦ Each state is responsible for the deployment of strategic national stockpile items in their state; interstate blood regions will have to coordinate with the appropriate state public health agencies. ♦ Personal protective equipment policies and provisions should be clear and consistent. ♦ Risks of exposure must be clearly communicated to blood donors by facility staff. ♦ A clear strategy is needed regarding the impact of the use of antivirals before the outbreak. ♦ Facilities must coordinate with vendors to ensure supply chain viability. ♦ Better data needs to be developed on the impact of an influenza pandemic on donation and transfusion patterns. ♦ Greater support is needed for scientific research (viremia in donors, convalescent plasma).

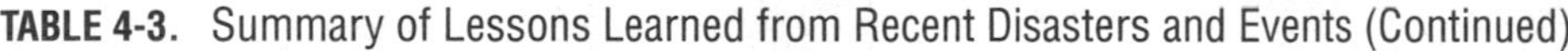

TABLE 4-3. Summary of Lessons Learned from Recent Disasters and Events (Continued)

Event	Lessons Learned
2008 Democratic National Convention (Denver)* 8/25/2008 - 8/28/2008 A United States Department of Homeland Security National Special Security Event involved more than 50,000 visitors a day, including presidential candidates, major political figures, congressional members, delegates, dignitaries, celebrities, media personnel, protestors, and volunteers.	◆ Attend and participate regularly in federal, state, and local emergency planning groups such as Metro Medical Response Systems, Urban Areas Security Initiatives, public health systems, and other hospital/medical/EMS groups. ◆ Consider adapting blood center disaster response plans to National Incident Management System/Incident Command System standards. ◆ Include health-care partners in blood center emergency response planning. ◆ Initiate contact with event planning committees far in advance of the actual event. ◆ Build hospital emergency blood component stockpiles over a defined period. ◆ Communicate stockpiling plans with hospitals, and ensure they have sufficient storage capacities. ◆ Be careful that stockpiling does not "dry up" the donor base. ◆ Determine postevent strategy for inventory return or use through normal use patterns. ◆ Consider delivery/courier mechanism issues in light of increased event security (eg, tamperproof tape, clearly marked boxes, courier credentialing). ◆ Consider the impact of street closures, parades, protests, etc, on scheduled blood drives.

*Information courtesy of Bonfils Blood Center.

NIH = National Institutes of Health; NHSBT = National Health Service Blood and Transport; NBS = National Blood Service; IT = information technology; FDA = Food and Drug Administration; FBI = Federal Bureau of Investigation; EMS = emergency medical services.

the aftermath of Hurricane Katrina, organizations that fail to be prepared or to respond quickly will be held strictly accountable and may suffer both successive loss of goodwill and a branded image. Blood collection and transfusion facilities are not immune to this reality and should therefore strive to maintain the highest standards of disaster preparedness. Above all else, the most important benefit of careful planning is assurance that blood and blood components are available to patients where and when needed.

KEY POINTS

1. Planning is the key to success during a real disaster. Disaster planning is not a one-time event; it is a continual review, exercise/practice, learn-and-change process.
2. Continuity of Operations Planning provides a framework for facilities to maintain or restore the critical functions necessary to collect, manufacture, store, and distribute blood components.
3. The cornerstone of an effective disaster plan is a thorough risk assessment of the probable hazards and resulting impact on critical operations. Risks can include internal events such as a broken pipe flooding a laboratory, or external events such as tornadoes and earthquakes.

4. It is the blood on the shelf that saves lives in an emergency. Blood has a finite shelf life and must be continually replaced.
5. The ability to communicate during a disaster determines much of the success of a response; facilities need well-developed and routinely tested communication plans.
6. Adequate cash reserves and insurance are essential for a blood center to survive a major disaster.
7. Coordination with local emergency management officials *before* the disaster is critical to success *during* a disaster.
8. Regulatory considerations during a disaster include assessment of the effect on the components on the shelf, the donors in the affected area, and operations.
9. Facilities should routinely reinforce the disaster plan by conducting information sessions with staff, volunteers and their families, suppliers, and hospital customers. The disaster plan should be tested by participation in local or regional disaster drills.
10. Facilities should use the resources of the AABB Interorganizational Task Force on Domestic Disasters and Acts of Terrorism in disaster management planning (ie, *Disaster Operations Handbook*) and incorporate the task force national response procedures into local plans.

REFERENCES

1. Disaster operations handbook: Coordinating the nation's blood supply during disasters and biological events. Version 2.0. Bethesda, MD: AABB, 2008. [Available at http://www.aabb.org/programs/disasterresponse/Pages/default.aspx#2 (accessed September 28, 2010).]
2. Comprehensive preparedness guide (CPG) 101: Developing and maintaining state, territorial, tribal, and local government emergency plans. Washington, DC: Federal Emergency Management Agency, 2009.
3. Multi-hazard identification and risk assessment: A cornerstone of the national mitigation strategy. Washington, DC: Federal Emergency Management Agency, 1996:325-9. [Available at http://www.fema.gov/library/viewRecord.do?id=2214 (accessed September 28, 2010).]
4. Emergency management guide for business and industry: A step-by-step approach to emergency planning, response, and recovery for companies of all sizes. FEMA 141/October 1993. Washington, DC: Federal Emergency Management Agency, 1993. [Available at http://www.fema.gov/business/guide/index.shtm (accessed September 28, 2010).]
5. State offices and agencies of emergency management. Washington, DC: Federal Emergency Management Agency, 2010. [Available at http://www.fema.gov/about/contact/statedr.shtm (accessed September 28, 2010).]
6. National response framework. (January 2008) Washington, DC: Department of Homeland Security, 2008. [Available at http://www.fema.gov/emergency/nrf (accessed September 28, 2010).]
7. Robert T. Stafford disaster relief and emergency assistance act (Public Law 93-288) as amended. Washington, DC: US Government Printing Office, 1993. [Available at http://www.fema.gov/about/stafact.shtm (accessed September 28, 2010).]
8. Homeland Security Advisory System. Washington, DC: Department of Homeland Security, 2010. [Available at http://www.dhs.gov/files/programs/Copy_of_press_release_0046.shtm (accessed September 28, 2010).]
9. National Incident Management System. Washington, DC: Federal Emergency Management Agency, 2010. [Available at http://www.fema.gov/emergency/nims/(accessed October 12, 2010).]
10. Public health emergency: National Disaster Medical System. Washington, DC: Department of Health and Human Services, 2010. [Available at http://www.phe.gov/Preparedness/responders/ndms/Pages/default.aspx (accessed October 12, 2010).]
11. Hess JR, Thomas MJG. Blood use in war and disaster: Lessons from the past century. Transfusion 2003;43:1622-33.
12. Linden JV, Davey RJ, Burch JW. The September 11, 2001, disaster and the New York blood supply. Transfusion 2002;42:1385-7.
13. Schmidt PJ. Blood and disaster—supply and demand. N Engl J Med 2002;346:617-20.

14. Klein HG. Earthquake in America. Transfusion 2001;41:1179-80.
15. Pandemic influenza update. Association bulletin #09-07. Bethesda, MD: AABB, 2009.
16. Open for business: A disaster planning toolkit for the small to mid-sized business owner. Tampa, FL: Institute for Business and Home Safety, 2006. [Available at http://www.ibhs.org/docs/OpenForBusiness.pdf (accessed September 28, 2010).]
17. Ready business: Prepare, plan, stay informed. Washington, DC: Federal Emergency Management Agency, 2010. [Available at http://www.ready.gov/business/index.html (accessed September 28, 2010).]
18. Federal continuity guidance circular 1 (CGC 1). Continuity guidance for non-federal entities (January 21, 2009). Annex I: Vital records management. Washington, DC: Federal Emergency Management Agency, 2009. [Available at http://www.fema.gov/pdf/about/org/ncp/coop/continuity_guidance_circular.pdf (accessed September 28, 2010).]
19. The Hartford. Business: Small business. Hartford, CT: The Hartford Financial Services Group, Inc., 2010. [Available at http://www.thehartford.com/servlet/Satellite?c=Page&cid=1150850367009&pagename=HIG%2FPage%2FLandingPage2 (accessed October 12, 2010).]
20. The conference on emergency response planning for your business. Mission, KS: SkillPath Seminars, 2002.
21. Carson TH, ed. Standards for blood banks and transfusion services. 27th ed. Bethesda, MD: AABB, 2011:2.
22. Comprehensive accreditation manual for hospitals. Oakbrook Terrace, IL: The Joint Commission, 2011.
23. CBBS Disaster response plan. Sacramento, CA:, California Blood Bank Society, 2008. [Available at http://www.cbbsweb.org/links/disaster_plan.html (accessed September 23, 2010).]
24. The smart approach to protecting your business: Managing your risk. Hartford, CT: The Hartford and the US Small Business Administration, 2002.
25. Myers KN. Manager's guide to contingency planning for disasters. New York: John Wiley and Sons, 1999.
26. Making educated decisions for your small business: Business insurance guide for the small business owner. Hartford, CT: The Hartford and the US Small Business Administration, 2004. [Available at http://clients.bn24.com/MediaRoomContent/Hartford/05-943/05-943_SBA/html/docs/SBA%20Course%20Brochure%20.pdf (accessed September 28, 2010).]
27. Gannon B. The best laid plans. Paper presented at America's Blood Centers 2006 Annual Meeting, Houston, TX, March 4-6, 2006.
28. IS-100.a introduction to incident command system, ICS-100 (interactive web-based course.) Emmitsburg, MD: FEMA Emergency Management Institute, 2010. [Available at http://training.fema.gov/EMIWeb/IS/IS100A.asp (accessed September 28, 2010).]
29. NS/EP [national security and emergency preparedness] priority telecommunications. Washington, DC: National Communications System, 2010. [Available at http://www.ncs.gov/services.html (accessed September 28, 2010).]
30. Blietz J. Disaster management: Sharing what we have learned over the past few years. CBBS Today 2006:XXIV:45-9.
31. Radio Amateur Civil Emergency Services (RACES). Arlington, VA: Virginia Office of Emergency Management, Emergency Support Function #2, 2010. [Available at http://www.usraces.org/ (accessed September 28, 2010).]
32. Salvation Army Team Emergency Radio Network (SATERN). [Available at http://www.satern.org (accessed September 28, 2010).]
33. ARRL, the national association for amateur radio. Newington, CT: ARRL, 2010. [Available at http://www.arrl.org (accessed September 28, 2010).]
34. Bell CA. Emergency communications: Who ya gonna call . . . and how? CBBS Today 2005;XXIII:19-22.
35. Ready America: Prepare. Plan. Stay informed. Washington, DC: Federal Emergency Management Agency, 2010. [Available at http://www.ready.gov/america/ (accessed September 28, 2010).]
36. IS-242: Effective communication (independent study course). Washington, DC: Federal Emergency Management Agency, 2005:6.5. [Available at http://training.fema.gov/EMIWeb/IS/is242.asp (accessed September 28, 2010).]
37. Pandemic influenza pre-event message maps. Washington, DC: US Department of Health andHuman Services, 2006. [Available at http://

pandemicflu.gov/news/pre_event_maps.pdf (accessed September 28, 2010).]

38. Emergency risk communication for public health professionals (online training course). Seattle, WA: Northwest Center for Public Health Practice, 2010. [Available at http://www.nwcphp.org/training/courses/risk-communication-competencies (accessed September 28, 2010).]
39. Preventing adverse events caused by emergency electrical power system failures. (September 6, 2006) Sentinel Event Alert #37. Oakbrook Terrace, IL: The Joint Commission, 2006.
40. Cybersecurity. Washington, DC: Department of Homeland Security, 2010. [Available at http://www.dhs.gov/files/cybersecurity.shtm (accessed October 12, 2010).]
41. Ready kids. Washington, DC: Federal Emergency Management Agency, 2010, [Available at http://www.ready.gov/kids/index.html (accessed September 28, 2010).]
42. Preparedness fast facts: Emergency-specific preparedness information. Washington, DC: American National Red Cross, 2010. [Available at http://www.redcross.org/portal/site/en/menuitem.86f46a12f382290517a8f210b80f78a0/?vgnextoid=92d51a53f1c37110VgnVCM1000003481a1 0aRCRD (accessed October 12, 2010).]
43. Disaster preparedness. New York: American Society for the Prevention of Cruelty to Animals, 2010. [Available at http://www.aspca.org/pet-care/disaster-preparedness/ (accessed September 28, 2010).]
44. Are You Ready? An in-depth guide to citizen preparedness. Washington, DC: Federal Emergency Management Agency, 2004. [Available at http://www.fema.gov/areyouready/ (accessed September 28, 2010).]
45. Federal Emergency Management Agency. Prepare for a disaster: Shelter. Guidelines for managing water supplies. Guidelines for managing food supplies. Washington, DC: FEMA, 2010. [Available at http://www.fema.gov/plan/prepare/shelter.shtm (accessed September 23, 2010).]
46. Emergency management guide. Function: Life safety. Shelter. Washington, DC: Federal Emergency Management Agency, 2010. [Available at http://www.fema.gov/business/guide/section2c.shtm#header4 (accessed September 28, 2010).]
47. Coping with shelter-in-place emergencies. Washington, DC: American National Red Cross, 2010. [Available at http://www.redcross.org/portal/site/en/menuitem.86f46a12f382290517a8f210b80f78a0/?vgnextoid=92d51a53f1c37110VgnVCM1000003481a10aRCRD (accessed October 12, 2010).]
48. State, provincial, and territorial psychological association directory. Washington, DC: American Psychological Association, 2010. [Available at http://www.apa.org/about/organizations/associations.aspx (accessed September 28, 2010).]
49. ACA divisions, regions, and branches. Alexandria, VA: American Counseling Association, 2010. [Available at http://www.counseling.org/AboutUs/DivisionsBranchesAndRegions/TP/Home/CT2.aspx (accessed September 28, 2010).]
50. TherapistLocator.net. Alexandria, VA: American Association for Marriage and Family Therapy, 2010. [Available at http://www.therapistlocator.net/ (accessed September 28, 2010).]
51. Homeland Security Presidential Directive 5: Management of domestic incidents. (February 28, 2003) Washington, DC: Department of Homeland Security, 2009. [Available at http://www.dhs.gov/xabout/laws/gc_1214592333605.shtm (accessed September 28, 2010).]
52. Homeland Security Presidential Directive 8: National preparedness. Washington, DC: Department of Homeland Security, 2008. [Available at http://www.dhs.gov/xabout/laws/gc_1215444247124.shtm (accessed September 28, 2010).]
53. Food and Drug Administration. Impact of severe weather conditions on biological products. Rockville, MD: CBER Office of Communication, Outreach, and Development, 2009. [Available at http://www.fda.gov/BiologicsBloodVaccines/SafetyAvailability/ProductSecurity/ucm147243. htm (accessed September 28, 2010).]
54. Radiological emergency response plan. Washington, DC: Food and Drug Administration.
55. Chemical and biological response plan. Washington, DC: Food and Drug Administration.
56. Food and Drug Administration. Impact of severe weather conditions on biological products. Rockville, MD: CBER Consumer Affairs Branch. [Available at http://www.fda.gov/BiologicsBloodVaccines/SafetyAvailability/ProductSecurity/ucm147243. htm (accessed February 2, 2011).]
57. Food and Drug Administration. FDA policy statement on urgent collection, shipment, and

use of whole blood and blood components intended for transfusion to address blood supply needs in the current disaster situation. (September 11, 2001) Rockville, MD: CBER Office of Communication, Outreach, and Development, 2001.

58. Food and Drug Administration. Guidance for industry: Recommendations for blood establishments: Training of back-up personnel, assessment of blood donor suitability, and reporting certain changes to an approved application. (November 2010) Rockville, MD: CBER Office of Communication, Outreach, and Development, 2010. [Available at http://www.fda.gov/downloads/BiologicsBloodVaccines/GuidanceComplianceRegulatoryInformation/Guidances/Blood/vcm190373.pdf (accessed February 2, 2011).]
59. FDA offers tips about medical devices and hurricane disasters. Washington, DC: Food and Drug Administration, 2010. [Available at http://www.fda.gov/MedicalDevices/Safety/EmergencySituations/ucm055987.htm (accessed September 28, 2010).]
60. IS-120. An orientation to community disaster exercises (FEMA independent study). Emmitsburg, MD: FEMA Emergency Management Institute, 2006. [Available at http://training.fema.gov/EMIWeb/IS/is120lst.asp (accessed September 28, 2010).]
61. Jett BW, LeBeau-Laird B, Lewis M. Flood, fire, wind and rain: Disasters and lessons learned. Presented at the AABB Annual Meeting, Miami, FL, October 24, 2006.
62. Hartwell B. The hospital and blood center partnership: Disaster response. Presented at the AABB National Blood Inventory Management Conference, Atlanta, GA, May 2002.
63. Doughty H, Allard S. Responding to major incidents: Lessons learnt from July 2005 bombings. Blood Matters, Autumn 2006.
64. Teague B. Surviving a devastating fire at a regional blood center. Presented at the AABB Annual Meeting, Seattle, WA, October 18, 2005.
65. Weales B. Hurricane Katrina: Before, during, and now. Presented at the AABB National Blood Inventory Management Conference, Dallas, TX, March 31-April 1, 2006.

◆ APPENDIX 4-1
Internet Resources Related to State and Local Organizations

- State and local emergency management agencies:
  http://www.fema.gov/about/contact/statedr.shtm
  https://www.disasterassistance.gov
  http://www.emergencymanagement.org/states
- State and local public health agencies:
  http://www.statepublichealth.org
  http://www.naccho.org
- State blood and hospital associations:
  http://www.aha.org/aha/resource_center/links.jsp#2
- Community-based disaster organizations:
  http://www.redcross.org/en/
  http://www.nvoad.org/
  http://www.salvationarmyusa.org/usn/www_usn_2.nsf

◆ APPENDIX 4-2
General Internet Resources for Disaster Management

- Disaster Help
  http://www.disasterassistance.gov/daip_en.portal
- FEMA Emergency Management Guide for Business and Industry
  http://www.fema.gov/business/guide/index.shtm
- FEMA mitigation resources
  http://www.fema.gov/plan/mitplanning/index.shtm
- Ready.gov
  http://www.ready.gov/
- Society for Risk Analysis
  http://www.sra.org/index.php
- ISO 31000 Risk management—principles and guidelines
  http://www.iso.org/catalogue_detail?csnumber=43170

Chapter 5

Allogeneic and Autologous Blood Donor Selection

Anne F. Eder, MD, PhD

THE PROCESS OF selecting blood donors aims to determine—to the extent possible—that the donor is in good general health to tolerate the collection procedure and is free of diseases that can be transmitted to patients by blood transfusion. Overlapping safeguards to protect both donor and recipient safety in the selection process use donor education, health history assessment and focused physical examination, additional instructions after the donation, and maintenance of records about ineligible (ie, deferred) donors.[1-2] Infectious disease testing of donations is also a critical part of the process. (See Chapter 8.)

Before blood is collected, individuals are provided with educational material that describes the donation process, and they are instructed not to donate if they are at increased risk of being infected with blood-borne pathogens. Potential donors are then given a focused physical examination and are questioned directly about specific risk behaviors as well as about medications, travel, and other factors that potentially affect recipient or donor safety. Donors are asked about risks related to infectious diseases for which sensitive tests are currently in place, for which tests are not universally used, and for which licensed screening tests are not yet available. (See Table 5-1.) To prevent future donation by ineligible donors, blood collection facilities maintain a confidential list of deferred donors to exclude individuals either for reactive test results, behavioral risks, or medical reasons. Deferrals may be for a defined interval of time, for an indefinite period, or permanent with no potential for reinstatement in the future. The selection criteria used for autologous donation are often less stringent than those for allogeneic donation, but the focus remains on providing the safest possible blood for transfusion to the donor-patient and on evaluating the risks that the collection procedure poses to his or her health.

Blood components for allogeneic transfusion are collected from volunteer, nonremunerated donors in the United States. Otherwise, they must be labeled as being from paid donors.[3] The blood center must determine donor eligibility on the day of collection, in accordance with federal and state regulations[1] and voluntary accreditation standards [AABB

Anne F. Eder, MD, PhD, Executive Medical Officer, American Red Cross, National Headquarters, Biomedical Services Medical Office, Holland Laboratory, Rockville, Maryland
The author has disclosed no conflicts of interest.

TABLE 5-1. Health History Assessment Questions for Infectious Diseases

Tests are available but may not detect early-stage or window-period infections	Tests are available but not used in all donor centers	No licensed laboratory tests are available for blood donor screening
Chagas disease Hepatitis (HBV, HCV) HIV-1, -2 Human T-cell lymphotropic viruses, types I and II West Nile virus	Human immunodeficiency virus (HIV) group O	Babesiosis Creutzfeldt-Jakob disease (CJD) Malaria Variant CJD

Standards for Blood Banks and Transfusion Services (Standards)].[2] Specific criteria used to select donors are established by the Food and Drug Administration (FDA) through the *Code of Federal Regulations* (CFR), guidance documents, or memoranda to industry. The AABB also develops professional standards for donor selection with which accredited blood establishments must comply. (See Appendices 5-1 and 5-2.)

Medical directors of blood collection facilities are responsible for determining donor eligibility on issues that are not covered by regulations or standards. Consequently, medical decisions regarding the same issue may differ among different blood centers or even among physicians at the same blood center. Considerable variability exists in national and international practice.[4-6] These disparate deferral policies may cause confusion, disenchantment, or anger among blood donors. Donors may also be puzzled by the relevance that certain questions have to their health or their ability to donate blood for transfusion to others. To minimize donor frustration and confusion, blood center staff should be able to explain the intended purpose of their center-specific eligibility screening practices and those of the AABB and the FDA. The most frequently asked questions about federal regulations defining blood donor eligibility are available to the public in the "Questions about Blood" section on the FDA website: http://www.fda.gov/BiologicsBloodVaccines/BloodBloodProducts/Questions aboutBlood/default.htm.

HISTORICAL PERSPECTIVE

Over the past several decades, the approach to blood safety has evolved. Progressive scientific advances have decreased the risk of transfusion-transmitted diseases but have also incrementally increased the cost, the operational complexity, and the redundancy of the process as more specific tests have been introduced without eliminating nonspecific measures.[7] The approach to transfusion-transmitted hepatitis and AIDS illustrates this progression. Before the etiologic hepatitis viruses were discovered, the first AABB donor card (used in 1953) to evaluate donor history included a question about a history of hepatitis and approximately 20 other conditions.[8] The recognition in the 1970s that the risk of hepatitis transmission was greatly increased if the blood was collected from paid or incarcerated donors led to measures to label the source of blood components as voluntary or paid and to eliminate collections at correctional institutions.[9] Studies clearly demonstrated that elimination of paid donors reduced the risk of hepatitis transmission through blood transfusion.[10] Specific testing for hepatitis B virus (HBV) was introduced in 1971; for hepatitis C virus (HCV), in 1990. The CFR continued to require permanent disqualification of all individuals with a history of viral hepatitis for many years before allowing an exception in 1992 to permit donation if the history of viral hepatitis occurred before the age of 11.[1] The current contribution to blood safety of questioning donors about a remote history of viral hepatitis, however, is unclear because of the advent of sensitive screening tests for the specific viruses responsible for transfusion-transmitted hepatitis.

Similarly, the recognition in the early 1980s that AIDS could be transmitted by blood transfusion led to the first donor screening methods for preventing transmission, before the human immunodeficiency virus (HIV) was identified as the etiologic agent. The initial effort relied on donor education and self-exclusion. Written material provided to blood donors at the collection site was modified to include a description of risk factors for AIDS, and direct questioning of blood donors regarding these risk behaviors was subsequently added. These measures effectively decreased donations from the populations at greatest risk for transmitting AIDS, and they decreased the risk of transfusion-transmitted HIV before specific tests were available.[11]

During the ensuing years, tests to detect exposure to HIV, HBV, and HCV were introduced and improved, such that the current residual risk of HIV and HCV transmission has fallen below 1 in 1 million donations.[12] The incremental value of continuing to evaluate behavioral risk factors in donor selection, in light of extremely sensitive tests for these infectious diseases, is difficult to assess. Theoretically, questioning donors may lower the prevalence of disease in the donor population and may reduce the likelihood that an infectious unit will ever reach the blood center for testing.[13] (See Table 5-2.) Furthermore, the donor interview may also eliminate donors who are potentially at increased risk for diseases for which there are no approved, appropriately sensitive, or operationally feasible tests, and may eliminate donors with very early-stage infections with pathogens that escape detection with current tests (eg, window-period infections). (See Table 5-3.) Finally, the screening process may reduce potential occupational risks to the collection and laboratory staff.

The AABB introduced the uniform donor history questionnaire to its members in 1992, but blood centers continued to add and modify questions each year. By 2000, the various health history questionnaires in use covered more than 70 items, and many included compound or multi-item questions, such that what was called the "uniform donor history questionnaire" was not being used in a standardized manner by blood centers around the country. The realization that the questionnaire had become onerous, complex, and possibly ineffective in eliciting reliable information from donors led to the formation of an interor-

TABLE 5-2. Prevalence and Incidence of Infectious Disease Markers Among ARC Blood Donors in 1999 Compared with Reported Rates for the US Population[7]

	Prevalence*		Incidence†	
	Donors	**US Overall**	**Donors**	**US Overall**
HBV (HBsAg)	84.4	420‡	4.5	114.4
HCV	386.3	1800	2.8	13.4
HIV	11.8	136	1.7	15.0

*Prevalence per hundred thousand first-time blood donors.

†Incidence per hundred thousand person-years among repeat donors.

‡As cited by McQuillan et al.[13]

ARC = American Red Cross; HBV = hepatitis B virus; HBsAg = hepatitis B surface antigen; HCV = hepatitis C virus; HIV = human immunodeficiency virus.

TABLE 5-3. Health History Assessment for Infectious Diseases*

Infectious Disease	Reported Transfusion-Transmitted Cases	Current Health History Deferrals
HIV group O†	None reported	Born or lived in African risk countries; sexual contact or blood transfusion in African risk countries (Cameroon, Benin, Central African Republic, Chad, Congo, Equatorial Guinea, Kenya, Gabon, Niger, Nigeria, Senegal, Togo, or Zambia)
Malaria *Plasmodia* sp.	0.6 per year‡	History of malaria—3 years Lived in endemic country—3 years Travel to endemic area—12 months
Babesiosis (*Babesia microti*)	3-6 per year§	History of babesiosis—indefinite deferral
Chagas disease (*Trypanosoma cruzi*)	7 to date	History of Chagas disease—indefinite deferral
vCJD	4 to date in United Kingdom	Geographic deferrals
CJD	No known cases associated with blood transfusion	Pituitary-derived growth hormone, dura mater transplant, blood relatives with CJD—indefinite deferral

*HIV-1,2 and hepatitis are not included but discussed in greater detail in the text.

†Questions are not necessary if a test licensed to detect HIV group O is used by the blood center for donor screening.

‡Cited by H. Nakhasi at FDA Workshop on Testing for Malarial Infections in Blood Donors, July 12, 2006.

§Reported to the American Red Cross, Hemovigilance Program.

HIV = human immunodeficiency virus; vCJD = variant Creutzfeldt-Jakob disease; CJD = classical CJD; FDA = Food and Drug Administration.

ganizational task force by the AABB, with representatives from the blood and plasma communities and the US government. The Donor History Questionnaire (DHQ) Task Force focused on streamlining the DHQ and on validating the simplified questions through focus groups and cognitive interviews to determine if donors understood the questions.[8] In October 2006, the FDA recognized the resulting DHQ (version 1.1) in a final guidance document, and the DHQ documents are currently used by the majority of blood centers in the United States.[14] The references in this chapter are to DHQ version 1.3 (May 2008), which the FDA officially recognized as acceptable DHQ documents in May 2010 with issuance of "Guidance for Industry: Revised Preventive Measures to Reduce the Possible Risk of Transmission of Creutzfeldt-Jakob Disease (CJD) and Variant Creutzfeldt-Jakob Disease (vCJD) by Blood and Blood Products." The FDA acknowledges the AABB DHQ documents as an effective donor screening tool that provides licensed and unlicensed facilities with one way to meet FDA requirements (21 CFR 640.3 and 640.63). The guidance document contains instructions for implementation of version 1.3 and reporting the changes to the FDA.

SELECTION OF ALLOGENEIC DONORS

Registration and Donor Identification

The blood donor should provide an acceptable form of identification, and each donor must be properly identified by the collection staff before each donation. Accurate donation records are essential to link a repeat donor to existing records and to prevent collection from a donor who is not currently qualified, as well as to ensure that the donor can be contacted in the weeks following the donation and informed of test results or other relevant information, if necessary.[2(pp13,16),15] There are no specific requirements for acceptable forms of identification, but most blood centers 1) require a government-issued photo identification, such as a driver's license or passport, or 2) assign a unique identifier to each blood donor and issue a donor-center-specific blood donor card, or 3) do both. Blood centers must make reasonable attempts to notify the donor within 8 weeks of the donation if any test results disqualify the individual from continued donation. Blood centers typically require an address and telephone number where the donor can be reached in this interval for counseling or other follow-up, if necessary.[15] Although some blood centers may still use US Social Security numbers (SSNs) to identify donors, federal and state legislation are expected in the near future that will restrict access and use of SSNs by US businesses and service establishments. The blood center should be able to determine if the donor has ever given blood under a different name, so that the link with all prior donations is maintained. Accurate donation records must be kept by the donor center for the requisite amount of time, according to current regulations and standards.

Educational Materials and Donor Consent

At each encounter, US blood centers provide all presenting blood donors with educational materials and give the donors an opportunity to ask questions. Prospective blood donors are informed of the risks of the procedures, of the clinical signs and symptoms associated with HIV infection, of behavioral risk factors for transmission of blood-borne pathogens, and of the importance of refraining from blood donation if they are at an increased risk of being infected. The DHQ process, discussed in greater detail below, incorporates all necessary elements for donor education required by federal regulations and AABB *Standards*.[2(pp15,56-61)]

At the time of each donation, the blood center staff should explain the collection procedure to the donor in terms the donor understands, and document the donor consent process to indicate that the donor has considered all the educational materials and has had an opportunity to ask questions.[2(pp15)] Either verbally or in the educational materials, the donor should be informed about possible risks of the procedure and the infectious disease tests that will be performed on his or her donation, as well as about the notification process for positive tests, about any reporting requirements to federal or state health authorities, and about the possibility of inclusion on the donor center's deferral registry and subsequent deferral from future donation. The individual donor should also be informed if investigational tests or other research may be performed on samples obtained from the donation by the collection facility.

Finally, the limitations of the tests to detect early infections and the possibility that a test may not be performed if samples are not adequate should be explained to the donor. Information about alternative HIV test sites or about options to obtain HIV tests should be provided to all prospective donors.[16] Most states in the United States allow blood donations by 17-year-old donors without parental permission; many states allow blood donations by 16-year-old donors with parental permission. Blood centers must comply with applicable state laws for obtaining permission from parents or guardians for minors or legally incompetent adults.[2(p15)] Moreover, AABB Standard 5.2.2 requires that the collection facility have a process to provide information concerning the donation process to the parent or legally authorized representative of the donor when parental permission is required.[2(p15)] All prospective donors must be able to give informed consent and an accurate health history.

Donor centers should make provisions for donors who are hearing- or vision-impaired, and may want to consider making provisions for those who are not fluent in English, or who are illiterate. Many US blood centers will not allow family members, business associates, or individuals known to the donor to serve as interpreters during the donor interview, because such a practice could compromise the integrity of the health history obtained from the donor. The Americans with Disabilities Act protects the rights of individuals with disabilities and requires that public accomodations ensure that their premises and services are readily accessible to, and usable by, individuals with disabilities.[17] Many blood centers feel an ethical and a moral obligation to accommodate blood donors who have disabilities, but the centers should also address unique safety considerations that always take priority to ensure the safety of the donor and maintain an adequate informed consent process.[5] The final authority for such decisions rests with the donor center's physician under whose supervision donor qualification and phlebotomy are performed.[2(p1)]

Physical Examination

Prospective blood donors must feel healthy and well on the day of donation and, in AABB-accredited facilities, must meet all AABB and FDA requirements for donor selection (see Appendices 5-1 and 5-2) as well as donor-center-specific criteria. (The deferral rates associated with these requirements in the American Red Cross blood system in 2008 are presented in Table 5-4.) The physical examination is intended to ensure that the donor is in good general health and will tolerate the collection procedure. The donor's temperature, skin inspection, and hemoglobin screening also have implications for the potency or safety of the collected component. The skin at the site of venipuncture must be free of lesions. Both of the donor's arms must be examined for multiple needle punctures (eg, small scars that may line up like "tracks") or for sclerotic veins as signs of injection drug use, which are a cause for indefinite deferral. Scars or pitting on the forearm associated with frequent blood donation should not be mistaken for evidence of injection drug use. Common and mild skin disorders are not a cause for deferral (eg, poison ivy rash) unless unusually extensive or with signs of localized infection, or if the condition interferes with proper skin disinfection in the antecubital site before phlebotomy. Individuals with hemorrhagic nodules suggestive of Kaposi's sarcoma should be deferred until definitive medical evaluation is performed.

Additional requirements are defined for apheresis donors (see Appendix 5-1); in addition, the donor must meet the specific weight and hemoglobin or hematocrit requirements as approved by the FDA for the automated collection device.

The most common reason for deferring blood donors is an unacceptable hemoglobin or hematocrit value on the day of donation (see Table 5-4). FDA-mandated screening criteria for hemoglobin and hematocrit in the United States are controversial and periodically debated, but they have remained unchanged for years. Hemoglobin or hematocrit screening is performed to prevent collection of blood from a donor with significant anemia, which could have implications for the health of the donor and the potency of the collected component. The FDA defines a single hemoglobin/hematocrit standard for all allogeneic blood donors, despite the factors that contribute to the variability of hemoglobin/hematocrit values in healthy populations.[18] The minimum acceptable hemoglobin level for both men and women is defined by the FDA as 12.5 g/dL, with the essentially equivalent hematocrit requirement of 38%.[19] Whether a single acceptance criterion for both men and women is appropriate from a donor safety perspective is debatable, because the distribution of normal hemoglobin values for a population is shifted to lower values for women than for men and is also influenced by race.[20] The practical significance of a single cutoff of 12.5 g/dL of hemoglobin for all donors is that women represent the vast majority of donors deferred for hemoglobin, most of whom likely have normal hemoglobin concentrations near this cutoff value (see Table 5-4.). In contrast, men with minimally acceptable hemoglobin for blood donation (eg, 12.5-13.6 g/dL) may be anemic.

Donor hemoglobin screening may also ensure a minimum content of hemoglobin in a

TABLE 5-4. Deferrals for Health History, American Red Cross (2008)*

Deferral Reason	Deferrals (Number)	Deferrals (% of Total Donor Presentations)
Physical Examination		
Hemoglobin	584,416	7.71
Men	51,727	0.68
Women	532,689	7.02
Blood pressure	48,777	0.64
Pulse	30,806	0.41
Other[†]	26,048	0.34
Total, Physical Examination	690,047	9.10
Health History		
Not healthy and well	11,232	0.15
Infection or antibiotics	25,400	0.33
Heart and lung disease	7,843	0.10
Blood or bleeding disorders	3,992	0.05
Cancer	10,816	0.14
Other medical conditions[‡]	7,128	0.09
Medications and vaccines[§]	12,492	0.16
Human immunodeficiency virus (HIV) or hepatitis risk (all reasons)	48,343	0.64
Hepatitis risk[‖]	1,426	0.02
Hepatitis, potential exposure[¶]	6,811	0.09
HIV risk[#]	902	0.01
HIV group O risk	1,444	0.02
Intravenous drug use	1,430	0.02
Male who has had sex with another male since 1977	3,424	0.05
Sexual contact with at-risk individual	2,357	0.03
Transfusion, transplantation, other blood exposure (eg, tattoos)	30,549	0.40

(Continued)

TABLE 5-4. Deferrals for Health History, American Red Cross (2008)* (Continued)

Deferral Reason	Deferrals (Number)	Deferrals (% of Total Donor Presentations)
Malaria risk (all reasons)	51,316	0.68
Malaria, past 3 years	51	<0.01
Lived in malaria-endemic country	3,727	0.05
Traveled to malaria area	47,538	0.63
Variant Creutzfeldt-Jakob disease (vCJD) risk		
Time spent in UK and Europe	9,689	0.13
CJD risk**	351	<0.01
Other	14,482	0.19
Total, Health History	203,084	2.68

*Total donor presentations = 7,583,371; data from Notari EP, ARCNET Data Center, American Red Cross, personal communication.

†Temperature, weight, arm inspection, age, date of last donation.

‡Pregnant in last 6 weeks; history of Chagas disease or babesiosis; other medical conditions.

§Medication Deferral List and vaccines with specific deferral periods.

||Viral hepatitis after age 11.

¶Lived with or had sexual contact with an individual with symptoms of viral hepatitis.

#Positive HIV test; history of sexually transmitted disease; accepted money or drugs for sex.

**Blood relative with CJD; received dura mater transplant or pituitary-derived human growth hormone.

unit of Red Blood Cells (RBCs), but currently neither the FDA nor the AABB define potency standards for RBC units prepared from whole blood collection. If a donor's hemoglobin is 12.5 g/dL, a 500-mL whole blood collection is expected to yield about 62.5 g of hemoglobin per unit of RBCs, but determining the final content of hemoglobin in an RBC unit prepared from whole blood is not required. AABB *Standards* defines apheresis RBC units as containing an average of 60 g of hemoglobin, with 95% of the units containing more than 50 g of hemoglobin.[2(p26)]

Neither the FDA nor the AABB specifies the test method or specimen type (capillary, venous blood) or the acceptable performance characteristics for tests used for hemoglobin/hematocrit screening. One exception is that a capillary sample collected from an earlobe puncture is not an acceptable specimen for hemoglobin/hematocrit screening for allogeneic[2(p56)] or autologous donors.[2(p18)] Earlobe capillary samples used to qualify donors were shown to yield hematocrit values approximately 5 percentage points higher on average than that of a venous sample, or the equivalent to nearly a 2-g/dL difference in hemoglobin, which led to concerns about the inappropriate acceptance of donors who may have significant anemia.[21] Much smaller differences have been observed between mean fingerstick and venous samples[22]; thus the use of fingerstick samples is acceptable for donor qualification in the United States. In contrast, venous samples are required in the United Kingdom.[23]

The methods to measure hemoglobin or hematocrit are generally selected for their ease of use in the mobile blood collection setting. The three methods historically or currently in widespread use are the copper sulfate density method (Method 6-1), the spun microhematocrit method, and the spectrophotometric measurement of hemoglobin with portable devices (eg, HemoCue Donor Hb Checker, HemoCue AB, Angelholm, Sweden; DiaSpect Hemoglobin, DiaSpect Medical AB, Uppsala, Sweden) or point-of-care hematology analyzers. The copper sulfate density method was widely used as a screening test in many blood centers because the method is rapid and inexpensive. However, state regulations regarding disposal of the reagent, which is an environmental and biologic hazard, added to its cost and inconvenience and led many centers to replace it with quantitative methods. The principle of the test is based on the relationship between the specific gravity of whole blood, which is determined primarily by the hemoglobin content, and a solution of copper sulfate. The copper sulfate method is a qualitative method, but it is capable of estimating hemoglobin to within approximately 0.5 g/dL using graded density solutions,[11] with a coefficient of variation (CV) of about 2%.[24] The spun hematocrit and HemoCue methods yield quantitative results, with CVs of 3.6% and 1.5%, respectively.[24] A typical automated analyzer measures hemoglobin on a venous sample with a CV ≤1.2%.[24]

Most quantitative methods currently in use will reliably measure hemoglobin within about 0.2 to 0.5 g/dL, and the vast majority of deferred donors will have hemoglobin or hematocrit values near the cutoff value. However, all test methods may give erroneous results in rare cases, leading to the acceptance of donors with significant anemia. Factors that increase the specific gravity of whole blood (eg, hyperproteinemia, hyperviscosity, or monoclonal gammopathy) will cause spuriously acceptable results when copper sulfate is used, despite hemoglobin values as low as 7 g/dL.[25,26] Markedly erroneous results are also possible with other test methods but are rare occurrences for donors with significant anemia without other apparent underlying disease.[26]

The screening algorithm to qualify donors should be sufficiently sensitive to detect donors with unacceptable hemoglobin levels but should achieve adequate specificity to limit erroneous rejection of donors with acceptable hemoglobin levels. Copper sulfate screening has been reported to have a relatively low false-acceptance rate (0.6%-1.2%) but a high false-rejection rate (50%-70%) of donors with acceptable hemoglobin.[27-29] Consequently, a confirmatory method such as spun microhematocrit is typically performed on donors deferred by copper sulfate to determine eligibility for donation. A novel approach to donor screening in Germany, relying on a venous hemoglobin result obtained on a previous donation, was deemed an acceptable alternative for performing donor hemoglobin screening.[30,31] However, this algorithm would require significant changes in the current regulatory environment in both the United States and Canada before the approach would be accepted.[30]

Hemoglobin screening does not ensure that the donor has an adequate store of iron. Hematologic recovery after whole blood or red cell donation depends on total body iron stores.[32,33] Current limitations on the donation interval and frequency reduce but do not eliminate the risk of iron depletion in repeat blood donors. Initially, the hemoglobin concentration is unaffected, but iron stores are inevitably depleted with increased frequency of blood donation. The physiologic consequences of low iron stores in the absence of anemia are controversial, with both beneficial and detrimental effects on health reported.[34-37] There are no formal recommendations in standards or regulations for iron supplementation after blood donation, but dietary advice including the use of iron-containing multivitamins is a relatively widespread practice in donor centers. Even casual use of iron supplementation has been shown to be advantageous to blood donors.[33]

Health History Assessment—Donor History Questionnaire

In October 2006, the FDA accepted the use of the material prepared by the interorganizational DHQ Task Force; such use provides adequate measures to meet FDA requirements related to donor health history assessment to determine eligibility. The DHQ has since been adopted by most blood centers in the United States. The FDA does not require licensed blood manufacturers to implement those DHQ documents, but the use of alternative procedures for collecting required information from blood donors is subject to FDA review and acceptance. In addition, the FDA acknowledges that the DHQ documents contain questions related to issues not addressed by any FDA requirement or recommendation, as follows: cancer; organ, tissue, or marrow transplants; bone or skin grafts; and pregnancy. Because the FDA does not require screening for these issues, blood centers can choose to eliminate the questions from the DHQ and will still be in compliance with FDA requirements. However, blood centers that eliminate these questions will be out of compliance with AABB *Standards*. The task force and the AABB recommend that blood centers implement the new donor screening materials in their entirety, which include the following documents:

- Full-length DHQ (Appendix 5-3).
- DHQ User Brochure, including glossary and references.
- Medication Deferral List (Appendix 5-4).
- Blood Donor Educational Materials (Appendix 5-5).

All DHQ documents that the FDA has recognized as acceptable are available from the FDA website at http://www.fda.gov/Biologics BloodVaccines/BloodBloodProducts/Approved Products/LicensedProductsBLAs/BloodDonor Screening/ucm164185.htm. The most current version is also available from the AABB website at http://www.aabb.org>Resource Center> Blood Donation Information>Donor History Questionnaires>Blood Donor History Questionnaire.

The questionnaire was evaluated for comprehension in focus groups and cognitive interviews; therefore, the wording, order, and text of the DHQ questions should not be changed. A collection facility may make minor changes to the time frame of a question on the DHQ only if the revision makes the question more restrictive (ie, the revision would result in the deferral of more donors). Blood centers may choose to add local questions, but local questions must be placed at the end of the DHQ. The task force prepared the DHQ documents so that the documents may be self-administered by the donor, but blood centers may choose to use direct oral questioning, self-administration, or a combination of both methods. Recent studies demonstrated that donors are more likely to provide information about HIV risk behavior [ie, injection drug use, males having sex with other males (MSM)] in self-administered interview formats (ie computer-assisted self-interviewing, or CASI) than they are to provide such sensitive information through direct verbal questioning.[38,39] The recent research findings contradict earlier studies conducted in the 1990s that favored direct, oral questions for eliciting HIV risk behavior. The recent research also provides the support for the current option to allow self-administration of the entire questionnaire.[40,41]

In addition, the DHQ User Brochure contains optional flow charts for each question to guide the health historian through the donor questionnaire process. If the eligibility decision is delimited by AABB or FDA guidance recommendations, the flow chart defines the risk period for the behavior, indicates the need to defer the donor, and provides the required deferral period. If AABB standards or FDA regulations do not address specific health conditions, the blood center must develop standard operating procedures (SOPs) for determining the criteria for donor acceptance or deferral criteria. A rational approach to donor health history assessment would balance the need to take appropriate precautions to protect the blood supply and the need to eliminate those measures that introduce unnecessarily restrictive blood donor deferral policies that could adversely affect blood availability without contributing to either recipient or donor safety. Decisions about donor eligibility should be based on available evidence to evaluate the risk that the medical condition or history poses to the blood donor and to transfusion recipients. If a potential exists for risk to the recipient or donor, the effectiveness and incremental benefit of screening donors by questioning should be evaluated, especially in light of other safeguards that protect the donor or other transfusion practices that mitigate potential risk to the recipient.

After a center receives postdonation information about a diagnosis or factor that is a cause for deferral, any subsequent actions such as product retrieval, market withdrawal, or consignee notification should be commensurate with the potential hazard and the likelihood of possible harm to the recipient. The center's approach to developing donor deferral criteria should take into account evidence as it becomes available to modify those decisions. Some of those issues that allow for medical judgment and for which questions exist in the DHQ are considered in greater detail later, but each donor center must develop and follow its own SOPs.

POSSIBLE MEASURES OF THE EFFECTIVENESS OF THE DONOR INTERVIEW

The contribution of the donor interview to blood safety is not known and is not readily amenable to study.[42] Donor education, self-exclusion, and health history screening may winnow out infected donors, as suggested by the lower prevalence of key infectious disease markers among first-time blood donors compared to the general US population. (See Table 5-2.) However, it may not be possible to define the extent to which the questions contribute to that difference. The demographics of the donor population are significantly different from those of the general population, and only a relatively small percentage of presenting donors are deferred for risk behaviors. (See Table 5-4.)

The questionnaire's effectiveness in eliminating donors considered to be at risk of infections has been used to evaluate the screening process. The National Heart, Lung, and Blood Institute (NHLBI) Retrovirus Epidemiologic Donor Study (REDS) sought to measure, through a series of anonymous blood donor mail surveys, the prevalence of blood donors who have risk factors that should have prevented their blood donations.[42-44] Donors who were identified as having deferrable risk through the survey mechanism represented the failures (false-negatives) of the screening process. The risk behavior that should have resulted in deferral is termed "deferrable risk." Deferrable risk prevalence among REDS donors at five blood centers was 1.9% in 1993 and 3.0% in 1998.[42-44]

Although the survey identified donors with deferrable risk factors that pose a potential risk and established the rate of failure in obtaining accurate answers to screening questions, this approach does not provide information as to how many of the deferred donors were infected or were capable of transmitting infection through their donated units. Zou et al addressed this issue by testing blood donors who were deferred either permanently or temporarily for hepatitis risk.[45,46] The blood donors who were indefinitely deferred for a history of hepatitis or intravenous drug use were more likely to have higher hepatitis marker rates than were those donors who were not deferred.[45] In contrast, blood donors who were deferred temporarily for questions related to potential risk for infection or exposure to hepatitis, but who returned to donate, did not appear to pose a higher risk compared to first-time or repeat donors.[46] These data demonstrate that temporarily deferred donors who return to donate pose no greater risk than do other donors, and the data may suggest that some questions can be safely eliminated.[46] Donors deferred even for short periods are less likely to ever return to donate.[46-48] Because the study could evaluate only the donors who returned to donate after having been deferred, definitive conclusions are not possible on the prevalence of infectious disease markers among all temporarily deferred donors.

Blood centers have reported experience with their transition to the DHQ and its effect on the screening process.[49-51] The broader question of the current contribution of the donor interview to blood safety or possible ways to improve the process remain unanswered. The value of retaining deferral criteria that have remained unchanged since their introduction two decades ago, which was before the availability of infectious disease tests (eg, remote history of risk behavior), has been described as scientifically unwarranted.[51] Regardless, an unwillingness to change the donor questionnaire perhaps reflects the profound and deeply ingrained concern that any modification could possibly introduce some degree of risk, however remote. Further research is warranted to define the value (or the lack of value) of donor questioning, with a view to eliminate or at least change some questions that do not contribute to the safety of the blood supply.

BLOOD-CENTER-DEFINED DONOR ELIGIBILITY CRITERIA

Unlike questions about potential infectious disease risks and most other recipient safety issues, questions directed primarily at protecting the safety of the donor are left to the discretion of the blood center's medical director. Consequently, acceptance criteria vary at different blood centers.[4-6] AABB *Standards* requires that the prospective donor appear to be in good health and be free of major organ disease (eg, heart, liver, lungs), cancer, or abnormal bleeding tendency, unless determined eligible by the medical director.[2(p57)] The rationale behind each deferral for medical conditions should be carefully considered, because even temporary deferrals will adversely affect the likelihood that individuals will return to donate blood.[46-48] Although few studies have been published, donor centers have successfully eliminated some questions and liberalized acceptance criteria without having an effect on donor reaction rates.[52] Because donors must feel healthy and well on the day of donation and because they are evaluated for cardiac and bleeding problems among other conditions, imposing additional arbitrary and rigid criteria that are ostensibly intended to protect the donor is unnecessary.

Cancer

Direct transmission of cancer through blood transfusion—although biologically plausible—is exceedingly unlikely and has not yet been documented to occur.[53] In contrast, the inadvertent transfusion of blood from donors with cancer occurs relatively frequently. A retrospective study examined the incidence of cancer among patients in Denmark and Sweden who received blood from donors with subclinical cancer at the time of donation. Of the 354,094 transfusion recipients, 12,012 (3%) were exposed to blood components from precancerous donors, yet there was no excess risk of cancer among recipients of blood from precancerous donors when compared with recipients of blood from donors without cancer.[54] The authors found no evidence of cancer transmission from blood donors who had incident cancer to transfusion recipients, and the authors concluded that if transmission does occur, it is so rare that it could not be captured in their large cohort, which included the total blood experience of two countries over several years.

Any residual risk of direct transmission of an oncogenic clone is likely mitigated by the lack of genetic similarity between transfusion recipients and the general donor population and by the metastatic inefficiency of circulating cancer cells. In addition, common transfusion practices such as leukocyte reduction and irradiation have been shown to remove circulating cancer cells or to render the cells incapable of dividing, respectively. Previously transfused patients may have a twofold increased risk for developing non-Hodgkin lymphoma when compared to untransfused individuals, which could reflect an immunosuppressive effect of allogeneic transfusion. However, the increased risk may also result from other coincident risk factors associated with transfusion.[55] Screening donors by asking them about a history of cancer is not an effective means to prevent individuals who have occult cancer from donating. Consideration could be given to eliminating the practice completely. Some degree of caution may still be warranted to allow sufficient time for donors to recover from cancer treatment. Because there currently are no US federal regulations or professional standards regarding the specific criteria that should be used to evaluate donors with a history of cancer, the blood center's medical director has considerable flexibility in determining donor eligibility policies. The vast majority of blood centers currently accept donors who report localized cancers after treatment, with no deferral period. These cancers include skin cancer (eg, basal cell or squamous cell carcinoma) and carcinoma in situ (eg, cervical) that have been fully excised and are considered cured.

Most blood centers will defer a donor with a history of a solid organ or nonhematologic malignancy for a defined period after completion of treatment, provided the donor remains symptom-free without relapse. The deferral period following completion of treatment for nonhematologic cancer ranges from 1 to 5 years.[53,56] Hematologic malignancy typically results in the permanent deferral of the donor, although exceptions were reported by some US blood centers who accept adults if they were successfully treated for childhood leukemia or lymphoma, after a defined cancer-free interval following completion of treatment.[53] Given the available evidence, these various deferral policies are currently defensible but should be reevaluated if additional information becomes available.

Bleeding Conditions or Blood Diseases

Bleeding conditions or blood diseases have the potential to affect donor safety as well as product potency, but there are no specific FDA regulations or recommendations regarding donor eligibility. Blood centers must define their procedures for handling donors with hematologic disorders. In general, prospective donors should be evaluated for bleeding conditions or blood diseases 1) that place the donors at risk for bleeding or thrombosis as a result of the collection procedure and 2) that may affect the hemostatic efficacy of their blood and suitability for transfusion to others.[5] Plasma components and Cryoprecipitated AHF should contain adequate amounts of functional coagulation factors and should not contain significant inhibitory or prothrombotic factors. Similarly, platelet components intended as the sole source for patients should contain platelets that have adequate function and that are not irreversibly impaired by the presence of inhibitors. Individuals with a history of significant bleeding are best counseled to avoid donation, although screening does not prevent rare but serious thrombotic or hemorrhagic complications in otherwise healthy blood donors. Compartment syndrome, which results from extensive antecubital bleeding, neurovascular compromise, and tissue necrosis, has been reported in two whole blood donors, neither of whom was reported to have underlying hemorrhagic diatheses.[57,58] Similarly, upper extremity deep vein thromboses have been reported in two whole blood donors and two apheresis donors, none of whom were found upon subsequent evaluation to have an underlying hypercoagulable state.[59-62]

Individuals with hemophilia, clotting factor deficiencies, or clinically significant inhibitors—all of which manifest with variable bleeding tendencies—require deferral for both donor safety and product potency considerations. The exception is Factor XII deficiency, which is not associated with either bleeding or thrombosis. Carriers of autosomal-recesssive or sex-linked recessive mutations in clotting factors usually are not at risk for bleeding. They typically have decreased factor levels but are accepted by most blood centers because of the normal, wide variability in clotting factor activity levels (50%-150%) compared to the much lower relative activity that is necessary to maintain hemostasis (5%-30%).[5] Individuals with von Willebrand disease are typically deferred by most blood centers, although some may allow individuals with mild disease and no history of bleeding to donate red cells.

Donors with thrombosis or thrombophilia taking anticoagulants to treat acute venous thromboembolism, or who are receiving lifelong therapy to prevent recurrence, are deferred for both donor safety and product potency considerations. Inherited hypercoagulable states are common in the general population and are associated with an increased but generally low lifetime risk of venous thromboembolism, which is only slightly higher than the risk to women taking oral contraceptives. Consequently, most donor centers accept women taking oral contraceptives as well as those individuals with Factor V Leiden, the prothrombin G20210A mutation, or hyperhomocysteinemia, as long as the individuals are not currently undergoing anticoagulant therapy.

Donors with a history of immune thrombocytopenia (ITP, formerly known as immune thrombocytopenic purpura) are accepted, after successful treatment, by most blood centers, although the definition of cure varies from center to center.[5] Criteria should include normal platelet counts after complete discontinuation of therapy and no history of splenectomy, which could be associated with persistent platelet antibodies despite normal platelet counts. Some blood collection agencies accept donors whose ITP resolved in childhood; others defer individuals with chronic ITP regardless of treatment outcome.[5]

Red cell disorders that impair the function or survival of transfused red cells are causes for deferral (eg, sickle cell disease). Most blood centers accept individuals with sickle cell trait, because these donors are typically healthy and because their blood is suitable for most transfusions. Red cell components that are positive for hemoglobin S (HbS) may not be selected for critically ill neonates and for patients with sickle cell disease, but the components can be screened for HbS to meet the special needs and medical preferences for transfusion to these patient subgroups.

Although hereditary hemochromatosis (HH) is a disorder of iron metabolism and not a blood disease, donors may voluntarily disclose a diagnosis of HH during the donor interview. The standard treatment to reduce iron levels for individuals with HH is regular therapeutic phlebotomy. The FDA allows blood centers to use blood collected from individuals during therapeutic phlebotomy but requires the conspicuous labeling of the units with the patient's condition,[63] which has proven a barrier to the use of the blood for transfusion in hospitals. Since August 1999, however, the FDA has allowed US blood centers to obtain variances to the regulations about labeling and about the frequency of collection from individuals with HH. The variance requires that blood centers provide therapeutic phlebotomy free of charge to all individuals with HH regardless of their eligibility as blood donors.[64] Estimates of the effect of hemochromatosis donor programs on the blood supply in the United States have been as high as an additional 2.3 million units, but more conservative estimates drawing on data collected from 18 blood centers suggest an increase of 58,000 units annually.[65,66] (The list of donor centers that provide the service is available on the FDA website at http://www.fda.gov/BiologicsBloodVaccines/BloodBloodProducts/RegulationoftheBloodSupply/Variances/ucm164649.htm.) Although the current contribution of hemochromatosis donor programs to the blood supply is not known with certainty, such programs likely augment the blood supply and offer other intangible value to the donor, the blood center, and the community.

Heart and Lung Conditions

Deferral policies for donors with a history of cardiac or pulmonary disease vary in different blood centers, but the deferral policies are presumably based on concerns reflecting the acute blood volume reduction, vasovagal reactions, or medical effects that may blunt the physiologic compensation to blood donation.[4] The low rate of severe reactions in autologous blood donors who are scheduled for cardiac surgery or transplantation has led many blood centers to eliminate stringent, blanket deferrals for all donors who have ever had cardiac disease. This allowance is important considering the burden of cardiovascular disease in the United States, which affects an estimated 79.4 million (1 in 3) Americans.[67] The collective, published experience with autologous donation by patients scheduled for cardiac procedures has demonstrated that adverse effects are not more frequent when compared to the experience of donors without a history of cardiac disease.[68-73] Vasovagal reactions occur in about 2% to 5% of whole blood donations by healthy donors; serious reaction and donor injury are uncommon.[74]

A rational approach to donors with a history of cardiac disease would allow the acceptance of donors who are asymptomatic on the day of donation, who have been medically evaluated, and who report no functional impairment or limitations on daily activity after being diagnosed or treated for cardiac disease. Some donor centers use 6 months as an appropriate interval for accepting allogeneic donors with a history of cardiac disease if they have been asymptomatic and are able to perform their usual daily activities. Causes for deferral may include recent symptoms, limitations on activity or functional impairment resulting from unstable angina, recent myocardial infarction, left main coronary disease, ongoing congestive heart failure, or severe aortic stenosis.

Medications

The DHQ Medication Deferral List contains the required deferrals specified by the AABB and the FDA. These criteria take into account the potential harm that a drug taken by the donor poses to a transfusion recipient or to a developing fetus; the criteria also identify individuals at risk for infection who take the following medications:

- Teratogens with long elimination half-lives that persist for extended periods in the circulation, such as the following:

    1. Finasteride (Proscar, Propecia), isotretinoin (Accutane, Amnesteem, Claravis, Sotret)—1-month deferral.
    2. Dutasteride (Avodart, Jalyn)—6-month deferral.
    3. Acitretin (Soriatane)—3-year deferral.
    4. Etretinate (Tegison)—permanent deferral.

- Growth hormone from human pituitary glands (permanent deferral) for the theoretical risk of transfusion-transmitted Creutzfeldt-Jakob disease (CJD) (no cases described to date).
- Bovine insulin if imported from countries with bovine spongiform encephalopathy (indefinite deferral) for potential variant CJD (vCJD) risk to recipients (no cases linked to bovine insulin have been described to date, although transmission of vCJD with blood transfusion has been demonstrated).
- Hepatitis B Immune Globulin (12-month deferral).
- Unlicensed vaccines (12-month deferral, unless determined eligible by the medical director).

The FDA has published additional guidance recommending evaluation of other medications for apheresis platelet donors.[75] The following are captured in DHQ version 1.3:

- Feldene (2-day deferral for platelet donors; does not affect whole blood donation).
- Plavix and Ticlid (14-day deferral for platelet donors; does not affect whole blood donation).

Antibiotics are addressed in a separate question in the DHQ, to determine if the donor is taking antibiotics to treat a bacterial infection that could be transmitted through blood transfusion. Most donor centers, however, will accept individuals who are taking preventive antibiotics for acne, rosacea, and other chronic conditions. Common medications such as antihypertensive drugs are not a cause for deferral, but the blood pressure measured on the day of donation must be acceptable. Nutritional supplements that are available over the counter typically are not a cause for deferral.

Although blood centers may elect to add requirements to the Medication Deferral List, many have chosen to use the list as presented by the FDA and the AABB or have added only a few drugs. The DHQ task force has encouraged blood centers to fully consider the rationale behind each local deferral and to keep such local practices to a minimum.[76] Local medication deferrals are often based on concerns about the reason for taking the medication and about the underlying medical condition rather than on any inherent threat posed by residual medication in the collected blood component. These considerations need to be evaluated in the context of all the other safeguards that are in place to protect the donor. Most drugs pose no harm to the recipient, and many factors should be considered when evaluating possible risk (eg, half-life, mean and peak plasma concentration, residual concentration in blood component, dilution with transfusion to recipient). Unnecessarily restrictive deferral policies for medications likely do not improve donor or recipient safety.

Almost universal additions to the Medication Deferral List have included heparin, warfarin, and certain other anticoagulants, because of the drugs' effects on the potency of plasma or platelet components and because of the potential for impaired hemostasis in the donor after the collection procedure. Many donors taking heparin and warfarin are otherwise ineligible because of the underlying disease that necessitates anticoagulation therapy. If the underlying disease is not a cause for deferral, an appropriate deferral period is still needed to ensure normal coagulation factor levels following discontinuation of the drugs. The specific deferrals for medications that irreversibly inhibit platelet function as currently defined by AABB and the FDA are limited to plateletpheresis[75] or use of the donor as the sole source of platelets.[2(p57)] Platelets prepared from whole blood donations cannot be labeled as being aspirin-free unless this history is obtained from each donor at the time of donation. For aspirin or aspirin-containing medications, plateletpheresis donors should be deferred for 48 hours after ingestion of aspirin.[75] For other medications that irreversibly inhibit platelet function, the medical director should define the deferral policy.

ABBREVIATED DONOR HISTORY QUESTIONNAIRE FOR FREQUENT DONORS

Blood centers have recognized for years that at every donation, frequent and repeat donors must answer the same questions about remote risk factors that are not likely to change—a situation that leaves many dedicated donors dissatisfied with the donation experience. A small number of US blood centers have received approval from the FDA to use an abbreviated DHQ (aDHQ) for donors who have successfully completed multiple administrations of the full-length questionnaire in use at the center and who have recently donated. The experience of these blood centers suggests that blood safety is not compromised by the abbreviated procedures and that donors perceive an improvement in the donation experience.[77] Given the extremely low risks of transfusion-transmitted infections, it is virtually impossible to prove conclusively that a change in the donor questionnaire did not affect donor safety. As a result, these concerns have hampered progress toward adoption of an abbreviated DHQ that is acceptable for use by the entire blood banking community.[78]

At the time of publication, the aDHQ, which was developed and validated by the same task force as the full-length DHQ, was under review by the FDA. Two "capture questions" about new diagnoses or treatments since the last donation replace 17 previous questions about remote risks (eg, blood transfusion, Chagas disease, babesiosis). To qualify for the aDHQ, a donor must have completed the full-length DHQ on two separate occasions in the past year, with at least one donation within the past 6 months, making it highly unlikely that the responses to these questions would have changed. Once the aDHQ is recognized by the FDA, a blood center that chooses to implement it must ensure that it is administered only to frequent donors who qualify for its use. The aDHQ may improve donors' satisfaction with the donation experience and may increase donors' willingness to continue to donate if the process becomes or is perceived as less onerous and time consuming. Although the aDHQ is only modestly shortened and restricted in use, it demonstrates that the blood banking organizations and the FDA are trying to improve the committed donor's experience.

POSTDONATION INSTRUCTIONS

After the collection procedure, blood donors are instructed to call the donor center if they have any concerns about the safety of their blood or if they believe that their blood should not be transfused. The postdonation instructions provide another opportunity to educate the donor and may contribute to blood safety. Although postdonation instruction is provided, a confidential unit exclusion (CUE) procedure is no longer used in most blood centers in the United States. CUE provided donors with a mechanism to indicate in a confidential manner whether or not the blood collected should be released for transfusion. The requirement for CUE was rescinded by the FDA in 1992, but it was still in use through 2005 by many blood centers. A study by Zou et al[79] provided a convincing demonstration of: 1) its minimal effectiveness in further reducing the transmission of infectious diseases through window-period units, 2) its association with errors in the selection of the CUE options by donors, and 3) the loss of large numbers of eligible donors.

RECIPIENT-SPECIFIC "DESIGNATED" OR "DIRECTED" BLOOD DONATION

Exceptional Medical Need

In certain clinical circumstances, a patient may benefit from blood components collected from a specific donor. As examples, 1) patients with multiple antibodies or with antibodies to high-incidence antigens may require units from donors whose red cells are negative for the corresponding antigens, or 2) an infant with neonatal alloimmune thrombocytopenia may require antigen-negative platelets from the mother.

Frequent donation by a specific donor for a specific patient with a medical need requires that the donor center have a procedure that typically calls for both a request from the patient's physician and approval by the donor center's physician. The donor must meet all allogeneic donor selection requirements, with the exception of the frequency of donation, which can be as often as every 3 days as long as the predonation hemoglobin meets or exceeds the minimum value for routine allogeneic blood donation. For frequent blood donors, the CFR allows for qualifying the donor by testing the first donation in each 30-day period.[80] Blood components can be released before infectious disease test results are available in appropriately documented emergency situations, provided that the units are labeled and managed in accordance with the CFR. Testing on the units must be completed as soon as possible after release or shipment, and results must be promptly reported to the hospital or transfusion service.[81]

Directed Donors

The ongoing demand from patients to choose specific donors who provide blood for their transfusions during scheduled surgeries likely still reflects the skewed perception among the general public of the risk for HIV associated with blood transfusion. Despite the lack of evidence of improved safety with directed donation, most blood centers and hospitals surmount the associated collection, storage, and tracking logistical difficulties to provide the service. Rates of positive tests for viral markers were lower in volunteer donors with a history of blood donation than in first-time blood donors and donors who provided recipient-specific blood.[82] There is no evidence that directed donors are safer to use than are volunteer community donors. Rather, directed donors may feel unduly pressured to give blood, and this could compromise the donor's interview and blood safety.[83,84] Regardless, directed donors must meet all of the same criteria as voluntary donors, and their blood can be used for other patients if not needed by the individual for whom the donations were initially intended. If collection of whole blood is required from a directed donor more than once in an 8-week period, the CFR requires that the donor be examined and certified by a physician on the day of donation to be in good health.[1]

The donor center should clearly communicate its procedures so that the expectations regarding availability of directed-donor units are known to the ordering physician and patient. The communication required includes defining the interval required between collection of the blood and its availability to the patient, mentioning the possibility that the patient will identify donors who are not ABO-compatible or not otherwise acceptable blood donors, and defining the policy for release of units for transfusion to other patients.

Selection of Autologous Donors

Autologous donations declined dramatically in the United States between 1992 and 1997, leveled off from 1997 to 2001, and decreased again from 2001 to 2008.[85] In 2008, US autologous collections comprised only 261,000 units, or 1.5% of total blood collections. Waning interest in autologous donations may reflect the decline in viral risk associated with allogeneic blood transfusion and consequently the minimal medical benefit and increased cost of autologous blood.[86-89] In general, the use of preoperative autologous blood donation alone provides only a relatively small benefit in reducing the probability of allogeneic transfusion and may actually increase the risk of lower postoperative hematocrits, with enhanced risk of ischemia.[89] As routine alternatives to allogeneic transfusion, preoperative autologous donations are often used in conjunction with other blood conservation methods such as acute normovolemic hemodilution, perioperative blood recovery, and pharmacologic strategies. (See the further discussion in Chapter 24.)

Despite the remarkable improvement in viral safety of the blood supply, the American public still erroneously perceives HIV to be the major risk of blood transfusion.[11,90] Autologous donation is an option that should be discussed with any patient as part of the consent process for a scheduled elective surgical procedure for which blood transfusion is likely. Such consent is mandated in California and other states, which specifically require documentation in the patient's medical record that the patient was informed of his or her transfusion options.[91] In selected patient groups, autologous donation has been reported to decrease allogeneic blood transfusion, preventing exposure in many cases.[87,92] However, the frequent observation of 1-unit transfusions suggests the limited utility of such programs,[87] as does the observation that patients who donated autologous blood were more likely to receive any blood transfusions (autologous, allogeneic, or both) than were those who did not.[88] Because ABO-incompatible transfusions related to medical error are among the most commonly reported causes of transfusion-related deaths, one could argue that autologous donation puts patients at greater risk for harm by increasing their chance of receiving an incompatible transfusion. Autologous donation cannot prevent other transfusion complications such as bacterial contamination of the unit, cytokine-mediated reactions, or circulatory overload.[86]

Although autologous blood currently represents only 1.5% of all blood collections, there may be renewed enthusiasm if new infectious diseases emerge to threaten the safety of the blood supply. Alternatively, autologous donations may become part of a strategy to augment the local blood supply if blood collection fails to keep pace with the demand for blood. Thus, judicious use of preoperative autologous blood donation in conjunction with other blood conservation methods remains an appropriate alternative for some patients.[92]

Autologous Donor Selection Criteria

Candidates for preoperative collection of autologous blood are patients who can tolerate phlebotomy and blood loss and who are scheduled for surgical procedures that are likely to require blood transfusion. The most common surgical procedures for which autologous blood is collected are total joint replacements, followed by other major orthopedic procedures, vascular surgery, and cardiac or thoracic surgery.[92] Autologous blood should not be collected for procedures that seldom (less than 10% of cases) require transfusion, such as cholecystectomy, herniorrhaphy, vaginal hysterectomy, and uncomplicated obstetric delivery.[92]

Patients identified as candidates for autologous donation are evaluated by the donor center. The following criteria are specified by the FDA, AABB, or both (see Appendix 5-1):

- Obtain a prescription or order from the patient's physician.

- ◆ Require a minimum hemoglobin concentration of 11 g/dL (hematocrit, 33%).
- ◆ Collect at least 72 hours before the anticipated surgery or transfusion.
- ◆ Defer for conditions presenting risk of bacteremia.
- ◆ Use only for the donor-patient. If exceptional circumstances warrant transfusion to a recipient other than the donor, the decision must be approved by the medical director on a case-by-case basis, and units shall not be issued for transfusion unless results of all infectious disease testing are negative.

Additional selection criteria are locally defined for other potential donor safety issues, such as heart and lung disease, bleeding conditions and blood disorders, cancer, and pregnancy. The risks associated with autologous blood collection for some patients with significant cardiac disease may be greater than the currently estimated risks for allogeneic donors because more liberal selection criteria are used. Contraindications for autologous blood donation should be defined by the blood center and may include those individuals thought to be at greatest risk from blood donation, such as individuals with 1) unstable angina, 2) recent myocardial infarction or cerebrovascular accident, 3) significant cardiac or pulmonary disease with ongoing symptoms but who have not been evaluated by the treating physician, or 4) untreated aortic stenosis.[92] Autologous collection in an uncomplicated pregnancy should not be performed unless circumstances exist that increase the risk of transfusion. However, both the ordering physician and the donor center physician need to carefully consider the risks of the collection procedure against any perceived benefit.[93] Similarly, autologous collection from pediatric patients has been reported, but a rational approach is strongly advocated.[94] Although hospital-based blood centers have offered preoperative autologous donation to very young children and even to infants, most non-hospital-affiliated blood centers either do not provide the service or accept only adolescents with adequate peripheral venous access who are old enough to understand and to cooperate fully with the standard collection procedure, and who are scheduled for surgical procedures that are expected to result in an acute loss of more than 15% to 20% of the total blood volume.

KEY POINTS

1. The Donor History Questionnaire (DHQ) and associated documents were developed by an AABB task force and are recognized by the Food and Drug Administration (FDA) as adequate measures to determine the eligibility of volunteers for allogeneic blood donation.
2. The most current versions of the DHQ and associated documents are available from the AABB website, and all DHQ documents that the FDA has recognized as acceptable are available from the FDA website (see Appendix 5-2).
3. Prospective blood donors are informed of the risks of blood donation, the clinical signs and symptoms associated with HIV infection, behavioral risk factors for transmission of bloodborne pathogens, and the importance of refraining from blood donation if they are at an increased risk of being infected.
4. To be accepted for blood donation, prospective blood donors must feel healthy and well on the day of donation and must meet all AABB and FDA requirements and criteria defined by the donor centers.
5. In certain clinical circumstances (eg, rare phenotype or antigen-negative RBC units needed), a patient may benefit from blood components collected from a specific donor who may not otherwise meet all the requirements for a volunteer donor. The blood center must have procedures and follow federal regulations for frequent donation by a specific donor for a designated patient with a medical need.

6. The ongoing demand from patients to choose specific donors who provide blood for their transfusions during scheduled surgeries, in the absence of a defined medical need, persists despite the lack of evidence of improved safety with directed donation.
7. Directed donors must meet all of the same criteria as voluntary donors, and their blood can be used for other patients if not needed by the individual for whom the donations were initially intended.
8. Autologous donations declined dramatically in the United States in the 1990s. In 2008, US autologous collections comprised only 261,000 units, or 1.5% of total blood collections.
9. Preoperative autologous donations today are most often used in conjunction with other blood conservation methods such as acute normovolemic hemodilution, perioperative blood recovery, and pharmacologic strategies.

REFERENCES

1. Code of federal regulations. Title 21, CFR 640.3. Washington, DC: US Government Printing Office, 2010 (revised annually).
2. Carson TH, ed. Standards for blood banks and transfusion services. 27th ed. Bethesda, MD: AABB, 2011.
3. Code of federal regulations. Title 21, CFR 606.121(c)(5). Washington, DC: US Government Printing Office, 2010 (revised annually).
4. Strauss RG. Rationale for medical director acceptance or rejection of allogeneic plateletpheresis donors with underlying medical disorders. J Clin Apher 2002;17:111-17.
5. Reik RA, Burch JW, Vassallo RR, Trainor L. Unique donor suitability issues. Vox Sang 2006;90:255-64.
6. Eder A, Goldman M, Rossmann S, et al. Selection criteria to protect the blood donor in North America and Europe: Past (dogma), present (evidence), and future (hemovigilance). Transfus Med Rev 2009;23:205-20.
7. Dodd RY. Germs, gels, and genomes: A personal recollection of 30 years in blood safety testing. In: Stramer SL, ed. Blood safety in the new millennium. Bethesda, MD: AABB, 2001:97-122.
8. Fridey JL, Townsend M, Kessler D, Gregory K. A question of clarity: Redesigning the AABB blood donor history questionnaire—a chronology and model for donor screening. Transfus Med Rev 2007;21:181-204.
9. Allen JG. The epidemiology of posttransfusion hepatitis. Basic blood and plasma tabulations. Stanford, CA: Commonwealth Fund, 1972.
10. Alter HJ, Houghton M. Hepatitis C virus and eliminating post-transfusion hepatitis. Nat Med 2000;6:1082-6.
11. Busch MP, Young MJ, Samson SM, et al. Risk of human immunodeficiency virus transmission by blood transfusions prior to the implementation of HIV antibody screening in the San Francisco Bay area. Transfusion 1991;31:4-11.
12. Zou S, Dorsey KA, Notari EP, et al. Prevalence, incidence, and residual risk of human immunodeficiency virus and hepatitis C virus infections among United States blood donors since the introduction of nucleic acid testing. Transfusion 2010; 50:1495-504.
13. McQuillan GM, Coleman PJ, Kruszon-Moran D, et al. Prevalence of hepatitis B infection in the United States: The National Health and Nutrition Examination Surveys, 1976 through 1994. Am J Public Health 1999;89:14-18.
14. Food and Drug Administration. Guidance for industry: Implementation of acceptable full-length donor history questionnaire and accompanying materials for use in screening donors of blood and blood components. (October 2006) Rockville, MD: CBER Office of Communication, Outreach, and Development, 2006. [Available at http://www.fda.gov/BiologicsBloodVaccines/GuidanceComplianceRegulatoryInformation/Guidances/Blood/ucm073445.htm (accessed October 1, 2010).]
15. Code of federal regulations. Title 21, CFR 630.6. Washington, DC: US Government Printing Office, 2010 (revised annually).
16. Food and Drug Administration. Memorandum: Revised recommendations for the prevention of human immunodeficiency virus (HIV) transmission by blood and blood products. (April 23, 1992) Rockville, MD: CBER Office of Communication, Outreach, and Development, 1992.

17. Americans with Disabilities Act of 1990, Pub. L. No. 101-336,104 Stat.327 as amended July 26, 1990 (see 42 U.S.C. 12101 et seq, 2000).
18. Beutler E, Waalen J. The definition of anemia: What is the lower limit of normal of the blood hemoglobin concentration? Blood 2006;107: 1747-50.
19. Code of federal regulations. Title 21, CFR 640.3(b)(3). Washington, DC: US Government Printing Office, 2010 (revised annually).
20. Fulwood F, Johnson CI, Bryner JD, et al. Hematological and nutritional biochemistry reference data for persons 6 months-74 years of age; United States, 1976-1980. Vital and health statistics, Series 11, No. 232. (PHS) 83-1682. Washington, DC: Public Health Service, National Center for Heath Statistics, Government Printing Office, 1982.
21. Wood EM, Kim DM, Miller JP. Accuracy of predonation Hct sampling affects donor safety, eligibility, and deferral rates. Transfusion 2001; 41:353-9.
22. Cable RG. Hemoglobin determination in blood donors. Transfus Med Rev 1995;9:131-44.
23. James V, Jones KF, Turner EM, Sokol RJ. Statistical analysis of inappropriate results from current Hb screening methods for blood donors. Transfusion 2003;43:400-4.
24. Cable RG. Hb screening of blood donors: How close is close enough? Transfusion 2003;43: 306-8.
25. Mannarino AD, Macpherson CR. Copper sulfate screening of blood donors: Report of a donor passing the test with less than 8 grams of hemoglobin. Transfusion 1963;3:398-400.
26. Newman B. Very anemic donors may pass copper sulfate screening tests. Transfusion 1997;37:670.
27. Kliman A. The microhematocrit test as a method for evaluating deferment by copper sulfate. Transfusion 1967;7:425-31.
28. Keating LJ, Gorman R, Moore R. Hemoglobin and hematocrit values of blood donors. Transfusion 1967;7:420-4.
29. Kline L, Baker N, Dodd RY. Effect of a quantitative hemoglobin test on donor deferral rates (abstract). In: Book of abstracts from the 1990 Joint Congress of ISBT and AABB. Arlington, VA: AABB, 1990:150.
30. Goldman MR. Another stab at donor hemoglobin screening. Transfusion 2005;45:1552-3.
31. Lotfi R, Wernet D, Starke U, et al. A noninvasive strategy for screening prospective blood donors for anaemia. Transfusion 2005;45: 1585-92.
32. Morse EE, Cable R, Pisciotto P, et al. Evaluation of iron status in women identified by copper sulfate screening as ineligible to donate blood. Transfusion 1987;27:238-41.
33. Simon TL, Garry PJ, Hooper EM. Iron stores in blood donors. JAMA 1981;245:2038-43.
34. Sempos CT, Looker AC, Gillum RF, Makuc DM. Body iron stores and the risk of coronary heart disease. N Engl J Med 1994;330:1119-24.
35. Meyers DG, Jensen KC, Menitove JE. A historical cohort study of the effect of lowering body iron through blood donation on incident cardiac events. Transfusion 2002; 42:1135-9.
36. Ascherio A, Rimm EB, Giovannucci E, et al. Blood donations and risk of coronary heart disease in men. Circulation 2001;103:52-7.
37. Murray-Kolb LE, Beard JE. Iron treatment normalizes cognitive functioning in young women (abstract). Am J Clin Nutr 2007; 85:778-87.
38. Katz LM, Cumming PD, Wallace EL, Abrams PS. Audiovisual touch-screen computer-assisted self-interviewing for donor health histories: Results from two years' experience with the system. Transfusion 2005;45:171-80.
39. Turner CF, Ku L, Rogers SM, et al. Adolescent sexual behavior, drug use, and violence: Increased reporting with computer survey technology. Science 1998;280:867-73.
40. Mayo DJ, Rose AM, Matchett SE, et al. Screening potential blood donors at risk for human immunodeficiency virus. Transfusion 1991;31: 466-74.
41. Gimble JG, Friedman LI. Effects of oral donor questioning about high-risk behaviors for human immunodeficiency virus infection. Transfusion 1992;32:446-9.
42. Kleinman S, Williams AE. Donor selection procedures: Is it possible to improve them? Transfus Med Rev 1998;12:288-302.
43. Williams AE, Thomson RA, Schreiber GB, et al. Estimates of infectious disease risk factors in US blood donors. JAMA 1997; 277:967-72.
44. Glynn SA, Smith JW, Schreiber GB, et al. Repeat whole-blood and plateletpheresis donors: Unreported deferrable risks, reactive screening tests, and response to incentive programs. Transfusion 2001;41:736-43.
45. Zou S, Fujii K, Johnson S, et al. Prevalence of selected viral infections among blood donors deferred for potential risk to blood safety. Transfusion 2006;46:1997-2003.

46. Zou S, Musavi F, Notari EP, et al. Prevalence of selected viral infections among temporarily deferred donors who returned to donate blood: American Red Cross blood donor study. Transfusion 2005;45:1593-600.
47. Halperin D, Baetens J, Newman B. The effect of short-term, temporary deferral on future blood donation. Transfusion 1998;38:181-3.
48. Piliavin JA. Temporary deferral and donor return. Transfusion 1987;27:199-200.
49. Katz LM. AABB UDHQ: New vs old (abstract). Transfusion 2005;45(3S):22A.
50. Zou S, Musavi F, Eder AF, et al. Changes in donor deferrals following implementation of the uniform donor history questionnaire at two blood centers (abstract). Transfusion 2005;45 (3S):22A.
51. Food and Drug Administration. Workshop on behavior-based deferrals in the NAT era (transcript). (March 8, 2006) Rockville, MD: Office of Communication, Outreach, and Development, 2006. [(Available at http://www.fda.gov/downloads/BiologicsBloodVaccines/NewsEvents/WorkshopsMeetingsConferences/TranscriptsMinutes/UCM054430.pdf (accessed October 1, 2010).]
52. Tomasulo PA, Anderson AJ, Paluso MB, et al. A study of criteria for blood donor deferral. Transfusion 1980;20:511-18.
53. Eder AF. Blood donors with a history of cancer. In: Eder AF, Bianco C, eds. Screening blood donors: Science, reason, and the donor history questionnaire. Bethesda, MD: AABB Press, 2007:77-92.
54. Edgren G, Hjalgrim H, Reilly M, et al. Risk of cancer after blood transfusion from donors with subclinical cancer: A retrospective cohort study. Lancet 2007;369:1724-30.
55. Vamvakas EC. Allogeneic blood transfusion as a risk factor for subsequent development of non-Hodgkin's lymphoma. Transfus Med Rev 2000;14:258-68.
56. Purdy E, Jensen K, Perry E, Gorlin J. Success of reinstating donors previously deferred five years for history of cancer (abstract). Transfusion 2005;45(Suppl):174a.
57. Newman B. Arterial puncture phlebotomy in whole-blood donors. Transfusion 2001;41:1390-2.
58. Gibble J, Ness PM. Compartment syndrome and hand amputation after whole blood phlebotomy: Report of a case (abstract). Transfusion 1999;39(Suppl):30S.
59. Covin RB, Rich NL, Asola A. Upper-extremity deep venous thrombosis complicating whole blood donation. Transfusion 2004;44:586-90.
60. Featherstone T, Bayliss AP. Deep venous thrombosis of the upper extremity—A case report. Angiology 1987;38:793-6.
61. Jones DA, Williams E, Riley SA, Makris M. Axillary vein thrombosis in a healthy donor following platelet apheresis. Br J Haematol 2002;116:390-1.
62. Llop I, Blanquer A, Larrea L, Chaves A. Axillar thrombosis after platelet apheresis procedure (abstract). Transfusion 2000;40(Suppl):47S.
63. Code of federal regulations. Title 21, CFR 640.3(d). Washington, DC: US Government Printing Office, 2010 (revised annually).
64. Food and Drug Administration. Guidance for industry: Variances for blood collection from individuals with hereditary hemochromatosis. (August 22, 2001) Rockville, MD: CBER Office of Communication, Outreach, and Development, 2001. [Available at http://www.fda.gov/BiologicsBloodVaccines/GuidanceComplianceRegulatoryInformation/Guidances/Blood/ucm076719.htm (accessed October 1, 2010).]
65. Leitman SF, Browning JN, Yau YY, et al. Hemochromatosis subjects as allogeneic blood donors: A prospective study. Transfusion 2003;43:1538-44.
66. Newman B. Hemochromatosis blood donor programs: Marginal for the red blood cell supply but potentially good for patient care. Transfusion 2004;44:1535-7.
67. AHA Statistics Committee and Stroke Statistics Subcommittee. Heart disease and stroke statistics—2007 Update. Circulation 2007;115:e69-e171.
68. Kasper SM, Ellering J, Stachwitz P, et al. All adverse events in autologous blood donors with cardiac disease are not necessarily caused by blood donation. Transfusion 1998;38:669-73.
69. Mann M, Sacks HJ, Goldfinger D. Safety of autologous blood donation prior to elective surgery for a variety of potentially high risk patients. Transfusion 1983;23:229-32.
70. Hillyer CD, Hart KK, Lackey DA III, et al. Comparable safety of blood collection in "high-risk" autologous donors versus non-high-risk autologous and directed donors in a hospital setting. Am J Clin Pathol 1994;102:275-7.
71. Klapper E, Pepkowitz SH, Czer L, et al. Confirmation of the safety of autologous blood donation by patients awaiting heart or lung

transplantation. A controlled study using hemodynamic monitoring. J Thorac Cardiovasc Surg 1995;110:1594-9.

72. Dzik WH, Fleisher AG, Ciavarella D, et al. Safety and efficacy of autologous blood donation before elective aortic valve operation. Ann Thorac Surg 1992;54:1177-80.
73. Popovsky MA, Whitaker B, Arnold NL. Severe outcomes of allogeneic and autologous blood donation: Frequency and characterization. Transfusion 1995;35:734-7.
74. Eder AF, Dy BA, Kennedy J, Notari E, et al. The American Red Cross donor hemovigilance program: Complications of blood donation reported in 2006. Transfusion 2008;48:1809-19.
75. Food and Drug Administration. Guidance for industry and FDA review staff: Collection of platelets by automated methods. (December 17, 2007) Rockville, MD: CBER Office of Communication, Outreach, and Development, 2007. [Available at http://www.fda.gov/BiologicsBloodVaccines/GuidanceComplianceRegulatoryInformation/Guidances/Blooducm073382.htm (accessed October 1, 2010).]
76. Townsend MJ. Donor history questionnaire Q&A. AABB News 2004;6:18-19.
77. Kamel HT, Bassett MB, Custer B, et al. Safety and donor acceptance of an abbreviated donor history questionnaire. Transfusion 2006; 46:1745-55.
78. Topic I: AABB abbreviated questionnaire (transcript). The 78th FDA Blood Products Advisory Committee meeting, Gaithersburg, MD, December 11, 2003. Rockville, MD: Office of Communication, Outreach, and Development, 2003. [Available at http://www.fda.gov/ohrms/dockets/ac/03/transcripts/4014T1.htm (accessed October 1, 2010).]
79. Zou S, Notari EP IV, Musavi F, Dodd RY. Current impact of the confidential unit exclusion option. Transfusion 2004;44:651-7.
80. Code of federal regulations. Title 21, CFR 610.40(c)(1)(i). Washington, DC: US Government Printing Office, 2010 (revised annually).
81. Code of federal regulations. Title 21, CFR 610.40(g). Washington, DC: US Government Printing Office, 2010 (revised annually).
82. Starkey JM, MacPherson JL, Bolgiano DC, et al. Markers for transfusion-transmitted disease in different groups of blood donors. JAMA 1989; 262:3452-4.
83. Yomtovian R. Is directed blood transfusion a good idea? Med Lab Obs 1992;24:31-4.
84. Pink J, Thomson A, Wylie B. Infectious disease markers in autologous and directed donations. Transfus Med 1995;4:135-8.
85. US Department of Health and Human Services. 2009 National blood collection and utilization survey report. Washington, DC: DHHS, 2011 (in press).
86. Brecher ME, Goodnough LT. The rise and fall of preoperative autologous blood donation. Transfusion 2002;42:1618-22.
87. Goldman M, Savard R, Long A, et al. Declining value of preoperative autologous donation. Transfusion 2002;42:819-23.
88. Schved JF. Preoperative autologous blood donation: A therapy that needs to be scientifically evaluated. Transfus Clin Biol 2005; 12:365-9.
89. Cohen JA, Brecher ME. Preoperative autologous blood donation, benefit or detriment: A mathematical analysis. Transfusion 1995; 35:640-4.
90. Ficucane ML, Slovic P, Mertz CK. Public perception of the risk of blood transfusion. Transfusion 2000;40:1017-22.
91. Paul Gann Blood Safety Act. California Health and Safety Code Section 1645b. 1990 (amended 1991).
92. Goodnough LT. Autologous blood donation. Anesthesiol Clin North Am 2005;23:263-70.
93. Sayers MH. Controversies in transfusion medicine: Autologous blood donation in pregnancy. Transfusion 1990;30:172-4.
94. Eder AF. Donor limitation for neonatal and pediatric transfusion. In: Herman JH, Manno CS, eds. Pediatric transfusion therapy. Bethesda, MD: AABB Press, 2002:193-215.

◆ APPENDIX 5-1
Requirements for Allogeneic and Autologous Donor Qualification

	Allogeneic (AABB Reference Standard 5.4.1A or as indicated*; 21 CFR 640.3)	Autologous (AABB Standard 5.4.4 or as indicated*)
General and Whole Blood Donation Requirements		
Age	Conform to applicable state law or ≥16 years. [Reference Standard 5.4.1A(1)]	In situations where requirements for allogeneic donor selection or collection are not applied, alternate requirements shall be defined and documented by the medical director. (5.4.4)
Whole blood volume collected	Maximum of 10.5 mL/kg donor weight, including samples [Reference Standard 5.4.1A(2)]	Collection volume may be adjusted, but the volume of blood drawn should be proportional to the amount of anticoagulant/preservative solution in the collection container. (5.6.4; see Chapter 6) Red Blood Cells Low Volume (see preparation requirements in 5.7.5.7)
Donation interval	8 weeks after whole blood donation [21 CFR 640.3(b); 21 CFR 640.3(f); more frequent donation is permitted as follows: "A person may serve as a source of whole blood more than once in 8 weeks only if at the time of donation the person is examined and certified by a physician to be in good health.")] 16 weeks after 2-unit red cell collection [FDA Guidance: Recommendations for Collecting Red Blood Cells by Automated Apheresis Methods (February 13, 2001)] 4 weeks after infrequent plasmapheresis [21 CFR 640.120 variance to 640.3(b) based on FDA Memorandum: Revision of FDA Memorandum of August 27, 1982: Requirements for Infrequent Plasmapheresis Donors (March 10, 1995)] >2 days after plasma-, platelet-, or leukapheresis [FDA Guidance for the collection of platelets by automated methods (December 17, 2007)]	All blood collection shall be completed more than 72 hours before the time of anticipated surgery or transfusion. (5.4.4.3)

◆ APPENDIX 5-1
Requirements for Allogeneic and Autologous Donor Qualification (Continued)

	Allogeneic (AABB Reference Standard 5.4.1A or as indicated*; 21 CFR 640.3)	**Autologous (AABB Standard 5.4.4 or as indicated*)**
Blood pressure	No specific requirement in AABB standards* [21 CFR 640.3(2): "Demonstration that systolic and diastolic blood pressures are within normal limits, unless the examining physician is satisfied that an individual with blood pressures outside these limits is an otherwise qualified donor under the provisions of this section."]	In situations where requirements for allogeneic donor selection or collection are not applied, alternate requirements shall be defined and documented by the medical director. (5.4.4)
Pulse	No specific requirement in AABB standards* or CFR for whole blood donors; Source Plasma donors: 50-100 bpm [21 CFR 640.63(c)]	In situations where requirements for allogeneic donor selection or collection are not applied, alternate requirements shall be defined and documented by the medical director. (5.4.4)
Temperature	≤37.5 C (99.5 F) if measured orally, or equivalent if measured by another method [Reference Standard 5.4.1A(4); 21 CFR 640.3(1): "normal temperature"]	Deferral for conditions presenting risk of bacteremia (5.4.4.4)
Venipuncture site	The venipuncture site shall be evaluated for lesions on the skin. [Reference Standard 5.4.1A(7); 21 CFR 640.3(b)(5): "Freedom from any infectious skin disease at the site of phlebotomy and from any such disease generalized to such an extent as to create a risk of contamination of the blood"; 21 CFR 640.3(b)(7): "Freedom of the arms and forearms from skin punctures or scars indicative of addiction to self-injected narcotics"]	In situations where requirements for allogeneic donor selection or collection are not applied, alternate requirements shall be defined and documented by the medical director. (5.4.4)
Hemoglobin/hematocrit	≥12.5 g/dL or a hematocrit value of ≥38% [Reference Standard 5.4.1A(5); 21 CFR 640.3(b)(3)]	≥11 g/dL or a hematocrit value of ≥33% [Standard 5.4.4.2; 21 CFR 640.3(b)(3)]

(Continued)

◆ APPENDIX 5-1

Requirements for Allogeneic and Autologous Donor Qualification (Continued)

	Allogeneic (AABB Reference Standard 5.4.1A or as indicated*; 21 CFR 640.3)	**Autologous (AABB Standard 5.4.4 or as indicated*)**
Apheresis and Special Donor Requirements		
Plateletpheresis	The results of platelet counts performed before or after a procedure may be used to qualify the donor for the next procedure. (Standard 5.5.3.4.2) Platelepheresis donors whose counts are <150,000/µL shall be deferred from plateletpheresis donation until a subsequent platelet count is at least 150,000/µL. [Standard 5.5.3.4.3; FDA Guidance for Industry and FDA Review Staff: Collection of Platelets by Automated Methods (December 17, 2007)]	
2-Unit red cell collection	In accordance with the device manufacturers' instructions.	In accordance with the device manufacturers' instructions.
Directed donation	Same as for general, volunteer donation.	Not applicable.

*Carson TH, ed. Standards for blood banks and transfusion services. 27th ed. Bethesda, MD: AABB, 2011.

◆ APPENDIX 5-2
The Donor History Questionnaire and Corresponding Regulations and Standards

The eligibility requirements for blood donation are defined in regulations issued by the Food and Drug Administration (FDA) and in voluntary standards of AABB. Specifically, the requirements originate from the *Code of Federal Regulations* (CFR) Title 21, Part 640.3; other FDA memoranda and guidance (as indicated throughout this appendix); and AABB *Standards for Blood Banks and Transfusion Services* [mostly from Reference Standard 5.4.1A (27th edition)]. The table on the following pages links each question in the donor history questionnaire (DHQ) with the corresponding AABB standards and FDA regulations that support it. FDA memoranda and guidance documents mentioned in the table may be accessed at http://www.fda.gov/BiologicsBloodVaccines/GuidanceComplianceRegulatoryInformation/Guidances/Blood/default.htm.

Note: The DHQ is available on both the AABB and FDA websites, where it may be updated as new versions arise. Version 1.3 (May 2008) was used to build this table; updates were included at the time of this writing. Please visit the following websites for the most recent version:

- AABB: http://www.aabb.org>Resource Center>Blood Donation Information>Donor History Questionnaires>Blood Donor History Questionnaire.
- FDA: http://www.fda.gov/BiologicsBloodVaccines/BloodBloodProducts/ApprovedProducts/LicensedProductsBLAs/BloodDonorScreening/ucm164185.htm.

(Continued)

◆ APPENDIX 5-2

The Donor History Questionnaire and Corresponding Regulations and Standards (Continued)

Donor History Questionnaire	AABB	Food and Drug Administration (FDA)
1. Are you feeling healthy and well today?	Reference Standard 5.4.1A(7)[1]: The prospective donor shall appear to be in good health and shall be free of major organ disease (eg, heart, liver, lungs), cancer, or abnormal bleeding tendency, unless determined eligible by the medical director. Standard 5.4.3[1]: On the day of donation and before collection, the prospective donor's history shall be evaluated and the donor examined to minimize donor risk.	21 CFR 640.3(a)(b)[2]: Donors shall be in good health. The suitability of a donor as a source of Whole Blood shall be determined by a qualified physician or by persons under his supervision and trained in determining suitability.
2. Are you currently taking an antibiotic?	Reference Standard 5.4.1A(6)[1]: Defer for other medications, such as antibiotics, as defined by the facility's medical director.	21 CFR 640.3(b)(6)[2]: Donors shall be . . . [free] from any disease transmissible by blood transfusion.
3. Are you currently taking any other medication for an infection?	See #2.	See #2

◆ APPENDIX 5-2

The Donor History Questionnaire and Corresponding Regulations and Standards (Continued)

Donor History Questionnaire	AABB	Food and Drug Administration (FDA)
4. Are you now taking or have you ever taken any medications on the Medication Deferral List?	Reference Standard 5.4.1A(6,10) (see also Appendix 3)[1]: ◆ Finasteride (Proscar, Propecia), isotretinoin, (Accutane, Amnesteem, Claravis, Sotret): **1-month** deferral. ◆ Dutasteride (Avodart): **6-month** deferral. ◆ Acitretin (Soriatane): **3-year** deferral. ◆ Etretinate (Tegison): **permanent** deferral. ◆ Bovine insulin manufactured in the UK: **indefinite** deferral. ◆ Piroxicam (Feldene): **2-day** (48-hour) deferral for platelet donors. ◆ Clopidogrel (Plavix) and ticlopidine (Ticlid): **14-day** deferral. ◆ Experimental medication or unlicensed (experimental) vaccine: **12-month** deferral unless otherwise indicated by medical director	FDA Memorandum of 7/28/93: Deferral of Blood and Plasma Donors Based on Medications[3]; FDA Guidance for Industry of May 2010: Revised Preventive Measures to Reduce the Possible Risk of Transmission of Creutzfeldt-Jakob Disease (CJD) and Variant Creutzfeldt-Jakob Disease (vCJD) by Blood and Blood Products,[4,5] and FDA Guidance for Industry and FDA Review Staff of 12/07/07: Collection of Platelets by Automated Method.[5] ◆ Finasteride (Proscar): **1-month** deferral. ◆ Isotretinoin (Accutane): **1-month** deferral. ◆ Etretinate (Tegison): **permanent** deferral. ◆ Human pituitary-derived growth hormone: **permanent** deferral. ◆ Other medications as determined by the medical director. ◆ Bovine insulin manufactured in the UK: **indefinite** deferral. ◆ Piroxicam (Feldene): **2-day** (48-hour) deferral for platelet donors. ◆ Clopidogrel (Plavix) and ticlopidine (Ticlid): **14-day** deferral.
5. Have you read the educational materials?	Standard 5.2.1(1,3)[1]: The blood bank shall have procedures to ensure that . . . ◆ Donors are given educational materials regarding infectious disease transmitted by blood transfusion. ◆ Donors acknowledge that the educational materials have been read.	FDA Memorandum of 4/23/92: Revised Recommendations for the Prevention of Human Immunodeficiency Virus (HIV) Transmission by Blood and Blood Products[6]: Donors should receive information about the safety of blood products in relation to AIDS epidemiology and high-risk behaviors. The educational material on AIDs should include a description of HIV-associated clinical signs and symptoms. The donation records should include a signed consent statement documenting that the donor acknowledged reviewing and understanding the information.

V. #1.3

(May 2008)
(Continued)

◆ **APPENDIX 5-2**
The Donor History Questionnaire and Corresponding Regulations and Standards (Continued)

Donor History Questionnaire	AABB	Food and Drug Administration (FDA)
In the past **48 hours:**		
6. Have you taken aspirin or anything that has aspirin in it?	Reference Standard 5.4.1A(6)[1]: Medications that irreversibly inhibit platelet function preclude use of the donor as sole source of platelets. ◆ Defer for 2 full days **(>48 hours)** after last dose of aspirin. ◆ Defer for other medications as defined by the facility's medical director.	No current regulations or recommendations for whole blood donation. FDA Guidance for Industry and FDA Review Staff: Collection of Platelets by Automated Method[5]: Donors who have recently taken medication containing aspirin, especially within **48 hours**, may not be suitable donors for platelet apheresis.
In the past **6 weeks:**		
7. Female donors: Have you been pregnant or are you pregnant now? (Males: check "I am male.")	Reference Standard 5.4.1A(8)[1]: Defer if pregnant within the last **6 weeks**.	No current regulations or recommendations on pregnancy.
In the past **8 weeks,** have you:		
8. Donated blood, platelets, or plasma?	Standards 5.5.2.1, 5.5.2.2, 5.5.3.1, 5.5.3.2, and Reference Standard 5.4.1A(3) (see exceptions throughout Standard 5.5)[1]: Donation interval requirements: ◆ **8 weeks** after whole blood donation. ◆ **4 weeks** after infrequent plasmapheresis. ◆ For plasmapheresis more frequently than once every 4 weeks, the FDA requirements for donor testing and evaluation by a physical examination shall be followed. ◆ **≥2 days** after platelet, granulocyte, or leukocyte donations.	21 CFR 640.3(f)[2]: Frequency of blood donation is every **8 weeks** unless—at the time of donation—the person is examined and certified by a physician to be in good health. FDA Guidance for Industry and FDA Review Staff: Collection of Platelets by Automated Method[5]: No more than 24 plateletpheresis procedures during a calendar year; with intervals of **48 hours between procedures**, a donor should not undergo more than **2 procedures within a 7-day period**.

V. #1.3 (May 2008)

8. (Continued)		See also: FDA Memorandum of 3/10/95: Revision of FDA Memorandum of August 27, 1982: Requirements for Infrequent Plasma Donors[7] FDA Memorandum of 12/04/95: Donor Deferral Due to Red Blood Cell Loss during Collection of Source Plasma by Automated Plasmapheresis[8]
9. Had any vaccinations or other shots?	Reference Standard 5.4.1A(10)[1]: **No deferral** for receipt of toxoids or synthetic or killed viral, bacterial, or rickettsial vaccines if donor is symptom-free and afebrile [Anthrax, Cholera, Diphtheria, Hepatitis A, Hepatitis B, Influenza, Lyme Disease, Paratyphoid, Pertussis, Plague, Pneumococcal polysaccharide, Polio (Salk/injection), Rabies, Rocky Mountain spotted fever, Tetanus, Typhoid (by injection)]. Defer for **2 weeks** for receipt of the following live attenuated viral and bacterial vaccines: Measles (rubeola), Mumps, Polio (Sabin/oral), Typhoid (oral), Yellow fever. Defer for **4 weeks** for receipt of the following live attenuated viral and bacterial vaccines: German measles (rubella), Chicken pox (varicella zoster). For receipt of Smallpox vaccine, refer to FDA Guidance. Defer for **12 months** unless otherwise indicated by medical director for receipt of other vaccines, including unlicensed vaccines.	21 CFR 640.3(b)(6)[2]: Donors shall be . . . [free] from any disease transmissible by blood transfusion . . . . Deferral recommendations on smallpox vaccine in FDA Guidance for Industry of 12/30/02 (corrected 2/04/03): Recommendations for Deferral of Donors and Quarantine and Retrieval of Blood and Blood Products in Recent Recipients of Smallpox Vaccine (Vaccinia Virus) and Certain Contacts of Smallpox Vaccine Recipients.[9]

(Continued)

◆ APPENDIX 5-2
The Donor History Questionnaire and Corresponding Regulations and Standards (Continued)

Donor History Questionnaire	AABB	Food and Drug Administration (FDA)
10. Had contact with someone who had a smallpox vaccination?	Reference Standard 5.4.1A(10)[1]: Refer to FDA Guidance.	FDA Guidance for Industry of 12/30/02 (corrected 2/04/03): Recommendations for Deferral of Donors and Quarantine and Retrieval of Blood and Blood Products in Recent Recipients of Smallpox Vaccine (Vaccinia Virus) and Certain Contacts of Smallpox Vaccine Recipients.[9]
In the past **16 weeks:**		
11. Have you donated a double unit of red cells using an apheresis machine?	Standard 5.5.3.5.1 and Reference Standard 5.4.1A(3)[1]: Defer for **16 weeks** after 2-unit red cell collection.	FDA Guidance for Industry of 2/13/01: Recommendations for Collecting Red Blood Cells by Automated Apheresis Methods[10]: All donors should be deferred for at least 16 weeks after undergoing a double [Red Blood Cell] collection procedure.
In the past **12 months**, have you:		
12. Had a blood transfusion?	Reference Standard 5.4.1A(9)[1]: Defer for **12 months** for receipt of blood or components.	FDA Memorandum of 4/23/92: Revised Recommendations for the Prevention of Human Immunodeficiency Virus (HIV) Transmission by Blood and Blood Products[6]: Persons who have received a transfusion of whole blood or a blood component within the past **12 months** should not donate blood or blood components.
13. Had a transplant such as organ, tissue, or bone marrow?	Reference Standard 5.4.1A(9)[1]: Defer for **12 months** for receipt of . . . human tissue.	No current regulations or recommendations on organ, tissue, or marrow transplants.

14. Had a graft such as bone or skin?	Reference Standard 5.4.1A(9)[1]: Defer for **12 months** for receipt of . . . human tissue. Defer **indefinitely** for receipt of dura mater.	No current regulations or recommendations on bone or skin grafts. FDA Guidance for Industry of 1/09/02: Revised Preventive Measures to Reduce the Possible Risk of Transmission of Creutzfeldt-Jakob Disease (CJD) and Variant Creutzfeldt-Jakob Disease (vCJD) by Blood and Blood Products[4]: Donors should be **permanently** deferred if they have an increased risk for CJD (ie, a dura mater transplant or human pituitary-derived growth hormone).
15. Come into contact with someone else's blood?	Reference Standard 5.4.1A(11)[1]: Defer for **12 months** from the time of mucous membrane exposure to blood. Defer **12 months** from time of nonsterile skin penetration with instruments or equipment contaminated with blood or body fluids other than the donor's own.	FDA Memorandum of 4/23/92: Revised Recommendations for the Prevention of Human Immunodeficiency Virus (HIV) Transmission by Blood and Blood Products[6]: Persons who have had any contact with blood and body fluids through percutaneous inoculation (such as injury or accidental needlestick) or through contact with an open wound, nonintact skin, or mucous membrane during the preceding **12 months** should be deferred.
16. Had an accidental needle-stick?	Reference Standard 5.4.1A(11)[1]: Defer for **12 months** from the time of: ◆ Mucous membrane exposure to blood. ◆ Nonsterile skin penetration with instruments or equipment contaminated with blood or body fluids other than the donor's own. Includes tattoos or permanent make-up unless applied by a state-regulated entity with sterile needles and ink that has not been reused.	See #15.

(May 2008)
(Continued)

◆ APPENDIX 5-2
The Donor History Questionnaire and Corresponding Regulations and Standards (Continued)

Donor History Questionnaire	AABB	Food and Drug Administration (FDA)
17. Had sexual contact with anyone who has HIV/AIDS or has had a positive test for the HIV/AIDS virus?	Reference Standard 5.4.1A(11)[1]: Defer for **12 months** from the time of sexual contact with an individual with HIV infection or at high risk of HIV infection.	FDA Memorandum of 4/23/92: Revised Recommendations for the Prevention of Human Immunodeficiency Virus (HIV) Transmission by Blood and Blood Products[6]: Persons who have had sex with persons with clinical or laboratory evidence of HIV infection in the preceding **12 months** must not donate blood or blood components.
18. Had sexual contact with a prostitute or anyone else who takes money or drugs or other payment for sex?	Reference Standard 5.4.1A(11)[1]: Defer for **12 months** from the time of sexual contact with an individual . . . at high risk of HIV infection.	FDA Memorandum of 4/23/92: Revised Recommendations for the Prevention of Human Immunodeficiency Virus (HIV) Transmission by Blood and Blood Products[6]: ◆ Men and women who have engaged in sex for money or drugs since 1977 and persons who have engaged in sex with such people during the preceding **12 months** should not donate blood or blood components. ◆ Persons who have had sex with any person who is a past or present intravenous drug user should not donate blood or blood components for **12 months**. ◆ Persons who have had sex with any person with hemophilia or related clotting disorders who have received clotting factor concentrates should not donate blood or blood components for **12 months.** ◆ Persons who have had sex with men who have had sex with another man—even one time since 1977—should not donate blood or blood components for **12 months**.

19. Had sexual contact with anyone who has ever used needles to take drugs or steroids or anything *not* prescribed by their doctor?	See #18.	See #18.
20. Had sexual contact with anyone who has hemophilia or has used clotting factor concentrates?	See #18.	See #18.
21. Female donors: Had sexual contact with a male who has ever had sexual contact with another male? (Males: check "I am male.")	See #18.	See #18.
22. Had sexual contact with a person who has hepatitis?	Reference Standard 5.4.1A(11)[1]: Defer for **12 months** for sexual contact or for having lived with an individual who ◆ Has acute or chronic hepatitis B (positive HBsAg and HBV NAT tests). ◆ Has symptomatic hepatitis C. ◆ Is symptomatic for any other viral hepatitis.	21 CFR 640.3(c)[2]: Defer for **12 months** after close contact with a person who has viral hepatitis.
23. Lived with a person who has hepatitis?	Reference Standard 5.4.1A(11)[1]: Defer for **12 months** for sexual contact or for having lived with an individual who ◆ Has acute or chronic hepatitis B (positive HBsAg and HBV NAT tests). ◆ Has symptomatic hepatitis C. ◆ Is symptomatic for any other viral hepatitis.	21 CFR 640.3(c)[2]: Defer for **12 months** after close contact with a person who has viral hepatitis.

(Continued)

◆ APPENDIX 5-2
The Donor History Questionnaire and Corresponding Regulations and Standards (Continued)

Donor History Questionnaire	AABB	Food and Drug Administration (FDA)
24. Had a tattoo?	Reference Standard 5.4.1A(11)[1]: ◆ Defer for **12 months** from the time of nonsterile skin penetration with instruments or equipment contaminated with blood or body fluids other than the donor's own. Includes tattoos or permanent make-up unless applied by a state-regulated entity with sterile needles and ink that has not been reused.	FDA Memorandum of 4/23/92: Revised Recommendations for the Prevention of Human Immunodeficiency Virus (HIV) Transmission by Blood and Blood Products[6]: Persons who have had any contact with blood and body fluids through percutaneous inoculation (such as injury or accidental needlestick) or through contact with an open wound, nonintact skin, or mucous membrane during the preceding **12 months** should be deferred. FDA memorandum of 4/23/92: Revised Recommendations for Testing Whole Blood, Blood Components, Source Plasma, and Source Leukocytes for Antibody to Hepatitis C Virus Encoded Antigen (anti-HCV) in Blood Establishments[11]: Individuals should be deferred from donating who within **1 year** of donation have undergone ear piercing or tattooing in which sterile procedures were not used.
25. Had ear or body piercing?	See #24.	See #24.
26. Had or been treated for syphilis or gonorrhea?	Reference Standard 5.4.1A(11)[1]: Defer for **12 months** or for longest applicable period in the following situations: ◆ Following the completion of treatment for syphilis or gonorrhea. ◆ Donor who has a reactive screening test for syphilis where no confirmatory testing was performed. ◆ A confirmed positive test for syphilis (FDA reentry protocol after 1 year applies).	FDA Memorandum of 12/12/91: Clarification of FDA Recommendations for Donor Deferral and Product Distribution Based on the Results of Syphilis Testing[12]: Persons who have had, or have been treated for, syphilis or gonorrhea during the preceding **12 months** should not donate blood or blood components. Persons with a positive serologic test for syphilis should be deferred for **12 months**.

27. Been in juvenile detention, lockup, jail, or prison for more than 72 hours?	Reference Standard 5.4.1A(11)[1]: **12-month** deferral from the time of incarceration in a correctional institution (including juvenile detention, lockup, jail, or prison) for more than 72 consecutive hours.	FDA Memorandum of 6/08/95: Recommendations for the Deferral of Current and Recent Inmates of Correctional Institutions as Donors of Whole Blood, Blood Components, Source Leukocytes, and Source Plasma[13]: Individuals who have been incarcerated for more than 72 consecutive hours during the previous 12 months should be deferred for **12 months** from the last date of that incarceration.
In the past **3 years**, have you:		
28. Been outside the United States or Canada?	Malaria Reference Standard 5.4.1A(11)[1]: ◆ Defer for **3 years** after departure from malaria-endemic area(s): individuals who have lived for at least 5 consecutive years in areas considered malaria endemic by the Malarial Branch, Centers for Disease Control and Prevention, US Department of Health and Human Services. ◆ Defer for **12 months** after departure: individuals who have traveled to an area where malaria is endemic. vCJD Reference Standard 5.4.1A(12)[1]: ◆ The prospective donor's travel history shall be evaluated for potential risks. ◆ Defer **indefinitely**: donors recommended for indefinite deferral for risk of vCJD, as defined in most recent FDA Guidance. Leishmaniasis ◆ AABB Association Bulletin #03-14[15] ◆ Defer for **12 months** from the last date of departure: prospective donors who have been to Iraq.	Malaria FDA Memorandum of 7/26/94: Recommendations for Deferral of Donors for Malaria Risk[14]: Travelers to an area considered endemic for malaria should not be accepted as donors of whole blood and blood components prior to **1 year** after departure. After 1 year, donors free of unexplained symptoms suggestive of malaria may be accepted whether or not they have received antimalarial chemoprophylaxis. Immigrants, refugees, and citizens of endemic countries should not be accepted as donors prior to **3 years** after departure. After 3 years, donors free of unexplained symptoms suggestive of malaria may be accepted. vCJD FDA Guidance for Industry of May 2010: Revised Preventive Measures to Reduce the Possible Risk of Transmission of Creutzfeldt-Jakob Disease (CJD) and Variant Creutzfeldt-Jakob Disease (vCJD) by Blood and Blood Products[4] (see for details).

(Continued)

◆ APPENDIX 5-2
The Donor History Questionnaire and Corresponding Regulations and Standards (Continued)

Donor History Questionnaire	AABB	Food and Drug Administration (FDA)
From **1980 through 1996:**		
29. Did you spend time that adds up to three (3) months or more in the United Kingdom? (Review list of countries in the United Kingdom.)	Reference Standard 5.4.1A(12)[1]: The prospective donor's travel history shall be evaluated for potential risks. Defer **indefinitely**: donors recommended for indefinite deferral for risk of vCJD, as defined in most recent FDA Guidance.	FDA Guidance for Industry of May 2010: Revised Preventive Measures to Reduce the Possible Risk of Transmission of Creutzfeldt-Jakob Disease (CJD) and Variant Creutzfeldt-Jakob Disease (vCJD) by Blood and Blood Products[4] (see for details).
30. Were you a member of the US military, a civilian military employee, or a dependent of a member of the US military?	See #29.	See #29.
From **1980 to the present,** did you:		
31. Spend time that adds up to five (5) years or more in Europe? (Review list of countries in Europe.)	Reference Standard 5.4.1A(12)[1]: The prospective donor's travel history shall be evaluated for potential risks. Defer **indefinitely**: donors recommended for indefinite deferral for risk of vCJD, as defined in most recent FDA Guidance.	FDA Draft Guidance of 8/08/06: Amendment (Donor Deferral for Transfusion in France Since 1980) to "Guidance for Industry: Revised Preventive Measures to Reduce the Possible Risk of Transmission of Creutzfeldt-Jakob Disease (CJD) and Variant Creutzfeldt-Jakob Disease (vCJD) by Blood and Blood Products"[4] (see for details).
32. Receive a blood transfusion in the United Kingdom or France? (Review list of countries in the United Kingdom.)	See #31.	See #31.

V. #1.3 (May 2008)

From 1977 to the present, have you:		
33. Received money, drugs, or other payment for sex?	Reference Standard 5.4.1A(11)[1]: Defer **indefinitely**: individuals as excluded by current FDA regulations and recommendations for the prevention of HIV transmissionby blood and components.	FDA Memorandum of 4/23/92: Revised Recommendations for the Prevention of Human Immunodeficiency Virus (HIV) Transmission by Blood and Blood Products[6]: Men and women who have engaged in sex for money or drugs since 1977 and persons who have engaged in sex with such people during the preceding **12 months** should not donate blood or blood components.
34. Male donor: Had sexual contact with another male, even once? (Female donors: check "I am female.")	Reference Standard 5.4.1A(11)[1]: Defer **indefinitely**: individuals as excluded by current FDA regulations and recommendations for the prevention of HIV transmission by blood and components.	FDA Memorandum of 4/23/92: Revised Recommendations for the Prevention of Human Immunodeficiency Virus (HIV) Transmission by Blood and Blood Products[6]: Men who have had sex with another man even once since 1977 should not donate blood or blood components **permanently**.
Have you **EVER**:		
35. Had a positive test for the HIV/AIDS virus?	Reference Standard 5.4.1A(11)[1]: Defer **indefinitely** for present or past clinical or laboratory evidence of infection with HIV . . . or as excluded by current FDA regulations and recommendations for the prevention of HIV transmission by blood and components.	FDA Memorandum of 4/23/92: Revised Recommendations for the Prevention of Human Immunodeficiency Virus (HIV) Transmission by Blood and Blood Products[6]: Persons with clinical or laboratory evidence of HIV infection must not donate blood or blood components.
36. Used needles to take drugs, steroids, or anything *not* prescribed by your doctor?	Reference Standard 5.4.1A(7)[1]: The venipuncture site shall be evaluated for lesions on the skin. Reference Standard 5.4.1A(11)[1]: ◆ Defer indefinitely if evidence or obvious stigmata of parenteral drug use. ◆ Defer indefinitely for use of a needle to administer nonprescription drugs.	21 CFR 640.3(b)(7)[2]: Donors must be free from skin punctures or scars indicative of addiction to self-injected narcotics. FDA Memorandum of 4/23/92: Revised Recommendations for the Prevention of Human Immunodeficiency Virus (HIV) Transmission by Blood and Blood Products[6]: Past or present intravenous drug users should not donate blood or blood components.

V. #1.3

(May 2008)
(Continued)

◆ APPENDIX 5-2
The Donor History Questionnaire and Corresponding Regulations and Standards (Continued)

Donor History Questionnaire	AABB	Food and Drug Administration (FDA)
37. Used clotting factor concentrates?	Reference Standard 5.4.1A(7)[1]: The donor shall be free of . . . abnormal bleeding tendency, unless determined eligible by the medical director. Reference Standard 5.4.1A(9)[1]: Defer for **12 months** for receipt of . . . plasma-derived clotting factor concentrates.	FDA Memorandum of 4/23/92: Revised Recommendations for the Prevention of Human Immunodeficiency Virus (HIV) Transmission by Blood and Blood Products[6]: Persons with hemophilia or related clotting disorders who have received clotting factor concentrates should not donate blood or components. Persons who have received . . . clotting factor concentrates within the past **12 months** should not donate blood or components.
38. Had hepatitis?	Reference Standard 5.4.1A(11)[1]: Defer **indefinitely** for history of viral hepatitis after 11th birthday.	21 CFR 640.3(c)(1)[2]: No individual with a history of hepatitis shall be a source of whole blood donation. There are exemptions for history of hepatitis before age 11. FDA Memorandum of 12/22/93: Donor Suitability Related to Laboratory Testing for Viral Hepatitis and a History of Viral Hepatitis[17] (see for details).
39. Had malaria?	Reference Standard 5.4.1A(11)[1]: Defer for **3 years** after becoming asymptomatic: prospective donors who have had a diagnosis of malaria.	FDA Memorandum of 7/26/94: Recommendations for Deferral of Donors for Malaria Risk[14]: Prospective donors who have had malaria should be deferred for **3 years** after becoming asymptomatic.
40. Had Chagas disease?	Reference Standard 5.4.1A(11)[1]: Defer **indefinitely** for history of . . . Chagas disease.	FDA Guidance of December 2010: Use of Serological Tests to Reduce the Risk of Transmission of *Trypanosoma cruzi* Infection in Whole Blood and Blood Components Intended for Transfusion.[18]

V. #1.3 (May 2008)

41. Had babesiosis?	Reference Standard 5.4.1A(11)[1]: Defer **indefinitely** for history of babesiosis.	21 CFR 640.3(b)(6)[2]: Donors shall be . . . [free] from any disease transmissible by blood transfusion.
42. Received a dura mater (or brain covering) graft?	Reference Standard 5.4.1A(9)[1]: Defer **indefinitely** for receipt of dura mater or pituitary growth hormone of human origin.	FDA Guidance for Industry of May 2010: Revised Preventive Measures to Reduce the Possible Risk of Transmission of Creutzfeldt-Jakob Disease (CJD) and Variant Creutzfeldt-Jakob Disease (vCJD) by Blood and Blood Products[4]: Persons who have received transplants or dura mater should be **permanently** deferred from donation.
43. Had any type of cancer, including leukemia?	Reference Standard 5.4.1A(7)[1]: The prospective donor shall appear to be in good health and shall be free of . . . cancer . . . unless determined eligible by the medical director. The venipuncture site shall be evaluated for lesions on the skin.	No current regulations or recommendations.
44. Had any problems with your heart or lungs?	Reference Standard 5.4.1A(7)[1]: The prospective donor shall appear to be in good health and shall be free of major organ disease (eg, heart, liver, lungs) . . . unless determined eligible by the medical director. The venipuncture site shall be evaluated for lesions on the skin.	21 CFR 640.3(b)(4)[2]: Donor must be free of acute respiratory disease.
45. Had a bleeding condition or a blood disease?	Reference Standard 5.4.1A(7)[1]: The prospective donor shall appear to be in good health and shall be free of . . . abnormal bleeding tendency, unless determined eligible by the medical director.	FDA Memorandum of 4/23/92: Revised Recommendations for the Prevention of Human Immunodeficiency Virus (HIV) Transmission by Blood and Blood Products[6]: Persons with hemophilia or related clotting disorders who have received clotting factor concentrates must not donate blood or blood components.

V. #1.3

(May 2008)
(Continued)

◆ APPENDIX 5-2
The Donor History Questionnaire and Corresponding Regulations and Standards (Continued)

Donor History Questionnaire	AABB	Food and Drug Administration (FDA)
46. Had sexual contact with anyone who was born or lived in Africa?*	Reference Standard 5.4.1A(11)[1]: Deferral for HIV risk . . . as excluded by current FDA regulations and recommendations for the prevention of HIV transmission by blood and components.	FDA Guidance for Industry of August 2009: Recommendations for Management of Donors at Increased Risk for Human Immunodeficiency Virus Type 1 (HIV-1) Group O Infection[18] (see for details). (Cameroon, Benin, Central African Republic, Chad, Congo, Equatorial Guinea, Kenya, Gabon, Niger, Nigeria, Senegal, Togo, or Zambia).*
47. Been in Africa?*	See #46.	See #46.
48. Had any relatives who had Creutzfeldt-Jakob disease?	Reference Standard 5.4.1A(7)[1]: Defer **indefinitely** for a family history of Creutzfeldt-Jakob disease.	FDA Guidance for Industry of May 2010: Revised Preventive Measures to Reduce the Possible Risk of Transmission of Creutzfeldt-Jakob Disease (CJD) and Variant Creutzfeldt-Jakob Disease (vCJD) by Blood and Blood Products[4]: Persons with a family history (blood relatives) of Creutzfeldt-Jakob disease (CJD) are to be **permanently** deferred from donation unless the diagnosis of CJD in the family member(s) is confidently excluded, CJD in the family member(s) is iatrogenic, the family member(s) is (are) not a blood relative(s), or laboratory testing (gene sequencing) shows that the donor does not have a mutation associated with familial CJD.

*The questions to detect donors at risk for HIV group O can be deleted from the DHQ if the blood center implements a licensed anti-HIV-1/2 test for donor screening that is specifically labeled in the "Intended Use" section of the package insert as sensitive for detection of HIV-1 group O antibodies.

1. Carson TH, ed. Standards for blood banks and transfusion services. 27th ed. Bethesda, MD: AABB, 2011.
2. Code of federal regulations. Title 21, CFR Part 640.3. Washington, DC: US Government Printing Office, 2010 (revised annually).
3. Food and Drug Administration. Memorandum: Deferral of blood and plasma donors based on medications. (July 28, 1993) Rockville, MD: CBER Office of Communication, Outreach, and Development, 1993.
4. Food and Drug Administration. Guidance for industry: Revised preventive measures to reduce the possible risk of transmission of Creutzfeldt-Jakob disease (CJD) and variant Creutzfeldt-Jakob disease (vCJD) by blood and blood products. (May 2010) Rockville, MD: CBER Office of Communication, Outreach, and Development, 2010.
5. Food and Drug Administration. Guidance for industry and FDA review staff: Collection of platelets by automated method. (December 17, 2007) Rockville, MD: CBER Office of Communication, Outreach, and Development, 2007.
6. Food and Drug Administration. Memorandum: Revised recommendations for the prevention of human immunodeficiency virus (HIV) transmission by blood and blood products. (April 23, 1992) Rockville, MD: CBER Office of Communication, Outreach, and Development, 1992.
7. Food and Drug Administration. Memorandum: Revision of FDA memorandum of August 27, 1982: Requirements for infrequent plasma donors. (March 10, 1995) Rockville, MD: CBER Office of Communication, Outreach, and Development, 1995.
8. Food and Drug Administration. Memorandum: Donor deferral due to red blood cell loss during collection of source plasma by automated plasmapheresis. (December 4, 1995) Rockville, MD: CBER Office of Communication, Outreach, and Development, 1995.
9. Food and Drug Administration. Guidance for industry: Recommendations for deferral of donors and quarantine and retrieval of blood and blood products in recent recipients of smallpox vaccine (vaccinia virus) and certain contacts of smallpox vaccine recipients. (December 30, 2002; corrected February 4, 2003) Rockville, MD: CBER Office of Communication, Outreach, and Development, 2003.
10. Food and Drug Administration. Guidance for industry: Recommendations for collecting Red Blood Cells by automated apheresis methods. (February 13, 2001) Rockville, MD: CBER Office of Communication, Outreach, and Development, 2001.
11. Food and Drug Administration. Memorandum: Revised recommendations for testing whole blood, blood components, source plasma, and source leukocytes for antibody to hepatitis C virus encoded antigen (anti-HCV) in blood establishments. (April 23, 1992) Rockville, MD: CBER Office of Communication, Outreach, and Development, 1992.
12. Food and Drug Administration. Memorandum: Clarification of FDA recommendations for donor deferral and product distribution based on the results of syphilis testing. (December 12, 1991) Rockville, MD: CBER Office of Communication, Outreach, and Development, 1991.
13. Food and Drug Administration. Memorandum: Recommendations for the deferral of current and recent inmates of correctional institutions as donors of whole blood, blood components, source leukocytes, and source plasma. (June 8, 1995) Rockville, MD: CBER Office of Communication, Outreach, and Development, 1995.
14. Food and Drug Administration. Memorandum: Recommendations for deferral of donors for malaria risk. (July 26, 1994) Rockville, MD: CBER Office of Communication, Outreach, and Development, 1994.
15. Deferral for risk of leishmaniasis exposure. Association bulletin #03-14. Bethesda, MD: AABB, 2003. [Available at (path) http://www.aabb.org>Resource Center>Publications>Association Bulletins>View past bulletins (accessed October 1, 2010).]
16. Food and Drug Administration. Memorandum: Donor suitability related to laboratory testing for viral hepatitis and a history of viral hepatitis. (December 22, 1993) Rockville, MD: CBER Office of Communication, Outreach, and Development, 1993.
17. Food and Drug Administration. Guidance for industry: Use of serological tests to reduce the risk of transmission of *Trypanosoma cruzi* infection in whole blood and blood components intended for transfusion. (December 2010) Rockville, MD: CBER Office of Communication, Outreach, and Development, 2010.
18. Food and Drug Administration. Guidance for industry: Recommendations for management of donors at increased risk for human immunodeficiency virus type 1 (HIV-1) group O infection. (August 2009) Rockville, MD: CBER Office of Communication, Outreach, and Development, 2009.

◆ APPENDIX 5-3
Full-Length Donor History Questionnaire (Version 1.3, May 2008)

	Yes	No	
Are you	☐	☐	
1. Feeling healthy and well today?	☐	☐	
2. Currently taking an antibiotic?	☐	☐	
3. Currently taking any other medication for an infection?	☐	☐	
Please read the Medication Deferral List.			
4. Are you now taking or have you ever taken any medications on the Medication Deferral List?	☐	☐	
5. Have you read the educational materials?	☐	☐	
In the past **48 hours**			
6. Have you taken aspirin or anything that has aspirin in it?	☐	☐	
In the past **6 weeks**			
7. Female donors: Have you been pregnant or are you pregnant now? (Males: check "I am male.")	☐	☐	☐ I am male
In the past **8 weeks have you**			
8. Donated blood, platelets or plasma?	☐	☐	
9. Had any vaccinations or other shots?	☐	☐	
10. Had contact with someone who had a smallpox vaccination?	☐	☐	
In the past **16 weeks**			
11. Have you donated a double unit of red cells using an apheresis machine?	☐	☐	
In the past **12 months have you**			
12. Had a blood transfusion?	☐	☐	
13. Had a transplant such as organ, tissue, or bone marrow?	☐	☐	
14. Had a graft such as bone or skin?	☐	☐	
15. Come into contact with someone else's blood?	☐	☐	

◆ APPENDIX 5-3

Full-Length Donor History Questionnaire (Version 1.3, May 2008) (Continued)

	Yes	No	
16. Had an accidental needle-stick?	☐	☐	
17. Had sexual contact with anyone who has HIV/AIDS or has had a positive test for the HIV/AIDS virus?	☐	☐	
18. Had sexual contact with a prostitute or anyone else who takes money or drugs or other payment for sex?	☐	☐	
19. Had sexual contact with anyone who has ever used needles to take drugs or steroids, or anything not prescribed by their doctor?	☐	☐	
20. Had sexual contact with anyone who has hemophilia or has used clotting factor concentrates?	☐	☐	
21. Female donors: Had sexual contact with a male who has ever had sexual contact with another male? (Males: check "I am male.")	☐	☐	☐ I am male
22. Had sexual contact with a person who has hepatitis?	☐	☐	
23. Lived with a person who has hepatitis?	☐	☐	
24. Had a tattoo?	☐	☐	
25. Had ear or body piercing?	☐	☐	
26. Had or been treated for syphilis or gonorrhea?	☐	☐	
27. Been in juvenile detention, lockup, jail, or prison for more than 72 hours?	☐	☐	
In the past **three years** have you			
28. Been outside the United States or Canada?	☐	☐	
From **1980 through 1996**,			
29. Did you spend time that adds up to three (3) months or more in the United Kingdom? (Review list of countries in the UK)	☐	☐	
30. Were you a member of the U.S. military, a civilian military employee, or a dependent of a member of the U.S. military?	☐	☐	
From **1980 to the present**, did you			
31. Spend time that adds up to five (5) years or more in Europe? (Review list of countries in Europe.)	☐	☐	
32. Receive a blood transfusion in the United Kingdom or France? (Review list of countries in the UK.)	☐	☐	

(Continued)

◆ APPENDIX 5-3
Full-Length Donor History Questionnaire (Version 1.3, May 2008) (Continued)

	Yes	No	
From **1977 to the present**, have you			
33. Received money, drugs, or other payment for sex?	☐	☐	
34. Male donors: Had sexual contact with another male, even once? (Females: check "I am female.")	☐	☐	☐ I am female
Have you **EVER**			
35. Had a positive test for the HIV/AIDS virus?	☐	☐	
36. Used needles to take drugs, steroids, or anything not prescribed by your doctor?	☐	☐	
37. Used clotting factor concentrates?	☐	☐	
38. Had hepatitis?	☐	☐	
39. Had malaria?	☐	☐	
40. Had Chagas disease?	☐	☐	
41. Had babesiosis?	☐	☐	
42. Received a dura mater (or brain covering) graft?	☐	☐	
43. Had any type of cancer, including leukemia?	☐	☐	
44. Had any problems with your heart or lungs?	☐	☐	
45. Had a bleeding condition or a blood disease?	☐	☐	
46. Had sexual contact with anyone who was born in or lived in Africa?	☐	☐	
47. Been in Africa?	☐	☐	
48. Have any of your relatives had Creutzfeldt-Jakob disease?	☐	☐	

◆ **APPENDIX 5-3**

Full-Length Donor History Questionnaire (Version 1.3, May 2008) (Continued)

Use this area for additional questions	Yes	No

◆ APPENDIX 5-4
Medication Deferral List for the Donor History Questionnaire (Version 1.3, May 2008; revised Sept 2010)

Please tell us if you are now taking or if you have EVER taken any of these medications:

- ☐ **Proscar (finasteride)** – usually given for prostate gland enlargement
- ☐ **Avodart, Jalyn (dutasteride)** – usually given for prostate enlargement
- ☐ **Propecia (finasteride)** – usually given for baldness
- ☐ **Accutane, Amnesteem, Claravis, Sotret (isotretinoin)** – usually given for severe acne
- ☐ **Soriatane (acitretin)** – usually given for severe psoriasis
- ☐ **Tegison (etretinate)** – usually given for severe psoriasis
- ☐ **Growth Hormone from Human Pituitary Glands** – used usually for children with delayed or impaired growth
- ☐ **Insulin from Cows (Bovine, or Beef, Insulin)** – used to treat diabetes
- ☐ **Hepatitis B Immune Globulin** – given following an exposure to hepatitis B.
  NOTE: This is different from the hepatitis B vaccine which is a series of 3 injections given over a 6 month period to prevent future infection from exposures to hepatitis B.
- ☐ **Plavix (clopidogrel) and Ticlid (ticlopidine)** – inhibits platelet function; used to reduce the chance for heart attack and stroke.
- ☐ **Feldene** – given for mild to moderate arthritis pain
- ☐ **Experimental Medication or Unlicensed (Experimental) Vaccine** – usually associated with a research protocol

IF YOU WOULD LIKE TO KNOW WHY THESE MEDICINES AFFECT YOU AS A BLOOD DONOR, PLEASE KEEP READING:

- ◆ If you have taken or are taking **Proscar, Avodart, Jalyn, Propecia, Accutane, Soriatane, or Tegison,** these medications can cause birth defects. Your donated blood could contain high enough levels to damage the unborn baby if transfused to a pregnant woman. Once the medication has been cleared from your blood, you may donate again. Following the last dose, the deferral period is one month for Proscar, Propecia and Accutane, six months for Avodart and Jalyn, and three years for Soriatane. Tegison is a permanent deferral.

- ◆ **Growth hormone from human pituitary glands** was prescribed for children with delayed or impaired growth. The hormone was obtained from human pituitary glands, which are found in the brain. Some people who took this hormone developed a rare nervous system condition called Creutzfeldt-Jakob Disease (CJD, for short). The deferral is permanent.

- ◆ **Insulin from cows (bovine, or beef, insulin)** is an injected material used to treat diabetes. If this insulin was imported into the US from countries in which "Mad Cow Disease" has been found, it could contain material from infected cattle. There is concern that "Mad Cow Disease" is transmitted by transfusion. The deferral is indefinite.

- ◆ **Hepatitis B Immune Globulin (HBIG)** is an injected material used to prevent infection following an exposure to hepatitis B. HBIG does not prevent hepatitis B infection in every case, therefore persons who have received HBIG must wait 12 months to donate blood to be sure they were not infected since hepatitis B can be transmitted through transfusion to a patient.

- ◆ **Feldene** is a non-steroidal anti-inflammatory drug that can affect platelet function. A donor taking Feldene will not be able to donate platelets for 2 days; however, its use will not affect whole blood donations.

- ◆ **Plavix and Ticlid** are medications that can decrease the chance of a heart attack or stroke in individuals at risk for these conditions. Since these medications can affect platelets, anyone taking Plavix or Ticlid will not be able to donate platelets for 14 days after the last dose. Use of either medication will not prohibit whole blood donations.

- ◆ **Experimental Medication or Unlicensed (Experimental) Vaccine** is usually associated with a research protocol and the effect on blood donation is unknown. Deferral is one year unless otherwise indicated by Medical Director.

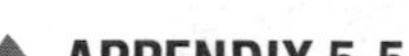

APPENDIX 5-5
Blood Donor Educational Materials: Making Your Blood Donation Safe (Version 1.3, May 2008)

Thank you for coming in today! This information sheet explains how **YOU** can help us make the donation process safe for yourself and patients who might receive your blood. **PLEASE READ THIS INFORMATION <u>BEFORE</u> YOU DONATE! If you have any questions now or anytime during the screening process, please ask blood center staff.**

ACCURACY AND HONESTY ARE ESSENTIAL!

Your **complete honesty** in answering all questions is very important for the safety of patients who receive your blood. **All information you provide is confidential.**

DONATION PROCESS:

To determine if you are eligible to donate we will:

- Ask questions about health, travel, and medicines
- Ask questions to see if you might be at risk for hepatitis, HIV, or AIDS
- Take your blood pressure, temperature and pulse
- Take a small blood sample to make sure you are not anemic

If you are able to donate we will:

- Cleanse your arm with an antiseptic **(If you are allergic to Iodine, please tell us!)**
- Use a new, sterile, disposable needle to collect your blood

DONOR ELIGIBILITY – SPECIFIC INFORMATION

Why we ask questions about sexual contact:

Sexual contact may cause contagious diseases like HIV to get into the bloodstream and be spread through transfusions to someone else.

Definition of "sexual contact":

The words "have sexual contact with" and "sex" are used in some of the questions we will ask you, and apply to <u>any</u> of the activities below, whether or not a condom or other protection was used:

1. Vaginal sex (contact between penis and vagina)

2. Oral sex (mouth or tongue on someone's vagina, penis, or anus)

3. Anal sex (contact between penis and anus)

HIV/AIDS RISK BEHAVIORS AND SYMPTOMS

AIDS is caused by HIV. HIV is spread mainly through sexual contact with an infected person OR by sharing needles or syringes used for injecting drugs.

DO NOT DONATE IF YOU:

- Have AIDS or have ever had a positive HIV test
- Have ever used needles to take drugs, steroids, or anything not prescribed by your doctor
- Are a male who has had sexual contact with another male, even once, since 1977
- Have ever taken money, drugs or other payment for sex since 1977
- Have had sexual contact in the past 12 months with anyone described above
- Have had syphilis or gonorrhea in the past 12 months
- In the last 12 months have been in juvenile detention, lockup, jail or prison for more than 72 hours

(Continued)

◆ APPENDIX 5-5
Blood Donor Educational Materials: Making Your Blood Donation Safe (Version 1.3, May 2008) (Continued)

– Have any of the following conditions that can be signs or symptoms of HIV/AIDS:
  - Unexplained weight loss or night sweats
  - Blue or purple spots in your mouth or skin
  - Swollen lymph nodes for more than one month
  - White spots or unusual sores in your mouth
  - Cough that won't go away or shortness of breath
  - Diarrhea that won't go away
  - Fever of more than 100.5 F for more than 10 days

Remember that you CAN give HIV to someone else through blood transfusions even if you feel well and have a negative HIV test. This is because tests cannot detect infections for a period of time after a person is exposed to HIV. **If you think you may be at risk for HIV/AIDS or want an HIV/AIDS test, please ask for information about other testing facilities.** ***PLEASE DO NOT DONATE TO GET AN HIV TEST!***

Travel to or birth in other countries

Blood donor tests may not be available for some contagious diseases that are found only in certain countries. If you were born in, have lived in, or visited certain countries, you may not be eligible to donate.

WHAT HAPPENS AFTER YOUR DONATION

To protect patients, your blood is tested for hepatitis B and C, HIV, certain other infectious diseases, and syphilis. If your blood tests positive it will not be given to a patient. You will be notified about test results that may disqualify you from donating in the future. **Please do not donate to get tested for HIV, hepatitis, or any other infections!**

Thank you for donating blood today!
(Donor Center Name)
(Telephone Number)

Chapter 6

Whole Blood Collection and Component Processing at Blood Collection Centers

Ram Kakaiya, MD, MBBS; Colleen A. Aronson, MT(ASCP)SBB; and Jana Julleis, MBA, MT(ASCP)SBB

THE COLLECTION OF whole blood (WB) from the donor and subsequent processing of the donation into separate components are key links in the transfusion chain of events. Careful attention to proper technique is critical to ensure optimal care of both the donor and the recipient. This chapter describes WB collection and covers only those aspects of component preparation and processing that predominantly take place at the blood centers.

WHOLE BLOOD COLLECTION

The phlebotomy staff involved in WB collection should be trained in proper collection technique to minimize contamination of the donated unit and to minimize phlebotomy-related local complications such as hematoma or nerve injury. Phlebotomists and other (collection) staff perform those functions under the direction of the medical director through the use of approved standard operating procedures (SOPs). Phlebotomy should be performed only after the donor has been found to be eligible for blood donation (Chapter 5) and the following items have been properly labeled using a unique unit identification (ID) number label: the blood donor record, the primary and satellite containers, and the sample tubes. A final check of appropriate labeling before phlebotomy ensures that the donor history data, laboratory data, and other manufacturing data are assigned to the right blood components. The final check can be documented by having the staff initial the donor record.

Ram Kakaiya, MD, MBBS, Medical Director, LifeSource Blood Services, Glenview, Illinois; Colleen A. Aronson, MT(ASCP)SBB, Blood Bank Quality Program Coordinator, Northshore University Health System, Evanston, Illinois; and Jana Julleis, MBA, MT(ASCP)SBB, Director, Manufacturing Processes, Blood Systems, Inc, Scottsdale, Arizona

The authors have disclosed no conflicts of interest.

Blood Containers

Desirable Properties

Blood containers or collection sets used for WB collection must be approved by the Food and Drug Administration (FDA), and they should be pyrogen-free and identified by a lot number. The desired properties of storage containers include the following: easily formed and processed, flexible, tough, kink resistant, and scratch resistant. In addition, the container's material should be able to withstand sterilization by gamma irradiation, ethylene oxide, electron beam, or all three. The plastic should allow adequate gas exchange for oxygen and carbon dioxide yet prevent evaporation of water from the blood component.

Blood containers in use are often made of polyvinyl chloride (PVC) plastic that contains di-(2-ethylhexyl) phthalate (DEHP) to make the containers pliable. Butyryl-trihexyl-citrate (BTHC) containers do not contain DEHP and are available for some blood components. Latex-free plastic containers are available for transfusions to patients with latex allergy (see Table 6-1). Although PVC containers are widely used, they have one major disadvantage: PVC containers have a tendency to break when used for frozen components. For PVC, the glass transition phase is about –25 C to –30 C. At those temperatures, the frozen product containers should be treated as if they are glass and fragile enough to break during jarring that occurs in the course of transport and handling.

Configurations

Containers come in different configurations: single, double, triple, or quadruple bags. More recently, additional configurations for blood containers include in-line filters for removal of leukocytes from WB or Red Blood Cell (RBC) units. Approved anticoagulant-preservatives include acid-citrate-dextrose solution (ACD), citrate-phosphate-dextrose solution (CPD), citrate-phosphate-dextrose-dextrose solution (CP2D), and citrate-phosphate-dextrose-adenine solution (CPDA-1). Composition, pH, and approved shelf life of RBCs for those anticoagulants are described in Table 6-2 and Table 6-3. The container configuration is available with one bag containing an additive solution. The three forms of additive solution (AS) that are in use are AS-1, AS-3, and AS-5; their constituents are listed in Table 6-4. These solutions should be pyrogen-free. Blood containers are supplied in pouches or packages that, once opened, should be used within the time prescribed by the manufacturer. Unused containers should be stored within open packages until the expiration date or time. The opened pouches should be labeled with the date and time that they were opened.

Containers have ports that allow access into each bag for transfer of components between the bags. Dielectric sealing or a metal clamp may be used to prepare segments of tubing.

The base label on the container shows the name of the manufacturer. Base labels and any additional labels that are placed directly on the container must use FDA-approved adhesives. In accordance with the FDA guideline for the uniform labeling of blood and blood components issued in 1985, only those substances that are FDA approved as "indirect food additives" may be used in adhesives and coating components for labels placed over the base label. The FDA has additional standards for labels that are applied directly on plastic blood containers. Because of a lack of sufficient space for attaching labels directly to the container, tie tags may be used as an appropriate alternative, particularly for those items that do not have to be directly affixed to the container.

Diversion Pouch

Collection containers with a diversion pouch are required if platelets are going to be prepared.[1(p21)] The system allows diversion of the first 30 to 45 mL of blood being collected into a pouch instead of the collection bag. Blood in the pouch is subsequently used to fill sample tubes for donor testing. The diversion pouches effectively capture the "skin plug" cored by the phlebotomy needle, resulting in decreased bacterial contamination of blood components by as much as 50% (see "Phlebotomy" below).[2]

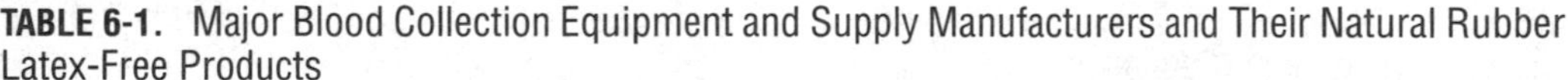

TABLE 6-1. Major Blood Collection Equipment and Supply Manufacturers and Their Natural Rubber Latex-Free Products

Manufacturer	Latex-Free Products	Comments
Pall Medical (East Hills, NY)	1. Leukotrap systems that have sample diversion pouch with the following configurations: RC PL and PL system; RC2D leukocyte reduction filter; WB system 2. Leukotrap SC RC leukocyte reduction filtration system for RBCs with BPF4 high efficiency filter 3. eBDS sample set 4. BPF4 high efficiency filter 5. Whole blood collection system with Nutricel Additive System (for non-leukocyte-reduced RBCs) 6. Acrodose PL and Acrodose PLus Systems	Personal communication (Karen Peterson-Doyle, Senior Director, Global Labeling Services, Pall Medical)
Terumo (Somerset, NJ)	1. TERUFLEX blood bags (with standard tubing; blood sampling arm with and without DonorCare; diversion blood sampling arm) 2. IMUFLEX blood bag 3. TERUFLEX dry blood bag (all sizes) 4. Straight-type blood administration set with 170-micron mesh filter 5. Plasma transfer set 6. Sampling site coupler 7. Medisystems apheresis needles, with MasterGuard anti-stick needle protector with and without clamp 8. VENOJECT multi-sample luer adapter 9. VENOJECT standard tube holder 10. DonorCare needle guard 11. Samp*lok* kit tube holder 12. Samp*lok* kit tube holder with luer adapter 13. Phlebotomy needle cap holder 14. Plasma separation stand 15. Green tubing clips 16. Blue slide clamp 17. Phlebotomy squeezers 18. Small multi pocket organizer 19. TERUSEAL tube sealer 20. SCD 312 sterile tubing welder 21. SCD IIB sterile tubing welder 22. TSCD sterile tubing welder 23. SCD welding wafers 24. Aluminum sealing clips	http://terumotransfusion.com/ Latex-free.aspx

(Continued)

TABLE 6-1. Major Blood Collection Equipment and Supply Manufacturers and Their Natural Rubber Latex-Free Products (Continued)

Manufacturer	Latex-Free Products	Comments
Haemonetics (Braintree, MA)	Haemonetics Patient Division disposable products contain no latex in the disposable sets or their packaging	Personal communication (Karen Elsner, Director of Product Marketing, Patient Division, Haemonetics Corp.)
Fenwal Blood Technologies (Lake Zurich, IL)	1. ALYX red cell collection kits 2. AMICUS apheresis kits for platelets 3. PLASMACELL-C disposable kits (except code S4R2278C) 4. BLOOD-PACK UNITS (except code 4R3202MC) 5. Bulk anticoagulant and blood processing solutions (such as sodium citrate and ACD-A) 6. TRANSFER PACK containers 7. Sterile-connect and bedside leukoreduction filter sets for red cells or platelets (except codes 4C2496 and 4C2497) 8. Transfer and administration sets (except code 4C2223) 9. Plasma pooling bottles 10. Ancillary products such as HEMATYPE segment device, hand sealers, sealer clips, and slide clamps	Personal communication (Bryan Blickman, Director, Engineering, and Tim Karlovsky, Senior Quality Engineer) Note: In a small number of applications, use of natural rubber latex components may be unavoidable. Examples of certain products that do contain natural rubber latex components: 1. Blood component infusion set, code 4C2223 2. Sample site coupler, code 4C2405 3. Bedside leukoreduction filter for platelets, codes 4C2496 and 4C2497 4. PLASMACELL-C disposable set, code S4R2278C 5. BLOOD-PACK UNIT for manual plasmapheresis, code 4R3203MC 6. Marrow collection kits (all codes) 7. Apheresis kits for the CS-3000 Blood Cell Separator Cautionary statements: These lists are not intended to be comprehensive. Consult directions for use for the particular product, and refer to Technical Information Document 1137810 for Fenwal's position regarding the term latex-free.

RBCs = Red Blood Cells; ACD-A = acid-citrate-dextrose formula A.

TABLE 6-2. Anticoagulant-Preservative Solutions (mg in 63 mL) for Collection*

Variable	CPD	CP2D	CPDA-1	ACD-A	ACD-B	4% Citrate
pH	5.3-5.9	5.3-5.9	5.3-5.9	4.5-5.5	4.5-5.5	6.4-7.5
Ratio (mL solution to blood)	1.4:10	1.4:10	1.4:10	1.5:10	2.5:10	0.625:10
FDA-approved shelf life (days)	21	21	35	Automated collection of RBCs, platelets, and FFP		Automated collection of plasma and for plasma exchange
Content						
Sodium citrate	1660	1660	1660	1386	832	2520
Citric acid	206	206	206	504	504	As needed for pH adjustment
Dextrose	1610	3220	2010	1599	956	
Monobasic sodium phosphate	140	140	140			
Adenine	0	0	17.3			

*For collection of 450 mL whole blood (or automated collections).
CPD = citrate-phosphate-dextrose; CP2D = citrate-phosphate-dextrose-dextrose; CPDA-1 = citrate-phosphate-dextrose-adenine; ACD-A = acid-citrate-dextrose formula A; ACD-B = acid-citrate-dextrose formula B; FDA = Food and Drug Administration; FFP = Fresh Frozen Plasma.

TABLE 6-3. Anticoagulant-Preservative Solutions (mg in 70 mL)*

Variable	CPD	CP2D	CPDA-1
pH	5.3-5.9	5.3-5.9	5.3-5.9
Ratio (mL solution to blood)	1.4:10	1.4:10	1.4:10
FDA-approved shelf life (days)	21	21	35
Content			
Sodium citrate	1840	1840	1840
Citric acid	209	229	229
Dextrose	1780	3570	2230
Monobasic sodium phosphate	155	155	155
Adenine	0	0	19

*For collection of 500 mL whole blood.
CPD = citrate-phosphate-dextrose; CP2D = citrate-phosphate-dextrose-dextrose; CPDA-1 = citrate-phosphate-dextrose-adenine; FDA = Food and Drug Administration.

TABLE 6-4. Content of Additive Solutions (mg/100 mL)

Constituent	AS-1 (Adsol)	AS-3 (Nutricel)	AS-5 (Optisol)
Dextrose	2200	1100	900
Adenine	27	30	30
Monobasic sodium phosphate	0	276	0
Mannitol	750	0	525
Sodium chloride	900	410	877
Sodium citrate	0	588	0
Citric acid	0	42	0

Container Modification by Sterile Connecting Device

Blood containers can be modified by using a sterile connecting device. FDA-approved indications for the use of a sterile connecting device are presented in Table 6-5.[3] Use of such a device is increasing rapidly, primarily for obtaining a sample from apheresis platelets for bacterial contamination testing; for attaching a leukocyte reduction filter to prepare prestorage leukocyte reduced RBCs and platelets; and for preparing pooled platelets and pooled cryoprecipitate, prestorage or prior to transfusion.

Donor and Blood Component Identification

Assignment of blood components and test results to the properly identified donor is critical to ensuring the transfusion recipient's safety. Those elements should match before blood collection can proceed, as well as during and after the collection.

Before phlebotomy, the donor is asked to present appropriate identification. Donor-identifying information commonly includes the donor's first name, middle name or initial, last name, and birth date. A donor's Social Security number is less commonly used as an identifier because of concern about identity theft. Contact information is obtained from each donor and is necessary for future recruitment and for notification of the donor about abnormal test results. The blood component ID process uniformly uses both a bar-coded and an eye-readable unique number that is assigned to each sample tube and each component prepared from the donation. The donor history form and blood sample tubes are similarly labeled with the unique number. Electronic records of the donation are also assigned the same number.

Phlebotomy

Vein Selection

The phlebotomist selects one arm for phlebotomy after inspecting both of the donor's arms. The arm is selected on the basis of the presence of a prominent, large, firm vein in the antecubital fossa to permit a single, readily accessible phlebotomy site that is devoid of scarring or skin lesions. Training arms are commercially available for use with new phlebotomy staff and are helpful in achieving simulated visual and tactile training for venous puncture.

A blood pressure cuff generally inflated at a pressure of between 40 and 60 mm Hg, or a tourniquet, is applied to enlarge the vein. Palpating the vein is also recommended before the phlebotomy site is prepared. The median vein is centrally located in the antecubital fossa and is the first choice because it is well anchored. The second choice is the cephalic vein that lies laterally (shoulder side) and is often superficial. The third and final choice is the

TABLE 6-5. Use of Sterile Connecting Devices for Modification of Collection Containers[3]

Use	Comment
To add a new or smaller needle to a blood collection set	If needle is added during the procedure, an approved device to weld liquid-filled tubing should be used.
To prepare components	Some examples include adding a fourth bag to make cryoprecipitate, adding solution to the RBC unit, or adding an in-line filter.
To pool blood products	Appropriate use of a sterile connecting device to pool platelets prepared from Whole Blood collection may obviate potential contamination from the spike and port entries commonly used.
To prepare an aliquot for pediatric use and divided units	FDA provides specific guidance if this activity is considered to be manufacturing new products.
To connect additional saline or anticoagulant lines during an automated plasmapheresis procedure	SOPs are required, although prior approval from the FDA is not required.
To attach processing solutions	Examples include washing and freezing RBCs.
To add an FDA-cleared leukocyte reduction filter	To prepare prestorage leukocyte-reduced RBCs.
To remove samples from blood product containers for testing	Label may need revision if cell count of the product is affected.

FDA = Food and Drug Administration; SOPs = standard operating procedures.

basilic vein, which lies on the underside of the antecubital fossa; the basilic vein is not well anchored and may roll during phlebotomy. Excessive probing with the needle should be avoided to prevent nerve injury. Although the Occupational Safety and Health Administration (OSHA) provides specific exemption from the requirements for having to wear gloves during phlebotomy of volunteer blood donors, some blood collection centers require their employees to wear gloves for phlebotomy of all donors.

Methods of Disinfection of Venipuncture Site

Specific instructions in the product insert for the use of FDA-approved agents should be followed for arm and phlebotomy site preparation (Method 6-2). Those methods provide surgical cleanliness, but none of the methods can achieve an absolutely aseptic site. An absence of any bacterial colonies on culture after disinfection with povidone-iodine or isopropyl alcohol plus iodine tincture is seen in approximately 50% of cases.[4] Bacterial growth with low colony numbers (1 to 100) may be seen in about half of the cases.[4] More than 100 colonies is rare (1%) in such cultures.[4]

During phlebotomy, a small plug of donor skin can enter the needle and can flow into the collected blood. Bacteria residing deep within skin layers are not accessible to disinfectants. Therefore, if the skin plug enters the collection bag, it can result in contamination. Concern over contamination is supported by venipuncture data on pigskin. Pigskin epidermal cells were detectable in the lavage fluid in 1 out of 150 punctures.[5] Whether human skin fragments or epidermal cells are carried into the bag during routine blood donation has not been studied in detail. Nonetheless, AABB *Standards for Blood Banks and Transfusion Services* (*Standards*) requires the use of collection containers that divert the first 30 to 45 mL of blood into a diversion pouch to retain skin plugs to prevent contamination when platelet components will be prepared from the collection.[1(p21)]

Blood Collection Process

Blood should be collected into an approved container with a single venipuncture that allows rapid flow. Method 6-3 describes steps for blood collection and sample collection for processing and compatibility tests. The average time in which 500 mL of blood is collected is less than 10 minutes. A draw time longer than 15 to 20 minutes may render the unit unsuitable for platelets or plasma for transfusions. In some countries where the average donor weight is low, the average collection volume may be 200 to 250 mL. AABB *Standards* permits collection of 10.5 mL of blood per kilogram (kg) of the donor's weight for each donation.[1(p56)]

Clotted and EDTA-anticoagulated specimens for testing are collected from the diversion pouch according to the time limits established by the manufacturer. Other methods include the following: cutting the withdrawal tubing and allowing blood to drip into tubes; using specially designed, integrated, Y-shaped, bifurcation line adapters; and using the collection needle to transfer blood from the containers into specimen tubes. A second phlebotomy may also be performed if the donated unit is collected satisfactorily but the sample quantity for testing is insufficient. The second phlebotomy should occur immediately after the blood collection.[6,7] Generally three to four tubes are collected for testing. Facilities that send their samples for testing to a distant location sometimes collect an extra tube to retain on-site. Blood collection container design now includes safety devices such as the sliding sheath needle guard to prevent accidental needle-stick injuries. These devices allow retraction of the needle into a safety guard at the completion of blood collection. Capping of needles should be avoided to prevent injuries.

Amount of Blood Collected

FDA-approved container labels indicate the amount of blood that can be collected depending on the amount of anticoagulant present in the container. In the United States, the volume of blood collected during routine phlebotomy is typically either 450 ± 10% (405-495 mL) or 500 mL ± 10% (450-550 mL). The volume of blood collected can be assessed in terms of gram weight by multiplying the volume collected by the specific gravity of blood (1.053). For 500-mL collection, weight limits of collected blood are 474 to 579 g. Those limits for 450-mL collection are 427 to 521 g. The weight of the bag and that of the retention segments are added to the blood volume's weight to obtain the total weight of the collected unit. With the maximum permissible donation volume of 10.5 mL/kg, a donor who weighs 100 lb (45 kg) can donate 473 mL, which is greater than the lower limit of the allowable collection. Overweight collections include units that exceed the volume of 550 mL (579 g) for the 500-mL containers. For autologous donors weighing >50 kg, the 450-mL collection bag is usually used instead of the 500-mL bag, in case the donor cannot give a full unit. If a low-volume (300-405 mL) unit is collected, the red cells are suitable for storage and subsequent autologous transfusion. The plasma from low-volume units cannot be transfused because of the abnormal anticoagulant/plasma ratio. Under-collected units (<300 mL) may be suitable for autologous use with approval of the medical director. For patients weighing <50 kg, there should be a proportional reduction in the volume of blood collected. Regardless of donor weight, the volume collected should not exceed 10.5 mL/kg of the donor's estimated body weight, including the samples for testing.

Red cell survival is not significantly affected by the volume of blood collected, as described below.[8] Red cell survival (average) after 21 days of storage in CPD was reported to be acceptable (approximately 80%) when only 300 g (285 mL) of blood was collected. Survival was more than 90% when 400 g (380 mL) of blood was collected and stored for 21 days. Similarly, as much as 600 g (570 mL) of blood collected in a standard 450-mL CPD container and stored for 21 days had normal red cell survival.[8] Undercollected units (275 mL or 290 g) in CPDA-1 and stored for 35 days had a mean 24-hour survival of 88%.[9] These data show that for undercollected and overcollected units, variability in the amount of collection does not adversely affect red cell storage for 21 to 35 days.

Specific Gravity of Blood Cells and Blood Components

Specific gravities of principal blood cells and blood components are described in Table 6-6. In practice, knowledge of the specific gravity of different blood cells is helpful in developing centrifugal conditions for optimal cell separation and collection. In addition, the values for the blood components are needed to convert weight of the component in grams to the volume in milliliters. For instance, as mentioned above, for WB, gram weight is divided by the specific gravity of the WB (1.053) to get the volume of WB in a bag. It should be noted that several factors affect the specific gravity, including temperature, measurement method, protein concentration, cell size, and hemoglobin level. The values provided in Table 6-6 are generally accepted values, and for some, the applicable regulatory documents provide a specific number for use.

TABLE 6-6. Density (Specific Gravity) of Principal Blood Cells and Components

Blood Cell or Component	Specific Gravity	Source
Cells		Council of Europe[10]
Platelets	1.058	
Monocytes	1.062	
Lymphocytes	1.070	
Neutrophils	1.082	
Red cells	1.100	
Components		
Red cells collected by automated methods with additive solution	1.06	FDA guidance[11]
Red cells collected by automated methods without additive solution	1.08	FDA guidance[11]
Apheresis Platelets	1.03	FDA guidance[12]
Plasma		Dependent on manufacturer of plasma or plasma derivatives
Octapharma AG*	1.026	
CSL Plasma†	1.027	
Fenwal (Amicus Cell Separator)‡	1.027	
Whole blood	1.053	FDA guide for inspection of blood banks[13]

*Octapharma AG, Lachen, Switzerland.

†CSL (previously ZLB) Plasma, Boca Raton, FL.

‡Fenwal, Lake Zurich, IL.

Donor Care After Phlebotomy

Immediately after collection, the needle is withdrawn into a protective sleeve to prevent accidental injuries. Local pressure is applied by hand to the gauze placed directly over the venipuncture site while the donor's arm is kept elevated. Pressure is applied until hemostasis is achieved, which may require more time for some donors who are taking anticoagulants or antiplatelet drugs. Once hemostasis is evident, a bandage or a tape may be applied.

Postphlebotomy care includes observing the donor for signs or symptoms of reactions. If the donor tolerates a sitting position without problems, the donor may be allowed to proceed to the canteen area and is encouraged to drink fluids while waiting to be released. Local or state laws may specify the amount of time that the donor must wait after the donation and before leaving the collection area. The donor is encouraged to drink more fluids for the next few hours, to avoid alcohol ingestion for several hours, and to refrain from smoking for some period following the donation. The donor is also instructed to apply local pressure to the phlebotomy site if any bleeding recurs and to call the blood center if the bleeding does not stop with pressure. A telephone number is provided so the donor can report if he or she feels that the donated unit should not be used, has any reactions, or experiences any signs or symptoms of infection.

Adverse Donor Reactions

On donor follow-up surveys, minor reactions, such as a dime-sized hematoma at the phlebotomy site, are reported by as many as one-third of all donors.[14] Adverse reactions are seen at the time of donation or reported later in about 3.5% of donations, on average. Reactions that need medical care after the donor has left the donation site are seen in 1 in 3400 donors. In a study of 7,000,000 WB donations, incidence numbers for different types of donor reactions were calculated and are summarized in Table 6-7.[14]

Systemic Reactions

Vasovagal reaction complex includes dizziness, sweating, nausea, vomiting, weakness, apprehension, pallor, hypotension, and bradycardia. In severe cases, syncope and convulsions may be observed. The pulse rate is often low during vasovagal reactions, while the rate is often high during volume depletion. Some donors with severe reactions or those with prolonged recovery times may need short-term observation, intravenous fluid adminis-

TABLE 6-7. The Incidence of Whole-Blood Donor Complications and Outside Medical Care[14]

Variable	Incidence: Observation or Donor Complaint	Incidence: Observations and Postdonation Interview	Donors Needing Outside Medical Care
Local: Bruise, sore arm, hematoma, nerve irritation, nerve injury, local allergy, arterial puncture, thrombophlebitis, and local infection	Approximately 0.002% for thrombophlebitis to 0.35% for hematoma	Approximately 0.9% for nerve irritation or injury to 22.7% for a bruise reported by the donor	Approximately 1:20,000 for hematoma or nerve injury; 1:225,000 for local infection
Systemic: Fatigue, vasovagal reaction, syncope with or without injury, nausea, vomiting, and vascular events	Approximately 0.01% for syncope with injury to 2.5% for vasovagal reaction	Approximately 0.4% for nausea or vomiting to 7.8% for fatigue	Approximately 1:9000 for vasovagal reaction

tration in the emergency room, or both. A protocol for a telephone follow-up of donors who have experienced severe reactions is helpful to assess the donors for any residual symptoms. Donors experiencing severe reactions generally defer themselves from future allogeneic donations although they may consider preoperative autologous donations.

Approximately 60% of systemic reactions are seen in the canteen area.[14] The reactions are more common in young donors, low-weight donors, female donors, and first-time donors. Ingestion of antihypertensive medications does not appear to be a risk factor.[15] Nonsyncopal reactions are 25 times more common than syncopal reactions.[14] About 15% of reactions occur away from the donation site and usually within 1 hour of donation.[14] In donors experiencing a reaction, an injury to head, face, or extremity may occur. The staff should be vigilant to detect reactions early and to prevent injuries as much as possible.

Phlebotomy should be stopped, and the donor should be placed in a recumbent position as soon as any reaction is suspected. Application of cold wet towels to the donor's neck and shoulder area and the loosening of the donor's clothes can assist in symptom management.

During automated component collection, the donor is given saline as a replacement—generally in equal volume to what is collected and therefore possibly reducing the frequency of donor reactions. Similarly, oral fluid intake before and soon after the nonautomated WB donation appears to reduce the frequency of systemic reactions.[16] Coffee ingestion can reduce the frequency of reactions, but it may also reduce blood flow during collection because of its vasoconstrictive effect.

Bruise or Hematoma

Bruising or hematomas are common after phlebotomy but generally do not prevent donor return.

Fatigue

First-time donors and females are more likely to report fatigue after donation. Donor return is reduced by one-third among those donors experiencing this symptom.[14]

Local Nerve Injury

Nerve injuries may be unavoidable because nerves cannot be palpated. In 40% of cases of nerve injuries, phlebotomy was performed without any difficulty.[14] Donors may complain of sensory changes away from the phlebotomy site, such as in the forearm, wrist, hand, upper arm, or shoulder. Those injuries are almost always transient, and recovery is almost always seen; however, in 7% of injured donors, it may take 3 to 9 months.[14] In severe cases, a neurologist referral may be indicated.

Arterial Puncture

Bright red blood, rapid collection (within 4 minutes), and pulsating needle suggest arterial puncture. The hematoma rate is higher with arterial puncture. When puncture is recognized early, the needle should be pulled out immediately, and local pressure should be applied for an extended period. Most donors recover quickly and completely, but some might present with waxing and waning hematomas and should be evaluated for pseudoaneurysm by ultrasound studies.

Upper Extremity Deep Vein Thrombosis

Only one case of this thrombosis has been reported in the literature.[14] Symptoms include pain; antecubital fossa tenderness; swelling of the arm; and a prominent, palpable, cord-like thickening of the thrombosed vein. Medical referral of donors who are experiencing deep vein thrombosis should not be delayed so that treatment with anticoagulant can begin promptly.

Postdonation Mortality

The FDA requires that blood establishments report deaths caused by blood donation. Between 1976 and 1985, three deaths were reported to the FDA. Most deaths seen after blood donation are coincidentally related to the donation rather than caused by it.[14]

BLOOD COMPONENT PREPARATION AND PROCESSING

WB is separated into components so that treatment-specific components can be provided to multiple recipients. Blood centers should plan and coordinate the type of container configurations to use at each collection site so that a desired mix of components is produced each day. The collected WB is transported to the component laboratory where differential centrifugation is used to prepare the components.

The FDA requires that blood be collected in pyrogen-free, sterile, uncolored, and transparent containers. Plastic collection containers that are hermetically sealed allow component manufacturing to take place in a closed system. The blood container should not be entered before issue except for the purposes of blood collection or transferring of components to a different container. The container material should not have an adverse effect on the safety, purity, or potency of the blood. In some cases, open-system manufacturing becomes necessary, although use of sterile connecting devices (approved by the FDA) are available and their use is encouraged.[3] Examples include preparation of prestorage pooled cryoprecipitate, washed RBCs or platelets, or deglycerolized RBCs. Components prepared with an open system may require a reduction in their expiration time.

The goal of blood component preparation is to separate WB into its major components while reducing the content of other components. For example, reduction of unwanted leukocytes in a unit of RBCs is a desirable goal. In Europe, leukocyte reduction is partially achieved by routine preparation of buffy-coat-depleted red cells. In North America, the primary method for leukocyte reduction is by filtration. In addition to the various methods popular in Europe and North America, many other collection and component preparation parameters affect the quality of products. Those variables are summarized in Table 6-8. A recent development is the increase in automated collection of components at the donor sites [eg, leukocyte-reduced (LR) RBCs, platelets, and plasma products]. Automated component collection reduces the need for centralized component manufacturing. Increasing use of prestorage leukocyte reduction is causing the component laboratories to look at complex technologies such as flow cytometry for performing residual leukocyte counts. More quality control (QC) testing of LR blood components has become necessary, resulting in an increase in the resources needed for QC. The number of procedures that require use of a sterile connecting device is also increasing the complexity of tasks performed in the laboratory. Pooling of platelets for 5-day storage and bacterial-contamination testing of platelets are also changing the nature of work being performed in the laboratory.

Transportation of Whole Blood

WB that is collected at mobile blood drives or at fixed collection sites should be transported as soon after collection as possible to the central component preparation laboratory. Regulatory and quality requirements dictate the postcollection temperature and time in which the blood must be transported. By the time phlebotomy is completed, the blood has air-cooled to about 30 C.[18] If such units are left at the ambient temperature, the cooling rate is quite slow and about 6 hours more are needed for units to reach 25 C.[18] Units are typically placed in specific storage environments depending on the component that will be prepared. For example, units from which platelets will be made are cooled toward room temperature (20-24 C). Some centers use cooling plates that provide rate-controlled cooling toward 20 C. Those cooling plates contain melting 1,4-butandiol wax that has a melting temperature of 20 C and serves as a heat absorber. With the cooling plates, about 2 hours are needed for the collected blood to reach 20 C.[18] If platelets will not be prepared the WB is generally placed in a storage environment that contains ice.

Shipping containers used for transportation should be validated to ensure that proper temperature is maintained. Validation is performed with various quantities of units in the

TABLE 6-8. Variables during Blood Collection, Processing, and Component Preparations That Affect Product Quality

Variable	Example/Comment
Collection containers	Gas exchange properties permit different storage length of components (eg, platelets).
Type of blood mixing	Automated mixing may reduce interruption in mixing.
Collection or draw time	Prolonged draw time (15 to 20 minutes) may not be suitable for platelet or plasma products.
Amount of blood collected	An alteration in the ratio of blood to anticoagulant may affect storage of RBCs.
Primary anticoagulant-preservative: ACD, CPD, CPDA-1, additive solutions	Permitted length of storage for RBCs varies with the type of preservative.
Temporary storage of whole blood before centrifugation	Labile coagulation factor levels decrease during room temperature or refrigerated storage. Platelets are better preserved when whole blood is stored at ambient temperature rather than at 4 C.
Centrifugation conditions	Major factors include temperature, duration of centrifugation, maximum *g*-force achieved, balancing of centrifuge cups, degree of braking.
Method of separation of cellular and plasma components	Automated methods may reduce variability in red cell contamination of platelets and may permit increased extraction of plasma. Buffy-coat removal allows reduction in leukocytes in cellular components.
Timing of RBC processing	Time limits exist during which leukocyte reduction must take place for prestorage leukocyte-reduced RBCs.
Freezing of plasma	Faster freezing may allow improved recovery of coagulation Factor VIII.

Modified from Heaton et al.[17]

RBCs = Red Blood Cells; ACD = acid-citrate-dextrose; CPD = citrate-phosphate-dextrose; CPDA-1 = citrate-phosphate-dextrose-adenine.

transport container and with a fixed amount of ice or gel-pack to determine the number of units that can be stored and transported while maintaining the desired temperature. Portable temperature monitors are available to record the temperature continuously.

Platelet-rich plasma (PRP) should be separated from RBCs within the time frame specified in the directions for use of the blood collection, processing, and storage system. In Europe, a 24-hour hold at 20 to 24 C is permitted to prepare platelets using the buffy-coat method.[10] Units destined for Fresh Frozen Plasma (FFP) are transported with ice to allow them to cool toward 1 to 10 C. FFP should be separated from the WB and frozen within the time frame specified in the directions for use of the blood collection, processing, and storage system. In the United States, plasma that is separated from WB collection and placed in the freezer within 8 to 24 hours after collection of WB can be labeled as "Plasma Frozen Within 24 Hours After Phlebotomy." In Europe, if the WB is refrigerated, plasma may be separated within 18 hours; if the WB is held at 20 to 24 C for platelet production, plasma can be separated within 24 hours, frozen, and labeled as FFP.[10]

Primary Separation by Centrifugation

The first step in preparing the three major blood components—RBCs, platelets, and plasma—is centrifugation of WB (primary separation). Methods 6-4, 6-10, and 6-13 describe preparation of those three components from WB.

The three major variables that affect the recovery of cells from WB by differential centrifugation are rotor size, centrifuge speed, and duration of centrifugation. Published papers often refer to relative centrifugation force (g-force) that is derived from the radius of the centrifuge rotor and the revolutions of the rotor.

More than one combination of these parameters can provide the optimal yield of platelets in platelet concentrates. For a given centrifuge, the rotor size is generally not variable. Therefore, the other two variables (centrifuge speed and duration) can be altered in a stepwise fashion in a Simplex strategy to determine the optimal conditions for preparing PRP.[19] The Simplex strategy can also be used to identify the optimal conditions of centrifugation for platelet concentrates when QC data show that the platelet counts in the platelet concentrates are not satisfactory. Method 8-4 describes a process of functional calibration of the centrifuge to maximize platelet yield.

After PRP and RBCs are separated by the first centrifugation step (soft spin), the supernatant PRP is removed into another container. Most laboratories use manual methods to express the supernatant plasma from the RBCs, although semiautomated devices are also available (see below).

Secondary Separation by Centrifugation

The PRP container undergoes secondary centrifugation using higher *g*-forces to pellet the platelets (hard spin). The resulting supernatant platelet-poor plasma (PPP) is transferred to another container, leaving approximately 40 to 70 mL of PPP with the pellet. The platelet pellet is allowed to remain undisturbed for a minimum of 1 hour and then is resuspended in the plasma. Once platelets are resuspended, they are stored at room temperature (between 20 to 24 C) with continuous agitation during storage per FDA requirements. In Europe, the buffy-coat method involves a "hard spin" for primary separation and thus allows greater plasma recovery.[17]

On the day of preparation, some units may contain clumps that are composed of platelet aggregates.[20] In routine practice, precise determination of the number and size of clumps is not possible. Visual inspection is adequate to determine the degree of clumping subjectively and to ensure that units with excessive clumping are not released for labeling. Most of the clumps seen on day 0 disappear on day 1 of storage with continuous agitation, particularly those showing light to moderate clumping.[20] The temperature at which platelets are prepared may influence clumping; platelets prepared at 24 C appear to show the least amount of clumping compared to those prepared at less than 24 C.[20] Visual inspections after the platelet concentrates are prepared have shown an absence of visible red cells in the vast majority of units, which implies that the units contain fewer than 0.4×10^9 red cells.[21] Generally, the number of red cells in a unit of platelets does not exceed 1.0×10^9.[21]

Automated Blood Component Processing

Blood component extractors are available for making components in a semiautomated manner. After primary centrifugation, WB is placed in the extractor, and a pressure plate creates an outflow of components from the container. Outflow can occur from the top or the bottom of the container, depending on the device. When a cellular interface is detected by an optical sensing device, outflow tubing is automatically clamped at an appropriate level. Such devices may improve the standardization of components, but they are not widely used in the United States.

An automated system is available in Europe that performs multiple functions to prepare pooled platelet concentrates derived from WB by the buffy-coat method. Steps that are automated include pooling, rinsing, centrifugation, transfer, filtration, and sealing.

DESCRIPTIONS OF MAJOR BLOOD COMPONENTS

Whole Blood

When an anticoagulant-preservative is present, the minimum hematocrit in Whole Blood units is usually around 33%. WB is most often separated into components and is rarely used for transfusion directly. Labile coagulation factors diminish as the storage interval increases. WB may be reconstituted by combining RBCs with FFP to achieve a desired hematocrit level—for example, when used for neonatal exchange transfusions. Further information about the preparation of reconstituted Whole Blood is provided in Chapter 9.

Red Blood Cells

CPD- or CP2D-preserved RBCs have a shelf life of 21 days and a hematocrit of 65% to 80%. CPD-preserved RBCs <7 to 10 days old are commonly provided for neonatal or pediatric transfusions. AS can be added to CPD or CP2D RBCs to extend their shelf life to 42 days. AS should be added to RBCs according to the manufacturer's instructions—generally within 72 hours of the blood collection. These preservatives are designed to minimize hemolysis during storage to less than 1%. The amount of AS added to RBCs from a 450-mL WB collection is 100 mL; for a 500-mL collection, the amount added is 110 mL. Mannitol is present in AS-1 and AS-5 but not in AS-3. The residual plasma in a unit of AS RBCs is generally <50 mL. The hematocrit of these units ranges from 55% to 65%. Such a hematocrit level facilitates excellent flow rates during transfusion, obviating the need to add saline to the bag. RBCs can also be collected and preserved in CPDA-1 (hematocrit <80%) with a shelf life of 35 days. (See Chapter 9, Table 9-1, for expiration dates of selected blood components currently in use.)

RBCs can be leukocyte reduced by filtering WB with an in-line leukocyte reduction filter or by attaching a filter with a sterile connecting device (see Method 6-5). In either case, residual leukocytes should not exceed 5×10^6 per unit in the United States or 1.0×10^6 per unit in Europe. The majority of RBC units are leukocyte reduced within 72 hours and always within 120 hours of collection per recommendations of the leukocyte reduction filter manufacturer.

The hemoglobin content per unit of RBCs is variable because hemoglobin levels vary from donor to donor. In the United States, a lower limit on the amount of hemoglobin that must be present in a unit has not been established. For a standard unit of RBCs in Europe, the lower limit is 45 g per the Council of Europe's standards.[10] Although a unit of RBCs prepared from a 450- or 500-mL WB collection typically contains a minimum of 45 g of hemoglobin, that amount is reduced to about 40 g in LR components.[22] The amount of hemoglobin per unit is determined for each automated component collection system and is based on the donor's hemoglobin level and weight. The amount of hemoglobin present in RBC units collected by automated methods is much more consistent than in units derived from WB collection. Some have advocated that the amount of hemoglobin per RBC unit be standardized at 50 g.[22]

RBCs that are labeled as low-volume units are made available for transfusion when 300 to 404 mL of WB is collected into an anticoagulant volume calculated for 450 ± 45 mL, or when 333 to 449 mL of WB is collected into an anticoagulant volume calculated for 500 ± 50 mL. Although the resulting RBCs may be transfused, other components such as platelets, FFP, and cryoprecipitate should not be prepared from low-volume units.

Each container is attached to a tubing that is divided into 13 to 15 segments. Segments may be used for crossmatching or for further investigation of adverse events of transfusion. A unique number is imprinted on each segment. A printed donation ID number is wrapped around the segment archived for investigative purposes in case any transfusion reactions occur. Retention segments are held at the blood center for 7 days after the expiration date of the unit and also at the hospital transfusion service for 7 days after the transfusion. Hemolysis identified in a segment by visual inspection often does not correlate to the presence of hemolysis in the unit.[23] In one study, approximately three-fourths of the visual assessments did not agree with the hemoglobin levels measured by chemical methods, indicating a high percentage of false-positive rates with visual assessment.[23]

Visual inspection of RBC units can detect white particulate matter, abnormal color caused by bacterial contamination, hemolysis, and clots. Abnormal color caused by bacterial contamination may be observed in segments that may appear lighter than the color of the bag content. The bag content may look purple with or without hemolysis, and large clots may be evident. The unit can be centrifuged to facilitate inspection of the supernatant in the case of suspected bacterial contamination, and visual inspection of the supernatant may reveal murky, brown, or red fluid.[24] However, visual inspection will not detect all contaminated units.

Blood clots in RBC units are often too small to be detected by visual inspection. Clots are sometimes revealed during transfusion when they cause clogging of the filter or in the component laboratory when the units are filtered through a leukocyte-reduction filter. Units known to have clots should not be released for transfusion.

Platelets

Two major methods are used in preparing Platelets from WB. The first is the PRP method, consisting of a soft spin followed by a hard spin (described above). The need for "resting" the resulting platelet pellet in plasma before resuspension, which is the accepted methodology, has recently been questioned.[25] In that study, resting times of 0 to 5 minutes, 1 hour, and 4 hours were compared. Both in-vitro properties and in-vivo viability were comparable between the three resting periods. Platelets are normally suspended in 40 to 70 mL of plasma, although studies have shown good recovery and survival rates when platelets were stored in plasma volumes of 35 to 40 mL.[26,27] The plasma contained in platelets does provide some coagulation factors, although labile coagulation Factor V and Factor VIII are diminished with storage, as shown in Table 6-9.

The second (buffy-coat) method consists of a hard spin of WB that enables removal of the supernatant PPP from the top of the container and the RBCs from the bottom into transfer packs. The buffy coat that remains in the primary container is used to harvest platelets. Platelets can be prepared using this method from WB stored at room temperature (not less than 20 C) for up to 24 hours. The PRP method is almost universally used in the United States, and the buffy-coat method is used in Europe and Canada.[29] One advantage of the buffy-coat method is that there is less activation of platelets than in the PRP method because in the buffy-coat method platelets are cushioned against red cells during the hard spin. Both approaches are described in Method 6-13. Platelets prepared by the PRP method result in 21% of the plasma and 19% of the platelets remaining with the red cells.[18] Therefore, the hematocrit of the packed RBCs produced with the PRP method is lower (51%) than in the buffy-coat method (60%).[18] Buffy-coat depletion also results in a 13% loss of the donated red cells. If leukocyte reduction by filtration is added to the RBCs prepared by the buffy-coat method, the loss of donated red cells is approximately 15%.[17] Plasma units prepared from buffy-coat-depleted units have approximately 41 mL more plasma than plasma units prepared by the PRP method.[17] Platelets prepared by the PRP method or the buffy-coat method can be further processed to reduce leukocytes by using a leukocyte reduction filter as described in Method 6-13.

Platelets must be continuously agitated during storage at a temperature between 20 and 24 C. However, platelets are not agitated during transport to hospitals from the blood center's distribution department nor during long-distance air transport when components are exchanged between blood centers. In-vitro studies showed that platelets are not damaged when stored without agitation for 24 hours, nor were platelets damaged when they were stored at 37 C for 6 hours followed by room-

TABLE 6-9. Coagulation Factor Values (%) in Platelet Concentrates[28]

Factor/Protein	Normal Range	Day 0	Day 1	Day 2	Day 3	Day 4	Day 5
II	78-122	104	91-96	96	85-94	90	90
V	47-153	78-98	69-78	50	36-47	28	24-35
VII	51-168	108	93-117	88	80-103	75	72
VIII	48-152	68-126	85-99	76	68-76	75	39-70
IX	62-138	72-105	100-106	95	91-98	93	63-97
X	58-142	66-101	93-94	92	85-88	84	60-83
XI	52-148	91-111	106-108	103	96-98	101	86-110
XII	46-126	117	107-112	116	106-123	123	131
Protein C	57-128	106	102	101	98	99	100
Protein S	83-167	95	75	61	40	32	31
Antithrombin	88-126	103	99	101	102	103	97
Plasminogen	60-140	140	133	126	122	124	117
Ristocetin cofactor	50-150	106	124	125	133	116	127
Fibrinogen (mg/dL)	198-434	217-308	278-313	310	265-323	302	221-299

Note: Coagulation factor % = 100 × coagulation factor units/mL.

temperature storage without agitation for an additional 18 hours.[30]

Platelets may need to be transported to distant regions during cold weather and may therefore be exposed to temperatures lower than 20 C. Studies have shown that storage at 18.5 C for 3 days is associated with decreased platelet survival when compared to storage at 21.5 C.[31] Platelets stored at 12 C for 17 hours resulted in a decrease in in-vivo recovery from 48% to 38%. Similarly, platelets stored at 16 C for 17 hours resulted in a decrease in recovery from 49% to 42%.[32] Furthermore, platelet survival has been shown to decrease to 2 days at 12 C and to 3.5 days at 16 C. Thus, proper steps should be taken to maintain the required range of temperature during storage at the blood center and during transport.

Fresh Frozen Plasma

In the United States, FFP is plasma separated from WB and placed in the freezer within 8 hours of WB collection or as directed by the manufacturer's instructions for use of the blood collection, processing, and storage system. FFP has a shelf life of 12 months while stored at –18 C or colder. According to AABB *Standards*,[1(p54)] FFP that is stored at –65 C may be stored for 7 years, but such storage requires FDA approval. The Council of Europe allows storage for up to 36 months if the FFP is stored at –25 C or colder, and 3 months if the FFP is stored within the –18 to –25 C temperature range.[10] Methods of FFP preparation listed in the Council of Europe's standards include the following: 1) plasma that is separated within 6 to 18 hours after collection if the unit is refrigerated, and 2) plasma that is separated from WB units held at a temperature between 20 and 24 C for up to 24 hours.[10] Rapid freezing of plasma can be accomplished using a blast freezer, dry ice, or a mixture of dry ice with either ethanol or antifreeze.

If continuous temperature monitoring of the component during storage is not possible, the FDA requires that the component be stored in such a manner as to allow detection of thawing. To recognize inadvertent thawing, the liquid plasma bag can be "indented" by placing a rubber band around the bag or by pressing a tube against the bag before freezing. The indentation will subsequently disappear if thawing has occurred. A plasma bag frozen in the horizontal position and then stored upright will also permit detection of thawing by tracking the air bubble that will be located at the top of the bag if thawing has occurred.

The volume of plasma per unit varies according to the method used to collect the plasma. In the past several years, many blood centers in the United States have increased the amount of WB collected from 450 to 500 mL, resulting in a higher amount of plasma per unit. A unit can contain 500 to 800 mL of plasma when collection is performed by automated (single-donor) plasmapheresis.

FFP contains normal amounts of all coagulation factors, antithrombin, and ADAMTS13.[33,34] The number of white cells present in FFP varies according to the centrifugation method used. Viable lymphocytes in thawed FFP have been documented. With the soft-spin method, the number of viable lymphocytes is 0.04 to 3.6×10^6; the hard-spin method gives 0.47 to 45.4×10^6; and with the second-spin method, the number is 0.4 to 37.2×10^6 white cells.[35] Moreover, for the hard-spin and second-spin methods, 92% and 86% of bags had counts of $>5 \times 10^6$, respectively.[35] Leukocyte-reduced FFP (LR-FFP) prepared using a filter can achieve counts of $<2.0 \times 10^5$; up to 5 units can be processed per filter.[35] Disadvantages of LR-FFP include reduced levels of some coagulation factors (Factors V, VIII, IX, XI, and XII), a volume loss of 5% to 10% during filtration, and some activation of coagulation factors.[36,37] FFP, once thawed, has a shelf life of 6 hours at 1 to 6 C. Extension of shelf life from 6 hours to 24 hours postthaw requires a variance from 21 CFR 606.122(m)(3). However, at the end of that interval, the plasma can be relabeled as Thawed Plasma, which can be stored for an additional 4 days at 1 to 6 C. Thawed Plasma prepared from FFP and stored for 5 days contains reduced levels of Factor V (>60%) and Factor VIII (>40%). ADAMTS13 levels are well maintained for 5 days at 1 to 6 C in Thawed Plasma.[34] FFP that is not used for transfusion can be used for fractionation to manufacture plasma derivatives.

Plasma Frozen Within 24 Hours After Phlebotomy

Plasma that is frozen within 24 hours of collection can be labeled as "Plasma Frozen Within 24 Hours After Phlebotomy" (PF24). Once thawed, PF24 has a shelf life of 6 hours at 1 to 6 C. Extension of the shelf life from 6 hours to 24 hours after thawing requires a variance from 21 CFR 606.122(m)(3). However, at the end of that interval, the plasma can be relabeled as Thawed Plasma, which can be stored for an additional 4 days at 1 to 6 C. This component contains normal amounts of Factor V, but it has somewhat reduced levels of Factor VIII, as shown in Table 6-10.[46] Additional information about Thawed Plasma is provided in Chapter 9.

Plasma Cryoprecipitate Reduced

Plasma Cryoprecipitate Reduced is a by-product of cryoprecipitate production and has a shelf life of 12 months from the date of collection at –18 C storage. The product contains a normal level of Factor V (85%); even after the removal of cryoprecipitate, the product has a fibrinogen level of about 200 mg/dL.[40] Plasma Cryoprecipitate Reduced is used to treat patients with thrombotic thrombocytopenic purpura. The levels of the following coagulation factors have been demonstrated to be normal: I, VII, X, α_2-antiplasmin, antithrombin, protein C, and protein S.[47] Factor VIII, the von Willebrand factor (vWF) antigen, vWF activity, fibrinogen, and Factor XIII are decreased.[47]

Liquid Plasma

Liquid plasma for transfusion can be separated from Whole Blood at any time during storage and stored at 1-6 C for up to 5 days after the expiration date of Whole Blood.

TABLE 6-10. Labile Coagulation Factors in Plasma Frozen Within 24 Hours After Phlebotomy and in Thawed Plasma

Reference	Product Type	Storage Interval	Average Factor V Level (%)	Average Factor VIII Level (%)
Smith[38]	24-hour plasma	Immediately after thawing	Not tested	75
Kakaiya[39]	24-hour plasma	Immediately after thawing	111	55
Smak Gregoor[40]	Fresh Frozen Plasma (FFP)	Immediately after thawing 3 days 7 days	88 76 70	
O'Neill[41]	24-hour plasma	Immediately after thawing	100	64
Smith[42]	24-hour plasma	Immediately after thawing	101	76
Downes[43]	FFP thawed and stored	1 day 2 days 3 days 4 days 5 days	79 75 71 68 66	70-107 51-76 43-71 43-67 41-67
Nifong[44]	24-hour plasma—thawed and stored	1 day 2 days 3 days 4 days 5 days	118 129 116 103 89	90 69 58 58 59
Cardigan[45]	24-hour plasma	Immediately after thawing	80	77

24-hour plasma = Plasma Frozen Within 24 Hours After Phlebotomy.

Recovered Plasma

Blood centers often convert plasma and liquid plasma to an unlicensed component, "Recovered Plasma (plasma for manufacture)," which is usually shipped to a fractionator and processed into derivatives such as albumin and/or immune globulins. To ship recovered plasma, the collecting facility must have a "short supply agreement" with the manufacturer.[1(p55)] Because recovered plasma has no expiration date, records for this component should be retained indefinitely. Storage conditions for recovered plasma are established by the fractionator.

Pathogen-Inactivated Plasma

Plasma can be treated to inactivate microbial agents for pathogen reduction. Three such methods are available and are in use in Europe but not in the United States: the methylene blue, psoralen (amotosalen), and solvent/detergent treatments.

Methylene blue (approximately 0.085 mg/unit of plasma) can be added to thawed FFP, followed by activation using white light. After removal of methylene blue with a filter (residual concentration: 0.3 μmol), plasma can be frozen. Methylene-blue-treated plasma contains approximately 15% to 20% less Factor VIII and fibrinogen.

Plasma prepared from WB or by automated methods can be treated with 15 mL of amotosalen per 250 mL of plasma, followed by illumination with ultraviolet A light (320 to 400 nm) with 3.0 J/cm^2. After amotosalen is removed by exposing treated plasma to an adsorption device, the unit is frozen for storage at –18 C. Average activity values for coagulation and antithrombotic factors are reported to be within reference ranges found in untreated plasma.

Solvent/detergent-treated plasma (SD plasma) is prepared from a pool of plasma from many donors (no more than 2500) that undergoes treatment with 1% tri-n-butyl phosphate (TNBP) and 1% Triton X-100 for pathogen reduction. The treatment has been shown to significantly inactivate lipid-enveloped viruses. SD plasma is manufactured in facilities that can manage large-scale production rather than in blood centers. Each unit contains 200 mL of plasma that is stored frozen at –18 C with an expiration date of 12 months.[36] All coagulation factors are reduced by 10% in SD plasma, except for Factor VIII, which is reduced by 20%.[48] Also, SD plasma contains 50% less functional protein S in comparison to the nontreated FFP.[49] The product is labeled with the ABO blood group and, once thawed, should be used within 24 hours. SD plasma is available in Europe, but it is no longer distributed by the manufacturer in the United States.

Cryoprecipitated Antihemophilic Factor (AHF)

Cryoprecipitated AHF is prepared from FFP. Cold-insoluble protein that precipitates when FFP is thawed to 1 to 6 C is collected by centrifugation; supernatant plasma (Plasma cryoprecipitate reduced) is transferred into a satellite container; and the precipitate is resuspended in a small amount of residual plasma, generally 15 mL, and then is refrozen as described in Method 6-11. Thawing of FFP to prepare Cryoprecipitated AHF can be performed by placing the FFP in a refrigerator (1 to 6 C) overnight or in a circulating waterbath of 1 to 6 C. An alternate method that uses microwaves for thawing has been described.[50] The Cryoprecipitated AHF is frozen within 1 hour of its preparation for storage at –18 C for 12 months from the original collection date.

AABB *Standards* requires that Cryoprecipitated AHF contain at least 80 international units (IU) of Factor VIII and 150 mg of fibrinogen per unit, although generally the average fibrinogen content is 250 mg.[51] More current preparations are reported to have much higher amounts of fibrinogen (median, 388 mg/unit).[52] It also contains the vWF ristocetin cofactor activity (approximately 170 units/bag), Factor XIII (approximately 60 units/bag), and fibronectin. Units containing 15 mL or more of plasma are often referred to as "wet cryoprecipitate," while "dry cryoprecipitate" generally has less than 10 mL of plasma per unit.[53] Dry cryoprecipitate may contain lower amounts of fibrinogen in comparison to wet cryoprecipitate (90 vs 140 mg/bag).[54] Rapid freezing of FFP is found to increase the Factor VIII yield in Cryoprecipitated AHF.[55] ADAMTS13 levels are normal in Cryoprecipitated AHF.[34] Anti-A and anti-B are known to be present in Cryoprecipitated AHF, but the combined amount of those antibodies from the unit of plasma is only 1.15% of the total.[56] Thawed Cryoprecipitated AHF is stored at room temperature (20-24 C), during which the mean rates of decline of Factor VIII levels at 2, 4, and 6 hours are approximately 10%, 20%, and 30%, respectively.[57] Cryoprecipitated AHF from blood groups A and B has higher levels of Factor VIII when compared to that derived from blood group O donors (about 120 vs 80 IU per bag, respectively).[54]

Cryoprecipitated AHF products can be prepared for transfusion in three ways.

1. Single units can be stored for 6 hours after thawing.[46]
2. Units pooled using an "open" system (a sterile connecting device is not used) can be stored for 4 hours after thawing.[46]

3. Units pooled by a "closed" system (a sterile connecting device is used) either before storage or after thawing can be stored for 6 hours after thawing or post-thaw pooling.[46]

Granulocytes

Granulocytes can be prepared from WB collections.[58] WB units that are less than 24 hours old are rested for 1 hour after 60 mL of hydroxyethyl starch (HES) is added to the unit. Gravitational force settles the red cells at the bottom, and the plasma remains at the top. The buffy coat, which contains granulocytes, is located at the interface between the plasma and the red cells. The plasma and the buffy coat are transferred to a satellite bag after the sedimentation. Subsequently, the plasma is centrifuged at 5000 × *g* for 5 minutes at 22 C, and 90% of the plasma is expressed back into the bag containing the red cells. Approximately 20 mL of the supernatant plasma is left with the granulocytes. Such a method gives 1.25×10^9 granulocytes per product and has an average hematocrit of 4%. Granulocytes are stored at 20 to 24 C without agitation and expire 24 hours after collection.[1(p52)] The FDA has not provided any guidance about Granulocytes; therefore, the requirements are based on AABB *Standards* only. There is a general decline in the clinical use of Granulocytes, and the use of Granulocytes prepared from single WB units is even rarer. Single unit-derived Granulocytes are most often used for neonates because the number of granulocytes per unit is quite low. The granulocyte yield is much higher with an apheresis collection.

Granulocytes are typically collected by apheresis from donors who are stimulated with corticosteroids. These units contain platelets, about 1.0×10^{10} granulocytes, and 20 to 50 mL of red cells and have an approximate volume of 200 to 300 mL. Granulocyte colony-stimulating factor (G-CSF) administration at a parenteral dose of 5 to 10 µg/kg along with oral dexamethasone (8-12 mg) or prednisone (60 mg) 12 hours before apheresis provides an optimal yield of granulocytes.[59] With G-CSF and corticosteroid stimulation together, the expected yield is 5 to 7×10^{10} granulocytes per product. Corticosteroid stimulation alone yields 1 to 2×10^{10} granulocytes per product. Generally, the yield is lower than 1.0×10^{10} without stimulation. Because G-CSF is not approved for donor stimulation, it is not generally administered in collection centers. The patient's family members may be stimulated with G-CSF by the patient's physician, and the stimulated donors may subsequently donate at the collection center. Apheresis platelet donors who have donated successfully in the past 1 to 2 months are often selected to donate granulocytes because those donors are familiar with apheresis donation and have been recently screened for infectious diseases. The latter attribute is important because it is necessary to transfuse Granulocytes before testing for infectious diseases can be completed. Authorization from the patient's physician is obtained to permit the transfusions before completion of testing.

Recently, concerns have been raised regarding stimulation of donors with corticosteroids. In a small study of 11 donors, 4 donors were found to have a posterior subcapsular cataract (PSC).[60] However, a multicenter study published subsequently found PSCs in only 6 of 89 (6.7%) granulocyte donors and in 4 of 89 (4.5%) apheresis platelet donors. The multicenter study concluded that corticosteroid stimulation of granulocyte donors is not associated with an increased risk of developing a PSC.[61] A cause-and-effect relationship between administration of corticosteroid to the donor and the development of a PSC has not been established. Drawing on the concerns for donor safety, the Council of Europe discourages the use of corticosteroids or G-CSF for granulocyte collection.[10]

BLOOD COMPONENT MODIFICATION

Prestorage Leukocyte Reduction by Filtration

A major difference exists between the US standards and the Council of Europe's standards regarding the number of residual leukocytes in prestorage LR blood components.[10] For RBCs that are leukocyte reduced, the United States requires a residual number of less than 5.0×10^6 leukocytes per unit. The Council of Europe requires that the residual number be less than 1×10^6 per unit.[10] In the United States, leukocyte reduction by filtration of RBCs should result in a component that contains at least 85% of the original red cell content. The Council of Europe's standards require a minimum of 40 g of hemoglobin to be present in each unit after leukocyte reduction.[10]

For whole-blood-derived platelets, AABB *Standards* requires that the leukocyte reduction process ensure that 95% of the platelet units sampled contain $<8.3 \times 10^5$ leukocytes per unit, at least 75% of the units sampled contain 5.5×10^{10} platelets, and at least 90% of the units sampled have a pH 6.2 at the end of the allowable storage period.[1(p28)] The number in the Council of Europe's standards is $<0.2 \times 10^6$ residual leukocytes per unit of platelets from WB.

In practice, approximately 1% of RBC components do not achieve the levels of $<1 \times 10^6$ residual leukocytes in the component. Sickle cell trait of red cells is the most common cause of filter failure. Approximately 50% of the RBC units with the sickle cell trait fail to filter. Although the other 50% do filter, the residual leukocyte content may be higher than the allowable limits.[62]

No standards exist in the United States for the residual number of leukocytes or platelets per FFP unit. The Council of Europe's standards require that the maximum number of leukocytes and platelets per unit be $<0.1 \times 10^9$/L and $<50.0 \times 10^9$/L, respectively.[10] FFP produced during the preparation of LR platelet concentrates will typically have a residual leukocyte count of $<5.0 \times 10^6$.

Prestorage leukocyte reduction is generally performed soon after WB collection and is always performed within 5 days of collection, per current manufacturers' instructions. Inline WB filters are available in collection sets that permit preparation of LR RBCs and FFP. WB filters that will spare platelets are now available also. If WB is collected without the in-line leukocyte-reduction filter, a filter can be attached to the tubing by a sterile connection device. The number of platelets in LR platelet concentrates is generally lower than the number of platelets in non-LR platelet concentrates.

Methods that measure residual leukocytes include Nageotte hemocytometry, flow cytometry, and microfluorimetry (see Method 8-8). In a multicenter study, flow cytometry and microfluorimetry gave better results than Nageotte hemocytometry when freshly prepared samples (within 24 hours) were tested.[63] For instance, at a concentration of 5 white cells per µL for RBC units, the intersite coefficient of variation (CV) was 4.9% for flow cytometry, 15.2% for microfluorimetry, and 54% for Nageotte hemocytometry.[63] In general, Nageotte hemocytometry tends to underestimate the number of white cells when compared to flow cytometry and microfluorimetry.[63]

Red Blood Cell Cryopreservation

RBCs can be frozen with a cryoprotective agent and can be stored for prolonged periods. Glycerol is the most commonly used agent and is added to RBCs within 6 days of collection. Glycerol is used at either a high concentration or a low concentration to cryopreserve the RBCs. Table 6-11 shows differences between the high-glycerol and the low-glycerol methods. For all practical purposes, only the high-glycerol method (40% weight/volume) is in use, because it is simpler and does not require liquid nitrogen. Two commonly used protocols for the high-glycerol method are described in Methods 6-7 and 6-8. Frozen RBCs must be stored at –65 C or colder and will expire after 10 years.[1(p49)] Polyolefin bags are commonly used for the high-glycerol method because the bags are less brittle at –80 C. Rare frozen units may be used beyond the expiration date, but only after medical review and approval that are based on the patient's needs and the availability of other rare compatible units. The units should be handled with care because the containers may crack if bumped or handled roughly. The containers are also known to crack during transportation.

TABLE 6-11. Comparison of Two Methods of Red Blood Cell Cryopreservation

Consideration	High-Concentration Glycerol	Low-Concentration Glycerol
Final glycerol concentration (wt/vol)	Approximately 40%	Approximately 20%
Initial freezing temperature	–80 C	–196 C
Freezing rate	Slow	Rapid
Freezing rate controlled	No	Yes
Type of freezer	Mechanical	Liquid nitrogen
Storage temperature (maximum)	–65 C	–120 C
Change in storage temperature	Can be thawed and refrozen	Critical
Type of storage bags	Polyvinyl chloride; polyolefin	Polyolefin
Shipping	Dry ice	Liquid nitrogen
Deglycerolizing equipment required	Yes	No
Hematocrit	55%-70%	50%-70%

The units should be thawed at 37 C and generally take about 10 minutes to thaw completely. Glycerol must be removed after thawing and before transfusion.[1(p25)] This removal is generally accomplished by instruments that allow the addition and removal of sodium chloride solutions. In most cases, addition of the glycerol and its removal (deglycerolization) require the system to be opened; for this reason, thawed and deglycerolized units can be stored only for 24 hours at 1 to 6 C. The final solution in which cells are suspended is 0.9% sodium chloride and 0.2% dextrose. Dextrose serves to provide nutrients and has been shown to support satisfactory posttransfusion viability for 4 days of storage after deglycerolization.[64] For QC, determining the volume of red cells in the unit after deglycerolization and examining the last wash for hemolysis are recommended (see Method 6-9).

Recently, automated addition and removal of glycerol to RBCs in a closed system has become available. With this system, glycerol is added within 6 days of WB collection. Postthaw red cells prepared in this manner are suspended in AS-3 and can be stored for 14 days at 4 C.[65] Post-wash units have a hematocrit of 51% to 53% and contain a mean of about 9.0×10^6 leukocytes per unit.[66] RBCs stored for 42 days in AS-1, AS-3, or AS-5 and then rejuvenated, frozen, and washed in a closed system can subsequently be stored for 24 hours at 1 to 6 C based on a satisfactory survival after autologous transfusion.[66] At the time of this writing, rejuvenation solution is not available for use in the United States. Red cells that are irradiated, stored at 1 to 6 C for 6 days, and then frozen and deglycerolized had posttransfusion recovery of 81% compared to 85% recovery of the simultaneously studied nonirradiated red cells.[67]

Platelet Cryopreservation

Cryopreservation of platelets is not widely available because the procedures for cryopreservation are complex and are not routinely practiced at most blood centers. Also, the platelet recovery is quite low after transfusion. In addition to those factors, the procedure is costly because of the expense related to labor, equipment, and reagents. As a result of those considerations, the cryopreservation procedure is used only occasionally for autologous transfusions for a few selected patients. The product is not licensed by the FDA.

Several cryoprotectants have been described for platelet cryopreservation.[68,69] However, 5% or 6% dimethylsulfoxide (DMSO) is most commonly used, mainly for autologous platelet transfusions in patients who are refractory to allogeneic platelets. Generally, platelets are collected by apheresis, stored at room temperature for 24 hours, and frozen. Sufficient DMSO is added to achieve a final concentration of 5% or 6%, and the cryoprotectant-containing platelets are placed in a mechanical freezer at –80 C. Rate-controlled freezing is not necessary. Cryopreserved platelets can be stored for at least 2 years. After thawing, platelet recovery in vitro is about 75%, which may be reduced further if thawed platelets are centrifuged to remove the DMSO before transfusion. DMSO removal is performed to reduce the DMSO toxicity to the recipient. In-vivo recovery after transfusion of thawed, DMSO-reduced platelets is about 33%. In vivo, the platelets that survive after transfusion are hemostatically effective.

Recently, the combination of reduced-concentration DMSO (2%) and a platelet storage solution has been described and has been used for autologous platelet cryopreservation for patients with malignancies before initiating chemotherapy.[70] In that procedure, the storage solution containing the DMSO is added to apheresis-collected platelets in a 1:50 ratio with the aim of achieving a final DMSO concentration of 2%. The storage solution for that procedure consists of a mixture of amiloride, adenosine, and nitroprusside. Following the DMSO addition, the platelets are incubated for 1 to 2 hours at room temperature. Platelets used for cryopreservation can also include a pool of 5 units of whole-blood-derived platelet concentrates. The platelet and autologous plasma bags are placed in an aluminum container, which is placed horizontally in a –80 C freezer. When platelets are needed for transfusion, they are thawed at 37 C. Thawed platelets are centrifuged to remove the cryoprotectant. The platelets are subsequently resuspended in 50 to 100 mL of the autologous plasma and transfused within 2 to 3 hours after removal from the freezer. After autologous transfusion, the median corrected count increment at 1 hour and at 24 hours is 15,700 and 13,000, respectively.

Irradiation

Cellular blood components can be irradiated for prevention of graft-vs-host disease (GVHD). Frozen plasma components such as FFP and Cryoprecipitated AHF do not need irradiation because they are considered noncellular components and because the small number of leukocytes present in the components may not survive the freeze-thaw cycle.

The irradiation sources in use include gamma rays—from either cesium-137 or cobalt-60 sources—and x-rays produced by radiation therapy linear accelerators or standalone units. Both sources achieve satisfactory results in rendering T lymphocytes inactive. Freestanding instruments that allow the use of each of those sources are commercially available for blood bank use. The US Nuclear Regulatory Commission recently increased the number of controls for the radioactive material license, which is required in order to have a gamma irradiator and its source on-site.[71] The increased controls are designed to reduce the risk of unauthorized use of radioactive materials.[71] The licensee is now required to secure any area where radioactive source is present so that only approved individuals who require access to perform their duties may enter. Only trustworthy and reliable individuals who are approved in writing by the licensee may have unescorted access to the radioactive material. For individuals employed by the blood bank fewer than 3 years, verifications of employment history, education, and personal references are mandatory. For portable devices, two independent physical controls must form tangible barriers to prevent the material from unauthorized removal. The recent increase in the number of regulations regarding radioactive sources is causing some blood banks to switch from gamma-ray irradiation instruments to those using x-rays.

The radiation dose to the center of the irradiation field must be at least 25 Gy (2500 cGy) and no more than 50 Gy (5000 cGy).[72] During dosimetry, the delivered dose of 2500 cGy is targeted to the internal midplane of the container. Moreover, the minimum delivered dose to any portion of the blood components must be at least 1500 cGy in a fully loaded canister.[73]

Several quality assurance steps are necessary to ensure proper irradiation of blood components. Those measures are designed to show that the instruments in use are working properly and that irradiation of the components actually occurred. Each instrument must be routinely monitored to ensure that an adequate dose is delivered to the container that houses the blood components during irradiation. Dose mapping is used to monitor the instrument's function. For this purpose, irradiation-sensitive films or badges that monitor the delivered dose are used for QC of the irradiators. Several systems consisting of irradiation films or badges are commercially available.[72] Verification of the delivered dose must be performed annually for the cesium-137 source and semiannually for the cobalt-60 source. For x-ray irradiators, the dosimetry should be performed in accordance with the manufacturer's recommendations. The dose verification is also required after major repairs and after relocation of the irradiator. For gamma irradiators, the turntable operation, the timing device, and the lengthening of irradiation time caused by source decay should also be monitored periodically.

Another important quality assurance step is the demonstration that the product that was irradiated received the desired amount of irradiation. For that reason, irradiation-sensitive labels are used to demonstrate that irradiation of each batch of units was accomplished.

RBCs can be irradiated up to the end of their storage shelf life. Regulatory requirements restrict the maximum permissible storage interval after irradiation. For RBCs, irradiated units can be stored for 28 days or up to the original expiration date, whichever is sooner. Platelets can be irradiated up to their expiration date, and the postirradiation expiration date is the same as the original expiration date.

Irradiation of RBCs followed by storage does result in some decrease in percentage of recovery after transfusion (± 10%). In addition, an increased efflux of potassium from red cells causes the potassium levels to rise approximately twofold compared to nonirradiated units. Platelets are not damaged by an irradiation dose as high as 5000 cGy.[73]

Pooling

The sterile connecting device offers a great degree of flexibility in component manufacturing. For instance, the device allows the addition of extra bags to a container system so that pooling of blood components can be performed in a closed system. Preformulated, multitubing, manifold systems that contain a pooling bag are available to perform the pooling. Manifold configurations are commercially available that permit pooling of 4, 5, 6, 8, or 10 units.

Platelets that are pooled have an expiration time of 4 hours from the time of opening the system for pooling. More recently, a closed system for prestorage pooling of platelets has been licensed by the FDA. The FDA-approved system permits the storage of pooled platelets for up to 5 days from the time of WB collection. From 4 to 6 LR or non-LR platelet units that are ABO identical can be pooled using a set that consists of a multilead tubing manifold for sterile connection. If non-LR units are pooled, they are then filtered as part of the pooling process. The shortest expiration date of the pooled units determines the expiration date of the pool. In the United States, each pool prepared from LR platelets must have $<5.0 \times 10^6$ residual leukocytes. The approved pooling set also allows sampling of the pool for detection of bacterial contamination. A record of the unique ID number for each individual member of the pool must be available. The pool must be labeled with the approximate total volume, the ABO/Rh of the units in the pool, and the number of units in the pool. Many countries in Europe prepare prestorage pools of buffy-coat platelets that are preserved in platelet additive solution or in the plasma from one of the units from which platelets are prepared.[29] Instruments that automate the pooling process are increasingly used in Europe. In a few countries in Europe, a system for prestorage pooling of buffy-coat-derived platelets followed by pathogen-reduction treatment with amotosalen has become available. The latter system is not yet licensed by the FDA.

Individual cryoprecipitate units expire 6 hours after thawing. Cryoprecipitated AHF units pooled immediately before transfusion in an "open" system have an expiration time of 4 hours at 20 to 24 C storage. Prestorage pools can also be prepared in an "open" or "closed" system and stored for 12 months at –18 C as described in Method 6-12. Thawed pools from an open system have an expiration time of 4 hours at 20 to 24 C storage. Prestorage pools are often prepared with the use of a sterile connecting device. When the device is used to produce a closed system, the post-thaw expiration time is 6 hours. The number of units pooled may vary and can consist of 4, 5, 6, 8, or 10 units. After prestorage pooling, cryoprecipitates must be placed in a freezer within 1 hour. The potency of the pool is calculated by assuming that each unit in the pool contains 80 IU of coagulation Factor VIII and 150 mg of fibrinogen multiplied by the number of units in the pool. If normal saline is used to rinse the bags during preparation of the pool, the amount of saline in the pool must be stated on the label.

Poststorage pooling of platelet concentrates and cryoprecipitate are described in Chapter 9.

Volume-Reduced Platelets

Volume-reduced platelets may be needed for patients in whom the amount of plasma in platelet units may cause cardiac overload or for patients who are transfused with ABO-incompatible platelets. Volume-reduced platelets are also used for neonates and for intrauterine transfusion. The amount of plasma is reduced by centrifugation of the platelet units to pellet the platelets. Supernatant plasma is removed, and the pelleted platelets are subsequently resuspended into a smaller volume of plasma compared to the starting volume described in Method 6-14.

Platelets derived from WB containing an average plasma volume of 50 mL/unit can be prepared in the manner just described, which results in a final volume of 15 to 20 mL/unit after the volume reduction. In-vitro properties such as platelet morphology, mean platelet volume, hypotonic shock response, synergistic aggregation, and platelet factor 3 activity appear to be maintained in the volume-reduced platelets stored for 5 days.[74] The in-vitro recovery of platelets is about 85% after the volume-reduction step. Platelets from WB that are volume reduced by centrifugation ($580 \times g$ for 20 minutes) from an approximate volume of 60 mL to between 35 and 40 mL yield a high platelet count ($>2.3 \times 10^9$/L).[75] The volume-reduced platelets may be stored in either 10-mL or 15-mL capacity plastic syringes for up to 6 hours. Under such storage conditions, the platelet concentrate pH seems to be maintained above 6.0 for up to 6 hours of storage.

Apheresis Platelets can also be volume reduced in a manner similar to that described for whole-blood-derived platelet concentrates. For Apheresis Platelets, the volume reduction from 250 mL to 90 mL by centrifugation has been shown to cause a mild increase in platelet activation and an impaired aggregation response to adenosine diphosphate (ADP) but not to collagen.[76] In these experiments, the platelet count before the volume reduction was 1.0×10^9/mL; after the reduction, the count was 1.9×10^9/mL.[77]

Recent developments include refinements in collection protocols for apheresis instruments that result in collection of platelets in a high concentration that may, therefore, obviate the need for volume reduction. New programs for apheresis instruments have been developed that permit platelet collections at concentrations as high as 3.0 to 4.0×10^9/L.[76,78] Further, the highly concentrated platelets may be suspended in a platelet additive solution with the autologous plasma at a ratio of 5:1 to 3:1. Platelet units prepared in this manner contain much lower amounts of plasma compared to the standard apheresis platelets.[78] Recently, the FDA has approved an additive solution for apheresis platelets.

Posttransfusion platelet increments have been satisfactory after transfusion of volume-reduced platelets.[74] However, the overall in-vivo survival data for volume-reduced platelets are limited. If an open system is used, the maximum allowable storage time is 4 hours. For a closed system, the maximum allowable storage time is not established.

Rejuvenation

Storage of RBCs causes reduction in the intracellular levels of 2,3-diphosphoglycerate (2,3-DPG) and adenosine triphosphate (ATP). Those levels can be restored to normal if an FDA-approved rejuvenation solution is added to the stored RBCs as described in Method 6-6. Each 50 mL of the rejuvenation solution contains 550 mg of sodium pyruvate, 1.34 g of inosine, 0.034 g of adenine, 0.50 g of dibasic sodium phosphate (anhydrous), and 0.20 g of monobasic sodium phosphate (monohydrate) in water for injection, and each has a pH of 6.7 to 7.4. The product insert for rejuvenation solution (Rejuvesol, Cytosol Opthalmics, Braintree, MA) provides the following information: 1) RBCs preserved in CPD or CPDA-1 can be rejuvenated up to 3 days after the expiration date of the RBCs as long as the storage conditions are met; 2) RBCs preserved in AS-1 may be rejuvenated until 42 days, but not after the expiration date; 3) rejuvenated CPD or CPDA-1 RBCs can be maintained in frozen storage for 10 years; and 4) AS-1 RBCs can be stored frozen for only 3 years. The rejuvenation solution is not approved by the FDA for RBCs preserved in CP2D, AS-3, and AS-5. However, satisfactory postrejuvenation survival of RBCs preserved in CP2D AS-3, CPD AS-3, and CPD AS-5 has been shown.[66,79] Rejuvesol is not available as of this writing.

Before transfusion, rejuvenated RBCs are washed to remove the rejuvenation solution. Another option is to freeze the rejuvenated unit with glycerol for long-term storage. At the time of transfusion, deglycerolization is performed, which accomplishes the removal of the rejuvenation solution and the glycerol. The Deglycerolized Rejuvenated RBCs have an expiration time of 24 hours.

QUARANTINE

All units of blood collected should be immediately placed in quarantine in a designated area until donor information and donation records have been reviewed, the current donor information has been compared against the previous information, the donor's previous deferrals have been examined, and all laboratory testing has been completed. Because of the limited amount of time after collection that is permitted for component separation, WB units may be separated into components before all of the earlier processes have been completed. Separated components are quarantined at the appropriate temperature until all the suitability steps have been completed and reviewed.

According to FDA requirements, all blood and blood components that are found unsuitable for transfusion or for further manufacturing must be stored in a separate quarantine area from blood and components for which testing has not been completed and from blood and components that are suitable for distribution. Computer software is also often used to prevent labeling of components until all the donor information and the current test results are reviewed and found acceptable. Special quarantine flags may be placed on each component computer record to prevent erroneous releases. Often, the physical quarantine and the electronic quarantine are used simultaneously.

Certain blood components from previous donations by donors whose more recent donations test positive for infectious disease also will require quarantine and appropriate disposition, as will units identified to be unsuitable for transfusion because of postdonation information.

Other components may need quarantine so that the QC samples can be taken and analyzed. For instance, if a sample for bacterial contamination testing is obtained, the component is held in quarantine for some preset amount of time and then released if the test results are negative at that time.

A thorough understanding of the quarantine process is needed to prevent erroneous release of unsuitable blood components. Components may be removed from the quarantine area, labeled, and released for distribution if all the donor information, previous donor records, and current test results are satisfactory. Some nonconforming autologous blood components may be released for autologous use only.

Some blood components require emergency release because of a very short storage time. Such is the case for granulocytes. Emergency release requires physician approval and a label or tie tag to indicate that testing was incomplete at the time of release.

Despite the widespread use of computer software for the control of manufacturing processes, instances of the failure of quarantine and of the release of unsuitable products continue to be reported to the FDA. For instance, during the fiscal year 2009, the FDA received 49,519 reports of blood product deviations from the manufacturers. Of those reports, 2,260 (4.6%) involved labeling, and another 506 (1.0%) involved the component preparation.

LABELING

Blood component labeling should be performed in a quiet area to prevent disruption of the process and errors caused by distraction. A number of items must be reviewed at the time of labeling. Any hold that is placed on the donation because of a donor's medical history should be resolved before labeling. Examples of holds that are placed on blood components include potential duplicate donor records and failure on the part of the donor to answer medical history questions. Donor demographic information on the current donation that differs from data on previous records should also be reviewed and resolved before labeling. Some WB donations may be designated as "not for components (platelet concentrate, fresh frozen plasma, or both)" because of prolonged draw time. All infectious disease tests should be nonreactive or negative before labeling occurs. Data on equipment maintenance and QC of equipment, supplies, reagents, and products should all be satisfactory to proceed with the labeling. Bar-coded and eye-readable labels are applied to the components, and a verification step is performed to ensure that correct labels have been used.

All purchased labels should be placed in quarantine until they undergo careful quality assurance steps to make certain that the labels are acceptable. If acceptable, the purchased labels are moved out of quarantine for routine use. The distribution of labels to the operating units should be controlled, and all distributed labels should be accounted for. If label templates are changed for any reason, the previous version should be identified and removed from operations. Many blood centers produce on-demand labels by in-house printers; this label production is controlled by computer software. Final visual inspections of the components and all attached labels are performed before the components are physically and electronically transferred to the distribution inventory.

The FDA requirements for labeling of blood and components are detailed in the "Guidelines for Uniform Labeling of Blood and Blood Components," published in 1985.[80] Additional guidance was issued in 2006.[81] In accordance with the *Code of Federal Regulations* [21 CFR 606.121(c)(13)], blood component labels must contain certain information encoded in a format that is machine readable and approved for use by the FDA. Machine-readable information that was approved by the FDA in 1985 was Codabar, which is a specific bar-code symbology. Subsequently, the FDA approved the International Society of Blood Transfusion (ISBT) 128 symbology, version 1.2.0 in 2000 and version 2.0.0 in 2006.[81] AABB *Standards* requires that accredited facilities use ISBT 128 labels.[1(p12)]

The FDA rule noted above that requires certain information on all blood components to be labeled with a bar-coded label became effective April 26, 2006. The rule requires that, at a minimum, the label contain bar-coded information about the following four items: 1) the unique facility identifier (eg, registration number), 2) the lot number relating to the donor, 3) the product code, and 4) the ABO group and Rh type of the donor. Those four pieces of information must also be present in eye-readable format. That rule applies to the blood centers that collect and prepare blood components. The rule also applies to the hospital transfusion services that prepare pooled cryoprecipitate and to those that prepare divided units or aliquots of RBCs, platelets, and plasma for pediatric use.

At present, the FDA does not permit other alternative automatic ID technology for blood component containers. In the future, component identification may make use of radio frequency ID chips or a two-dimensional symbology instead of the linear bar code that is currently in use.

The FDA has established clear requirements for label size, for the location where labels must be placed, for certain color combinations to use, and for the type of information to include on the label for different components.

One more major part of the labeling is the information circular. The circular must be made available to all those who are involved in transfusion of blood components. The *Circular of Information for the Use of Human Blood and Blood Components*[46] is produced by AABB, America's Blood Centers, the American Red Cross, and the Armed Services Blood Program and is recognized as acceptable by the FDA. The *Circular* provides important information for each blood component and should be consulted for information not included in this chapter.

Blood component containers may also be affixed with special message labels. The labels may include one or more of the following indications: 1) hold for further manufacturing, 2) for emergency use only, 3) for autologous use only, 4) not for transfusion, 5) irradiated, 6) biohazard, 7) from a therapeutic phlebotomy, and 8) screened for special factors [eg, HLA type or cytomegalovirus (CMV) antibody status]. ISBT 128 allows incorporation of special attributes of the component, such as CMV antibody status. Additional information on the container can be conveyed using a tie tag. Tie tags are especially useful for autologous and directed donations. Tie tags include the patient's identifying information, the name of the hospital where the patient will be admitted for surgery, the date of surgery, and other information that may be helpful to the hospital transfusion service.

Additional requirements for container labels are noted below and are fully described in Title 21 of the *Code of Federal Regulations,* Parts 606.120, 606.121, and 606.122, which should be consulted for comprehensive information.

- **Component Name and Identification.** The label must include the proper name of the component, including any qualifier, if applicable. Each component must also bear a unique ID number that can be traced back to the blood donor. If components are pooled, a pool number must allow tracing to the individual units within a pool.
- **Manufacturer.** The name and the FDA registration number of the manufacturer must be included in the label. For licensed products, the facility's license number is required. If there is more than one manufacturer, the registration number of all manufacturers must be present on the label or available through associated component records. The FDA considers hospital facilities to be hospital transfusion services if they 1) prepare only RBCs or Recovered Plasma from Whole Blood, 2) pool platelets or Cryoprecipitated AHF for ease of transfusion, or 3) use bedside leukocyte-reduction filters with blood components, and such activities do not necessitate FDA establishment registration [See 21 CFR 607.65(f) exemptions for blood product establishments]. However, hospitals that irradiate units or collect blood (autologous, directed, and allogeneic) and that prepare components from these collections are considered to be hospital blood banks and are required to register with the FDA.
- **Expiration Date.** The expiration date must include the day, the month, and the year. For components with an expiration date of 72 hours or less, the hour of expiration must also be indicated. (For components with an expiration date greater than 72 hours, expiration time is the midnight of the last day of shelf life.) ISBT 128 can en-

code not only the expiration date but also the expiration time. For Recovered Plasma, the collection date is used rather than the expiration date.

- **Type of Donor.** For components for transfusion, the label must indicate either a "paid donor" or a "volunteer donor."
- **Amount of Blood Components and Anticoagulant-Preservative.** The volume of the component within (±) 10% must be described. Each component has a numeric product code; within this numeric code is a digit that provides information about the "standard content." An example of the standard content is RBCs prepared from 450-mL or 500-mL WB collection. Content may be written on the label for certain plasma products, for pooled platelets, and for aliquoted units. The product code contains a digit that corresponds with the type of anticoagulant-preservative used. An exact amount of anticoagulant is not required on the label for certain components (eg, frozen, deglycerolized, rejuvenated, or washed RBCs).
- **Test Results.** ABO group and Rh type are required on the label. For Cryoprecipitated AHF, Rh type may be omitted. Special attributes such as CMV antibody negative, hemoglobin S-negative, the presence of unexpected red cell antibodies, and red cell phenotype are indicated by a special label or tie tag. For autologous units, any positive infectious disease markers require biohazardous and "For Autologous Use Only" labels. The *Circular of Information* describes testing for infectious disease agents.[46]
- **Statements.** The following statements must be present, if applicable: 1) for components for transfusion, "℞ only"; 2) "See *Circular of Information* for indications, contraindications, cautions, and methods of infusion"; 3) "Properly identify intended recipient"; 4) "For emergency use only by ____" if applicable; 5) for Recovered Plasma, "Caution: for manufacturing use only"; 6) "For autologous use only" if applicable; and 7) for components that are not suitable for transfusion, "Not for transfusion."
- **Autologous Units.** Label must include the name of the autologous donor, the blood group, the hospital, and the ID number.

ISBT 128

ISBT 128 bar-code symbology was created in 1994, and many countries have already implemented this symbology for blood component labeling. In the United States, the FDA approved the use of ISBT 128 in 2000. AABB member institutions were required to implement ISBT 128 by May 1, 2008. Several issues regarding conversion from Codabar to ISBT 128 were identified and resolved during implementation in AABB member institutions. For instance, cross-reference tables between the two symbologies were created, allowing for insertion of product codes into the new systems that correlated with hospital medical records and billing systems. AABB also provided prepared letters for member institutions to use in requesting FDA approval of ISBT 128 use in their facilities. Several software and hardware vendors modified their products to permit ISBT 128 use with existing systems. Capacity to use dual symbologies may be needed for the near future for labeling some components, such as Frozen RBCs, and for shipping blood components between countries until all countries have uniformly implemented ISBT 128. For those groups planning to implement ISBT 128, an important source of information is ICCBBA (formerly known as the International Council for Commonality in Blood Banking Automation). This organization's website (http://www.iccbba.org) lists future updates and a revised list of product codes.

Some of the benefits of ISBT 128 include the following:

- Uniform labels applied on blood components manufactured by different collection centers.
- Better traceability of components.
- Improved self-checking features per character.
- Encoding of entire ASCII character set that includes alphanumeric and special characters.

TABLE 6-12. Comparison of Requirements for Quality Control of Blood Components by the AABB, the FDA, and the Council of Europe

Component	AABB[1(pp24-29)]	FDA	Council of Europe
Whole Blood	None	None	Test a minimum 4 units per month; minimum hemoglobin 45 g/unit (WB collection = 450 mL), hemolysis at end of storage <0.8%. Test 1% of all units for volume: 450 mL ± 10%.
Red Blood Cells	RBCs without additive solutions shall be prepared using a method known to result in a final hematocrit of ≤80%.	None	Test a minimum 4 units per month; minimum hemoglobin 45 g/unit (WB collection = 450 mL), hematocrit 65%-75%, and hemolysis <0.8% of red cell mass. Test 1% of all units for volume: 280 ± 50 mL.
RBCs, buffy coat removed	None	None	Test a minimum 4 units per month: minimum hemoglobin 43 g/unit, hematocrit 65%-75%, hemolysis <0.8% of red cell mass, and leukocyte content $<1.2 \times 10^9$/unit. Test 1% of all units for volume: 250 ± 50 mL.
RBCs in additive solution	None	None	Test a minimum 4 units per month: minimum hemoglobin 45 g/unit, hematocrit 65%-75%, and hemolysis <0.8% of red cell mass. Test 1% of all units for volume. Volume range differs by additive solution used.
RBCs, buffy coat removed, in additive solution	None	None	Test a minimum 4 units per month: minimum hemoglobin 43 g/unit, hematocrit 50%-70%, hemolysis <0.8% of red cell mass, and leukocyte content $<1.2 \times 10^9$/unit. Test 1% of all units for volume. Volume range differs by additive solution used.

(Continued)

TABLE 6-12. Comparison of Requirements for Quality Control of Blood Components by the AABB, the FDA, and the Council of Europe (Continued)

Component	AABB[1(pp24-29)]	FDA	Council of Europe
Washed RBCs	None	None	Test all units: minimum hemoglobin 40 g/unit, hematocrit 65%-75%, hemolysis <0.8% of red cell mass, protein content of final supernatant <0.5 g/unit.
RBCs Leukocytes Reduced	Leukocyte-reduced blood and components shall be prepared by a method known to reduce the leukocyte number to $<5 \times 10^6$ for RBCs in at least 95% of the units sampled and retain 85% of red cells after filtration.	Test 1% of all units from WB (with a minimum of 4 units/month) for each method of leukocyte reduction for residual leukocytes $<5 \times 10^6$/unit.	Test 1% of all units (with a minimum of 10 units/month) for residual leukocyte count $<1 \times 10^6$/unit; 1% of all units with a minimum of 4 units/month for hemoglobin (40 g/unit) and hematocrit (50%-70%); 1% of all units for volume; and a minimum 4 units/month for hemolysis <0.8% of red cell mass.
Deglycerolized RBCs	Deglycerolized RBCs shall be prepared by a method known to ensure adequate removal of cryoprotective agents, result in minimal free hemoglobin in the supernatant solution, and yield a mean recovery of ≥80% of the preglycerolized red cells following the deglycerolization process.	None	Test all units for volume >185 mL, supernatant hemoglobin <0.2 g/unit, hematocrit 65%-75%, and minimum hemoglobin >36 g/unit. Test 1% of all units (minimum 4 units/month) for osmolality <340 mOsm/L, leukocytes $<0.1 \times 10^9$/unit, and sterility.
Apheresis RBCs Leukocytes Reduced	Ensure a final component contains a mean hemoglobin of ≥51 g (or 153 mL red cell volume) and $<5 \times 10^6$ residual leukocytes per unit. At least 95% of units sampled shall have >42.5 g of hemoglobin (or 128 mL red cell volume).	Same as RBCs Leukocytes Reduced for residual leukocyte determination. Also test 1% of the units or minimum 50 units per month from each collection site for hemoglobin mass.	Test 1% of all units for volume (limits defined by the system used). Test 4 units/month for hematocrit (65%-75% without additive solution; 50%-70% with additive solution). Test 4 units for hemoglobin (minimum 40 g/unit). Test 1% of all units or a minimum of 10 units/month for residual leukocytes ($<1 \times 10^6$/unit). Test 4 units/month for hemolysis <0.8% of red cell mass.

TABLE 6-12. Comparison of Requirements for Quality Control of Blood Components by the AABB, the FDA, and the Council of Europe (Continued)

Component	AABB[1(pp24-29)]	FDA	Council of Europe
Platelets	Demonstrate that at least 90% of units sampled contain ≥5.5 × 10^{10} platelets and have a pH ≥6.2 at the end of allowable storage.	Test 4 units each month at the end of storage interval for pH (≥6.2). Also, centrifugation conditions must ensure platelet count of ≥5.5 × 10^{10}/unit in 75% of the units.	Test volume for all units (>40 mL per 60 × 10^9 platelets). Test 1% of units for platelet count (>60 × 10^9/single unit equivalent in at least 75% of the units tested). Test 1% of all units for residual leukocytes before leukocyte reduction (if prepared from PRP, <0.2 × 10^9/single unit equivalent, and if prepared from buffy coat, <0.05 × 10^9/single unit equivalent in at least 75% of the units tested). Test 1% of all units or minimum of 10 units/month for residual leukocytes after leukocyte reduction (<0.2 × 10^6/single unit equivalent in 90% of the units tested). Test 1% of all units or minimum of 4 units/month for pH (6.4 to 7.4 in 90% of the units tested).
Apheresis Platelets	Demonstrate that at least 90% of units sampled contain ≥3.0 × 10^{11} platelets and that at least 90% of units have a pH ≥6.2 at the end of allowable storage. At a minimum, 95% of units sampled shall contain a residual leukocyte count <5 × 10^6 for leukocyte-reduced units.	Number of units to test must be sufficient to allow 95% confidence that 75% of component's platelet yield is ≥3.0 × 10^{11}/unit. Similarly, test sufficient number for pH ≥6.2 and residual WBCs <5.0 × 10^6/unit (for leukocyte-reduced units) to achieve 95% confidence that 95% of components will meet the requirements.	Test all units for volume (>40 mL per 60 × 10^9 platelets). Test 1% of all units or a minimum of 10 units per month for platelet count (>200 × 10^9/unit in at least 90% of the units tested) and residual leukocytes for leukocyte-reduced units (<1.0 × 10^6 leukocytes/unit in at least 90% of the units tested). Test 1% of all units or a minimum of 4 units/month for pH (pH between 6.4 and 7.4).

(Continued)

TABLE 6-12. Comparison of Requirements for Quality Control of Blood Components by the AABB, the FDA, and the Council of Europe (Continued)

Component	AABB[1(pp24-29)]	FDA	Council of Europe
Fresh Frozen Plasma (FFP)	None	None	Test all units for volume (± 10% of stated volume). Every 3 months, measure Factor VIII levels in 10 randomly selected units that are in their first month of storage (Factor VIII level ≥70% of the freshly collected plasma unit). Test 1% of all units or a minimum of 4 units/month for residual red cells ($<6.0 \times 10^9$/L), leukocytes ($<0.1\times 10^9$/L), and platelets ($<50 \times 10^9$/L). Cell counting is performed before freezing. For Factor VIII measurement, exact number of units to be tested could be determined by statistical process control.
Cryoprecipitated AHF	Minimum of 150 mg of fibrinogen and a minimum of 80 IU of coagulation Factor VIII. In tests on pooled components, the pool shall contain a minimum of 150 mg fibrinogen and 80 IU of coagulation Factor VIII times the number of components in the pool.	Test 4 representative units each month for Factor VIII (≥80 IU/unit).	Test all units for volume (30 to 40 mL); test every 2 months a pool of 6 units of mixed blood group during first month of storage and also during the last month of storage (Factor VIII ≥70 IU/unit). Test 1% of all units or a minimum of 4 units for fibrinogen (≥140 mg/unit). Test every 2 months a pool of 6 units of mixed blood groups during first month of storage and also during last month of storage (von Willebrand factor >100 IU/unit).
Plasma Cryoprecipitate Reduced	None	None	Test all units for volume (± 10% stated volume).
Apheresis Platelets Cryopreserved	None	None	Test all units for volume (50 to 200 mL). Test all units for platelet count (>40% of the prefreeze count). Test all units for residual leukocytes before freezing ($<1.0 \times 10^6$/dose).

TABLE 6-12. Comparison of Requirements for Quality Control of Blood Components by the AABB, the FDA, and the Council of Europe (Continued)

Component	AABB[1(pp24-29)]	FDA	Council of Europe
Apheresis Granulocytes	Unless prepared for neonates, each granulocyte unit must have a minimum of 1.0×10^{10} granulocytes in at least 75% of the units tested.	None	Test all units for volume (<500 mL) and test all units for granulocyte count (1×10^{10}/unit). (Note: Pretreatment of donors with corticosteroids and granulocyte colony-stimulating factor is discouraged.)

WB = Whole blood; RBCs = Red Blood Cells; PRP = platelet-rich plasma; WBCs = white blood cells.

- Improved accuracy from reducing the number of misreads during scanning of the bar-coded information.
- Double-density coding of numeric characters, which permits encoding of more information in a given space.
- A larger number of product codes, which allows more detailed description of the blood components.
- Enhanced scanning, which permits more facile auditing of movements of blood components from one location to another.
- Ability to add information for autologous donations.
- Ability to read more than one bar code with a single sweep (concatenation).
- Less laborious importation of "foreign" inventory into "own" inventory via the availability of uniform systems for donation identification numbers and product codes.

In the future, ISBT 128 is expected to permit information transfer by radio-frequency ID tags or by other means of electronic data transmission.

QUALITY CONTROL OF BLOOD COMPONENTS

QC testing of blood components is necessary to meet FDA requirements and other regulatory requirements. Those requirements are minimum standards, and an individual manufacturer may establish more stringent standards. QC failures can serve as an indicator of unexpected suboptimal reagents or material. Furthermore, QC data can reveal previously unrecognized variations from validated procedures. The timely detection provides a proactive approach to early identification and resolution of a manufacturing problem.

Limitations of QC are demonstrated, for example, in QC failures that are not process failures but are associated with donor-related variables that cannot be controlled. Examples of donor-associated variables include occult donor bacteremia or viremia and leukocyte-reduction filter failure resulting from the presence of sickle hemoglobin trait.

In the United States, the FDA provides specific instructions for which QC measures must be applied. Information in Table 6-12 shows major differences in QC requirements between the United States and Europe. For certain blood components, it may be impractical to perform the QC steps. For example, the FDA or the Council of Europe does not require QC of bedside leukocyte-reduction filters.

Equipment QC is necessary to ensure that blood components achieve desired properties in a consistent manner. Suggested QC steps for standard equipment in component laboratories are described in Chapter 1 and are listed in Appendix 1-4.

A statistical process control has been suggested for QC. Such an approach is expected to provide definition of product conformance to a standard with a given probability. This approach also allows a limit to be established for nonconformance, facilitates implementation of corrective actions, and permits QC to be individualized for different blood components.

KEY POINTS

1. Modern blood containers are composed of soft plastic and identified by a lot number. They should be pyrogen-free and flexible, yet tough and kink- and scratch-resistant. During frozen storage, each plastic has a set temperature for glass transition when it becomes brittle and therefore susceptible to breakage during transportation.
2. The initial 30 to 45 mL of blood drawn is allowed to collect into a diversion pouch located at the collection tubing. The pouch reduces bacterial contamination of collected blood by retaining bacteria that may have otherwise entered the collection. Blood in this pouch is used for laboratory tests.
3. The average rate of adverse donor reactions after donation is 3.5%. Most are mild and require no further medical care. These reactions can be systemic (eg, fainting) or local (eg, hematoma). About 1 in 3400 donors experience a reaction after leaving the donation site and may need medical care.
4. Regarding centrifugation for component preparation, primary variables that affect cell separation and cell recoveries are rotor size, centrifuge speed, and duration. The platelet-rich plasma method is used in the United States for platelet concentrate preparation, and the buffy-coat method is more predominant in Canada and Europe.
5. In the United States, the residual leukocyte count for red cells after filtration must not exceed 5.0×10^6/unit; Europe's requirement is 1.0×10^6/unit.
6. In plasma separated from whole blood as "Plasma Frozen Within 24 Hours After Phlebotomy," the levels of all the coagulation factors are similar to Fresh Frozen Plasma except for some decrease in coagulation Factor VIII.
7. Platelet freezing is not widely used because the procedures available to freeze platelets are complex and not approved by the US Food and Drug Administration (FDA).
8. Irradiated cellular blood components are prepared by exposure to a dose of at least 25 Gy, not to exceed 50 Gy. RBC units have a maximum of 28 days shelf life after irradiation (not to exceed the permitted total storage days for a given preservative). Platelet shelf life (5 days) is not reduced after irradiation.
9. Container labels are increasingly using the International Society of Blood Transfusion symbology (ISBT 128). ISBT 128 offers a number of advantages over the Codabar symbology, including identification of the manufacturer throughout the world, more product codes, improved accuracy as a result of reduced misreads during scanning, and enhanced conveyance of other labeling information.
10. Variable approaches to perform quality control of blood components have been promulgated by the AABB, the Council of Europe, and the US FDA.

REFERENCES

1. Carson TH, ed. Standards for blood banks and transfusion services. 27th ed. Bethesda, MD: AABB, 2011.
2. McDonald CP, Roy A, Mahajan P, et al. Relative values of the interventions of diversion and improved donor-arm disinfection to reduce the bacterial risk from blood transfusion. Vox Sang 2004;86:178-82.
3. Food and Drug Administration. Guidance for industry: Use of sterile connecting devices in blood bank practices. (November 22, 2000) Rockville, MD: CBER Office of Communication, Outreach, and Development, 2000. [Available at http://www.fda.gov/BiologicsBloodVaccines/GuidanceComplianceRegulatoryInformation/Guidances/Blood/ucm076779.htm or .pdf (accessed October 8, 2010).]
4. Goldman M, Roy G, Fréchette N, et al. Evaluation of donor skin disinfection methods. Transfusion 1997;37:309-12.

5. Buchta C, Nedorost N, Regele H, et al. Skin plugs in phlebotomy puncture for blood donation. Wien Klin Wochenschr 2005; 117:141-4.
6. Siemens HJ, Klüter H, Brückner S, et al. Evaluation of two new integrated adapters for blood drawing in closed blood bag systems: Influence on different molecular coagulation markers. Transfus Med 1998;8: 325-32.
7. Shinar E, Michlin H. SampLink: A new system for the collection of donor blood samples. Transfus Med 1996;6:149-53.
8. Button LN, Orlina AR, Kevy SV, Josephson AM. The quality of over- and undercollected blood for transfusion. Transfusion 1976;16:148-54.
9. Davey RJ, Lenes BL, Casper AJ, Demets DL. Adequate survival of red cells from units "undercollected" in citrate-phosphate-dextrose-adenine-one. Transfusion 1984; 24:319-22.
10. Council of Europe. Guide to the preparation, use and quality assurance of blood components. 12th ed. Strasbourg, France: Council of Europe Publishing, 2006.
11. Food and Drug Administration. Guidance for industry: Recommendations for collecting Red Blood Cells by automated apheresis methods—technical correction February 2001. (February 13, 2001) Rockville, MD: Office of Communication, Outreach, and Development, 2001. [Available at http://www.fda.gov/BiologicsBloodVaccines/GuidanceCompliance RegulatoryInformation/Guidances/Blood/default.htm (accessed October 4, 2010).]
12. Food and Drug Administration. Guidance for industry and FDA review staff: Collection of platelets by automated methods. (December 17, 2007) Rockville, MD: Office of Communication, Outreach, and Development, 2007. [Available at http://www.fda.gov/Biologics BloodVaccines/GuidanceComplianceRegula toryInformation/Guidances/Blood/default.htm (accessed October 4, 2010).]
13. Food and Drug Administration. Compliance programs (CBER). 7342.001. Inspection of licensed and unlicensed blood banks, brokers, reference laboratories, and contractors. Rockville, MD: Office of Compliance and Biologics Quality, 2010. [Available at http://www.fda.gov/BiologicsBloodVaccines/GuidanceCom plianceRegulatoryInformation/Compliance Activities/Enforcement/CompliancePro grams/ucm095226.htm (accessed April 4, 2011).]
14. Newman BH. Blood donor complications after whole-blood donation. Curr Opin Hematol 2004;11:339-45.
15. Pisciotto P, Sataro P, Blumberg N. Incidence of adverse reactions in blood donors taking antihypertensive medications. Transfusion 1982; 22:530-1.
16. Hanson SA, France CR. Predonation water ingestion attenuates negative reactions to blood donation. Transfusion 2004;44:924-8.
17. Heaton WA, Rebulla P, Pappalettera M, Dzik WH. A comparative analysis of different methods of routine blood component preparation. Transfus Med Rev 1997;11:116-29.
18. Högman CF, Knutson F, Lööf H. Storage of whole blood before separation: The effect of temperature on red cell 2,3-DPG and the accumulation of lactate. Transfusion 1999;39:492-7.
19. Reiss RF, Katz AJ. Optimizing recovery of platelets in platelet-rich plasma by the Simplex strategy. Transfusion 1976;16:370-4.
20. Welch M, Champion AB. The effect of temperature and mode of agitation on the resuspension of platelets during preparation of platelet concentrates. Transfusion 1985;25:283-5.
21. Berseus O, Högman CF, Johansson A. Simple method of improving the quality of platelet concentrates and the importance of production control. Transfusion 1978; 18:333-8.
22. Högman CF, Meryman HT. Red blood cells intended for transfusion: Quality criteria revisited. Transfusion 2006;46:137-42.
23. Janatpour KA, Paglieroni TG, Crocker VL, et al. Visual assessment of hemolysis in red blood cell units and segments can be deceptive. Transfusion 2004;44:984-9.
24. Kim DM, Brecher ME, Bland LA, et al. Visual identification of bacterially contaminated red cells. Transfusion 1992;32:221-5.
25. Moroff G, Kline L, Dabay M, et al. Reevaluation of the resting time period when preparing whole blood-derived platelet concentrates with the platelet-rich plasma method. Transfusion 2006;46:572-7.
26. Holme S, Heaton WA, Moroff G. Evaluation of platelet concentrates stored for 5 days with reduced plasma volume. Transfusion 1994;34: 39-43.
27. Ali AM, Warkentin TE, Bardossy L, et al. Platelet concentrates stored for 5 days in a reduced volume of plasma maintain hemostatic function and viability. Transfusion 1994;34:44-7.
28. Brecher ME. Collected questions and answers. 6th ed. Bethesda, MD: AABB, 2000.

29. Murphy S. Platelets from pooled buffy coats: An update. Transfusion 2005;45:634-9.
30. Moroff G, George VM. The maintenance of platelet properties upon limited discontinuation of agitation during storage. Transfusion 1990;30:427-30.
31. Gottschall JL, Rzad L, Aster RH. Studies of the minimum temperature at which human platelets can be stored with full maintenance of viability. Transfusion 1986;26:460-2.
32. Moroff G, Holme S, George VM, Heaton WA. Effect on platelet properties exposure to temperatures below 20 degrees C for short periods during storage at 20 to 24 degrees C. Transfusion 1994;34:317-21.
33. Mintz PD, Blatt PM, Kuhns WJ, Roberts HR. Antithrombin III in fresh frozen plasma, cryoprecipitate, and cryoprecipitate-depleted plasma. Transfusion 1979; 19:597-8.
34. Scott EA, Puca KE, Pietz BC, et al. Analysis of ADAMTS13 activity in plasma products using a modified FRETS-VWF73 assay (abstract). Blood 2005;106(Suppl):165a.
35. Willis JI, Lown JA, Simpson MC, Erber WN. White cells in fresh-frozen plasma: Evaluation of a new white cell-reduction filter. Transfusion 1998;38:645-9.
36. Hellstern P, Haubelt H. Manufacture and composition of fresh frozen plasma and virus-inactivated therapeutic plasma preparations: Correlation between composition and therapeutic efficacy. Thromb Res 2002;107(Suppl 1):S3-S8.
37. Cardigan R, Sutherland J, Garwood M, et al. The effect of leucocyte depletion on the quality of fresh-frozen plasma. Br J Haematol 2001; 114:233-40.
38. Smith JK, Snape TJ, Haddon ME, et al. Methods of assessing factor VIII content of stored fresh frozen plasma intended for preparation of factor VIII concentrates. Transfusion 1978; 18:530-7.
39. Kakaiya RM, Morse EE, Panek S. Labile coagulation factors in thawed fresh frozen plasma prepared by two methods. Vox Sang 1984;46: 44-6.
40. Smak Gregoor PJH, Harvey MS, Briet E, Brand A. Coagulation parameters of CPD fresh-frozen plasma and CPD cryoprecipitate-poor plasma after storage at 4 C for 28 days. Transfusion 1993;33:735-8.
41. O'Neill EM, Rowley J, Hansson-Wicher M, et al. Effect of 24-hour whole-blood storage on plasma clotting factors. Transfusion 1999;39: 488-91.
42. Smith JF, Ness PM, Moroff G, Luban NLC. Retention of coagulation factors in plasma frozen after extended holding at 1-6° C. Vox Sang 2000;78:28-30.
43. Downes KA, Wilson E, Yomtovian R, Sarode R. Serial measurement of clotting factors in thawed plasma stored for five days (letter). Transfusion 2001;41:570.
44. Nifong TP, Light J, Wenk RE. Coagulant stability and sterility of thawed S/D-treated plasma. Transfusion 2002;42:1581-4.
45. Cardigan R, Lawrie AS, Mackie IJ, Williamson LM. The quality of fresh frozen plasma produced from whole blood stored at 4C overnight. Transfusion 2005;45:1342-8.
46. AABB, America's Blood Centers, American Red Cross, Armed Services Blood Program. Circular of information for the use of human blood and blood components. (revised December 2009) Bethesda, MD: AABB, 2009.
47. Yarraton H, Lawrie AS, Mackie IJ, et al. Coagulation factor levels in cryosupernatant prepared from plasma treated with amotosalen hydrochloride (S-59) and ultraviolet A light. Transfusion 2005;45:1453-8.
48. Sharma AD, Sreeram G, Erb T, Grocott HP. Solvent-detergent-treated fresh frozen plasma: A superior alternative to standard fresh frozen plasma? J Cardiothorac Vasc Anesth 2000;14: 712-17.
49. Murphy K, O'Brien P, O'Donnell J. Acquired protein S deficiency in thrombotic thrombocytopenic purpura patients receiving solvent/detergent plasma exchange. Br J Haematol 2003;122:518-19.
50. Bass H, Trenchard PM, Mustow MJ. Microwave-thawed plasma for cryoprecipitate production. Vox Sang 1985;48:65-71.
51. Ness PM, Perkins HA. Fibrinogen in cryoprecipitate and its relationship to factor VIII (AHF) levels. Transfusion 1980;20:93-6.
52. Callum JL, Karkouti K, Yulia L. Cryoprecipitate: The current state of knowledge. Transfus Med Rev 2009;23:177-88.
53. Hoffman M, Jenner P. Variability in the fibrinogen and von Willebrand factor content of cryoprecipitate. Implications for reducing donor exposure. Am J Clin Pathol 1990;93:694-7.
54. Hoffman M, Koepke JA, Widmann FK. Fibrinogen content of low-volume cryoprecipitate. Transfusion 1987;27:356-8.

55. Farrugia A, Prowse C. Studies on the procurement of blood coagulation factor VIII: Effects of plasma freezing rate and storage conditions on cryoprecipitate quality. J Clin Pathol 1985; 122:686-92.
56. Smith JK, Bowell PJ, Bidwell E, Gunson HH. Anti-A haemagglutinins in factor VIII concentrates. J Clin Pathol 1980;33:954-7.
57. Pesquera-Lepatan LM, Hernandez FG, Lim RD, Chua MN. Thawed cryoprecipitate stored for 6 h at room temperature: A potential alternative to factor VIII concentrate for continuous infusion. Haemophilia 2004;10:684-8.
58. Rock G, Zurakowski S, Baxter A, Adams G. Simple and rapid preparation of granulocytes for the treatment of neonatal septicemia. Transfusion 1984;24:510-12.
59. Bishton M, Chopra R. The role of granulocyte transfusions in neutropenic patients. Br J Haematol 2004;127:501-8.
60. Ghodsi Z, Strauss RG. Cataracts in neutrophil donors stimulated with adrenal corticosteroids. Transfusion 2001;41:1464-8.
61. Burch JW, Mair DC, Meny GM, et al. The risk of posterior subcapsular cataracts in granulocyte donors. Transfusion 2005;45: 1701-8.
62. Schuetz AN, Hillyer KL, Roback JD, Hillyer CD. Leukoreduction filtration of blood with sickle cell trait. Transfus Med Rev 2004;18:168-76.
63. Dzik S, Moroff G, Dumont L. A multicenter study evaluating three methods for counting residual WBCs in WBC-reduced blood components: Nageotte hemocytometry, flow cytometry, and microfluorimetry. Transfusion 2000; 40:513-20.
64. Valeri CR. Simplification of the methods for adding and removing glycerol during freeze-preservation of human red blood cells with high or low glycerol methods: Biochemical modification prior to freezing. Transfusion 1975;15:195-218.
65. Valeri CR, Ragno G, Pivacek LE, et al. A multicenter study of in vitro and in vivo values in human RBCs frozen with 40-percent (wt/vol) glycerol and stored after deglycerolization for 15 days at 4°C in AS-3: Assessment of RBC processing in the ACP 215. Transfusion 2001;41: 933-9.
66. Valeri CR, Pivacek LE, Cassidy GP, Ragno G. The survival, function, and hemolysis of human RBCs stored at 4°C in additive solution (AS-1, AS-3, or AS-5) for 42 days and then biochemically modified, frozen, thawed, washed, and stored at 4°C in sodium chloride and glucose solution for 24 hours. Transfusion 2000; 40:1341-5.
67. Suda BA, Leitman SF, Davey RJ. Characteristics of red cells irradiated and subsequently frozen for long-term storage. Transfusion 1993;33: 389-92.
68. Alving BM, Reid TJ, Fratantoni JC, Finlayson JS. Frozen platelets and platelet substitutes in transfusion medicine. Transfusion 1997;37: 866-76.
69. Lee DH, Blajchman MA. Novel platelet products and substitutes. Transfus Med Rev 1998; 12:175-87.
70. Vadhan-Raj S, Kavanagh JJ, Freedman RS, et al. Safety and efficacy of transfusions of autologous cryopreserved platelets derived from recombinant human thrombopoietin to support chemotherapy-associated severe thrombocytopenia: A randomised cross-over study. Lancet 2002;359:2145-52.
71. Nuclear Regulatory Commission Security Orders. Holders of material licenses authorized to possess radioactive material quantities of concern. Rockville, MD: Nuclear Regulatory Commission, 2005. [Available at http://www.nrc.gov/reading-rm/doc-collections/enforcement/security/#8 (accessed October 8, 2010).]
72. Moroff G, Leitman SF, Luban NLC. Principles of blood irradiation dose validation, and quality control. Transfusion 1997;37:1084-92.
73. Voak D, Chapman J, Finney RD, et al. Guidelines on gamma irradiation of blood components for the prevention of transfusion-associated graft-versus-host disease. Transfus Med 1996;6:261-71.
74. Moroff G, Friedman A, Robkin-Kline L, et al. Reduction of the volume of stored platelet concentrates for use in neonatal patients. Transfusion 1984;24:144-6.
75. Pisciotto P, Synder EL, Napychank PA, Hopper SM. In vitro characteristics of volume-reduced platelet concentrate stored in syringes. Transfusion 1991;31:404-8.
76. Dumont LJ, Krailadsiri P, Seghatchian J, et al. Preparation and storage characteristics of white-cell-reduced high-concentration platelet concentrates collected by an apheresis system for transfusion in utero. Transfusion 2000; 40:91-100.
77. Schoenfeld H, Muhm M, Doepfmer UR, et al. The functional integrity of platelets in volume-reduced platelet concentrates. Anesth Analg 2005;100:78-81.

78. Ringwald J, Walz S, Zimmerman R, et al. Hyperconcentrated platelets stored in additive solution: Aspects of productivity and in vitro quality. Vox Sang 2005;89:11-18.
79. Lockwood WB, Hudgens RW, Szymanski IO, et al. Effects of rejuvenation and frozen storage on 42-day-old AS-3 RBCs. Transfusion 2003; 43:1527-32.
80. Food and Drug Administration. Guideline for the uniform labeling of blood and blood components. (August 1985) Rockville, MD: CBER Office of Communication, Outreach, and Development, 1985. [Available at http://www.fda.gov/BiologicsBloodVaccines/GuidanceComplianceRegulatoryInformation/Guidances/Blood/default.htm (accessed October 4, 2010).]
81. Food and Drug Administration. Guidance: Industry consensus standard for the uniform labeling of blood and blood components using ISBT 128 version 2.0.0, November 2005. (September 22, 2006) Rockville, MD: CBER Office of Communication, Outreach, and Development, 2006. [Available at http://www.fda.gov/BiologicsBloodVaccines/GuidanceComplianceRegulatoryInformation/Guidances/Blood/default.htm (accessed October 4, 2010).]

Chapter 7

Blood Component Collection by Apheresis

James W. Smith, MD, PhD

APHERESIS, PHERESIS, hemapheresis, or any of the various terms used for automated blood component collection procedures are derived from the Greek *aphairos,* meaning "to take from." Both centrifugal and membrane-based apheresis techniques were under development in the late 19th and early 20th centuries. By the 1970s, multiple technologies had begun to develop for the separation of blood components from donors or patients.

The status of donor apheresis at present parallels the evolution in technology. In the United States, centrifugal technology has been developed for apheresis applications. Other parts of the world, primarily Europe and Japan, have seen the additional development of membrane filtration technology for some donor procedures.

The development of automated, online, centrifugal technologies was linked with the development of the first devices to allow donor apheresis in large-scale applications. Early device developments allowed the donation of platelets, plasma, and granulocytes. As the technology continued to develop, equipment, disposables, and software programs became increasingly sophisticated for the separation of these components as well as others. The collection of various combinations of components by apheresis is now possible (see Table 7-1). This chapter discusses the technology and instrumentation used in the collection of these components, with special consideration given to the regulatory aspects involved with donors, products, testing, and other requirements specifically related to apheresis.

COMPONENT COLLECTION

Collection of components by apheresis follows many of the same rules and guidelines that apply to whole blood donation. For instance, like whole blood donors, donors who are to undergo a procedure involving apheresis must be given information so that their consent to donate is informed. Although apheresis collection and preparation processes differ from those used for whole-blood-derived components, the storage conditions, transportation requirements, and some quality control steps are the same for both. Yet another similarity is that the facility must maintain written procedures and protocols for all types of

James W. Smith, MD, PhD, Medical Director, Oklahoma Blood Institute, Oklahoma City, Oklahoma
The author has disclosed no conflicts of interest.

TABLE 7-1. Components That Can Be Collected from Various Instruments

Instrument	GRAN	PLT	cRBC	2-RBC	PLASMA	cPLASMA
Fenwal ALYX			X	X		X
Fenwal Amicus		X	X			X
Fenwal Autopheresis C					X	
Fresenius AS104	X					
Caridian (COBE) Spectra	X	X				X
Caridian Trima V-4		X	X	X		X
Caridian Trima Accel		X	X	X		X
Haemonetics Cymbal				X		
Haemonetics MCS+ LN9000	X	X				X
Haemonetics MCS+ LN8150			X	X		X
Haemonetics PCS-2					X	

GRAN = granulocytes; PLT = plateletpheresis (single, double, triple); cRBC = concurrent 1-unit RBC; 2-RBC = double unit of RBCs; PLASMA = 1-unit plasma; cPLASMA = concurrent plasma; concurrent = more than one product can be collected; V-4 = software version 4.

collections used and must keep records for each procedure as required by AABB *Standards for Blood Banks and Transfusion Services* (*Standards*).[1(pp62-67)] The circumstances unique to apheresis collection are addressed in the sections that follow.

Platelets

Apheresis platelet collections are used to obtain platelets from volunteer donors, from patients' family members, or from donors with HLA or platelet-antigen-compatible phenotypes. By design, apheresis procedures are intended to collect large numbers of platelets from an individual, thereby providing a more consistent product with fewer donor exposures for the patient. AABB *Standards* requires that an apheresis platelet component contain at least 3×10^{11} platelets in 90% of sampled units.[1(pp28-29)] With newer technology and more efficient processes, higher yields of platelets may be obtained from one donor, and the original apheresis unit may be split into multiple units, each of which must meet minimum standards. Some instruments are programmed to calculate the yield from the donor's hematocrit, platelet count, height, and weight. For alloimmunized patients who are refractory to random allogeneic platelets, platelets from an apheresis donor selected on the basis of a compatible platelet crossmatch or matched for HLA antigens may be the only way to achieve a satisfactory posttransfusion platelet increment. In the United States, the use of apheresis platelets has been steadily increasing over the past 25 years. It is estimated that 86% of therapeutic platelet doses transfused in the United States are apheresis platelets.[2]

Donor Selection and Monitoring

Plateletpheresis donors may donate more frequently than whole blood donors but must meet all other donor criteria. The interval between donations should be at least 2 days, and donors should not undergo plateletpheresis more than twice in a week or more than 24 times in a year.[1(p19),3] If the donor donates a unit of whole blood, or if it becomes impossible to return the donor's red cells during plateletpheresis, at least 8 weeks should elapse before a subsequent plateletpheresis procedure unless the extracorporeal red cell volume is less than 100 mL. Platelets may be collected from donors who do not meet these requirements only if the component is expected to be of particular value to a specific intended recipient and if a physician certifies in writing that the donor's health will not be compromised by the donation. Donors who have taken antiplatelet medications that irreversibly inhibit platelet function are deferred for specific intervals before donation (aspirin/aspirin-containing medications, 48 hours; Feldene, 48 hours; Plavix/clopidogrel, 14 days; Ticlid/ticlopidine, 14 days) because apheresis platelets are often the sole source of platelets given to a patient.[1(p57),3]

Plateletpheresis donors should meet the same usual qualifications as allogeneic blood donors, with the exception of the donation interval (ie, hemoglobin or hematocrit level). Platelet count is not required before the first apheresis collection; however, triple collections of platelets may not be drawn from first-time donors unless a qualifying platelet count is obtained from a sample collected before the procedure. If the donation interval is less than 4 weeks, many facilities prefer that the donor's platelet count be above 150,000/µL before subsequent plateletpheresis occurs, to prevent a postdonation count of less than 100,000/uL. AABB *Standards* permits qualifying the donor with a platelet count from a sample collected immediately before the procedure or from a sample obtained either before or after the previous procedure.[1(p20)] Exceptions to these laboratory criteria should be approved in writing by the apheresis program physician, based on documented medical need. The Food and Drug Administration (FDA) specifies that the total volume of plasma collected should be no more than 500 mL (or 600 mL for donors weighing more than 175 lb) or the volume described in the labeling for the automated blood cell separator device (which may be more or less than the 500-mL or 600-mL volume previously stated). The platelet count of each unit should be kept on record but need not be written on the component label. Units containing less than 3.0×10^{11} platelets should be labeled with the actual platelet count.[3]

It is possible to collect plasma concurrently with the collection of platelets. Such collection is discussed further in the section about donor plasmapheresis. With regard to donor reactions, vasovagal and hypovolemic reactions are rare in apheresis donors but may occur. Paresthesias and other reactions to citrate anticoagulant are not uncommon. [Reactions (of recipients) are discussed with those for whole blood in Chapter 27.] Serious reactions occur less often among apheresis donors than among donors of whole blood.[4]

Laboratory Testing

Tests for ABO group, for Rh type, for unexpected alloantibodies, and for markers for transfusion-transmitted diseases must be performed by the collecting facility in the same manner as for other blood components. Each unit must be tested unless the donor is undergoing repeated procedures to support a specific patient, in which case testing for infectious disease markers needs to be repeated only at 30-day intervals.

If red cells are visible in a product, the hematocrit should be determined. AABB *Standards*[1(p35)] requires that if the component contains more than 2 mL of red cells, the red cells must be ABO compatible with recipient plasma and be crossmatched. In such cases, a sample of donor blood for compatibility testing is attached to the container. In some instances it may be desirable for the donor plasma to be ABO compatible with the recipient's red cells (eg, if the recipient is a child or an ABO-mismatched allogeneic progenitor cell transplant recipient). In the United States, to be considered leukocyte reduced, apheresis platelets must contain fewer than 5×10^6 leukocytes per unit, and platelets must meet the specifications of the apheresis device manufacturer.[3] In Europe, the guideline for leukocyte-reduced components is fewer than 1×10^6 white cells (WBCs) per unit.

Record-Keeping

Complete records must be kept for each procedure. All adverse reactions occurring during collection procedures (or transfusion) should be documented along with results of thorough investigations. Records of all laboratory findings and collection data must be periodically reviewed by a knowledgeable physician and must be found to be within acceptable limits. FDA guidelines require a periodic review of donor records to monitor platelet counts.[3] Facilities must have policies and procedures in place to ensure that donor red cell loss during each procedure does not exceed acceptable limits.

Plasma

Apheresis devices can be used to collect plasma as transfusable Fresh Frozen Plasma (FFP) or as Source Plasma for subsequent manufacturing. The FDA has provided guidance with regard to the volume of plasma that is allowed to be collected using automated devices. The distinction is made between infrequent plasmapheresis, in which the donor undergoes plasmapheresis no more frequently than once every 4 weeks, and serial plasmapheresis (or Source Plasma collection, the process to collect plasma for fractionation into plasma components), in which the donation is more frequent than once every 4 weeks. For donors in infrequent plasmapheresis programs, donor selection and monitoring requirements are the same as those for whole blood donation, and plasma obtained by these processes is intended for direct transfusion.

For serial plasma collection (Source Plasma collection), using either automated instruments or manual techniques, the following principles apply[5]:

1. Donors must give consent for the procedure, and they must be observed closely during the procedure. Emergency medical care must always be available.
2. Red cell losses related to the procedure, including samples collected for testing, must not exceed 25 mL/week so that no more than 200 mL of red cells are removed in 8 weeks. If the donor's red cells cannot be returned during an apheresis procedure, hemapheresis or whole blood donation should be deferred for 8 weeks.
3. For manual collection systems, a mechanism must exist to ensure safe reinfusion of the autologous red cells. Before the blood container is separated from the donor for processing, there should be two separate, independent means of identification, so that both the donor and the phlebotomist can ascertain that the contents are those of the donor. Often, the donor signature is one identifier along with a unique identification number.
4. In manual procedures for donors weighing 110 to 175 lb, no more than 500 mL of whole blood should be removed at one time or no more than 1000 mL during a session or within a 48-hour period. The limits for donors who weigh ≥175 lb are 600 mL and 1200 mL, respectively. For automated procedures, the allowable volume has been determined for each instrument by the FDA.
5. At least 48 hours should elapse between successive procedures. Donors should not undergo more than two procedures within a 7-day period. However, exceptions are permissible when plasma is expected to have special therapeutic value for a specific recipient.
6. At the time of initial plasmapheresis and at 4-month intervals for donors undergoing serial (large-volume) plasmapheresis (donors undergoing plasmapheresis more often than once every 4 weeks), serum or plasma must be tested for total protein and for serum protein electrophoresis or for quantitative immunoglobulins. Results must be within normal limits. This requirement applies to donors undergoing large-volume plasma collections, where the total annual volume of plasma collected exceeds 12 L (14.4 L for donors weighing more than 175 lb) or if the donor is a frequent (more often than once every 4 weeks) plasma donor.

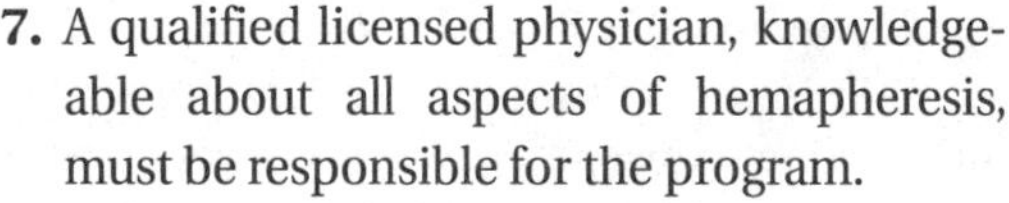

7. A qualified licensed physician, knowledgeable about all aspects of hemapheresis, must be responsible for the program.

Red Blood Cells and Multicomponent Donations

Both AABB *Standards* and FDA guidance documents address the removal of red cells by automated apheresis methods. A guidance document issued in 2001 by the FDA finalized recommendations for Red Blood Cells (RBCs) to be collected by automated apheresis.[6] The guidance document included the use of automated apheresis equipment that involved collection protocols for the following[6]:

- A single unit of RBCs and plasma.
- A single unit of RBCs and platelets.
- A single unit of RBCs, platelets, and plasma.
- A double unit of RBCs only.

The guidance document notes FDA regulations requiring that equipment perform in a manner for which it was designed for collecting or processing blood and components. Standard operating procedures, including device manufacturers' instructions for use and maintenance of current records, are described. The following sections present the information in the guidance document.[6]

Donor Selection and Monitoring

The FDA requires that an adequate hemoglobin level be determined by a quantitative method for predonation hemoglobin or for hematocrit of donors undergoing double RBC collection. The procedure is limited to persons who are larger and have higher hematocrits than the minimum standards for whole blood donations (for males: minimum weight = 130 lb, height = 5′ 1″; for females: minimum weight = 150 lb, height = 5′ 5″; minimum hematocrit = 40% for both genders). Donors of small stature and minimum weight criteria, as established by the FDA in device operator's manuals, should be further evaluated. Those donors must also meet all appropriate FDA criteria for allogeneic or autologous whole blood donation. Donors giving a single unit of RBCs with platelets or plasma, or both, should be deferred for at least 8 weeks. The exception to this deferral is when a donor serves as a plateletpheresis donor or a donor of platelets with plasma by-products within 8 weeks, if the extracorporeal red cell volume of the procedure is <100 mL.

Donors should be deferred for at least 16 weeks after a double RBC donation. If an apheresis procedure is discontinued before completion and if absolute red cell loss is <200 mL, the donor may return to donate within 8 weeks if all donor eligibility criteria are met.

If there is a second red cell loss of <100 mL during a subsequent donation within 8 weeks, the donor should be deferred for 8 weeks. If the total absolute red cell loss within 8 weeks is >300 mL, the donor should be deferred for 16 weeks from the date of the last red cell loss.

If an apheresis procedure is discontinued and the absolute red cell loss is >200 mL but <300 mL, the donor should be deferred for 8 weeks. If an apheresis procedure is discontinued and total absolute red cell loss is ≥300 mL, the donor should be deferred for 16 weeks.

Saline infusion is used to minimize volume depletion.

Quality Control Issues

The FDA has promulgated quality control (QC) programs for RBC units collected by apheresis. There are two phases:

- Phase I QC consists of 100 consecutive RBC units that are tested to determine the expected or target RBC volume in accordance with the specifications set forth in the device operator's manual. Target values are compared with the actual values to determine product acceptability. After the completion of satisfactory QC, which includes having at least 95% of the units meet product specifications, the establishment may proceed to Phase II.
- Phase II QC consists of monthly testing of a representative sample of the manufactured product. This testing includes a requirement that each month a minimum of 50

units be tested for each collection center. At least 1 unit from a single RBC protocol or both units from a double RBC protocol device used at the center should be included. At least 95% of the products tested should meet product specifications as described in the device operator's manual.

Record Requirements

US blood establishments must update their blood establishment registrations and product listing forms with the FDA in order to collect red cells using automated methods. Implementation of automated RBC collection is a change that has a substantial potential to have an adverse effect on the identity, strength, quality, purity, or potency of a product. Blood establishments that are approved to manufacture RBCs with one manufacturer's device and that wish to change to another manufacturer's device must submit a prior approval supplement and must receive approval before distribution of the product manufactured on the new device. A number of records are described that must be available for FDA inspection in relation to RBC or multicomponent collection. These records and forms include those addressing donor consent, donor eligibility, product collection, and QC for the product.

Granulocytes

The use of granulocyte transfusions has been controversial for a number of years. Analysis of randomized controlled trials of granulocyte transfusions in adults has indicated that an acceptable minimum dose (>1 × 10^{10} granulocytes/day) and crossmatch compatibility (no recipient antibodies to granulocyte antigens) have a major bearing on effectiveness. Recently, there has been renewed interest in granulocyte transfusion therapy because much greater cell doses may be obtained from donors who have received recombinant colony-stimulating factors.

Agents Administered to Increase Yields

A daily dose of at least 1 × 10^{10} granulocytes is necessary to achieve a therapeutic effect in adult patients. For infants and children, a dose of 10 to 15 mL/kg may provide adequate granulocytes per dose. To collect this number of cells in a unit of granulocytes, one must administer drugs or sedimenting materials to the donor. The donor's consent must include specific permission for any of these drugs or sedimenting agents to be used.

HYDROXYETHYL STARCH. A common sedimenting agent, hydroxyethyl starch (HES), causes red cells to aggregate, thereby sedimenting them more completely. Sedimenting agents enhance granulocyte harvest by causing increased sedimentation of the red cells, thereby enhancing the interface in the collection device and resulting in minimal red cell content in the final product. Because HES can be detected in donors as long as a year after infusion, AABB *Standards*[1(p22)] requires facilities performing granulocyte collections to have a process to control the maximum cumulative dose of any sedimenting agent administered to the donor in a given interval. HES is a colloid, which acts as a volume expander. Donors who receive HES may experience headaches or peripheral edema because of expanded circulatory volume.

CORTICOSTEROIDS. Corticosteroids can double the number of circulating granulocytes by mobilizing granulocytes from the marginal pool. The common protocol is to use 60 mg of oral prednisone as a single or divided dose before donation in order to collect significant numbers of granulocytes with minimal systemic steroid activity. Another protocol uses 8 mg of oral dexamethasone. Donors should be questioned about relevant medical history (hypertension, diabetes, cataracts, or peptic ulcer can be relative to absolute contraindications) before they use systemic corticosteroids.

GROWTH FACTORS. Recombinant hematopoietic growth factors, specifically granulocyte colony-stimulating factor (G-CSF), can effectively increase granulocyte yields. Hematopoietic growth factors given alone can result in collection of up to 4 to 8 × 10^{10} granulocytes per apheresis procedure. Typical doses of

G-CSF are 5 to 10 µg/kg given 8 to 12 hours before collection. Preliminary evidence suggests that in-vivo recovery and survival of these granulocytes are excellent and that growth factors are well tolerated by donors.

Laboratory Testing

Testing for ABO and Rh, for red cell antibodies, and for infectious disease markers is required on a sample drawn at the time of phlebotomy. Red cell content in granulocyte products is inevitable; the red cells should be ABO compatible with the recipient's plasma. If >2 mL of red cells are present, the component should be crossmatched. Both Rh compatibility and HLA compatibility are recommended.

Storage and Infusion

Granulocyte function deteriorates rapidly during storage, and concentrates should be transfused as soon as possible after preparation. AABB *Standards* mandates a storage temperature of 20 to 24 C for no longer than 24 hours.[1(p52)] Agitation during storage is undesirable. Irradiation is required for immunodeficient recipients and is indicated for nearly all recipients because their primary diseases are likely to involve deficiencies in their immune systems. Use of a microaggregate or leukocyte reduction filter is contraindicated because it will remove the collected granulocytes.

INSTRUMENTS AND SYSTEMS FOR DONOR APHERESIS COLLECTIONS

The following is a list of equipment that is available for use in the United States for the respective blood components collected by automated techniques. A brief description is given for each instrument; more detailed information can be found in other resources.[7,8] [Note: The CS3000 and CS3000+ (Fenwal, Lake Zurich, IL) have not been included because the company has discontinued the sale of these devices in the United States (although disposables are still available at the time of this writing). The devices are capable of collecting platelets, concurrent plasma, and granulocytes.]

Plasma

Fenwal Autopheresis C

The Autopheresis C (Fenwal) is an instrument designed to collect plasma only.[9] It uses a rotating cylindrical filter to separate the plasma from the cellular elements of blood. Because of the high efficiency of the rotating filter, a small filter is used and the extracorporeal volume (ECV) of the system is approximately 200 mL. The Autopheresis C is a single-access system, and saline replacement can be administered. It is considered an open system and can collect several units of plasma. According to FDA definition, an open system requires that plasma outdates 4 hours after thawing and cannot be converted to thawed plasma.

Haemonetics PCS-2

The PCS-2 (Haemonetics, Braintree, MA) is designed specifically for plasma collection.[9] The PCS-2 is a simplified version of the MCS Plus. The PCS-2 uses a blow-molded (grenade-shaped) centrifuge bowl to separate plasma from the cellular elements. Depending on the degree of cell reduction required, one of three versions of the PCS-2 bowl can be used: standard, filter core, and high separation core. The standard bowl uses centrifugal force to remove the plasma from the top of the bowl. To increase cell reduction, the filter core and high separation core bowls allow plasma to pass through the core, one covered with a filter membrane (it has the highest cell reduction but has not been released in the United States at this time).[10-12] The ECV of the PCS-2 is variable depending on the hematocrit of the donor, ranging from 491 mL (38% hematocrit) to 385 mL (50% hematocrit). The PCS-2 is a single-access system, and saline replacement can be administered. It is considered an open system. The PCS-2 can collect several units of plasma.

Equipment for Concurrent Plasma Collection

Plasma can be collected as a concurrent product during collection of apheresis platelets or automated RBCs. The amount that can be collected is determined by the volume of platelets, red cells, or both, that are being collected and by the maximum volume that can be removed from the donor. Equipment capable of concurrent plasma collection includes Haemonetics MCS+ LN9000, Haemonetics MCS+ LN8150, Fenwal Amicus, Fenwal ALYX, Caridian (COBE) Spectra (CaridianBCT, Lakewood, CO), Caridian Trima, and Caridian Trima Accel.

Platelets

Caridian (COBE) Spectra

The Caridian (COBE) Spectra is capable of collecting single, double, or triple apheresis platelet units as well as concurrent plasma, depending on the size and platelet count of the donor.[7,13-16] It uses a dual-stage (different radius) channel to collect leukocyte-reduced platelets. Leukocyte reduction to $<5 \times 10^6$ WBCs can be obtained in approximately 85% of the collections for software versions less than 5.0.[17] Software versions 5.0 and 7.0 are able to more consistently obtain products containing $<1.0 \times 10^6$ WBCs by using the Leukocyte Reduction System (LRS), which uses a cone in the centrifuge and saturated, fluidized, particle-bed filter technology to remove residual WBCs leaving the second stage of the channel.[7,13-16] The Spectra is capable of single- or double-access procedures. The ECV of the single-access kit is 361 mL, and that of the double-access kit is 272 mL. It should be noted that the Spectra is being replaced by the more efficient Caridian Trima or Trima Accel.[8]

Caridian Trima and Trima Accel

The Caridian Trimas were designed as automated donor collection machines for platelets, plasma, and RBCs only. The Caridian Trima (Version 4) uses a smaller, modified, dual-stage channel and LRS cone to consistently collect leukocyte-reduced platelets ($<1.0 \times 10^6$ WBCs). To increase platelet yields, the Trima Accel (Versions 5.0, 5.01, and 5.1) uses a single-stage, donut-shaped channel and larger LRS cone to consistently collect leukocyte-reduced platelets.[18] The Trimas use single-access kits only. The ECV of the Trimas is 182 to 196 mL. They are capable of collecting single, double, or triple units of apheresis platelets as well as concurrent plasma and RBCs, depending on donor size, platelet count, and hematocrit.[18-20]

Fenwal Amicus

The Amicus is capable of collecting single, double, or triple apheresis platelets as well as concurrent plasma and RBCs (single-access kit only), depending on the donor's size, platelet count,[7,13,19,21] and hematocrit. The Amicus uses centrifugal force and a double compartment belt wrapped around a spool to separate the platelets. The platelets accumulate in the collection chamber and are transferred to the final collection bags at the end of the procedure. The Amicus is capable of single- or double-access procedures. The ECV of the double-access kit is 210 mL, and the ECV of the single-access kit is 209 mL plus the whole blood bag (adjustable). Consistent leukocyte reduction is accomplished without external filtration, and this process is approved for submission of a prior approval supplement.

Haemonetics MCS+ LN9000

The Haemonetics MCS+ LN9000 system is capable of several different apheresis procedures, including apheresis platelet collection. It uses the Latham conical bowl, plasma-controlled hematocrit, and plasma surge technique to build up the platelets and float them off the bowl with rapid plasma infusion. Although this technique results in leukocyte-reduced platelets, the use of an online leukocyte-reduction filter ensures consistency in leukocyte reduction.[7,22-25] The LN9000 uses a single-access kit, and the ECV is variable from 480 mL (38% hematocrit) to 359 mL (52% hematocrit). The LN9000 is capable of collecting single, double, or triple units of apheresis platelets as well as concurrent plasma, depending on donor size and platelet count.[7,22-25]

Red Blood Cells

Caridian Trima and Trima Accel

As previously mentioned, the Trima can collect a single unit of RBCs concurrently with platelets.[8,20,26] There is also a kit to collect a double unit of RBCs with or without concurrent plasma, depending on the donor's size and hematocrit. The Trima uses the single-stage channel for the double RBC collection, and saline is returned to the donor during the collection. Addition of the preservative solution and the leukocyte reduction by filtration are performed manually and offline after the collection is complete, for both the single and double units of RBCs.

Fenwal ALYX

The Fenwal ALYX was developed as an automated, double RBC collection system only. Recently, it has been approved to also collect concurrent plasma. The ALYX uses a rigid, cylinder-shaped chamber in the centrifuge to separate the plasma from the cells. The plasma is collected in one bag, with the red cells in a separate bag. During reinfusion, the plasma and saline are returned to the donor. When collection is complete, the ALYX automatically adds the preservative solution and pumps the red cells through an online leukocyte-reduction filter into the final storage bags. The ALYX uses a single-access kit only, and the ECV is approximately 110 mL. The ALYX is capable of collecting 2 units of RBCs or 1 unit of RBCs and concurrent plasma, depending on donor size and hematocrit.[8,25-27]

Fenwal Amicus

As mentioned previously, the Fenwal Amicus can collect a single unit of RBCs concurrently with plateletpheresis, but only with the single-access kit.[8,28] Addition of the preservative solution and leukocyte reduction by filtration are performed manually and offline after the collection is complete.

Haemonetics Cymbal

The Cymbal is a collection system that uses an expanding, variable-volume bowl; has a small ECV; and collects a double RBC unit.[29]

Haemonetics MCS+ LN8150

The Haemonetics MCS+ LN8150 was designed as a donor instrument only, for collection of RBCs and concurrent plasma. The LN8150 uses the blow-molded bowl that is also used for plasma collection. It uses a single-access kit and the ECV is variable depending on the donor's hematocrit, from 542 mL (38% hematocrit) to 391 mL (54% hematocrit). The LN8150 is capable of collecting a single or double unit of RBCs with or without concurrent plasma, depending on the donor's size and hematocrit.[8,26,30] The addition of preservative and the leukocyte reduction by filtration are performed manually and offline after the collection is complete.

Granulocytes

Caridian (COBE) Spectra

The Spectra is capable of collecting granulocytes.[8,31,32] It uses the donut-shaped, single-stage channel in the centrifuge to isolate the granulocytes that are continuously collected in the final storage bag. It uses a double-access kit (only), and the ECV is 285 mL.

Fresenius AS 104

The Fresenius AS 104 is capable of collecting several components, including granulocytes.[8,33] It uses a donut-shaped, single-stage channel to separate the granulocytes. The granulocytes are allowed to build up in the centrifuge and are harvested into the final collection bag intermittently. The AS 104 uses a double-access kit, and the ECV is 175 mL.

Haemonetics MCS+ LN9000

The LN9000 can also be used to collect granulocytes. It uses the conical Latham bowl for separation, and then the buffy coat is transferred to one of two bags. The red cells are allowed to settle to the bottom of the bag before being returned to the donor. The LN9000 switches from one bag to another to return the red cells. A single- or double-access kit can be used for granulocyte collection, and the ECV is variable based on the hematocrit of the donor, from 480 mL (38% hematocrit) to 359 mL (52% hematocrit).

KEY POINTS

1. Apheresis components must meet many of the same basic regulatory requirements (eg, donor consent, storage conditions, transportation requirements, etc) as whole-blood-derived components, although more specific requirements apply for each type of apheresis component collection.
2. The majority of platelets transfused in the United States are apheresis platelets.
3. Plasma can be collected by apheresis as transfusable Fresh Frozen Plasma or as Source Plasma for subsequent manufacturing. The Food and Drug Administration has provided guidance with regard to the volume of plasma that is allowed to be collected using automated devices.
4. In multicomponent donations, a variety of components or combinations of components may be collected with apheresis technology. Regulations specific to this practice apply to donor selection and monitoring, quality control, and records.
5. Red cells can be removed concurrently with other components, or a double unit of red cells may be collected.
6. Several instruments and systems have been developed and/or adapted for apheresis collection of blood components, using different technologies. Some are appropriate for collection of only one type of component, and others can collect multiple components.
7. Granulocyte collection differs from that of other components. Specific techniques and conditions should be considered for the optimal collection of granulocytes by apheresis.

REFERENCES

1. Carson TH, ed. Standards for blood banks and transfusion services. 27th ed. Bethesda, MD: AABB, 2011.
2. US Department of Health and Human Services. 2009 National blood collection and utilization survey report. Washington, DC: DHHS, 2011 (in press).
3. Food and Drug Administration. Guidance for industry and FDA review staff: Collection of platelets by automated methods. (December 17, 2007) Rockville, MD: CBER Office of Communication, Outreach, and Development, 2007. [Available at http://www.fda.gov/cber/guidelines.htm (accessed November 22, 2010).]
4. Wiltbank TB. Donor reaction rates: A preliminary comparison of automated vs whole blood procedures (abstract). Transfusion 2002;42 (Suppl):67S.
5. Code of federal regulations. Title 21, CFR Part 640, Subpart G—Source Plasma. Washington, DC: US Government Printing Office, 2010 (revised annually).
6. Food and Drug Administration. Guidance for industry: Recommendations for collecting red blood cells by automated apheresis methods. (January 30, 2001; Technical Correction February 2001) Rockville, MD: CBER Office of Communication, Outreach, and Development, 2001. [Available at http://www.fda.gov/cber/guidelines.htm (see technical correction, February 13, 2001; accessed November 22, 2010).]
7. Burgstaler EA. Current instrumentation for apheresis. In: McLeod BC, Szczepiorkowski ZM, Weinstein R, Winters JL, eds. Apheresis: Principles and practice. 3rd ed. Bethesda, MD: AABB Press, 2010:71-110.
8. Burgstaler EA. Blood component collection by apheresis. J Clin Apher 2006;21:142-51.
9. Hood M, Mynderup N, Doxon L. Evaluation of Haemonetics PCS-2 and Fenwal Auto-C plas-

mapheresis collection systems (abstract). J Clin Apher 1996;11:99.

10. Burkhardt T, Kappelsberger C, Karl M. Evaluation of a new combined centrifugation/filtration method for the collection of plasma via plasmapheresis (abstract). Transfusion 2001; 41(Suppl):50S.
11. Burnouf T, Kappelsberger C, Frank K, Burkhardt T. Protein composition and activation markers in plasma collected by three apheresis procedures. Transfusion 2003;43:1223-30.
12. Burnouf T, Kappelsberger C, Frank K, Burkhardt T. Residual cell content in plasma produced by three apheresis procedures. Transfusion 2003;43:1522-6.
13. Burgstaler EA, Pineda AA, Bryant SC. Prospective comparison of plateletapheresis using four apheresis systems on the same donors. J Clin Apher 1999;14:163-70.
14. Perseghin P, Mascaretti L, Riva M, et al. Comparison of plateletapheresis concentrates produced with Spectra LRS version 5.1 and LRS Turbo version 7.0 cell separators. Transfusion 2000;40:789-93.
15. Zingsem J, Glaser A, Weisbach V. Evaluation of a platelet apheresis technique for the preparation of leukocyte-reduced platelet concentrates. Vox Sang 1998;74:189-92.
16. Zingsem J, Zimmermann R, Weisbach V, et al. Comparison of COBE white cell-reduction and standard plateletapheresis protocols in the same donors. Transfusion 1997; 37:1045-9.
17. Maresh S, Randels M, Strauss R, et al. Comparison of plateletapheresis with a standard and an improved collection device. Transfusion 1993;33:835-7.
18. McAteer M, Kagen L, Graminske S, et al. Trima Accel improved platelet collection efficiency with the merging of single stage separation technology with leukoreduction performance of the LRS chamber (abstract). Transfusion 2002;42(Suppl):37S.
19. Burgstaler EA, Winters JL, Pineda AA. Paired comparison of Gambro Trima Accel vs Baxter Amicus single-needle plateletapheresis. Transfusion 2004;44:1612-20.
20. Elfath MD, Whitley P, Jacobson MS, et al. Evaluation of an automated system for the collection of packed RBCs, platelets, and plasma. Transfusion 2000;40:1214-22.
21. Yockey C, Murphy S, Eggers L, et al. Evaluation of the Amicus separator in the collection of apheresis platelets. Transfusion 1999;38:848-54.
22. Valbonesi M, Florio G, Ruzzenenti MR, et al. Multicomponent collection (MCC) with the latest hemapheresis apparatuses. Int J Artif Organs 1999;22:511-15.
23. Paciorek L, Holme S, Andres M, et al. Evaluation of the continuous filtration method with double platelet products collected on the MCS+ (abstract). J Clin Apher 1998;13:87.
24. Ford K, Thompson C, McWhorter R, et al. Evaluation of the Haemonetics MCS+ LN9000 to produce leukoreduced platelet products (abstract). J Clin Apher 1996;11:104.
25. Rose C, Ragusa M, Andres M, et al. Evaluation of the MCS + LN9000 in-line leukoreduction filter (abstract). Transfusion 1996;36(Suppl): 85.
26. Picker SM, Radojska SM, Gathof BS. Prospective evaluation of double RBC collection using three different apheresis systems. Transfus Apher Sci 2006;35:197-205.
27. Snyder EL, Elfath MD, Taylor H, et al. Collection of two units of leukoreduced RBCs from a single donation with a portable multiple-component collection system. Transfusion 2003; 43:1695-705.
28. Moog R, Frank V, Müller N. Evaluation of a concurrent multicomponent collection system for the collection and storage of WBC-reduced RBC apheresis concentrates. Transfusion 2001;41:1159-64.
29. Nussbaumer W, Grabmer C, Maurer M, et al. Evaluation of a new mobile two unit red cell apheresis system (abstract). J Clin Apher 2006; 21:20.
30. Smith JW. Automated donations: Plasma, red cells, and multicomponent donor procedures. In: McLeod BC, Szczepiorkowski ZM, Weinstein R, Winters JL, eds. Apheresis: Principles and practice. 3rd ed. Bethesda, MD: AABB Press, 2010:125-40.
31. Worel N, Kurz M, Peters C, Höcker P. Serial granulocyte apheresis under daily administration of rHuG-CSF: Effects on peripheral blood counts, collection efficiency, and yield. Transfusion 2001;41:390-5.
32. Dale DC, Lises WC, Llewellyn C, et al. Neutrophil transfusions: Kinetics and functions of neutrophils mobilized with granulocyte colony-stimulating factor and dexamethasone. Transfusion 1998;38:713-21.
33. Kretschmer V, Biehl M, Coffe C, et al. New features of the Fresenius blood cell separator AS104. In: Agishi T, Kawamura A, Mineshima M, eds. Therapeutic plasmapheresis (XII): Pro-

ceedings of the 4th International Congress of the World Apheresis Association and the 12th Annual Symposium of the Japanese Society for Apheresis, June 3-5, 1992, Sapporo, Japan. Utrecht, the Netherlands: VSP, 1993:851-5.

Chapter 8

Infectious Disease Screening

Susan A. Galel, MD

BLOOD COMPONENTS, LIKE all other medications in the United States, are regulated by the Food and Drug Administration (FDA). The FDA requires medication manufacturers to verify the suitability of every raw material.[1] For biologic pharmaceuticals, the donor is the key ingredient whose suitability must be scrutinized.

Blood banks test a sample of blood from each donation in order to identify donors and donated components that might harbor infectious agents. This screening process is critically important because many blood components (eg, red cells, platelets, plasma, and cryoprecipitate) are administered intravenously into recipients without pasteurization or sterilization or other treatments to inactivate infectious agents. Thus, an infectious agent that is in a donor's blood at the time of donation and not detected by the screening process would be transmitted directly to the recipient.

HISTORICAL OVERVIEW OF BLOOD DONOR SCREENING

The first infectious disease test performed on blood donations in the United States was a test for syphilis, implemented in the 1940s and mandated since the 1950s. This was the only test required for many years. In the 1960s, posttransfusion hepatitis (PTH) was recognized to occur in more than 30% of multitransfused recipients.[2] Once the hepatitis B surface antigen (HBsAg) was identified, HBsAg testing demonstrated that hepatitis B virus (HBV) accounted for approximately 25% of the PTH cases.[2] These studies also noted that posttransfusion cases of both HBV and non-A, non-B (NANB) hepatitis occurred more frequently in recipients of blood from commercial (paid) blood donors than in recipients of blood from volunteer donors. By the mid-1970s, widespread implementation of sensitive HBsAg donor screening tests and nearly universal changeover to a volunteer donor supply resulted in a dramatic reduction in the posttransfusion incidence of both HBV and NANB hepatitis. Still, NANB PTH continued to occur in approximately 6% to 10% of multiple-transfusion recipients.[2,3]

In the absence of a specific test for the causative agent of NANB PTH, investigators searched for surrogate markers that could be used to identify donations associated with NANB hepatitis. The presence of antibody to

Susan A. Galel, MD, Associate Professor of Pathology, Stanford University School of Medicine, and Director of Clinical Operations, Stanford Blood Center, Palo Alto, California

The author has disclosed no conflicts of interest.

hepatitis B core antigen (anti-HBc) and/or the presence of elevated alanine aminotransfersase (ALT) in blood donors were shown to be associated with an increased risk of NANB PTH.[4-7] However, concerns about the nonspecific nature of these tests led to a delay in their implementation for donor screening.

The concept of using surrogate tests was revisited when concerns arose about the transmission of AIDS by transfusions, before the identification of its causative agent. Case reports from 1982 to 1984 suggested that the agent causing AIDS was most likely transmissible by transfusion, although the prevalence of infection among donors was initially thought to be low.[8] In an effort to reduce the potential transmission of AIDS by transfusion, some blood banks implemented donor testing for anti-HBc (as this antibody was noted to be highly prevalent in populations at increased risk of AIDS) or donor screening for inverted CD4/CD8 T-cell ratio (an immune abnormality found in both AIDS patients and those with the pre-AIDS lymphadenopathy syndrome).[9] After the human immunodeficiency virus (HIV) was isolated and identified as the causative agent of AIDS, a specific donor screening test for antibody to this agent was rapidly developed and implemented in 1985.

Once the HIV antibody test became available and cases of HIV were recognized both in prior donors and transfusion recipients, it became clear that the risk of transmitting HIV via blood transfusion had been underestimated.[10] Furthermore, the HIV experience highlighted the possibility that an infectious agent associated with a long asymptomatic carrier state could be present in the blood supply for years without being recognized. In the wake of this realization, the approach to donor screening was extended beyond screening for known agents. Current donor history evaluations and testing now include screening for, and exclusion of, donors with an increased risk of exposure to blood-borne or sexually transmitted diseases. The intention is to reduce the likelihood that the blood supply will contain other, as yet unidentified agents potentially transmissible by blood.

The initial donor screening tests for HIV had some deficiencies. There appeared to be a delay of weeks or months between the time a person was exposed to HIV and the time the donor screening test for antibody showed positive results.[11] Blood donated during this "window period" would contain HIV but would not be detected by the donor screening tests. One approach to protect the blood supply from window-period donations was to exclude potential donors who had an increased likelihood of exposure to HIV. Through interviews of individuals diagnosed with HIV, the US Centers for Disease Control and Prevention (CDC) identified behaviors that were associated with an increased risk of HIV infection. The FDA initially recommended that blood banks provide informational materials to donors, listing the HIV risk activities and requesting that individuals not donate if they had engaged in these activities. Later, in 1990, the FDA recommended direct questioning of each donor about each risk activity, as this was determined to be a more effective method of screening donors, and in 1992 the FDA issued a comprehensive guidance detailing this questioning.

In the years since the discovery of HIV, the risk of transfusion-transmitted disease has been progressively reduced through a variety of measures:

1. Use of donor education and screening questions to minimize window-period donations.
2. Use of questions and tests that exclude donors at increased risk of blood-borne or sexually transmitted infections.
3. Shortening of the window period for each agent by improving and/or adding tests to detect earlier stages of infection.
4. Use of donor questioning to screen for infections for which there is no available test.
5. Surveillance for transfusion-transmissible diseases and implementation of new donor screening tests, when available.

The current donor screening process for infectious diseases involves a combination of 1) donor education and self-deferral, 2) donor questioning, and 3) testing. The approach used to screen for a specific agent depends on whether risk factors are identifiable and whether donor screening tests are available. Table 8-1 lists the types of screening approaches used for different infectious agents.

DONOR SCREENING TESTS: GENERAL ASPECTS

The donor infectious disease tests required by the FDA are specified in Title 21, Section 610.40, of the *Code of Federal Regulations* (CFR).[1] The process of amending the CFR is slow; therefore, the FDA initially communicates changes in its recommendations by issuing guidance publications. Although FDA guidance documents do not constitute legal requirements, they effectively define the expected standard of practice in the United States. The AABB also issues recommendations to the blood banking community, and these are communicated either by inclusion in AABB standards for accreditation or through *Association Bulletins*. AABB recommendations do not have the force of law, with the exception that one US state (California) has incorporated some AABB standards as state law. AABB standards are often considered throughout the United States as defining a standard of practice in the blood banking community, and therefore these recommendations are widely implemented.

Since 1985, the FDA and AABB have issued a series of recommendations for additional screening tests in addition to the longstanding donor screens for syphilis and HBsAg. Table 8-2 summarizes the chronology of changes in donor infectious disease testing since 1985, and Table 8-3 lists the donor screening tests that are currently performed by US blood banks.

Logistics of Testing

With one exception, all infectious disease testing is performed on tubes that are collected at the time of donation and then sent to the donor testing laboratory. In contrast, the testing of platelets for bacterial contamination is performed on the platelet component itself, and is typically performed by the component manufacturing facility.

The laboratories that perform the FDA-mandated donor testing must be registered with the FDA as biologics manufacturers be-

TABLE 8-1. Approaches to Donor Screening

Approach	Situation for Use	Example(s)
Questioning only	Agents with defined risk and no sensitive and/or specific test	Malaria, prions
Testing only	Donor test is available, but no question can distinguish individuals at risk of infection	West Nile virus
Questioning and testing	Agents for which there are both identified risk factors and effective tests	Human immunodeficiency virus, hepatitis B and C viruses
Use of test-negative blood for specific recipients	Agents have high prevalence in donors, but an identifiable subset of recipients can benefit from test-negative blood	Cytomegalovirus
Testing of blood component itself	Agent not detectable in donor samples	Bacteria

TABLE 8-2. Changes in US Donor Testing for Infectious Diseases Since 1985

Year First Implemented	Screening Test	FDA Licensed at Time of Initial Implementation?	Comments
1985	Antibody to HIV ("anti-HTLV-III")	Yes	The initial name for HIV, the virus that causes AIDS, was HTLV-III. The first antibody test was called "anti-HTLV-III."
1986-1987	ALT and anti-HBc	No. Testing was recommended by AABB as surrogate screens for NANB hepatitis.	The AABB recommendation for donor ALT testing was dropped in 1995 after antibody testing for HCV was in place. Anti-HBc was licensed and required by the FDA in 1991.
1988	Anti-HTLV-I	Yes	HTLV-I is a retrovirus transmissible by transfusion. Although infection is usually asymptomatic, a small percentage of infected individuals develop leukemia, lymphoma, or a neurologic disease.
1990	Antibody to HCV, version 1 (anti-HCV 1.0)	Yes	HCV was identified as the cause of most cases of NANB hepatitis.
1991	Anti-HBc	Yes	Anti-HBc was previously recommended by AABB as a surrogate screen for NANB hepatitis and is now required by the FDA as an additional screen for HBV.
1992	Anti-HCV 2.0	Yes	This version is an improved test for antibody to HCV.
1992	Anti-HIV-1/2	Yes	New HIV antibody tests with improved detection of early infection and expanded range of detection to include HIV-2 in addition to HIV-1.
1996	HIV-1 p24 antigen test	Yes	This test was found to detect HIV-1 infection 6 days earlier than the antibody test.
1997-1998	Anti-HTLV-I/II	Yes	New HTLV antibody tests expanded detection to include HTLV-II in addition to HTLV-I.

1999	HIV-1 and HCV nucleic acid tests (detect HIV and HCV RNA)	Implemented initially as investigational assays; licensed by the FDA in 2002.	These were found to detect infection earlier than antibody or antigen assays. (Note: The FDA permitted discontinuation of HIV-1 p24 antigen testing with implementation of a licensed HIV-1 nucleic acid test.)
2003	West Nile virus nucleic acid test (detects WNV RNA)	Implemented initially as investigational assays; licensed by the FDA during 2005-2007.	Testing of individual donations (rather than minipools) is recommended at times of increased WNV activity in the region, according to the AABB in 2004 and the FDA in 2009.
2004	Sampling of platelet components to detect bacterial contamination	Some tests are approved by the FDA as quality control tests.	Testing was recommended by the AABB in 2004. As of 2011, the AABB accepts only FDA-approved tests or those of equivalent sensitivity.
2006-2007	Antibody to *Trypanosoma cruzi*	Yes	Widespread testing was implemented in 2007 after FDA licensure of a donor screening test. The rarity of seroconversion in US residents led many blood banks to switch to testing each donor only once. FDA guidance issued late in 2010 recommends one-time donor screening.
2007-2009	HBV nucleic acid test (detects HBV DNA)	Yes	Testing is not required by the FDA or recommended by the AABB as of December 2010. Some blood banks have implemented automated multiplex assays that screen for HIV RNA, HCV RNA, and HBV DNA simultaneously.

FDA = Food and Drug Administration; HIV = human immunodeficiency virus; HTLV = human T-cell lymphotropic virus; ALT = alanine aminotransferase; anti-HBc = antibody to hepatitis B core antigen; NANB = non-A, non-B (hepatitis); HCV = hepatitis C virus; HBV = hepatitis B virus; HIV-1/2 = test for HIV types 1 and 2.

TABLE 8-3. Donor Screening Tests Performed by US Blood Banks

Agent	Marker Detected	Test Method	Confirmatory or Supplemental Assays*
HBV	◆ Hepatitis B surface antigen	ChLIA or EIA	Neutralization (c)
	◆ IgM and IgG antibody to hepatitis B core antigen	ChLIA or EIA	
	◆ HBV DNA (optional)[†‡]	TMA or PCR	
HCV	◆ IgG antibody to HCV peptides	ChLIA or EIA	RIBA (c)
	◆ HCV RNA[†]	TMA or PCR	
HIV-1/2	◆ IgM and IgG antibody to HIV-1/2	ChLIA or EIA	HIV-1: IFA or Western blot (c) HIV-2: EIA (c)
	◆ HIV-1 RNA[†]	TMA or PCR	
HTLV-I/II	◆ IgG antibody to HTLV-I/II	ChLIA or EIA	IFA or line immunoblot
Syphilis	◆ IgG or IgG + IgM antibody to *Treponema pallidum* antigens OR ◆ Nontreponemal serologic test for syphilis (eg, rapid plasma reagin)	Microhemagglutination or EIA Solid-phase red cell adherence or particle agglutination	*T. pallidum* antigen-specific immunofluorescence or agglutination assays
WNV	◆ WNV RNA[†]	TMA or PCR	
Trypanosoma cruzi	◆ IgG antibody to *T. cruzi* (one time)[§]	ChLIA or EIA	RIPA

*Supplemental assays noted with "(c)" are FDA-required confirmatory assays. Other supplemental assays listed are not required but may be useful for donor counseling. HIV or HCV antibody confirmation may not be required if donor's RNA test result is positive (only some RNA tests are approved for this purpose).
[†]Screening for RNA or DNA is usually performed on minipools of 6 to 24 donor samples.
[‡]HBV DNA testing is not required as of December 2010.
[§]*T. cruzi* antibody testing may be limited to one-time testing of each donor.
HBV = hepatitis B virus; ChLIA = chemiluminescent immunoassay; EIA = enzyme immunoassay; Ig = immunoglobulin; TMA = transcription-mediated amplification; PCR = polymerase chain reaction; HCV = hepatitis C virus; RIBA = recombinant immunoblot assay; HIV-1/2 = test for HIV types 1 and 2; IFA = immunofluorescence assay; HTLV-I/II = human T-cell lymphotropic virus, types I and II; WNV = West Nile virus; RIPA = radioimmunoprecipitation assay; FDA = Food and Drug Administration.

cause this "qualification of raw materials" is considered part of the blood component manufacturing process. The infectious disease tests and the testing equipment used to screen donors must be specifically approved and licensed for this purpose by the FDA Center for Biologics Evaluation and Research (CBER). The tests must be performed exactly as specified in the manufacturers' package inserts. Tests and test platforms that are approved only for diagnostic use may *not* be used for donor screening.

Serologic Testing Process

Typically, the process for serologic testing (testing to detect antibody or antigen) involves performing each required screening test one time on each donor sample. Most of the screening tests are enzyme immunosorbent assays or chemiluminescent immunoassays. If the screening tests are nonreactive, the test result is considered "negative" (ie, there is no evidence of infection). If a test is reactive during the first round of testing ("initially reactive"), the package insert for the test typically requires that the test be repeated in duplicate. If both of the repeat results are nonreactive, the final interpretation is nonreactive or negative, and the unit may be used. If one or both of the repeat results is reactive, the donor sample is interpreted as "repeatedly reactive," and the corresponding blood unit is not permitted to be used for allogeneic transfusion. (It should be noted, however, that in the case of cellular therapy products, there are some circumstances in which repeatedly reactive donations may be used. See "Considerations in Testing HCT/P Donors," later in this chapter.)

A repeatedly reactive result does not necessarily indicate that the donor is infected. The infectious disease tests that are approved for donor screening have cutoff points chosen to make the test highly sensitive. They are designed to detect almost all infected individuals and minimize false-negative results. However, to achieve this sensitivity, the assays also react with samples from some individuals who are not infected (false-positive results). Because the blood donor population is preselected by questioning to be at low risk for infection, the vast majority of repeatedly reactive results in donors do not represent true infections. In order to determine whether a repeatedly reactive result represents a true infection rather than a false-positive result, additional, more specific testing may be performed on the donor sample.

For some agents, the FDA has licensed additional, more specific tests as "confirmatory" assays. FDA-licensed confirmatory assays are currently available only for HIV type 1 (HIV-1) antibody, hepatitis C virus (HCV) antibody, and HBsAg. FDA approval of a test as a confirmatory assay typically requires that repeatedly reactive specimens be evaluated by that test. If no licensed confirmatory assay is available, unlicensed supplemental tests or retesting of the donor sample on a second licensed screening test may be helpful for the purpose of donor counseling. Table 8-3 displays the available confirmatory and supplemental assays.

It is important to emphasize that a donation that is repeatedly reactive on a screening test is not permitted to be used for allogeneic transfusion, regardless of the results of confirmatory or supplemental testing. The syphilis screening assay [eg, rapid plasma reagin (RPR) test] represents the only situation in which negative supplemental test results can, in some circumstances, permit use of a reactive unit. This situation is discussed more fully in the syphilis section.

Nucleic Acid Testing

The process of screening donor samples for viral nucleic acid (RNA or DNA) is somewhat different than the serologic screening process. Nucleic acid testing (NAT) requires the extraction of nucleic acid from donor plasma, followed by use of a nucleic acid amplification test to amplify and detect viral genetic sequences. The test systems that were initially developed in 1999 to screen donors for HIV and HCV RNA were only semiautomated and had insufficient throughput to allow testing of each donor sample individually. It was believed that there would be little loss of sensitivity if donor plasma samples were tested in small pools ("minipools" or MP), because levels of HIV and HCV RNA are typically high in the blood of infected individuals, and NAT assays are exquisitely sensitive. Thus, in the initially approved NAT donor screening systems, minipools of 16 to 24 donor samples were tested together. If a pool tested negative, all donations contributing to that pool were considered negative for HIV and HCV RNA. If a pool showed reactivity on the viral nucleic acid test, further testing of smaller pools and ultimately individual samples was performed to determine which donation was responsible for the reactive test. Donations that were nonreactive on this additional testing could be released for transfusion. Donations reactive at the individual sample level were considered positive for viral nucleic acid and could not be released for transfusion.

In recent years, fully automated NAT systems have been developed. The two FDA-approved automated test platforms for donor screening use multiplex assays that detect HIV RNA, HCV RNA, and HBV DNA in one reaction chamber. These systems are approved for testing of individual donations and pools of 6 to 16 donor samples, depending on the platform. The availability of fully automated NAT platforms raises the possibility of moving to routine screening of individual donor samples [individual donation (ID) screening], rather than testing of pools (MP-NAT). However, it is not clear that ID-NAT screening of the entire US blood supply would be logistically feasible on the available platforms. Furthermore, it has been estimated that ID-NAT screening would minimally increase detection of infected donors, whereas the associated testing cost would be significantly increased.[12] An additional important concern is that donors would be deferred for false-positive results much more frequently with ID-NAT screening than pooled screening. In contrast to serologic testing policies, repeat testing is not permitted by the FDA for an individually reactive NAT sample to determine whether the initially reactive result represents a true-positive result. If an individual (unpooled) specimen is reactive on a NAT screen for HIV or HCV, the FDA requires that the corresponding blood component be discarded and the donor be deferred permanently.

In the case of NAT for West Nile virus (WNV) RNA, ID-NAT screening rather than MP-NAT screening is recommended when WNV activity is increased in a specific geographic area. Circulating levels of viral RNA are often low during WNV infection. When donor samples are combined into minipools, the RNA from a WNV-infected sample may become diluted below the detectable level. It has been estimated that MP-NAT screening for WNV RNA may fail to detect 20% to 30% of infected donations.[13,14] Therefore, both the FDA and AABB have recommended ID-NAT screening for WNV RNA at times of high WNV activity in a region.[15,16]

Implications of Reactive Test Results

A repeatedly reactive result on a donor screening test (or individually reactive NAT result) typically results in mandatory discard of the reactive donation. Most blood bank computer systems contain controls that prevent labeling and/or release of products from donations with reactive test results. A reactive test result may also indicate that the donor should be prohibited from making future donations, because many infections are persistent. Furthermore, past donations may also be considered suspect, because the exact date of onset of a donor's infection cannot be determined.

Both the FDA and AABB make recommendations as to whether reactive test results affect a donor's eligibility for future donations, whether components from prior donations should be retrieved (and how far back), and whether patients who previously received components from that donor should be notified. These recommendations are often guided by the results of supplemental or confirmatory testing performed on the donor sample. Many of these recommendations have evolved over time.

Because these recommendations are complex, blood bank laboratories typically create checklists that list each of the actions to be performed after a specific reactive test result is observed. Staff use these checklists to document completion of each action as they perform it.

Table 8-4 lists FDA regulations, FDA guidance documents, AABB standards, and AABB *Association Bulletins* that contain recommendations regarding management of donors with reactive test results, retrieval of other components, and notification of prior recipients. These recommendations are described briefly below.

Donor Eligibility

FDA regulation 21 CFR 610.41 addresses donors with reactive screening test results. FDA guidance documents and AABB *Association Bulletins* contain more detailed recommendations regarding additional testing, donor eligibility, and donor counseling for these and other tests. Donors should be notified of any test results that affect their eligibility or that are of importance to their health. Blood banks should have systems that prevent future collections from ineligible donors and that prevent release of any components inadvertently collected from such individuals.

For donors deferred for reactive screening tests, FDA regulation 21 CFR 610.41 provides for reinstatement by means of FDA-defined requalification algorithms. The FDA has issued guidance documents that define reentry pathways for donors deferred for reactivity on HIV, HCV, HBsAg, anti-HBc, and syphilis tests. Most of the pathways require that the donor have negative results on specified tests after a defined waiting period. Blood banks that desire to reenter donors must follow the FDA-defined algorithms explicitly. Table 8-4 indicates the FDA guidance documents that discuss reentry algorithms.

Retrieval of Prior Donations and Notification of Prior Recipients ("Look-Back")

The FDA and AABB offer guidance with regard to the appropriate management of previously collected blood components from donors whose current donation is repeatedly reactive (or, in the case of a NAT test, individually reactive) on an infectious disease screening test. These recommendations address the concern that at the time of the previous donation, the donor could have been in the window period of an early infection when the screening test results were negative.

In the case of HIV and HCV tests, the algorithms for managing prior donations and recipients of prior donations are spelled out in 21 CFR 610.46 and 21 CFR 610.47. For other agents, recommendations for the management of previously donated components may be found in the FDA guidance documents or AABB *Association Bulletins* (or both) listed in Table 8-4.

In most cases, the FDA and AABB recommend retrieval and quarantine of any remaining components from prior donations of that donor. It is essential that the retrieval of indated components be initiated immediately after the repeatedly reactive result is found, rather than waiting until confirmatory testing is completed. The FDA requires initiation of retrieval within 3 calendar days of a reactive HIV or HCV test, and within 1 week of reactive HBsAg, anti-HBc, or anti-HTLV screening tests. If confirmatory test results on the current donation are negative, the FDA, in some circumstances, permits rerelease of the prior donations. However, in many cases, some or all of the components from prior donations have been transfused. For some infectious agents, the FDA and AABB recommend that the recipients of prior donations from confirmed positive donors be notified of their possible exposure to the infectious agent.

Recommendations for notification of prior recipients (as part of "look-back") are now usually issued by the AABB or FDA, or both, at the time a new test is implemented, but these recommendations may evolve as confirmatory tests become available or as medical treatments are developed for the infection in question. Look-back (notification of prior recipients) is required by law only for HIV and HCV (21 CFR 610.46 and 21 CFR 610.47). In the case of an HIV look-back investigation involving a deceased prior recipient, the next of kin must be notified. The CFR spells out very specific

TABLE 8-4. FDA and AABB Recommendations for Donor Testing and Actions Following Reactive Results*

		Topics Discussed				
Document	**Agent/Test**	**Donor Testing**	**Donor Management**	**Product Retrieval**	**Recipient Notification**	**Donor Reentry**
21 CFR 610.40	HIV-1/2, HBV, HCV, HTLV-I/II, syphilis	X				
21 CFR 610.41	HIV-1/2, HBV, HCV, HTLV-I/II, syphilis		X			
21 CFR 610.46, 610.47, 610.48	HIV, HCV			X	X	
FDA Guidance, December 2010[17]	HCV			X	X	
FDA Guidance, December 2010[18]	*Trypanosoma cruzi*	X	X	X	X	
FDA Guidance, May 2010[19]	HIV, HCV	X	X	X	X	X
FDA Guidance, May 2010[20]	Anti-HBc					X
FDA Guidance, Nov 2009[16]	WNV	X	X	X		
FDA Guidance, Aug 2009[21]	HIV-1 group O	X	X			X
FDA Guidance, July 2009[22]	Parvovirus B19[†]					
FDA Guidance, June 2005[23]	WNV		X	X	X	
FDA Guidance, Oct 2004[24]	NAT for HIV-1 and HCV	X				
FDA Guidance, Aug 1997[25]	HTLV	X	X	X		

FDA Memorandum, July 1996[26]	HBsAg, anti-HBc[‡]			X		
FDA Memorandum, Dec 1991[27]	Syphilis	X	X	X[§]	X[§]	X
FDA Memorandum, Dec 1987[28]	HBsAg	X	X			X
AABB Standard 5.8.4[29]	Required donor tests for HIV, HCV, HBV, HTLV, WNV, syphilis	X				
AABB Standards 5.1.5.1, 5.1 5.1.1, 5.1.5.2, 7.1.3[29]	Bacteria	X		X[‖]		
Association Bulletin #10-05[30]	Bacteria	X		X[‖]		
Association Bulletin #08-03[15]	WNV	X				
Association Bulletin #06-08[31]	*Trypanosoma cruzi*		X	X	X	
Association Bulletin #05-02[32]	Bacteria		X			X
Association Bulletin #04-07[33]	Bacteria	X		X	X	
Association Bulletin #99-9[34]	HTLV	X	X			

*Recommendations in effect as of December 2010. Blood centers may be bound by additional requirements—for example, specifications in Recovered Plasma contracts.

[†]Plasma for further manufacture only.

[‡]Memorandum also includes recommendations regarding HCV and HTLV, but these have been superseded by subsequent documents.

[§]Not recommended.

[‖]Cocomponents of current donation.

FDA = Food and Drug Administration; CFR = *Code of Federal Regulations*; 21 CFR 610.40 = Title 21, CFR Part 610.40; HIV-1/2 = test for human immunodeficiency virus, types 1 and 2; HBV = hepatitis B virus; HCV = hepatitis C virus; HTLV-I/II = human T-cell lymphotropic virus, types I and II; anti-HBc = antibody to hepatitis B core antigen; WNV = West Nile virus; NAT = nucleic acid testing; HBsAg = hepatitis B surface antigen.

timelines for component retrieval and recipient notification. It also specifies how far back in time (ie, to which donations) the retrieval and notification should extend. For other agents, such as WNV and *Trypanosoma cruzi*, recommendations regarding retrieval and recipient notification have been included in FDA guidance documents and AABB *Association Bulletins*. Table 8-4 indicates which of these address product retrieval or recipient notification.

In the absence of published guidance, it is not always obvious whether or when it is appropriate to notify prior recipients of their possible exposure to infection. If there is no confirmatory assay available, it may be difficult to determine whether a repeatedly reactive screening test result in a donor represents a true infection. Furthermore, if there is no effective treatment for the particular infection, there may be no obvious benefit to the recipient of being told that he or she might have been exposed. There could, however, be a public health benefit from such a notification. Specifically, a recipient who was alerted of potential exposure could be tested and, if results are positive, could take precautions to avoid further spread of the infection.

Testing of Products for Selected Recipient Populations: Immunocompromised Recipients

Some common infections cause relatively innocuous illnesses in immunocompetent individuals but can cause severe disease in immunocompromised patients. Such is the case with cytomegalovirus (CMV).

CMV is a lipid-enveloped DNA virus in the *Herpesvirus* family. Like other herpesviruses, CMV causes lifelong infection, typically in latent state, with the potential for reactivation. The majority of adult blood donors have CMV antibodies, indicating previous exposure and latent infection. Primary CMV infection in immunologically competent individuals is mild, with symptoms ranging from none to an infectious mononucleosis-type syndrome. In immunosuppressed or immunodeficient patients, however, both primary infection and reactivation disease can be overwhelming and even fatal. CMV can be transmitted by blood transfusion, primarily through intact white cells contained in cellular blood components. Frozen/thawed plasma components do not appear to transmit infection. Immunocompromised patients who are at increased risk of transfusion-transmitted disease include fetuses, low-birthweight premature infants who are born to CMV-seronegative mothers, and CMV-seronegative recipients of solid organ or allogeneic hematopoietic cell transplants from seronegative donors.[35]

Because the majority of blood donors have had prior exposure to CMV, it would not be possible to produce an adequate supply of blood if all CMV-antibody-positive donations were discarded. It is possible, however, to minimize CMV transmission to patients at risk of severe CMV disease, such as those described above. These patients should be supported with cellular blood components that have a reduced risk of transmitting CMV. Reduced-risk options include blood components obtained from donors who are CMV antibody negative, or components that have been effectively leukocyte reduced. The literature suggests that these two methods are similar in efficacy but not identical, with an estimated transmission risk by seronegative components of 1% to 2%, vs a transmission risk of 2% to 3% with leukocyte-reduced components.[35-37] Given that many of these at-risk patients are monitored closely for CMV infection, treated early with anti-CMV drugs, or both, it is not clear that there is a measurable clinical benefit to using CMV-seronegative, as compared to leukocyte-reduced, blood components.

Autologous Donations

The FDA requires infectious disease testing of autologous donations that are shipped from one facility to another. If the receiving facility does not permit autologous donations to be crossed over to the general inventory, the FDA requires testing of only the first donation in each 30-day period [21 CFR 610.40(d)]. The labeling of the unit must be consistent with its testing status. Units from donors with repeatedly reactive tests must be labeled with biohazard labels. Some hospitals have policies that prohibit acceptance of autologous units with positive results on some tests because there is a potential for an infectious unit to be transfused to the wrong patient. The AABB has warned that refusal of test-positive units could be interpreted to violate the Americans with Disabilities Act.[38]

Considerations in Testing HCT/P Donors

The FDA rules for screening donors of human cells, tissues, and cellular and tissue-based products (HCT/Ps) are different from those for screening blood donors. Both the questions and tests required for HCT/P donors differ from those for blood donor screening, and screening requirements may vary with the type of tissue. Blood bank laboratories that perform testing on samples from HCT/P donors must take care to check package inserts for HCT/P testing methods; a package insert may require a different testing method for HCT/P donors than for blood donors. For example, NAT for most types of HCT/P donors must be performed on individual donor samples; MP-NAT is not permitted for most HCT/P donor categories.

In some cases, FDA regulations permit the use of HCT/P donations that are reactive on infectious disease screening tests. These exceptions are listed in 21 CFR 1271.65; specific labeling, storage, and notification requirements apply to these tissues.

International Variation in Donor Testing

Although this chapter focuses on infectious disease screening in the United States, the general approach to donor screening is similar in other countries. However, the specific donor questions and tests vary from country to country, according to the regional epidemiology of infections and the tests available in each country. For example, most countries where WNV is not endemic do not test for this agent, although they may question donors about travel to the United States or Canada during WNV season. Countries where HBV is hyperendemic cannot exclude donations from individuals who test positive for anti-HBc. The AABB Standards Program Units, in conjunction with a subcommittee for the Evaluation of International Variances, consider variance applications from facilities in countries where national practices and available tests differ from those in the United States.

RESIDUAL INFECTIOUS RISKS OF TRANSFUSION

Despite donor screening, blood components may still transmit infections. The residual risk of transmission varies according to the incidence of the infection in the donor population and the nature of the donor screening processes that are in place.

Agents for Which Blood Is Tested

Transfusion-transmission of HIV, HCV, and HBV is now so rare that the rate of transmission cannot be measured by prospective clinical studies. The risk can only be estimated by theoretical modeling.

One theoretical source of risk is a virus strain that the current test kits do not detect. The CDC maintains surveillance for such emerging strains, and over time the FDA has required that test manufacturers expand detection capabilities to include new strains. A second potential cause of transmission is a quarantine failure (ie, a blood bank's failure to quarantine a unit that tests positive). Quarantine errors are thought to occur rarely in blood banks that use electronic systems to control blood component labeling and release, as these systems are designed to prevent release of any unit with incomplete testing or a positive test result. In contrast, erroneous releases appear to occur more frequently in blood banks that rely on manual records and quarantine processes.[39]

The primary cause of residual transmissions, however, is thought to be related to donations made by individuals in the window period of early infection, before test results are positive.

Figure 8-1 displays the sequence in which different types of donor screening tests demonstrate reactivity. Over time, the window periods have been shortened by implementation of donor screening tests that detect earlier infection. However, because there is no test that will give a positive result instantly after an individual acquires an infection, the window period remains. With NAT, the average duration of the window period for HIV and HCV infections is estimated to be 9.0 and 7.4 days, respectively.[12] The window period for HBV is longer, as discussed in the HBV section below.

The likelihood that a blood donation has been obtained from a donor in the window period can be estimated mathematically using a simple formula[40]:

Probability a donation was made during the window period =
Length of window period × Incidence of infections in the donor population

The incidence of infections in donors is an important element in the risk calculation. This can be measured by two different approaches. First, it can be calculated from the observed number of donors who test negative on one donation but positive on a subsequent donation (ie, seroconverting donors). This method measures incidence rates in only repeat donors and does not permit assessment of the likelihood that first-time donors might be in the window period. Second, there are alternative methods that permit measurement of new infection rates in both first-time and repeat donors. These methods use tests that differentiate new infections from established infection. Such tests include nucleic acid tests (ie, donors who have HIV or HCV RNA but not antibody most likely have very early infection) and "sensitive/less sensitive" antibody testing.[12,40-43] Using these alternative methods, it has been found that new HIV and HCV infections are two to four times more common among first-time donors compared to repeat

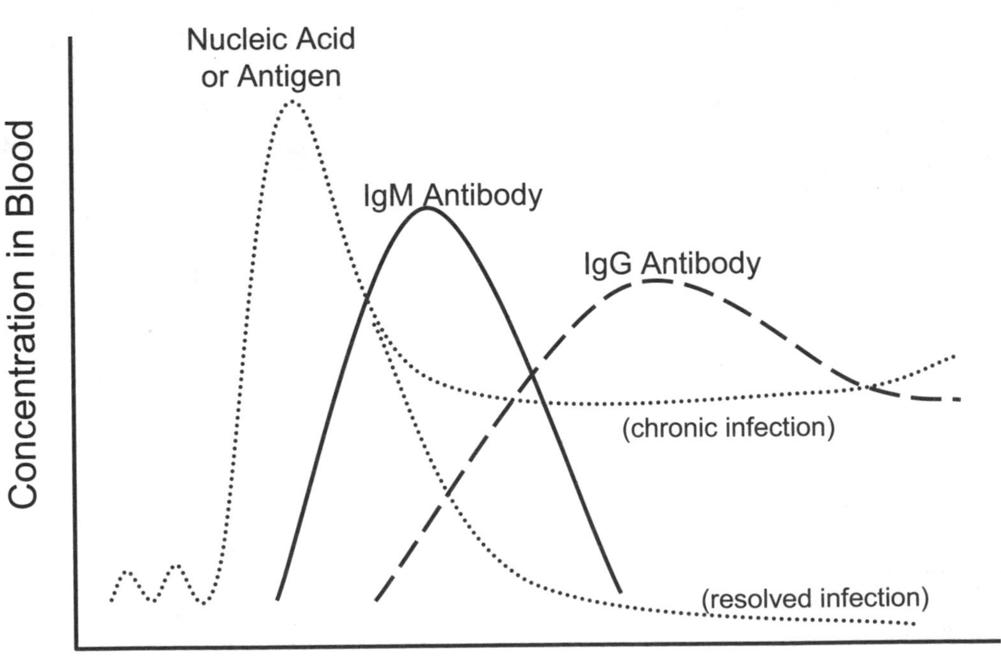

FIGURE 8-1. Time sequence of the appearance of various markers of infection.

donors.[40-42] However, both of these donor populations have significantly lower infection rates than the general population. The continued importance of using donor questioning to select a donor population that has a low incidence of infection is explored in more detail in the HIV section below.

The current estimated risks of HIV, HCV, and HBV transmission, based on window-period and incidence calculations, are shown in Table 8-5.[40,44]

Agents for Which There Are No Donor Screening Tests

Essentially any infectious agent that could circulate in the blood of an apparently healthy person could be transmitted by transfusion. It is impossible to estimate the risk of transmission for each of the infinite number of infectious agents for which donors are not tested. However, transfusion-transmitted infections are rarely identified. Infections most likely to be recognized as transfusion-transmitted would be those that have a distinctive clinical presentation and are otherwise rare in the United States. Recognition of an infection as transfusion transmitted is enhanced if the infection is usually associated with a behavioral risk that the transfusion recipient lacks (eg, when malaria develops in a transfusion recipient who has not traveled outside of the United States). Many transfusion-transmitted infections may go unrecognized.

If a life-threatening agent is recognized as a potential threat to the blood supply, both the AABB and FDA typically consider whether a donor screening question could be used to exclude potentially exposed donors in the absence of a donor screening test. Donor questioning regarding travel to and residence in endemic areas is currently the only means of protecting the US blood supply from malaria and variant Creutzfeldt-Jakob disease (vCJD). Most agents, however, do not have such clear geographic risk areas. In general, it is difficult to design donor questions that are both sensitive (ie, would detect most infected individuals) and specific (ie, would exclude only infected individuals).

An alternative method of protecting the blood supply from infectious agents is pathogen inactivation or pathogen reduction. This refers to processes that inactivate or remove residual pathogens from blood components. Indeed, heat inactivation, solvent/detergent treatment, nanofiltration, chromatography, cold ethanol fractionation, and others are used to inactivate or remove residual pathogens in plasma derivatives. Pathogen reduction systems are not yet available for transfusable US blood components but are in use in some other countries for platelets, plasma, or both.

TABLE 8-5. Estimated Risks of Transfusion-Transmitted Infection Based on Window-Period and Incidence Estimates, 2007-2008*

Agent	Window Period (days)†	Incidence of New Infections in Repeat Donors (per 100,000 person years)	Estimated Risk per Unit Transfused
Human immunodeficiency virus	9.0	2.16	1:1,467,000
Hepatitis C virus	7.4	2.98	1:1,149,000
Hepatitis B virus	38	2.49	1:280,000

*Estimates for HIV and HCV risk are based on figures from Zou et al.[40] The estimated risk calculations include an adjustment for the proportion of units obtained from first-time donors, whose incidence of infection is two to four times higher than that of repeat donors. The estimate for HBV risk is based on the analysis by Zou et al.[44]

†Window-period estimates assume minipool nucleic acid testing for HIV and HCV and no HBV DNA testing.

These systems are discussed later in this chapter.

The AABB Transfusion Transmitted Disease Committee recently compiled an extensive review of 68 infectious agents that have been evaluated as possible threats to the blood supply.[45] Potential mitigation strategies are discussed for each agent, including the documented or theoretical efficacy of pathogen reduction processes. The agents deemed to pose the highest threats, from either a scientific or public perspective, will be briefly discussed in this chapter. (See the full supplement to *TRANSFUSION*[45] and updates on the AABB website for a more thorough review of these potential infectious risks.)

SCREENING FOR SPECIFIC AGENTS

Human Immunodeficiency Virus

HIV-1, a lipid-enveloped, single-stranded RNA virus, was identified in 1984 as the causative agent of AIDS, and blood donor screening for antibodies to this virus was implemented in the United States in 1985. In 1992, donor screening tests were modified to include detection of antibodies to HIV-2, a closely related virus identified initially in West Africa.

HIV can be transmitted sexually, parenterally, and perinatally from infected mothers to their infants. Although heterosexual and vertical spread of HIV predominate in some parts of the world, new HIV cases in the United States continue to be largely concentrated in males who have sex with other males (MSM) and individuals with high-risk heterosexual contact (defined as contact with an individual who is HIV positive or who is in an identified risk group for HIV such as MSM or injection drug users).[46]

Current donor screening for HIV includes NAT testing for HIV-1 RNA and serologic testing for antibodies to HIV. The antibody tests approved for donor screening detect both IgM and IgG antibody to both HIV-1 and HIV-2. Some of the approved tests also detect antibody to the HIV-1 group O strain, a strain of HIV-1 found primarily in central and West Africa.[21] If the antibody test used by a donor center does not have an HIV-1 group O detection claim, the donor center must use donor questioning to exclude individuals who have resided in, received medical treatment in, or had sex partners from HIV-1 group O endemic areas.[21]

The average lag from HIV-1 exposure to test detection (window period) is currently estimated to be 9 days for MP-NAT.[12] Based on window period and incidence rate calculations, the current risk of acquiring HIV from transfusion is estimated to be approximately 1 in 1.5 million units (Table 8-5).

In the United States, blood donor screening questions exclude very broadly defined populations at increased risk of HIV. Given the short delay of only days between exposure and detection of infection by NAT, it has been questioned whether donor interviews and exclusion of donors with increased risk remain medically necessary.[47] The continued importance of a low-risk donor population becomes evident if different HIV incidence figures are entered into the blood safety calculation. For example, HIV incidence rates as high as 1% to 8% have been observed in some high-risk populations, such as young urban MSM.[48,49] If an individual from a population with a 1% incidence of HIV were to donate blood, the likelihood that this individual would be in the window period and the component would transmit HIV can be calculated as follows:

Risk that the donation is in window period =
Length of window period ×
Incidence of infection in donor population =
(9.0 days/365 days/year) ×
(1/100 person-years) = 1/4100.

This is the likelihood that a unit from this high-risk donor would harbor HIV but be missed by the current donor screening. This risk is clearly much higher than the estimated HIV transmission risk of 1 in 1.5 million for a unit of blood obtained from the current donor population. Thus, despite the short window period with current testing, inclusion of donors with a high risk of acquiring HIV would have a profoundly adverse impact on blood safety. Accordingly, questioning of donors for risk and temporarily excluding those at increased risk to minimize window-period donations continue to be critical for preserving blood safety.

Despite the efficacy of current donor questioning approaches, there has been great interest in developing a more specific donor screening algorithm for MSM that would exclude only those individuals who are truly at increased risk of HIV. Although more specific donor screening criteria for MSM are desirable, the FDA states that no algorithm has yet been demonstrated that reliably identifies MSM whose HIV risk is as low as that of current blood donors.[50]

A frequently asked question is, What is FDA's rationale for *permanently* excluding MSM from donation? Most other high-risk populations are excluded only temporarily (for 1 year after the risk activity). The FDA's rationale for excluding MSM beyond 1 year appears to be based on two concerns. One is "quarantine release errors," that is, the risk that a blood center would inadvertently release a test-positive unit. However, based on current electronic controls used by most US blood centers, these release errors appear to be extremely rare. Mathematical modeling suggests that the deferral period for MSM could be shortened without a substantial increase in risk to recipients.[39] The other concern that has been raised is that there are other potentially transfusion-transmissible infections that are more prevalent in MSM populations (such as human herpesvirus 8, the causative agent of Kaposi sarcoma), and donors are not tested for all of these infections.[47] A US Department of Health and Human Services advisory committee recently concluded that "currently available scientific data are inadequate to support change to a specific alternative policy."[51]

Hepatitis B Virus

HBV is a lipid-enveloped, double-stranded DNA virus. Like HIV, HBV is transmitted parenterally, sexually, and perinatally. Jaundice is noted in only 25% to 40% of adult cases and in a smaller proportion of childhood cases. A large percentage of perinatally acquired cases result in chronic infection, but most HBV infections acquired in adulthood are cleared. HBV is highly prevalent in certain parts of the world such as the Far East and Africa, where perinatal transmission and resultant chronic infection have perpetuated infection in the population. In the United States, the incidence of acute HBV infection has decreased in association with implementation of childhood vaccination programs. Perinatal screening and newborn treatment have also been effective in reducing perinatal transmission.

During HBV infection, viral envelope material (HBsAg) is typically detectable in circulating blood, with plasma levels of incomplete virions (spheres and tubules) greatly exceeding those of intact virus. This overproduced envelope material can be detected by HBsAg serologic tests. Antibody to the core antigen is produced soon after appearance of HBsAg, initially in the form of IgM antibody, then IgG. As infected individuals produce antibody to the surface antigen (anti-HBsAg), the HBsAg is cleared.

The FDA requires donor screening for HBsAg and for anti-HBc (IgM and IgG antibody). Published estimates of the residual risk of HBV transmission based on the window-period/incidence modeling have varied from approximately 1/220,000[42,43] to 1/357,000 units.[44] It has been difficult to apply the window-period/incidence model to estimate HBV risk because neither the window-period duration nor the incidence of donor HBV infection is precisely known. The incidence of donor HBV infections has been estimated by using observed rates of HBsAg in donors and adjusting this figure for the transience of HBsAg detectability and for the proportion of donor HBsAg results that are thought to represent false-positive results rather than true infections.[42,44] The duration of the infectious window period before HBsAg detectability is also not absolutely known. Published estimates have varied because of differences in the sensitivity of various HBsAg assays and differing assumptions regarding the level of viremia in the donor required for infectivity.[52] The duration of the infectious window period before HBsAg detectability by the Abbott PRISM (Abbott Laboratories, Abbott Park, IL) has recently been estimated at 30 to 38 days.[52] Using this as the window-period estimate along with mathematically adjusted HBsAg incidence figures, a recent publication estimated US HBV transfusion-transmission risk to be between 1/280,000 and 1/357,000 units.[44]

It is not clear to what degree donor screening for HBV DNA would reduce the risk of HBV transmission. During the infectious window period before HBsAg detection, HBV DNA levels may be below the limits of detection of MP-NAT assays.[52] Later in infection, following the clearance of HBsAg, HBV NAT may detect persistent infection,[53] but donations from individuals with persistent infection are already interdicted in the United States by the donor screening test for anti-HBc. Although HBV NAT assays for donor screening are currently available in the United States, they are not yet required. One surprising finding in US clinical studies of HBV NAT has been the detection through MP-NAT of acute HBV infections in donors who were previously vaccinated.[54,55] These donations were HBsAg negative but DNA positive. The infectivity of such donations is not known, as these units contain vaccine-induced antibodies to HBsAg in addition to HBV. If these units are infectious, the US risk of transfusion-transmitted HBV would be higher than previously estimated, as HBsAg-negative, vaccine-breakthrough infections were not included in the risk estimate model. Routine HBV DNA screening of US blood donations would detect at least some of these infections.

Hepatitis C Virus

HCV is a lipid-enveloped, single-stranded RNA virus. HCV was shown to have been the cause of up to 90% of cases previously called NANB transfusion-related hepatitis.[56] The majority of HCV infections are asymptomatic. However, HCV infection is associated with a high risk of chronicity, which can result in liver cirrhosis and hepatocellular carcinoma. HCV is thought to be transmitted primarily through blood exposure. In the United States, about 50% of HCV infections are associated with injection drug use, but the risk factors for the remainder of the infections are not clear.[57] Sexual and vertical transmission are uncommon, although coinfection with HIV may increase transmission by these routes.

Current donor screening for HCV includes NAT testing for HCV RNA and serologic testing for antibodies to HCV. The average window period between exposure and detection of infection by MP-NAT is estimated to be 7.4 days.[12] The serologic test detects only IgG antibody, a relatively late marker of infection, and therefore there may be a significant lag (1.5 to 2 months) between detection of RNA and detection of antibody.[58] Donor questioning has limited potential to exclude individuals who may be harboring HCV infection because a large proportion of infected individuals are asymptomatic and have no identifiable risk. Despite this limitation, the current estimated US risk of HCV transmission by transfusion is extremely low—approximately 1 in 1.1 million (Table 8-5).

Human T-Cell Lymphotropic Virus, Types I and II

HTLV-I is a lipid-enveloped RNA virus. It was the first human retrovirus identified, isolated in 1978 from a patient with cutaneous T-cell lymphoma. A closely related virus, HTLV-II, was later isolated from a patient with hairy cell leukemia. Both viruses infect lymphocytes and cause lifelong infections, but most of these infections are asymptomatic. Approximately 2% to 5% of HTLV-I-infected individuals develop adult T-cell leukemia/lymphoma, after a lag of 20 to 30 years. A smaller percentage develop a neurologic disease called HTLV-associated myelopathy (HAM) or tropical spastic paraparesis (TSP). HTLV-II disease associations remain unclear. Both infections are thought to be spread through blood, sexual contact, and breastfeeding. HTLV-I infection is endemic in certain parts of the world, including regions of Japan, South America, the Caribbean, and Africa. In the United States, infections are found in immigrants from endemic areas, injection drug users, and the sexual partners of these individuals. Approximately one-half of the HTLV infections in US blood donors are HTLV-II.[59,60]

The only FDA-approved donor tests for HTLV infection are screening assays for IgG antibody to HTLV-I and HTLV-II. Units reactive on the screening assay cannot be released for transfusion. Because there is no FDA-approved confirmatory assay and the majority of reactive donor samples are thought to represent false-positive results, the FDA does not require permanent deferral of donors after one reactive donation. Donors are permanently excluded only if the donor reacts again on a subsequent donation (21 CFR 610.41). Unlicensed supplemental tests such as immunoblots or immunofluorescence assays may be very helpful in counseling donors about the likelihood that the screening test reactivity represents a true infection. Some of these supplemental assays can also differentiate between HTLV-I and HTLV-II infection.[59,60] Rather than use unlicensed supplemental tests, some blood centers retest reactive samples on a different FDA-licensed donor screening assay; samples nonreactive on the alternative screening assay most likely represent false-positive results. Donors whose samples are reactive on the second screen, however, must be counseled and deferred.[25]

Risk estimates for transfusion-transmitted HTLV are somewhat uncertain, given the absence of well-defined window periods for the current HTLV antibody tests and absence of confirmatory assays to definitively measure true case rates in donors.[42] Like CMV, HTLV is thought to be transmitted only by white-cell-containing blood components and not by frozen/thawed plasma components.[59,60]

Syphilis

Syphilis is caused by the spirochete bacterium *Treponema pallidum*. Donor screening for syphilis has been performed for more than 60 years. Donors were initially screened by nontreponemal serologic tests that detect antibody to cardiolipin (eg, RPR). In recent years, however, most blood banks have converted to tests that detect specific antibodies to *T. pallidum*, as these tests can be performed on automated testing instruments.

The vast majority of reactive donor test results do not represent active cases of syphilis. Most reflect either biologic false-positive results or persistent antibody in previously treated individuals (the latter are detected by the treponemal-specific antibody screening tests). The FDA has permitted use of additional, treponemal-specific, confirmatory assays (eg, fluorescent treponemal antibody absorption test, or FTA-ABS) to guide management of both donors and components. Specifically, the FDA has permitted release of units from donors who have reactive screening test results and negative confirmatory results if the units are labeled with both test results.[1,27] If, however, the result of the treponemal-specific confirmatory test is positive, or if no additional testing is performed, the donor must be deferred for at least 12 months.

The current value of donor screening for syphilis is controversial,[61-63] and the FDA has considered eliminating this requirement. Although numerous cases of transfusion-transmitted syphilis were reported before World War II, no cases have been reported in the US for more than 40 years. The low transmission risk is probably related to a declining incidence of syphilis in donors as well as the limited survival of the *T. pallidum* spirochete during blood storage. One issue that has been considered is whether the syphilis screen improves blood safety by serving as a surrogate marker of high-risk sexual activity. However, studies have demonstrated that donor screening for syphilis does not provide incremental value for detection of other blood-borne and sexually transmitted infections such as HIV, HBV, HCV, or HTLV.[63]

Other Bacteria

Bacterial contamination of blood components (mainly platelets) is a major cause of transfusion-related fatalities, following only transfusion-related acute lung injury and hemolytic reactions in frequency.[64] Bacteria are reportedly present in approximately 1 in 3000 cellular blood components.[65] The source of the bacteria can be either the donor's skin or asymptomatic bacteremia in the donor. The level of bacteria in components just after collection is generally too low to detect or to cause symptoms in the recipient. However, bacteria can multiply during component storage, particularly in platelet components, which are kept at room temperature. Bacteria proliferate to a lesser extent in refrigerated Red Blood Cells, and septic reactions occur much less commonly with these components. In order to reduce the risk of septic transfusion reactions associated with platelets, the AABB in 2004 implemented a requirement for processes to limit and detect bacterial contamination in all platelet components. (Subsequently, the requirement was modified to "limit and detect or inactivate.")

To limit blood component contamination by bacteria from donor skin, two elements of the blood collection process are critical. Before venipuncture, the donor skin must be carefully disinfected using a method with demonstrated efficacy. Most of these methods involve two-stage processes using iodophors, chlorhexidine, or alcohol.[66] Second, diversion of the first 10 to 40 mL of donor blood away from the collection container (eg, into a sample pouch) further reduces the likelihood that skin contaminants will enter the component.[66,67] The AABB has required since 2008 that collection sets with diversion pouches be used for all platelet collections, including whole blood collections from which platelets are made.[29(p21)]

A variety of technologies are available for detection of bacteria in platelet components. None of these methods is sensitive enough to detect bacteria just after collection. All methods require a waiting time for bacteria contaminants to multiply before the component is sampled. The process most commonly used in the United States to screen apheresis platelets is the BacT/ALERT culture system manufactured by bioMérieux (Marcy L'Etoile, France). This system, approved by the FDA as a quality control test, requires that platelet components be stored for 24 hours before sampling. After that time, 4 to 8 mL of the platelet component are withdrawn and inoculated into either one aerobic culture bottle or both aerobic and anaerobic bottles. The bottles are then incubated in the BacT/ALERT culture system. If the culture remains negative after the first 12 to 24 hours of culture, the component is released for transfusion, but the culture is continued for the shelf life of the unit. If the culture tests positive after the component is released, the blood center should attempt to retrieve it. If the component has not been transfused, resampling of the product for culture is very informative, as approximately two-thirds of the initially positive signals are determined to be caused by either contamination of the bottle (and not the component) or false signals from the BacT/ALERT system.[66,67] All positive cultures should be sent for identification of the organism. If a true-positive result is related to an organism that is not a skin contaminant, the donor should be notified and advised to seek medical consultation.[32]

Other methods approved in the United States for platelet quality control testing early in the storage period include the Pall eBDS system (Pall Corp., Port Washington, NY), a culture-based system, and ScanSystem, manufactured by Hemosystem (Marseille, France), which uses optical scanning to detect bacteria. All of these methods are approved for testing of leukocyte-reduced apheresis platelets, and some are approved for testing of pools of leukocyte-reduced whole-blood-derived platelets. None of these methods is practical for routine screening of individual whole-blood-derived platelet concentrates.

Since the implementation of routine bacterial screening of apheresis platelets, the frequency of FDA-reported fatalities from contaminated apheresis platelets has declined.[64] However, some contaminated apheresis platelets escape detection by this early testing, presumably because bacterial concentrations are below limits of detection at the time of sampling; thus, septic, and even fatal, reactions do still occur.

Other tests can be applied to platelet components just before issue. One, the Platelet PGD test manufactured by Verax Biomedical (Worcester, MA), is a rapid strip immunoassay for bacterial antigens. It has been approved by the FDA both as an adjunct (time-of-issue) screen for apheresis platelets previously screened by another method and as the sole bacteria test to screen pools of whole-blood-derived platelet concentrates that are pooled just before issue. Low-technology methods for screening platelets just before issue—such as visually inspecting the platelets for swirling, or testing them for low glucose or pH—have been used by some facilities, but these have been demonstrated to be of little clinical utility, lacking both sensitivity and specificity.[66] The use of these latter methods has ceased to fulfill the AABB standard for bacteria detection.[29(p11),30]

All of the above methods are cumbersome and provide incomplete assurance of bacteria detection. None of these methods is practical for screening of the red cell inventory. Pathogen-reduction methods, which impair proliferation of bacteria in the blood component, are theoretically an alternative approach that could be used to reduce the risk of septic reactions from bacteria in blood components. Indeed, in some regions outside of the United States, pathogen reduction has replaced bacteria detection testing for platelets, but these technologies have not been approved for use in the United States.

Infections Transmitted by Insect Vectors

Until recently, malaria was the only vector-transmitted disease that was widely recognized as having the potential for secondary transmission by transfusion. Malaria is rare in the United States, and the blood supply has been effectively protected by questions that exclude donors who recently traveled to or resided in malaria-endemic regions. In the past decade, however, other vector-transmitted infections have been recognized as threats to the US blood supply, and these are the infections targeted by the newest blood donor screening assays.

West Nile Virus

WNV is a lipid-enveloped RNA virus in the *Flaviviridae* family. First detected in the United States in 1999, it subsequently spread through North America, appearing as annual epidemics during the summer and autumn. Birds are thought to be the primary reservoir for WNV, with infection spreading to humans through the bite of a mosquito. Approximately 80% of human cases are asymptomatic, 20% are associated with a self-limited febrile illness, and fewer than 1% are associated with severe neuroinvasive disease such as meningoencephalitis.

Transfusion transmission of WNV was first recognized in 2002 and traced to blood donations containing viral RNA but not antibody. Thus NAT, rather than serologic testing, was required to protect the blood supply. Donor screening was widely implemented in 2003 using investigational NAT assays. Donor tests for WNV RNA are now FDA approved and required by both the FDA and AABB.[16,29(p30)] The predominant method of testing is in minipools. However, as discussed in the NAT section above, circulating levels of viral RNA are frequently low during WNV infection, and a donor sample containing a low concentration of RNA may escape detection if mixed with other donor samples for MP-NAT testing. Therefore, both the AABB and FDA have recommended that donor screening for WNV RNA be performed on individual donor samples, rather than pooled donor samples, when WNV activity is high in a particular collection region.[15,16] Regional WNV activity can be monitored through active communications between neighboring blood collection agencies with regard to viremic donors detected, as well as by monitoring public health reports of clinical WNV cases in the area. The two most recently documented cases of WNV transmission by transfusion were traced to donations screened by MP-NAT during periods when neighboring blood collection facilities were screening donors by ID-NAT.[68] It is possible that some WNV transmissions have escaped recognition because most WNV infections lack distinctive symptoms.

Trypanosoma cruzi

T. cruzi, the protozoan parasite that causes Chagas disease, is endemic in portions of Mexico, Central America, and South America. It is transmitted to humans by an insect vector, the reduviid bug. Acute infection is usually self-limited but may be severe in immunocompromised patients. Most infections become chronic but asymptomatic. Decades after the initial infection, 10% to 40% of infected individuals develop late-stage manifestations, including intestinal dysfunction or cardiac disease, which can be fatal. Transfusion transmission of *T. cruzi* from the blood of chronically infected, asymptomatic donors has been reported in endemic areas.

A blood donor screening enzyme immunoassay for antibodies to *T. cruzi* was approved by the FDA for US use in December 2006. Although not initially required by the FDA, the test was widely implemented by US blood centers during 2007. There is no FDA-licensed confirmatory assay, but supplemental testing of reactive specimens by radioimmunoprecipitation assay (RIPA) is very helpful for guiding donor counseling. Based on the results of this latter assay, only about 25% of the reactive US donors appear to be truly infected.[31,69,70] All donors reactive on the screening assay, however, should be permanently deferred, regardless of the results of the supplemental testing.[18,31]

The vast majority of US blood donors who are positive by RIPA were born in *T. cruzi*-endemic areas. Other RIPA-positive donors appear to represent congenitally acquired infections (ie, the donor's mother is from a *T. cruzi*-endemic area), and only a small number of donor infections appear to have been acquired from vector exposure within the United States (true autochthonous cases). In the first 2 years of US donor screening, no donor seroconversions were seen, raising the possibility that testing donors only once, on their first donation, could be sufficient to protect the US blood supply.[31,69,70] In December 2010, the FDA issued guidance recommending one-time screening of every donor.[18]

While the epidemiology of *T. cruzi* infections in donors was being characterized during the first few years of testing, the risk of *T. cruzi* transmission by transfusion in the United States was also evaluated. Before implementation of donor screening, seven cases of transfusion-transmitted *T. cruzi* had been identified in the United States and Canada; all that had available data were linked to platelet transfusion. Since implementation of donor screening, RIPA-positive donors have been identified throughout the United States, and recipients of their prior donations have been notified and tested. Thus far, only two prior recipients (of platelets from one donor) appear positive by testing. Thus, despite reported transmission rates of 10% to 20% from components from infected donors in endemic areas, no *T. cruzi* transmissions by red cells in the United States have been documented to date. The lower infectivity of US red cell components compared to those in endemic areas may be at least partly attributable to more frequent use of fresh whole blood in endemic areas.

Babesia

Babesia are intraerythrocytic parasites. Cases of transfusion-transmitted babesiosis are being identified with increasing frequency, and some have been fatal.[64,71,72] There is no FDA-approved donor screening test for this infection.

Human *Babesia* infections are zoonotic, usually acquired through the bite of an infected tick. In the northeastern and midwestern United States, the most common *Babesia* species is *B. microti.* The vector is *Ixodes scapularis,* the same tick that transmits Lyme disease. Human infection with *B. microti* appears to be increasing in frequency. In the western United States, *Babesia* infections appear to be less common, and a different species, *B. duncani,* appears to be predominant. The insect vector for *B. duncani* has not been clearly defined. *Babesia* infection is usually asymptomatic, even though parasites can circulate for months to years. In some individuals, however, *Babesia* infection presents as a severe malaria-like illness that can be fatal. Immunocompromised, elderly, and asplenic patients are at increased risk of severe disease.

In patients, *Babesia* infection is diagnosed when the intraerythrocytic parasites are seen on a blood smear. If a patient is suspected of having acquired the infection by transfusion, donors of the patient's components can be recalled and tested for antibodies to *Babesia* using an immunofluorescence assay (IFA); the presence of high-titer antibody in the donor is suggestive of recent infection. Most of the donors implicated in transfusion-transmitted cases have been residents of endemic areas, although some were residents of nonendemic areas who were apparently exposed to *Babesia* during travel to endemic areas.[72]

Studies in Connecticut have found *B. microti* antibodies in approximately 1% of blood donors, suggesting that *B. microti* infections are highly prevalent in the population of this state and grossly underrecognized.[73] In the absence of FDA-approved tests for blood donor screening, there have been discussions regarding the potential investigational use of IFA or NAT assays to attempt to reduce transfusion risk in the most highly endemic regions.[71,73,74]

Malaria

Malaria is caused by an intraerythrocytic parasite of the genus *Plasmodium*. Infection is transmitted to humans through the bite of a mosquito. Four species account for most human infections: *P. falciparum, P. vivax, P. malariae,* and *P. ovale.*

No FDA-approved test is available to screen US blood donors for malaria infection. Screening is accomplished solely by donor questioning. Individuals are excluded from donating blood for 1 year after traveling to malaria-endemic areas, and for 3 years after recovery from clinical malaria or after long-term residence (5 years or more) in malaria-endemic areas. Donor questioning is remarkably effective at preventing transfusion-transmitted malaria in the United States, with only four cases of transfusion-transmitted malaria reported between 1999 and 2010. All four cases were linked to donors who had emigrated from Africa; on reinterview, three of the four donors were verified to have met acceptance criteria, but one had emigrated less than 3 years before donation.[75-78]

This level of transfusion safety has been achieved at substantial cost in terms of donor loss; malaria-related questions have excluded hundreds of thousands of otherwise acceptable US donors annually. Although travel to Mexico has accounted for the largest proportion of deferred donors, the risk of acquiring malaria during tourist travel to Mexico is exceedingly low.[79] Recently, the FDA Blood Products Advisory Committee recommended to the FDA that travelers to Quintana Roo, Mexico, a popular tourist destination, be permitted to donate blood.[80] The CDC subsequently declared most resort areas in Mexico to be without malaria risk, eliminating the need for some of these deferrals.[81]

Some other countries that exclude donors after travel to malarious areas permit reinstatement of these donors if they test negative for malaria antibodies 4 to 6 months after completion of travel. Thus far, such a "test-in" reinstatement strategy has not been accepted by the FDA. One barrier to US implementation of this strategy is that there is not yet a test that includes antigens for all four of the clinically important malaria species.

Other Vector-Transmitted Infections

There are many other vector-transmitted infections that could be secondarily transmitted by transfusion. These agents and potential intervention strategies are reviewed in a *TRANSFUSION* supplement on emerging infectious diseases.[45] Two of these, dengue and chikungunya viruses, have received recent attention because donations containing viral nucleic acid have been documented during epidemics outside of the continental United States. Dengue activity has also been documented within the southern United States.[82] The degree to which these agents threaten the US blood supply is unclear.[83]

Prions

Prions are proteinaceous infectious particles that induce disease by triggering conformational changes in naturally occurring protein counterparts. These agents cause fatal infections of the nervous system called transmissible spongiform encephalopathies (TSEs).

Classical CJD is a TSE with both a sporadic form and a familial form, occurring with an incidence of about 1 per million. CJD has been transmitted iatrogenically by infusion or implantation of products that were extracted from infected central nervous system tissues. Blood components do not appear to transmit classical CJD. Nevertheless, blood donations are not accepted from donors who are at increased risk of this disease.[84]

Another TSE with the descriptor "variant" (vCJD) does appear to be transmissible by blood transfusion. This TSE is caused by the same prion that causes bovine spongiform encephalopathy (BSE) or "mad cow disease." As of October 2010, four cases of vCJD transmission by transfusion had been reported in the United Kingdom, the area in which BSE was most endemic. In addition, one latent vCJD infection was identified in a hemophiliac in the United Kingdom who died of other causes. This patient had received UK-plasma-derived Factor VIII including material from one donor who later developed vCJD, suggesting possible transmission of vCJD by clotting factor concentrates.[45] vCJD infection is extremely rare in the United States. The few reported cases have been in individuals who most likely acquired their infections elsewhere, and no US transfusion-transmitted cases have been reported.

There are no FDA-approved donor screening tests for prion infections. Blood donors in the US are screened solely by questioning and are excluded if they have increased risk for either CJD or vCJD. CJD exclusions are for family history of disease, receipt of human growth hormone derived from pituitary glands, or receipt of a dura mater tissue graft. vCJD exclusions are for residence in the United Kingdom or Europe for specified times when BSE was endemic, receipt of a transfusion in the United Kingdom or France, or receipt of UK bovine insulin.[84] It is thought that plasma derivative manufacturing processes remove substantial amounts of TSE infectivity.[84]

In-Process Screening for Plasma Derivatives: Parvovirus B19

Commercial plasma derivatives are prepared from large pools of plasma derived from thousands of donors. Before the incorporation of specific pathogen-reduction processes, contamination of these large pools with viral agents was common. Today, plasma derivative manufacturing processes incorporate methods that have been demonstrated to inactivate most known pathogens—methods such as prolonged heat or solvent/detergent treatment. The latter inactivates lipid-enveloped agents such as HIV, HCV, and HBV. Pathogen infectivity may also be reduced by nanofiltration, chromatography, and cold ethanol fractionation, which are used in the production of certain products. Not all infectious agents, however, are removed or inactivated by these processes. One agent that can persist in plasma derivative products is human parvovirus B19.

Human parvovirus B19 is a small nonenveloped DNA virus that is extremely resistant to physical inactivation. Acute infection is typically mild and self-limited; clinical manifestations include "fifth disease" (erythema infectiosum) and polyarthropathy. Acute infection is associated with a transient red cell aplasia; this may be of clinical importance for individuals with underlying hemolytic processes. Red cell aplasia can be prolonged in immunodeficient individuals, and intrauterine infection is associated with severe fetal anemia and hydrops fetalis. Parvovirus B19 infection is very common; most adults have antibodies to this agent, indicating previous exposure. Levels of viral DNA during acute infection may exceed 10^{12} IU/mL, decreasing over weeks to months in association with production of antibody. Viral DNA, mostly at low concentrations, has been detected in approximately 1% of blood donations and in essentially all lots of pooled plasma derivatives. Transmission of parvovirus B19 by transfusion has been linked only to blood components or plasma products that contain high concentrations of viral DNA; no transmissions have been documented with products containing less than 10^4 IU/mL.[85,86]

Currently, there is no FDA-approved test to screen fresh blood donations for infection. However, plasma derivative manufacturers require screening of incoming plasma units for the presence of high-titer parvovirus B19. This is performed by NAT of plasma donations, with sensitivity adjusted to detect only units with a high concentration of virus. By excluding high-titer units from the plasma pools, the final titer in the plasma pool is kept below 10^4 IU/mL.

PATHOGEN REDUCTION TECHNOLOGY

Donor screening reduces, but cannot eliminate, the infectious risks of blood transfusion. The efficacy of blood donor testing is limited by a number of factors, including the following:

1. It is not logistically feasible to test donors for every infection that is conceivably transmissible by transfusion.
2. For every test, there is a lag between the time a person becomes infected and the time the test will detect infection (window period).
3. Every test has a limitation in sensitivity (the concentration of the target marker that can be detected by the test).
4. Developing a donor test is a long, multiphase process that includes identification of the infectious agent, selection of the type of test that would be effective in interdicting infectious donations (eg, serology vs NAT), development of a test suitable for donor screening, performance of clinical trials, and regulatory approval. During this development process, infections can be transmitted.

Pathogen reduction technology (PRT) presents an attractive alternative to relying on donor testing to interdict all infectious donations. PRT refers to processes that reduce the infectivity of residual pathogens in blood components. This approach could reduce transmission of agents for which there are no donor screening tests and further reduce the residual transmission risks of known agents.

As discussed above, PRT is now an essential component of the plasma derivative manufacturing process. A variety of technologies incorporated into these manufacturing processes are highly effective in reducing the infectivity of plasma pools; these processes include prolonged heat, solvent/detergent treatment, and ultrafiltration. None of these processes, however, can be applied to cellular blood components.

At the time of writing, no PRT processes were available in the United States for treatment of individual blood components, although some technologies were in use outside of the United States. Processes that are available or are in development have been recently reviewed in detail[45,87,88] and are summarized in Table 8-6.

Currently, the quantifiable infectious risks of transfusion in the United States are low, and the benefit to be gained from PRT is largely theoretical. Therefore, it is critically important to demonstrate that PRT treatments do not introduce new hazards to patients. Rigorous preclinical and clinical studies are required for US regulatory approval of PRT. Toxicology studies are critical, as most of these agents act by crosslinking nucleic acid, raising the theoretical potential of carcinogenicity and mutagenicity. Treated products should be assessed for neoantigen formation and the impact of the PRT on the clinical efficacy of the final product. The evaluation process for PRT in North America was the subject of a recent consensus conference.[89] Documented transmission of new infectious agents for which there are no donor screening tests could influence the risk/benefit assessment of PRTs. It is important, though, to keep in mind that not all agents are inactivated by PRTs. Pooled solvent/detergent plasma, for example, would carry a reduced risk of transmitting most infectious agents but a potentially increased risk of transmitting an agent that lacks a lipid envelope.

TABLE 8-6. Pathogen Reduction Technologies for Transfusible Blood Components

Component	Technology	Manufacturer
Plasma: commercially prepared pools	Solvent/detergent treatment	Octapharma
Plasma: individual units	◆ Amotosalen (psoralen) + UV light	Cerus
	◆ Riboflavin (vitamin B2) + UV light	CaridianBCT
	◆ Methylene blue + light	MacoPharma
Platelets	◆ Amotosalen (psoralen) + UV light	Cerus
	◆ Riboflavin (vitamin B2) + UV light	CaridianBCT
	◆ UV light	MacoPharma
Red Blood Cells	◆ Frangible nucleic acid crosslinker	Cerus
	◆ Riboflavin (vitamin B2) + UV light	CaridianBCT

UV = ultraviolet.

SUMMARY

The current level of safety of blood components is based on two critical elements of donor screening: donor questioning, which serves as the sole method of screening for certain agents such as malaria and prions, and donor testing. Testing must be performed carefully and in accordance with manufacturers' instructions, and facilities must have robust systems for quarantining components of donations that test positive and for retrieving prior donations from test-positive donors. Current quantifiable risks of infectious disease transmission are very low, with HIV transmission risk estimated at 1 in 1.5 million, and HCV transmission, about 1 in 1.1 million. However, it is critical to remain vigilant for evidence of new agents and to implement mitigation measures as quickly as feasible. PRT may, in the future, provide some protection against emerging agents for which no screening is in place.

KEY POINTS

1. Infectious disease screening of donors is accomplished by 1) questioning of potential donors and exclusion of individuals with an increased risk of infection and 2) testing of donated blood.
2. There is a delay between the time an individual is exposed to an infection and the time the donor screening test for the infection becomes positive. Blood donated during this window period could transmit infection.
3. The estimated window period for human immunodeficiency virus (HIV) and hepatitis C virus (HCV) with nucleic acid testing (NAT) of donor samples is less than 10 days.
4. The residual risk of transfusion-transmitted infection is a function of the length of the window period and the incidence of infection in the donor population. Maintaining a donor population that has a low incidence of infection continues to play a key role in preserving blood safety.

5. Based on window period and incidence calculations, the current risk of HIV transmission by transfusion in the United States is approximately 1 in 1.5 million units, and the risk of HCV transmission is approximately 1 in 1.1 million units.
6. There are no donor screening tests approved by the Food and Drug Administration (FDA) for malaria or variant Creutzfeldt-Jakob disease. Donor questioning for potential exposure is the sole means of protecting the US blood supply from these diseases.
7. The AABB requires blood banks to have processes that limit and detect or inactivate bacteria in platelet components. Methods for pathogen reduction have replaced bacteria testing in some regions outside of the United States.
8. Infections transmitted to humans by insect vectors are increasingly recognized as a potential source of transfusion-transmitted infection. These include West Nile virus, *Trypanosoma cruzi*, *Babesia* species, and dengue virus.
9. Pathogen-reduction technologies (PRTs) may reduce transmission of agents for which there are no donor screening tests, and they may further reduce the residual transmission risks of known agents. Some PRT systems are available outside of the United States for treatment of platelet and plasma components, but these systems are not currently approved for US use.
10. Blood banks must have processes in place to ensure that test-positive donations are not released for transfusion. In some circumstances, 1) prior donations from those donors must also be retrieved and quarantined, and 2) recipients of prior donations must be notified of their possible exposure to infection.

REFERENCES

1. Code of federal regulations. Title 21, CFR Parts 211 and 610. Washington, DC: US Government Printing Office, 2010 (revised annually).
2. Alter HJ, Klein HG. The hazards of blood transfusion in historical perspective. Blood 2008; 112:2617-26.
3. Seeff LB, Wright EC, Zimmerman HJ, McCollum RW. VA cooperative study of post-transfusion hepatitis, 1969-1974: Incidence and characteristics of hepatitis and responsible risk factors. Am J Med Sci 1975;270:355-62.
4. Alter HJ, Purcell RH, Holland PV, et al. Donor transaminase and recipient hepatitis. Impact on blood transfusion services. JAMA 1981;246: 630-4.
5. Aach RD, Szmuness W, Mosley JW, et al. Serum alanine aminotransferase of donors in relation to the risk of non-A, non-B hepatitis in recipients: The transfusion-transmitted viruses study. N Engl J Med 1981; 304:989-94.
6. Alter HJ, Holland PV. Indirect tests to detect the non-A, non-B hepatitis carrier state. Ann Intern Med 1984;101:859-61.
7. Stevens CE, Aach RD, Hollinger FB, et al. Hepatitis B virus antibody in blood donors and the occurrence of non-A, non-B hepatitis in transfusion recipients. An analysis of the Transfusion-Transmitted Viruses Study. Ann Intern Med 1984;101:733-8.
8. American Red Cross, AABB, and Council of Community Blood Centers. Joint statement on directed donations and AIDS (June 22, 1983). Arlington, VA: AABB, 1983.
9. Galel SA, Lifson JD, Engleman EG. Prevention of AIDS transmission through screening of the blood supply. Annu Rev Immunol 1995;13:201-27.
10. Busch MP, Young MJ, Samson SM, et al. Risk of human immunodeficiency virus (HIV) transmission by blood transfusions before the implementation of HIV-1 antibody screening. The Transfusion Safety Study Group. Transfusion 1991;31:4-11.
11. Ward JW, Holmberg SD, Allen JR, et al. Transmission of human immunodeficiency virus (HIV) by blood transfusions screened as negative for HIV antibody. N Engl J Med 1988;318: 473-8.
12. Busch MP, Glynn SA, Stramer SL, et al. A new strategy for estimating risks of transfusion-transmitted viral infections based on rates of detection of recently infected donors. Transfusion 2005;45:254-64.
13. Stramer SL, Foster GA, Townsend RL, et al. Evaluation of the yield of triggering and detrig-

gering criteria for West Nile virus (WNV) NAT (abstract). Transfusion 2009;49(Suppl 3):30A.
14. Busch MP, Caglioti S, Robertson EF, et al. Screening the blood supply for West Nile virus RNA by nucleic acid amplification testing. N Engl J Med 2005;353:460-7.
15. West Nile virus—revised recommendations for triggering individual donation nucleic acid testing and use of communication plans. Association bulletin #08-03. Bethesda, MD: AABB, 2008.
16. Food and Drug Administration. Guidance for industry: Use of nucleic acid tests to reduce the risk of transmission of West Nile virus from donors of whole blood and blood components intended for transfusion. (November 2009) Rockville, MD: CBER Office of Communication, Outreach, and Development, 2009. [Available at http://www.fda.gov/downloads/BiologicsBloodVaccines/GuidanceComplianceRegulatoryInformation/Guidances/Blood/UCM189464.pdf (accessed December 8, 2010).]
17. Food and Drug Administration: Guidance for industry: "Lookback" for hepatitis C virus (HCV): Product quarantine, consignee notification, further testing, product disposition, and notification of transfusion recipients based on donor test results indicating infection with HCV. (December 2010) Rockville, MD: CBER Office of Communication, Outreach, and Development, 2010. [Available at http://www.fda.gov/downloads/BiologicsBloodVaccines/GuidanceComplianceRegulatoryInformation/Guidances/Blood/UCM238488.pdf (accessed January 2, 2011).]
18. Food and Drug Administration. Guidance for industry: Use of serological tests to reduce the risk of transmission of *Trypanosoma cruzi* infection in whole blood and blood components intended for transfusion. (December 2010) Rockville, MD: CBER Office of Communication, Outreach, and Development, 2010. [Available at http://www.fda.gov/downloads/BiologicsBloodVaccines/GuidanceComplianceRegulatoryInformation/Guidances/Blood/UCM235960.pdf (accessed January 2, 2011).]
19. Food and Drug Administration. Guidance for industry: Nucleic acid testing (NAT) for human immunodeficiency virus type 1 (HIV-1) and hepatitis C virus (HCV): Testing, product disposition, and donor deferral and reentry. (May 2010) Rockville, MD: CBER Office of Communication, Outreach, and Development, 2010. [Available at http://www.fda.gov/downloads/BiologicsBloodVaccines/GuidanceComplianceRegulatoryInformation/Guidances/Blood/UCM210270.pdf (accessed December 8, 2010).]
20. Food and Drug Administration. Guidance for industry: Requalification method for reentry of blood donors deferred because of reactive test results for antibody to hepatitis B core antigen (Anti-HBc). (May 2010) Rockville, MD: CBER Office of Communication, Outreach, and Development, 2010. [Available at http://www.fda.gov/downloads/BiologicsBloodVaccines/GuidanceComplianceRegulatoryInformation/Guidances/Blood/UCM210268.pdf (accessed December 8, 2010).]
21. Food and Drug Administration. Guidance for industry: Recommendations for management of donors at increased risk for human immunodeficiency virus type 1 (HIV-1) group O infection. (August 2009) Rockville, MD: CBER Office of Communication, Outreach, and Development, 2009. [Available at http://www.fda.gov/BiologicsBloodVaccines/GuidanceComplianceRegulatoryInformation/Guidances/Blood/ucm180817.htm (accessed December 8, 2010).]
22. Food and Drug Administration. Guidance for industry: Nucleic acid testing (NAT) to reduce the possible risk of parvovirus B19 transmission by plasma-derived products. (July 2009) Rockville, MD: CBER Office of Communication, Outreach, and Development, 2009. [Available at http://www. fda.gov/BiologicsBloodVaccines/GuidanceComplianceRegulatoryInformation/Guidances/Blood/ucm071592.htm (accessed December 8, 2010).]
23. Food and Drug Administration. Guidance for industry: Assessing donor suitability and blood and blood product safety in cases of known or suspected West Nile virus infection. (June 2005) Rockville, MD: CBER Office of Communication, Outreach, and Development, 2005. [Available at http://www.fda.gov/BiologicsBloodVaccines/GuidanceComplianceRegulatoryInformation/Guidances/Blood/ucm074111. htm (accessed December 8, 2010).]
24. Food and Drug Administration: Guidance for industry: Use of nucleic acid tests on pooled and individual samples from donors of whole blood and blood components (including Source Plasma and Source Leukocytes) to adequately and appropriately reduce the risk of transmission of HIV-1 and HCV. (October 2004) Rockville, MD: CBER Office of Commu-

nication, Outreach, and Development, 2004. [Available at http://www.fda.gov/BiologicsBloodVaccines/GuidanceComplianceRegulatoryInformation/Guidances/Blood/ucm074934.htm (accessed December 8, 2010).]

25. Food and Drug Administration: Guidance for industry: Donor screening for antibodies to HTLV-II. (August 1997) Rockville, MD: CBER Office of Communication, Outreach, and Development, 1997. [Available at http://www.fda.gov/BiologicsBloodVaccines/GuidanceComplianceRegulatoryInformation/Guidances/Blood/ucm170786.htm (accessed December 8, 2010).]
26. Food and Drug Administration. Memorandum to all registered blood and plasma establishments: Recommendations for the quarantine and disposition of units from prior collections from donors with repeatedly reactive screening tests for hepatitis B virus (HBV), hepatitis C virus (HCV) and human T-lymphotropic virus type I (HTLV-I). (July 1996) Rockville, MD: CBER Office of Communication, Outreach, and Development, 1996. [Available at http://www.fda.gov/downloads/BiologicsBloodVaccines/GuidanceComplianceRegulatoryInformation/OtherRecommendationsforManufacturers/MemorandumtoBloodEstablishments/UCM062600.pdf (accessed December 8, 2010).]
27. Food and Drug Administration. Memorandum to all registered blood establishments: Clarification of FDA recommendations for donor deferral and product distribution based on the results of syphilis testing. (December 1991) Rockville, MD: CBER Office of Communication, Outreach, and Development, 1991. [Available at http://www.fda.gov/downloads/BiologicsBloodVaccines/GuidanceComplianceRegulatoryInformation/OtherRecommendationsforManufacturers/MemorandumtoBloodEstablishments/UCM062840.pdf (accessed December 8, 2010).]
28. Food and Drug Administration. Memorandum to all registered blood establishments: Recommendations for the management of donors and units that are initially reactive for hepatitis B surface antigen (HBsAg). (December 1987) Rockville, MD: CBER Office of Communication, Outreach, and Development, 1987. [Available at http://www.fda.gov/downloads/BiologicsBloodVaccines/GuidanceComplianceRegulatoryInformation/OtherRecommendationsforManufacturers/MemorandumtoBloodEstablishments/UCM063011.pdf (accessed December 8, 2010).]
29. Carson TH, ed. Standards for blood banks and transfusion services. 27th ed. Bethesda, MD: AABB, 2011.
30. Suggested options for transfusion services and blood collectors to facilitate implementation of BB/TS Interim Standard 5.1.5.1.1. Association bulletin #10-05. Bethesda, MD: AABB, 2010.
31. Information concerning implementation of a licensed test for antibodies to *Trypanosoma cruzi*. Association bulletin #06-08. Bethesda, MD: AABB, 2006.
32. Guidance on management of blood and platelet donors with positive or abnormal results on bacterial contamination tests. Association bulletin #05-02. Bethesda, MD: AABB, 2005.
33. Actions following an initial positive test for possible bacterial contamination of a platelet unit. Association bulletin #04-07. Bethesda, MD: AABB, 2004.
34. Dual enzyme immuno assay (EIA) approach for deferral and notification of anti-HTLV-I/II EIA reactive donors. Association bulletin #99-9. Bethesda, MD: AABB, 1999.
35. Blajchman MA, Goldman M, Freedman JJ, Sher GD. Proceedings of a consensus conference: Prevention of post-transfusion CMV in the era of universal leukoreduction. Transfus Med Rev 2001;15:1-20.
36. Vamvakas EC. Is white blood cell reduction equivalent to antibody screening in preventing transmission of cytomegalovirus by transfusion? A review of the literature and meta-analysis. Transfus Med Rev 2005; 19:181-99.
37. Bowden RA, Slichter SJ, Sayers M, et al. A comparison of filtered leukocyte-reduced and cytomegalovirus (CMV) seronegative blood products for the prevention of transfusion-associated CMV infection after marrow transplant. Blood 1995;86:3598-603.
38. The ADA, HIV, and autologous blood donation. Association bulletin #98-5. Bethesda, MD: AABB, 1998.
39. Anderson SA, Yang H, Gallagher LM, et al. Quantitative estimate of the risks and benefits of possible alternative blood donor deferral strategies for men who have had sex with men. Transfusion 2009;49:1102-14.
40. Zou S, Dorsey KA, Notari EP, et al. Prevalence, incidence, and residual risk of human immunodeficiency virus and hepatitis C virus infections among United States blood donors since

the introduction of nucleic acid testing. Transfusion 2010; 50:1495-504.

41. Stramer SL, Glynn SA, Kleinman SH, et al. Detection of HIV-1 and HCV infections among antibody-negative blood donors by nucleic acid-amplification testing. N Engl J Med 2004; 351:760-8.
42. Dodd RY, Notari EP, Stramer SL. Current prevalence and incidence of infectious disease markers and estimated window-period risk in the American Red Cross blood donor population. Transfusion 2002;42:975-9.
43. Glynn SA, Kleinman SH, Wright DJ, Busch MP. International application of the incidence rate/window period model. Transfusion 2002; 42:966-72.
44. Zou S, Stramer SL, Notari EP, et al. Current incidence and residual risk of hepatitis B infection among blood donors in the United States. Transfusion 2009;49:1609-20.
45. Stramer SL, Hollinger FB, Katz LM, et al. Emerging infectious disease agents and their potential threat to transfusion safety. Transfusion 2009;49(Suppl 2):1S-235S.
46. Centers for Disease Control and Prevention. HIV/AIDS surveillance report, 2007. Vol. 19. Atlanta, GA: CDC, 2009;19:1-63. [Available at http://www.cdc.gov/hiv/topics/surveillance/resources/reports/ (accessed December 8, 2010).]
47. Food and Drug Administration. Proceedings of the FDA workshop on behavior-based donor deferrals in the NAT era, Bethesda, MD, March 8, 2006. Rockville, MD: CBER Office of Communication, Outreach, and Development, 2006. [Available at http://www.fda.gov/downloads/BiologicsBloodVaccines/NewsEvents/WorkshopsMeetingsConferences/TranscriptsMinutes/UCM054430.pdf (accessed December 8, 2010).]
48. HIV prevalence, unrecognized infection, and HIV testing among men who have sex with men—five U.S. cities, June 2004-April 2005. MMWR Morb Mortal Wkly Rep 2005;54:597-601.
49. Truong HM, Kellogg T, Klausner JD, et al. Increases in sexually transmitted infections and sexual risk behaviour without a concurrent increase in HIV incidence among men who have sex with men in San Francisco: A suggestion of HIV serosorting? Sex Transm Infect 2006;82: 461-6.
50. Food and Drug Administration. Blood donations from men who have sex with other men questions and answers. Rockville, MD: CBER Office of Communication, Outreach, and Development, 2009. [Available at http://www.fda.gov/BiologicsBloodVaccines/BloodBloodProducts/QuestionsaboutBlood/ucm108186.htm (accessed December 8, 2010).]
51. US Department of Health and Human Services. HHS Advisory Committee on Blood Safety and Availability (report). Committee recommendations. (June 2010) Washington, DC: HHS, 2010. [Available at http://www.hhs.gov/ash/bloodsafety/advisorycommittee/recommendations/06112010_recommendations.pdf (accessed January 2, 2011).]
52. Kleinman SH, Busch MP. Assessing the impact of HBV NAT on window period reduction and residual risk. J Clin Virol 2006;36(Suppl 1):S23-9.
53. Stramer SL. Pooled hepatitis B virus DNA testing by nucleic acid amplification: Implementation or not. Transfusion 2005;45:1242-6.
54. Stramer SL, Townsend RL, Foster GA, et al. HBV NAT yield and donor characteristics in US blood donors; impact of vaccine breakthrough infection (VBI) and correlation with modeled yield (abstract). Transfusion 2009;49(Suppl 3):1A-2A.
55. Linauts S, Saldanha J, Strong DM. PRISM hepatitis B surface antigen detection of hepatits B virus minipool nucleic acid testing yield samples. Transfusion 2008;48:1376-82.
56. Alter HJ. Descartes before the horse: I clone, therefore I am: The hepatitis C virus in current perspective. Ann Intern Med 1991;115:644-9.
57. Daniels D, Grytdal S, Wasley A. Surveillance for acute viral hepatitis—United States, 2007. MMWR Surveill Summ 2009;58:1-27.
58. Page-Shafer K, Pappalardo BL, Tobler LH, et al. Testing strategy to identify cases of acute hepatitis C virus (HCV) infection and to project HCV incidence rates. J Clin Microbiol 2008;46: 499-506.
59. Guidelines for counseling persons infected with human T-lymphotropic virus type I (HTLV-I) and type II (HTLV-II). Centers for Disease Control and Prevention and the U.S.P.H.S. Working Group. Ann Intern Med 1993;118:448-54.
60. Vrielink H, Zaaijer HL, Reesink HW. The clinical relevance of HTLV type I and II in transfusion medicine. Transfus Med Rev 1997;11:173-9.

61. Orton S. Syphilis and blood donors: What we know, what we do not know, and what we need to know. Transfus Med Rev 2001;15:282-92.
62. Katz LM. A test that won't die: The serologic test for syphilis. Transfusion 2009;49:617-19.
63. Zou S, Notari EP, Fang CT, et al. Current value of serologic test for syphilis as a surrogate marker for blood-borne viral infections among blood donors in the United States. Transfusion 2009;49:655-61.
64. Food and Drug Administration. Fatalities reported to FDA following blood collection and transfusion: Annual summary for fiscal year 2009. Rockville, MD: CBER Office of Communication, Outreach, and Development, 2010. [Available at http://www.fda.gov/downloads/BiologicsBloodVaccines/SafetyAvailability/ReportaProblem/TransfusionDonationFatalities/UCM205620.pdf (accessed December 8, 2010).]
65. Hillyer CD, Josephson CD, Blajchman MA, et al. Bacterial contamination of blood components: Risks, strategies, and regulation: Joint ASH and AABB educational session in transfusion medicine. Hematology Am Soc Hematol Educ Program 2003:575-89.
66. Ramirez-Arcos SM, Goldman M, Blajchman MA. Bacterial infection: Bacterial contamination, testing and post-transfusion complications. In: Hillyer CD, Silberstein LE, Ness PM, et al, eds. Blood banking and transfusion medicine: Basic principles and practice. 2nd ed. Philadelphia: Churchill Livingstone, 2007:639-51.
67. Eder AF, Kennedy JM, Dy BA, et al. Limiting and detecting bacterial contamination of apheresis platelets: Inlet-line diversion and increased culture volume improve component safety. Transfusion 2009;49:1554-63.
68. Centers for Disease Control and Prevention. West Nile virus transmission via organ transplantation and blood transfusion—Louisiana, 2008. MMWR Morb Mortal Wkly Rep 2009;58:1263-7.
69. Otani MM, Vinelli E, Kirchhoff LV, et al. WHO comparative evaluation of serologic assays for Chagas disease. Transfusion 2009;49:1076-82.
70. Food and Drug Administration. Potential testing strategies for *T. cruzi* infection in blood donors. FDA Blood Products Advisory Committee meeting materials, 94th Meeting, Rockville, MD, April 1, 2009. Rockville, MD: CBER Office of Communication, Outreach, and Development, 2009. [Available at http://www.fda.gov/downloads/AdvisoryCommittees/CommitteesMeetingMaterials/BloodVaccinesandOtherBiologics/BloodProductsAdvisoryCommittee/UCM155597.pdf (accessed December 8, 2010).]
71. Gubernot DM, Nakhasi HL, Mied PA, et al. Transfusion-transmitted babesiosis in the United States: Summary of a workshop. Transfusion 2009;49:2759-71.
72. Tonnetti L, Eder AF, Dy B, et al. Transfusion-transmitted *Babesia microti* identified through hemovigilance. Transfusion 2009;49:2557-63.
73. Johnson ST, Cable RG, Tonnetti L, et al. Seroprevalence of *Babesia microti* in blood donors from Babesia-endemic areas of the northeastern United States: 2000 through 2007. Transfusion 2009;49:2574-82.
74. Food and Drug Administration. Proceedings of the Blood Products Advisory Committee meeting, Gaithersburg, MD, July 26, 2010. Rockville, MD: CBER Office of Communication, Outreach, and Development, 2010. [Available at http://www.fda.gov/downloads/AdvisoryCommittees/CommitteesMeetingMaterials/BloodVaccinesandOtherBiologics/BloodProductsAdvisoryCommittee/UCM225388.pdf (accessed December 8, 2010).]
75. Mali S, Steele S, Slutsker L, Arguin PM. Malaria surveillance—United States, 2007. MMWR Surveill Summ 2009;58(SS-2):1-16.
76. Eliades MJ, Shah S, Nguyen-Dinh P, et al. Malaria surveillance—United States, 2003. MMWR Surveill Summ 2005;54(SS-2):25-39.
77. Purdy E, Perry E, Gorlin J, et al. Transfusion-transmitted malaria: Unpreventable by current donor guidelines? (abstract) Transfusion 2003;43(Suppl):79A.
78. Kessler D, Grima KM, Hillyer CD. A case of malaria transfusion transmission (abstract). Transfusion 2010;50(Suppl 2):199A-200A.
79. Spencer B, Steele W, Custer B, et al. Risk for malaria in United States donors deferred for travel to malaria-endemic areas. Transfusion 2009;49:2335-45.
80. Food and Drug Administration. Blood donor deferral for malaria risk associated with travel to Mexico. FDA Blood Products Advisory Committee meeting materials, 96th meeting, Bethesda, MD, November 16-17, 2009. Rockville, MD: CBER Office of Communication, Outreach, and Development, 2009. [Available at http://www.fda.gov/downloads/AdvisoryCommittees/CommitteesMeetingMaterials/BloodVaccinesandOtherBiologics/BloodProd

uctsAdvisoryCommittee/UCM189010.pdf (accessed December 8, 2010).]

81. Centers for Disease Control and Prevention. CDC health information for international travel 2010. Atlanta, GA: CDC, 2010.
82. Centers for Disease Control and Prevention. Locally acquired dengue—Key West, Florida, 2009-2010. MMWR Morb Mortal Wkly Rep 2010;59:577-81.
83. Petersen LR, Busch MP. Transfusion-transmitted arboviruses. Vox Sang 2010;98:495-503.
84. Food and Drug Administration. Guidance for industry: Revised preventive measures to reduce the possible risk of transmission of Creutzfeldt-Jakob disease (CJD) and variant Creutzfeldt-Jakob disease (vCJD) by blood and blood products. (May 2010) Rockville, MD: CBER Office of Communication, Outreach, and Development, 2010. [Available at http://www.fda.gov/downloads/biologicsbloodvaccines/guidancecomplianceregulatoryinformation/guidances/UCM213415.pdf (accessed December 8, 2010).]
85. Brown KE, Simmonds P. Parvoviruses and blood transfusion. Transfusion 2007;47:1745-50.
86. Kleinman SH, Glynn SA, Lee TH, et al. A linked donor-recipient study to evaluate parvovirus B19 transmission by blood component transfusion. Blood 2009;114:3677-83.
87. McCullough J. Pathogen inactivation: A new paradigm for preventing transfusion-transmitted infections. Am J Clin Pathol 2007;128:945-55.
88. AuBuchon J, Prowse C, eds. Pathogen Inactivation: The penultimate paradigm shift. Bethesda, MD: AABB Press, 2010.
89. Klein HG, Anderson D, Bernardi MJ, et al. Pathogen inactivation: Making decisions about new technologies. Report of a consensus conference. Transfusion 2007;47:2338-47.

Chapter 9

Storage, Monitoring, Pretransfusion Processing, and Distribution of Blood Components

William B. Lockwood, PhD, MD; Jill Leonard, MT(AMT); and Sandy L. Liles, MT(ASCP)SBB

BLOOD COMPONENT manufacturing processes following collection have undergone marked changes in selected areas in the past few years, yet they have remained relatively unchanged in other areas. New technology in automated component preparation, new regulatory and minimal acceptable final component requirements, and new computer capabilities have influenced the quality-oriented procedures that blood centers, blood banks, and transfusion services use in today's manufacturing model. This model incorporates Food and Drug Administration (FDA) current good manufacturing practice (cGMP) regulations, originally published for drugs[1] and revised to include biologics,[2] from receipt to issue of the blood and blood component.

The common thread that is found in cGMP and other regulatory bodies' rules (Clinical Laboratory Improvement Amendments, state laboratory statutes) or volunteer laboratory accrediting organization policies (College of American Pathologists, AABB, The Joint Commission, American Osteopathic Association) is maintaining the safety, quality, potency, purity, and identity of blood and blood components. The manufacturing facility demonstrates that it is following these concepts through the utilization of policies, processes, and procedures found in written standard operating procedures and associated records. Review of these documents assists these agencies, and the facility, in determining that cGMP compliance in storing, monitoring, pretransfusion processing, and distributing blood and blood components is achieved (see Chapter 3 for additional regulatory details).

William B. Lockwood, PhD, MD, Clinical Professor (retired), Department of Pathology and Laboratory Medicine, and Director, Transfusion Services and Tissue/Bone Bank, University of Louisville Hospital and Norton-Kosair Children's Hospitals; Jill Leonard, MT(AMT), Administrative Supervisor, Clinical Laboratory, University of Louisville Hospital; and Sandy L. Liles, MT(ASCP)SBB, Technical Specialist, Transfusion Services, Norton Hospital, Louisville, Kentucky

The authors have disclosed no conflicts of interest.

BLOOD AND BLOOD COMPONENT STORAGE

Proper storage requirements must be followed on receipt of the blood or blood component from the collection area or blood supplier. Storage requirements and expiration dates vary depending on the particular blood unit as a result of the in-vitro cellular metabolism in storage medium or plasma protein stabilization (see Table 9-1). Failure to adhere to these storage and expiration requirements could result in decreased transfusion efficacy, potential harm to the recipient, or both.

Temperature requirements during transport of blood or blood components differ from those of storage.[4] Transport of whole blood and red cell components from the collection site to the processing facility is considered to relate to short-term conditions, and use of validated transport containers (boxes, coolers) allows the temperature to be decreasing toward 1 to 10 C (providing that platelet concentrates will not be manufactured from a whole blood unit, which would require the temperature to be cooling toward 20 to 24 C). However, should the red cell component require prolonged storage, the red cells must be maintained at 1 to 6 C.

It is recommended that all red cell transport containers be validated to maintain a temperature of 1 to 6 C for a specified period to ensure compliance with the transport and storage requirements for Red Blood Cells (RBCs).

Monitoring of Storage Temperatures

Refrigerators, freezers, and platelet incubators for blood component storage are available with continuous temperature monitoring devices that would be able to detect a temperature deviation before blood components might be affected. Automated electronic monitoring devices that are available include, but are not limited to, the following: 1) a weekly pen and chart recorder, 2) a set of hard-wired or radio frequency temperature recording devices, or 3) a centralized temperature monitoring system. Thermometers or thermocouplers are strategically placed in the equipment for optimal temperature monitoring. Daily checks of the temperature recordings should be performed to ensure proper operation of the equipment and recorder. Deviations from acceptable temperature ranges should be annotated on the temperature recording chart, as well as dated and initialed by the person noting the deviation. Most equipment also has audible alarms to alert personnel that temperature ranges are approaching unacceptable levels. Central alarm monitoring allows facilities that do not have personnel in the vicinity of the equipment to alert the designated staff at another location (or even send a page transmission to a selected individual) when an alarm is activated. Because platelets must be gently agitated during storage, and horizontal flatbed or elliptical rotators are used to prevent pH from decreasing below 6.2, alarm systems should also alert when the agitator has malfunctioned.

If an automated temperature recording device is not used, then temperatures of the blood component storage environment must be recorded manually every 4 hours.[3(p14)] This requirement includes ambient room temperature monitoring if blood components such as platelets are not stored in a platelet chamber or incubator.

Transfusion services may elect to have blood storage refrigerators located in other areas of the hospital to allow immediate access to blood components in emergencies. Such a policy of having externally located refrigerators will require that the same blood monitoring standards are met. The best scenario would be to have transfusion service personnel responsible for monitoring these refrigerators.

In the event that an equipment failure occurs and that the failure prevents acceptable temperature ranges from being maintained, the facility should have policies, processes, and procedures in place to relocate the blood components. The secondary storage location may be another on-site refrigerator or freezer, validated storage boxes or coolers appropriate for the blood component and potential prolonged storage time, areas in which the ambi-

TABLE 9-1. Storage and Expiration Requirements for Blood Components[3(pp48-55)]

Component	Storage	Expiration
Whole Blood Requirements		
Whole Blood	1-6 C. If intended for room temperature components, store at 1-6 C within 8 hours of collection	ACD/CPD/CP2D: 21 days CPDA-1: 35 days
Whole Blood Irradiated	1-6 C	Original expiration or 28 days from date of irradiation, whichever is sooner
Red Blood Cell Components		
Red Blood Cells (RBCs)	1-6 C	ACD/CPD/CP2D: 21 days CPDA-1: 35 days Additive solution (AS-1, AS-3, AS-5): 42 days Open system: 24 hours
RBCs Irradiated	1-6 C	Original expiration or 28 days from date of irradiation, whichever is sooner
RBCs Leukocytes Reduced	1-6 C	ACD/CPD/CP2D: 21 days CPDA-1: 35 days Additive solution (AS-1, AS-3, AS-5): 42 days Open system: 24 hours
Washed RBCs	1-6 C	24 hours
Apheresis RBCs	1-6 C	CPDA-1: 35 days Additive solution (AS-1, AS-3, AS-5): 42 days Open system: 24 hours
Apheresis RBCs Leukocytes Reduced	1-6 C	CPDA-1: 35 days Additive solution (AS-1, AS-3, AS-5): 42 days Open system: 24 hours
Frozen RBCs 40% glycerol or 20% glycerol	–65 C if 40% glycerol, or as FDA approved; –120 C if 20% glycerol, or as FDA approved (not in AABB *Standards*)	10 years, or a policy shall be developed if rare frozen units are to be retained beyond this time
Deglycerolized RBCs	1-6 C	Open system: 24 hours or as FDA approved Closed system: 14 days or as FDA approved
Rejuvenated RBCs	1-6 C	CPD/CPDA-1: 24 hours AS-1: freeze after rejuvenation at 42 days (time not specified in AABB *Standards*)

(Continued)

TABLE 9-1. Storage and Expiration Requirements for Blood Components[3(pp48-55)] (Continued)

Component	Storage	Expiration
Washed Rejuvenated RBCs	1-6 C	24 hours (not in AABB *Standards*)
Frozen Rejuvenated RBCs	–65 C	CPD,CPDA-1: 10 years AS-1: 3 years A policy shall be developed if rare frozen units are to be retained beyond this time
Deglycerolized Rejuvenated RBCs	1-6 C	24 hours or as approved by FDA
Platelet Components*		
Platelets	20-24 C with continuous gentle agitation	24 hours to 5 days depending on collection system
Platelets Irradiated	20-24 C with continuous gentle agitation	No change from original expiration date
Platelets Leukocytes Reduced	20-24 C with continuous gentle agitation	Open system: 4 hours Closed system: No change from original expiration date
Pooled Platelets	20-24 C with continuous gentle agitation	Open system: 4 hours Closed system: Expiration date should be earliest expiration date in pool
Pooled Platelets Leukocytes Reduced	20-24 C with continuous gentle agitation	Open system: within 4 hours of opening the system Closed system: 4 hours after pooling or 5 days following collection using an approved FDA system
Apheresis Platelets	20-24 C with continuous gentle agitation	24 hours to 5 days depending on collection system
Apheresis Platelets Irradiated	20-24 C with continuous gentle agitation	No change from original expiration date
Apheresis Platelets Leukocytes Reduced	20-24 C with continuous gentle agitation	Open system: within 4 hours of opening the system Closed system: 5 days
Granulocyte Components*		
Apheresis Granulocytes	20-24 C without agitation	24 hours
Apheresis Granulocytes Irradiated	20-24 C without agitation	No change from original expiration date
Plasma Components		
Fresh Frozen Plasma (FFP)	–18 C or –65 C	<–18 C: 12 months <–65 C: 7 years[†]

TABLE 9-1. Storage and Expiration Requirements for Blood Components[3(pp48-55)] (Continued)

Component	Storage	Expiration
FFP (after thawing)‡	1-6 C	If issued as FFP: 24 hours
Plasma Frozen Within 24 Hours After Phlebotomy (PF24)	–18 C	12 months from original collection date
Plasma Frozen Within 24 Hours After Phlebotomy (after thawing)‡	1-6 C	If issued as PF24: 24 hours
Thawed Plasma	1-6 C	5 days from date original product was thawed Can be prepared from FFP (whole-blood-derived FFP or collected in an apheresis closed system) or PF24 Label must be modified, as Thawed Plasma Is not an FDA-licensed component
Apheresis FFP	–18 C	12 months from original collection date (not in AABB *Standards*)
Thawed Apheresis FFP‡	1-6 C	If issued as FFP: 24 hours If issued as Thawed Plasma: 5 days from date original product was thawed (closed system) Label must be modified, as Thawed Plasma Is not an FDA-licensed component (not in AABB *Standards*)
Cryoprecipitated AHF	–18 C	12 months from original collection date
Cryoprecipitated AHF (after thawing)	20-24 C	Pooled without sterile connecting device: 4 hours Single unit: 6 hours Pooled prestorage or postthaw with sterile connecting device: 6 hours
Plasma Cryoprecipitate Reduced	–18 C	12 months
Plasma Cryoprecipitate Reduced (after thawing)	1-6 C	5 days
Liquid Plasma	1-6 C	5 days after expiration of Whole Blood
Recovered Plasma, liquid or frozen	Refer to short supply agreement (21 CFR 601.22).	Refer to short supply agreement (21 CFR 601.22).

*Platelet and granulocyte component storage temperatures presume that all reasonable steps are taken to maintain the temperature at 20-24 C as required by 21 CFR 600.15.

†FDA approval is required to store longer than 12 months.

‡FDA variance needed for storage of thawed plasma longer than 6 hours.

ACD = acid-citrate-dextrose; CPD = citrate-phosphate-dextrose; CP2D = citrate-phosphate-dextrose-dextrose; CPDA-1 = citrate-phosphate-dextrose-adenine-1; RBCs = Red Blood Cells; AS-1 = additive solution 1; FDA = Food and Drug Administration; AHF = antihemophilic factor; CFR = *Code of Federal Regulations.*

ent room temperature is monitored, or off-site locations. Because the safety, quality, purity, and potency of the blood components may be affected by delay in relocating to a secondary storage location, it is recommended that the relocation occur *before* the upper or lower acceptable storage temperature is exceeded. This can be accomplished by setting the alarm points of the storage devices just short of the acceptable storage threshold.

Some facilities may choose to use temperature monitoring indicators applied to each blood component container. Such indicators (depending on the type of various temperature-sensitive labels available) typically monitor the liquid temperature of the immediate inner blood bag, not the liquid core temperature in the unit.[5] However, a conservative approach is to use the indicator temperature in deciding component acceptability. The policies, processes, and procedures should specify how the facility will determine the disposition of these blood components. By following a blood banker's philosophy of "when in doubt, throw it out," noncompliance issues can be minimized.

Biochemical Changes of Stored Blood

Red Cells

Because blood components are stored in plastic bags of different types with a variety of added anticoagulants and additive solutions, the cellular and protein environment is modified from its natural state. During storage, biochemical and morphologic changes occur to red cells, producing a "storage lesion," which is one of the factors determining how long components may be stored (see Table 9-2). Changes include acidosis and decreased adenosine triphosphate (ATP) (both affecting red cell morphology), decreased 2,3-diphosphoglycerate (2,3-DPG), and oxidative and apoptotic changes as well as accumulation of lysophospholipids and potassium. Although the level of 2,3-DPG is markedly reduced at the end of storage times, the transfused red cell reestablishes normal levels within 12 to 24 hours following transfusion.[6] Supernatant potassium levels are increased during storage, but because of the small plasma volume in the additive units, even most neonates can tolerate routine transfusion of 15 mL/kg without adverse events.[7] At the end of storage, at least 75% of the transfused red cells must be present in circulation at 24 hours after transfusion, with less than 1% hemolysis. A 2% increment in 24-hour in-vivo survival is seen if the blood is leukocyte reduced at the time of initial processing. Leukocyte reduction tends to decrease hemolysis by 50%.[5,8]

Platelets

Platelet biochemical changes relate to the glycolytic production of lactic acid and oxidative metabolism of free fatty acids, resulting in production of carbon dioxide.[9] With the advent of newer plastic bags for platelets, pH is maintained above 6.2 by buffering of lactic acid by bicarbonate and promotion of oxidative metabolism by diffusion of oxygen into and carbon dioxide out of the bag during agitation.[9] Platelet shelf life is limited by functional changes during storage and the risk of bacterial growth.

Bacterial contamination has been addressed by the requirement to monitor for the presence of bacterial organisms in platelet concentrates and apheresis platelets. All such components must be tested using various techniques to identify bacterial contamination.[3(p11),10] Platelet manufacturers may wish to apply to the FDA to use a specific protocol that includes specific testing for bacterial contamination and allows for a 7-day expiration of the platelets.[11]

Plasma Components

Plasma from whole blood donation may be prepared from the primary centrifugation of whole blood into red cells and plasma or from platelet-rich plasma (PRP) following a second, harder centrifugation (see Method 6-13). Plasma prepared from whole blood donations may be frozen within either 1) 8 hours of whole blood collection (Fresh Frozen Plasma, or FFP) or 2) 24 hours of whole blood collection (Plasma Frozen Within 24 Hours After Phlebotomy, commonly referred to as PF24). FFP prepared

TABLE 9-2. Biochemical Changes in Stored Nonleukocyte-Reduced Red Blood Cells*

	CPD		CPDA-1				AS-1	AS-3	AS-5
Variable	**Whole Blood**		**Whole Blood**	**Red Blood Cells**	**Whole Blood**	**Red Blood Cells**	**Red Blood Cells**	**Red Blood Cells**	**Red Blood Cells**
Days of storage	0	21.00	0	0	35.00	35.00	42.00	42.00	42.00
% Viable cells (24 hours after transfusion)	100.00	80.00	100.00	100.00	79.00	71.00	76.00 (64-85)	84.00	80.00
pH (measure at 37 C)	7.20	6.84	7.60	7.55	6.98	6.71	6.60	6.50	6.50
ATP (% of initial value)	100.00	86.00	100.00	100.00	56 (± 16)	45 (± 12)	60.00	59.00	68.50
2,3-DPG (% of initial value)	100.00	44.00	100.00	100.00	<10.00	<10.00	<5.00	<10.00	<5.00
Plasma K+ (mmol/L)	3.90	21.00	4.20	5.10	27.30	78.50†	50.00	46.00	45.60
Plasma hemoglobin	17.00	191.00	82.00	78.00	461.00	658.00†	N/A	386.00	N/A
% Hemolysis	N/A	N/A	N/A	N/A	N/A	N/A	0.50	0.90	0.60

*Reprinted from Vengelen-Tyler V, ed. Technical manual. 12th ed. Bethesda, MD: AABB. 1999:164.

†Values for plasma hemoglobin and potassium concentrations may appear somewhat high in 35-day stored Red Blood Cell units; however, the total plasma in these units is only about 70 mL.

CPD = citrate-phosphate-dextrose; CPDA-1 = citrate-phosphate-dextrose-adenine-1; AS-1 = additive solution formula 1; ATP = adenosine triphosphate; 2,3-DPG = 2,3-diphosphoglycerate; N/A = not applicable.

from apheresis plasma collection may be frozen within 6 hours of collection or according to device manufacturers' instructions (also called FFP). The labile coagulation factors (Factor V and Factor VIII) as well as the stable factors are maintained well above 50% of donor levels in all three frozen components.[12]

FFP or PF24, thawed at 30 to 37 C, expires as FFP (thawed) or PF24 (thawed) 24 hours after thawing if stored at 1 to 6 C.[13] (A variance from 21 CFR 606.122(m)(3) is required in order to keep thawed FFP and PF24 for 24 hours.)

These products can be converted to Thawed Plasma as long as they were originally collected in closed systems. Thawed Plasma, although not licensed by the FDA, is included in the AABB *Standards for Blood Banks and Transfusion Services*[3] and the *Circular of Information for the Use of Human Blood and Blood Components.*[13]

If FFP or PF24 (after thawing) are converted to Thawed Plasma, the component label must be modified. Because Thawed Plasma is considered by the FDA as an unlicensed product, if the product remains in house, a facility may choose to label thawed FFP or PF24 as Thawed Plasma at the initial time of thawing. Thawed Plasma expires 5 days after thawing if stored at 1 to 6 C.[13] Thawed Plasma has a reduced concentration of Factor VIII, so it is not suitable for Factor VIII replacement when antihemophilic factor (AHF) derivatives are unavailable. Concentrations of remaining factors are clinically adequate for transfusion to other patients.[12] By maintaining Thawed Plasma as part of a plasma inventory, a transfusion service can reduce wastage from unused FFP or PF24 (after thawing).[14] Blood centers have found it useful to prepare PF24 when operational logistics do not allow for plasma to be frozen in 6 to 8 hours in order to be labeled as FFP. The use of PF24 by transfusing facilities may also increase their frozen plasma inventory.

Cryoprecipitated AHF

Cold precipitation at 1 to 6 C of insoluble glycoproteins in whole-blood-derived FFP produces Cryoprecipitated AHF (hereinafter referred to as CRYO). After precipitation, the supernatant fluid (Plasma Cryoprecipitate Reduced) is removed, leaving approximately 15 mL of CRYO, which is refrozen within 1 hour of preparation. CRYO contains ≥80 IU of Factor VIII and >150 mg of fibrinogen. Coagulation Factor XIII is approximately two- to threefold enriched in CRYO.[15] Also present are von Willebrand factor multimers and fibronectin. After thawing, individual units of CRYO may be pooled using small quantities of 0.9% Sodium Chloride, Injection (USP) for rinsing the contents of the bag into the final container. Thawed CRYO is stored at 20 to 24 C. Thawed CRYO in an open system or pool expires 4 hours from thawing. Thawed CRYO as a single unit or pooled using an FDA-approved sterile connecting device before storage or after thawing expires 6 hours from thawing.[13]

Transfusion facilities have access to prepooled CRYO from many blood suppliers (see Chapter 6 for more information on CRYO preparation). This component is available in frozen unit quantities (usually 5 pooled CRYO units) and alleviates the need for the transfusion facility to thaw and pool individual units of CRYO on site.

The supernatant fluid removed in the processing of CRYO is frozen to manufacture Plasma Cryoprecipitate Reduced. This component has reduced levels of the precipitated glycoproteins but contains other enzymatic clotting proteins (Factors II, V, VII, IX, X, XI). It has been used mostly as replacement fluid for thrombotic thrombocytopenic purpura (TTP) patients, although its clinical efficacy is similar to FFP and PF24, as all contain similar levels of ADAMTS13, the protein that is reduced in TTP.

Granulocytes

Granulocytes are collected by apheresis techniques in the United States, although a buffy-coat collection from a whole blood donation may be useful for neonates. The minimal granulocyte yield of Apheresis Granulocytes should be $\geq 1 \times 10^{10}$ but is difficult to achieve unless the donor has been pretreated with steroids, granulocyte colony-stimulating factor, or both. Lower-yield components are adequate for transfusion to neonates, who are becoming the major recipients of granulocytes. Granulocytes are fragile, deteriorate rapidly in vitro, should not be agitated during storage (granulocytes should never be stored in a refrigerated environment but at 20-24 C), contain abundant platelets (10^{11}), and must not be leukocyte reduced. Therefore, granulocytes should be transfused as soon after collection as possible to gain increased clinical efficacy. Because of the requirement to transfuse granulocytes within 24 hours of collection, most blood centers maintain a list of donors who are willing to donate on an emergency basis and who have had negative infectious disease marker tests on multiple prior donations.

PRESTORAGE PROCESSING

Differential Centrifugation

With the advent of plastic blood bags and the refrigerated centrifuge in blood component manufacturing in the early 1950s, separation of whole blood into various blood components became the norm. Depending on the "collection set" being used, blood centers can choose the set design required to meet the inventory requirements (doubles, triples, quads). Again, depending on the collection sets being used, several methods of component preparation are available.

Because of the physical properties of each cellular and liquid constituent in whole blood or blood components, separation can be achieved using differential centrifugation.[16] Method 8-4 describes the procedure for centrifuge calibration for platelet preparation, but each cellular or liquid constituent will require modifications of the procedure that are appropriate to manufacture each component. Quality control of the centrifuge should be monitored as part of the quality plan and good laboratory practice (see Chapters 1, 3, and 6).

Care should be used to properly pack and balance the centrifuge heads because of the bulky collection sets now being used. These sets may have an integral leukocyte-reduction filter (or filters), and improper centrifugation may lead to less-than-optimal component separation or cause bag or tubing compromise. Also, an improperly balanced or packed centrifuge may not only pose safety concerns for the operator but also cause potential damage to the centrifuge.

Prestorage Filtration

Leukocyte reduction with the use of blood filters may be performed either with integral filters or by the use of sterile connection of the appropriate component filters to the selected component. Whole blood filters currently allow recovery of leukocyte-reduced red cells and plasma with retention (depending on the filter manufacturer) of platelets. The manufacturer's directions should be followed as to timing and temperature of filtration for acceptable leukocyte reduction. Current practice is for the blood suppliers to leukocyte reduce the cellular component soon after collection and before storage (prestorage leukocyte reduction). This practice provides the best leukocyte reduction efficiency.[17]

Most automated collection devices have the capability for leukocyte reduction during the collection process unless double RBC units are collected where leukocyte reduction filters are required. Computerized settings that conform to the manufacturer's instructions should be programmed on the basis of each donor's total blood volume, hematocrit, and platelet count. Quality control documentation of instrument settings, outcome measures, and adverse events is required. With proper operation techniques, a leukocyte-reduced cellular component having $<1 \times 10^6$ white cells per collection can be achieved depending on the donor's precollection white cell count and quality of access.

POSTSTORAGE PROCESSING

Thawing FFP and Cryoprecipitated AHF

FFP may be thawed in waterbaths at temperatures of 30 to 37 C or in other FDA-approved devices. Thawing in a waterbath will require the container to be in a plastic overwrap before insertion into the water to prevent contamination of the container entry ports. There should be a procedure for quality control of indicated functions for any thawing device. (Refer to Method 6-12 for thawing Cryoprecipitated AHF.)

Thawing and Deglycerolizing RBCs

The freezing canister in which the RBC unit has been stored is placed in a 37 C dry heater or, after overwrapping, is placed in a 37 C waterbath. If the red cells have been frozen in the primary blood container, the container should be thawed at 42 C.[18] Thawing should be complete within 40 minutes.

The glycerol cryopreservative must be removed before the component is transfused. This removal should be accomplished in a slow "deglycerolization" process to minimize hemolysis. Deglycerolization is performed using a stepwise decreasing osmolar solution of saline (see Methods 6-7 through 6-9). Several vendors of deglycerolization instruments offer batch or continuous-flow washing techniques. Manufacturer's instructions should be followed to ensure maximal red cell recovery and minimal hemolysis.

Integrally attached tubing should be filled with the deglycerolized red cells and sealed appropriately so that a segment may be detached and available for crossmatch testing. The tubing is labeled not only with the name of the collecting facility but also with the name of the deglycerolization facility (when different from the collecting facility).

Shelf life of Deglycerolized RBCs will depend on the type of system used for deglycerolization. Closed system devices allow storage for up to 14 days, but components prepared using open systems would expire within 24 hours of deglycerolization.

Irradiating

Cellular components are required to be irradiated for certain patient populations to prevent transfusion-associated graft-vs-host disease. Irradiation may be accomplished with the use of gamma irradiators (cesium-137 and cobalt-60 radioisotopes), linear accelerators, ultraviolet-A irradiation (photoluminescence), and other nonradioisotope equipment (x-rays). The current gamma irradiation dose recommended to prevent proliferation of donor T lymphocytes in the recipient is a minimum of 25 Gy (2500 cGy/rads) to the central point of the blood container and 15 Gy (1500 cGy/rads) to any other part of the container.[3(p24)] The expiration date of irradiated RBCs is 28 days after irradiation or the original expiration date, whichever date is earliest.[3(p49)]

Confirmation that the blood container has received an adequate irradiation dose can be achieved with the use of commercially available radiographic film labels. A label may be affixed to the blood bag before irradiation and may be read following irradiation according to the manufacturer's instructions. Alternatively, a radiographic indicator label may be placed in the irradiator canister with the blood components and read after irradiating the single or multiple units. Several transfusion services have begun to universally irradiate platelets because platelets sustain minimal damage after irradiation and because the possibility of not irradiating a component to be transfused to a patient in need of irradiated components is eliminated.

Washing

There are very few clinical indications for washing red cell or platelet components [multiple progressive allergic reactions, antibodies against immunoglobulin A (IgA) in the recipient when IgA-deficient cellular components are not available, presence of maternal antibodies (anti-HPA-1), complement removal]. Washing is accomplished with the use of 1 to 2 L of sterile normal saline (preferably using automated equipment). Up to 20% of the red cell yield or 33% of the platelet yield may be lost during the washing procedure. Because washing creates an "open system" and removes anticoagulant-preservative solutions, washed RBC units expire 24 hours after washing. Washed platelets expire 4 hours after washing.

Pooling

Pooling of certain blood components (whole-blood-derived platelets, red cells or washed red cells pooled with plasma, and CRYO) may be required to provide clinically effective transfusion therapy without the need to transfuse multiple single components. Larger volumes of FFP for use as therapeutic plasma exchange fluid are best provided as "jumbo" plasma units (600 mL), which eliminates the need to pool FFP units.

Pooled platelets contain a significant number of red cells; therefore, units selected for the pool should preferably be type-specific or type-compatible. A unique pool number should be affixed to the final container, and electronic or manual records must document all units included in the pool. If whole-blood-derived platelets are pooled using an open system, the expiration is 4 hours from the start of pooling, with storage at 20-24 C. A commercial prestorage pooling bag is available, which allows for culture-based bacteria detection during the pooling process. Prestorage pools in this system maintain the expiration date of the oldest component in the pool (up to 5 days).

Reconstituted Red Blood Cells (RRBCs, often referred to as Reconstituted Whole Blood) are red cells to which plasma has been added. RRBCs can be stored at 1 to 6 C for 24 hours with an expiration date and time that corresponds to the earlier expiration date and time of the two components. Current FDA uniform labeling guidelines should be followed when labeling the RRBCs.[19] If modifiers apply they should be printed before the proper name (Reconstituted Red Blood Cells). For example, if the red cells were washed, the name of the product becomes Washed Reconstituted Red Blood Cells. Whether to label the RRBCs with a unique pool number or the donor identification number of the RBCs is a facility decision. Regardless of which labeling method is chosen, traceability of both the RBCs and plasma must be ensured. When creating a RRBC unit for neonatal exchange transfusion, the conventional approach by many facilities is to combine group O (Rh compatible with the neonate) RBCs and group AB FFP to achieve a 50% ± 5% hematocrit of the final product. The volumes of the two components, before pooling, can be adjusted to achieve a desired hematocrit level. Alternatively, sufficient plasma may be removed from RRBCs to achieve the desired final hematocrit. Table 9-3 provides information for the amount of plasma to remove for a given hematocrit of the whole blood.

Pooling of single CRYO components after thawing is accomplished in a similar manner as that used for platelets. A unique pool number should be affixed to the final container,

TABLE 9-3. Removing Plasma from Units of Whole Blood (to Prepare RBCs in Anticoagulant-Preservative with a Known Hematocrit)

Hematocrit of Segment from WB Unit (%)	Volume of Plasma to Be Removed (450-mL WB units)	Volume of Plasma to Be Removed (500-mL WB units)	Final Hematocrit of RBC Unit (%)
40	150	163	56
39	150	166	55
38	160	175	55
37	165	179	54
36	170	190	54
35	180	200	54
34	195	217	55
33	200	228	55

RBC = Red Blood Cells; WB = Whole Blood.

and electronic or manual records must document all units in the pool. The expiration date of pooled CRYO concentrates will depend on the method chosen for pooling. Open pooling systems have an expiration of 4 hours following pooling because the pooled component is stored at 20 to 24 C; thawed single concentrates and pooled concentrates using sterile connecting devices expire 6 hours from thawing and are stored at 20 to 24 C.

Volume Reduction of Platelets

Decreasing the supernatant substances of platelets (whole-blood-derived or apheresis platelets) may be clinically required to reduce the total transfusion volume to prevent transfusion-associated circulatory overload (TACO) or to partially remove incompatible ABO alloantibodies. Volume reduction performed using an open procedure reduces the expiration date of the platelets to 4 hours. If a sterile connection device is used, it is not necessary to impose the 4-hour expiration interval required for entered platelets, but the transfusion should be completed as soon as possible because of the minimal amount of plasma remaining in the component. Volume reduction may also be performed using a closed system (sterile connecting device). If a sterile connecting device is used, the transfusion should be completed as soon as possible because of the minimal amount of plasma remaining in the component. Volume-reduced platelets are stored at 20 to 24 C.

Platelet Gel

The term platelet "gel" (or platelet glue) is applied to products with a consistency of gelatin-like material, which is generated when thrombin and calcium are added to PRP.[20] Liquid supernatant from platelets that are activated by thrombin or damaged from a freeze-thaw cycle contains bioactive material, referred to as the "releasate." The gel matrix is able to retain bioactive substances produced from the trapped platelets, and these substances are slowly released from the gel. Platelet gel is used for oral and maxillofacial surgeries and also in reconstructive and orthopedic procedures.

Platelet gel and releasate are prepared at the bedside and are not stored for any length of time. The source of PRP could be allogeneic platelet concentrates from a blood bank, whole blood collected from the patient before the surgery, or the PRP prepared in the operating room immediately before or during surgery by automated instruments from whole blood or apheresis platelet collections. The ratio of PRP to the calcified thrombin varies from 5:1 to 10:1. Thrombin solution is prepared by dissolving 10,000 units of thrombin in 10 mL of 10% calcium chloride, which results in a thrombin concentration of 1000 U/mL.[21] In practice, up to 50 mL of PRP is needed for platelet gel preparation. Once calcified thrombin is added to the PRP, a firm gel is produced within 10 to 15 seconds and is used immediately. For firmer consistency, CRYO may be added to the above mixture.

Precise quality control criteria for platelet gels are not established but may include determining the platelet count of the PRP, measuring the strength of the clot generated, and analyzing the composition of the gel. The rate of in-vivo degradation of the gel may also be important. Viscoelastographic properties of platelet gel can be measured with thromboelastographs. With that approach, clots that are produced by varying concentrations of the thrombin showed similar viscoelastographic properties.[22] Facilities providing this component should refer to the current edition of the AABB *Standards for Perioperative Autologous Blood Collection and Administration* for guidance and quality assurance oversight in the manufacturing processes of platelet gel.

Aliquoting

Certain transfusion recipients requiring very-low-volume transfusion (eg, neonates) will necessitate aliquoting small volumes (10-30 mL) into syringes from the original unit. Use of a sterile connecting device and syringe set makes the process easy to perform (see Fig 9-1). A sterile connecting device may also be used to "split" primary blood containers into

One Aliquot (one syringe)

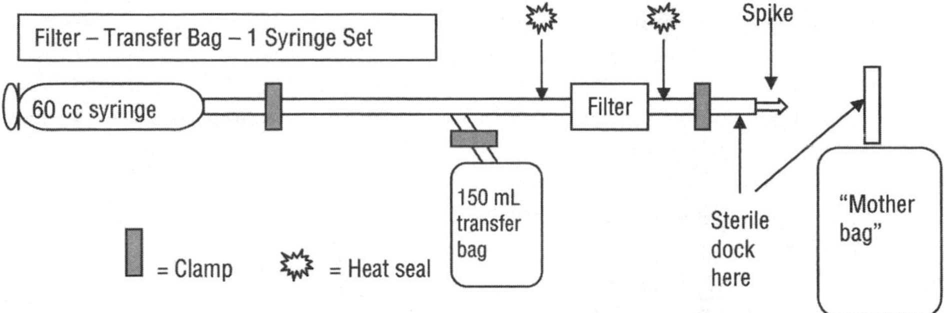

Two Aliquots (two syringes) Drawn at the Same Time

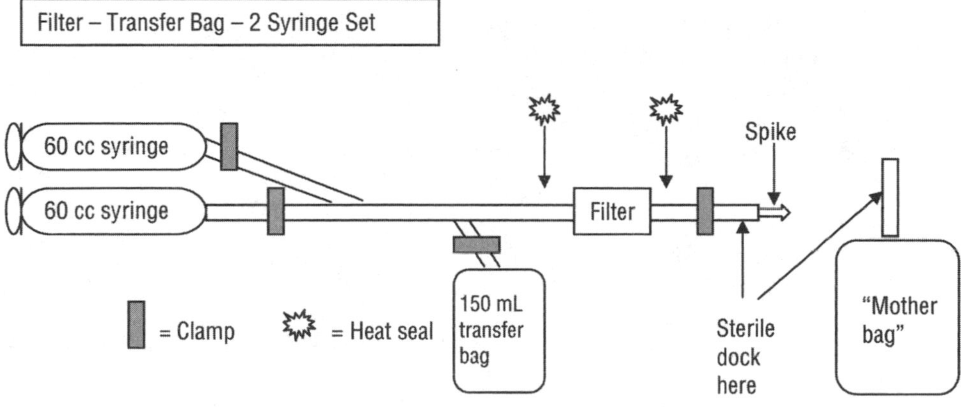

FIGURE 9-1. Schematic diagrams of syringe aliquoting devices. Single-syringe and double-syringe sets are depicted showing points of sterile welding to original container, points of clamping tubing for transferring component to transfer bag and then to the syringe (or syringes), and final heat sealing points before detaching from original component bag.

smaller transfer bags for larger recipients to minimize TACO. If a sterile connecting device is used to prepare the aliquot, the expiration date is dependent on the storage container used for the aliquot. Cellular components stored in syringes have an expiration of 4 hours, but if stored in an FDA-approved transfer bag, the expiration remains the same as that of the "mother" unit. After the aliquot is retrieved, the disposable needle is discarded; the syringe is capped and then dispensed to the newborn nursery in a plastic zippered bag. The syringe can be attached to an auto-syringe infusion pump to complete the transfusion within 4 hours of filling the syringe.

Divided RBC units are sometimes used for patients in whom extra fluid infusion causes concerns of fluid or cardiac overload. Patients with severe chronic anemia, overt heart failure, or moderate to severe renal failure may be candidates for transfusions of divided RBC units. Divided RBC and plasma units can be stored in the standard transfer containers and do not require specialized bags for their storage. However, such is not the case for storing divided platelet units. Storage properties of platelets are influenced by the plastic properties of the bag, the number of platelets in the bag, and the amount of plasma in which platelets are suspended. Therefore, split-platelet products should be stored in bags that are approved for platelet storage. Nonetheless, short-term (2 to 4 hours) storage of aliquots of apheresis platelets in standard polyvinyl chloride (PVC) plastic containers has been described. In the short term, approximately 30 to 60 mL of apheresis platelets that are aliquoted into 150-mL PVC bags seem to maintain acceptable metabolism.[23] Even during short storage intervals, platelets may adhere to the new containers, which can result in decreased numbers of platelets available for transfusion.[23]

Platelets derived from whole blood may be leukocyte reduced and then stored for up to 6 hours at 22 C in a 30-mL polypropylene syringe without agitation and will retain satisfactory in-vitro storage properties.[24] The 6-hour expiration time is acceptable for syringe aliquoting using a closed system. Between 12 and 30 mL of platelet concentrate can be stored in that manner in plastic syringes at room temperature (20-24 C) but not at 37 C (the temperature often used in isolette incubator beds in neonatal intensive care units).[24]

Aliquoting volumes multiple times from the primary container may be appropriate to minimize waste and to reduce donor exposure. The facility should have policies, processes, and procedures on the minimum threshold volume of the primary container after which the component may not be transfused as a "whole" unit.

Rejuvenation

The use of an FDA-licensed solution of pyruvate-inosine-phosphate-adenine (PIPA) has been shown to restore the decreased levels of 2,3-DPG and ATP to near-normal levels in stored red cells. This solution (Rejuvesol) has been licensed for use with citrate-phosphate-dextrose (CPD) and citrate-phosphate-dextrose-adenine-1 (CPDA-1) RBC units within 3 days after the expiration date of the original component[25] or at the 42-day expiration of CPD/additive solution (AS)-1.[26] Studies have shown that the addition of PIPA to CPD/AS-3 and CPD/AS-5 (although not licensed for this use) provides similar results.[27,28] The rejuvenated RBCs may be glycerolized and frozen for additional storage time (see Method 6-6). The thawed rejuvenated component must be deglycerolized before immediate transfusion or stored for up to 24 hours at 1 to 6 C. At the time of this writing, Rejuvesol is not available in the United States.

INSPECTION, SHIPPING, RECEIVING INTO INVENTORY, DISPOSITION, AND ISSUE

Inspection

A major critical control point in blood component manufacturing, on receipt from another facility, or before issue for transfusion is inspection of the component before disposition.[3(pp13,14,31-32,39)] Proper electronic or manual documentation of this process includes the following: 1) date of inspection, 2) donor identifying number, 3) description of any visual abnormalities, 4) action taken, and 5) identity of the staff performing the inspection. Any questionable component inspection requires the component to be quarantined until final disposition is determined.

Visible abnormalities may include segments appearing lighter or darker in color than the primary bag contents, purple color to the red cells, clots, white particulate matter in the primary container, supernatant fluid that is discolored from normal appearance, gross lipemia, and foreign objects in the primary container or ports. Green-colored plasma resulting from increased α_2 globulin (ceruloplasmin) associated with birth-control pills is not considered a reason for quarantine[29] but should be distinguished from a green color caused by bacterial contamination (eg, *Pseudomonas* species) or a green-brown color associated with liver or pancreatic disease. A conservative approach would be to quarantine or return to the blood supplier those components that have questionable color.

Current requirements for screening platelet components for bacteria should reduce the possibility of moderate or severe bacterial contamination. Other components that appear suspect should be quarantined and cultured. Positive cultures may be related to the donor's arm (eg, scarring, skin disease such as psoriasis), donor arm preparation, contamination during microbiology processing, handling or pooling of the component, or infection in the donor. If it is determined that a bacterially contaminated component exists, then the component manufacturer should be notified so an immediate investigation can take place. Other components prepared from that collection should be quarantined until the investigation is completed. If the component has been transfused, the recipient's attending physician should be informed, and consultation with the medical director is recommended.

Shipping

Validation of all shipping or transport containers is required before they are placed into use. The containers must be able to maintain the proper transport temperature that is appropriate for the component. Shipping transit time, mode of transport, climatic conditions to which the container may have been exposed, presence of residual wet or dry ice upon receipt, appearance of the component(s), and expiration date of the component(s) should be evaluated. Any deviation from routine shipping or component conditions should be reported to the shipping facility and documented according to each location's policies, processes, and procedures. Similar evaluation of blood components transported between blood centers, between hospitals, and between blood centers and hospitals should be performed by the receiving facility.

Whole Blood, RBCs, and Plasma Products (After Thawing)

Whole Blood, RBCs, and plasma products (after thawing) must be transported at a temperature of 1 to 10 C. Bagged wet ice, commercial cooling packs, or specially designed containers may be used to maintain acceptable transport temperatures. In order to avoid hemolysis, the Whole Blood, RBCs, and segments should never come into direct contact with the bagged ice or cooling pack.

Blood components transported at 1 to 10 C or stored at 1 to 6 C may need to be removed from those temperatures for manipulation (eg, entering into inventory, irradiating). The maximum number of units that can be manipulated before the component reaches a temperature greater than 10 C should be determined and not exceeded. Validation of this process may be accomplished using manual temperature monitoring indicators affixed to the blood components, or electronic devices that can measure the temperature of the blood components without entering the bag.

Platelets, Thawed CRYO, and Granulocytes

Platelets, thawed CRYO, and granulocytes must be transported at a temperature of 20 to 24 C. Well-insulated containers with appropriate coolant are recommended. If the transit time will be >24 hours for platelet shipment or if extreme climate conditions are anticipated, then double-insulated containers or room-temperature coolant bags should be used.

Frozen Components

Frozen components should be packaged to minimize breakage and to maintain the components in a frozen state. Dry ice in a suitable container is routinely used for shipping these components. The amount of dry ice is dependent on the container, the distance for transport, and the ambient temperature that will be encountered. The dry ice may be layered by starting on the bottom of the container and then spreading a layer of dry ice over each component layer, ending with dry ice on the top of the final component layer.

Receiving into Inventory and Disposition

The receiving facility should notify the shipping facility of any deviation from normal appearance of the shipped blood components or absence of wet or dry ice. Documentation of the abnormal condition should be performed according to each facility's policies, processes, and procedures. Any blood component not meeting the facility's policies, processes, and procedures should be physically and, if applicable, electronically quarantined. Only after investigation of the deviation and determination that the component meets acceptable criteria may the component be removed from quarantine and released into the general blood inventory.

Tracking the disposition of blood and blood components is required from collection to either transfusion or discard. Electronic or manual records should be generated indicating compliance with policies, processes, and procedures. Any deviation is recorded, and blood components not meeting requirements should be quarantined or discarded as biohazardous material. Deviations are investigated to determine possible corrective actions, and results of the corrective action are reported to the blood supplier as needed. Inventory management should consist of routine determination that all blood components have been disposed of properly and that there are no "lost products."

Additionally, policies, processes, and procedures for hospital transfusion services must include ABO retyping before transfusion of red cell components and Rh typing of RBC units labeled as Rh negative (confirmatory testing for weak D is not required).[3(p33)] Granulocytes must also be ABO retyped, and Rh retyped if labeled as Rh negative (confirmatory testing for weak D is not required), because this component contains 20 to 50 mL of red cells.

Inventory

A sufficient number of ABO- and Rh-compatible units should be placed into inventory for each patient who might need blood. Planning for adequate blood and blood component inventory depends on using surgical blood order schedules that are set to meet the anticipated transfusion requirements of at least 90% of the patients undergoing the scheduled surgeries. The blood bank should maintain a reserve of ABO-compatible RBCs, should have a reliable emergency blood delivery system from its blood supplier, and should prepare for the unexpected, because blood loss can significantly exceed what is expected in an individual patient as well as in the case of mass casualties. Drills to simulate unexpected situations with massive blood usage in hemorrhage, disaster, or both should be carried out periodically (see Chapter 4).

Routine Surgical Blood Orders

Blood ordering levels for common elective procedures can be developed from previous records of blood use. Because surgical requirements vary among institutions, routine blood orders should be based on local transfusion utilization patterns. The surgeons, the anesthesiologists, and the medical director of transfusion services should all agree on the number of units required for each procedure. Transfusion medicine practices should always be supported by current transfusion medicine guidelines published in peer-reviewed journals. Routine blood order schedules (also called maximum surgical blood order schedules, or MSBOS) are successful when there is cooperation and confidence among the professionals involved in setting and using the guidelines.[30] Once a surgical blood ordering schedule has been established, the transfusion service routinely crossmatches the predetermined number of units for each patient undergoing the designated procedures. Routine orders may need to be modified for patients with anemia, bleeding disorders, or other conditions in which increased blood use is anticipated. As with other circumstances that require rapid availability of blood, the transfusion service staff should be prepared to provide additional blood if the need arises.

Labeling of Blood and Blood Components with the Recipient's Information

The following activities are required at the time of issue[3(pp38,39)]:

- A tag or label indicating the recipient's two independent identifiers, the donation identification number, and the compatibility test interpretation (if performed) must be attached securely to the blood container.
- A final check of records maintained in the blood bank for each unit of blood or component must include the following:

  1. Two independent identifiers, one of which is usually the patient's name.
  2. The recipient's ABO group and Rh type.
  3. The donation identification number.
  4. Donor's ABO group and, if required, Rh type.
  5. The interpretation of the crossmatch tests (if performed).
  6. The date and time of issue.
  7. Special transfusion requirements (eg, cytomegalovirus reduced-risk, irradiated, or antigen-negative components).
  8. Expiration date and, if applicable, time.

- A process must exist to confirm that the identifying information, the request, the records, and the blood or component are all in agreement and that any and all discrepancies have been resolved before issue.

Additional records that may be useful include those that identify the person issuing the blood, the person to whom the blood was issued, and the destination of the unit. After the transfusion, a record of the transfusion shall be made a part of the patient's medical record. That information may be part of a computer record or a paper form. Records must contain the identification of the person(s) performing the testing and, if blood is issued before the resolution of compatibility problems, the final status of the serologic findings. Before issuing a unit of blood or component, personnel must inspect the blood or component to ensure that it is acceptable for use, that it does not have an abnormal color or appearance, that its container is not leaking, and that it is not outdated. Final identification of the transfusion recipient and the component rests with the transfusionist, who identifies the patient and donor unit and who certifies that identifying information on forms, tags, and labels is in agreement.

Transfusion Service Issuing of Components

Ensuring that the correct blood component is being issued to the correct patient is paramount in preventing a transfusion mishap. Systems should be in place, either electronic or manual processes, to check the recipient's name and another patient identifier, the recipient's blood type, the component's unique unit number, the component's blood type and expiration date, the crossmatch status or other serologic information (eg, cytomegalovirus antibody-negative). There should be documentation of visual inspection, the time and date of issue, and the person (or location if sending by pneumatic tube) to whom (or where) it is issued. When the component is issued to an individual, that individual should conduct a second check on the correctness of the component information (label, computer or manual log information) and manually provide a signature or use an electronic badge or personnel identification number. If all checks are correct, the unit may be issued.

Issue of a component to more than one patient at any one time is not recommended; issue of multiple components for multiple patients at any one time is also not recommended. If more components for immediate transfusion are required, use of a validated cooler is an acceptable alternative to help prevent component-recipient mix-ups before transfusion.

Blood Administered in Urgent Situations

When blood is urgently needed, the patient's physician must weigh the risk of transfusing uncrossmatched or partially crossmatched blood against the risk of delaying transfusion until compatibility testing is complete. Ideally, a transfusion service physician should provide consultation. The risk that the transfused unit might be incompatible may be judged to be less than the risk of depriving the patient of oxygen-carrying capacity during that transfusion. (See Chapter 20.)

When blood is released before pretransfusion testing is complete, the records must contain a signed statement from the requesting physician indicating that the clinical situation was sufficiently urgent to require release of blood.[3(p40)] Such a statement does not need to be obtained before issuing lifesaving transfusions, nor does it absolve blood bank personnel from their responsibility to issue properly labeled donor blood that is ABO compatible with the patient. When urgent release is requested, transfusion service personnel should take the following actions:

1. Issue uncrossmatched blood:
   a. Use group O RBCs if the patient's ABO group is unknown. It is preferable to give D-negative blood if the recipient's D type is unknown, especially if the patient is a female of childbearing potential. In massive transfusion cases many facilities will routinely provide D-positive RBCs to adult males and all females greater than 50 years of age.
   b. Issue ABO- and Rh-compatible blood if there has been time to test a current specimen.
2. Indicate in a conspicuous fashion on the attached tag or label that compatibility testing was *not* completed at the time of issue.
3. Begin compatibility tests and complete them promptly (for massive transfusion, see below). If incompatibility is detected at any stage of testing, the patient's physician and the transfusion service medical director should be notified immediately.

Massive Transfusion

There are several different definitions of massive transfusion. In this chapter, massive transfusion is defined either as the administration of 8 to 10 RBC units to an adult patient in less than 24 hours, or as the acute administration of 4 to 5 RBC units in 1 hour. Exchange transfusion of an infant is also considered a massive transfusion.

Following massive transfusion, the pretransfusion specimen no longer represents the blood currently in the patient's circulation. If possible, in the massive transfusion setting, an abbreviated crossmatch such as a computer crossmatch or an IS crossmatch should be performed to confirm ABO compatibility of units administered. If a more limited pretransfusion testing protocol is used in these situations, the protocol should be described in a written procedure.

Some facilities stop crossmatching RBC units (and routinely issue uncrossmatched RBCs) as soon as a patient has received 10 RBC units in less than 24 hours. These facilities justify the practice by stating that most of the circulating blood has been diluted with transfused blood and any antibodies capable of causing a hemolytic reaction have also been diluted.

Blood Administration After Non-Group-Specific Transfusion

Transfusion services must sometimes release group O RBC units for transfusion during emergencies before a pretransfusion specimen is received in the laboratory. Once a specimen is received, the patient's ABO group and Rh type can be quickly determined, and group-specific components can begin to be released. Group O AS-1, AS-3, and AS-5 RBC units contain minimal residual plasma, which minimizes concerns regarding passive transfusion of anti-A and anti-B. In this case, switching to ABO-identical RBC components can be done safely, although an occasional patient may exhibit a transient positive direct antiglobulin test. In some cases, when large volumes of red cells are transfused, or when small children or infants receive transfusions, passively acquired ABO antibodies may be detected in the patient's serum/plasma.[31] If that should occur, transfusion with red cells that lack the corresponding ABO antigen should be continued. If a patient receives blood of an Rh type different from his or her own, it may become difficult to determine the patient's true Rh type. If there is any question about the patient's true Rh type, it may be prudent to administer D-negative blood, especially if the patient is a female of childbearing potential. The use of Rh Immune Globulin prophylaxis may be considered when D-positive components are transfused to D-negative patients. (See Chapter 20.)

Return of Blood Components and Reissue

The transfusion service may receive back into the blood component inventory those units that meet acceptance specifications. These conditions include the following:

1. The primary container has not been entered.
2. The component has been maintained at the appropriate temperature.
3. At least one sealed segment remains integrally attached to the container of RBCs.
4. Documentation is made indicating that the component has been inspected and is acceptable for reissue.

If individual unit temperature indicators or temperature reading devices are not being used, or if the blood components are not being returned in validated transport containers, acceptable time frames for returning blood components to inventory should be validated by individual facilities. The validation should demonstrate that for the defined period the appropriate temperature of the blood component can be maintained.

Platelets returned to the transfusion service after issue may be placed back into inventory following a visual inspection of the component, providing the component has not been out of agitation for longer than 24 hours. The presence of swirling platelets in the platelet bag correlates with pH values and is one criterion for adequate platelet in-vivo viability.[32] The platelet bag can be held in front of a light source and gently squeezed to check the "swirling" appearance of the platelets. If "swirling" is evident and there is no visible clumping of the platelets, they may be returned into inventory.

Documentation of all acceptable or unacceptable conditions must be carried out. Depending on the criterion not met, the component may be either placed in quarantine for further investigation or discarded in a biohazard container. If the component is accepted, it may be returned to the general blood inventory and reissued.

KEY POINTS

1. Temperature requirements during transport of blood or blood components differ from those of storage. The Food and Drug Administration considers coolers used to store blood and components in the operating room to be a storage situation. It is recommended that all red cell transport containers be validated to maintain a temperature of 1 to 6 C for a specified period to meet the requirements for Red Blood Cells (RBCs).
2. At the end of their 24-hour shelf life as Fresh Frozen Plasma (FFP) (thawed) and Plasma Frozen Within 24 Hours After Phlebotomy (PF24) (thawed), these components can be converted to Thawed Plasma (with an additional 4 days before expiration) as long as they were originally collected in closed systems. If they were collected in an open system, they cannot be converted to Thawed Plasma.
3. Thawed Cryoprecipitated AHF (CRYO) in an open system or pool expires 4 hours from thawing. Thawed CRYO as a single unit or pooled before storage or after thawing using a sterile connection device expires 6 hours from thawing.
4. Reconstituted Red Blood Cells (RRBCs, often referred to as Reconstituted Whole Blood) refers to red cells to which plasma has been added. Whether to label the RRBCs with a unique pool number or the donor identification number of the RBCs is a facility decision. Regard-

less of which labeling method is chosen, traceability of both the RBCs and plasma must be ensured.

5. Divided RBC and plasma units can be stored in the standard transfer containers and do not require specialized bags for their storage. However, such is not the case for storing divided platelet units. Split-platelet products should be stored in bags that are approved for platelet storage. Short-term (2 to 4 hours) storage of aliquots of apheresis platelets in standard polyvinyl chloride plastic containers has been described.
6. Blood components transported at 1 to 10 C or stored at 1 to 6 C may need to be removed from those temperatures for manipulation (eg, entering into inventory, irradiating). The maximum number of units that can be manipulated before the component reaches a temperature greater than 10 C should be determined and not exceeded. Validation of this process may be accomplished using manual temperature monitoring indicators affixed to the blood components or electronic devices that can measure the temperature of the blood components without entering the bag.
7. Acceptable time frames for returning blood components to inventory after issue should be validated by individual facilities if individual unit temperature indicators or temperature reading devices are not being used or if the blood components are not being returned in validated transport containers, The validation should demonstrate that for the defined time period, the appropriate temperature of the blood component can be maintained.

REFERENCES

1. Food and Drug Administration. Drugs; current good manufacturing practice in manufacture, processing, packing, or holding. Docket No. 63-6336. (June 19, 1963) Fed Regist 1963;133: 6385-7.
2. Code of federal regulations. Title 21, CFR Parts 210 and 211. Washington, DC: US Government Printing Office, 2010 (revised annually).
3. Carson TH, ed. Standards for blood banks and transfusion services. 27th ed. Bethesda, MD: AABB, 2011.
4. Clarification offered for storage versus transport of blood components in monitored coolers. AABB Weekly Report 2006;12:4-5.
5. Beutler E. Red cell metabolism and storage. In: Anderson KC, Ness PM, eds. Scientific basis of transfusion medicine. Philadelphia: WB Saunders, 1994:188-202.
6. Heaton A, Keegan T, Holme S. In vivo regeneration of red cell 2,3-diphosphoglycerate following transfusion of DPG-depleted AS-1, AS-3, and CPDA-1 red cells. Br J Haematol 1989;71:131-6.
7. Strauss GS. Additive solutions and product age in neonatal blood transfusions. In: Hermann JH, Manno CS, eds. Pediatric transfusion therapy. Bethesda, MD: AABB Press, 2002:131-9.
8. Vassallo R. Preparation, preservation, and storage of platelet concentrates. In: Simon TL, Snyder EL, Solheim B, et al, eds. Rossi's principles of transfusion medicine. 4th ed. Bethesda, MD: AABB Press, 2009:187-98.
9. Zimrin AB, Hess JR. Current issues to the transfusion of red blood cells. Vox Sang 2009; 96:93-103.
10. Brumit MC, Hay SN, Brecher ME. Bacteria detection. In: Brecher ME, ed. Bacterial and parasitic contamination of blood components. Bethesda, MD: AABB Press, 2003:57-82.
11. Beaudoin J. Baxter collaborates with Gambro BCT on 7-day platelet study to speed adoption (press release). (May 17, 2006) Deerfield, IL: Baxter Healthcare, 2006.
12. Downes KA, Wilson E, Yomtovian R, Sarode R. Serial measurement of clotting factors in thawed plasma stored for 5 days (letter). Transfusion 2001;41:570.
13. AABB, American Red Cross, and America's Blood Centers. Circular of information for the use of human blood and blood components. Bethesda, MD: AABB, 2009.
14. Werhli G, Taylor NE, Haines, AL, et al. Instituting a thawed plasma procedure: It just makes sense and saves cents. Transfusion 2009;49: 2625-30.
15. Caudill JSC, Nichols WL, Plumhoff EA, et al. Comparison of coagulation Factor XIII content

and concentration in cryoprecipitate and fresh-frozen plasma. Transfusion 2008;49:765-70.
16. Calhoun L. Blood product preparation and administration. In: Petz LD, Swisher SN, Kleinman S, et al, eds. Clinical practice of transfusion medicine. 3rd ed. New York: Churchill Livingstone, 1996:305-33.
17. Leukocyte reduction. Association bulletin #99-07. Bethesda, MD: AABB, 1999.
18. Meryman HT, Hornblower M. A method for freezing and washing RBCs using a high glycerol concentration. Transfusion 1972;12:145-56.
19. Food and Drug Administration. Guidance: Industry consensus standard for the uniform labeling of blood and blood components using ISBT 128 version 2.0.0, November 2005. (September 22, 2006) Rockville, MD: CBER Office of Communication, Outreach, and Development, 2006.
20. Borzini P, Mazzucco L. Platelet gels and releasates. Curr Opin Hematol 2005;12:473-9.
21. Wajon P, Gibson J, Calcroft R, et al. Intraoperative plateletpheresis and autologous platelet gel do not reduce chest tube drainage or allogeneic blood transfusion after reoperative coronary artery bypass graft. Anesth Analg 2001; 93:536-42.
22. Ellis WC, Cassidy LK, Finney AS, et al. Thromboelastograph (TEG) analysis of platelet gel formed with different thrombin concentrations. J Extra Corpor Technol 2005;37:52-7.
23. Strasser EF, Stachel DK, Schwarzkopf P, et al. Platelet function in variable platelet split products intended for neonatal transfusion. Transfusion 2006;46:757-65.
24. Pisciotto PT, Snyder EL, Snyder JA, et al. In vitro characteristics of white-cell-reduced single-unit platelet concentrates stored in syringes. Transfusion 1994;34:407-11.
25. Valeri CR, Zaroules CG. Rejuvenation and freezing of outdated stored human red cells. N Engl J Med 1972;287:1307-13.
26. Szymanski IO, Teno RA, Lockwood W, et al. Effect of rejuvenation and frozen storage on 42-day AS-1 red cells. Transfusion 2001;41:550-5.
27. Lockwood WB, Hudgens RW, Symanski IO, et al. Effects of rejuvenation and frozen storage on 42-day-old AS-3 RBCs. Transfusion 2003; 43:1527-32.
28. Valeri CR, Pivacek LE, Cassidy GP, Ragno G. The survival, function, and hemolysis of human RBCs stored at 4 C in additive solution (AS-1, AS-3, or AS-5) for 42 days and then biochemically modified, frozen, thawed, washed, and stored at 4 C in sodium chloride and glucose solution for 24 hours. Transfusion 2000; 40:1341-5.
29. Elkassabany NM, Meny GM, Doria MT, Marcucci C. Green plasma-revisited. Anesthesiology 2008;108:764-5.
30. Boral LI, Dannemiller FJ, Standard W, et al. A guideline for anticipated blood usage during elective surgical procedures. Am J Clin Pathol 1979;71:680-4.
31. Garratty G. Problems associated with passively transfused blood group antibodies. Am J Clin Pathol 1998;109:169-77.
32. Bertoloni F, Murphy S. A multicenter inspection of the swirling phenomenon in platelet concentrates prepared in routine practice. Transfusion 1996;36:128-32.

Chapter 10

Molecular Biology and Immunology in Transfusion Medicine

James C. Zimring, MD, PhD, and Steven L. Spitalnik, MD

THIS CHAPTER DESCRIBES the fundamental principles for analyzing deoxyribonucleic acid (DNA), ribonucleic acid (RNA), and protein. In transfusion medicine, these techniques are used to 1) detect infectious pathogens, 2) determine genotype and phenotype of red cell antigens, 3) detect and identify red cell and platelet antibodies, 4) determine HLA type, and 5) perform relationship testing. In addition to the principles behind these analyses, potential problems with the assay systems that may lead to erroneous results are described. Also addressed are the basic mechanisms by which the immune system initiates a response to foreign antigens, as well as the effector mechanisms by which immunity eliminates infectious pathogens and foreign cells. Entire textbooks have been written to describe these processes, and it is outside the scope of this chapter to provide a detailed and comprehensive explanation of them. Instead, the focus is on topics immediately relevant to transfusion serology and, moreover, predominantly on humoral immunity, because cellular immunity is thus far of unknown consequence in transfusion medicine and only seldom of consequence in the pathophysiology of hemolytic transfusion reactions. Specific assay protocols are not provided. Rather, this chapter conveys a detailed understanding of the scientific principles underlying the molecular biology and immunologic assays used in transfusion medicine.

NUCLEIC ACID ANALYSIS

The utility of nucleic acid analysis in transfusion medicine lies in detecting infectious pathogens and genotyping blood donors and recipients. The human genome is encoded in polymers of DNA. Likewise, many pathogens use DNA to encode their genome. In addition, multiple viral pathogens encode their genome as RNA. With the possible exception of prion-

James C. Zimring, MD, PhD, Associate Professor, Emory University Hospital, Atlanta, Georgia, and Steven L. Spitalnik, MD, Professor of Pathology and Cell Biology, and Director of Clinical Laboratories, Columbia University, New York, New York

J. Zimring has disclosed a financial relationship with Immucor Inc. S. Spitalnik has disclosed no conflicts of interest.

associated disorders, either DNA or RNA encodes all genetic material relevant to transfusion medicine.

Basic Chemistry and Structure of Nucleic Acids

DNA is a nucleic acid polymer, which consists of long chains of nucleotides linked together.[1] The general structure of a nucleotide consists of a pentose (a carbohydrate with 5 carbon atoms), a phosphate group attached to carbon number 5 (designated C5) of the pentose, and a base group attached to C1 [Fig 10-1(A)]. Variation in the chemistry of the base group gives rise to the four different nucleotides that compose DNA, the purines (adenine and guanine) and the pyrimidines (cytosine and thymine). In addition, C3 of the pentose is modified by a hydroxyl group [Fig 10-1(A)]. The individual nucleotides form DNA polymers when the phosphate group on C5 of one nucleic acid forms a covalent bond with the free hydroxyl group on C3 of another nucleic acid [Fig 10-1(B)]. DNA molecules vary from each other based on the sequence of nucleotides that are incorporated into the strand. Each strand of DNA has a terminal 5 end, which contains a free phosphate (attached to C5), and a termi-

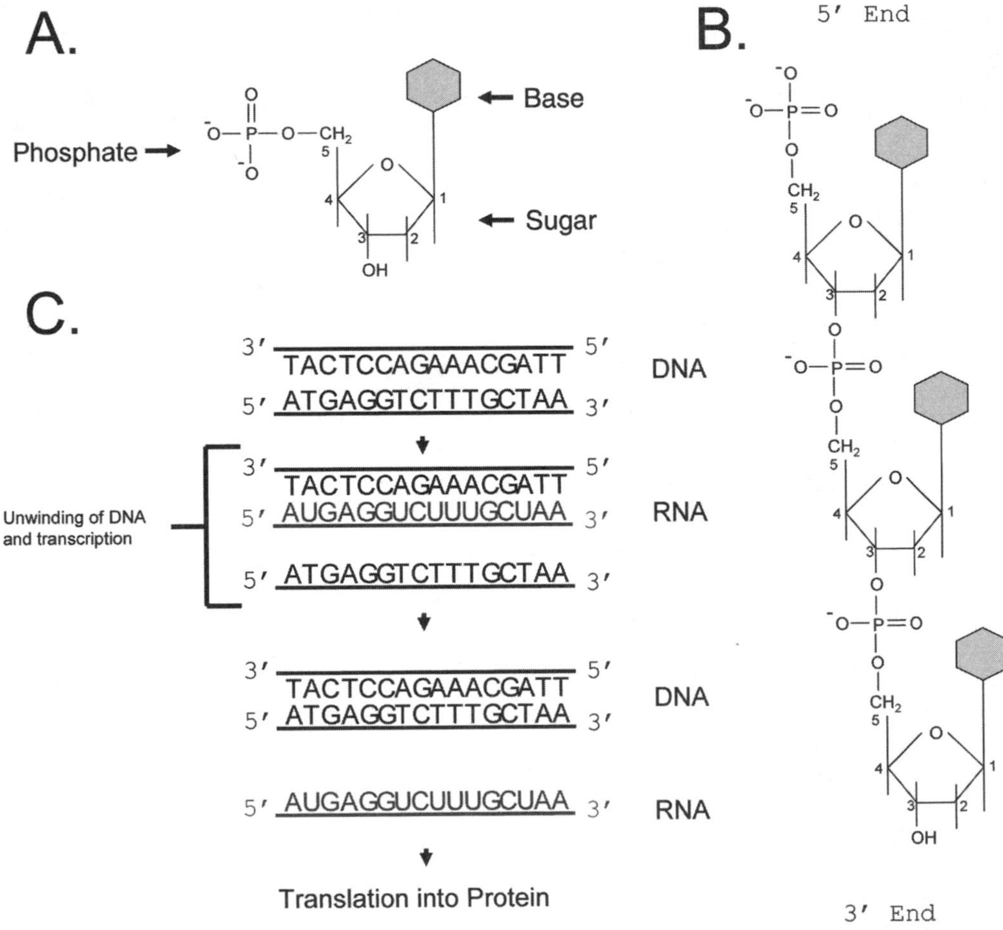

FIGURE 10-1. Chemical structure of nucleic acids and DNA.

nal 3 end, which has a free hydroxyl group (attached to C3).

The human genome consists of double-stranded DNA. The bases contained within a single strand of DNA have the ability to form hydrogen bonds to complementary bases on another strand of DNA. In particular, thymidine binds to adenine, and guanine binds to cytosine. When two strands have complementary sequences, they can hybridize to each other to form a double-stranded molecule [Fig 10-1(C)]. The strands hybridize such that the 5 and 3 ends of complementary molecules are in opposite orientation and form a double helix in which the phosphodiester backbone is on the outside and the hydrogen-bond paired bases are on the inside.

When individual human genes are expressed, the DNA encoding a given gene is transcribed into RNA [Fig 10-1(C)]. The structure of RNA is similar to DNA, with the following exceptions: 1) individual ribonucleotides (see the description of nucleic acids above) have an additional hydroxyl group on C2 of the pentose sugar (thus forming ribose), 2) uracil takes the place of thymine, and 3) RNA is typically single stranded. Several different classes of RNA exist in human cells; the specific type described in this paragraph, which is subsequently translated into protein, is messenger RNA (mRNA). When a gene is expressed, the transcription machinery unwinds the DNA double helix, synthesizes an RNA strand of complementary sequence to the transcribed DNA strand, and rehybridizes the DNA in its wake [Fig 10-1(C)]. In this way, the RNA is essentially a copy of the sequence found in the DNA. RNA is synthesized only in the 5 to 3 direction, and thus only a single strand of the DNA is transcribed into RNA. After synthesis in the nucleus, the RNA is processed and exported to the cytoplasm, where ribosomes translate the RNA into protein.

Isolation of Nucleic Acids

The first step in most DNA and RNA analyses is the isolation of nucleic acids. All nucleated cells of an individual contain essentially identical genomic DNA, with some notable exceptions (eg, rearranged genes in mature T and B cells). Thus, for most analyses genomic DNA can be isolated from readily obtainable sources, such as peripheral blood leukocytes and buccal swabs. However, mRNA types are distinct in different cell populations because their expression patterns are important in defining the phenotype of those cells. For mRNA analysis then, the choice of starting cell type is critical. Several manufacturers offer reagents that simplify and expedite isolation of cellular DNA and/or mRNA and help purify virus-associated nucleic acids from plasma. Depending on the type of analysis that will be performed, the quality of the resulting nucleic acids—based on the relative purity of DNA or RNA—and the absence of contaminating proteins may be important.

Hybridization-Based Methods of Nucleic Acid Detection

Before the advent of techniques that allowed the amplification of a specific nucleic acid sequence (see below), detection of nucleic acids was dependent on hybridization-based methods. Probes with a particular sequence of nucleotides were synthesized and were labeled with one of a variety of detectable markers. Such a probe could then hybridize to complementary sequences of DNA or RNA on the basis of the hydrogen-bonding effect described above. This approach provided the ability to both detect and quantify the targets to which the probe hybridized. It could be performed in either the solid phase (ie, Southern[2] and Northern blots[3]) or the fluid phase (ie, RNAse protection assay[4] or S1 protection assay[5]) or as a result of enzymatic extension (ie, primer extension assay).

Compared to amplification-based techniques, hybridization-based methods have limited sensitivity. When abundant sample is available, such as in genotyping an individual from whom one can obtain reasonably large amounts of blood, these techniques are quite adequate. However, because the amount of virus or bacteria that constitutes an infectious inoculum is far below the limits of hybridization-based detection, such methods are insufficient for screening donors and donor products for infectious microbes. In addition, hybridization-based methods are less amenable to automation than amplification methods. Therefore, although hybridization-based methods are quite useful in the basic research setting and still play a minor role in some diagnostic laboratories, most diagnostic analyses of nucleic acids are carried out by amplification-based methods.

The Polymerase Chain Reaction

Nucleic acid detection, analysis, and molecular engineering were revolutionized by the invention of the polymerase chain reaction (PCR). PCR, initially described by Mullis and Faloona,[6] was the first amplification-based technique for analyzing nucleic acids. In addition to the widespread use of PCR itself, the use of amplification-based systems has grown to include multiple other techniques and applications (detailed below). As a result of the overwhelming impact of PCR on molecular biology and molecular diagnostics, Mullis was awarded the Nobel Prize in chemistry in 1993.

A PCR consists of the following components: 1) a DNA sample to be analyzed, 2) gene-specific primers, 3) a thermostable DNA polymerase, and 4) the required components that allow the DNA polymerase to enzymatically synthesize DNA, such as individual nucleotide building blocks and the proper salts and buffer. The PCR is then subjected to a heating and cooling procedure called thermocycling, which allows DNA amplification to occur. This reaction is carried out in an instrument called a thermocycler, which can rapidly change temperature with great accuracy and precision. The general order of the thermocycling reaction is 1) melting, 2) primer annealing, and 3) extension. This procedure is continued for multiple cycles, typically 20 to 40 depending on the abundance of the template and the required sensitivity of the assay.

An overview of the PCR process is presented in Fig 10-2. The example presented begins with a single copy of a double-stranded DNA template. The DNA is denatured by heating to near boiling temperatures (typically 94-95 C), which disrupts the hydrogen bonds between complementary bases, thereby separating the two strands. The temperature is then lowered (annealing reaction) to allow gene-specific primers to anneal to their complementary target. Typically an annealing temperature of 5 C below the melting temperature of the primers increases their specificity to the correct target sequence. The exact melting temperature of a given primer will depend upon its length, the abundance of guanines and cytosines in the sequence (ie, GC content), and any mismatches with the target. At this point, the temperature is raised to the optimal temperature at which the DNA polymerase can function enzymatically (typically 72 C), and the primers are extended along the length of the DNA by the incorporation of the correct complementary nucleotides. Consequently, at the end of extension there are two copies of the DNA. This process repeats itself with denaturing, annealing, and extension, and with each subsequent cycle, an exponential increase in DNA copy number occurs. PCR results in a geometric expansion of a selected DNA "amplicon," defined as the sequence that is flanked by the two chosen primers.

In actuality, PCR is typically carried out on complex mixtures of long nucleic acids (eg, chromosomes isolated from human cells). In this case, a slightly more complicated series of events at the beginning lead to the synthesis and amplification of the desired amplicon (Fig 10-3). Two primers are used that flank the desired region to be amplified and that bind to opposite strands in opposite orientations (Fig 10-3, cycle 1C). Using the primer as a starting point, the DNA polymerase then extends in the 5 to 3 direction. In the first cycle, this extension will continue as long as the polymerase is allowed to continue synthesizing DNA (genomic extension). In the second cycle, the genomic extension products are once again melted, and annealing is allowed to take place (cycle 2E). In addition to priming a second round of genomic extension by priming the original genomic DNA, this also results in priming of the previous genomic extension products. The new DNA synthesized off the genomic extension from the first cycle results in

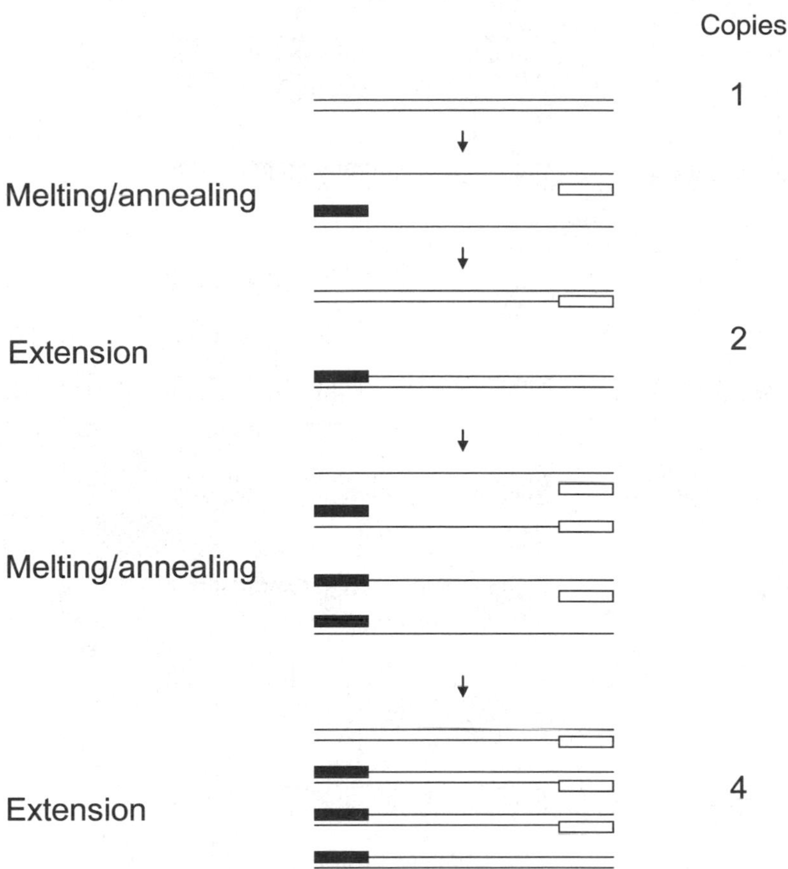

FIGURE 10-2. Graphical overview of the polymerase chain reaction.

a smaller piece of DNA (the amplicon), which is flanked on each end by the gene-specific primers. Because the amplicon has two strands, each of which gives rise to a new amplicon with each cycle, the amplicon undergoes a geometric amplification with subsequent rounds of thermocycling, as described above in Fig 10-2.

Problems with PCR

Although PCR is a robust and reliable method of detecting nucleic acids, as with all methods, there are technical problems that can affect PCR and other amplification-based technologies.

SPECIMEN PROCESSING AND TEMPLATE DEGRADATION. DNA is a stable chemical entity that can withstand various conditions before processing. However, as with all analytes, attention must be paid to proper specimen transport, processing, and storage. In the case of amplification techniques that detect RNA, sample integrity is much more of a concern, as RNA is far less stable than DNA and is susceptible to autocatalytic destruction and degradation by RNAse enzymes found in many biologic specimens.

INHIBITORS. Because the PCR amplification process depends on the enzymatic activity of a DNA polymerase, PCR can be inhibited by any substance that negatively affects synthesis by DNA polymerase. For example, heparin found in clinical specimens can inhibit PCR in some situations.[7] In addition, hemoglobin or lactoferrin, released from erythrocytes or leukocytes, can also inhibit PCR.[8] Most analytic sys-

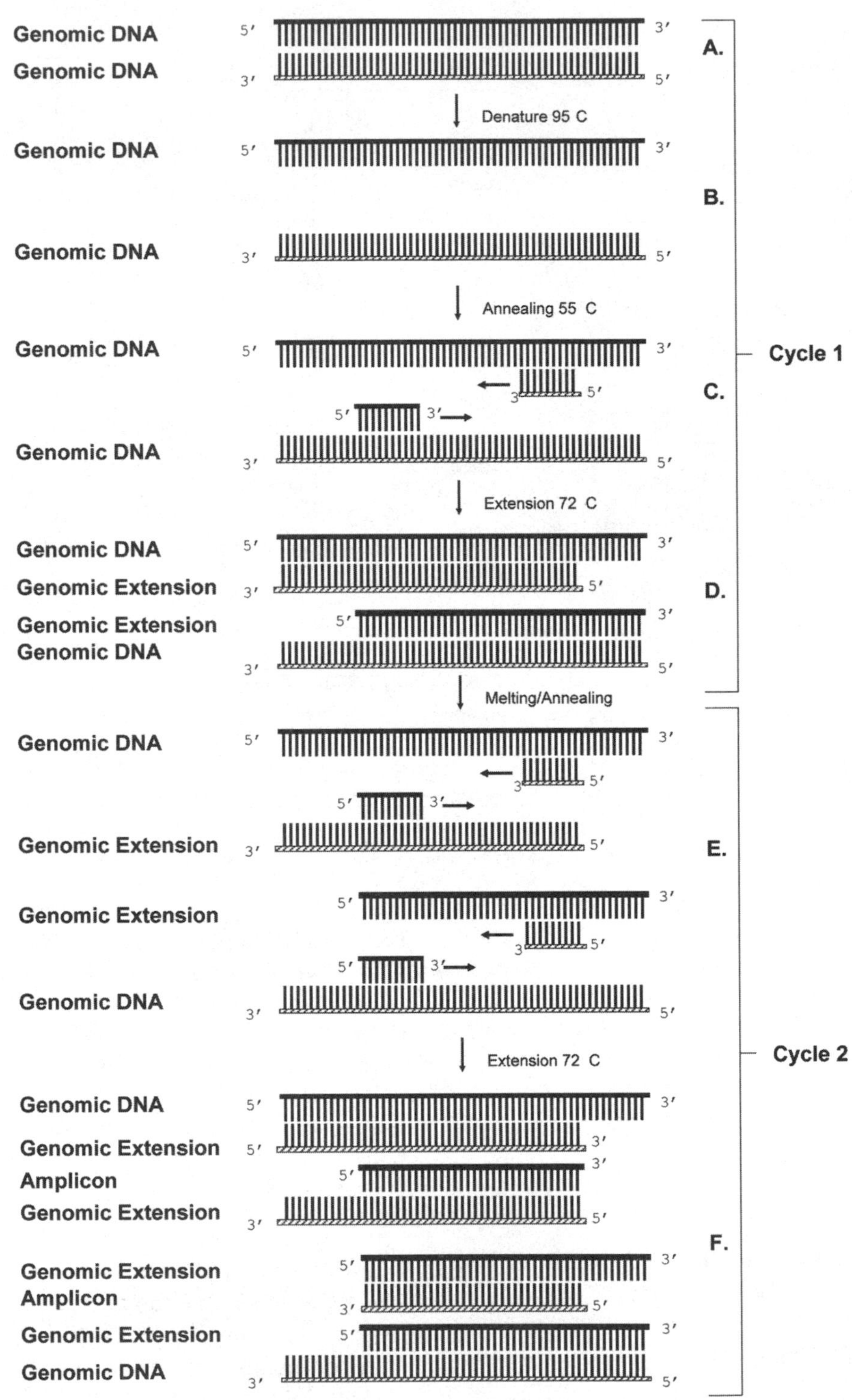

FIGURE 10-3. Detailed representation of initial cycles of genomic polymerase chain reaction.

tems are optimized such that the risk of interference by an inhibitor is minimized. Nevertheless, care should be taken not to deviate from established protocols; doing so may introduce unintended inhibitory substances. In addition, amplifying ubiquitous target sequences that should be in all samples (ie, conserved genomic DNA or housekeeping genes) and/or spiking the specimens being analyzed with an internal positive control can help in assessing whether inhibitors are present.

PRIMER DEFECTS. Defects in primer function should not be a concern in the context of commercially available tests. Nevertheless, a thorough understanding of issues regarding primer design is important in troubleshooting assays, and primer design is a key component in developing PCR-based assays for new targets. Although the ideal primers will hybridize to a target that is found in only one location in the entire genome, given the complexity of human DNA, this is not always possible. Accordingly, cross-annealing to unintended targets can occur, which can result in amplification of unintended sequences if the primers bind to opposite strands close enough for adequate extension to occur. This can clearly happen with a combination of two primers; however, even a single primer can prime both ends of an amplicon. Because the majority of nonspecific annealing occurs at distant sites, no cross-amplification is typically observed. Nonetheless, even this scenario still results in ongoing consumption of primers with each cycle, thereby decreasing the analytical sensitivity of the assay.

In addition to cross-annealing, primers can have intrinsic defects. Thus, it is possible for two primers to anneal to each other in such a fashion that they can form a short amplicon. For example, if the 3 ends of two primers can bind to each other, the polymerase will fill in the 5 overhangs [Fig 10-4(A)]. This results in even stronger binding of the primers to each other. In addition, although a primer so modified may be still able to anneal to its target sequence, the additional bases added to the 3 end will no longer anneal and so prohibit proper extension. This occurrence, commonly called "primer-dimer formation," takes place between either two different primers in a reaction or two molecules of the same primer [Fig 10-4(B)]. Finally, primers can form hairpin loops and thereby anneal to themselves [Fig

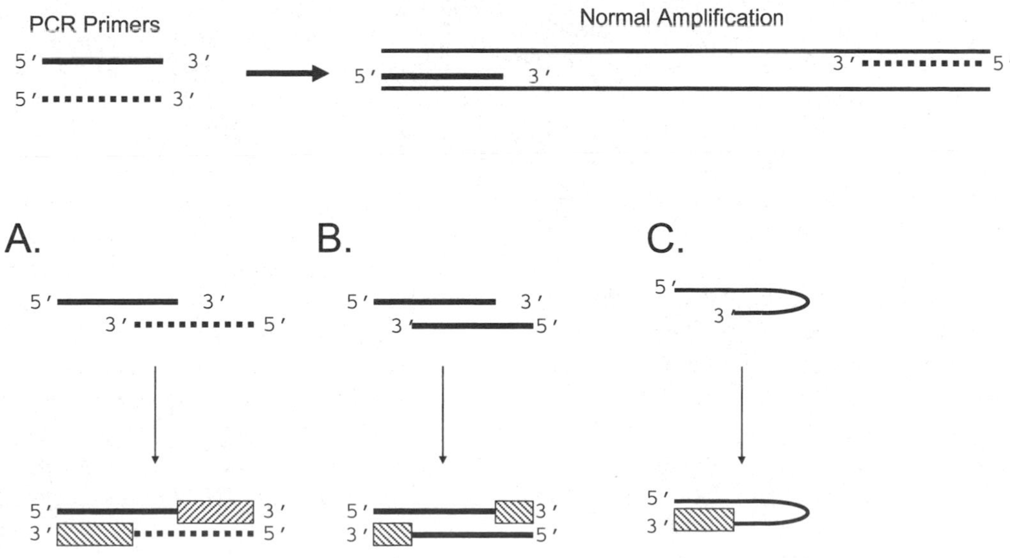

FIGURE 10-4. Potential problems in primer design that may inhibit polymerase chain reaction.

10-4(C)]. When a self-complementary sequence in a primer allows this to occur, the thermodynamics of this reaction are favored because of its intramolecular nature. If self-annealing results in a 5 overhang, the molecule can self-prime, with the polymerase extending off the 3 end to be complementary to the 5 end. In addition to increasing the tendency of this primer to self-anneal, as described above with primer dimers, the presence of the additional sequence prevents amplification of the authentic amplicon.

CONTAMINATION BETWEEN SPECIMENS. One of the greatest strengths of PCR-based approaches is the ability to amplify very small amounts of genetic material. In theory, single-copy sensitivity can be achieved. In practice, detection of 10 copies of DNA or fewer is not uncommon. However, this level of sensitivity also makes the assay susceptible to false-positive results because of contamination. This can occur from contamination between specimens being analyzed, and special care must be taken to avoid cross-contamination, as even a small amount can lead to a false-positive result. An even more likely source of contamination is amplicons generated in previous amplification reactions. Beginning with just 10 molecules of DNA, 30 rounds of amplification in a PCR will yield more than 1×10^{10} amplicons. Thus, if only 0.0000001% of a previous reaction is inadvertently introduced onto a pipette used to set up a subsequent reaction, a false-positive result may occur. Hence, the possibility of contaminating subsequent reactions with previously amplified material is considerable.

To minimize the potential for contamination, PCR laboratories are routinely set up for samples to proceed in only one direction. In the best of situations, PCR reactions are assembled in one room, amplified in a second room, and opened for analysis (if required) in a third room. There should be no retrograde flow, and no materials or instruments that are used in the amplification or analysis rooms should make their way into the PCR setup room. Also, filter tips that minimize both pipette contamination and sample aerosolization are routinely used.

In addition to controlling the flow of materials through the laboratory, there are other ways to minimize potential contamination. For example, many laboratories add deoxyuridine triphosphate (dUTP) to their PCRs. dUTP does not occur naturally in humans, but polymerases will incorporate dUTP in place of deoxythymidine triphosphate (dTTP). Uracil-DNA glycosylase (UNG) is an enzyme that specifically cleaves DNA containing uracil but does not cleave normal DNA or RNA.[9] Adding UNG to PCRs destroys amplicons generated from previous amplifications but not native DNA found in the specimen. The UNG is heat-inactivated during the initial denaturation step of the PCR, allowing amplification of the new sample. This maneuver can be carried out for both PCR and reverse transcriptase PCR (RT-PCR), described below.

Reverse Transcriptase PCR

In contrast to DNA PCR as described above, in a number of contexts, the object in reverse transcriptase (RT)-PCR is to detect RNA. Because DNA polymerases used for PCR do not amplify RNA, a special modification is used to adapt PCR to detect RNA. The RT enzyme, which will synthesize DNA from an RNA template,[10,11] is used. Like DNA polymerase, RT synthesizes in the 5 to 3 direction and requires the annealing of a primer to initiate transcription. When RNA is reverse transcribed, the resulting DNA is a single-stranded complementary copy of the RNA and is referred to as complementary DNA (cDNA). The cDNA is then a suitable substrate for PCR, as described above.

The choice of primers used to initiate reverse transcription is an important consideration in the design of an RT-PCR assay. For example, the downstream primer used in the PCR can prime reverse transcription. In this case, only the specific RNA species recognized by the primer is converted to cDNA. However, reverse transcription has additional considerations that may make it suboptimal to use the same primer as that used for PCR. First, RT typically functions at 42 C, a much lower temperature than that for the DNA polymerase used in PCR, and considerably lower than the annealing temperature of most PCR primers. This lower temperature makes the formation of primer dimers and hairpin loops more likely (see above). In addition, it is also more likely that the primer will cross-hybridize to unintended sequences. Because the primer will become fully incorporated into such sequences, authentic primer binding sites will exist in subsequent PCR cycles, which may give rise to undesired amplicons. Thus, although RT-PCR conditions can be found in which the same downstream primer is used for the RT reaction and the subsequent PCR amplification, sometimes this is not possible.

Often, separate primers are used for the RT reaction and subsequent DNA PCR. To make a generally applicable primer, two main approaches have been taken. Because the vast majority of eukaryotic mRNA transcripts have a 3 sequence of consecutive adenine residues (the poly-A tail), a primer consisting of a run of thymidine residues (oligo dT) can reverse-prime off the poly-A tail [Fig 10-5(A)]. Because priming by oligo dT begins at the far 3 end of the mRNA molecule, the entire RNA may be converted to cDNA. Although the oligo dT approach is widely used, it does have several disadvantages. For example, certain RNA species do not have poly-A tails and are thus not susceptible to RT using oligo dT. In addition, RNA is a fairly labile chemical entity that is susceptible to rapid degradation, which may separate the poly-A tail from the portion of the RNA of interest. Finally, RNA has much more secondary structure than DNA, especially at 42 C. This secondary structure can present a barrier to RT, thus preventing RT from transcribing the whole mRNA molecule.

Random hexamers are used as an alternate priming strategy that can circumvent many of the problems of oligo dT. In this case, a mixture of primers is synthesized in which all four nucleic acid bases are randomly incorporated for six cycles of DNA synthesis. The resulting mixture of primers containing a sequence of six bases (hexamers) will hybridize at multiple points along RNA molecules. When

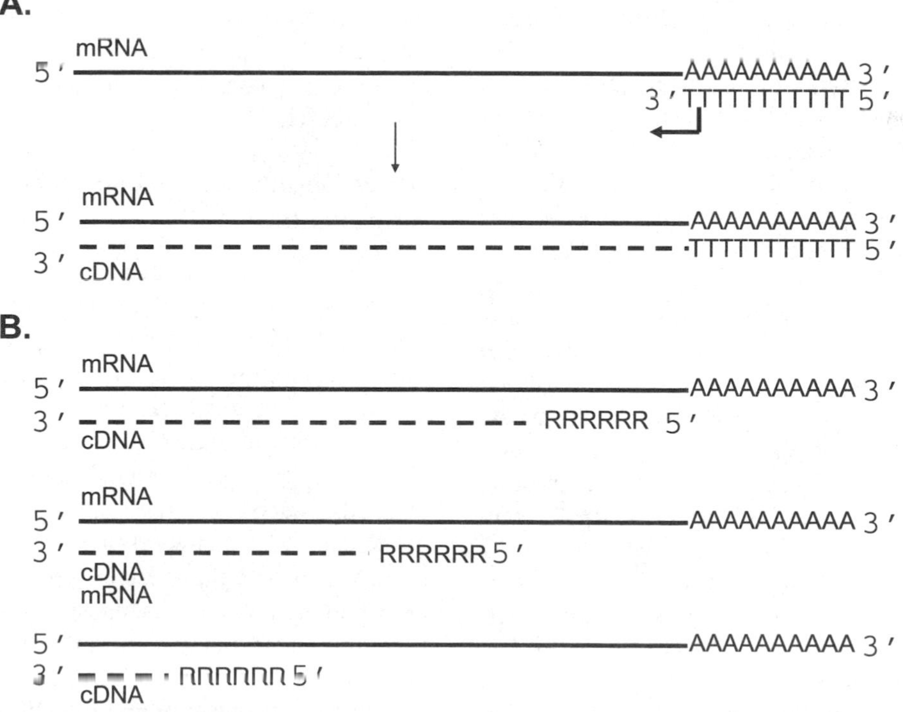

FIGURE 10-5. Methods of priming reverse transcriptase.

reverse transcription occurs in this situation, multiple partial cDNAs will be synthesized at different points along each RNA molecule [Fig 10-5(B)]. Such random priming largely circumvents issues of secondary structure, as priming will occur all along the RNA molecule. In addition, in the case of partial degradation, the whole RNA molecule will still be reverse transcribed, just in different pieces. However, as degradation is largely random, some cDNA containing the desired amplicon will likely be synthesized. The disadvantage to random hexamer priming is that it heavily favors synthesis of the 5 end of mRNA molecules. Thus, if the sequence to be amplified by the subsequent PCR is contained in the 3 end of the molecule, random hexamers will result in underrepresentation of the relevant transcript, leading to decreased analytical sensitivity.

Transcription-Mediated Amplification and Nucleic Acid Sequence-Based Amplification

Since the advent of PCR, several additional nucleic acid amplification strategies have been devised. Among the most useful are two highly related techniques, transcription-mediated amplification (TMA) and nucleic acid sequence-based amplification (NASBA).[12,13] Although TMA and NASBA have some differences (see below), they are conceptually similar and thus are described together. Currently, TMA plays a large role in nucleic acid testing (NAT) for human immunodeficiency virus (HIV), hepatitis C virus (HCV), and West Nile virus [ie, the Gen-Probe system (Gen-Probe Inc., San Diego, CA)]. For both techniques, the target of amplification is RNA. The reaction contains two primers, reverse transcriptase, DNA polymerase, RNAse H, and T7 polymerase. The reaction begins when a specific downstream primer hybridizes to the 3 end of the target RNA and reverse transcriptase synthesizes a cDNA copy (Fig 10-6, step 1). Not only does the first primer (primer 1) contain a complementary sequence at its 3 end that hybridizes to the target RNA, but the 5 end also encodes a bacteriophage T7 promoter. The RNA template is degraded either by RT with TMA or by RNAse H in an additional step with NASBA (Fig 10-6, step 2). A second upstream primer then binds to the newly synthesized cDNA (Fig 10-6, step 3) and uses DNA polymerase to synthesize a double-stranded DNA (Fig 10-6, step 4). The resulting double-stranded DNA molecule has a T7 promoter at one end; T7 polymerase then drives transcription of RNA. Because T7 polymerase is in the reaction mixture, multiple copies of RNA are synthesized from the DNA template, and these are antisense to the original target RNA (Fig 10-6, step 5). This results in significant amplification, as numerous transcripts are synthesized from a single DNA template. These new RNA molecules can reenter the amplification cycle, with primer 2 initiating reverse transcription, followed by RNA degradation and subsequent synthesis of DNA using primer 1 and DNA polymerase. This leads to additional amplification, with ongoing cycles of transcription and template synthesis. One distinct advantage of NASBA and TMA as compared to PCR is that nucleic acid denaturation is not required. Therefore, NASBA amplifies RNA sequences in an isothermal reaction, which does not require a thermocycler.

Other Methods of Nucleic Acid Amplification

In addition to the amplification methods described above, several additional technologies use nucleic acid polymerizing or ligating enzymes to amplify DNA and/or RNA. These include strand displacement amplification (SDA)[14,15] and the ligase chain reaction (LCR).[16] There are also probe/signal amplification methods such as the cleavase-invader, branched DNA, and hybrid capture assays. Although these techniques have been adapted to detect different pathogens, they are not widely used in transfusion medicine and are thus not described further here. However, they are summarized elsewhere[17] and may be applied to transfusion medicine in the future.

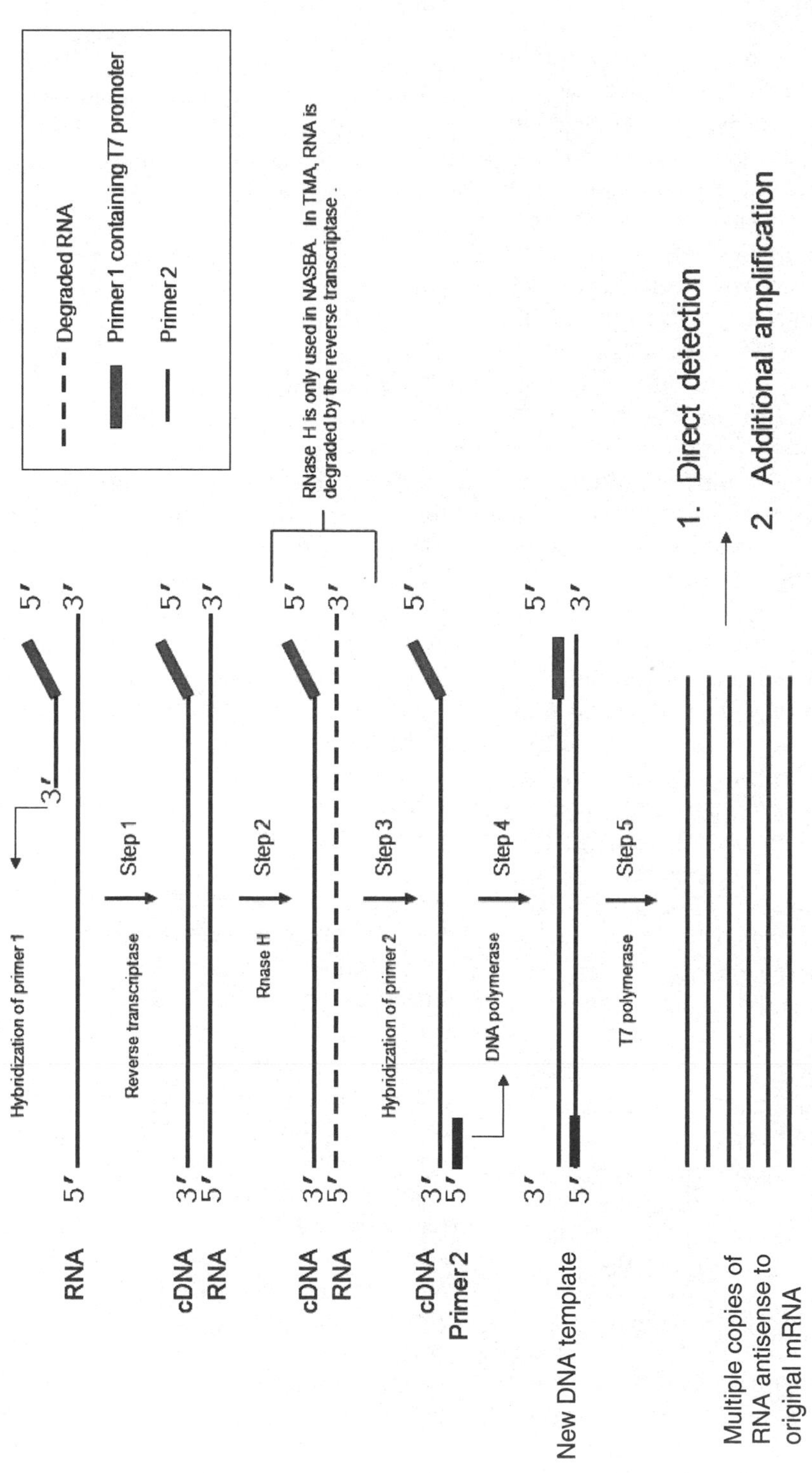

FIGURE - 0-6. Schematic overview of transcription-mediated amplification (TMA) and nucleic acid sequence-based amplification (NASBA). cDNA = complementary DNA; mRNA = messenger RNA.

Detection of Nucleic Acid Amplification Products

PCR, RT-PCR, TMA, and NASBA each result in the amplification of specific nucleic acid sequences. However, methods are still required to detect the amplified sequences. Traditionally, this was accomplished by separating the amplification reactions by gel electrophoresis in the presence of a fluorescent dye (eg, ethidium bromide) that made the nucleic acids visible in the gel using an ultraviolet lamp. This allows visualization of the bands, and if appropriate standards are included in the gels, it also provides a molecular weight by which one can distinguish amplicons of the correct size from cross-reactive products of different sizes. Further confirmation that the amplified nucleic acids are the correct sequences can be obtained by subjecting the products of the amplification reaction to restriction endonucleases and observing the sizes of the resulting molecules. Because the sequence of the amplicon is known, one can predict the correct restriction sites [this technique is known as restriction fragment length polymorphism (RFLP) analysis]. Even greater specificity can be achieved through hybridization analysis. Thus, after electrophoresis, the amplified products are transferred to nitrocellulose paper, which is then hybridized with DNA probes specific for the amplified sequences. Each of these analyses requires gel electrophoresis, which can be time consuming, not compatible with the throughput needs of donor testing laboratories, and not easily automated. Moreover, this approach requires opening the tubes containing the amplification reactions and manipulating the products, which increases the risk of contamination of reagents and false-positive results in subsequent samples.

Fluorescent Methods

More recently developed techniques for detecting amplification products rely heavily on the chemistry of fluorescent molecules. In such settings, probes that fluoresce only when the correct amplicon is present are included in the amplification reactions. By including a fluorescence spectrophotometer in the thermocycler, the generation of amplification products can be measured at each cycle. This approach, referred to as real-time PCR, is highly sensitive and much more quantitative than gel electrophoresis-based methods. In addition, with the use of multiple reporter dyes with distinct fluorescence spectra, detection of multiple targets in a single reaction (so-called multiplex nucleic acid amplification) is feasible. Moreover, including fluorescent probes in the reaction allows the analysis to be performed without ever opening the tube containing the amplification products, which decreases the risk of laboratory contamination with amplicons and false-positive results.

Two of these fluorescent methods rely on the juxtaposition of a fluorescent molecule with a quencher molecule that prevents fluorescence. In the Taqman system, a sequence-specific probe has the fluorescent molecule at one end and the quencher at the other. When the probe hybridizes to its target, it essentially blocks the DNA polymerase that is synthesizing the next round of DNA by extending from the primer. When the DNA polymerase encounters the hybridized probe, it degrades the probe, thus separating the fluorescent and quencher molecules [Fig 10-7(A)]. Because this only occurs when the probe hybridizes to its target, fluorescence is generated as a function of amplicon generation. The other approach uses molecular beacons that also have a fluorescent molecule on one end of a DNA probe and a quencher molecule on the other end. In this case, the sequence-specific probe is flanked with two sequences complimentary to each other that form a hairpin loop, thus juxtaposing the fluorescent molecule with its quencher. However, when the probe hybridizes to its target, the hairpin loop unfolds, separating the quencher from the fluorescent molecule and allowing fluorescence to occur [Fig 10-7(B)].

An alternate approach is to have two molecules that do not fluoresce unless they are in close proximity to each other. These molecules are linked to two separate DNA probes that hybridize to adjacent sequences on the amplicon. If the amplicon is present, the probes an-

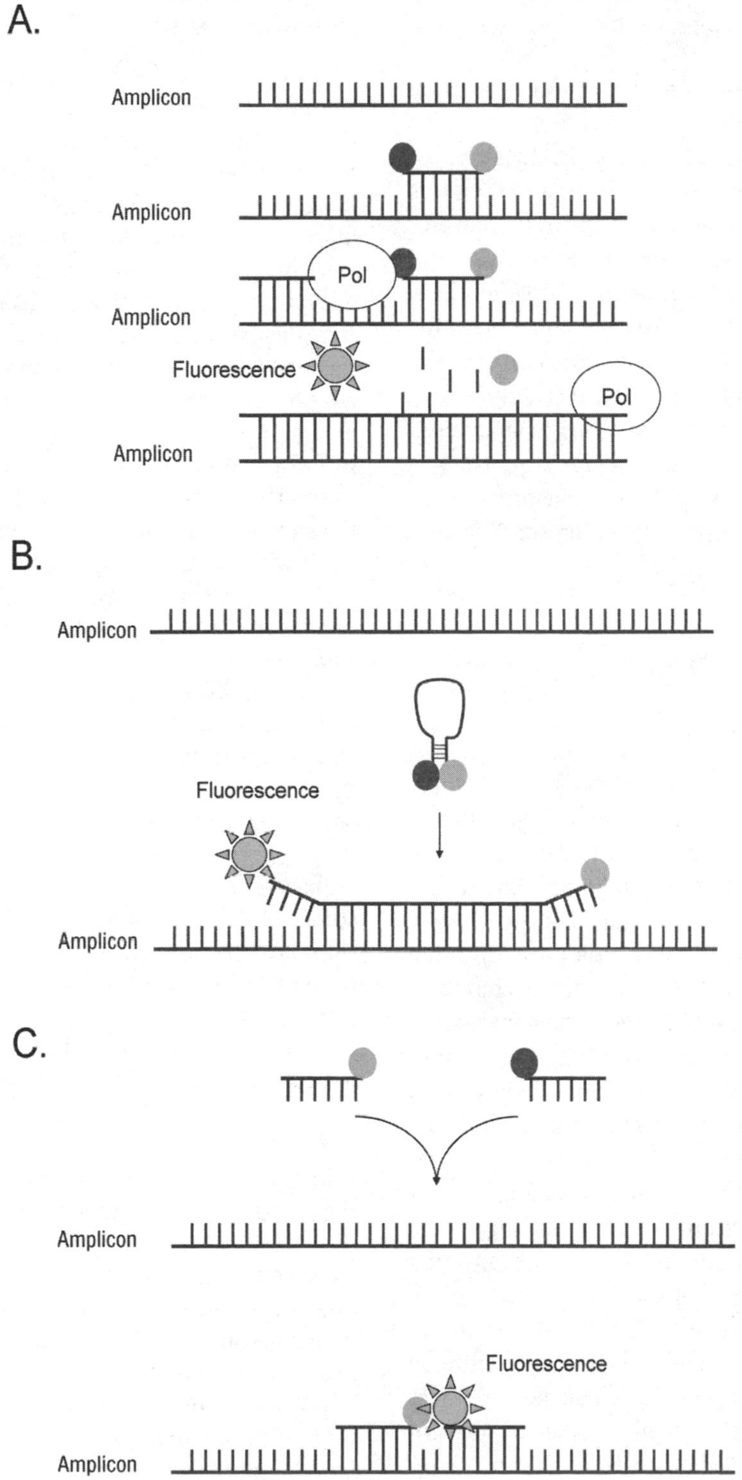

A.
Amplicon
Amplicon
Pol
Amplicon
Fluorescence
Pol
Amplicon
B.
Amplicon
Fluorescence
Amplicon
C.
Amplicon
Fluorescence
Amplicon

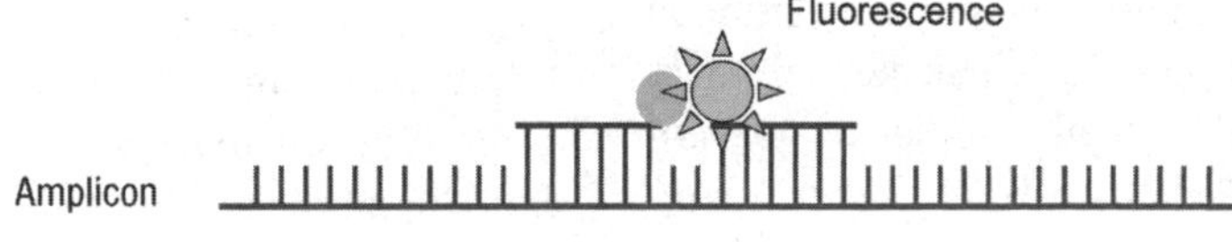

FIGURE 10-7. Methods of detection by sequence-specific probes during real-time polymerase chain reaction. Pol = polymerase.

neal in such a way that the two molecules are in close proximity, providing a fluorescent signal [Fig 10-7(C)].

A fourth method of real-time detection uses cyber-green dye that fluoresces when bound to double-stranded DNA. Cyber-green is not a sequence-specific probe and therefore detects all amplicons. However, authentic amplicons can be distinguished from cross-reactive products using a melting-curve analysis. Because the melting curve is a function of the size and GC content of the amplicon, and the size and sequence of the correct amplicon is known, the correct melting curve can be used to confirm the identity of the amplicon. As with PCR, the above fluorescent-probe techniques can be applied to other amplification technologies, such as TMA.

DNA and RNA Microarray Hybridization

The advent of microarray technology allows for the simultaneous analysis of multiple genes or gene products from a single sample. The chemistry behind this technology is the same as with other hybridization-based systems, such as Northern and Southern blots. However, in microarrays multiple probes are spotted onto small surfaces, often referred to as gene chips. The specimen being analyzed is then incubated with the gene chip, and amplified nucleic acids in the sample hybridize to their complementary sequences on the chip. The presence of hybridization can be detected by several different methods, including surface plasmon resonance and labeling of the specimen with fluorescent dyes.[18] By detecting hybridization at each specific position on the chip, which contains a probe of known sequence, one can determine the composition of the specimen. Gene chips can be manufactured to contain a small number of relevant probes for focused analysis, or they can contain tens of thousands of probes to provide a broad canvas of multiple genes, gene products, or both.

Analysis of Single Nucleotide Polymorphisms

The techniques described above detect the presence or absence of a given DNA or RNA sequence. This is most relevant for screening the blood supply for specific infectious microbes because in such situations, the question being asked is whether the infectious agent is present or absent. However, the vast majority of blood group antigens consist of small polymorphisms; therefore, assays identifying the presence or absence of an entire gene product are not informative for most blood group antigen genotyping. The gene product is present in most people, but the difference that determines the identity of the blood group antigen is a small change in sequence, often of a single nucleotide. In this case, it is necessary to use methods that can detect single nucleotide polymorphisms (SNPs) that differ between samples.

Some SNPs destroy or create recognition sites for restriction endonucleases. In this case, PCR-amplified material can be digested by restriction enzymes and then analyzed by agarose electrophoresis to observe the breakdown products. This approach of RFLP analysis (see above) was an early method by which some SNPs were discovered. However, it is slow, has low throughput, and depends on the presence of an SNP that alters restriction patterns.

More recently, several different methods for detecting SNPs have been developed, consisting mostly of modifications of PCR or microarray technologies. In these cases, the primers or probes are engineered such that their hybridization depends on the presence of the correct SNP. In particular, both multiplex PCR[19] and microarray systems[20] have been reported that can determine the genotype regarding the blood group antigens in individual specimens.

Genotyping of red cell antigens may be more efficient than traditional serologic typing. In addition, when a patient has been transfused with multiple units of Red Blood Cells (RBCs) and it is not possible to distinguish the patient's own red cells from transfused cells, genotyping of the patient's DNA may be the only reliable way to determine the patient's red cell phenotype. Despite these advantages, there are several scenarios in which genotyping may not correlate with phenotype. It is worth noting that genotyping typically focuses on known polymorphisms but does not provide the entire sequence of the gene or its regulatory regions. Therefore, several circumstances in which genotype might not predict phenotype include 1) new, hitherto unknown polymorphisms in the coding region that alter protein structure; 2) new polymorphisms in the promoter or enhancer regions that prevent gene expression despite the presence of the correct coding sequence; or 3) epigenetic alterations in the epitope (ie, modification by bacterial enzymes), when epitopes depend on posttranslational modification. Thus, considerable work still remains before SNP genotyping becomes a routine method for red cell typing.

PROTEIN ANALYSIS

Nucleic acid analysis, as described above, detects the presence of DNA or RNA that encodes genomic material and/or measures gene expression at the level of RNA. However, as a result of regulation at the level of protein translation, the presence of mRNA does not always correlate with the presence of the encoded protein. Moreover, multiple serologically defined blood group antigens require posttranslational modifications (eg, glycosylation); the presence of these types of antigens requires the coordinate expression of several different gene products. Finally, the detection of antibodies, which are proteins, cannot be determined by detecting or measuring nucleic acids. Accordingly, measuring protein-protein and protein-carbohydrate interactions provides relevant biologic information in transfusion medicine that may not be obtainable by nucleic acid analysis.

Fluid-Phase Assays (Agglutination-Based Methods)

Depending on antibody isotype, immunoglobulins have between two and 10 antigen-binding sites per molecule. Because each antibody can bind more than one target molecule, antibodies can crosslink antigens present in multiple copies on particulate substances, such as red cells or beads. This crosslinking can result in an aggregation of particles that have the relevant antigen on their surface, a process known as agglutination. Agglutination reactions are an old but still reliable serologic method for detecting antibody-antigen interactions, and they are used extensively in transfusion medicine.

Agglutination can be detected by several different methods. In many cases, the antigen is present as multiple copies on the red cell surface. This principle is used for serologic crossmatching (donor red cells incubated with recipient serum), screening plasma for unexpected antibodies (reagent red cells of known blood group antigen composition incubated with patient serum), and blood group antigen phenotyping of donor or recipient (patient red cells incubated with monoclonal antibodies or reagent-quality antisera of known specificity). Because red cells are easily visible by their red color, several different systems were devised to detect agglutination. These include 1) tube testing in which agglutination is visually detected by the adhesion of red cells to one another in the postcentrifuge pellet (also called a button), 2) passive agglutination in microtiter plates where agglutination is detected by the spread pattern of red cells in individual wells, and 3) gel testing in which unagglutinated red cells pass through a matrix but agglutinated complexes are retained at the top of the matrix because of their increased size.[21] In addition to blood bank serology, red cells can be used to detect antibodies against other antigens by linking these particular antigens to the red cell surface. Agglutination-based assays can also be engineered using particles other than red cells, such as latex beads. Each of these techniques uses the same basic principles and has broad applicability in clinical diagnostic testing.

Although agglutination reactions are very sensitive and easy to perform, the formation of agglutinates depends on the proper stoichiometric ratio of antibody to antigen. When the ratio of antigen to antibody is in a range such that agglutination readily occurs, it is referred to as the zone of equivalence. In this case, a reaction in which each arm of the antibody binds to a different particle is favored, and a network (or lattice) of linked particles results in agglutination [Fig 10-8(B)]. However, a false-negative result can occur if the stoichiometric ratio is outside the zone of equivalence at either extreme.

An instance of antibody excess is called the prozone effect. When a prozone effect occurs, such a high concentration of antibody is present that the statistical likelihood of an antibody being able to bind to two separate particles is diminished [Fig 10-8(A)]. Accordingly, a very high antibody titer can give a false-negative agglutination reaction. This is seen most commonly with non-red-cell-based agglutination assays, such as the rapid plasma reagin screening test for syphilis serology. Although prozone effects are unusual in classical red cell serology, they have been observed when titers of red cell antibodies are very high. In particular, discrepant reverse ABO typing caused by prozone effects has been reported.[22,23] If a prozone effect is present, a dilution of the serum being tested will provide a positive result. In addition, the use of EDTA-containing diluents decreases the likelihood of prozone effects. One reason that prozone effects are uncommon in red cell serology is that the use of antihuman globulin (AHG) largely overcomes these problems. However, a secondary "prozone-like" effect occurs if there is inadequate washing before the addition of AHG.[24] In this

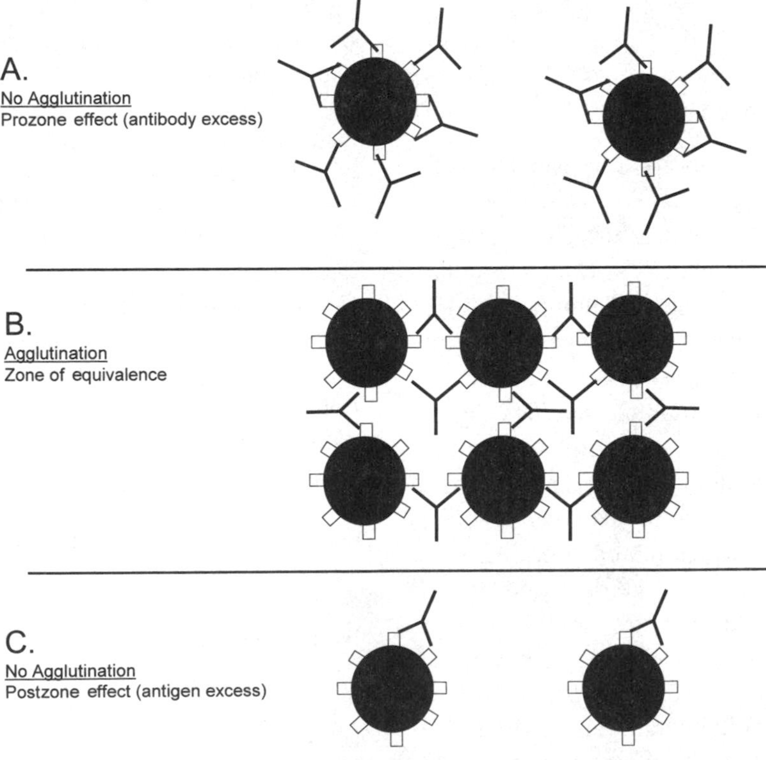

FIGURE 10-8. Effects of relative concentrations of antigen and antibody on the outcome of agglutination reactions.

case, residual IgG in solution will bind the AHG and compete for AHG binding to IgG on the red cell. This may occur with very high titers of blood group antibodies or even in the presence of highly increased levels of polyclonal antibodies, as in hypergammaglobulinemia. In this setting, additional washing steps remove the problem.[24]

In theory, one can also obtain a false-negative agglutination reaction from a postzone effect, in which the antigen is in excess [Fig 10-8(C)]. In this case, every antibody binds to multiple epitopes on the same particle, thereby preventing the crosslinking that leads to agglutination. This could occur in red cell serology if a large excess of red cells were used, but it is easily controlled by careful attention to methods and is not a common problem in transfusion medicine. Postzone effects can also theoretically occur as a result of highly increased antigen density on red cells. However, antigen densities on red cells are not typically elevated to supraphysiologic levels.

Solid-Phase Assays

Various solid-phase assays all use the same general principle. As opposed to fluid-phase assays such as agglutination, where the reaction occurs in a solution or suspension, in solid-phase assays the antigen or antibody being studied is immobilized on a solid matrix. The analyte is then incubated with the coated solid phase, and the adherence of the analyte to the solid phase is measured. Several different combinations of adherence and detection approaches have been described.

Solid-Phase Assays for Phenotyping Red Cells

In this case, antibodies specific for known blood group antigens are coated onto round-bottom microtiter plates [Fig 10-9(A)]. The red

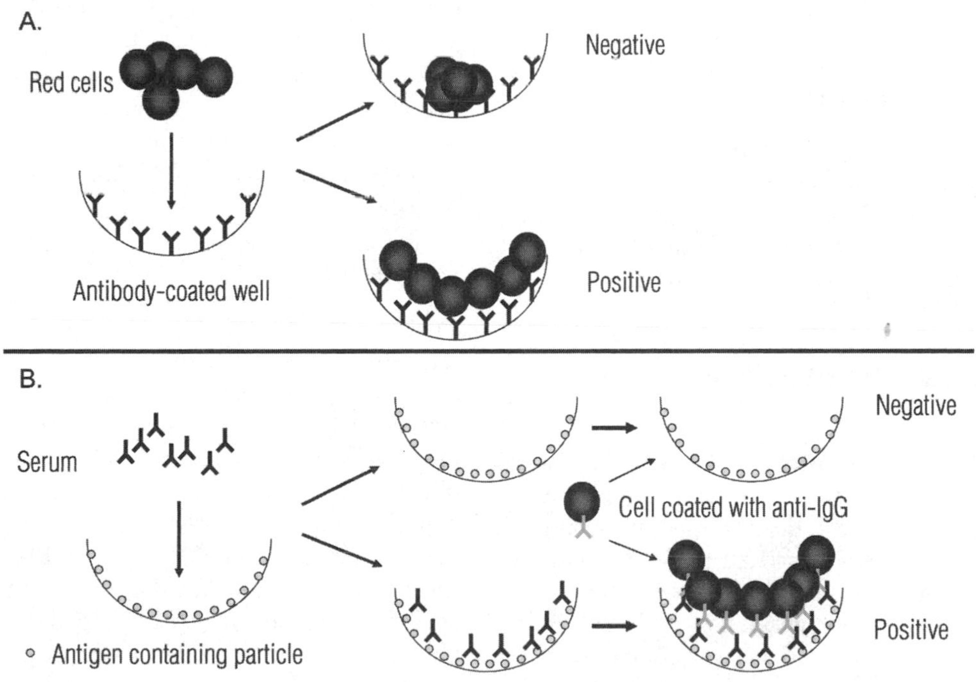

FIGURE 10-9. Schematic representation of (A) phenotyping red cells and (B) detecting antibodies by solid-phase assay.

cells being analyzed are then added to the microtiter plates and allowed to adhere. If no binding occurs (negative reaction), the red cells all cluster together as a "button" at the bottom of the well. In contrast, specific binding results in diffuse sticking of the red cells over the surface of the well (positive reaction). Thus, a positive reaction indicates the presence of the antigen on the cells being tested.

Solid-Phase Assays for Detecting Antibodies to Red Cell Antigens

Antigen-coated particles consisting of red cells or red cell fragments are coated onto microtiter plate wells [Fig 10-9(B)]. Patient serum is then added to each well, followed by incubation and then washing. If the patient serum has antibodies against the red cell antigens coated on the well, the antibodies will bind. Indicator red cells coated with antihuman IgG are then added, and a positive reaction is demonstrated by diffuse adherence of the indicator cells to the well, and a negative reaction is characterized by indicator cells clustering in a button.

Solid-Phase Assays for Typing Antigens on Cells Other Than Red Cells

Solid-phase red cell adherence (SPRCA) technology has also been adapted to detect antigens on platelets, such as human platelet antigen (HPA)-1a, as well as antibodies against platelet antigens using the approaches described above.[25]

Enzyme-Linked Immunosorbent Assay

The enzyme-linked immunosorbent assay (ELISA), also referred to as enzyme immunoassay (EIA), can detect either antibodies or antigens. In each case, an ELISA generates a signal via an enzyme linked to a secondary antibody or antigen, which converts a substrate to a measurable product (eg, a color change or a chemiluminescent reaction). For this reason, ELISAs have considerable signal amplification and are significantly more sensitive than fluid-phase agglutination or SPRCA assays. In most cases, ELISAs use purified or recombinant antigens or antibodies, depending on the analyte requiring detection. However, whole red cells can be used as antigen to screen for red cell antibodies; this is referred to as the enzyme-linked antiglobulin test.[26]

Detection of Antibodies by ELISA (Indirect ELISA)

To detect antibodies against a given antigen, the antigen is coated onto individual wells of a microtiter plate [Fig 10-10(A)]. The test sample is then added to the well, incubated, and extensively washed. If antibodies against the antigen are present, they will be bound to the antigen-coated well and not washed away. Bound antibodies are then detected by incubating the well with a secondary antibody, consisting of an immunoglobulin antibody (eg, anti-IgG) linked to an enzyme (eg, alkaline phosphatase or horseradish peroxidase). After further washing, enzyme substrate is added, which is typically converted to a detectable colored product if enzyme is present. Quantification is performed using a standard curve and a spectrophotometer to measure the absorbance at the wavelength appropriate for that enzyme product. In some cases, samples may need to be diluted to ensure that they yield absorbance values in the linear range of the assay.

Detection of Antigens by ELISA

SANDWICH ELISA. In sandwich ELISAs, two separate antibodies are used that bind to different epitopes on the same target antigen; the antibodies bind to the target without interfering with each other. Typically, this is accomplished using monoclonal antibodies. Microtiter plate wells are coated with one antibody, the "capture antibody" [Fig 10-10(B)]. The specimen is then incubated in the well; if the antigen is present, it will bind to the solid-phase antibody coated in the well. The plate is then washed, and the wells are incubated with the second antibody, which is linked to a reporter enzyme, the "conjugate." Because the second antibody is specific for the target anti-

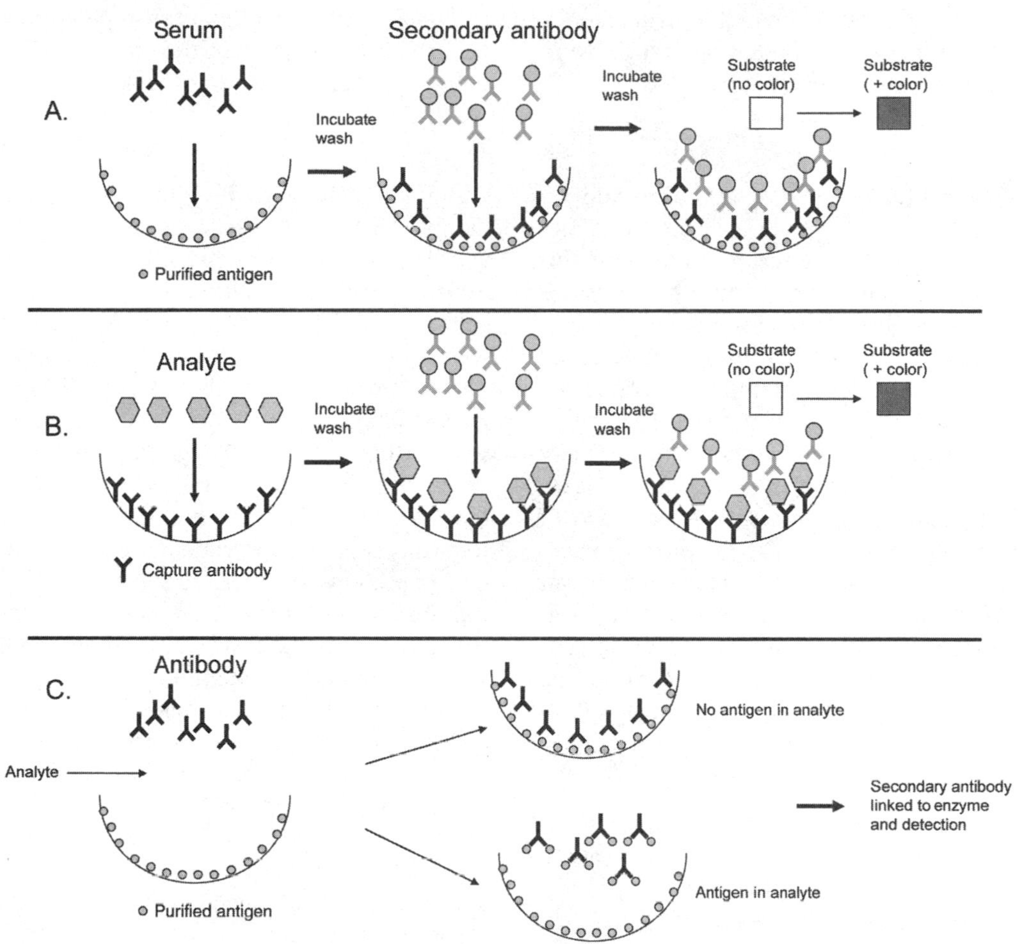

FIGURE 10-10. Schematic representation of (A) indirect enzyme-linked immunosorbent assay (ELISA), (B) sandwich ELISA, and (C) competitive ELISA.

gen, it will bind to the microtiter plate well only if antigen is bound to the capture antibody. After additional washing, enzyme substrate is added and converts to a detectable color if enzyme is present.

COMPETITIVE ELISA. Competitive ELISAs are similar to the indirect ELISA in that the antigen itself is already bound to the microtiter plate well. The test sample is incubated with antibody, and this mixture is then added to the well [Fig 10-10(C)]. If no antigen is present in the specimen, the reagent antibodies will bind to the solid-phase antigen. If antigen is present in the specimen, it will prevent the antibodies from binding the solid-phase antigen by competing for the antibody-binding sites. Therefore, the more soluble antigen in the specimen, the less antibody that is free to bind to the solid-phase antigen. In this case, the weaker the signal, the more soluble antigen present in the specimen. Competitive ELISA can also be performed for antibody detection. In this case, the test sample along with a labeled antibody is added to an antigen-coated well. Both patient antibody and labeled antibody compete for antigen-binding sites in the well, and again, a higher signal is generated if the antibody concentration in the sample is low or absent. Although slightly more difficult to optimize, competitive ELISAs have a distinct advantage over sandwich ELISAs in not requiring two separate antibodies against different epitopes on the target antigen.

Technical Problems with ELISAs

Typically, ELISAs are straightforward and robust assay systems. Although decreased signals are possible as a result of enzymatic inhibitors in the analyte, and false-positive signals can occur from enzymatic activity in the analyte, proper controls and washing should prevent these problems. Problems can also occur if the amount of the antigen being measured exceeds the amount of antibody present. This phenomenon, called the "hook effect," underestimates the concentration of the antigen. Moreover, like the prozone effect (see above), excess amounts of the analyte can cause the signal to decrease in some sandwich ELISAs in which the analyte and detection antibody are added simultaneously. Hook effects can be overcome by diluting the analyte.

Protein Microarrays

Microarray technology has dramatically increased the number of substrates that can be simultaneously assayed by solid-phase methods. By spotting numerous different protein substances on a small chip, a single specimen can be assayed for binding activity to multiple substances (in some cases, thousands) simultaneously. For example, patient serum could be tested for antibodies to blood group antigens by making a microarray chip with different blood group antigens and then incubating it with patient serum. Although microarray approaches are very promising, like ELISA they require that the antigens being tested be spotted on a chip in a pure form that maintains the structural conformation required for recognition. In the case of carbohydrate antigens or linear protein epitopes, this is fairly easily achieved. However, with a multipass transmembrane protein that requires membrane insertion to have proper conformation (eg, the Rh antigens), it is considerably more difficult to manufacture the purified epitopes for use on chips. Although the application of protein microarrays to blood bank serology is still in early stages of development, it represents an evolving technology with tremendous potential.

Western Blotting

The ELISA techniques described above can be highly sensitive. However, because the antigens used may not be pure (eg, lysates of viruses grown in tissue culture), false-positive results are possible as a result of cross-reactivity with other components in the antigen preparation. Western blotting is conceptually similar to ELISA, except that instead of coating a well with the antigen, the (glyco)protein antigen mixture (eg, viral lysate) is first separated by high-resolution protein electrophoresis (typically using polyacrylamide gels). The separated proteins are then transferred to nitrocellulose paper (or another suitable medium), which serves as the solid phase to be probed with an antibody-containing patient sample. In this case, one can determine the molecular weight of the antigens recognized by antibodies in the patient sample. In addition, although not often used clinically, other gel electrophoresis methods can be used to separate antigens based on physical properties other than size, such as using isoelectric focusing, which separates proteins of different charges over a pH gradient. Because the likelihood of having a cross-reactive antigen with the same physical characteristics as the authentic antigen is small, Western blotting provides additional specificity as compared to ELISA testing. Accordingly, Western blots are often used as confirmatory tests for screening serologic assays, especially for serologic tests for infectious agents such as HIV. Similar techniques have been developed using recombinant or otherwise purified proteins for the detection of other infectious disease agents, such as HCV.

Flow Cytometry

Over the past several decades, flow cytometry has revolutionized the molecular analysis of cell populations. The basic principle is that antibodies against cell surface molecules are labeled with fluorescent tags. Cell populations are incubated with the antibodies and these "stained" cells are then passed through a flow cytometer. The individual cells being analyzed are exposed to lasers that excite the fluorochromes, causing fluorescent emission at known wavelengths, which is then detected by sensors in the flow cytometer. The amount of fluorescence is determined on a cell-by-cell basis, allowing not only the quantification of the cell surface molecules on each cell but also the visualization of small populations of cells within a complex mixture. Clinical flow cytometry has been applied primarily to the diagnosis of neoplasia, particularly for hematologic malignancies. However, flow cytometry can also be applied to red cell serology. For example, red cells can be phenotyped using labeled antibodies of known specificity. Alternatively, antibody screens or crossmatching can be performed by mixing red cells of known phenotype with patient antisera and then staining with a secondary antihuman immunoglobulin (eg, anti-IgG) that is coupled to a fluorescent molecule. Although flow cytometry has not been widely applied to blood bank serology or phenotyping, it is a sensitive and specific technology that can be useful for these purposes. It has the advantages of high sensitivity, the ability to make small populations visible that might be missed in transplanted or heavily transfused patients, and the lack of potential problems or idiosyncrasies of agglutination (eg, the prozone effect). In addition, it has high throughput and the potential for automation. A drawback of this approach is that the instrumentation required for flow cytometry is expensive.

BASIC IMMUNOLOGIC PRINCIPLES UNDERLYING TRANSFUSION MEDICINE

The Generation of Antibody Responses: Afferent Immunity

The generation of an antibody response is a complicated process that necessitates coordinated interaction of at least three different cell types (Fig 10-11). Antigen-presenting cells (APCs) process proteins and present them to the immune system; T cells regulate whether or not the immune response occurs; and B cells synthesize antibodies. Immunization typically takes place in specialized anatomic compartments that are specifically designed for this process. In the context of transfused red cells and platelets, lymphatics and lymph nodes are largely excluded, and most responses occur in the spleen and liver.

Antigen Processing and Presentation

APCs (mostly macrophages and dendritic cells) continually sample proteins in the body by ingesting them and then proteolytically digesting them into small peptides ("antigen processing"). These peptides are loaded onto antigen-presenting proteins: major histocompatibility complex Class I and II (MHC I and MHC II). MHC/peptide complexes represent a sampling of all proteins in the host and are present on the APC surface. Thus, when a foreign antigen enters the body and is consumed by APCs, peptides from that antigen are presented by MHC I and MHC II molecules.

For humoral immunity, MHC II is the most relevant MHC, and its interaction with the T-cell receptor (TCR) on CD4+ T cells is of central importance. Most human blood group antigens are single amino acid polymorphisms of red cell surface proteins that may differ between donor and recipient. For this theoretical discussion, the donor polymorphism is designated as "D" and the recipient polymorphism as "R" (for donor and recipient), indicating generic blood group antigens. When the recipient is transfused with red cells expressing the D alloantigen, two events occur simultaneously: 1) B cells are activated that encode immunoglobulin genes specific for epitopes determined by the three dimensional structure of the D antigen (see Fig 10-11 and below), and 2) APCs ingest red cells expressing D, process red cell proteins into peptides, and present some of these peptides on MHC II. For this discussion, the peptides containing the D polymorphism are loaded on and fit into the peptide-binding pocket of the recipient's MHC II molecules (Fig 10-11).

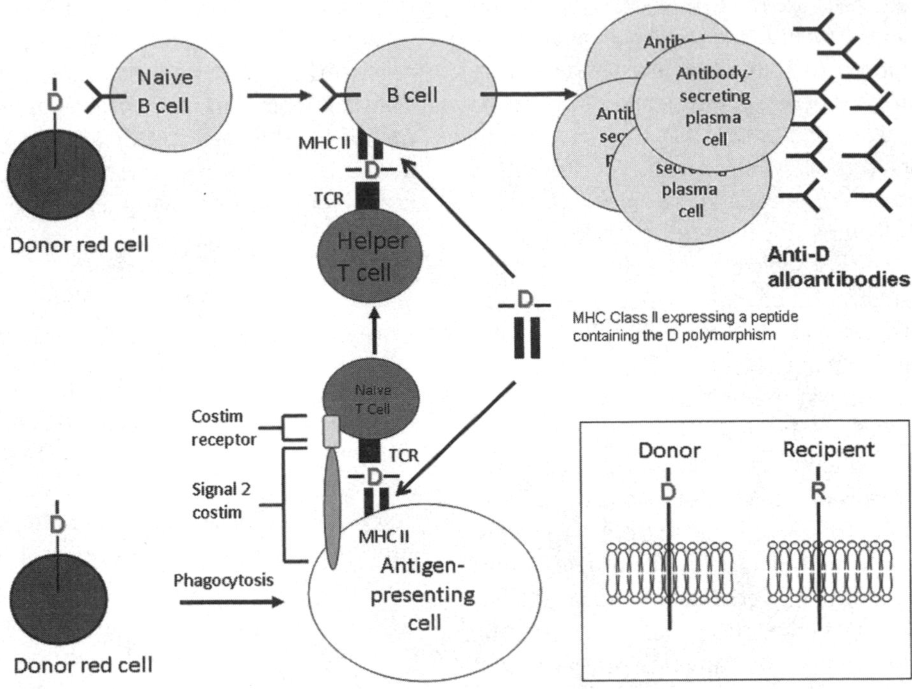

FIGURE 10-11. Diagram of humoral alloimmunization to a theoretical blood group antigen. "D" and "R" represent polymorphisms on donor and recipient antithetical blood group antigens, respectively.
MHC II = major histocompatibility complex Class II; TCR = T-cell receptor.

CD4+ T-Cell Activation

T cells specific for a given MHC/peptide complex become activated if they encounter an APC presenting the peptide they recognize, and if the microenvironment is correct for activation. For the most part, APCs do not distinguish between foreign proteins and self-proteins. Thus, peptides derived from both self-proteins and foreign proteins will be presented by MHC II. Any given T cell recognizes MHC/peptide complexes through its TCR. Because the TCRs are recombinant genes, every T cell expresses a unique TCR. The vast majority of T cells that have high affinity for peptides derived from self-proteins (ie, autoreactive CD4+ T cells) are deleted during development in the thymus. For this reason, most mature T cells recognize foreign antigens. Although some autoreactive CD4+ T cells are not deleted and thus increase the risk of autoimmunity, they can also play an active role in peripheral tolerance if they have phenotypes that suppress immune responses to autoantigens (ie, suppressor T cells or regulatory T cells).

Inflamed microenvironments favor T-cell activation, whereas quiescent states can favor tolerance. Although recognition of the MHC II/peptide complex on the APC surface is required for CD4+ T-cell activation (Fig 10-11), this stimulus through the TCR (known as signal 1) is not sufficient to stimulate the T cell to differentiate into an effector phenotype; additional stimulation, such as signaling by costimulatory molecules on the APC (signal 2), is required. Secretion of certain proinflammatory cytokines may be an additional factor in some settings (signal 3). If signals 1 and 2 are delivered simultaneously, CD4+ T cells typically differentiate into helper T cells. However, if signal 1 is encountered without signals 2 and/or 3, CD4+ T cells fail to become helper T cells; they are deleted, become anergic, or differentiate into suppressor/regulatory phenotypes. The complexity of this system is compounded by the presence of both positive and negative regulators of the signal 2 and signal 3 pathways in both APCs and CD4+ T cells.

The regulation of stimulatory signals 2 and 3 in APCs is currently an area of intense research. In general, conditions that induce inflammation (eg, infection or injury) favor stimulatory signals 2 and 3 and thus helper CD4+ T-cell differentiation. However, this is an oversimplification because different types of inflammation have different effects. Nevertheless, for this discussion it is sufficient to conclude that generating helper CD4+ T cells requires recognition of a foreign peptide on an MHC II molecule presented by an APC in an immune stimulatory context.

Generation of Plasma Cells That Secrete Antigen-Specific Antibodies

Each B cell expresses its own particular immunoglobulin genes on the cell surface in the form of a functional signaling complex: the B-cell receptor (BCR). The BCR allows the B cell to detect antigens (eg, the theoretical donor "D" antigen discussed in "Antigen Processing and Presentation" above) recognized by its particular immunoglobulin. Thus, if the BCR binds an antigen with sufficient affinity, the B cell then internalizes the BCR, along with the antigen, by receptor-mediated endocytosis. The ingested antigen is processed into peptides and loaded on the B cell's MHC II (see Fig 10-11). Because this B-cell MHC II/peptide complex is identical to the MHC II/peptide complex on the APC that activated a CD4+ T cell, that helper CD4+ T cell specifically recognizes the activated B cell. In doing so, the CD4+ T cell provides "help," which allows the B cell to differentiate. This help is highly specific to B cells that encode immunoglobulins recognizing the antigen in question, as only they will endocytose the antigen and present the relevant peptide. B cells with antibodies that do not recognize the antigen will never engulf the protein in question, will not present peptides on MHC II, and will thus not be able to receive help from CD4+ T cells specific to peptides containing the "D" polymorphism.

When the BCR of a given B cell encounters its antigen, in addition to presenting peptides on MHC II, the B cell becomes activated so that it is receptive to CD4+ T-cell help. If CD4+ T-cell help is available (in the form of both CD40/CD40L interactions and soluble cytokines), the B cell then undergoes class switching (IgM converts to IgG and other isotypes); proliferates extensively, geometrically increasing the number of B cells expressing that particular immunoglobulin; and finally differentiates into plasma cells that secrete large quantities of that immunoglobulin. Interestingly, some antigens directly activate B cells without T-cell help ("T-independent antigens"), which precludes efficient class switching; these can be nonspecific B-cell mitogens or long polymeric repetitive antigens that activate the BCR so strongly that T-cell help is not required. The latter often consists of carbohydrates, likely explaining why most carbohydrate antibodies are predominantly IgM (eg, antibodies to ABO antigens). However, for most protein antigens, including most blood group antigens, CD4+ T-cell help is required.

Generation of Immune Diversity

The above description of the generation of a humoral immune response focuses on the specificity of a given CD4+ T cell and a given B cell. It is essential to note that the genomic DNA encoding both the TCR and the BCR consists of a complex array of different variable genetic sequences that recombine at random to produce a vast number of different TCR and BCR products. Additional diversity is provided by the introduction of random or mutated nucleic acid sequences into the recombined TCR and BCR gene segments. The result is that the TCR or BCR in every T or B cell, respectively, is essentially unique. This provides a vast repertoire of different TCR and immunoglobulin specificities, estimated at 10^{15} different TCRs and greater than 10^{10} different BCRs (or antibodies). This process unfolds during normal development of the immune system, even before any foreign antigen is encountered. Moreover, this is an ongoing process. B cells expressing various immunoglobulin genes are continuously generated in the marrow. Finally, after an immune response is under way, additional somatic hypermutation of immunoglobulin genes in B cells provides further increases in diversity, favoring development of higher affinity antibodies over time (termed "affinity maturation"). Somatic hypermutation has not been detected in T cells.

Once activated, T and B cells undergo rapid and extensive proliferation, spreading effector cells throughout the body. Moreover, some activated cells differentiate into long-lived memory cells, which reactivate more easily than the initial naive cells when antigen is encountered a second time. Thus, every naive T and B cell encodes a different TCR or immunoglobulin gene product; however, when a given cell encounters an antigen, numerous copies of that cell are subsequently produced.

At first glance, randomly rearranging genes at the TCR and immunoglobulin loci might seem like a massive waste of resources because the vast majority of the T and B cells will then encode TCRs and immunoglobulins that will never encounter their cognate antigen(s). There is also a substantial danger of generating autoreactive T and B cells, which could cause autoimmune disease. However, extensive editing of T and B cells in the thymus and marrow removes most autoreactive T cells and many autoreactive B cells (see below). Thus, constructing the immune system in this fashion provides a state of universal readiness where all possible TCRs and antibodies are formed and available for activation if a foreign antigen is detected. Although the vast majority of T and B cells encode irrelevant TCRs and antibodies, there will always be a few preformed cells available in case they are required for host defense.

Mechanistic Explanations for the Evolution of Helper T Cells

The cellular interactions in the humoral immune system (depicted in Fig 10-11) may appear unnecessarily convoluted and complex. For example, one is tempted to ask why CD4+ helper T cells are even involved in this process. After all, B cells are activated only once they encounter an antigen recognized by their BCR (ie, the immunoglobulin they encode). Thus, why not simply have B cells differentiate into plasma cells and secrete large amounts of immunoglobulin when they encounter the antigen they recognize? The theoretical explanation for this phenomenon relates to maintaining immunologic tolerance. Because immunoglobulin genes rearrange randomly, many of the resulting antibodies recognize self-antigens (ie, are autoreactive) and, if expressed, could cause autoimmune disease. To avoid this fate, the B cell initially expresses its unique immunoglobulin rearrangement on the cell surface as a rudimentary BCR. If the BCR is crosslinked at this stage (presumably by encountering self-antigen), that B cell is rapidly eliminated or rendered nonreactive. Although this process ("central B-cell tolerance") is very efficient, it is restricted to antigens encountered during B-cell development. Thus, only cell surface antigens expressed in the marrow, where B cells mature and develop, efficiently induce central B-cell tolerance. In contrast, this process cannot affect autoreactive B cells recognizing either cytoplasmic proteins in marrow cells or proteins expressed by nonhematopoietic tissues.

Similar to the process with B cells, T cells expressing TCRs with high affinity for self-antigen are eliminated during development. However, unlike B cells, autoreactive T cells are deleted in the thymus. Because TCRs on CD4+ T cells recognize peptides presented by MHC II, they tolerate both cell surface and cytoplasmic proteins. Moreover, a transcription factor expressed by thymic epithelium ("autoimmune regulator gene," or AIRE) induces at least low levels of expression of essentially every gene product in the genome. Thus, these factors provide for very efficient removal of autoreactive T cells.

Taken together, the activation of B cells encoding autoreactive antibodies is minimized by linking B-cell activation to T-cell help. In effect, this confers B-cell tolerance to essentially all proteins expressed in the host genome regardless of tissue distribution or cellular location. Indeed, patients with a genetic defect in AIRE exhibit substantial autoimmunity (autoimmune polyglandular syndrome type 1). Nonetheless, despite the protection conferred by linking B-cell responses to CD4+ T-cell help, humoral autoimmunity does occur. Although several mechanisms are probably involved, the removal of autoreactive CD4+ T cells, despite being highly efficient, fails in some instances.

Summary of Afferent Immunity

The process by which the immune system synthesizes an effective antibody is complex and highly regulated. The regulatory complexity is probably a result of the difficult task assigned to the humoral immune system. In particular, the goal is to synthesize antibodies against every possible foreign antigen expressed by every possible pathogen that may endanger the host. However, at the same time, it is essential to prevent immune responses to self-antigens expressed by the host's own tissues.

The Effect of Established Immunity: Efferent Immunity

The efferent processes by which antibodies destroy their targets are distinct from the afferent processes by which the immune system regulates antibody synthesis. Once plasma cell differentiation occurs, immunoglobulins are secreted and distributed throughout the body. If antibodies encounter their targets, the target cells can be destroyed by several mechanisms, as described below.

Antibody Structure

The general structure of antibodies can be described by dividing them into several different domains. At its simplest, an antibody is a tetramer of two identical heavy chains and two identical light chains (Fig 10-12). The heavy and light chains are encoded by different DNA sequences; each contains a distinct variable region (shown as dark) that represents the recombinant part of the molecule that varies from antibody to antibody and also binds antigen. In addition, light chains encode a constant region. Two light-chain constant regions exist in the genome (kappa and lambda), and any given antibody has either kappa or lambda light chains. Likewise, heavy chains have one of several different constant regions depending on the isotype (see below).

Immunoglobulins can be functionally divided into two domains. The Fab domain con-

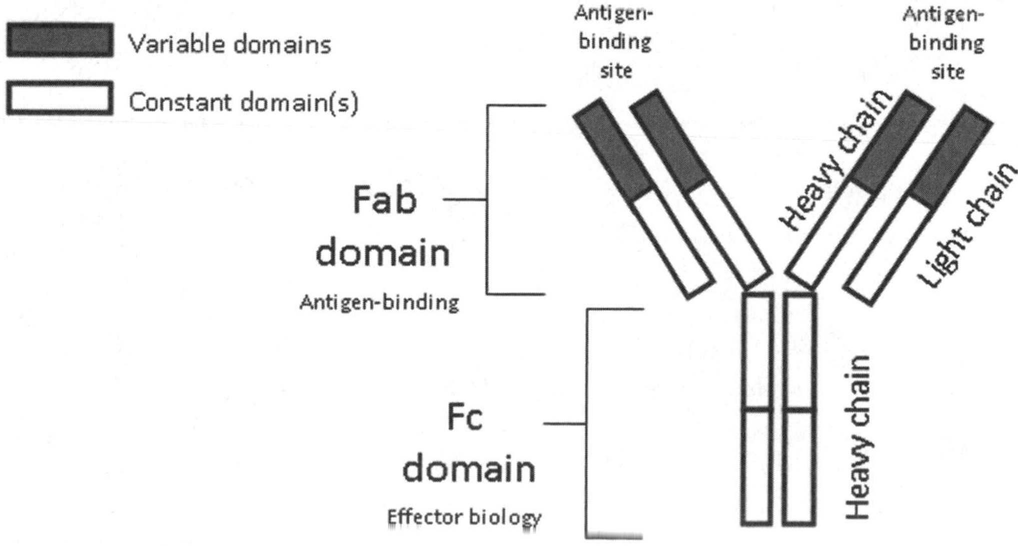

FIGURE 10-12. General structure of a monomeric immunoglobulin.

sists of the heavy- and light-chain variable regions, the light-chain constant region, and one heavy-chain constant region. The Fab domain binds antigen but does not activate effector mechanisms. In contrast, the Fc domain, consisting only of heavy-chain constant regions, activates effector mechanisms, allowing destruction of the antibody target (see below). Additionally, Fc constant regions differ based on antibody isotype and subclass.

There are five different antibody isotypes: IgM, IgG, IgE, IgA, and IgD. In general, IgM and IgG cause hemolysis during transfusion reactions and autoimmune hemolytic anemia. Antibody isotypes differ in the number of Fab domains per molecule and the number and potency of their Fc domains (Fig 10-13). The number of Fab domains per antibody affects binding avidity for antigen. For example, IgM has high avidity because of its 10 antigen-binding Fab domains, resulting from five identical immunoglobulins that are connected by an additional protein (the J chain) and extensive disulfide bonding. The high avidity of IgM compensates for the typically low affinity of its Fab domains; IgM molecules are expressed early in an immune response before the onset of affinity maturation. Treatment with dithiothreitol can destroy IgM binding because it reduces disulfide bonds, thereby eliminating the high avidity of IgM. IgM potently activates complement by changing its three-dimensional structure upon antigen binding. Although an IgM-specific Fc receptor has long been suspected and was recently cloned, its function is not yet known.

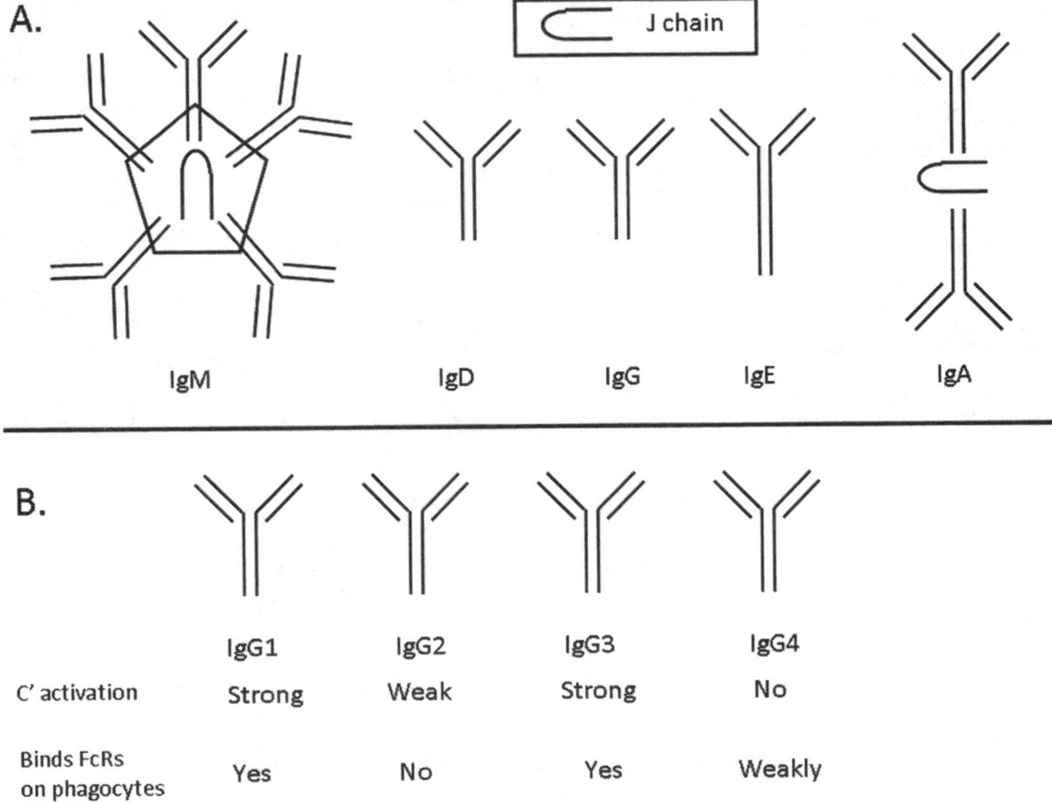

FIGURE 10-13. Immunoglobulin isotypes (A) and IgG subclasses and their relative activation of complement and binding to Fc gamma receptors (B).

IgG antibodies are important in mature humoral immune effector function and are divided into four subclasses: IgG1 through IgG4. Each subclass has a different constant region, constituting distinct Fc domains. Each Fc domain has a differential capacity to activate complement and/or interact with Fc receptors on phagocytes (Fig 10-13). IgG1 and IgG3 are generally most potent in these regards, IgG2 only weakly activates complement, and IgG4 largely lacks effector activity. Consistent with these observations, patients with IgG4 subclass red cell autoantibodies do not exhibit hemolysis. In contrast, IgG1, IgG2, and IgG3 red cell antibodies can each induce hemolysis.

IgA is the primary antibody isotype secreted at mucosal surfaces; therefore, it is largely responsible for neutralization of pathogens encountered in the gastrointestinal, genitourinary, and respiratory tracts. Although IgA exists in either monomeric or dimeric forms (a dimer is shown in Fig 10-13), it is often monomeric in serum. IgA is further divided into IgA1 and IgA2 subclasses (not shown). In its dimeric form, IgA monomers are connected by the J chain, similar to IgM. In rare instances, IgA red cell antibodies cause hemolysis. It is important to note that most antiglobulin (ie, direct antiglobulin test, or DAT) reagents do not detect IgA; thus, the potential presence of IgA red cell antibodies must be considered when analyzing a patient with DAT-negative hemolysis.

IgE antibodies bind to Fc receptors on mast cells and induce histamine release when they encounter antigen; thus, IgE antibodies are the predominant cause of allergic and anaphylactic responses (type I hypersensitivity). IgD primarily remains membrane bound on the B-cell surface, with only minimal levels in serum; the functions of IgD remain unknown.

The Role of Fc Receptors in Target Destruction

The Fc domains of bound IgGs are recognized by a specific family of Fc receptors—Fc gamma receptors (FcRs). There have been at least four FcRs described to date, each of which has subtly different properties and can have opposite functions. For example, FcR2a and FcR3 promote phagocytosis of targets that are bound by multiple antibodies. In contrast, FcR2b is an inhibitory receptor that prevents phagocytosis. FcR1 has an unusually high affinity and thus binds to monomeric IgG. The result of this is that FcR1 binds IgG whether it has recognized its target or not; the function of this activity is currently unclear. Thus, FcR biology is complicated by the fact that any given IgG-bound cell or particle may simultaneously activate multiple and potentially antagonistic receptors. The biology is further complicated by the fact that each of the four different subtypes of IgG (IgG1, IgG2, IgG3, and IgG4) has a different affinity for the different FcRs (Fig 10-13). Thus, a particle or cell bearing a foreign antigen may be bound by a mixture of IgG subclasses (1 through 4), and the net effect on opsonization or inhibition of phagocytosis will be the result of the relative bindings of different IgG subtypes and interactions with different FcRs. Suffice it to say that direct binding of Fc domains to FcRs can promote red cell consumption in many cases, but not necessarily in every event.

The Role of Complement in Target Cell Destruction and Opsonization

In addition to serving as ligands for FcRs, the Fc domains of IgG antibodies can activate complement. The complement system consists of a cascade of proteases that, once activated, amplify the initial signal into a large number of effector molecules. Although there are several complement activation pathways, the current discussion focuses on the "classical pathway," initiated by antibody Fc domains. Because of its multimeric structure, IgM is highly efficient in activating complement. However, to avoid indiscriminant activation, the IgM structure undergoes a conformational shift upon binding antigen, thereby exposing complement binding sites. This interaction is so potent that in theory, a single antigen-bound IgM molecule is sufficient to lyse a target. In contrast, IgG does not require a conformational change to bind complement, but complement activation does require clustered binding of multiple IgG molecules to the same target. This requirement prevents indiscriminate activation of complement by unbound circulating IgG.

Once activated, the complement system provides at least two distinct mechanisms of target destruction. The first mechanism involves target opsonization by complement components. During early events in complement activation, C3 covalently attaches to the antigen surface by thioester bonds, providing multiple copies of C3b, which are recognized by the CR1 and CRIg complement receptors on phagocytes. When a phagocyte encounters a C3b-coated molecule, it ingests and destroys it. C3b also rapidly degrades sequentially into iC3b, C3c, and C3dg. Because C3dg is recognized by complement receptor CR2, which is not on phagocytes, complement can degrade past the point that it can promote phagocytosis. In the second mechanism, downstream of C3 activation, the cascade assembles the membrane attack complex (MAC). The MAC consists of complement proteins C5b through C9 arranged into a structure resembling a hollow tube inserted into the membrane of the target cell. This provides a nonselective channel between the inside of a target cell and its external environment, resulting in osmotic lysis of the target (if it is sensitive to osmotic shock).

Specific Outcomes Resulting from MAC Assembly, C3 Opsonization, and Fc Opsonization of Antibody-Coated Red Cells

The effector mechanisms induced by antibody binding have different effects on bacteria, viruses, particles, and various human tissues. In general, once an IgG antibody is bound to a red cell, the target red cell may undergo FcR-mediated phagocytosis by phagocytes (Fig 10-14). If the antibody can initiate the complement cascade, then C3b deposition on the red cell surface will contribute to opsonization, leading to phagocytosis mediated by the CR1 and CRIg complement receptors. Finally, if complement activation is complete, the MAC

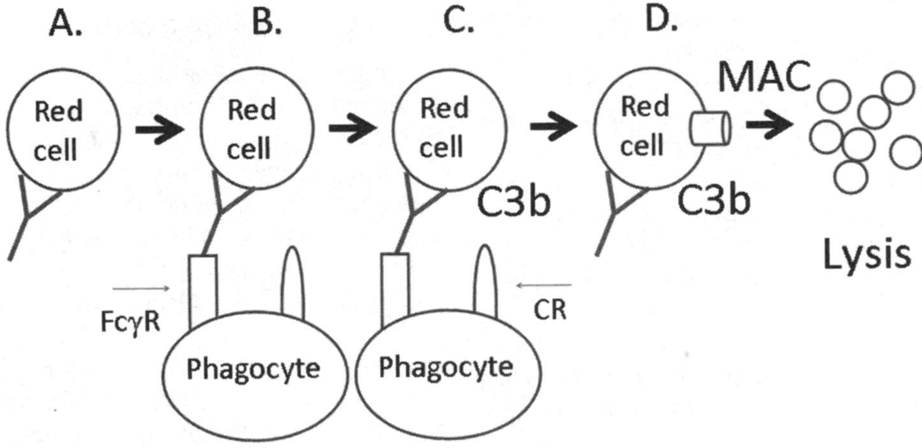

FIGURE 10-14. Mechanisms of red cell destruction by antibody binding. Upon binding (A), an IgG represents a ligand for Fc gamma receptors (FcRs) on phagocytes (B). If the red cell avoids FcR-mediated phagocytosis, opsonization may be increased by activation of complement with deposition of C3b (C). Should the combined opsonization of FcR binding and C3b not be sufficient to mediate clearance, completion of the complement cascade may lead to insertion of the membrane attack complex (MAC) into the red cell surface, resulting in lysis (D). In reality, these processes are likely occurring simultaneously, with the ultimate outcome being the aggregate effect of competing pathways.
CR = complement receptor.

will be inserted into the red cell membrane, causing osmotic lysis. The relative contributions of each of these pathways will vary based on the relative amounts of antibody isotype and subclass and on the nature of the antigen (eg, antigen density, linkage to cytoskeleton, etc). The sections below describe what is known about these processes with regard to red cell destruction and the clinical manifestations of hemolysis.

EXTRAVASCULAR HEMOLYSIS. Consumption of antibody- and/or C3b-bound red cells by phagocytes in the reticuloendothelial system (RES; predominantly in the spleen and liver) is referred to as extravascular hemolysis because the red cells are destroyed outside of their normal compartment: the intravascular space. This process is also commonly referred to as a delayed hemolytic transfusion reaction (DHTR) because it is often not clinically recognized until days after transfusion, as compared to intravascular hemolysis (see below), which is recognized acutely during the transfusion [eg, an acute hemolytic transfusion reaction (AHTR)]. The delayed kinetics for recognizing DHTRs are the result of the milder clinical manifestations of extravascular hemolysis and/or the need for the implicated antibodies to develop or increase in titer before the onset of significant red cell destruction. The term hemolysis in this context can lead to confusion for health-care providers not accustomed to blood bank terminology because they typically think of hemolysis as the rupture of red cells within the circulation (ie, intravascular hemolysis). Instead, in the case of extravascular hemolysis, the red cells undergo hemolysis in the digestive compartment (ie, lysosomes) of phagocytes. This is a very important distinction because phagocytes in the RES consume a substantial number of senescent, autologous red cells each day in the normal process of red cell turnover. Thus, red cell consumption in this fashion uses a pathway that specifically evolved to break down and recycle red cell contents (eg, hemoglobin and iron) in a safe manner that avoids tissue damage. This does not mean, however, that extravascular removal of antibody-coated red cells is biologically equivalent to clearance of normal, senescent red cells. On the contrary, DHTRs can cause substantial morbidity and occasional mortality; indeed, in murine models of incompatible transfusion, rapid clearance of antibody-coated red cells induces systemic inflammation and cytokine storm. Nonetheless, extravascular hemolysis is different from intravascular hemolysis; in extravascular hemolysis red cell contents are directly released into the circulating blood (see below).

It is not clear why some red cell antibodies preferentially promote opsonization and phagocytosis instead of osmotic lysis by the MAC. Substantial evidence indicates that the antibody type, the topographical arrangement of the target antigen on the red cell, or both are important. In addition, although complement may be activated, the aggregate opsonization of red cells by C3b and antibody may result in phagocytosis before MAC-induced lysis occurs. Consistent with these explanations is the observation that extravascular hemolysis is typically induced by IgG red cell antibodies, whereas intravascular hemolysis is typically induced by IgM red cell antibodies; the latter is much more efficient at fixing complement and promoting MAC formation.

INTRAVASCULAR HEMOLYSIS. In some cases of incompatible red cell transfusion, the MAC rapidly assembles and lyses the red cell before C3b and/or IgG opsonization can induce phagocytosis. Because these red cells lyse while still circulating inside blood vessels, this is termed intravascular hemolysis. In addition, because alloantibody-mediated intravascular hemolysis occurs at a brisker pace than extravascular hemolysis (or at least is more quickly noticed because of dramatic signs and symptoms), it is called acute (ie, AHTR). As discussed above, AHTRs are typically caused by IgM antibodies, which efficiently activate complement, leading to rapid formation of the MAC. Although an IgM-specific Fc receptor has been described (ie, FcR), it is predominantly expressed on nonphagocytic lymphocytes; thus, it is unlikely to promote phagocytosis of IgM-coated red cells. Nonetheless, complement activation by IgM red cell antibodies can produce opsonization by C3b, leading to CR1- and CRIg-mediated phagocytosis. Taken together then, it is not surprising that IgMs predominantly induce intravascular hemolysis.

Intravascular hemolysis, unlike extravascular hemolysis, is a decidedly unnatural event that does not normally occur at any appreciable level. The release of red cell contents directly into the circulation can be highly toxic, with free hemoglobin inducing perhaps the greatest insult. Although much free hemoglobin is scavenged by haptoglobin, this system is easily overwhelmed. AHTRs often result in tea-colored urine (ie, hemoglobinuria), which can induce renal dysfunction. Moreover, the signs and symptoms of AHTRs can be very dramatic, including disseminated intravascular coagulation, shock, and death. This type of reaction most often occurs as a result of a clerical error leading to an ABO-incompatible transfusion, and much of current immunohematology practice has developed to prevent ABO-incompatible AHTRs.

NONHEMOLYTIC RED CELL ANTIBODIES. Given the redundant pathways that lead to destruction of antibody-coated red cells, it is not surprising that transfusions of crossmatch-incompatible RBCs can lead to hemolysis. However, somewhat surprisingly, the vast majority of red cell antibodies are not hemolytic. For some blood group antigens, hemolysis is never, or only very rarely, observed following incompatible transfusion (eg, JMH, Chido, and Rogers antigens). Indeed, approximately 1% of healthy blood donors have a positive DAT, indicating that IgG autoantibodies are bound to their own red cells, yet there is no evidence of hemolysis in these donors. Even for antigens known to be involved in antibody-mediated hemolysis (eg, in the Rh, Kell, Kidd, Duffy, and Ss systems), hemolysis is variable. In fact, retrospective analysis of patients mistakenly transfused with ABO-incompatible RBCs shows that even for this robustly hemolytic antigen-antibody combination, no clinically significant hemolysis is seen in 50% of cases.

Several explanations may account for the lack of hemolysis during incompatible transfusions. For antigens essentially never involved in hemolysis, the antigen density or surface topography may prevent hemolysis from occurring. For antigens that are variably involved in hemolysis, idiosyncrasies concerning a given recipient's antibodies may play a role (ie, titer, affinity, isotype, or IgG subclass). Based on these properties, different antibodies (of the same antigenic specificity) may have different capacities for activating complement. This is the rationale behind including the anti-C3b component in the antiglobulin reagent: it provides information regarding whether an antibody can fix complement. A number of different genetic polymorphisms and/or deficiencies may also regulate hemolysis vs red cell survival on a patient-by-patient basis, including perturbations in complement, complement regulatory proteins, and allelic polymorphisms in FcRs. Thus, in some cases, regulation of hemolysis may be independent of the nature of the antibody.

From a practical standpoint, crossmatch-incompatible RBCs may be issued for transfusion if the offending entity is a "clinically insignificant antigen," especially if the antigen is of very high frequency and antigen-negative blood is difficult or impossible to obtain. The blood bank should be prepared to address appropriate concerns from the health-care providers managing these patients. Also from a practical standpoint, although clinically significant antigens may demonstrate variable hemolysis from patient to patient, currently there are only very limited means of predicting whether hemolysis will occur in a given recipient. Thus, it is imperative that RBCs never be issued for transfusion that are crossmatch incompatible for clinically significant antigens—unless there is no other choice and, as a lifesaving procedure, such transfusion is specifically requested by the managing physician. For example, in some cases if compatible RBCs are unavailable, it might be determined that hemolysis occurring over several days (eg, in the case of a DHTR) is less dangerous than the consequences of the patient's severe anemia. Close and frequent communication between managing physicians and the blood bank is required in these cases.

Summary of Efferent Immunity

In aggregate, when an antibody binds a red cell, multiple pathways are activated that can lead to red cell destruction. Complement activation promotes phagocytosis, through the opsonizing properties of C3b, and direct red cell lysis, through assembly of the MAC. The presence of IgG Fc domains promotes red cell phagocytosis by ligating FcRs on the phagocyte surface. The relative contributions of these different pathways vary depending on the nature of the target antigen and the properties of the cognate antibodies. Moreover, the immune activation events that occur and the toxicity of the released red cell products can produce a scenario in which the negative effects of immune destruction of transfused red cells extend far beyond loss of efficacy of the transfused cells. Indeed, substantial toxicity can occur, leading to morbidity and, in some cases, mortality. (For more fine mechanistic detail of immunobiology and the immune response, see the suggested readings at the end of this chapter.)

KEY POINTS

1. Hybridization-based methods can be used to detect genes, gene products, and polymorphisms, but they lack sensitivity.
2. Amplification-based methods are highly sensitive but are also susceptible to problems with contamination, inhibitors, or both because of the nature of geometric amplification involved.
3. The presence of nucleic acids predicts, but does not always equate to, expression of the corresponding protein or antigen structure.
4. Analysis of protein expression directly detects the actual gene product(s) and thus does not encounter the problems of nucleic acid testing (ie, by which antigen is only predicted).
5. Protein analysis is less sensitive than nucleic acid testing because no amplification is involved, but it is also less susceptible to contamination and inhibition, which can lead to false-positive and false-negative results.
6. Methods of detecting protein are hindered by nonamplification-based artifacts (ie, heterophilic antibodies, prozone effects, hook effects) that can lead to erroneous results.
7. Variability can be substantial in detecting antigens and antibodies with different methods.
8. Most antibodies to blood group antigens are IgG (excluding antibodies to ABO and other carbohydrate antigens).
9. Formation of IgG antibodies typically requires CD4+ T-cell help. Generation of CD4+ T-cell help requires processing and presentation of antigen as T-cell epitopes (peptides on the major histocompatibility complex) by antigen-presenting cells. This process, which is required for most IgG alloimmunization, is not detected by existing clinical assays.
10. Immunoglobulins can cause destruction of red cells by several different mechanisms, based largely on the antigen recognized and the antibody structure.
11. Most IgG antibodies that cause red cell destruction induce extravascular hemolysis by promoting consumption of red cells by phagocytes (through Fc receptors and/or complement-based opsonization). This typically presents as a delayed hemolytic transfusion reaction.
12. IgM (and in some rare cases, IgG) antibodies that cause red cell destruction typically induce intravascular hemolysis by activation of complement and, in turn, the membrane attack complex. This typically presents as an acute hemolytic transfusion reaction.
13. Despite the serious nature of hemolysis caused by incompatible transfusion, many antibodies to red cell antigens are clinically insignificant and do not result in destruction of red cells. Incompatibility is best avoided whenever possible, but when compatible blood is not available, incompatible red cells can often be safely used when the antigens are known to be clinically insignificant. Such maneuvers should be carefully considered on a case-by-case basis.

REFERENCES

1. Alberts B, Bray D, Lewis J, et al. Molecular biology of the cell. 3rd ed. New York: Garland Science, 1994:98-105.
2. Southern EM. Detection of specific sequences among DNA fragments separated by gel electrophoresis. J Med Biol 1975;98:503-17.
3. Alwine JC, Kemp DJ, Stark GR. Method for detection of specific RNAs in agarose gels by transfer to diazobenzyloxymethyl-paper and hybridization with DNA probes. Proc Natl Acad Sci U S A 1977;74:5350-4.
4. Melton DA, Krieg PA, Rebagliati MR, et al. Efficient in vitro synthesis of biologically active RNA and RNA hybridization probes from plasmids containing a bacteriophage SP6 promoter. Nucleic Acids Res 1984;12:7035-56.
5. Berk AJ, Sharp PA. Sizing and mapping of early adenovirus mRNAs by gel electrophoresis of S1 endonuclease-digested hybrids. Cell 1977; 12:721-32.
6. Mullis KB, Faloona FA. Specific synthesis of DNA in vitro via a polymerase-catalyzed chain reaction. Methods Enzymol 1987;155:335-50.
7. Masukawa A, Miyachi H, Ohshima T, et al. [Monitoring of inhibitors of the polymerase chain reaction for the detection of hepatitis C virus using the positive internal control]. Rinsho Byori 1997;45:673-8.
8. Al-Soud WA, Radstrom P. Purification and characterization of PCR-inhibitory components in blood cells. J Clin Microbiol 2001;39:485-93.
9. Pang J, Modlin J, Yolken R. Use of modified nucleotides and uracil-DNA glycosylase (UNG) for the control of contamination in the PCR-based amplification of RNA. Mol Cell Probes 1992;6:251-6.
10. Temin HM, Mizutani S. RNA-dependent DNA polymerase in virions of Rous sarcoma virus. Nature 1970;226:1211-13. [Erratum appears in Nature 1970;227:102.]
11. Baltimore D. RNA-dependent DNA polymerase in virions of RNA tumour viruses. Nature 1970;226:1209-11.
12. Compton J. Nucleic acid sequence-based amplification. Nature 1991;350:91-2.
13. Kwoh DY, Davis GR, Whitfield KM, et al. Transcription-based amplification system and detection of amplified human immunodeficiency virus type 1 with a bead-based sandwich hybridization format. Proc Natl Acad Sci U S A 1989;86:1173-7.
14. Walker GT, Fraiser MS, Schram JL, et al. Strand displacement amplification—an isothermal, in vitro DNA amplification technique. Nucleic Acids Res 1992;20:1691-6.
15. Walker GT, Little MC, Nadeau JG, Shank DD. Isothermal in vitro amplification of DNA by a restriction enzyme/DNA polymerase system. Proc Natl Acad Sci U S A 1992;89:392-6.
16. Wu DY, Wallace RB. The ligation amplification reaction (LAR)—amplification of specific DNA sequences using sequential rounds of template-dependent ligation. Genomics 1989;4: 560-9.
17. Zimring JC, Nolte FS. Polymerase chain reaction and other amplification technologies. 20th ed. Philadelphia: WB Saunders, 2001: 1287-95.
18. Schaferling M, Nagl S. Optical technologies for the read out and quality control of DNA and protein microarrays. Anal Bioanal Chem 2006; 385:500-17.
19. Denomme GA, Van Oene M. High-throughput multiplex single-nucleotide polymorphism analysis for red cell and platelet antigen genotypes. Transfusion 2005;45:660-6. [See comment.]
20. Bugert P, McBride S, Smith G, et al. Microarray-based genotyping for blood groups: Comparison of gene array and 5-nuclease assay techniques with human platelet antigen as a model. Transfusion 2005;45:654-9. [See comment.]
21. Langston MM, Procter JL, Cipolone KM, Stroncek DF. Evaluation of the gel system for ABO grouping and D typing. Transfusion 1999;39: 300-5.
22. Voak D. Observations on the rare phenomenon of anti-A prozone and the non-specific blocking of haemagglutination due to C1 complement fixation by IgG anti-A antibodies. Vox Sang 1972;22:408-19.
23. Judd WJ, Steiner EA, O'Donnell DB, Oberman HA. Discrepancies in reverse ABO typing due to prozone. How safe is the immediate-spin crossmatch? Transfusion 1988;28:334-8.
24. Salama A, Mueller-Eckhardt C. Elimination of the prozone effect in the antiglobulin reaction by a simple modification. Vox Sang 1982;42: 157-9.
25. Procter JL, Vigue F, Alegre E, et al. Rapid screening of platelet donors for PIA1 (HPA-1a) alloantigen using a solid-phase microplate immunoassay. Immunohematology 1998;14:141-5.

26. Leikola J, Perkins HA. Enzyme-linked antiglobulin test: An accurate and simple method to quantify red cell antibodies. Transfusion 1980; 20:138-44.

SUGGESTED READING

Kindt TJ, Osborne BA, Goldsby RA. Kuby immunology. 6th ed. New York: WH Freeman and Company, 2007.

Murphy K, Travers P, Walport M, Janeway C. Janeway's immunobiology. 7th ed. New York: Garland Science, 2008.

Chapter 11

Blood Group Genetics

Christine Lomas-Francis, MSc, FIBMS

THE SCIENCE OF genetics is the study of heredity, that is, the mechanisms by which particular characteristics are passed from parents to offspring. This chapter describes the genetics of blood groups. The term "blood group," in its broadest sense, could be applied to any detectable, variable characteristic of a component of the blood, such as platelet and white cell groups, serum groups, red cell enzymes, and hemoglobin variants. However, in common usage and for the purpose of this chapter, the term "blood group" is restricted to antigens on the surface of the red cell membrane that are defined serologically by an antibody.

That blood groups are inherited characteristics was first shown by von Dungern and Hirszfeld in 1910, 10 years after Landsteiner's discovery of the ABO blood group.[1] As more blood groups were identified, their value for use in human genetics grew, and blood groups have played an important role in demonstrating that the principles of genetics established in other species also apply to humans. Blood groups became an ideal tool for geneticists because they could be identified by specific antibodies in simple hemagglutination tests, and once identified, their inheritance could easily be followed in family studies. Hence, red cell antigens were (and still are) valuable as **markers** (a detectable characteristic to recognize the presence of a gene) in genetic and anthropologic studies as well as in relationship testing.

The detection of inherited differences on the red cells from different people is the basis of safe blood transfusion. Therefore, an understanding of the principles of human genetics (including the patterns of inheritance, the language, and the terminology in use) is an important aspect of immunohematology and transfusion medicine. The aim of this chapter is to outline the fundamental principles of genetics as they apply to red cell antigens and to relate them to examples relevant to the blood bank. This requires the use of numerous genetic terms that may not be familiar to all readers. Therefore, each genetic term, when first used or when later fully described, will be in **bold** text and usually closely followed by a definition.

In this age of molecular genetics, inheritance can also be studied at the nucleic acid level, and genes can be cloned and sequenced.[2] Knowledge of the fundamental principles of genetics allows for a deeper un-

Christine Lomas-Francis, MSc, FIBMS, Technical Director, Immunohematology and Genomics Laboratory, New York Blood Center, New York, New York

The author has disclosed no conflicts of interest.

derstanding and appreciation of the molecular aspects of genetics of individual blood groups (addressed in Chapter 10), but the reverse is also true.

FUNDAMENTAL PRINCIPLES OF GENETICS

In the second half of the 19th century, Gregor Mendel established the basic techniques of genetic analysis when, in 1865, he published his meticulous (and now classic) breeding experiments with pea plants. Mendel's observations led him to conclude that there is a "factor" or unit of inheritance (now known as a gene, the term introduced by the Danish biologist Johannsen in 1909) that is passed from one generation to another according to two simple rules: the principles of independent segregation and independent assortment (see "Mendel's Laws" later). Early in the 20th century it was realized that genes are carried by structures called chromosomes that are located in the nucleus of a cell. The existence of chromosomes had been recognized toward the end of the 19th century because they could be visualized with the aid of a light microscope in the cell nucleus during cell division. Another milestone was reached in 1944 when studies on bacteria showed that the chromosomal material (often referred to as chromatin) is primarily made up of nucleic acids and associated proteins.[2,3]

The publishing of Mendel's findings in 1865 was the start of a fascinating journey of discovery that has made genetics relevant to most medical specialties. The 20th century witnessed many genetic discoveries, too many to detail here. Many excellent texts offer a greater knowledge of classical genetics.[2-5] This chapter focuses on the fundamental principles of genetics and is intended only as a foundation on which to build the more detailed and specialized information of blood group genetics.

Genes (Alleles) and Chromosomes

A **gene** is a segment of deoxyribonucleic acid (DNA) that encodes a particular protein. It is the basic unit of inheritance of any **trait** (defined as a genetically determined characteristic or condition), including blood group antigens. Each gene occupies a specific location on a chromosome (see below), known as the **gene locus.** A locus may be occupied by one of several alternative forms of the gene; these alternatives are called **alleles.** For example, the gene that encodes the protein carrying the Jk^a antigen is an alternative form (allele) of the one that encodes the Jk^b antigen. The terms "gene" and "allele" can be used interchangeably.

A brief introduction to gene and allele terminology, which will be expanded upon later, is required before proceeding further. In compliance with accepted terminology, the gene or allele name will be italicized—for example, *RHD* for the gene encoding the RhD protein, or *A* for the allele encoding the A blood group antigen. The name will not be italicized when the word "gene" or "allele" follows the name: for example, "RHD gene," or "A allele."

Chromosomes are the gene-carrying structures, composed of chromatin, that are visible during nuclear division as thread-like bodies in the nucleus of the cell; they contain the genetic material (DNA) necessary to maintain the life of the cell and the organism. **Chromatin** is the name given by scientists at the end of the 19th century to the material present in the cell nucleus that stains most strongly with chromosome-specific dyes; thus, it corresponds to the chromosomes. The term "chromatin" is frequently used to denote the physical and structural organization of DNA and proteins in the chromosomes. In most chromosomes, the chromatin consists of DNA (40%) bound to protein (60%) that is primarily responsible for packaging the DNA in a regular fashion within the chromosome.

The number of chromosomes and their morphology are specific for each species. A human somatic cell contains a total of 46 chromosomes that make up 23 pairs; each chromosomal pair has one paternally and one maternally derived chromosome. In both males and females, 22 of the pairs are alike or **homologous chromosomes** (a pair of chromosomes in which males and females carry equivalent genes) and are referred to as the **autosomes** (any chromosome that is not a sex chromosome); the remaining pair is different (nonhomologous) in males and females and consists of the **sex chromosomes** that determine the sex (gender) of a person. The sex-determining chromosomes of the male are X and Y, whereas in the female there are two X chromosomes. The particular array, or chromosome complement, of a person is referred to as the **karyotype**; this is written as 46,XY and 46,XX for a normal male and female, respectively. The hereditary information carried by the chromosomes is passed on from a parent cell to a daughter cell during somatic cell division and from parents to future offspring (children) by the gametes during reproduction.

Techniques to visualize and analyze chromosomes have greatly advanced since chromosomes were first observed in the 1880s with the aid of a light microscope by the German embryologist Flemming. Chromosomes are best studied during cell division (mitosis; see later section) when they become visible as discrete structures in the nucleus. All chromosomes have some common morphologic features but differ in other characteristics, including size, location of the centromere, and staining properties. Each chromosome has two sections or arms that are joined at a central constriction called the **centromere** (Figs 11-1 and 11-2). Chromosomes are distinguished by their length and the position of the centromere; this provides the basis for numbering the autosomes 1 through 22 such that chromosome 1 is the largest and chromosome 22 the smallest (Fig 11-3). To facilitate discussion among geneticists, an internationally recognized terminology is used to describe chromosomes.[7]

The chromosomal arms are of different length, although the difference in length between the arms of chromosome 1 is not obvious (see Fig 11-2). The "p" (or petite) arm is the shorter of the two segments and, in diagrams, is at the top of the chromosome. The longer arm is termed "q" and forms the bottom portion of the chromosome (Fig 11-2). For example, the short arm of chromosome 1 is referred to as 1p, and the long arm of chromosome 4 is

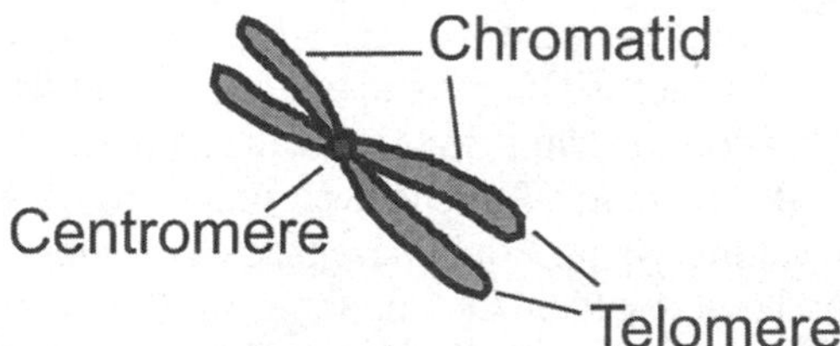

FIGURE 11-1. Diagram of a metaphase chromosome. At the metaphase stage of the cell cycle, the chromosomes have condensed and become visible by light microscopy. As shown in the diagram, metaphase chromosomes have replicated in preparation for cell division so that each chromosome consists of two sister chromatids connected by the centromere. The telomere is the end or terminal part of a chromosome.

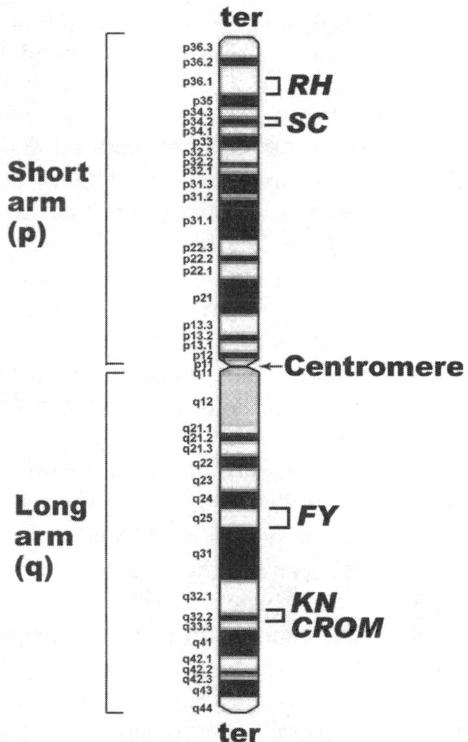

FIGURE 11-2. Morphology and banding pattern of a Giemsa-stained human chromosome 1. The locations of the genes controlling the expression of antigens for the Rh *(RH)*, Scianna *(SC)*, Duffy *(FY)*, Knops *(KN)*, and Cromer *(CROM)* blood group systems are shown.

4q. The terminal portion of a chromosome is referred to as "ter"; pter and qter represent the terminus of the short (p) and long (q) arms, respectively.

Staining techniques provide a more detailed means to distinguish individual chromosomes because selected dyes do not stain chromosomes uniformly. For example, as shown in Figs 11-2 and 11-3, Giemsa staining of chromosomes reveals a specific banding pattern of dark and light bands for each chromosome pair. The dark Giemsa-stained bands are the G bands; the bands that are the reverse of the G bands are called the reverse or R bands. Quinacrine, used to stain chromosomal preparations for fluorescence microscopy, results in fluorescent bands equivalent to the dark G bands seen in light microscopy. The G bands are dark bands of condensed DNA known as heterochromatin and may represent areas of little genetic activity. The lighter bands, known as euchromatin, may correspond to the active regions of DNA. The bands are numbered from the centromere outward (Fig 11-2). Using chromosome 1 as an example, the region closest to the centromere on the short or long arm would be numbered 1p1 or 1q1, respectively. Each region is subdivided by finer bands (eg, 1p11 and 1p12); more refined staining techniques allow for even further distinction (eg, 1p11.1 and 1p11.2). Genes can be individually mapped to a specific band location (Fig 11-2), and the genes encoding the 30 blood group systems have been located on specific chromosomes (Fig 11-3).[7-9]

Cell Division

Cells multiply by cell division. As a cell divides, its chromosomes must be replicated so that each daughter cell receives a full complement of genetic material. In somatic cells, this occurs through mitosis; in reproductive cells, a similar but different process, called meiosis, takes place. A feature common to both types of cell division is that, before the start of the process, each chromosome will replicate itself to form two daughter chromatids that are attached to each other through the centromere (Fig 11-1). The centromere, in addition to being the structure that holds the chromatids together, also plays an important role in cell division by being the point of attachment for the fiber that draws the dividing chromosomes apart.

Mitosis

Somatic cells divide for growth and repair by **mitosis**; through this process of cell division, a single cell (the parent or mother cell) gives rise to two daughter cells. The daughter cells, like the parent cell, are **diploid (2N)**; that is, they contain 46 chromosomes in 23 pairs and have all the genetic information of the parent cell. Mitosis is a continuous process, but for convenience of description, it can be divided into four stages: prophase, metaphase, anaphase, and telophase (Fig 11-4).

Meiosis

Meiosis occurs only in germ (or primordial) cells that are intended to become gametes (sperm and egg cells). It is a cycle of two nuclear divisions that begins with a diploid cell containing 46 chromosomes and results in four gametes, each of which is **haploid** [having half the chromosomal complement **(1N)** of a somatic cell; ie, 23 chromosomes]. Thus, **meiosis** is a process of cell division and replication that leads to the formation of haploid gametes. As with mitosis, each meiotic division can be divided into separate phases for ease of description (Fig 11-5).

The formation of haploid gametes is essential because sperm and egg cells fuse at fertilization to form a zygote. If each gamete carried a diploid (2N) set of 46 chromosomes, the resulting zygote would have 92 chromosomes, and this would be incompatible with life. Meiosis ensures genetic diversity through two mechanisms: independent assortment and crossing-over (discussed in more detail later). Through independent assortment, each daughter cell randomly receives either maternally or paternally derived homologous chromosomes during the first division of meiosis. Chromosomal crossing-over allows for an exchange of genetic material between homologous chromosome pairs. Such shuffling of ge-

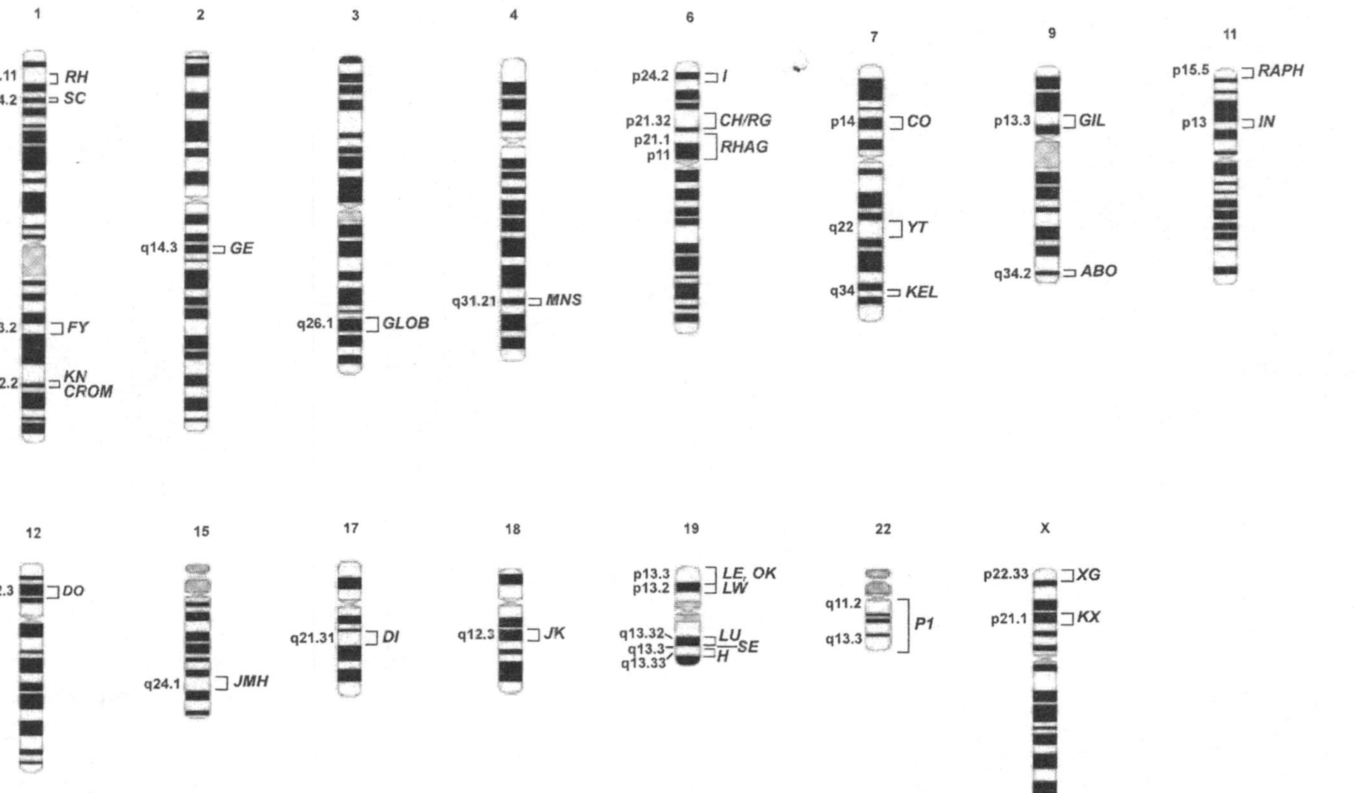

FIGURE 11-3. Diagram of the 14 autosomes and the X chromosome that encode, or influence the expression of, the human blood group systems. Shown are the differences in size and banding patterns and the chromosomal locations of the genes controlling expression of the 30 blood group systems. Also shown is *SE*, the gene involved in synthesis of Lewis and ABH antigens. The italicized symbol for each blood group gene [using the traditional name and not the Human Gene Nomenclature Committee (HGNC) name] is given to the right of each chromosome, and the banding location is given to the left of the chromosome. A range is given for *P1*; however, the gene encoding P1 has now been more precisely located to chromosome 22q13.2.

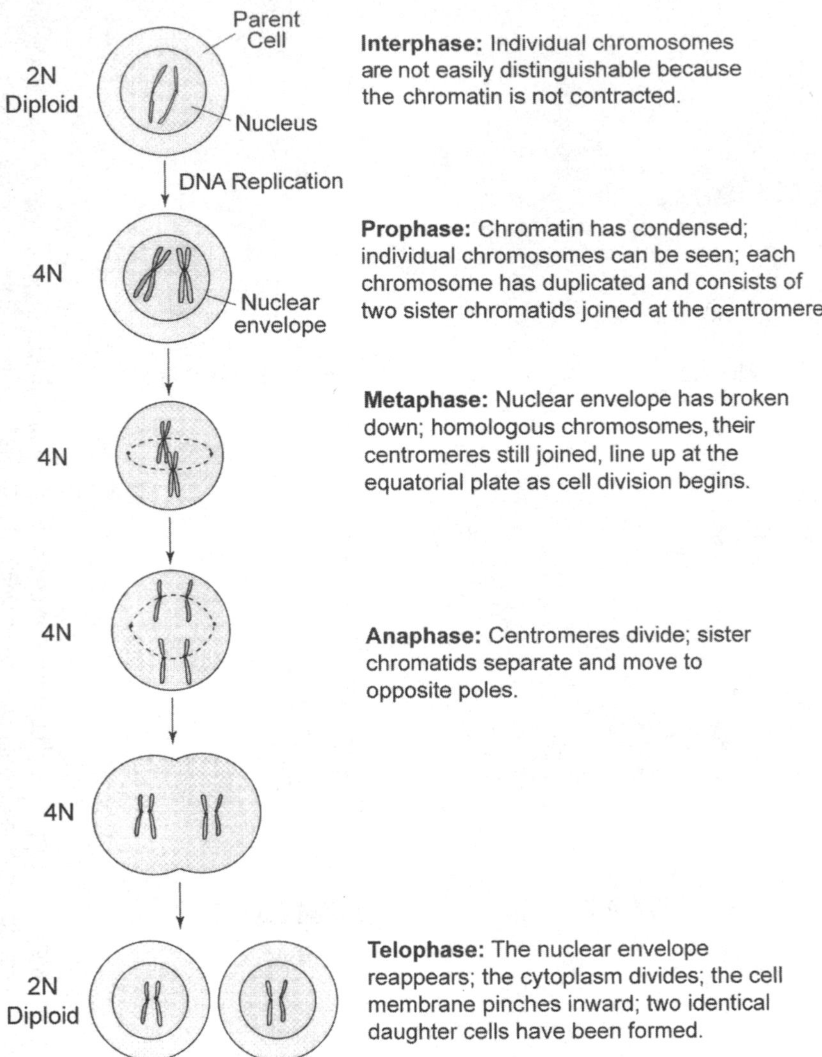

FIGURE 11-4. Diagram showing mitosis.

netic material ensures diversity and produces genetically unique gametes that fuse to produce a unique zygote.

X Chromosome Inactivation (Lyonization)

Females have two X chromosomes and thus have two copies of X-borne genes in their somatic cells. Male somatic cells have only one X chromosome and thus only one copy of X-borne genes. As most X-borne genes do not have a homolog on the Y chromosome, there is a potential imbalance in the dosage of X-borne genes between males and females. This difference is compensated for by **X chromosome inactivation**, formerly known as lyonization (after Mary Lyon and the Lyon hypothesis), a process through which most of the genes on one of the two X chromosomes in each female somatic cell are inactivated at a very early stage of embryonic development.[10] The inactivated X can be visualized in the interphase cell nucleus as darkly staining X-chromatin (previously referred to as the Barr body). It is a matter of chance whether the maternal or paternal

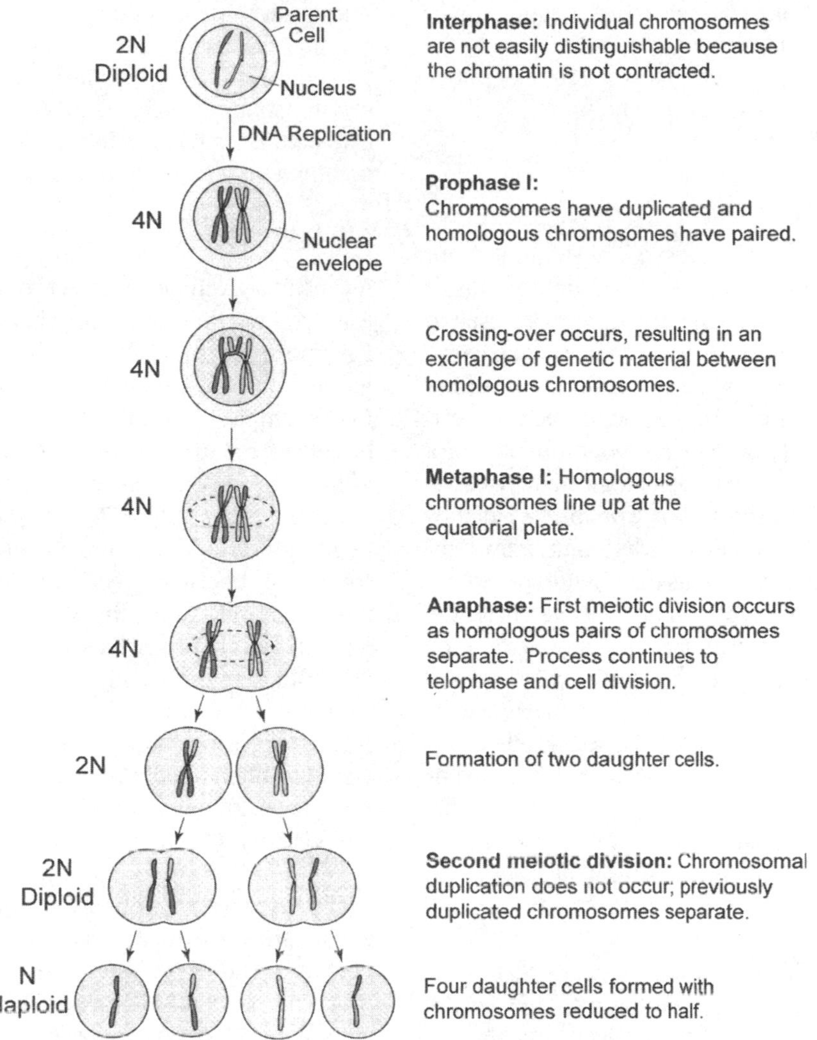

FIGURE 11-5. Diagram showing meiosis.

X chromosome is inactivated in any one cell, but once inactivation has occurred, all descendants of that cell will have the same inactive X chromosome. Some X-borne genes (at least 20 of them) escape inactivation; the first found to escape inactivation was *XG*, the gene encoding the antigens of the Xg blood group system. Most of the genes that escape inactivation, like *XG*, are located on the extreme tip of the short arm of the X chromosome, but several of the genes are clustered in regions on the short and long arms of the chromosome.[11(pp374-386),12]

The XK gene, which encodes the antigens of the Kx blood group system, is the only other X-borne gene that encodes blood group antigens. Changes or deletions in *XK* result in McLeod phenotype red cells that lack Kx antigens and have reduced expression of Kell antigens.[13,14] The XK gene, unlike *XG*, is subject to X chromosome inactivation, with the result that a female who is a **carrier** (a person who carries one gene for a recessive trait and one normal gene) of a gene responsible for the McLeod phenotype can have a dual population of Kx+ and Kx– red cells. This mixed-cell population is often easier to demonstrate by flow cytometry than by hemagglutination and reflects the randomness of whether the maternal or paternal X is inactivated in any one somatic cell lineage.[11(pp295-323),12-14]

Genotype and Phenotype

The **genotype** of a person is the complement of genes inherited by each person from his or her parents; the term is frequently also used to refer to the set of alleles at a single gene locus. Whereas the genotype of a person is his or her genetic constitution, the **phenotype** is the observable expression of the genes inherited by a person and reflects the biologic activity of the gene(s). Thus, the presence or absence of antigens on the red cells, as determined by serologic testing, represents the phenotype. Sometimes the genotype can be predicted from the phenotype; for example, when a person's red cells react with anti-A and anti-B (blood group AB), the presence of A and B genes (*A/B* genotype) can be inferred. Similarly, red cells with a Jk(a+b+) phenotype indicate a Jk^a/Jk^b genotype. Frequently, the phenotype provides only a partial indication of the genotype; for example, red cells that are group B reflect the presence of a B gene, but the genotype may be *B/B* or *B/O*. Previously, family studies were often the only way to determine a genotype, but advances in the understanding of the genetic bases for blood group antigens mean that most antigens can now be defined at the DNA level, thereby reducing the need for extensive family studies to determine genotype. Although not as challenging as a family study, determination of the true genotype can be complex and time consuming, and requires sequencing of the entire gene of interest. Polymerase chain reaction/restriction fragment length polymorphism (PCR-RFLP) analysis can be used to target a portion of the gene (and the polymorphism) of interest; this procedure is simpler than gene sequencing and is useful to predict a partial phenotype. Mature red cells have lost their DNA, but answers can be obtained by analysis of DNA extracted from white cells obtained from peripheral blood samples, or by analysis of DNA extracted from buccal swab samples or urine sediment. In certain circumstances—for example, if the person was the recipient of an allogeneic stem cell transplant—the result obtained from DNA extracted from white cells will differ from that obtained from a buccal swab sample.

Alleles

A gene at a given locus on a chromosome may exist in more than one form, that is, be allelic. Each person has two alleles for a trait, one maternally derived, the other paternally derived. At the simplest level, the ABO gene locus can be considered to have three alleles: *A*, *B*, and *O*. With three alleles, there are six possible genotypes (*A/A*, *A/O*, *A/B*, *B/B*, *B/O*, and *O/O*). Depending on the parental contribution, a person could inherit any combination of two of the alleles and express the corresponding antigens on their red cells. For example, *A/A* and *A/O* would result in group A red cells, or *A/B* would result in group AB red cells, or *B/B* and *B/O* would result in group B red cells, or *O/O* would result in group O red cells.

When identical alleles for a given locus are present on both chromosomes, the person is said to be **homozygous** for the particular allele, whereas when different (ie, not identical) alleles are present at a particular locus, the person is said to be **heterozygous**. For example, a person with K–k+ red cells is homozygous at the *KEL* locus (the locus encoding antigens of the Kell blood group system) for the allele encoding the k antigen. A person who is heterozygous for *K* and *k* would have red cells that are K+k+. Antigens that are encoded by alleles at the same locus are said to be **antithetical** (meaning "opposite"); thus, K and k are a pair of antithetical antigens. When the K antigen is encoded by an allele, k antigen will not be encoded by that allele and vice versa. It is incorrect to refer to red cells that are K–k+ or Kp(a–b+) as being homozygous for the k or Kp^b antigen; rather, it should be said that the cells have a double dose of the antigen in question and that they are from a person who is homozygous for the particular allele. Thus, genes are allelic but not antithetical, whereas antigens are antithetical but not allelic.

The quantity of antigen expressed on red cells (the antigen density) is influenced by whether a person is heterozygous or homozygous for an allele; the antigen density is greater when a person is homozygous for an allele. In some blood group systems, this difference in antigen density is manifested by antibodies giving stronger reactions with cells that have a double dose of the antigen. Red cells with the Jk(a+b–) phenotype have a double dose of the Jk^a antigen and are likely to react more strongly with anti-Jk^a than those that are Jk(a+b+) and have only a single dose of the Jk^a antigen. Similarly, M+N– red cells tend to react more strongly with anti-M than do M+N+ red cells. Antibodies that are weakly reactive may not be detected if tested with red cells expressing a single dose of the particular antigen. This observable difference in strength of reaction, based on homozygosity or heterozygosity for an allele, is termed the **dosage effect**. The dosage effect is not observed with all blood group antigens or with all antibodies of a given specificity. Antibodies in the Rh, MNS, Kidd, Duffy, and Lutheran blood group systems frequently demonstrate dosage. It is because of the dosage effect that red cells expressing a double dose of the pertinent antigen(s) should be used for antibody detection and identification.

Polymorphism

The first genetic polymorphism to be defined in humans was that of the ABO blood group system, identified by Landsteiner in 1900. Since then, blood groups have consistently played an important part in the study of human polymorphism. There are numerous definitions for "polymorphism" in the scientific literature. An acceptable definition suitable for blood group genetics defines **polymorphism** as the occurrence, in the same population, of two or more alleles at one locus, each with appreciable (greater than 1%) frequency. Based on current knowledge, some blood group systems (Rh and MNS for example) appear highly polymorphic and have many more alleles at a given locus than other systems such as Kidd, Duffy, and Colton.[6] An allele that is polymorphic in one population is not necessarily so in all populations; for example, the Fy allele (*FY*0*) is polymorphic in populations of African ethnicity, with a prevalence of greater than 70%, but outside of populations of African ethnicity, the Fy allele does not occur. This phenomenon can result in the inappropriate usage of the term "polymorphism" when an allele is not universally polymorphic. A particular gene polymorphism may represent an evolutionary advantage for a population, and a polymorphic population is likely to be able to adapt to evolutionary change more rapidly than if there were genetic uniformity. It is not yet understood what, if any, evolutionary advantages were derived from the extensive polymorphism displayed by red cell antigens, but many publications exist that associate resistance or susceptibility for a particular disease with a particular blood type.[15]

The difference between one allele and another is the result of a permanent change in the DNA. In traditional genetics an event that leads to the production of an altered gene and a new allele or polymorphism that did not exist in the biologic parents is referred to as a **mutation**. A mutation is essentially a mistake that occurs as the DNA is being copied, and although this occurs constantly in genetic systems, it is a rarely observed event; the mutation rate of expressed genes resulting in a new phenotype has been estimated to be less than 10^{-5} (<1 in 100,000) in humans, and a mutation has to occur in the germ cells (gametes) for it to be inherited. A mutation can occur spontaneously or can be brought about by agents such as radiation (eg, ultraviolet rays or x-rays) or chemicals. A mutation may occur within a gene or in the intergenic regions. It may be **silent**—that is, have no discernible effect on the encoded protein—or it may alter the gene product and cause an observable effect in the phenotype. In the context of an allele that encodes a protein that carries red cell antigens, any genetically induced change must be recognized by a specific antibody before an allele can be said to encode a new antigen.

Numerous genetic events that generate red cell antigens and phenotypes have been identified; they are summarized in Table 11-1. The event can occur at the level of the chromo-

TABLE 11-1. Molecular Events that Give Rise to Blood Group Antigens and Phenotypes

- Missense nucleotide change (by far the most common)
- Nonsense nucleotide change
- Nucleotide changes in motifs involved in transcription
- Alternative splicing
- Deletion of a gene, exon, or nucleotide(s)
- Insertion of an exon or nucleotide(s)
- Alternative initiation
- Chromosome translocation
- Single cross-over
- Gene conversion
- Other gene recombination events

some (eg, deletion or translocation of part of a chromosome), the gene (eg, deletion, conversion, or rearrangement), the exon (eg, deletion or duplication), or the nucleotide (eg, deletion, substitution, or insertion). An event can induce alternative splicing or initiation, or affect transcription of the gene. Based on the findings of the Human Genome Project, the mechanism that has given rise to most diversity in the human genome is single nucleotide polymorphism (SNP), that is, a single nucleotide change in the DNA.[16-18] Accordingly, the majority of polymorphic blood group antigens are the result of SNPs. Details of these events and the molecular genetic bases of red cell antigens are beyond the scope of this chapter; several reviews that address this topic are available.[19-22]

DNA analysis can be used to successfully predict the red cell phenotype. However, because of a variety of molecular events the results obtained by DNA analysis do not always agree with hemagglutination results (Table 11-2). The majority of these cases involve rare occurrences such as a grossly normal gene that is not expressed, resulting in a null phenotype.[19,20,22]

TABLE 11-2. Examples of Some Molecular Events Where Analysis of Gene and Phenotype Will Not Agree

Molecular Event	Mechanism	Observed Blood Group Phenotype
Transcription	Nt change in GATA box	Fy(b–)
Alternative splicing	Nt change in splice site Partial/complete skipping of exon Deletion of nts	S–s–; Gy(a–) Dr(a–)
Premature stop codon	Deletion of nt(s) → frameshift Insertion of nt(s) → frameshift Nt change	Fy(a–b–); D–; Rh_{null}; GE:–2,–3,–4; Gy(a–); K_0; McLeod D–; Co(a–b–) Fy(a–b–); r′; Gy(a–); K_0; McLeod
Amino acid change	Missense nucleotide change	D–; Rh_{null}; K_0; McLeod
Reduced amount of protein	Missense nucleotide change	Fy^X; Co(a–b–)
Hybrid genes	Cross-over Gene conversion	GP.Vw; GP.Hil; GP.TSEN GP.Mur; GP.Hop; D– –; R_0^{Har}
Interacting protein	Absence of RhAG Absence of Kx Absence of aas 59 to 76 of GPA Absence of protein 4.1	Rh_{null} Weak expression of Kell antigens Wr(b–) Weak expression of Ge antigens
Modifying gene	*In(Lu)* *In(Jk)*	Lu(a–b–) Jk(a–b–)

Nt = nucleotide.

INHERITANCE OF GENETIC TRAITS

A genetic trait is the observed expression of one (or more than one) gene. Examples of traits are the expression of a blood group antigen, a clotting factor deficiency such as Factor VIII in hemophilia, and eye color. The inheritance of any genetic trait (and therefore red cell antigens) in a family follows a certain pattern and is determined by whether the gene responsible is located on an autosome or on the X chromosome and whether the trait is dominant or recessive. There are four basic patterns of inheritance: autosomal dominant (which includes autosomal codominant), autosomal recessive, sex-linked dominant, and sex-linked recessive. A trait is said to be dominant if it is expressed when only one member of a pair of autosomes carries the gene (heterozygous state) for the trait (eg, *A* in *A/O*); it is said to be codominant when each member of an autosomal pair carries a different allele (also a heterozygous state), each of which produces an observable trait (eg, *A* and *B* in *A/B*). A recessive trait is one that is not expressed by heterozygotes (eg, *O* in *A/O* or *B/O*) but requires the gene to be present on both members of an autosomal pair (homozygous state; *O/O*). Thus the alleles at the ABO locus include allelic pairs that display dominant-recessive inheritance and others that display codominance.

An observable trait is equivalent to the phenotype, and in the context of the blood bank, the phenotype refers to detectable red cell antigen(s). It may be possible to infer the genotype from the phenotype, especially if family studies are performed; however, often the phenotype does not reflect the genotype, and antigen typing may not be sufficient for genotype determination.

Pedigrees

A family study follows the inheritance of a genetic character—say, an allele encoding the expression of a red cell antigen—as it is transmitted through a kinship. The result of such a study can be analyzed by plotting the findings on a "map" that shows how the different family members are related. Such a "map" of family relationship is termed a **pedigree**, or a **pedigree chart** (also known as a **family tree**). A review of a pedigree should reveal the pattern or type of inheritance for the trait, or antigen, of interest. The finding of a person **affected** (ie, expressing the gene as evidenced by the presence of the condition) by a particular condition or a genetic disease of interest may initiate a family study; in the case of red cell antigens, perhaps a person with an unusual, or a null, phenotype is identified. Conventions apply to the construction of pedigrees and their analysis. The person in the pedigree who first caused the family to be investigated is considered the index case (indicated by an arrow on a pedigree) and is often referred to as the **proband** or **propositus**. The term propositus is used when referring to a male (in the singular form) index case or when referring to an index case (singular) regardless of the person's gender. The plural male form and also the plural form regardless of gender is **propositi**. When referring to a female index case (in the singular form), the correct form is **proposita**, and **propositae** is its plural form. Details of the conventions that apply and the symbols used for the construction of pedigrees are provided in Figs 11-6 and 11-7.

Autosomal Dominant Inheritance

An antigen (or any trait) that is inherited in an **autosomal dominant** manner is always expressed when the relevant allele is present, regardless of whether a person is homozygous or heterozygous for the allele. The antigen will appear in every generation and occur with equal frequency in both males and females. A person who carries an autosomal dominant trait will, on average, transmit it to half of his or her children. The pedigree in Fig 11-8 is representative of autosomal dominant inheritance and can be used to illustrate the expected inheritance pattern in a family with group B and group O blood types. Analysis of the ABO types of the family shows that the B allele is dominant over *O*; this is explained in detail in the figure legend.

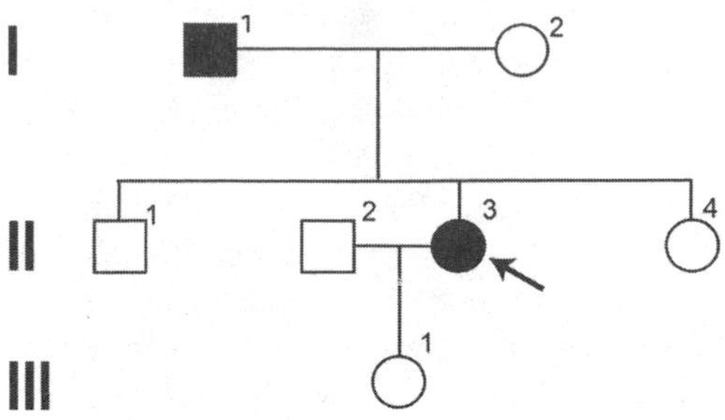

FIGURE 11-6. An example of a pedigree. Males are denoted by squares and females by circles, and each different generation in a pedigree is identified by Roman numerals. Persons in each generation are identified by Arabic numbers; the numbering is sequential from left to right, with the eldest child for each family unit being placed on the left of any series of siblings. Closed symbols represent family members affected by the trait, whereas open symbols are unaffected members.

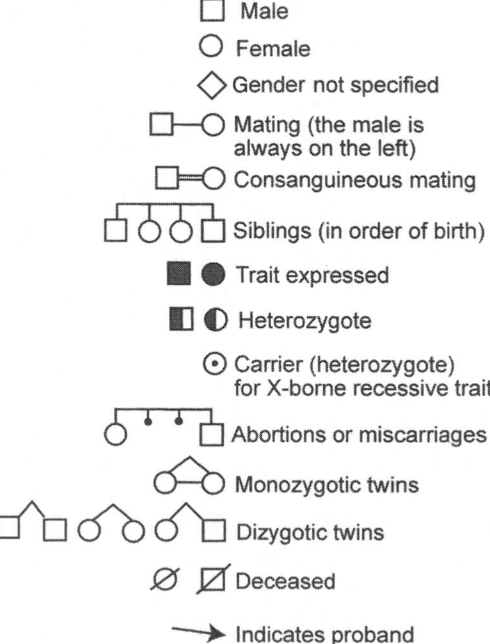

FIGURE 11-7. Symbols, and their significance, used in the construction of pedigrees.

Autosomal Codominant Inheritance

Blood group antigens that appear to be autosomal dominant may be encoded by alleles that are inherited in a **codominant** manner—that is, when two different alleles are present (the heterozygous condition), the products of both alleles are expressed. Thus, when red cells have the S+s+ phenotype, the presence of one allele encoding S and another allele encoding s (or an *S/s* genotype) can be inferred; similar reasoning can be applied when red cells are K+ and k+ (*K/k* genotype). Figure 11-9 demonstrates the autosomal codominant inheritance of the alleles encoding the Jk^a and Jk^b antigens and the codominant phenotypic expression of the antigens.

Autosomal Recessive Inheritance

A trait with autosomal recessive inheritance is expressed only in a person who is homozygous for the relevant allele and thus has inherited the recessive allele from both parents. When a person inherits a single copy of a recessive allele in combination with a silent or deleted (null) allele—that is, a nonfunctioning allele or one that encodes a product that cannot be detected—the recessive trait will be expressed, and the person will appear to be homozygous for that allele. It is often difficult to distinguish such a combination from homozygosity for the recessive allele. Recessive traits are transmitted with equal frequency to males and females. A mating between two heterozygous carriers will result in one in four of the children being homozygous for the trait. The parents of a child homozygous for a recessive trait must be obligate carriers of the trait and, depending on the prevalence of the trait in the general population, may or may not express the trait. If the frequency of the allele for the recessive trait is low, the condition will be rare and usually will be found only among siblings (that is, brothers and sisters of the person) and not other relatives of the affected person. The condition will not be found in preceding or successive generations unless consanguineous mating (ie, a mating between blood relatives) occurs. When a recessive allele is rare, the parents of an affected person are most likely consanguineous because a rare allele is more likely to occur in blood relatives than in unrelated persons in a random population. However, the appearance of a rare recessive trait does not always imply consanguinity because a recessive trait may remain unexpressed for many generations. In such cases, research into the family ethnicity and geographic origin may be interesting and informative. When a recessive trait is one that is common, consanguinity is not a prerequisite for homozygosity; for example, the O allele of the ABO system, although recessive, is not rare, and persons homozygous for *O* are easily found in the random population.

In blood group genetics, a recessive trait or condition is almost always equivalent to red cells expressing a null phenotype [eg, the Lu(a–b–) or Rh_{null} or O phenotypes] because of homozygosity for a **silent** or **amorphic gene**, a gene that either results in no product or encodes an ineffective product. The family in Fig 11-10 demonstrates the inheritance of the recessive silent gene *Lu,* which in the homozygous state results in the Lu(a–b–) phenotype. In this family, the red cells of persons who are heterozygous Lu/Lu^b can be distinguished from the red cells of those who are homozygous for Lu^b/Lu^b by the strength of the Lu^b antigen expressed (single-dose expression vs double-dose expression), although dosage studies with anti-Lu^b are not always definitive. The proband, II-3, who was multitransfused, was identified because of the presence of anti-Lu3 (an antibody to a high-prevalence Lutheran antigen) in his plasma. Because his Lu(a–b–) phenotype is the result of recessive inheritance, any potential donors in the family will be found by testing his **sibs** (ie, siblings). About 25%, or one in four of the offspring of the mating between I-1 and I-2, would be expected to have the Lu(a–b–) phenotype; in this case, only the proband has Lu(a–b–) red cells. For this and any other recessively inherited phenotype, there is no value in testing the proband's parents or children for potential donors (unless the family is extensively inbred).

Sex-Linked Inheritance

A **sex-linked** trait is one that is encoded by a gene located on the X or Y chromosome and, thus, also can be referred to as being X- or Y-borne. The Y chromosome carries few func-

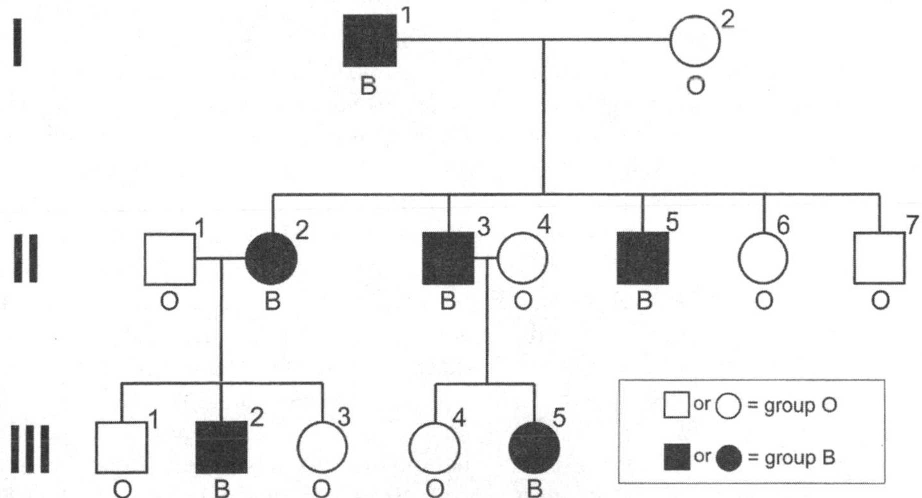

FIGURE 11-8. Autosomal dominant inheritance of the ABO alleles. Based on the ABO groups of his children, I-1 would be expected to have a *B/O* rather than a *B/B* genotype (showing that the B allele is dominant over *O)* because two of his children (II-6 and II-7) are group O and must have inherited an O allele from their father (I-1) in addition to the O allele inherited from their mother (I-2). Similarly, II-2 and II-3 are *B/O*, based on the ABO type of their children again, showing the dominance of *B* over *O.*

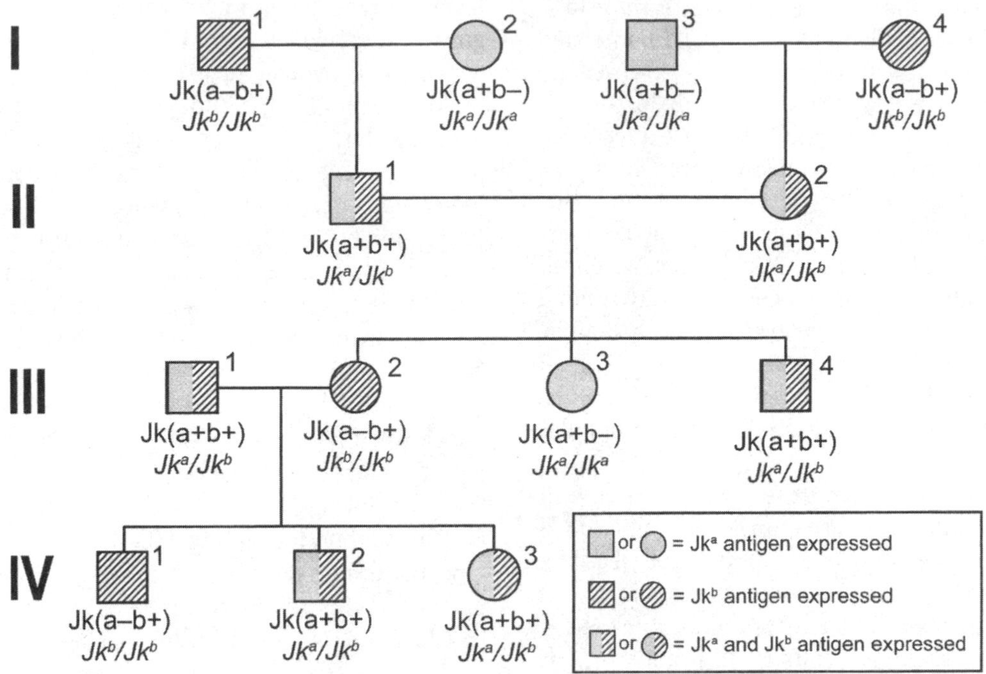

FIGURE 11-9. Autosomal codominant inheritance of the alleles encoding Jk^a and Jk^b antigens. I-1 and I-4 each have Jk(a–b+) red cells; that is, they are homozygous for *Jk^b* and express a double dose of the Jk^b antigen. I-2 and I-3 are homozygous for *Jk^a*. When offspring inherit a Jk^a allele from one parent and a Jk^b allele from the other parent, the antigens encoded by either allele are expressed, showing codominant expression of *Jk^a* and *Jk^b*.

tional genes, and those that are active are mostly responsible for determining features that are associated with "maleness." Therefore, discussion of sex-linked inheritance generally focuses on, and tends to be synonymous with, inheritance of X-borne genes. Females have two X chromosomes; therefore, the inheritance of X-borne genes, like the inheritance of genes carried on the autosomes, can be dominant or recessive. Males, by contrast, have one X chromosome (always maternally derived) and one Y chromosome (always paternally derived) and are **hemizygous** for genes on the X or Y chromosome because only one chromosome (and thus one copy of a gene) is present. Most X-borne genes do not have a **homolog** (a similar sequence of DNA) on the Y chromosome. As a consequence, inheritance of an X-borne dominant trait will be the same in males and females, but an X-borne trait that is recessive in females will be expressed by all males who carry the gene for the trait. The most striking feature of both dominant and recessive X-linked inheritance is that there is no male-to-male transmission, that is, the trait is never transmitted from father to son.

The MIC2 gene, which encodes the CD99 antigen of the Xg blood group system, is unusual in that it is located on the tips of the short arms of both the X and Y chromosomes in a region called the pseudoautosomal region. During meiosis in the male, the X and Y chromosomes segregate into separate gametes (sperm) and undergo pairing during the first meiotic division, as in the autosomes. This pairing involves only the telomeric (the terminal) portions of the short and long arms of the X and Y. Within the pairing region, crossing-over and recombination can occur. Genes located in the pairing region may not follow the rules of X-borne inheritance and could be mistaken for autosomal genes; therefore, these

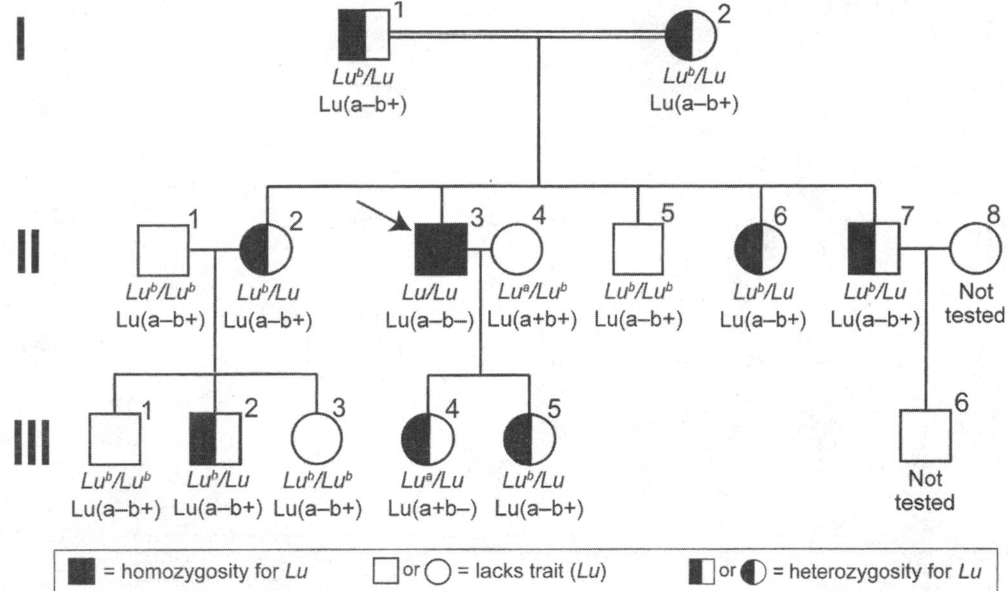

FIGURE 11-10. Autosomal recessive inheritance. The mating between II-3, the Lu(a–b–) proband, and II-4, his Lu(a+b+) wife, serves to demonstrate that *Lu* is recessive to Lu^a and Lu^b and that the presence of the silent Lu allele is masked by the product of Lu^a or Lu^b at the phenotype level.

pairing regions on the X and Y chromosomes were named **pseudoautosomal**.

Sex-Linked Dominant Inheritance

A trait encoded by an X-borne allele that has **sex-linked dominant** inheritance is expressed by hemizygous males and by both heterozygous and homozygous females. A male must pass his single X chromosome to all his daughters, making them obligate recipients of any trait, and all daughters must express the condition or trait. When a female is heterozygous for an allele encoding a dominant trait, each of her children, whether male or female, has a 50% chance of inheriting the trait. When a female is homozygous for an X-borne allele with dominant inheritance, the encoded trait will be expressed by all her children.

The Xg^a antigen (Xg blood group system) is encoded by an allele on the X chromosome and is inherited in a sex-linked dominant manner. The first indication that the Xg^a antigen is X borne came from the observation that the prevalence of the Xg(a–) and Xg(a+) phenotypes differed noticeably between males and females: the Xg^a antigen has a prevalence of 89% in females and only 66% in males.[6] Figure 11-11 shows the inheritance of the Xg^a antigen in a three-generation family. In generation I, the father (I-1) is Xg(a+), and as would be expected, he has transmitted Xg^a (the allele encoding the Xg^a antigen) to all his daughters but to none of his sons. His eldest daughter (II-2) must be heterozygous Xg^a/Xg; that is, she received the allele encoding the Xg^a antigen from her Xg(a+) father and a silent allele, *Xg*, from her Xg(a–) mother. II-2 has transmitted Xg^a to half her children, either sons or daughters. The family in Fig 11-11 does not include a woman homozygous for Xg^a; however, such a woman would be expected to transmit Xg^a to all her children. In this example, there is insufficient information to determine if II-8 is homozygous or heterozygous for Xg^a.

Aneuploidy and Xg^a

Any deviation from the normal chromosome number is termed **aneuploidy**. An abnormality in the number of chromosomes occurs be-

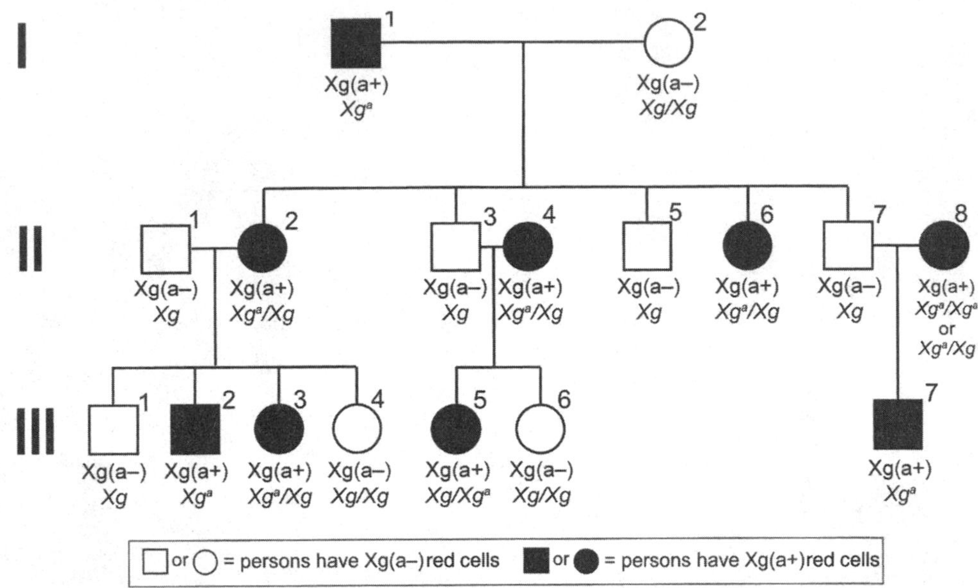

FIGURE 11-11. Sex-linked dominant inheritance. The Xg^a antigen is encoded by an allele on the tip of the short arm of the X chromosome. This family demonstrates the sex-linked dominant inheritance of the Xg^a antigen.

cause two chromosomes fail to separate (nondisjunction) during meiosis, resulting in gametes with either extra or missing chromosomes. If such gametes produce zygotes, the resulting offspring, if viable, can have mild to profound abnormalities—for example, trisomy (three copies) of chromosome 21, resulting in a person with Down syndrome. Nondisjunction can also involve the sex chromosomes, producing persons with abnormal karyotypes such as 47,XXX; 47,XXY; 47,XYY; and 45,XO. Family studies following the inheritance of the X-borne Xg^a antigen were very informative about the basis for aneuploidy, and it was frequently possible to determine at which meiotic division the nondisjunction occurred.

Sex-Linked Recessive Inheritance

A trait encoded by an **X-borne recessive** allele is carried, but not expressed, by a heterozygous female. A male will inherit the allele for the trait from his mother, who is usually a carrier, but occasionally a mother can be homozygous for the trait if she is the offspring of a mating between a male who expresses the trait (ie, is affected) and a carrier female for the trait. An affected male will transmit the trait to all of his daughters, who in turn will transmit the trait to approximately half of their sons. Therefore, the prevalence for the expression of an X-borne recessive trait is much higher in males than in females. A carrier female, when mating with a male lacking the trait, will transmit the trait to one half of her daughters (who will be carriers) and to one half of her sons (who will be affected). If the mating is between an affected male and a female who lacks the trait, all of the sons will lack the trait and all of the daughters will be carriers. If an X-borne recessive trait is rare in the population, the trait will be expressed almost exclusively in males; the more frequently a trait occurs in the population, the greater the chance that an affected male will mate with a carrier female, with the result that half of their daughters are likely to be homozygous for the trait.

The classic example of a gene with X-borne recessive inheritance is that for hemophilia A, but an example of relevance to blood group genetics is *XK*, the gene that encodes the Kx protein that carries the high-prevalence red cell antigen Kx. Mutations in *XK* result in red cells with the McLeod phenotype; such red cells lack Kx and have reduced expression of Kell antigens (McLeod syndrome). McLeod syndrome is inherited as a sex-linked recessive condition and is found only in males; this is demonstrated by the family in Fig 11-12. Because *XK* is subject to X chromosome inactivation, a mixed population of red cells, made up of those that are Kx+ and those that are Kx– with weakened Kell antigen expression, can often be demonstrated in carrier females.

Mendel's Laws

Mendel was the first to document that the passing of a trait from one generation to the next follows certain patterns, or principles, of inheritance. The principles established by him, based on his breeding experiments with pea plants (*Pisum sativum*), are still valid today and are relevant to the study of blood group genetics. One such principle is the Law of Independent Segregation, which was derived from Mendel's Law of Segregation (also known as Mendel's First Law). The **Law of Independent Segregation** governs the transmission of a trait (or allele) from parent to offspring and states that during gamete formation, allelic pairs of chromosomes separate during meiosis and are distributed into different gametes. Only one member of an allelic pair is passed on to the next generation, and each gamete has an equal probability of receiving either member of a parental homologous allelic pair. The allelic chromosomes are randomly united at fertilization and thus segregate independently from one generation to the next. The family in Fig 11-13 demonstrates the independent segregation of chromosome 9, on which the ABO alleles are located, from parent to offspring. The father (I-1) is blood group B and the mother (I-2) is blood group A at the phenotypic level, but their ABO genotype, which can be determined from their offspring, is *B/O* and *A/O*, respectively. The four

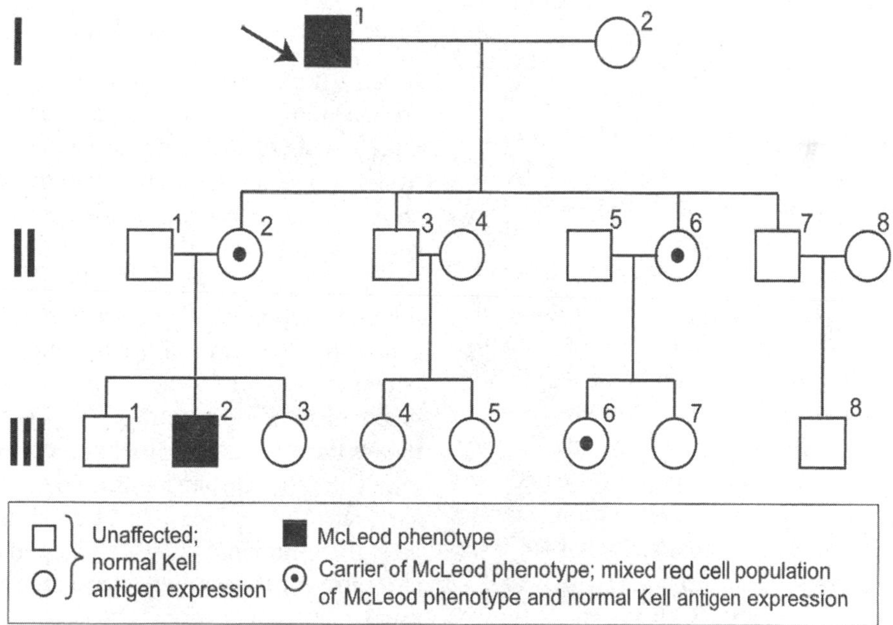

FIGURE 11-12. Sex-linked recessive inheritance. This family demonstrates that a sex-linked trait that is recessive in females will be expressed by any male who inherits the trait. Homozygosity for such a trait is required for it to be expressed in females. The trait skips one generation and is carried through females.

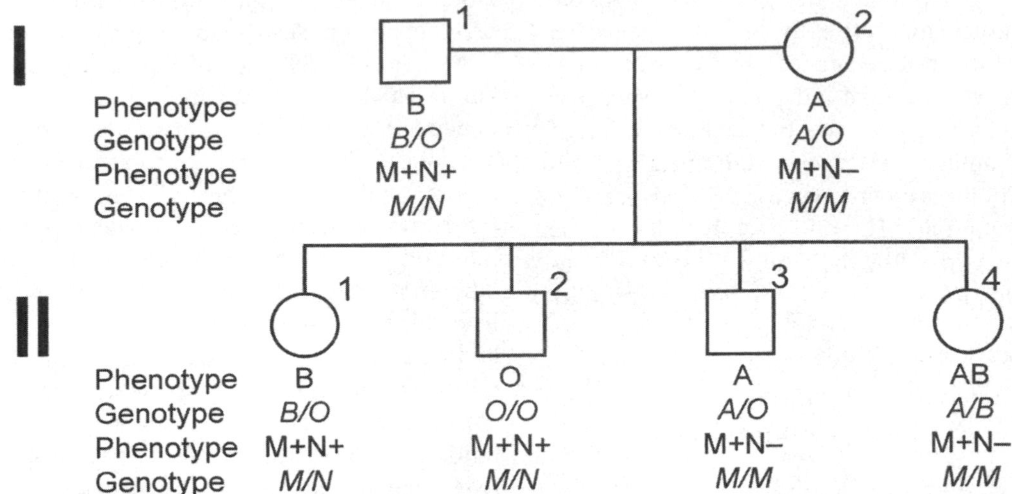

FIGURE 11-13. Mendel's laws of independent segregation and independent assortment are illustrated by the inheritance of blood group alleles in one family. Parental ABO alleles were randomly transmitted **(independent segregation),** and each child has inherited a different combination. The family also illustrates that the alleles encoding antigens of the ABO and MNS blood group systems are inherited independently from each other **(independent assortment).**

offspring have each inherited a different combination of paternally and maternally derived alleles (*B/O, O/O, A/O, A/B*), thereby demonstrating random transmission, or independent segregation, of each ABO allele.

Another important principle is Mendel's Second Law, the **Law of Independent Assortment**, which states that alleles determining various traits are inherited independently from each other. In other words, the inheritance of one allele (eg, a B allele encoding B antigens) does not influence the inheritance of another allele (eg, an M allele encoding M antigens). This is demonstrated by the family in Fig 11-13 for alleles that encode the antigens of the ABO and MNS systems. The alleles for these two blood group systems are located on different chromosomes: *ABO* on chromosome 9 and *MNS* on chromosome 4. The father, I-1, has contributed *B* with *N* to II-1, *O* with *N* to II-2, *O* with *M* to II-3, and *B* with *M* to II-4, showing the independent inheritance of *ABO* and *MNS* and, thus, independent assortment of these alleles into the gametes. The maternal allele combination (*A/O* with *M/M*) is not suitable to demonstrate the concept of independent assortment.

Linkage and Crossing-Over

Because there are many more genes than there are chromosomes, some genes must display linkage. **Linkage** is the physical association between two genes that are located on the same chromosome; based on Mendel's Second Law, genes located on the same chromosome should not assort independently. However, in the early 1900s it became obvious that some genes on the same chromosome did assort independently, and this can be explained by the mechanism of crossing-over. **Crossing-over** is the exchange of genetic material between homologous chromosome pairs and occurs at an early stage of meiosis (Fig 11-5). In this process, the chromatids of a homologous pair of chromosomes become intertwined; at the point of contact (referred to as a **chiasma**), breakage occurs, and a segment from one chromatid (and any associated genes) changes places with the corresponding part of the other chromatid (and its associated genes); the segments are rejoined, and some genes will have switched chromosomes. Thus, crossing-over is a means to shuffle genetic material. Because crossing-over can result in new gene combinations on the chromosomes involved, it is also referred to as **recombination**, and the rearranged chromosomes can be referred to as **recombinants**. Crossing-over and recombination, using chromosome 1 as an example, are explained in Fig 11-14.

Although all genes located on the same chromosome are linked, whether or not linkage between two genes becomes apparent depends, in part, on the closeness of the loci: the farther apart they are, the more likely it is that linkage will be broken by crossing over; that is, they will appear like genes on separate chromosomes and often assort independently. Two gene loci carried by the same chromosome that are not closely linked are referred to as being **syntenic**. For example, the loci for *RH* and *FY*, both located on chromosome 1, are syntenic because the distance between them (*RH* on the short arm and *FY* on the long arm) is great enough for them to be assorted and inherited independently following crossing-over. When two genes, or the antigens encoded by them, are inherited as a unit (eg, *RHD* and *RHCE*, the alleles encoding the antigens of the Rh system) more often than would be expected by chance alone, they are said to be linked; thus, linked loci do not assort independently.

The frequency of crossing-over involving two genes on the same chromosome is a measure of the distance [measured in centimorgans (cM), after Thomas Hunt Morgan (see below)] between them; the greater the distance between two loci, the greater the probability that crossing-over (and recombination) will occur, whereas genes located very close together (linked) tend to be transmitted together without recombination occurring. The degree of crossing-over between two genes can be calculated by analyzing pedigrees of families informative for the genes of interest and observing the extent of recombination. For example, if family analysis shows that recombination between two linked genes occurs in 6% of meioses, the recombination fraction is 0.06, and the map distance between the genes is 6 cM. When the distance between two loci is so great that the probability of crossing-over occurring between them reaches 0.5 (50% recombination), linkage is no longer detectable and the loci are not considered linked, even though they are on the same chromosome. Linkage is confirmed or ruled out by statistical pedigree analysis, and the traditional method of linkage analysis requires the use of lod (logarithm of the odds) scores; their application is explained by Race and Sanger.[23] Computer programs are available for calculating linkage from family data. Linkage analysis was the basis through which chromosomes were mapped and the relative position and distance between genes of interest were established.

The phenomena of linkage and crossing-over were established by Thomas Hunt Morgan from his work with fruit flies (*Drosophila*

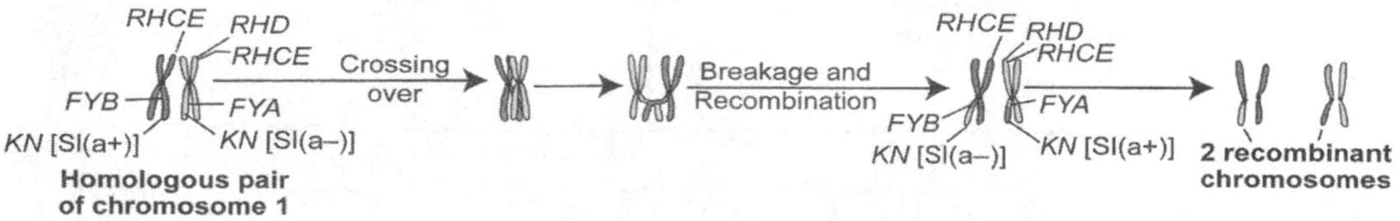

FIGURE 11-14. Crossing-over and recombination. In the diagram, chromosome 1 is used as an example. The very closely linked RH genes, *RHD* and *RHCE*, are located near the tip of the short arm of chromosome 1. The loci for *FY* and *KN* are on the long arm of the chromosome and are not linked. During meiosis, crossing-over occurs between this homologous chromosome pair, and portions of chromosome break and become rejoined to the partner chromosome. Crossing-over of the long arm of chromosome 1 results in recombination between the loci for *FY* and *KN* such that the gene encoding Fy^b antigen is now traveling with a gene that encodes the Sl(a–) phenotype of the Knops system.

melanogaster). Linkage between the locus for Lutheran (*LU*) and that controlling ABH secretion (*SE* or *FUT2*) was the first recognized example of autosomal linkage in humans and is explained in Fig 11-15. Proof of linkage between two loci establishes that the loci are located on the same chromosome but does not provide any information about which chromosome carries the linkage group. Study of the *LU-SE* linkage group contributed to the recognition that in humans, the rate of crossing-over at meiosis is higher in females than in males. This is because the duration of meiosis is longer in females than in males.

Although crossing-over occurs more readily between distant genes, rare examples of recombination have been documented for genes that are very closely linked or adjacent on a chromosome. The genes encoding the MN (*GYP*A*) and Ss (*GYP*B*) antigens are contiguous (adjacent) on chromosome 4 and are linked. Thus, as determined from family studies, if a person is known to carry *M* with *S* on one chromosome 4 and *N* with *s* on the other chromosome 4, generally *MS* or *Ns* is passed from parent to offspring as a set or **haplotype** (a combination of alleles at two or more closely linked loci on the same chromosome). Even for such closely linked loci, recombination, presumably as a result of crossing-over, is occasionally observed. In a family reported by Chown, Lewis, and Kaita [reviewed by Daniels[11(pp99-174)]], the MNS phenotypes were as follows: father, Ns; mother, MNSs; three children, Ns; and three children, MNSs (which indicates the father's genotype is *Ns/Ns* and the mother's is *MS/Ns*). However, one child (whose paternity was not at issue) was MNs (*Ms/Ns*), indicating that recombination between *MS* and *Ns* had most probably occurred.

Linkage Disequilibrium

Genes at closely linked loci tend to be inherited together and constitute a haplotype. As described in the previous section, the MNS antigens are encoded by two very closely linked genes, *GYP*A* and *GYP*B,* and the alleles are inherited as four haplotypes: *MS, Ms, NS,* or *Ns.* Because linked genes do not assort independently, the antigens encoded by each of these haplotypes occur in the population with a different prevalence than would be expected if the genes were not linked. If *M* and *S* were not linked, the expected prevalence for the M and S antigens in the population would be 17% (from frequency calculations), whereas the actual or observed prevalence (obtained from testing and analyzing families) of the *MS* haplotype is 24%.[11(pp99-174)] This constitutes

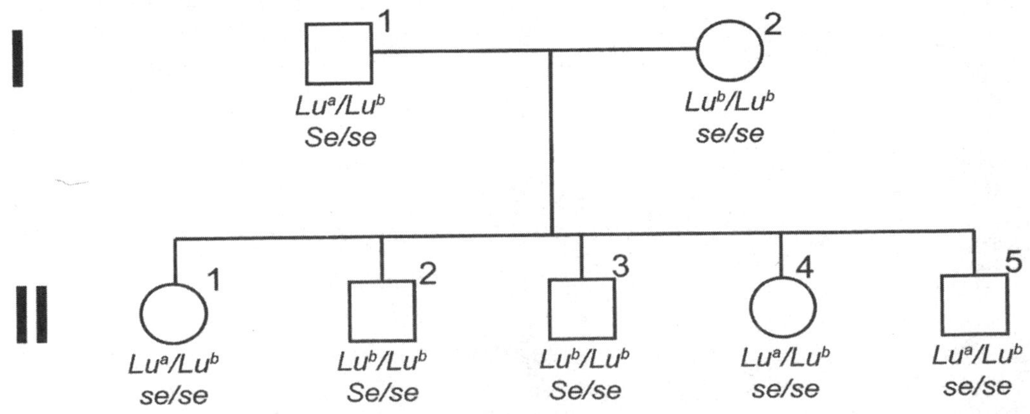

FIGURE 11-15. Linkage between *LU* and *SE*. I-2 is homozygous for Lu^b and *se* and must transmit these alleles to all her offspring. I-1 is doubly heterozygous (Lu^a/Lu^b and *Se/se*). He has transmitted Lu^b with *Se* and Lu^a with *se*, showing linkage between *Lu* and *Se*. Several such informative families would need to be analyzed to statistically confirm linkage.

linkage disequilibrium, which is the tendency of specific combinations of alleles at two or more linked loci to be inherited together more frequently than would be expected by chance. In contrast, genes are said to be in **linkage equilibrium** when alleles at two loci associate according to their individual frequencies in the population.

Gene Interaction and Position Effect

When alleles are carried on the same chromosome, they are referred to as being in *cis* position. When on opposite chromosomes of a homologous pair, genes are in *trans* position. The meaning of *cis* and *trans* is similar to "coupling" and "repulsion"; alleles that are in *cis* and linked demonstrate "coupling" by always being inherited together on the same chromosome, whereas genes in *trans* appear to demonstrate "repulsion" by being capable of independent segregation. Historically, the Rh blood group system was used to explain the meaning of *cis* and *trans*. For example, the *DCe/DcE* genotype was described as having C and e alleles in *cis* in the *DCe* haplotype, with c and E alleles in *cis* in the partner *DcE* haplotype, whereas *C* and *E* and also *c* and *e* are in opposing haplotypes and are in *trans*. In this alignment, *C* and *e*, for example, will always be inherited together, but *C* and *E* will not. The preceding explanation, which implies that one gene encodes C and c antigens while another linked gene encodes E and e antigens, is based on the Fisher-Race theory of three genes at the Rh locus. Although this is useful for the interpretation of serologic results, molecular analysis indicates that one gene (*RHCE*), with four alleles (*RHCE*Ce*, *RHCE*cE*, *RHCE*ce*, and *RHCE*CE*), encodes one protein that carries the CE series of antigens. Thus, for a *Ce* haplotype (*C* and *e* are in *cis*), the antigens are encoded by an RHCE*Ce allele, and similarly for a *cE* haplotype (*c* and *E* are in *cis*), the antigens are encoded by an RHCE*cE allele.

The expression of red cell antigens may be modified or affected by gene interactions that can manifest in several ways. One example in which the haplotype on one chromosome affects the expression of the haplotype on the paired chromosome is commonly referred to as the position effect and can be observed with Rh antigen expression. When a *Ce* haplotype (note the absence of *RHD*) is in *trans* to a D antigen-encoding haplotype, the expression of D is dramatically reduced and a weak D phenotype results. When the same D-encoding haplotype is inherited with either *ce* or *cE*, D antigen is normally expressed. More E antigen appears to be encoded by the *cE/ce* genotype than by *DcE/ce*, and in general, the presence of *D* in *trans* often has a depressing effect on the amount of C, E, and e antigen expressed compared to the absence of *D* in *trans*. The cause of this reduced antigen expression is not known. In the presence of the Kell system antigen Kp^a, expression of other inherited Kell system antigens encoded by the same haplotype is suppressed to varying degrees (cis-modifier effect). This is best observed in persons who have K^0 (a $Kell_{null}$ gene) in *trans*. The change that results in the expression of Kp^a adversely affects trafficking of the Kell glycoprotein to the red cell surface, with the result that the quantity of Kp^a-carrying Kell glycoprotein that reaches the red cell surface is greatly reduced.[24]

Suppressor or modifier genes affect the expression of another gene, or genes, through gene interaction by mechanisms that are not fully understood. For example, a rare type of the Jk(a–b–) phenotype is the result of Kidd antigen suppression by *In(Jk)*, a dominant gene that is independent from *JK*.[11(pp342-351)] In the Lutheran blood group system, two of the three types of the Lu(a–b–) phenotype are caused by suppressor genes. The dominant gene *In(Lu)* not only suppresses all Lutheran antigens, such that red cells appear to be Lu(a–b–), but also suppresses the expression of antigens in several other systems. Singleton et al[25] have shown that the antigen suppression is the result of heterozygosity of an altered KLF1 gene in the presence of a normal KLF1 allele. *KLF1* encodes the transcription factor erythroid Krüppel-like factor (EKLF) that is essential for terminal differentiation of red cells. Another factor essential for erythroid and megakaryocyte differentiation is the transcription factor GATA-1 that is encoded by the X-borne GATA-1 gene. Changes in this gene have been shown to be associated with the X-linked type of Lu(a–b–) phenotype.[26]

In the past, independent, unidentified modifier or regulator genes were postulated as the basis of a number of null or variant phenotypes when a silent or inactive (nonfunctioning) gene was not evident. For example, the regulator type (as opposed to the amorph type) of Rh_{null} resulted from the silencing of the RH genes. This regulator gene, termed *X°r*, was shown to be independent of *RH* through family studies. Because of recent advances in our understanding of the molecular basis of the expression of many antigens, the bases for some of the modifying effects have been identified. For example, the basis of the regulator type of Rh_{null} has been associated with various silencing changes in *RHAG*, a gene located on chromosome 6 (and thus independent of *RH*) that encodes the Rh-associated glycoprotein RhAG, which is required in the red cell membrane for Rh antigen expression. Similarly, molecular analysis indicates that the modifying gene that causes the Rh_{mod} phenotype is a mutated *RHAG*. The Rh_{mod} phenotype could be mistaken for Rh_{null} because of the suppressed Rh antigen expression. Through DNA analysis, it is possible to detect grossly normal but silenced genes as the basis of null phenotypes. A null phenotype often has more than one molecular basis.

Several red cell antigens require the interaction of the products of two or more independent genes for their expression. Assignment of the high-prevalence antigen Wr^b to the Diego blood group system took many years because the only red cells that lacked Wr^b were rare MNS null phenotypes [En(a–) and M^kM^k], yet Wr^a, the antigen antithetical to Wr^b, was clearly independent of MNS. This anomaly was resolved when it was understood that GPA (or more precisely, amino acids 59 to 76), which carries MN antigens, must be present in the red cell membrane for Wr^b expression. Wr^a/Wr^b polymorphism is encoded by *DI* and carried on band 3, whereas GPA is the product of *GYP*A*, a gene independent of *DI*. An absence of RhD and RhCE protein (Rh_{null}) results in red cells that lack LW antigens and lack or have reduced expression of U and S or s antigens, again demonstrating the interaction of the products of two or more independent genes.

The sequential interaction of genes at several loci is required for the expression of ABO, H, Lewis, and I antigens on red cells and in secretions. These antigens are carbohydrate determinants carried on glycoproteins or glycolipids, and the genetics of these antigens is more complex than that of protein-based antigens. When the antigen is the result of a protein polymorphism (eg, antigens of the Kell system), each allele encodes a protein that expresses antigen. By contrast, the carbohydrate antigens are carried on oligosaccharide chains that are built up by the stepwise addition of monosaccharides. Therefore, ABO genes and the genes encoding the other carbohydrate-based antigens do not encode membrane proteins but encode an enzyme, a glycosyltransferase, that catalyzes the sequential transfer of the appropriate immunodominant monosaccharide. Each monosaccharide structure is transferred by a separate glycosyltransferase, such that two genes are required for a disaccharide, three for a trisaccharide, and so on. An inactivating change at one locus can prevent or modify the expression of the other gene products. The product encoded by the H gene is the biosynthetic precursor for A and B antigen production; if the H gene is silenced, A or B antigens cannot be produced. A mutated A or B allele may result in a glycosyltransferase that is inactive or that causes more or less antigen to be expressed. Details of the biosynthesis of the ABO, H, Lewis, and I antigens may be found in Chapter 12.

POPULATION GENETICS

Population genetics is the study of the distribution patterns of genes and of the factors that maintain or change gene (or allele) frequencies. It is the statistical application of genetic principles to determine genotype occurrence and phenotype prevalence using gene frequency. A basic understanding of population genetics, probability, and the application of simple algebraic calculations is important for relationship (identity) testing. In blood banking, the knowledge can be applied to clinical situations such as predicting the likelihood of finding compatible blood for a patient who has made antibody(ies) to red cell antigens.

Before continuing, it may be helpful to define three commonly used words so that their appropriate use is understood. **Frequency** is used to describe prevalence at the genetic level, that is, the occurrence of an allele (gene) in a population. **Prevalence** is used to describe the occurrence of a permanent inherited characteristic at the phenotypic level—for example, a blood group—in any given population. **Incidence** is the appropriate term to use when describing the rate of occurrence in a population for a condition that changes over time, such as a disease, and is thus not suitable for use with blood groups.

Phenotype Prevalence

The prevalence of a blood group antigen or phenotype is determined by testing red cells from a large random sample of people of the same race or ethnicity with a specific antibody and calculating the percentage of positive and negative reactions. The larger the cohort being tested, the more statistically significant is the result. In a given blood group system, the sum of the percentages for the prevalence of the phenotypes should equal 100%. For example, in the Duffy blood group system, the prevalence in a random population of African ethnicity for the Fy(a+b–), Fy(a–b+), Fy(a+b+), and Fy(a–b–) phenotypes is 9%, 22%, 1%, and 68%, respectively; together, they total 100%. Similarly, for any given red cell antigen, the sum of the percentages for the prevalence of the presence or absence of a particular antigen should equal 100%. If the red cells from 1000 donors of European ethnicity are tested with anti-c, and 800 of the samples are positive and 200 are negative for the Rh antigen c, the prevalence of the c+ phenotype is 80% and that of the c– phenotype is 20%. Thus, in this donor population, approximately 20% of ABO-compatible units of blood, or 1 in 5, should be compatible with the serum from a patient who has made anti-c.

Calculations for Antigen-Negative Phenotypes

When providing blood for a patient with antibodies directed at one or more red cell antigens, a simple calculation can be used to estimate the number of units that would need to be tested to find the desired antigen combination. To calculate the prevalence of the combined antigen-negative phenotype, the prevalence for each of the individual antigens is multiplied together because the antigens are inherited independently of each other, unless the antigens are encoded by alleles that are so closely linked that they demonstrate linkage disequilibrium, with the result that sets of antigens are inherited as haplotypes (eg, the M, N, S, s and C, c, E, e antigens; see previous section). If a patient with antibodies to K, S, and Jk^a antigens requires 3 units of blood, for example, the prevalence of the antigen-negative phenotype and the number of units that need to be tested to find them can be calculated using the following information: the prevalence of K– donors is 91%; of these K– donors, 48% are expected to be S–, and 23% of these are expected to be Jk(a–). The percentage of donors negative for the individual antigens is expressed as a decimal and multiplied: 0.91(K–) × 0.48(S–) × 0.23[Jk(a–)] = 0.10 or 10%. Thus, 1 out of 10 Red Blood Cell (RBC) units would be expected to match the desired phenotype profile, and 10 ABO-compatible donors would need to be tested to find 1 crossmatch-compatible RBC unit. The patient in question requires 3 units, so on average, 30 units would need to be tested to fulfill the request. Based on these statistics, a hospital blood bank would be able to determine the likelihood of having the requested units in house.

The prevalence of a particular antigen (or phenotype) can vary with race, and the prevalence for a combined antigen-negative phenotype calculation should be selected on the basis of the predominant race found in the donor population. Tables that provide the antigen-negative rates for common polymorphic antigens are available in some books[6] or can be easily compiled by staff in the blood bank.

Gene (Allele) Frequency

The **gene frequency** is the frequency with which persons in a population possess a particular gene. It differs from **allele frequency** in that allele frequency refers exclusively to the frequency of the allele in a population and not directly to the frequency of individual genotypes. The frequency of an allele is the proportion that it contributes to the total pool of alleles at a particular gene locus in a given population at a given time. This frequency can be calculated from the prevalence of each phenotype observed in a population. The sum of allele frequencies at any given locus must equal 100% (or 1 at the level of algebraic calculation) in the population sample tested.

The Hardy-Weinberg Equilibrium

Gene frequencies tend to remain constant from generation to generation in any relatively large population unless influenced by factors such as selection, mutation, migration, or nonrandom mating, any of which would have to be rampant to have a discernible effect. According to the principles and conditions independently, but almost simultaneously, proposed by the British mathematician Hardy and the German physician Weinberg, gene frequencies reach equilibrium. This equilibrium can be expressed in algebraic terms by the Hardy-Weinberg formula or equation:

$$p^2 + 2pq + q^2 = 1$$

If two alleles, classically referred to as A and a, have gene frequencies of p and q, the homozygotes and heterozygotes are present in the population in the following proportions:

$$AA = p^2 \quad Aa = 2pq \quad aa = q^2$$

In such a two-allele system, if the gene frequency for one allele, say p, is known, q can be calculated by $p + q = 1$.

The Hardy-Weinberg equation permits estimation of genotype frequencies from the phenotype prevalence observed in a sampled population and, reciprocally, allows the determination of genotype frequency and phenotype prevalence from the gene frequency. The equation has a number of applications in blood group genetics, and its use is demonstrated below. In a population of European ethnicity, the frequencies for the two alleles *K* and *k* can be determined as follows:

Frequency of the K allele = p
Frequency of the k allele = q
Frequency of the *KK* genotype = p^2
Frequency of the *Kk* genotype = 2pq
Frequency of the *kk* genotype = q^2

The K antigen is expressed on the red cells of 9% of people of European ethnicity; therefore:

$p^2 + 2pq$ = the frequency of people who carry *K* and are K+

Thus, $p^2 + 2pq = 0.09$

$q^2 = 1 - (p^2 + 2pq)$ = the frequency of people who carry *kk* and are K–

$q^2 = 1 - 0.09$
$q^2 = 0.91$
$q = \sqrt{0.91}$
$q = 0.95$ = the frequency of *k*

Because the sum of the frequencies of both alleles must equal 1.00:

$p + q = 1$
$p = 1 - q$
$p = 1 - 0.95$
$p = 0.05$ = the frequency of *K*

Having calculated the allele frequencies for *K* and *k*, it is possible to calculate the percentage of k+ (both K+k+ and K–k+) and K+ (both K+k– and K+k+) people:

Prevalence of k+ $= 2pq + q^2$
$= 2(0.05 \times 0.95) + (0.95)^2$
$= 0.9975 \times 100$
= a calculated prevalence of 99.75% (the observed prevalence of the k+ phenotype is 99.8%)

Prevalence of K+ $= 2pq + p^2$
$= 2(0.05 \times 0.95) + (0.05)^2 = 0.0975$
$= 0.0975 \times 100 =$ a calculated prevalence for K+ of 9.75% (the observed prevalence of the K+ phenotype is 9%)

The Hardy-Weinberg equation also can be applied to calculate the frequencies of the three possible genotypes *KK*, *Kk*, and *kk* from the gene frequencies *K* (p) = 0.05 and *k* (q) = 0.95:

$p^2 + 2pq + q^2 = 1$
Frequency of *KK* $= p^2 = 0.0025$
Frequency of *Kk* $= 2pq = 0.095$
Frequency of *kk* $= q^2 = 0.9025$

If antibodies are available to test for the products of the alleles of interest (in this example, anti-K and anti-k), the allele frequencies also can be obtained by direct counting as demonstrated in Table 11-3. The allele frequencies obtained by direct testing are the **observed frequencies** for the particular population being sampled, whereas those obtained by gene frequency calculations (above) are the **expected frequencies**. The various calculations above, when applied to a two-allele situation, are relatively simple; dealing with three or more alleles greatly increases the complexity and is beyond the scope of this chapter.

For a given population, if the prevalence of one genetic trait, such as the presence of a red cell antigen, is known, the Hardy-Weinberg equation can be applied to calculate allele and genotype frequencies. The Hardy-Weinberg equilibrium principle is valid only under certain conditions. It applies, above all, only when the population is sufficiently large that chance alone cannot alter an allele frequency and when the mating is random. A lack of selective advantage or disadvantage of a particular trait and other influencing factors, such as mutation or migration in or out of the population, are assumed to be absent when applying the Hardy-Weinberg equilibrium principle. When all these conditions are met, the gene pool is in equilibrium and allele frequencies will not change from one generation to the next. If the conditions are not met, changes in allele frequencies may occur over a few generations and may explain many of the differences in allele frequencies between populations.

RELATIONSHIP TESTING

Polymorphisms are inherited characters or genetic markers that can distinguish between people. The blood groups with the greatest number of alleles (greatest polymorphism) have the highest power of discrimination and

TABLE 11-3. Allele Frequencies of *K* and *k* Calculated Using Direct Counting (Assuming the Absence of Null Alleles)

Phenotype	No. of Persons	No. of Kk Alleles	*K*	*k*
K+k–	2	4	4	
K+k+	88	176	88	88
K–k+	910	1820	0	1820
Totals	1000	2000	92	1908
Allele frequency			0.046	0.954

In a random sample of 1000 people tested for K and k antigens, there are a total of 2000 alleles at the *Kk* locus because each person inherits two alleles, one from each parent. Therefore, the two persons with a K+k– phenotype (each with two alleles) contribute a total of four alleles. To this are added 88 K alleles from the K+k+ group, for a total of 92 K alleles or an allele frequency of 0.046 (92 ÷ 2000). The frequency of the k allele is 0.954 (1908 ÷ 2000).

are the most useful for determining relationships. Blood is a rich source of inherited characters that can be detected, including red cell antigens, HLA antigens, platelet antigens, serum groups, red cell enzymes, and hemoglobin variants. Red cell and HLA antigens are easily identifiable, are polymorphic, and follow Mendelian laws of inheritance. The greater the polymorphism of a system, the less chance there is of finding two people who are identical. The extensive polymorphism of the blood group systems and of the HLA system has made them valuable tools for relationship testing. The polymorphisms of the HLA system alone allow the exclusion of over 90% of falsely accused men in cases of disputed paternity.

The traditional methods of identity testing mostly have been surpassed and replaced by DNA-based assays[27] (frequently referred to as DNA fingerprinting, DNA profiling, or DNA typing) that were pioneered by Jeffreys and colleagues.[28-30] The targets of such DNA analyses are regions of genomic DNA with great allelic variability that can be studied by RFLP mapping and PCR-based tests. Tandemly repeated sequences of DNA of varying lengths occur predominantly in the noncoding genomic DNA, and they are classified into groups depending on the size of the repeat region. The extensive variation of these tandemly repeated sequences between individuals makes it unlikely that the same number of repeats will be shared by two individuals, even if related. Minisatellite (also referred to as variable number of tandem repeat, or VNTR) loci have tandem repeat units of nine to 80 base pairs, whereas microsatellite (also referred to as short tandem repeat, or STR) loci consist of two to five base pair tandem repeats.[31] Microsatellites and minisatellites are reviewed by Bennett.[32] Assays for VNTR and STR sequences involve the electrophoretic separation of DNA fragments according to size. Initially, DNA profiling was performed by RFLP analysis, but this is being replaced by amplification of selected, informative VNTR and STR loci using locus-specific oligonucleotide primers with the subsequent measurement of the size of the produced PCR products. Hundreds of STR loci have been mapped throughout the human genome, and many have been applied to identity testing. Analysis of different STR loci (usually at least 12) is used to generate a person's DNA profile that is virtually guaranteed to be unique to that person (or an identical twin). DNA fingerprinting is a powerful tool not only for identity testing and population genetics but also for monitoring chimerism after marrow transplantation.[33,34] STR profiles of donor and recipient are established before the transplant procedure, and distinguishing loci are monitored for engraftment after transplantation and early detection of graft rejection or disease relapse. STR analysis also has been used to monitor for graft-vs-host disease after organ transplantation, particularly for liver transplants.[35]

Red cell antigens, many of which are inherited as codominant alleles, are still useful in cases of disputed paternity. If maternity is assumed, paternity can be excluded by either direct or indirect exclusion. In a **direct exclusion**, the child has inherited a genetic marker that is not found in the mother or alleged father. For example:

	Alleged Father	Mother	Child
Blood group phenotype	O	O	A
Presumed genotype	*O/O*	*O/O*	*A/O*

The child has inherited an A allele that was not present in the alleged father or in the mother, assuming that neither the mother nor the alleged father have the rare Bombay (O_h) or para-Bombay phenotypes. Based on the phenotypes of the mother and child, the A allele must have been inherited from the biologic father and is thus called a paternal obligatory gene. In this case, the alleged father is excluded from being this child's father.

In an **indirect exclusion**, the child lacks a genetic marker that the father, based on his observed phenotype, should have transmitted to all his offspring. For example:

	Alleged Father	Mother	Child
Blood group phenotype	Jk(a+b–)	Jk(a–b+)	Jk(a–b+)
Presumed genotype	Jk^a/Jk^a	Jk^b/Jk^b	Jk^b/Jk^b

The alleged father appears to be homozygous for Jk^a and should have transmitted Jk^a to the child; however, the child did not inherit Jk^a. This is an indirect exclusion because the child lacks a genetic marker that the father should have transmitted to all his offspring. The failure to find an expected gene in the child when the father appears to be homozygous for the gene (indirect exclusion) is not as conclusive as a direct exclusion. An apparent indirect exclusion can occasionally result from the presence of a silent (amorph) or null allele. In this example, the alleged father could have one silent Jk allele (Jk/Jk^a) that was transmitted to the child, and the child's genotype could be the rare Jk/Jk^b instead of the far more common Jk^b/Jk^b. For this reason, indirect exclusions are not used as the only marker to exclude paternity. However, the finding of indirect exclusion in two independent systems is usually sufficient evidence to show nonpaternity. Although this example is illustrative of indirect exclusion using blood group antigens, from a practical perspective, the Kidd locus or any other single blood group locus is rarely used for relationship testing.

If an alleged father cannot be excluded from paternity, the probability of his paternity can be calculated. The calculation compares the probability that the alleged father transmitted the paternal obligatory genes with the probability that any other randomly selected man from the same racial or ethnic group could have transmitted the genes. The result is expressed as a likelihood ratio (paternity index) or as a percentage. The AABB has developed standards and guidance documents for laboratories that perform relationship testing.[36]

BLOOD GROUP GENE MAPPING

Gene mapping is the process through which a gene locus is assigned to a location on a chromosome. Much of the initial mapping of blood group genes was accomplished through testing many families (the larger the family, the better) for selected red cell antigens. The results of such testing were transcribed onto pedigrees that were analyzed for evidence of recombination between the genes of interest to rule out or establish linkage of a blood group with another marker, frequently one that was disease related, with a known chromosomal location. Currently, 30 blood group systems are recognized by the International Society of Blood Transfusion (ISBT). The genes for all of them have been assigned to their respective chromosomes, and all have been cloned. The chromosomal location and the gene names are shown in Figs 11-2 and 11-3 and in Table 11-4.

The gene encoding the antigens of the Duffy blood group system was the first to be assigned to a chromosome, by showing that the gene is linked to an inherited deformity of chromosome 1 that is visible under the microscope. This was made possible by the development of chromosomal staining techniques that revealed a unique pattern of bands for each chromosome. The chromosomal locations provided in Table 11-4 are based on the banding pattern; traditionally, genes were mapped to chromosomes according to the metaphase banding patterns produced when staining with Giemsa (G banding) or quinacrine (Q banding). Increasingly, mapping has related more to the positions of other genetic markers on a chromosome and not to metaphase banding patterns.

Other methods used in chromosome mapping have included deletion mapping (partial or total loss of a chromosome related to presence or absence of a gene), exclusion mapping (gathering information that excludes a gene from being located on a particular chromosome), somatic cell hybridization (human-rodent hybrid cell lines randomly shed human chromosomes, permitting the association of a trait with the presence or ab-

TABLE 11-4. Blood Group Systems

ISBT System Name (Number)	Gene Name ISBT (HGNC)*	Chromosome Location	Gene Product and Component Name [CD number]	Associated Blood Group Antigens [Null phenotype]
ABO (001)	*ABO* (*ABO*)	9q34.2	Glycosyltransferase, carbohydrate	A; B; A,B; A1 [Group O]
MNS (002)	*MNS* (*GYP*A* *GYP*B* *GYP*E*)	4q31.21	Glycophorin A (GPA) [CD235a] Glycophorin B (GPB) [CD235b]	M, N, S, s, U, He, Mi^a, Vw + 38 more [En(a–); U–; M^kM^k]
P1PK (003)	*P1* (*4GALT*)	22q13.2	Galactosyltransferase, carbohydrate	P1, P^k
Rh (004)	*RH* (*RHD* *RHCE*)	1p36.11	RhD [CD240D] RhCE [CD240CE]	D, G, Tar C, E, c, e, V, Rh17 + 43 more [Rh_{null}]
Lutheran (005)	*LU* (*LU*)	19q13.32	Lutheran glycoprotein; B-cell adhesion molecule [CD239]	Lu^a, Lu^b, Lu3, Lu4, Au^a, Au^b + 14 more [Recessive Lu(a–b–)]
Kell (006)	*KEL* (*KEL*)	7q34	Kell glycoprotein [CD238]	K, k, Kp^a, Kp^b, Ku, Js^a, Js^b + 25 more [K_0 or K_{null}]
Lewis (007)	*LE* (*FUT3*)	19p13.3	Fucosyltransferase, carbohydrate (Adsorbed from plasma)	Le^a, Le^b, Le^{ab}, Le^{bh}, ALe^b, BLe^b [Le(a–b–)]
Duffy (008)	*FY* (*DARC*)	1q23.2	Duffy glycoprotein [CD234]	Fy^a, Fy^b, Fy3, Fy5, Fy6 [Fy(a–b–)]
Kidd (009)	*JK* (*SLC14A1*)	18q12.3	Human urea transporter (HUT) Kidd glycoprotein	Jk^a, Jk^b, Jk3 [Jk(a–b–)]
Diego (010)	*DI* (*SLC4A1*)	17q21.31	Band 3, Anion Exchanger 1 [CD233]	Di^a, Di^b, Wr^a, Wr^b, Wd^a, Rb^a + 16 more
Yt (011)	*YT* (*ACHE*)	7q22	Acetylcholinesterase	Yt^a, Yt^b
Xg (012)	*XG (XG)* (*MIC2*)	Xp22.33 Yp11.3	Xg^a glycoprotein CD99 (*MIC2* product)	Xg^a CD99
Scianna (013)	*SC* (*ERMAP*)	1p34.2	ERMAP	Sc1, Sc2, Sc3, Rd + 3 more [Sc:–1,–2,–3]

TABLE 11-4. Blood Group Systems (Continued)

ISBT System Name (Number)	Gene Name ISBT (HGNC)*	Chromosome Location	Gene Product and Component Name [CD number]	Associated Blood Group Antigens [Null phenotype]
Dombrock (014)	*DO* *(ART4)*	12p12.3	Do glycoprotein; ART 4 [CD297]	Do^a, Do^b, Gy^a, Hy, Jo^a + 2 more [Gy(a–)]
Colton (015)	*CO* *(AQP1)*	7p14	Aquaporin 1 (AQP1)	Co^a, Co^b, Co3, Co4 [Co(a–b–)]
Landsteiner-Wiener (016)	*LW* *(ICAM4)*	19p13.2	LW glycoprotein Intracellular adhesion molecule 4 (ICAM4) [CD242]	LW^a, LW^{ab}, LW^b [LW(a–b–)]
Chido/ Rodgers (017)	*CH/RG (C4A, C4B)*	6p21.32	Complement component: C4A; C4B	Ch1, Ch2, Rg1 + 6 more [Ch–Rg–]
H (018)	*H* *(FUT1)*	19q13.33	Fucosyltransferase, carbohydrate [CD173]	H [Bombay (O_h)]
Kx (019)	*XK* *(XK)*	Xp21.1	XK glycoprotein	Kx [McLeod phenotype]
Gerbich (020)	*GE* *(GYPC)*	2q14.3	Glycophorin C (GPC) [CD236] Glycophorin D (GPD)	Ge2, Ge3, Ge4 + 8 more [Leach phenotype]
Cromer (021)	*CROM* *(CD55)*	1q32.2	DAF [CD55]	Cr^a, Tc^a, Tc^b, Tc^c, Dr^a, Es^a, IFC + 9 more [Inab phenotype]
Knops (022)	*KN* *(CR1)*	1q32.2	CR1 [CD35]	Kn^a, Kn^b, McC^a, Sl^a, Yk^a + 4 more
Indian (023)	*IN* *(CD44)*	11p13	Hermes antigen [CD44]	In^a, In^b + 2 more
Ok (024)	*OK* *(BSG)*	19p13.3	Neurothelin, basigin [CD147]	Ok^a, OKGV, OKGM
Raph (025)	*RAPH (CD151)*	11p15.5	CD151	MER2 [Raph–]
JMH (026)	*JMH* *(SEMA7A)*	15q24.1	Semaphorin 7A [CD108]	JMH + 5 more [JMH–]
I (027)	*IGNT* *(GCNT2)*	6p24.2	Glucosaminyltransferase, carbohydrate	I [I– or i adult]
Globoside (028)	*GLOB* *(3GALT3 or GalNAcT1)*	3q26.1	Transferase, carbohydrate (Gb_4, globoside)	P [P–]

(Continued)

TABLE 11-4. Blood Group Systems (Continued)

ISBT System Name (Number)	Gene Name ISBT (HGNC)*	Chromosome Location	Gene Product and Component Name [CD number]	Associated Blood Group Antigens [Null phenotype]
Gill (029)	*GIL* *(AQP3)*	9p13.3	Aquaporin 3 (AQP3)	GIL [GIL–]
Rh-associated glycoprotein (030)	*RHAG*	6p21-qter	Rh-associated glycoprotein [CD241]	Duclos, Ol^a, DSLK† [Rh_{null} (regulator type)][37]

*If the genetic information is obtained by blood group typing, the gene name used should be the italic form of the of the blood group system ISBT symbol. For example, *SLC14A1* would be written as *JK*A* and *JK*B* or *Jk^a* and *Jk^b*.

†Provisionally numbered by the ISBT because of limited genetic evidence.

ISBT = International Society of Blood Transfusion; HGNC = Human Gene Nomenclature Committee; ERMAP = erythroid membrane-associated protein.

sence of a chromosome), in-situ hybridization (use of fluorescent DNA probes with a preparation of intact chromosomes), and chromosome walking (a technique to clone a gene from its known closest markers). Details of gene mapping procedures are beyond the scope of this chapter, but reviews are available.[11(pp533-548)] The early gene maps were genetic maps, that is, maps that express the distance of linked loci by their frequency of recombination. Advances in biochemical, microbiologic, and molecular genetic technology as well as information generated through the Human Genome Project (http://www.ornl.gov/sci/techresources/Human_Genome/home.shtml) are making it feasible to construct a physical gene map that refers to the absolute position of gene loci and for which the distance between loci is expressed by the number of base pairs of DNA.

CHIMERISM

The observation that a sample gives mixed-field agglutination is not an unusual one in the blood bank. Mostly, this is the result of artificially induced chimerism through the transfusion of donor red cells or through a stem cell transplant. On rare occasions, the observation of mixed-field agglutination identifies a true **chimera**, that is, a person with a dual population of cells derived from more than one zygote. Indeed, the first example of a human chimera was a female blood donor discovered through mixed-field agglutination during antigen typing. Most human chimeras can be classified as either twin chimeras or tetragametic (dispermic) chimeras. Chimerism is not a hereditary condition.[38,39]

Twin chimerism occurs through the formation of placental blood vessel anastomoses, which results in the mixing of blood between two fetuses. This vascular bridge allows hematopoietic stem cells to migrate between twins and to take root in the marrow of the opposite twin. Each twin may have two distinct populations of cells (red cells and leukocytes), that of their true genetic type and that of their twin. However, the percentage of the two cell lines in each twin tends to vary; the major cell line is not necessarily the autologous cell line, and the proportions of the two cell lines may change throughout life. Chimeric twins have immune tolerance; they do not make antibody against the A or B antigens that are absent from their own red cells but present on the cells of the engrafted twin. This tolerance extends beyond red cells to negative mixed lymphocyte cultures and the mutual acceptance of skin grafts.

In twin chimeras, the dual cell population is strictly confined to blood cells. Tetragametic or dispermic chimeras present chimerism in all tissues and are more frequently identified because of infertility and rarely because of mixed populations of red cells. The exact mechanism(s) leading to the development of tetragametic chimeras is unknown, but it is known that they arise through the fertilization of two maternal nuclei by two sperm followed by fusion of the two zygotes and development into one person containing two cell lineages.

More commonly, chimeras occur through medical intervention and arise from the transfer of actively dividing cells, for example through hematopoietic transplantation.[39] However, chimerism may be more prevalent than once thought. DNA analysis, to confirm the Rh-negative status of Northern European blood donors, identified a donor with a dual red cell population of which 95% was Rh negative and 5% was Rh positive. The donor was confirmed to be a chimera. Chimerism was found to be the cause of a discrepancy observed when determining ABO, and news headlines were made by a case of disputed maternity when a woman was falsely excluded as the mother of her children because of chimerism.[40,41]

BLOOD GROUP TERMINOLOGY

Although the principles of classic Mendelian genetics apply to the inheritance of blood group antigens, the terminology did not follow classic Mendelian convention. Starting with the ABO and Rh systems, different researchers have used different names for the same set of antigens. As a consequence, blood group terminology is inconsistent and can be confusing to the user. Antigens were named using an alphabetical (eg, A/B, C/c) notation, or they were named after the proband whose red cells carried the antigen or who made the first known antibody (eg, Duclos). A symbol with a superscript letter (eg, Lu^a, Lu^b; Jk^a, Jk^b) was used, and a numerical (eg, Fy3, Jk3, Rh32) terminology was introduced. Some blood group systems have antigens named using more than one scheme (eg, the Kell blood group system: K, k, Js^a, Js^b, K11, K17, TOU). To convert the results of antigen typing to a phenotype can be equally confusing; if a person were to be positive for all the Kell antigens listed in the last sentence, the phenotype would be: K+ k+ Js(a+b+) K11+ K17+ TOU+ or K+ k+ Js(a+b+) K:11,17, TOU+.

These inconsistencies are also evident when interpreting antigen expression to the level of the gene or allele; Mendelian convention denotes the allele encoding a dominant trait (*T*) by an italicized uppercase letter, and the allele encoding the recessive trait (*t*) with the corresponding lowercase letter. By contrast, blood group alleles are denoted in multiple ways: the codominant ABO alleles *A* and *B* are denoted by an uppercase letter as is the recessive O allele. The O allele, although recessive to *A* and *B*, is an amorph or silent (null) allele; it does not encode an active product. Silent alleles are sometimes designated by use of a lowercase letter (*le* for the amorph of the Lewis system) and sometimes by the system symbol without the superscript letter (*Lu* for Lutheran, *Jk* for Kidd, or *Co* for Colton). Uppercase letters combined with the corresponding lowercase letter have been used to indicate allelic relationships regardless of the fact that the alleles are codominant; for example, *S* and *s* of the MNS system and *E* and *e* of the Rh system. Another way codominant alleles are differentiated is through the use of superscripts; for example, Jk^a and Jk^b, or Do^a and Do^b. For some allelic pairs, the superscript "a" represents the low-frequency allele (Js^a vs Js^b), but for other allelic pairs, the "a" represents the high-frequency allele (Co^a vs Co^b). As these selected examples demonstrate, no single convention was originally applied to the terminology used for blood group genes other than that they are written in italics or, in lieu of italics, the gene or allele is underlined (eg, <u>RHD</u>).

In 1980, the ISBT established its Working Party on Terminology for Red Cell Surface Antigens. There was concern that the lack of a standardized terminology would hinder the use of computers for storage of results and the electronic exchange of information and results. The working party was charged to develop a uniform nomenclature that would be "both eye and machine readable" and "in keeping with the genetic basis of blood groups." Therefore, the devised terminology was based primarily around the blood group systems.

A blood group system consists of one or more antigens under the control of a single gene locus or of two or more homologous genes that are so closely linked that virtually no recombination occurs between them. Thus, each blood group system is genetically independent from every other blood group system. The independence of a particular system can be ascertained by various means: by family analyses to show that the genes of any two systems segregate independently of each other at meiosis; by the ability to assign the genes to separate chromosomes or discrete parts of the same chromosome (eg, through deletion or exclusion mapping); and more recently by biochemical and molecular techniques. The failure of an antibody to react with red cells of a particular null phenotype is not sufficient for assignment of the corresponding antigen to a system. Some null phenotypes are the result of inhibitor or modifying genes that may suppress the expression of antigens from more than one system [eg, the Rh_{null} phenotype lacks not only Rh antigens but also LW system antigens, Fy5 antigen (Duffy system), and sometimes U (MNS system) antigen]. Similarly, a blood group antigen must be shown to be inherited, either through family studies or by DNA analysis, to be assigned antigen status by the ISBT terminology working party. A blood group antigen must be defined serologically by an antibody; a polymorphism that is detectable only by DNA analysis and for which there is no corresponding antibody cannot be called a blood group antigen.

A terminology consisting of uppercase letters and Arabic numbers to represent blood group systems and antigens was established by the working party.[42,43] Each system can also be identified by a set of numbers (eg, ABO system = 001; Rh system = 004), and similarly each antigen in the system is assigned a number (eg, A antigen = 001; B antigen = 002; D antigen = 001). Thus, 001001 identifies the A antigen, or 004001 identifies the D antigen. Alternatively, the sinistral zeros may be omitted so that the A antigen becomes 1.1 and the D antigen becomes 4.1. Each system also has an alphabetical symbol (Table 11-4); KEL represents the Kell system, the Rh system is represented by RH, and an alternative name for the D antigen is RH1. This alphanumeric terminology, which was designed primarily for computer use, is not ideal for everyday communication, and in order to achieve uniformity, a recommended list of user-friendly alternative names was compiled. This "traditional" alternative terminology uses many of the names and symbols identical to those originally published, and there are recommended formats for describing phenotypes in the alternative terminology.

The ISBT working party meets periodically to assign names and numbers to new antigens and discuss aspects of terminology. Two monographs have been published in addition to shorter papers summarizing the decisions made at the meetings. Criteria for the terminology; tables listing the systems, antigens, and phenotypes; and other information is available on the website for the ISBT terminology working party. The following information is taken from the website[44]:

> *Symbols for designations of new specificities will consist of 3-6 on-line capital letters and must not duplicate, alphabetically or phonetically, any current or obsolete symbols shown in the tables. Also, symbols used in related fields, such as those used for platelet and leucocyte antigens, must be avoided. Symbols for specificities that may herald new blood group systems, and thus new genes, have the further constraint that they must differ from any symbols given to genes by the Human Genome Organisation (HUGO) Gene Nomenclature Committee (http://www.genenames.org/).*

A comprehensive review of the terminology and its usage is found in Garratty et al.[45] Examples of the traditional and ISBT terminology as they apply to alleles, genotypes, phenotypes, and antigens are shown in Table 11-5.

TABLE 11-5. Examples of Allele, Genotype, Phenotype, and Antigen Terminology

	Traditional	ISBT*
Kell System		
Allele	*K, k, Js^a, Js^b, K11*	*KEL*1, KEL*2, KEL*6, KEL*7, KEL*11*
Genotype/haplotype	*kJs^b/kJs^b*	*KEL*2,7/KEL*2,7*
Phenotype	K– k+ Js(b+)	KEL:–1,2,7
Antigen	K, k, Js^a, Js^b, K11	KEL1, KEL2, KEL6, KEL7, KEL11
Duffy System		
Allele	*Fy^a, Fy^b, Fy3, Fy*	*FY*1* or *FY*A*, *FY*2* or *FY*B*, *FY*3*, *FY*0* or *FY*
Genotype/haplotype	*Fy^a/Fy^b*	*FY*A/FY*B* or *FY*1/FY*2*
Phenotype	Fy(a+b+)	FY:1,2
Antigen	Fy^a, Fy^b	FY1, FY2

*Genes are designated by the ISBT system symbol, followed by an asterisk, followed by the antigen number, all italicized (eg, *FY*1*). Genotypes have the ISBT system symbol, followed by an asterisk, followed by alleles or haplotypes separated by a slash, all italicized (eg, *KEL*2,7/KEL*2,7*). Use of the traditional terminology is also acceptable. It is recommended that one or the other terminology is used unless only one name exists.

Guidelines for human gene nomenclature were devised and regulated for many years at Human Gene Mapping (HGM) meetings. The HGM nomenclature committee published a summary titled "International System for Human Gene Nomenclature" (ISGN).[46] HGM was succeeded by HUGO, which in turn has formed a gene nomenclature committee, and this group is now responsible for naming all genes based on ISGN.[47]

With the increasing application of DNA testing for the prediction of blood group phenotypes, the name of the working party was changed to the ISBT Working Party on Red Cell Immunogenetics and Blood Group Terminology in 2009. The terms of reference of the working party were expanded, and it is now also charged to develop, maintain, and monitor a terminology for blood group genes and their alleles.[43] A subgroup was established to devise a terminology for the multitude of alleles encoding blood group phenotypes; the allele names will be readily recognizable and for use by transfusion medicine practitioners. In due course there will be a mechanism for obtaining ISBT names for newly identified alleles, similar to that in place for blood group antigens.

KEY POINTS

1. Genetics is the study of heredity, that is, the mechanisms by which a particular characteristic, such as a blood group, is passed from parents to offspring.
2. A gene is a segment of DNA and is the basic unit of inheritance; it occupies a specific location on a chromosome (the gene locus). Alleles are alternative forms of a gene at the same gene locus (eg, alleles *JK*A* and *JK*B* respectively encode the Jk^a and Jk^b antigens).

3. A human somatic (body) cell is diploid, containing 46 chromosomes in 23 pairs: 22 pairs are alike (homologous) in males and females and are termed autosomes; the remaining pair is the sex chromosomes: X and Y for males, or two X chromosomes for females.
4. Somatic cells divide for growth and repair by mitosis. Mitosis replicates the chromosomes and produces two identical nuclei in preparation for cell division. The new cells are diploid, like the parent cell, and have all the genetic information of the parent cell.
5. Meiosis is the process by which germ cells divide to become gametes (sperm and egg cells); diploid cells undergo DNA replication and two divisions to form four gametes, each of which is haploid and has half the chromosomal complement of the parent somatic cell.
6. The four basic patterns of inheritance for genes are autosomal dominant (which includes autosomal codominant), autosomal recessive, sex-linked dominant, and sex-linked recessive.
7. The term "genotype" traditionally refers to the complement of genes inherited by each person from his or her parents; the term is also used to refer to the set of alleles at a single gene locus. Whereas the genotype of a person is his or her genetic constitution, the phenotype is the observable expression of the genes and reflects the biologic activity of the gene(s). Thus, the presence or absence of antigens on the red cells, as determined by serologic testing, represents the phenotype. In some cases the genotype can be predicted from the phenotype.
8. When identical alleles for a given locus are present on both chromosomes, a person is homozygous for the particular allele, whereas when nonidentical alleles are present at a particular locus, the person is heterozygous. Antigens encoded by alleles at the same locus are said to be antithetical. Thus, genes are allelic but not antithetical, whereas antigens are antithetical but not allelic.
9. The expression of blood group antigens on the red cell may be modified or affected by gene interaction (eg, position effect, suppressor or modifier genes).
10. A blood group system consists of one or more antigens under the control of a single gene locus (eg, *KEL* encodes the Kell blood group antigens) or of two or more homologous genes (eg, *RHD* and *RHCE* encode the Rh blood group antigens) so closely linked that virtually no recombination occurs between them; thus, each blood group system is genetically independent. Currently, 30 blood group systems are recognized.

REFERENCES

1. Levine P. A review of Landsteiner's contributions to human blood groups. Transfusion 1961;1:45-52.
2. Brown TA. Genetics: A molecular approach. 3rd ed. Newman, GA: Hippo Books, 1992.
3. Passarge E. Color atlas of genetics. 2nd ed. New York: Georg Thieme Verlag Stuttgart, 2001.
4. Johnson GB, Raven PH. Biology. 7th ed. Boston: McGraw-Hill, 2005.
5. Nussbaum RL, Thompson MW, McInnes RR, Willard HF. Thompson & Thompson genetics in medicine. 6th ed. Philadelphia: Saunders, 2004.
6. Reid ME, Lomas-Francis C. Blood group antigen factsbook. 2nd ed. San Diego: Academic Press, 2004.
7. An international system for human cytogenetic nomenclature. Report of the Standing Committee on Human Cytogenetic Nomenclature (1978) ISCN (1978). Cytogenet Cell Genet 1978; 21:309-404.
8. Lewis M, Zelinski T. Linkage relationships and gene mapping of human blood group loci. In: Cartron J-P, Rouger P, eds. Molecular basis of major human blood group antigens. New York: Plenum Press, 1995: 445-75.
9. Lögdberg L, Reid ME, Zelinski T. Human blood group genes 2010: Chromosomal locations and cloning strategies revisited. Transfus Med Rev 2011;25:36-46.
10. Lyon MF. X-chromosome inactivation. Curr Biol 1999;9:R235-R237.

11. Daniels G. Human blood groups. 2nd ed. Oxford: Blackwell Science, 2002.
12. Clemson CM, Hall LL, Byron M, et al. The X chromosome is organized into a gene-rich outer rim and an internal core containing silenced nongenic sequences. Proc Natl Acad Sci U S A 2006;103:7688-93.
13. Redman CM, Reid ME. The McLeod syndrome: An example of the value of integrating clinical and molecular studies. Transfusion 2002;42:284-6.
14. Russo DCW, Lee S, Reid ME, Redman CM. Point mutations causing the McLeod phenotype. Transfusion 2002;42:287-93.
15. Garratty G. Blood groups and disease: A historical perspective. Transfus Med Rev 2000;14: 291-301.
16. Thorisson GA, Stein LD. The SNP Consortium website: Past, present and future. Nucleic Acids Res 2003;31:124-7.
17. Blumenfeld OO, Patnaik SK. Allelic genes of blood group antigens: A source of human mutations and cSNPs documented in the Blood Group Antigen Gene Mutation Database. Hum Mutat 2004;23:8-16.
18. US Department of Energy and National Institutes of Health. Human Genome Project. Washington, DC: US Department of Energy Genome Programs, Office of Biological and Environmental Research, 2010. [Available at http://www.ornl.gov/sci/techresources/Human_Genome/home.shtml (accessed December 29, 2010).]
19. Reid ME. Molecular basis for blood groups and function of carrier proteins. In: Silberstein LE, ed. Molecular and functional aspects of blood group antigens. Bethesda, MD: AABB, 1995:75-125.
20. Storry JR, Olsson ML. Genetic basis of blood group diversity. Br J Haematol 2004;126:759-71.
21. Reid ME, Yazdanbakhsh K. Molecular insights into blood groups and implications for blood transfusions. Curr Opin Hematol 1998;5:93-102.
22. Reid ME. Applications of DNA-based assays in blood group antigen and antibody identification. Transfusion 2003;43:1748-57.
23. Race RR, Sanger R. Blood groups in man. 6th ed. Oxford: Blackwell, 1975.
24. Yazdanbakhsh K, Lee S, Yu Q, Reid ME. Identification of a defect in the intracellular trafficking of a Kell blood group variant. Blood 1999; 94:310-18.
25. Singleton BK, Burton NM, Green C, et al. Mutations in EKLF/KLF1 form the molecular basis of the rare blood group In(Lu) phenotype. Blood 2008;112:2081-8.
26. Singleton, BK, Roxby, D, Stirling, J, et al. A novel GATA-1 mutation (Ter414Arg) in a family with the rare X-linked blood group Lu(a–b–) phenotype (abstract). Blood 2009;114:783.
27. Pena SDJ, Chakraborty R. Paternity testing in the DNA era. Trends Genet 1994;10:204-9.
28. Jeffreys AJ, Wilson V, Thein SL. Hypervariable 'minisatellite' regions in human DNA. Nature 1985;314:67-73.
29. Jeffreys AJ, Wilson V, Thein SL. Individual-specific 'fingerprints' of human DNA. Nature 1985;316:76-9.
30. Jeffreys AJ. 1992 William Allan Award address. Am J Hum Genet 1993;53:1-5.
31. National Institute of Standards and Technology, Bioechemical Science Division. Short tandem repeat DNA internet database. [Available at http://www.cstl.nist.gov/div831/strbase/index.htm (accessed December 29, 2010).]
32. Bennett P. Demystified ... microsatellites. Mol Pathol 2000;53:177-83.
33. Khan F, Agarwal A, Agrawal S. Significance of chimerism in hematopoietic stem cell transplantation: New variations on an old theme. Bone Marrow Transplant 2004;34:1-12.
34. Thiede C, Bornhauser M, Ehninger G. Evaluation of STR informativity for chimerism testing—comparative analysis of 27 STR systems in 203 matched related donor recipient pairs. Leukemia 2004;18:248-54.
35. Domiati-Saad R, Klintmalm GB, Netto G, et al. Acute graft versus host disease after liver transplantation: Patterns of lymphocyte chimerism. Am J Transplant 2005;5:2968-73.
36. Baird ML, ed. Standards for relationship testing laboratories. 9th ed. Bethesda, MD: AABB, 2009.
37. Tilley L, Green C, Poole J, et al. A new blood group system, RHAG: Three antigens resulting from amino acid substitutions in the Rh-associated glycoprotein. Vox Sang 2010;98:151-9.
38. Daniels G. Human blood groups. 1st ed. Oxford: Blackwell, 1995:684-92.
39. Bluth MH, Reid ME, Manny N. Chimerism in the immunohematology laboratory in the molecular biology era. Transfus Med Rev 2007;21: 134-46.
40. Wagner FF, Frohmajer A, Flegel WA. *RHD* positive haplotypes in D negative Europeans. BMC Genet 2001;2:10.

41. Cho D, Lee JS, Yazer MH, et al. Chimerism and mosaicism are important causes of ABO phenotype and genotype discrepancies. Immunohematology 2006;22:183-7.
42. Daniels GL, Anstee DJ, Cartron J-P, et al. Blood group terminology 1995. ISBT Working Party on Terminology for Red Cell Surface Antigens. Vox Sang 1995;69:265-79.
43. Storry JR, Castilho L, Daniels G, et al. International Society of Blood Transfusion Working Party on Red Cell Immunogenetics and Blood Group Terminology: Berlin report (2010). Vox Sang 2011 (in press).
44. International Society of Blood Transfusion. Committee on Terminology for Red Cell Surface Antigens. Introduction to the terminology: Procurement of ISBT numerical designations. [Available at http://www. blood.co.uk/ibgrl/ISBT%20Pages/ISBT% 20Home.htm (accessed January 24, 2011).]
45. Garratty G, Dzik WH, Issitt PD, et al. Terminology for blood group antigens and genes: Historical origins and guidelines in the new millennium. Transfusion 2000;40:477-89.
46. Shows TB, Alper CA, Bootsma D, et al. International system of human gene nomenclature (1979) ISGN (1979). Cytogenet Cell Genet 1979; 25:96-116.
47. Wain HM, Bruford EA, Lovering RC, et al. Guidelines for human gene nomenclature. Genomics 2002;79:464-70.

Chapter 12

ABO, H, and Lewis Blood Groups and Structurally Related Antigens

◆12

Laura Cooling, MD, MS

THE ANTIGENS OF the ABO, H, Lewis, I, and P blood group systems are defined by small carbohydrate epitopes on glycoproteins and glycolipids. Because the epitopes represent posttranslational modifications, the synthesis of those antigens requires the action of several enzymes known as glycosyltransferases. Glycosyltransferases reside in the Golgi apparatus and are responsible for adding specific sugars, in a specific sequence and steric or anomeric linkage (α-linked or β-linked), to growing oligosaccharide chains on glycolipids and glycoproteins. Transcriptional regulation, coupled with the enzymatic specificity of those glycosyltransferases for both sugar donors [nucleotide sugars; eg, uridine diphosphate (UDP)-galactose] and acceptor substrates (eg, type 1 chain vs type 2 chain), is responsible for the tissue-specific distribution of many blood group antigens.[1-3] Because they are widely distributed on many tissues, including embryonic stem cells, such antigens are considered histo-blood group antigens.[2-6] Several studies have shown a role for these antigens in development, cell adhesion, malignancy, and infectious disease.[1-3]

ABO SYSTEM

The ABO system, initially described by Karl Landsteiner in 1900,[7] remains the most important blood group system in transfusion and organ transplantation medicine.[8] In blood, ABO antigens are found on red cells, platelets, and many circulating proteins. As histo-blood group antigens, ABO antigens are also present on many tissues, including the endothelium, kidney, heart, bowel, pancreas, and lung.[2,3] Transfusion of ABO-incompatible blood can be associated with acute intravascular hemolysis, renal failure, and death. Likewise, transplantation of ABO-incompatible organs is associated with acute humoral rejection.[8] Because of the dire clinical consequences associated with ABO incompatibilities, ABO typing and ABO compatibility testing remain the foundation of pretransfusion testing and an important component of typing before transplantation.

The ABO system contains four major ABO phenotypes: A, B, O, and AB. The four phenotypes are determined by the presence or absence of two antigens (A and B) on red cells (see Table 12-1). The ABO system is also char-

Laura Cooling, MD, MS, Associate Professor, Department of Pathology, and Associate Medical Director, Transfusion Medicine, University of Michigan, Ann Arbor, Michigan

The author has disclosed no conflicts of interest.

TABLE 12-1. Routine ABO Grouping

Reaction of Red Cells with Antisera (Red Cell Grouping)		Reaction of Serum with Reagent Red Cells (Serum Grouping)			Interpretation	Prevalence (%) in US Population	
Anti-A	**Anti-B**	**A_1 Cells**	**B Cells**	**O Cells**	**ABO Group**	**European Ethnicity**	**African Ethnicity**
0	0	+	+	0	O	45	49
+	0	0	+	0	A	40	27
0	+	+	0	0	B	11	20
+	+	0	0	0	AB	4	4
0	0	+	+	+	Bombay*	Rare	Rare

+ = agglutination; 0 = no agglutination.
*H null phenotype (see section on H antigen).

acterized by the presence or absence of naturally occurring antibodies, termed isohemagglutinins, directed against missing A and B antigens. As shown in Table 12-1, an inverse reciprocal relationship exists between the presence of A and/or B antigens on red cells and the presence of anti-A, anti-B, or both, in sera. For example, group O individuals, who lack A and B antigens on red cells, possess both anti-A and anti-B. It is believed that the immunizing sources for such naturally occurring antibodies are gut and environmental bacteria, such as the *Enterobacteriaceae*, which have been shown to possess ABO-like structures on their lipopolysaccharide coats.[9,10]

Biochemistry

The A and B antigens are defined by three sugar terminal epitopes on glycolipids and glycoproteins. As shown in Fig 12-1, the H antigen is characterized by a terminal $\alpha 1 \rightarrow 2$ fucose; it is the immediate biosynthetic precursor for both A and B antigens and is required for their expression.[11] In group A individuals, an *N*-acetylgalactosamine is added, in an $\alpha 1 \rightarrow 3$ linkage, to the subterminal galactose of H antigen to form the A antigen. In group B individuals, an $\alpha 1 \rightarrow 3$ galactose is added to the same subterminal galactose to form the B antigen. In group AB individuals, both A and B structures are synthesized. In group O individuals, neither A nor B antigens are synthesized as a result of a mutation in the ABO gene.[11,12] As a consequence, group O individuals express only H antigen. A and B antigens are also absent in the very rare Bombay phenotype because of the absence of the H-antigen precursor (see later section on the H system).

As terminal motifs, the A and B antigens can be displayed on a number of oligosaccharide scaffolds that differ in their size, composition, linkages, and tissue distribution. On red cells, ABH sites are present on *N*-linked (65%-75%) and *O*-linked (5%-15%) glycoproteins, polyglycosylceramides (10%-15%), and simpler glycosphingolipids (Fig 12-2). ABO antigens are subclassified by the carbohydrate sequence immediately upstream of the ABO motif. In mammals, six different oligosaccharide chains have been described (see Table 12-2).[3,12] On human red cells, the majority of endogenous ABH antigen synthesized is present on type 2 chain structures. The ability to synthesize and use different carbohydrate chains is genetically determined and can contribute to antigenic differences in weak ABO subgroups.[12-14] For instance, type 3 (repetitive A) and type 4 (globo-A) A antigens are present on A_1, but not on A_2, red cells. Differences in *cis* carbohydrate sequences upstream of the terminal ABO motif can also influence antibody

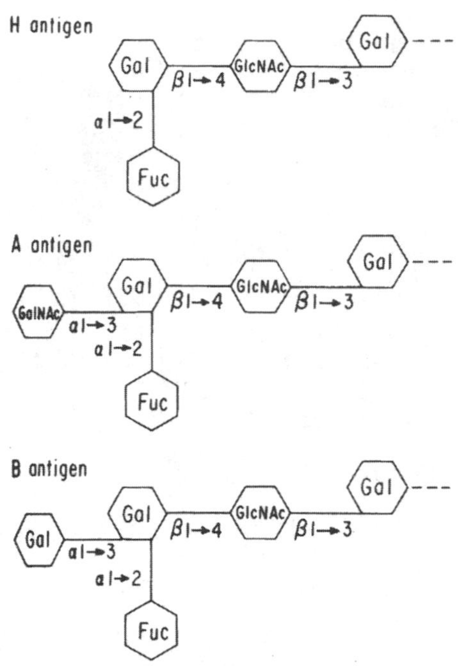

FIGURE 12-1. GalNAc added to the subterminal Gal confers A activity to the sugar; Gal added to the subterminal Gal confers B activity. Unless the fucose moiety that determines H activity is attached to the number 2 carbon, galactose does not accept either sugar on the number 3 carbon.

reactivity.[12,13] As an example, ABO antigens on type 1 chain substrates can be recognized by antibodies directed against both ABO and Le^b antigen (see later section on the Lewis system).[12,15]

ABO in Development and Aging

ABO antigens can be detected on red cells of embryos as early as 5 to 6 weeks of gestation.[15] The quantity of ABO antigens on cord red cells is less than that of adults, in part as the result of the immaturity of type 2 chain precursors on cord red cells (see discussion of I/i antigen). With increasing age, precursor chains become increasingly branched, thereby allowing more A and B antigen to be expressed. Adult levels of ABO expression are generally observed by age 2 to 4 years.[15]

Anti-A and anti-B are not present at birth or, if present, are of maternal origin. Endogenous synthesis of anti-A and anti-B can develop as early as age 3 to 6 months, with nearly all children displaying the appropriate isohemagglutinins in their sera at 1 year of age.[15,16] Titers of anti-A and anti-B continue to increase during early childhood and achieve adult levels within 5 to 10 years. Among healthy adults, ABO titers can naturally vary from 4 to 2048 or higher.[15,16] High-titer ABO antibodies can be observed in group O multiparous women and in patients taking certain bacteria-based nutritional supplements.[10,15] Although older reports indicated a fall in isoagglutinin titers in the elderly, more recent studies have disputed those findings.[15,16] In industrialized countries, isoagglutinin titers have generally decreased with increasing consumption of processed foods.[17]

Genetics

The ABO gene is located on chromosome 9q34. The ABO gene is fairly large, consisting of 7 exons spread over 18 kb.[11] The open reading frame of the protein is located primarily in exons 6 and 7. A study of the promoter region indicates that ABO gene expression is transcriptionally regulated by several mechanisms, including methylation, tissue-specific transcription factor binding proteins, antisense RNA, and possibly a minisatellite enhancer region 4 kb upstream of exon 1.[11,18,19] ABO expression is also regulated by the H gene, which is responsible for the synthesis of H antigen substrate, the precursor of A and B antigens. The H gene is tightly regulated in a tissue-specific manner through tissue-specific transcription factors and promoters.[20] In the absence of H, no A or B antigen is expressed regardless of *ABO* genotype (Bombay or O_h phenotype).[12]

A series of elegant studies over the past decade have identified the molecular basis for A, B, O, *cis*-AB, and weak ABO subgroups.[11,12,21] Fundamentally, three common ABO alleles are responsible for the A, B, and O phenotypes. The A and B consensus alleles are autosomal

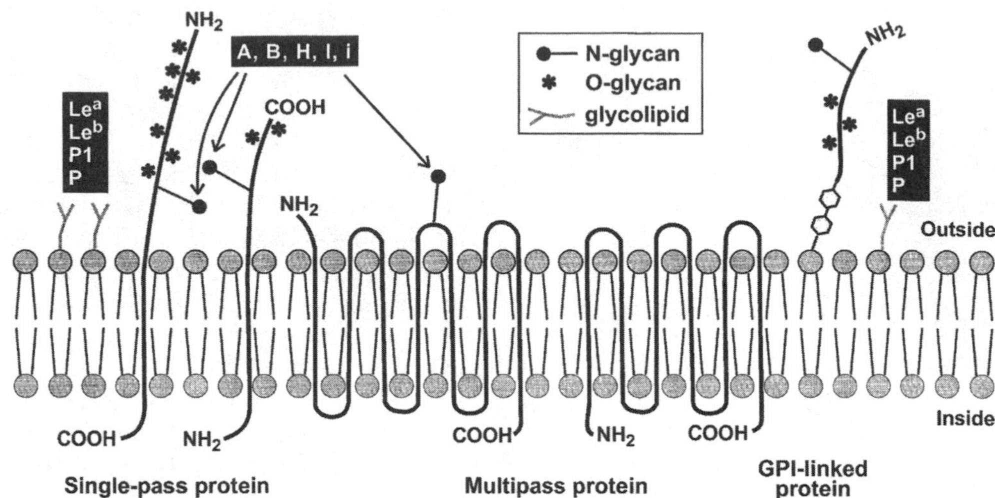

FIGURE 12-2. Schematic representation of the red cell membrane showing antigen-bearing glycosylation of proteins and lipids.
GPI = glycosylphosphatidylinositol. (Courtesy of ME Reid, New York Blood Center.)

codominant and differ by only seven nucleotides and four amino acids.[11] Three amino acids (A→B; Gly235Ser, Leu266Met, and Gly268Ala) are critical in determining whether the glycosyltransferase will use UDP-*N*-acetyl-D-galactosamine or UDP-D-galactose donor sugars to synthesize A or B antigens, respectively.[11] The rare *cis*-AB phenotype is a chimeric enzyme with a mix of A-specific and B-specific amino acids at those or other amino acid positions.[11,21] A plethora of mutations associated with weak A and B subgroups has been described, with some mutations linked to more than one subgroup. As an example, group A_2 (a weak A subgroup) is commonly the result of a nucleotide deletion and frameshift, resulting

TABLE 12-2. Chain Variants of A Antigen

Antigen	Oligosaccharide Sequence
A epitope	GalNAcα1-3(Fucα1-2)Galβ1-R
Type 1 A	GalNAcα1-3(Fucα1-2)<u>Galβ**1-3**GlcNAc</u>β1-3-R
Type 2 A	GalNAcα1-3(Fucα1-2)<u>Galβ**1-4**GlcNAc</u>β1-3-R
Type 3 A (repetitive A)	GalNAcα1-3(Fucα1-2)Galβ**1-3**GalNAcα1-3(Fucα1-2)Galβ**1-4**GlcNAcβ1-3-R
Type 4 A (globo-A)	GalNAcα1-3(Fucα1-2)Galβ**1-3**<u>GalNAcα1-4Galα1-4Gal</u>β1-4Glc-Cer
Type 5 A	GalNAcα1-3(Fucα1-2)<u>Galβ**1-3**Galβ1</u>-R
Type 6 A	GalNAcα1-3(Fucα1-2)<u>Galβ**1-4**Glcβ1</u>-Cer

Cer = ceramide; Fuc = fucose; Gal = galactose; GalNAc = *N*-acetylgalactosamine; Glc = glucose; GlcNAc = *N*-acetylglucosamine; R = upstream oligosaccharide.
Underlined sequences denote the critical differences between type 1, 2, 4, 5, and 6 chains. Boldface type indicates linkage and anomery (α-linked or β-linked) of the A antigen galactose.
Bracketed sequences denote repetitive A antigen characteristic of type 3 chain A antigen.

in an enzyme with an additional 21 amino acids at the C-terminus of the molecule.[11,12]

The O allele is an amorph, encoding a nonfunctional enzyme. The group O phenotype, therefore, is an autosomal recessive trait, representing inheritance of two nonfunctional ABO genes. Overall, more than 30 O alleles have been identified.[21,22] The two most common O alleles (*O01, O02*) contain a nucleotide deletion and frameshift, leading to a truncated, 117-amino-acid protein. Another common O allele is *O03 (or O^2)*, a group of nondeletional O alleles that contains a mutation at amino acid 268 (Gly268Arg), which is a critical residue for donor binding (UDP-galactose or UDP-N-acetyl-galactosamine). One German study found that *O03* and a related allele (*Aw08)* were responsible for 25% of all ABO typing discrepancies caused by reverse grouping problems in normal donors.[23] It was speculated that weak anti-A and anti-B could reflect weak residual glycosyltransferase activity; however, a recent study was unable to demonstrate A antigen or enzyme activity in *O03* individuals.[24]

ABO Subgroups

ABO subgroups are phenotypes that differ in the amount of A and B antigen carried on red cells and present in secretions. In general, A subgroups are more common than B subgroups. Clinically, the two most common subgroups encountered are A_1 and A_2. A_1 represents the majority of group A donors (80%) and is characterized by approximately 1 million A antigen epitopes per red cell. A_2 is the second most common subgroup (20%) and possesses only one fifth (2.2×10^5) the number of A antigen sites as A_1. Both A_1 and A_2 are strongly agglutinated by reagent anti-A in routine direct testing. A_1 can be distinguished from A_2 with the lectin *Dolichos biflorus*, which will agglutinate A_1 red cells, but not A_2 red cells. In addition, 1% to 8% of A_2 individuals and 25% of A_2B individuals possess an alloanti-A1 in their sera. Because the A_2 phenotype reflects the inefficient conversion of H→A antigen, A_2 red cells show increased reactivity with the anti-H lectin *Ulex europaeus*. Enzyme studies comparing A_1 and A_2 glycosyltransferase activity show that the A_1 enzyme is 5 to 10 times more active than the A_2 enzyme, resulting in quantitative and qualitative differences in A antigen expression.[12,15] The latter includes the synthesis of unusual type 3 and type 4 chain A antigen on A_1 red cells, which are not present on A_2 and weaker A subgroups.[12,13]

In addition to A_2, several weaker A subgroups have been described (eg, A_3, A_x, A_m, A_{el}). The extremely weak A (and B) subgroups are infrequently encountered and are usually recognized by apparent discrepancies between the red cell (forward) and serum (reverse) grouping results. The original descriptions of most weak A and B subgroups were made before the advent of monoclonal typing reagents and were based on reactivity with human polyclonal anti-A, anti-B, and anti-A,B reagents. Weak A subgroups are frequently nonreactive with human polyclonal anti-A (see Table 12-3) and can show variable reactivity with human polyclonal anti-A1, anti-A,B and murine monoclonal antibodies (not shown).[12,15,25] The degree of reactivity with commercial murine monoclonal reagents is clone dependent[25]; however, most commercially available anti-A will agglutinate A_3 red cells. Because of the reciprocal relationship between H and synthesis of A and B antigens, all weak A and B subgroups have increased H expression. Molecular testing has shown several mutations associated with weak ABO subgroups.[21] In clinical practice, it is seldom necessary to identify the specific A or B subgroup encountered. When performed, classification of weak A subgroups is typically based on the following:

1. Degree of red cell agglutination by anti-A and anti-A1.
2. Degree of red cell agglutination by human and some monoclonal anti-A,B.
3. Degree of H antigen expression (anti-H lectin, *Ulex europaeus*).
4. Presence or absence of anti-A1 (Method 2-9).
5. Presence of A and H in saliva (Method 2-10).
6. Adsorption and elution studies (Method 2-7).

TABLE 12-3. Serologic Reactions Observed in A and B Subgroups

Red Cell Phenotype	Red Cell Reactions with *Antisera or Lectins*				Serum Reactions with *Reagent Red Cells*			Saliva (Secretors)
	Anti-A	Anti-B	Anti-A,B	Anti-H	A_1 Cells	B Cells	O Cells	
A_1	4+	0	4+	0	0	4+	0	A & H
A_2	4+	0	4+	2+	0/2+*	4+	0	A & H
A_3	$2+^{mf}$	0	$2+^{mf}$	3+	0/2+*	4+	0	A & H
A_x	0/±	0	1-2+	4+	0/2+	4+	0	H
A_{el}	0	0	0	4+	0/2+	4+	0	H
B	0	4+	4+	0	4+	0	0	B & H
B_3	0	$1+^{mf}$	$2+^{mf}$	4+	4+	0	0	B & H
B_x	0	0/±	0/2+	4+	4+	0	0	H
B(A)	±/2+†	4+	4+	0	4+	0	0	B & H

1+ to 4+ = agglutination of increasing strength; ± = weak agglutination; mf = mixed-field agglutination; 0 = no agglutination.
*The occurrence of anti-A1 is variable in these phenotypes.
†Most often detected with anti-A clones containing the MHO4 clone.

7. Family (pedigree) studies.

B(A) and A(B) Phenotypes

The B(A) phenotype is an autosomal dominant phenotype characterized by weak A expression on group B red cells.[15,26] Serologically, red cells from B(A)-phenotype individuals react strongly with anti-B and weakly with monoclonal anti-A (<2+), and they possess a strong anti-A, reactive with both A_1 and A_2 red cells, in their sera. B(A) red cells can show varying reactivity with monoclonal anti-A reagents; however, most cases are detectable with monoclonal typing reagents containing the MHO4 clone. In general, the agglutination is weak with fragile, easily dispersed agglutinates. Testing the sample with polyclonal anti-A or a different monoclonal anti-A should resolve the discrepancy. Amino acid polymorphisms have been identified in some B(A) individuals near (Pro234Ala) or at critical amino acids (Ser235Gly).[11,12,21] The B glycosyltransferase in those individuals has an increased capacity to use UDP-*N*-acetylgalactosamine, in addition to UDP-galactose, resulting in detectable A antigen synthesis.

An A(B) phenotype has also been described with monoclonal anti-B. The A(B) phenotype was associated with elevated H antigen and plasma H-transferase activity.[15] It is hypothesized that the increased H precursor on those cells may permit the synthesis of some B antigen by the A glycosyltransferase.

Acquired B Phenotype

The acquired B phenotype phenomenon is an acquired, transient serologic discrepancy encountered in group A individuals and is a cause of red cell grouping discrepancies.[27] Acquired B should be suspected when a patient or donor who has historically typed as group A now presents with weak B expression on forward or red cell grouping. Serologically, the acquired B phenotype shows strong agglutination with anti-A, shows weak agglutination (2+ or less) with monoclonal anti-B, and contains a strong anti-B in serum. Despite reactivity of the patient's red cells with reagent anti-B, the patient's serum will not react with autologous red cells. Chemically, acquired B is the result of deacetylation of the A antigen's *N*-acetyl-galactosamine, yielding a B-like, galactosamine sugar.[12,28] In patients' samples, acquired B often occurs in the setting of infection by gastrointestinal bacteria. Many enteric bacteria possess a deacetylase enzyme capable of converting A antigen to a B-like analog.[28,29] Identification of the acquired B phenotype can also be influenced by reagent pH and specific monoclonal anti-B typing reagents.[27] In the past, anti-B reagents containing the ES-4 clone were associated with an increased incidence of acquired B. To resolve the patient's true red cell type and to confirm the presence of acquired B, red cells should be retyped using a different monoclonal anti-B or acidified (pH 6.0) human anti-B. Acidified human anti-B will not react with acquired B antigen. The ability of monoclonal anti-B to recognize acquired anti-B should be noted in the manufacturer's insert.

ABO Antibodies

Anti-A and Anti-B

IgM is the predominant isotype found in group A and group B individuals, although small quantities of IgG antibody can be detected. In group O serum, IgG is the major isotype for anti-A and anti-B. As a consequence, hemolytic disease of the fetus and newborn (HDFN) is more common among group O mothers because IgG can cross the placenta, while IgM cannot.

Both IgM and IgG anti-A and anti-B preferentially agglutinate red cells at room temperature (20 to 24 C) or cooler, and both can efficiently activate complement at 37 C. The complement-mediated lytic capability of these antibodies becomes apparent if serum testing includes an incubation phase at 37 C. Hemolysis caused by ABO antibodies should be suspected either when the supernatant serum is pink to red or when the cell button is decreased in size or is absent. Hemolysis must be interpreted as a positive result. The use of plasma for testing, or the use of reagent red cells suspended in solutions that contain EDTA, will prevent complement activation and hemolysis.

Anti-A,B

Sera from group O individuals contain an antibody designated as anti-A,B because it reacts with both A and B red cells. Such anti-A and anti-B reactivity cannot be separated by differential adsorption, suggesting that the antibody recognizes a common epitope shared by the A and B antigens. Saliva containing secreted A or B substance can inhibit the activity of anti-A,B against both A and B red cells.

Anti-A1

Anti-A1 occurs as an alloantibody in the serum of 1% to 8% of A_2 individuals and 22% to 35% of A_2B individuals.[15,29] Anti-A1 can sometimes be found in the sera of other weak A subgroups. Group O serum contains a mixture of anti-A and anti-A1. Anti-A1 can cause ABO discrepancies during routine testing and can lead to incompatible crossmatches with A_1 and A_1B red cells. Anti-A1 is usually of IgM isotype, reacting best at room temperature or below, and is usually considered clinically insignificant. Anti-A1 is considered clinically significant if reactivity is observed at 37 C. Group A_2 patients with an anti-A1 reactive at 37 C testing should be transfused with group O or A_2 red cells only; group A_2B patients should receive group O, A_2, A_2B, or B red cells.

Routine Testing for ABO

Donor blood samples are routinely typed for ABO at the time of donation and upon receipt of the Red Blood Cell (RBC) units in the hospital transfusion service (confirmatory typing). Recipient samples are typed before transfusion. ABO grouping requires both antigen typing of red cells for A and B antigen (red cell grouping or forward type) and screening of serum or plasma for the presence of anti-A and anti-B isoagglutinins (serum grouping or reverse type). Both red cell and serum or plasma grouping are required for donors and patients because each grouping serves as a check on the other. Reverse or serum grouping is not required in two circumstances—1) for confirmation testing of labeled, previously typed donor red cells and 2) in infants less than 4 months of age. As previously discussed, isoagglutinins are not present at birth and develop only after 3 to 6 months of age.

Commercially available anti-A and anti-B for red cell typing are extremely potent and will agglutinate most antigen-positive red cells directly, even without centrifugation. Most monoclonal typing reagents have been formulated to detect many weak ABO subgroups (see manufacturers' inserts for specific reagent characteristics). Additional reagents (anti-A1 and anti-A,B) and special techniques to detect weak ABO subgroups are not necessary for routine testing but are helpful in resolving ABO typing discrepancies.

In contrast to commercial ABO typing reagents, human anti-A and anti-B in the sera of patients and donors can be relatively weak, requiring incubation and centrifugation. Tests for serum grouping, therefore, should be performed by a method that will adequately detect human anti-A and anti-B. Several methods are available for determining ABO group, including slide, tube, microplate, and column agglutination techniques. Procedures for ABO grouping by slide, tube, and microplate tests, as well as for resolving ABO discrepancies, are described in the methods section of this book.

ABO Discrepancies

Table 12-1 shows the results and interpretations of routine red cell and serum tests for ABO. A discrepancy exists when the results of red cell tests do not agree with serum tests, usually caused by unexpected negative or unexpected positive results in either the forward or reverse typing (see Table 12-3). ABO discrepancies may arise from intrinsic problems with either red cells or serum, or technical errors in performing the test (see Table 12-4 and section on resolving ABO discrepancies).

When a discrepancy is encountered, the discrepant results must be recorded, but interpretation of the ABO group must be delayed until the discrepancy has been resolved. If the specimen is from a donor unit, the unit must be quarantined and cannot be released for transfusion. When an ABO discrepancy is identified in a patient, it may be necessary to transfuse group O red cells pending an investigation. It is important to obtain a sufficient pretransfusion blood sample from the patient to complete any additional studies that may be required.

Red Cell Testing Problems

ABO testing of red cells may give unexpected results for many reasons, including the following:

1. Weak ABO expression that results from inheritance of a weak ABO subgroup. Some patients with leukemia and other malignancies can also show weakened ABO expression.[29]
2. Mixed-field agglutination, with circulating red cells of more than one ABO group, following out-of-group red cell transfusion or hematopoietic progenitor cell (HPC) transplantation (eg, group O to group A). Mixed-field agglutination is also observed in some ABO subgroups (A_3), in blood group chimerism in fraternal twins, and in very rare cases of mosaicism arising from dispermy.
3. Neutralization of anti-A and anti-B typing reagents by high concentrations of A or B blood group substance in serum, resulting in unexpected negative reactions with serum- or plasma-suspended red cells.
4. Spontaneous agglutination or autoagglutination of serum- or plasma-suspended red cells caused by heavy coating of red cells by potent autoagglutinins.
5. Nonspecific aggregation of serum- or plasma-suspended red cells caused by abnormal concentrations of serum proteins or infused macromolecular solutions.
6. False-positive reactions caused by a pH-dependent autoantibody, a reagent-dependent antibody (eg, EDTA, paraben),[29] or rouleaux.
7. Anomalous red cell grouping resulting from acquired B, B(A), or A(B) phenotypes.
8. Polyagglutination (eg, T activation) resulting from inherited or acquired abnormalities of the red cell membrane, with expo-

TABLE 12-4. Possible Causes of ABO Typing Discrepancies

Category	Causes
Weak/missing red cell reactivity	ABO subgroup
	Leukemia/malignancy
	Transfusion
	Intrauterine fetal transfusion
	Transplantation
	Excessive soluble blood group substance
Extra red cell reactivity	Autoagglutinins/excess protein coating red cells
	Unwashed red cells: plasma proteins
	Unwashed red cells: antibody in patient's serum to reagent constituent
	Transplantation
	Acquired B antigen
	B(A) phenomenon
	Out-of-group transfusion
Mixed-field red cell reactivity	Recent transfusion
	Transplantation
	Fetomaternal hemorrhage
	Twin or dispermic (tetragametic) chimerism
Weak/missing serum reactivity	Age related (<4-6 months old, elderly)
	ABO subgroup
	Hypogammaglobulinemia
	Transplantation
Extra serum reactivity	Cold autoantibody
	Cold alloantibody
	Serum antibody to reagent constituent
	Excess serum protein
	Transfusion of plasma components
	Transplantation
	Infusion of intravenous immune globulin

sure of "cryptic autoantigens."[29] Because all human sera contain naturally occurring antibodies to such cryptic antigens, those abnormal red cells are agglutinated by sera from group A, B, and AB individuals. Monoclonal anti-A and anti-B reagents do not detect polyagglutination.

Problems with Serum or Plasma Testing

Problems may arise during ABO testing of serum or plasma, including the following:

1. Small fibrin clots in plasma or incompletely clotted serum that can be mistaken for red cell agglutinates.
2. Lack of detectable isoagglutinins in infants less than 4 to 6 months of age. Children do not develop isoagglutinins until 3 to 6 months of age. Isoagglutinins present at birth are passively acquired from the mother.
3. Unexpected absence of ABO agglutinins caused by a weak A or B subgroup (see Table 12-3).[8,11,22]
4. Unexpected absence of ABO agglutinins in children resulting from long-term parenteral and enteral nutrition, that are sterile and free of bacteria.[6,30]
5. ABO-incompatible HPC transplantation with induction of tolerance. For example, a group A patient receiving a group O marrow transplant will have circulating group O red cells but will produce only anti-B in serum. (Refer to Chapter 25 for more information on ABO-mismatched transplants.)
6. Severe hypogammaglobulinemia secondary to an inherited immunodeficiency or disease therapy. Hypogammaglobulinemia, with dilution of isoagglutinins, can also be encountered after several courses of plasma exchange with albumin replacement.
7. Cold alloantibodies (eg, anti-M) or autoantibodies (eg, anti-I) reacting with reverse grouping cells, leading to unexpected positive reactions.
8. Antibodies directed against constituents in the diluents used to preserve reagent A_1 and B red cells.
9. Nonspecific aggregation or agglutination caused by high-molecular-weight plasma expanders, rouleaux, high serum protein concentrations, or altered serum protein ratios.
10. Recent transfusion of out-of-group plasma-containing components (eg, a group A patient transfused with platelets from a group O donor, causing unexpected anti-A detectable in the patient's plasma).
11. Recent infusion of intravenous immune globulin (IVIG), which can contain ABO isoagglutinins.

Technical Errors

Technical problems with the sample or during testing can also lead to problems in ABO grouping. Such problems include the following:

1. Specimen mix-up.
2. Too heavy or too light red cell suspensions.
3. Failure to add reagents.
4. Missed observation of hemolysis.
5. Failure to follow the manufacturer's instructions.
6. Under- or overcentrifugation of tests.
7. Incorrect interpretation or recording of test results.

Resolving ABO Discrepancies

The first step in resolving an apparent serologic problem should be to repeat the test with the same sample to exclude the possibility of technical error during testing. Additional studies may include testing washed red cells; testing a new sample; testing to detect unexpected red cell alloantibodies; and reviewing the patient's medical record for conditions, medications, or recent transfusions that may contribute to conflicting test results (Method 2-4). Samples with apparent weak or missing ABO antigens or antibodies, or both, may require tests using methods to enhance antigen-antibody binding. Techniques include incubating red cells at 4 C (Method 2-5), using enzyme-treated red cells (Method 2-6), and adsorption and elution studies (Method 2-7). In some instances, it may be necessary to test for the secretion of ABO antigens in saliva (Method 2-8). Patients with suspected B(A), acquired B, and A(B) phenotypes should be retested using different monoclonal and human polyclonal reagents.

ABO discrepancies caused by unexpected serum reactions are not uncommon. Commonly encountered causes of serum grouping discrepancies include cold autoantibodies, rouleaux, cold-reacting alloantibodies (eg, anti-M), and weak A subgroups with an anti-A1. To resolve an ABO discrepancy caused by an anti-A1 in a group A individual, red cells should be tested with *Dolichos biflorus* lectin, which will agglutinate group A_1 but not A_2 and weaker A subgroups. The presence of an anti-A1 should be confirmed by testing serum against A_1, A_2, and O red cells (Method 2-9). Reverse grouping problems resulting from either a cold alloantibody (Method 2-10) or autoantibody can be uncovered with a room-temperature antibody detection test and a direct antiglobulin test (DAT). Techniques to identify ABO antibodies in the presence of cold autoantibodies include testing at 37 C without centrifugation (Method 2-11) and cold autoadsorption (Method 4-5). Serum or plasma properties can induce rouleaux formation that will look like agglutination with A1 and B red cells. Saline replacement or saline dilution (Method 3-4) can be used to distinguish rouleaux from agglutination and to identify ABO antibodies.

Cold autoantibodies can cause autoagglutination of red cells and unexpected reactions during red cell typing. Red cells heavily coated with autoantibodies can spontaneously agglutinate and cause false-positive reactions in tests with anti-A and anti-B. Usually, false-positive reactions caused by autoantibodies can be eliminated by washing red cells with warm saline (Method 2-17). Autoagglutination caused by IgM can also be inhibited or dispersed by incubating red cells in the presence of either dithiothreitol or 2-aminoethylisothiouronium bromide (AET) (Method 3-10). Those reagents reduce the disulfide bonds on IgM molecules, decreasing their polyvalency and ability to directly agglutinate red cells.

THE H SYSTEM

The H antigen is ubiquitously expressed on all red cells except the rare Bombay phenotype. Because H antigen serves as the precursor to both A and B antigens, the amount of H antigen on red cells depends on an individual's ABO type. H antigen is highly expressed on group O red cells, because group O individuals lack a functional ABO gene. In group A and B individuals, the amount of H antigen is considerably less, as H is converted to the A and B antigens, respectively. The amount of H antigen on red cells, based on agglutination with the anti-H lectin *Ulex europaeus*, is represented thus: $O>A_2>B>A_2B>A_1>A_1B$. H antigen is present on HPCs, red cells, megakaryocytes, and other tissues.[2,3,31] H antigen has been implicated in cell adhesion, in normal hematopoietic differentiation, and in several malignancies.[1-3]

Biochemistry and Genetics

The H antigen is defined by the terminal disaccharide, fucose $\alpha 1 \rightarrow 2$ galactose. Two different fucosyltransferase (FUT) enzymes are capable of synthesizing the H antigen: *FUT1* (H gene) and *FUT2* (Secretor gene). *FUT1* specifically fucosylates type 2 chain oligosaccharides on red cell glycoproteins and glycolipids to form type 2 chain H. In contrast, *FUT2* or Secretor recognizes type 1 chain precursors to form type 1 chain H and Le^b antigens in secretions (Fig 12-3).[12] Secretion of type 1 chain ABH antigens in saliva and other fluids requires a functional *FUT2* gene. *FUT2* is not expressed in red cells but is expressed in salivary glands, gastrointestinal tissues, and genitourinary tissues.[1-3] Type 1 chain ABH antigen present on red cells is passively adsorbed from circulating glycolipid antigen present in plasma (see Lewis system section).

Null Phenotypes

Bombay (O_h) Phenotype

Originally described in Bombay, India, the O_h or Bombay phenotype is a rare, autosomal recessive phenotype characterized by the ab-

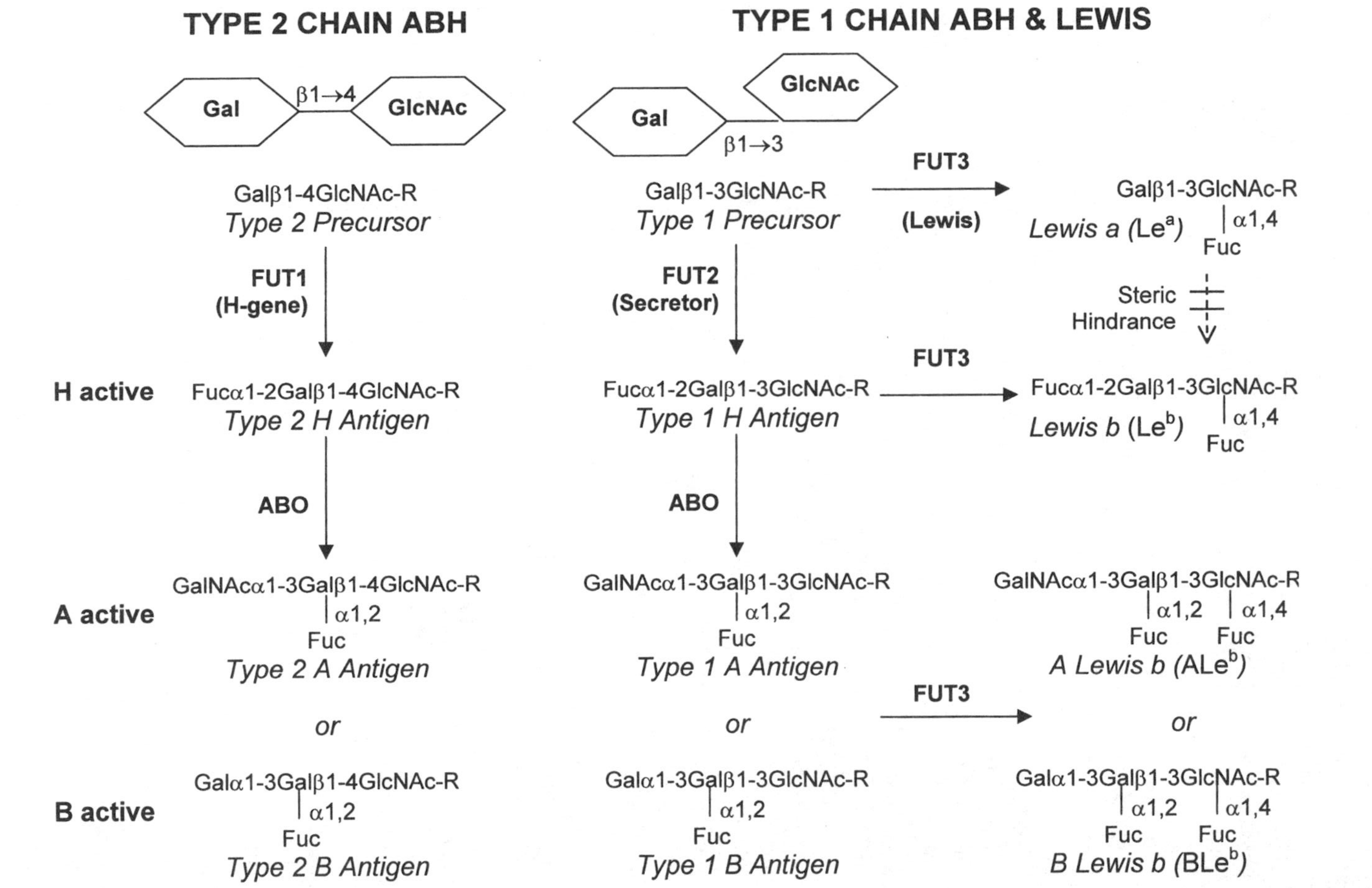

FIGURE 12-3. Synthesis of type 1 chain ABH and Lewis antigens by Secretor (*FUT2*), Lewis (*FUT3*), and ABO enzymes. Type 2 chain ABH antigen synthesis is also shown for comparison.
Fuc = fucose; Gal = galactose; GalNAc = *N*-acetylgalactosamine; GlcNAc = *N*-acetylglucosamine; R = other upstream carbohydrate sequence. Reproduced with permission from Cooling.[32]

sence of H, A, and B antigens on red cells and in secretions. Genetically, O_h individuals are homozygous for nonfunctional H (*hh*) and Secretor (*sese*) genes, resulting in a complete absence of type 1 and type 2 chain H, A, and B. O_h red cells will type as H negative with the anti-H lectin *Ulex europaeus* and monoclonal anti-H. Because these individuals lack a functional Secretor gene necessary for Le^b synthesis, O_h individuals also type as Le(b–) (see Lewis system). Genotyping studies have described a wide range of inactivating mutations in both the H and Secretor genes in O_h individuals.[12,21]

Because they lack all ABH antigens, O_h individuals possess natural isohemagglutinins to A, B, *and* H (see Table 12-1). In routine ABO typing, those individuals will initially type as group O. The O_h phenotype becomes apparent during antibody detection tests with group O red cells, which are rich in H antigen. The anti-H present in O_h individuals will strongly agglutinate all group O red cells and will sometimes demonstrate in-vivo hemolysis. The O_h phenotype can be confirmed by demonstrating an absence of H antigen on red cells and the presence of an anti-H in serum that is reactive with group O red cells but not with O_h red cells from other individuals.

Para-Bombay Phenotype

The para-Bombay phenotype describes individuals who are H-deficient secretors.[12,15,29] Genetically, those individuals are homozygous for a nonfunctional H gene (*hh*), but they have inherited at least one functional Secretor gene (*Se*). The red cells from H-deficient secretors lack serologically detectable H antigen but can carry small amounts of A and/or B antigen, because unlike classic Bombay, para-Bombay persons express type 1 chain ABH antigens in their secretions and plasma (Method 2-8). Type 1 chain A or B antigen in plasma is then passively adsorbed onto red cells, resulting in weak A or B antigen expression. Para-Bombay can also occur in group O individuals, as evidenced by trace type 1 chain H on red cells and in their secretions. Red cells from para-Bombay individuals are designated A_h, B_h, and AB_h.

In laboratory testing, red cells from para-Bombay individuals may (or may not) give weak reactions with anti-A and anti-B reagents. In some cases, A and B antigens may be detected only after adsorption and elution. Para-Bombay red cells are nonreactive with anti-H lectin, monoclonal anti-H, and human anti-H from O_h individuals. The sera of para-Bombay individuals contain anti-H, anti-HI, or both, and depending on their ABO type, anti-A and anti-B.

Anti-H

Alloanti-H (Bombay and Para-Bombay)

The anti-H observed in Bombay and para-Bombay phenotypes is clinically significant and is associated with acute hemolytic transfusion reactions. The antibody is predominantly of IgM isotype and exhibits a broad thermal range (4 to 37 C) with all red cells except O_h red cells. As with anti-A and anti-B, alloanti-H is capable of activating complement and causing red cell hemolysis.

Autoanti-H and Autoanti-HI

Autoantibodies to H and HI antigens can be encountered in normal individuals. When observed, those autoantibodies are most common in A_1 individuals, who have very little H antigen on their red cells. Autoanti-H and autoanti-HI are usually of IgM isotype and are reactive at room temperature.

Transfusion Practice

Alloanti-H is highly significant, capable of fixing complement and causing hemolytic transfusion reactions. As a result, patients with alloanti-H, caused by a Bombay or para-Bombay phenotype, must be transfused with H-negative (O_h) RBCs.

In contrast, autoantibodies against H and HI are generally clinically insignificant. In most patients, transfusion of either group-specific or group O RBCs should have a normal in-vivo survival. Occasionally, autoanti-HI can result in decreased red cell survival and hemolytic transfusion reactions after transfusion of group O RBCs.[12] In most instances, hemolysis follows transfusion of group O RBCs to a group A_1 or B patient with an unusually potent high-titer anti-HI that is reactive at 37 C.[29] In such patients, it may be advisable to transfuse group-specific (A_1, B, or AB) RBCs.

THE LEWIS SYSTEM

The Lewis blood group system consists of two main antigens, Le^a and Le^b, and three common phenotypes: Le(a+b–), Le(a–b+), and Le(a–b–). In addition to their presence on red cells, Lewis antigens are expressed on platelets, endothelium, and the kidney as well as on genitourinary and gastrointestinal epithelium.[2,3,29] Lewis antigens are not synthesized by red cells but are passively adsorbed onto red cell membranes from a pool of soluble Lewis glycolipid present in plasma. The gastrointestinal tract, which is rich in Lewis-active glycolipid and glycoprotein, is thought to be the primary source of Lewis glycolipid in plasma. Because Lewis antigens are passively adsorbed onto red cell membranes, Lewis antigens can be eluted from red cells after transfusion or by increases in plasma volume and circulating lipoproteins, which also adsorb Lewis glycolipid. For example, Lewis antigen is often decreased on red cells during pregnancy, with some women transiently typing as Le(a–b–). That marked decrease is the result of an increase in circulating plasma volume and a fourfold increase in lipoprotein.[29] Le^b expression and immunoreactivity are also influenced by ABH type[33] as a result of the synthesis of hybrid structures with both Lewis and ABH activity (Fig 12-3).[2,3,12,29]

Biochemistry and Synthesis

Lewis antigen synthesis depends on the interaction of two distinct fucosyltransferases (Fig 12-3): Lewis (*FUT3*) and Secretor (*FUT2*). Unlike *H* or *FUT1*, which is specific for type 2 chain substrates, Lewis and Secretor preferentially fucosylate type 1 chain substrates. Secretor (*FUT2*) can add a terminal $\alpha1\rightarrow2$ fucose to a type 1 chain precursor to form type 1 chain H antigen. The Lewis gene encodes an $\alpha1\rightarrow3/4$ fucosyltransferase that transfers a fucose, in an $\alpha1\rightarrow4$ linkage, to the penultimate *N*-acetyl-glucosamine of type 1 chain precursor ("Lewis c") to form Le^a antigen. Lewis (*FUT3*) can also add a second fucose to type 1 H antigen to form Le^b antigen. Note that Le^b cannot be formed from Le^a because the presence of a subterminal fucose on Le^a sterically inhibits binding by the Secretor enzyme. In individuals with both Lewis and Secretor enzymes, type 1 chain H is favored over Le^a synthesis. As a result, most of the Lewis antigen synthesized is Le^b [Le(a–b+) phenotype]. In group A_1 and B individuals, Le^b and type 1 chain H can be further modified by ABO glycosyltransferases to form ALe^b, BLe^b, type 1 A, and type 1 B antigens.[2,3] In group A_1 individuals, it has been shown that the majority of Lewis antigen in plasma is actually ALe^b.[34]

Genetics and Lewis Phenotypes

The three Lewis phenotypes commonly encountered represent the presence or absence of Lewis and Secretor enzymes (see Table 12-5). Le(a+b–) individuals have inherited at least one functional Lewis gene (*Le*) but are homozygous for nonfunctional Secretor alleles (*sese*). As a result, such individuals synthesize and secrete Le^a antigen but lack Le^b and type 1 chain ABH antigens. The Le(a–b+) phenotype reflects inheritance of both *Le* and *Se* alleles, leading to the synthesis of Le^a, Le^b, and type 1 chain ABH. Because most type 1 chain precursor is converted to Le^b in those individuals, they appear to type as Le(a–). A Le(a+b+) phenotype is transiently observed in infants, as Secretor activity increases with developmental age. A Le(a+b+) phenotype is also encountered in 16% of Japanese individuals as a result of inheritance of a weak Secretor gene (Se^w).[21] In the absence of a functional Lewis gene (*lele*), neither Le^a nor Le^b is synthesized, leading to a Le(a–b–) or null phenotype. Type 1 chain ABH antigens may still be synthesized and secreted in individuals who have inherited at least one functional *Se* allele (Method 2-8). The frequency of the Le(a–b–) phenotype is significantly higher in persons of African ethnicity.

TABLE 12-5. Adult Phenotypes and Prevalence in the Lewis System

Red Cell Reactions			Prevalence (%)		Genotype*		
Anti-Le^a^	Anti-Le^b^	Phenotype	Whites	Blacks	Lewis	Secretor	Saliva†
+	0	Le(a+b–)	22	23	*Le*	*sese*	Le^a^
0	+	Le(a–b+)	72	55	*Le*	*Se*	Le^a^, Le^b^, ABH
0	0	Le(a–b–)	6	22	*lele* *lele*	*sese* *Se*	Type 1 precursor Type 1 ABH
+	+	Le(a+b+)‡	Rare	Rare	*Le*	*Se^w^*	Le^a^, Le^b^

*Probable genotype at the Lewis (*FUT3*) and Secretor (*FUT2*) loci.

†Type 1 chain antigens present in saliva and other secretions.

‡Le(a+b+) is present in 16% of Japanese individuals and is also transiently observed in infants.

Le = gene encoding functional Lewis enzyme; *lele* = homozygous for gene encoding an inactive enzyme; *Se* = gene encoding active Secretor enzyme; *sese* = homozygous for gene encoding an inactive enzyme; *Se^w^* = gene encoding weak Secretor enzyme.

Several inactivating mutations have been identified in both Lewis and Secretor genes.[21] Many of the mutations are geographically and racially distributed, with many populations displaying a few predominant alleles. Of the nonfunctional *Le* alleles described, most have more than one mutation.[12,21]

Lewis Expression in Children

Table 12-5 shows the distribution of Lewis types in adults. In contrast, most newborns type as Le(a–b–) with human anti-Lewis typing reagents. Approximately 50% of newborns will subsequently type as Le(a+) after ficin treatment. The prevalence of Le^b antigen, however, is low relative to adults because of developmental delays in Secretor (*FUT2*) activity. A Le(a+b+) phenotype can be transiently observed in children as the level of Secretor activity approaches adult levels. A valid Lewis phenotype is not achieved until age 5 or 6.[15]

Lewis Antibodies

Antibodies against Lewis antigens are generally of IgM isotype and are naturally occurring. Clinically, Lewis antibodies are most often encountered in the sera of Le(a–b–) individuals and may contain a mixture of anti-Le^a, anti-Le^b, and anti-Le^{a+b}, an antibody capable of recognizing both Le(a+) and Le(b+) red cells. Because small amounts of Le^a are synthesized in the Le(a–b+) phenotype, Le(a–b+) individuals do not make an anti-Le^a. Anti-Le^b is observed infrequently in the Le(a+b–) phenotype. Lewis antibodies, accompanied by a transient Le(a–b–) phenotype, are reported during pregnancy. Finally, anti-Le^b can demonstrate ABO specificity (anti-Le^{bH}, anti-ALe^b, anti-BLe^b), reacting preferentially with Le(b+) red cells of a specific ABO group.[29,33] Anti-Le^{bH}, the most common reactivity, reacts more strongly with Le(b+) group O and A_2 red cells than with group A_1 and B red cells, which are low in H antigen. Anti-Le^{bL} reacts strongly with all Le(b+) red cells, regardless of ABO group.

Most examples of Lewis antibodies are saline agglutinins reactive at room temperature. Unlike ABO, the agglutination is relatively fragile and easily dispersed, requiring gentle resuspension after centrifugation. Agglutination is sometimes observed after 37 C incubation, but the reaction strength is typically weaker than that observed at room temperature. On occasion, Lewis antibodies can be detected in the antihuman globulin (AHG) phase. Such detection may reflect either IgG or bound complement (if polyspecific AHG reagent is used). Very rarely, Lewis antibodies can cause in-vitro hemolysis. Hemolysis is more often observed when testing fresh serum containing anti-Le^a or anti-Le^{a+b}, particularly when tested against enzyme-treated red cells.

Transfusion Practice

In general, Lewis antibodies are not considered clinically significant. Red cells that are compatible in tests at 37 C, regardless of Lewis phenotype, are expected to have normal in-vivo survival. It is not considered necessary to transfuse antigen-negative RBCs for most patients. Unlike ABO antigens, Lewis antigens are extrinsic glycolipid antigens that are readily eluted and shed from transfused red cells within a few days of transfusion. Furthermore, Lewis antigens present in transfused plasma can neutralize Lewis antibodies in the recipient. For these reasons, hemolysis is rare following the transfusion of either Le(a+) or Le(b+) red cells.

Lewis antibodies are not a cause of HDFN.[15] Lewis antibodies are predominantly of IgM isotype and do not cross the placenta. In addition, Lewis antigens are poorly expressed on neonatal red cells, with most newborns typing as Le(a–b–) with human Lewis antibodies (see above).

Disease Associations

The Le^b and H antigens are receptors for *Helicobacter pylori*, a gram-negative bacterium implicated in gastritis, peptic ulcer disease, gastric carcinoma, mucosa-associated lymphoma, and idiopathic thrombocytopenia.[35,36] Le^b and type 1 H antigens are also receptors for Norwalk virus, a common cause of acute gastroenteritis.[37] A Le(a–b–) phenotype is associated with an increased susceptibility to infections by *Candida* and uropathogenic *Escherichia coli*.[38,39]

I AND i ANTIGENS

The I and i antigens are ubiquitous, structurally related antigens present on all cell membranes. The minimum epitope common to both i and I is a terminal lactosamine (Galβ1→4GlcNAc) or type 2 chain precursor. The i antigen is a linear, nonbranched structure, whereas the I antigen is a polyvalent, branched glycan (Fig 12-4). Both i and I serve as substrate and scaffold for the synthesis of ABO, Lewis X [Galβ1-4(Fucα1-3) GlcNAc], and other type 2 chain antigens.[1-3] On red cells, i and I antigens are present on *N*-linked glycoproteins and glycolipids.

Phenotypes

Two phenotypes are recognized according to the presence or absence of I antigen: I and i (I–). The i phenotype is characteristic of neonatal red cells, whereas I+ is the common phenotype in adults. With increasing age, there is a gradual increase in I antigen, accompanied by a reciprocal decrease in i antigen, with most children achieving an adult I+ phenotype by age 2. An increase in i antigen can be observed in chronic hemolytic disorders and is a sign of stressed erythropoiesis.[40]

The i_{adult} phenotype (I–i+) is an autosomal recessive phenotype caused by mutations in the I gene *(IGnT* or *CGNT2*). Two genetic disorders are associated with an increase in i antigen. In Asian populations, the i_{adult} phenotype can be associated with congenital cataracts.[41] A marked increase in i antigen is also observed in HEMPAS (hereditary erythroblastic multinuclearity with a positive acidified serum lysis test). The latter is a genetic defect in Golgi transport and *N*-glycosylation and is associated with chronic hemolysis.[1,42]

Genetics

The I gene *(IGnT, CGNT2)* encodes a β1→6 *N*-acetyl-glucosaminyltransferase, which converts the linear i antigen into the branched I antigen.[29,41] The gene resides on chromosome 6p24 and contains five exons, including three tissue-specific exons (exons 1A, 1B, and 1C). As a result, three slightly different mRNA tran-

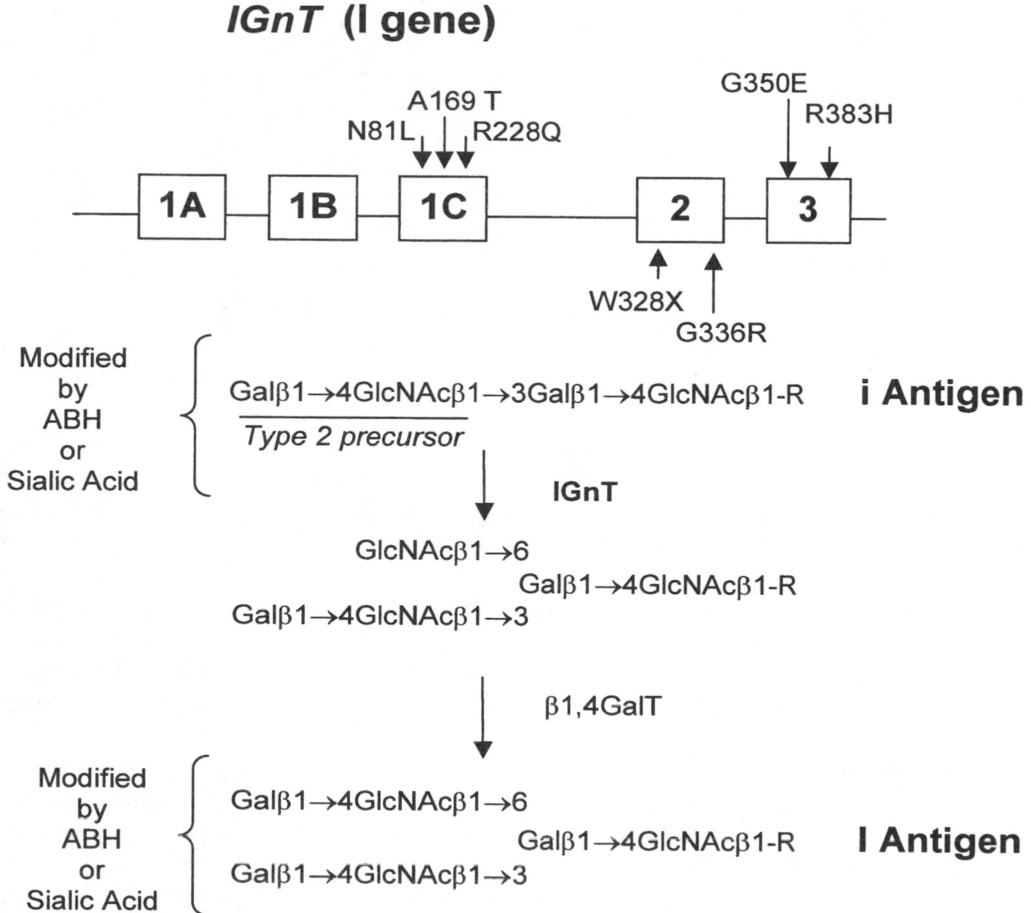

FIGURE 12-4. Structure and synthesis of I antigen and I gene (*IGnT*). Also shown are point mutations (arrows) associated with the i_{adult} phenotype.
Gal = galactose; GlcNAc = *N*-acetylglucosamine; R = other upstream carbohydrate sequence. Reproduced with permission from Cooling.[32]

scripts can be synthesized, depending on which exon 1 is used. In the i_{adult} phenotype without cataracts, there is a mutation in exon 1C, which is specific for I antigen synthesis in red cells. As a consequence, I antigen is missing on red cells but is still synthesized in other tissues that use either exon 1A or exon 1B. In the i_{adult} phenotype with cataracts, there is a loss of I antigen synthesis in all tissues, caused by either gene deletion or mutations in exons 2 and 3.[41]

Antibodies

Anti-I

Anti-I is a common antibody present in the serum of normal healthy individuals. Anti-I is usually of IgM isotype, reacting best at 4 C with titers of <64. Stronger examples may also be detectable at room temperature. Anti-I is identified by strong reactions with adult red cells but weak or no agglutination with cord red cells (see Table 12-6). Anti-I can be enhanced

TABLE 12-6. Comparative Serologic Behavior of the I/i Blood Group Antibodies with Saline Red Cell Suspensions

Temperature	Cell Type	Anti-I	Anti-i
4 C	I adult	4+	0-1+
	i cord	0-2+	3+
	i adult	0-1+	4+
22 C	I adult	2+	0
	i cord	0	2-3+
	i adult	0	3+

by 4 C incubation, by the presence of albumin, or by using enzyme-treated red cells. An alloanti-I can be seen in the i_{adult} phenotype.

Some examples of anti-I can demonstrate complex reactivity, reacting stronger with red cells of specific ABO, P_1, or Lewis phenotypes. Many of those antibodies appear to recognize branched oligosaccharides that have been further modified to express additional blood group antigens. Anti-IH is a common antibody encountered in the serum of A_1 individuals. Anti-IH reacts stronger with group O and group A_2 red cells, which are rich in H antigen, than with group A_1 red cells. Anti-IH is suspected when serum from a group A individual directly agglutinates all group O red cells but is compatible with most group A donor blood tested. Other examples of complex reactivity include anti-IA, -IP1, -IBH, and -ILe^{bH}.

Anti-i

Autoanti-i is a relatively uncommon cold agglutinin in normal sera. Like anti-I, anti-i is primarily of IgM isotype, reacting weakly at 4 to 10 C. Anti-i reacts most strongly with cord and i_{adult} red cells and weaker with I+ adult red cells (Table 12-6). Patients with infectious mononucleosis often have a transient but potent anti-i. As with anti-I, complex reactivity can sometimes be observed (eg, anti-iH).

Cold Agglutinin Syndrome

Autoanti-I and autoanti-i are pathologically significant in cold agglutinin syndrome (CAS) and mixed-type auto-immune hemolytic anemia. In those disorders, autoanti-I (or anti-i) behaves as a complement-binding antibody with a high titer and wide thermal range. Primary CAS is observed with lymphoproliferative disorders (Waldenström macroglobulinemia, lymphoma, and chronic lymphocytic leukemia). A potent autoanti-I can also be observed in the setting of infection. *Mycoplasma pneumoniae* infections are a common cause of autoanti-I and can be accompanied by a transient hemolysis. (See Chapter 17 for additional discussions of CAS.)

The specificity of the autoantibody in CAS may not be apparent when undiluted samples are tested. Titration studies and thermal amplitude studies may be required to discern the specificity of the autoantibodies and their potential clinical significance. Table 12-6 illustrates the serologic behavior of anti-I and anti-i at 4 C and 22 C. (See Chapter 17 and Method 4-7 for additional information regarding titration and thermal amplitude studies.)

Transfusion Practice

Autoanti-I can interfere with ABO typing, antibody screening, and compatibility testing. In laboratory testing, those antibodies can be reactive in the antiglobulin phase of testing, particularly when polyspecific AHG is used. Such reactions rarely indicate antibody activity at 37 C but are the consequence of antibody binding, followed by complement binding, at low temperatures. Usually, avoiding room-temperature testing and using anti-IgG-specific AHG will prevent detection of nuisance cold autoantibodies. For stronger antibody examples, autoantibody can be removed from serum by cold autoadsorption techniques (see Method 4-5). Cold autoadsorbed serum can also be used for ABO testing.

P BLOOD GROUPS/GLOB COLLECTION

The first antigen of the P blood group system was discovered by Landsteiner and Levine in 1927 in a series of experiments that also led to the discovery of M and N antigens. Originally called P, the name of the antigen was later changed to P1, and it is the only antigen officially assigned to the P blood group system. The P, P^k, and LKE antigens, which were previously considered part of the P system, are currently assigned to the GLOB, P1PK, and 028 collection.[12,21] P^k and P antigens are high-incidence antigens expressed on nearly all red cells except rare null phenotypes, which lack P (P^k phenotype) or both P and P^k antigens (p phenotype). (See Table 12-7.) Red cells are particularly rich in P antigen, which makes up nearly 6% of the total red cell lipid. P^k and P antigens are also widely expressed on nonerythroid cells, including lymphocytes; platelets; and plasma, kidney, lung, heart, endothelium, placenta, and synovium cells. In contrast, the P1 antigen is uniquely expressed on red cells.[43]

Phenotypes

The P_1 (P1+) and P_2 (P1–) phenotypes account for >99% of donors (see Table 12-7). Both phenotypes synthesize P^k and P antigens and differ only in the expression of the P1 antigen. Three rare, autosomal recessive phenotypes have been identified (p, P_1^k, P_2^k), as well as weak variants.[44] Analogous to the ABO system, the rare p and P^k phenotypes are associated with the presence of naturally occurring antibodies against missing antigens (anti-P1, anti-P, anti-PP1P^k).

Biochemistry

The synthesis of the P^k, P, and P1 antigens proceeds through the stepwise addition of sugars to lactosylceramide, a ceramide dihexose (CDH). (See Fig 12-5 and Table 12-8.) The first step is the synthesis of the P^k antigen, the ultimate precursor of all globo-type glycosphingolipids. To make the P^k antigen, α1,4 galactosyltransferase 1 (α4GalT1) adds a terminal galactose, in an α1→4 linkage, to CDH. The P^k antigen can then serve as a substrate for β1,3 *N*-acetylgalactosaminyltransferase I (β3GalNAcT1), which adds a β1→3 *N*-acetylga-

TABLE 12-7. Phenotypes and Prevalence in the P1PK and GLOB Group

Red Cell Reactions with Antisera						Prevalence (%)	
Anti-P1	Anti-P	Anti-P^k	Anti-PP1P^k	Antibodies in Serum	Phenotype	European Ethnicity	African Ethnicity
+	+	0	+	None	P_1	79	94
0	+	0	+	P1*	P_2	21	6
0	0†	0	0	PP1P^k (Tj^a)	p	Rare	Rare
+	0	+	+	P	P_1^k	Rare	Rare
0	0	+	+	P	P_2^k	Rare	Rare

*An anti-P1 is detected in approximately 25% of P_2 individuals.
†Usually negative. Some examples may be weakly-positive as a result of crossreactivity of anti-P with X_2 and sialosyl-X_2 glycolipid on p red cells.

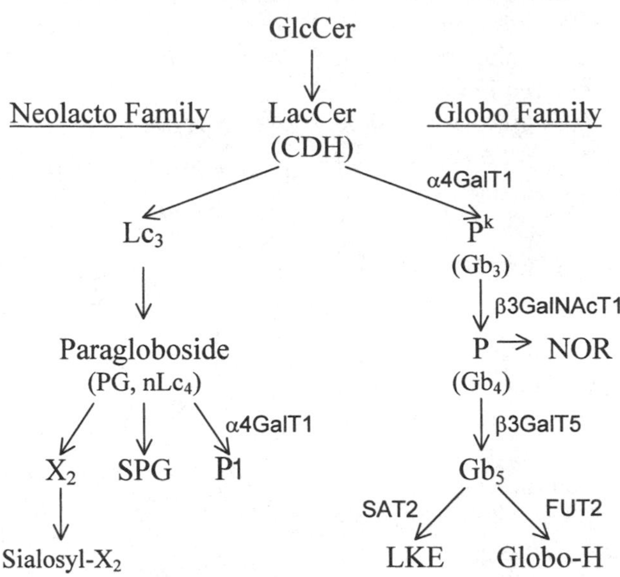

FIGURE 12-5. Synthesis of P1, P^k, P, and related glycosphingolipid antigens. Carbohydrate structures are shown in Table 12-8.

lactosamine to the terminal galactose of P^k (Gb_3) to form P antigen. In some cells, including red cells, the P antigen is further elongated to form additional, globo-family antigens such as Luke (LKE), type 4 chain ABH antigens (globo-ABH), and NOR. NOR, a rare polyagglutinable red cell phenotype, is the result of unusual globo-family antigens characterized by the addition of an α1→4 galactose to the terminus of P and related long chain globo-glycolipids (see Table 12-8).[45]

Unlike P^k and P antigens, the P1 antigen is not a globo-glycosphingolipid but is a member of the neolacto-family (type 2 chain glycosphingolipids). In P_1 individuals, it is hypothesized that α4GalT1 or P^k synthase is responsible for adding an α1→4 galactose to the terminus of paragloboside. The P1 antigen is not expressed on red cell glycoproteins.[46] The weak P-like activity found on some p red cells is believed to be X_2 and sialosyl-X_2, two related type 2 chain glycolipids.

Molecular Biology

Several inactivating mutations have been identified in both α4GalT1 and β3GALNAcT1.[44,47] The p phenotype is the consequence of mutations in the protein coding sequence of α4GalT1. In the absence of α4GalT1 activity, there is a loss of all globo-family antigens as well as a loss of P1 antigen synthesis. Those patients have a compensatory increase in type 2 chain glycolipid synthesis as evidenced by increased paragloboside, sialoparagloboside, and sialosyl-X_2. Mutations in β3GalNAcT1 give rise to the P^k phenotype, characterized by a loss of P and LKE antigens and by increased P^k expression. The absence of P1 antigen in P_2 individuals was initially thought to be the result of mutations in the α4GalT1 promoter; however, this has been challenged.[48] Instead, recent studies suggest that P1 synthesis may arise from an alternate start codon and α4GalT1 transcript.[49]

P Blood Group Antibodies

Anti-P1

Anti-P1 is a commonly encountered antibody in the sera of P_2 donors, occurring in one-quarter to two-thirds of P_2 individuals. Anti-P1 is a naturally occurring antibody of IgM isotype and is often detected as a weak, room-

TABLE 12-8. Structures of P1, GLOB, and Related Glycosphingolipids

Family*	Name	Oligosaccharide Structure
	CDH	Galβ1-4Glcβ1-1Cer
Globo (Gb)	Gb_3, P^k	Galα1-4Galβ1-4Glcβ1-1Cer
	Gb_4, P	GalNAcβ1-3Galα1-4Galβ1-4Glcβ1-1Cer
	Gb_5	Galβ1-3GalNAcβ1-3Galα1-4Galβ1-4Glcβ1-1Cer
	NOR1	Galα1-4GalNAcβ1-3Galα1-4Galβ1-4Glcβ1-1Cer
	Globo-H	Fucα1-2Galβ1-3GalNAcβ1-3Galα1-4Galβ1-4Glcβ1-1Cer
	LKE	NeuAcα2-3Galβ1-3GalNAcβ1-3Galα1-4Galβ1-4Glcβ1-1Cer
	NOR2	Galα1-4GalNAcβ1-3Galα1-4GalNAcβ1-3Galα1-4Galβ1-4Glcβ1-1Cer
Neolacto (nLc)	Lc_3	GlcNAcβ1-3Galβ1-4Glcβ1-1Cer
	nLc_4, PG	Galβ1-4GlcNAcβ1-3Galβ1-4Glcβ1-1Cer
	P1	Galα1-4Galβ1-4GlcNAcβ1-3Galβ1-4Glcβ1-1Cer
	SPG	NeuAcα2-3Galβ1-4GlcNAcβ1-3Galβ1-4Glcβ1-1Cer
	X_2	GalNAcβ1-3Galβ1-4GlcNAcβ1-3Galβ1-4Glcβ1-1Cer
	Sialosyl-X_2	NeuAcα2-3GalNAcβ1-3Galβ1-4GlcNAcβ1-3Galβ1-4Glcβ1-1Cer

*Glycosphingolipid family. Note: Neolacto are type 2 chain glycosphingolipids.
CDH = ceramide dihexose or lactosylceramide; Cer = ceramide; Gal = galactose; GalNAc = *N*-acetyl-galactosamine; Glc = glucose, GlcNAc = *N*-acetylglucosamine; NeuAc = N-acetyl-neuramanic acid (sialic acid); PG = paragloboside; SPG = sialosylparagloboside.

temperature agglutinin. Rare examples of anti-P1 are reactive at 37 C or show in-vitro hemolysis. Because anti-P1 is nearly always IgM, anti-P1 does not cross the placenta and is not reported to cause HDFN. Anti-P1 has only rarely been reported to cause in-vivo hemolysis. Anti-P1 titers are often elevated in patients with hydatid cyst disease or fascioliasis (liver fluke) and in bird fanciers. It is believed that P1-like substance in bird excrement can stimulate anti-P1 levels.[29] Some examples of anti-P1 also have I blood group specificity (anti-IP1).

P1 expression varies in strength between individuals and has been reported to decrease during in-vitro storage.[29] As a consequence, anti-P1 may not react with all P1+ red cells tested. Anti-P1 can be enhanced by incubation at lower temperatures (4 C) or by testing serum against enzyme-treated red cells. Anti-P1 reactivity can be inhibited in the presence of hydatid cyst fluid or P1 substance derived from pigeon eggs. Inhibition of P1 activity may be helpful when testing sera containing multiple antibodies.

Alloanti-PP1P^k and Alloanti-P

Anti-PP1P^k (historically known as anti-Tj^a) is a separable mixture of anti-P, anti-P1, and anti-P^k in the sera of p individuals. Alloanti-P is found in the sera of P_1^k and P_2^k individuals and is naturally occurring and predominantly of IgM isotype or a mixture of IgM and IgG (see Table 12-7). The antibodies are potent hemolysins and are associated with hemolytic transfusion reactions and occasionally HDFN. There is an association between anti-PP1P^k and early spontaneous abortion. The placenta, which is of fetal origin, is rich in P^k and P antigen and is a target for maternal cytotoxic IgG antibodies.

Autoanti-P (Donath-Landsteiner)

An autoantibody with P specificity is seen in patients with paroxysmal cold hemoglobinuria (PCH), a clinical syndrome most commonly observed in children following viral infection. In PCH, autoanti-P is an IgG biphasic hemolysin capable of binding red cells at colder temperatures, followed by intravascular hemolysis at body temperature. That characteristic can be demonstrated in vitro in the Donath-Landsteiner test. (See Chapter 17 and Method 4-11 for further details.)

Transfusion Practice

Alloanti-PP1P^k and alloanti-P are clinically significant antibodies associated with acute hemolytic transfusion reactions and spontaneous abortion. Rare individuals of p and P^k phenotypes should be provided antigen-negative, crossmatch-compatible RBCs for transfusion.

In general, anti-P1 is a clinically insignificant, room-temperature agglutinin. Patients with anti-P1, reactive only at room temperature or below, can be safely transfused with P1+ RBCs with normal red cell survival. It is not necessary to provide antigen-negative units for those patients. Very rarely, anti-P1 can cause decreased red cell survival and hemolytic transfusion reactions. Examples of anti-P1 that are capable of fixing complement at 37 C and that are strongly reactive in the AHG phase of testing are considered potentially clinically significant. In such rare instances, units selected for transfusion should be nonreactive at 37 C and in an indirect antiglobulin test with either polyspecific AHG or anti-C3.[29]

Disease Associations

The P^k antigen is a receptor for shiga toxins, the causative agent of shigella dysentery, and *E. coli*-associated hemolytic uremic syndrome.[43,44] The P^k antigen is also a receptor for *Streptococcus suis*, a species of bacteria that causes zoonotic illness capable of causing bacterial meningitis.[44] P^k expression may also modulate host-resistance to human immunodeficiency virus.[50] The P antigen is a receptor for parvovirus B19, the etiologic agent of erythema infectiosum (fifth disease). In some patients, B19 can cause a transient anemia or aplastic crisis. P1, P^k, P, and LKE antigens can all serve as receptors for P-fimbriated uropathogenic *E. coli*, a cause of chronic urinary tract infections.[39,44] LKE is a common oncofetal marker present on tumors and pluripotent embryonic, mesenchymal, and very small embryonic-like stem cells.[5,6]

KEY POINTS

1. The antigens of the ABO, H, Lewis, I, and P blood group systems are defined by small carbohydrate epitopes on glycoproteins and glycolipids, and they are widely distributed on many tissues, including embryonic stem cells. Such antigens are considered histo-blood group antigens.
2. The ABO system contains four major ABO phenotypes: A, B, O, and AB. The four phenotypes are determined by the presence or absence of two antigens (A and B) on red cells. An inverse reciprocal relationship exists between the presence of A and B antigens on red cells and the presence of anti-A, anti-B, or both, in sera.
3. ABO grouping requires both antigen typing of red cells for A and B antigen (red cell grouping, or forward type) and screening serum or plasma for the presence of anti-A and anti-B isoagglutinins (serum grouping, or reverse type).
4. The H antigen is ubiquitously expressed on all red cells except the rare Bombay phenotype.
5. Because H antigen serves as the precursor to both A and B antigens, the amount of H antigen on red cells depends on an individual's ABO group. H antigen is highly expressed on

group O red cells, because group O individuals lack a functional ABO gene. In group A and B individuals, the amount of H antigen is considerably less, as H is converted to the A and B antigens, respectively.

6. Lewis antigens are not synthesized by red cells but are passively adsorbed onto red cell membranes from a pool of soluble Lewis glycolipid present in plasma.

7. The three Lewis phenotypes commonly encountered represent the presence or absence of Lewis and Secretor enzymes.

8. With increasing age, there is a gradual increase in I antigen, accompanied by a reciprocal decrease in i antigen, with most children achieving an adult I+ phenotype by age 2.

9. Autoanti-I and autoanti-i are pathologically significant in cold agglutinin syndrome and mixed-type autoimmune hemolytic anemia.

10. The P_1 (P1+) and P_2 (P1–) phenotypes account for >99% of donors. Both phenotypes synthesize P^k and P antigens and differ only in the expression of the P1 antigen.

REFERENCES

1. Lowe JB, Marth JD. A genetic approach to mammalian glycan function. Annu Rev Biochem 2003;72:643-91.
2. Marionneau S, Cailleau-Thomas A, Rocher J, et al. ABH and Lewis histo-blood group antigens: A model for the meaning of oligosaccharide diversity in the face of a changing world. Biochimie 2001;83:565-73.
3. Holgersson J, Breimer ME, Samuelsson BE. Basic biochemistry of cell surface carbohydrates and aspects of the tissue distribution of histo-blood group ABH and related glycosphingolipids. APMIS 1992;100(Suppl 27):18-27.
4. Mölne J, Björquist P, Andersson K, et al. Blood group ABO antigen expression in human embryonic stem cells and in differentiated hepatocyte- and cardiomyocyte-like cells. Transplantation 2008;86:1407-13.
5. Gang EJ, Bosnakovski D, Figueiredo CA, et al. SSEA-4 identifies mesenchymal stem cells from bone marrow. Blood 2007;109:1743-51.
6. Ratajczak MZ, Zuba-Surma EK, Machalinski B, et al. Very small embryonic-like (VSEL) stem cells: Purification from adult organs, characterization and biological significance. Stem Cell Rev 2008;4:89-99.
7. Watkins WM. The ABO blood group system: Historical background. Transfus Med 2001;11: 243-65.
8. Stussi G, Halter J, Schanz U, Seebach JD. ABO-histo blood group incompatibility in hematopoietic stem cell and solid organ transplantation. Transfus Apher Sci 2006;35:59-69.
9. Springer GF. Blood-group and Forssman antigenic determinants shared between microbes and mammalian cells. Prog Allergy 1971;15:9-77.
10. Daniel-Johnson J, Leitman S, Klein H, et al. Probiotic-associated high-titer anti-B in a group A platelet donor as a cause of severe hemolytic transfusion reactions. Transfusion 2009;49:1845-9.
11. Yamamoto F. Review: ABO blood group system—ABH oligosaccharide antigens, anti-A and anti-B, A and B glycosyltransferases, and ABO genes. Immunohematology 2004;20:3-22.
12. Daniels G. Human blood groups. 2nd ed. Oxford: Blackwell Science, 2002.
13. Clausen H, Levery SB, Nudelman E, et al. Repetitive A epitope (type 3 chain A) defined by group A_1-specific monoclonal antibody TH-1: Chemical basis of qualitative A_1 and A_2 distinction. Proc Natl Acad Sci U S A 1985;82:1199-203.
14. Svensson L, Rydberg L, Hellberg A, et al. Novel glycolipid variations revealed by monoclonal antibody immunochemical analysis of weak ABO subgroups of A. Vox Sang 2005;89:27-38.
15. Klein HG, Anstee D. ABO, Lewis and P group and Ii antigens. In: Mollison's blood transfusion in clinical medicine. 11th ed. Oxford: Blackwell, 2005:114-62.
16. Auf Der Maur C, Hodel M, Nydegger UE, Rieben R. Age dependency of ABO histo-blood group antibodies: Reexamination of an old dogma. Transfusion 1993;33:915-18.
17. Mazda T, Yabe R, NaThalang O, et al. Differences in ABO antibody levels among blood donors: A comparison between past and present Japanese, Laotian, and Thai populations. Immunohematology 2007;23:38-41.

18. Kominato Y, Hata Y, Matsui K, et al. Transcriptional regulation of the human ABO histo-blood group genes is dependent on the N box upstream of the proximal promoter. Transfusion 2004;44:1741-9.
19. Hata Y, Kominato Y, Takizawa H. Identification and characterization of a novel antisense RNA transcribed from the opposite strand of the human blood group ABO gene. Transfusion 2007;47:842-51.
20. Koda Y, Soejima M, Kimura H. Changing transcription start sites in H-type α(1,2)fucosyltransferase gene (FUT1) during differentiation of the human erythroid lineage. Eur J Biochem 1998;256:379-87.
21. Reid ME, Lomas-Francis C. The blood group antigen factsbook. 2nd ed. San Diego, CA: Academic Press, 2004.
22. Roubinet F, Despiau S, Calafell F, et al. Evolution of the O alleles of the human ABO blood group gene. Transfusion 2004;44:707-15.
23. Wagner FF, Blasczyk R, Seltsam A. Nondeletional *ABO*O* alleles frequently cause blood group typing problems. Transfusion 2005;45:1331-4.
24. Yazer MH, Hult AK, Hellberg A, et al. Investigation into A antigen expression on O2 heterozygous group O-labeled red blood cell units. Transfusion 2008;48:1650-7.
25. Rouger P, Liberge G, Gane P, et al. Immunological properties of 31 anti-A monoclonal antibodies. Rev Fr Transfus Immunohematol 1987;30:413-20.
26. Beck ML, Yates AD, Hardman J, Kowalski MA. Identification of a subset of group B donors reactive with monoclonal anti-A reagent. Am J Clin Pathol 1989;92:625-9.
27. Garratty G, Arndt P, Co A, et al. Fatal hemolytic transfusion reaction resulting from ABO mistyping of a patient with acquired B antigen detectable only by some monoclonal anti-B reagents. Transfusion 1996;36:351-7.
28. Okubo Y, Seno T, Tanaka M, et al. Conversion of group A red cells by deacetylation to ones that react with monoclonal antibodies specific for the acquired B phenotype (letter). Transfusion 1994;34:456.
29. Issitt PD, Anstee DJ. Applied blood group serology. 4th ed. Durham, NC: Montgomery Scientific Publications, 1998.
30. Cooling LW, Sitwala K, Dake LR, et al. ABO typing discrepancies in children requiring long-term nutritional support (abstract). Transfusion 2007;47(3S):10A.
31. Hosoi E, Hirose M, Hamano S. Expression levels of H-type α(1,2)-fucosyltransferase gene and histo-blood group ABO gene corresponding to hematopoietic cell differentiation. Transfusion 2003;43:65-71.
32. Cooling L. Carbohydrate blood group antigens and collections. In: Petrides M, Stack G, Cooling L, Maes L. Practical guide to transfusion medicine. 2nd ed. Bethesda, MD: AABB Press, 2007:59-91.
33. Larson G, Svensson L, Hynsjo L, et al. Typing for the human Lewis blood group system by quantitative fluorescence-activated flow cytometry: Large differences in antigen presentation on erythrocytes between A_1, A_2, B, O phenotypes. Vox Sang 1999;77:227-36.
34. Lindstrom K, Breimer ME, Jovall P-A, et al. Non-acid glycosphingolipid expression in plasma of an A_1 Le(a–b+) secretor human individual: Identification of an ALe^b heptaglycosylceramide as major blood group component. J Biochem 1992;111:337-45.
35. Boren T, Falk P, Roth KA, et al. Attachment of *Helicobacter pylori* to human gastric epithelium mediated by blood group antigens. Science 1993;262:1892-5.
36. Kandulski A, Selgrad M, Malfertheiner P. *Helicobacter pylori* infection: A clinical overview. Digest Liver Dis 2008;40:619-26.
37. Hutson AM, Atmar RL, Marcus DM, Estes MK. Norwalk virus-like particle hemagglutination by binding to H histo-blood group antigens. J Virol 2003;77:405-15.
38. Hilton E, Chandrasekaran V, Rindos P, Isenberg HD. Association of recurrent candidal vaginitis with inheritance of Lewis blood group antigens. J Infect Dis 1995;172:1616-19.
39. Stapleton A, Nudelman E, Clausen H, et al. Binding of uropathogenic *Escherichia coli* R45 to glycolipids extracted from vaginal epithelial cells is dependent on histo-blood group secretor status. J Clin Invest 1992;90:965-72.
40. Navenot JM, Muller JY, Blanchard D. Expression of blood group i antigen and fetal hemoglobin in paroxysmal nocturnal hemoglobinuria. Transfusion 1997;37:291-7.
41. Yu LC, Twu YU, Chou ML, et al. The molecular genetics of the human I locus and molecular background explain the partial association of the adult i phenotype with congenital cataracts. Blood 2003;101:2081-8.
42. Schwarz K, Iolascon A, Verissimo F, et al. Mutations affecting the secretory COPII coat component SEC23B cause congenital dyserythro-

poietic anemia type II. Nat Genet 2009;41:936-40.

43. Cooling LW, Walker KE, Gille T, Koerner TAW. Shiga toxin binds human platelets via globotriaosylceramide (P^k antigen) and a novel platelet glycosphingolipid. Infect Immun 1998;66:4355-66.
44. Beadling W, Cooling L. Immunohematology. In: McPherson RA, Pincus MR, eds. Henry's clinical diagnosis and management by laboratory methods. 25th ed. Philadelphia: Saunders, 2007:618-68.
45. Duk M, Singh S, Reinhold VN, et al. Structures of unique globoside elongation products present in erythrocytes with a rare NOR phenotype. Glycobiology 2007;17:304-12.
46. Yang Z, Bergstrom J, Karlsson K-A. Glycoproteins with Galα4Gal are absent from human erythrocyte membranes, indicating that glycolipids are the sole carriers of blood group P activities. J Biol Chem 1994;269:14620-4.
47. Hellberg A, Ringressi A, Yahalom V, et al. Genetic heterogeneity at the glycosyltransferase loci underlying the GLOB blood group system and collection. Br J Haematol 2004;125:528-36.
48. Tilley L, Green C, Daniels G. Sequence variation in the 5′ untranslated region of the human A4GALT gene is associated with, but does not define, the P1 blood-group polymorphism. Vox Sang 2006;90:198-203.
49. Thuresson B, Westman JS, Olsson ML. Genetic typing of the P1/P2 histo-blood groups made possible by identification of a novel A4GALT exon (abstract). Transfusion 2009;49(3S):48A.
50. Lund N, Olsson ML, Ramkumar S, et al. The human P(k) histo-blood group antigen provides protection against HIV-1 infection. Blood 2009;133:4980-91.

Chapter 13

The Rh System

Stella T. Chou, MD, and

Connie M. Westhoff, PhD, MT(ASCP)SBB

13

RH IS THE MOST important blood group system after ABO in transfusion medicine. The Rh system is highly immunogenic and complex with numerous polymorphisms and clinically significant alleles. The history of the Rh system began with its discovery as the cause of severe jaundice and fetal death, referred to at the time as "erythroblastosis fetalis." The syndrome had complicated pregnancies for many decades, with the earliest recorded description dating to the 1600s from a French midwife who attended the delivery of a set of twins, one of whom was hydropic and the other was jaundiced and died of kernicterus.[1] The wide spectrum of fetal symptoms—ranging from mild jaundice, kernicterus, and anemia to severe and fatal hydrops—was not readily attributable to a single agent. When it was realized that an immunologic process might be responsible, the target antigen was initially suggested to be fetal hemoglobin. Then, in 1941, Levine made a key observation that the delivery of a stillborn fetus and an adverse transfusion reaction in the mother to a blood transfusion from the father were related.[2] These findings led to the realization that an immune reaction to a paternal antigen was responsible for the syndrome, now referred to as hemolytic disease of the fetus and newborn (HDFN).

The naming of the system "Rh" for Rhesus was the result of confusion with the LW antigen, named for Landsteiner and Wiener, who were studying an antiserum produced by immunizing guinea pigs and rabbits with red cells of the Rhesus macaque. When the antiserum was diluted (to eliminate anti-species reactivity), it agglutinated approximately 85% of human red cells tested. The reactivity of this "anti-Rhesus" appeared to parallel the reactivity of sera from women who had delivered a fetus suffering from hemolytic disease; thus, the blood group became associated with anti-Rhesus, that is, Rh. The confusion resulted because the LW antigen is present on Rh-positive red cells in greater amounts than on Rh-negative red cells, thus explaining the reactivity pattern observed with the diluted antiserum.

Stella T. Chou, MD, Assistant Professor, Department of Pediatrics, Division of Hematology, University of Pennsylvania, and Connie M. Westhoff, PhD, MT(ASCP)SBB, Director of Immunohematology and Genomics, New York Blood Center, New York, New York, and Adjunct Assistant Professor, Department of Pathology and Laboratory Medicine, University of Pennsylvania, Philadelphia, Pennsylvania

The authors have disclosed no conflicts of interest.

For many years there was controversy over who actually discovered the blood group responsible for HDFN. Landsteiner and Wiener never accepted credit for identifying the LW antigen; to do so would diminish their claim to having determined the cause of hemolytic disease.[3] In retrospect, credit for the discovery of the Rh system appropriately goes to many different groups whose collective observations unlocked the mystery of the pathogenesis of the disease.

"Rh positive" and "Rh negative" refer to the presence or absence of the D antigen. By the mid-1940s four additional Rh antigens, the antithetical C and c, and E and e, had been recognized. These were named by Fisher for the next letters of the alphabet, according to the precedent set with the naming of A and B blood groups. The five principal Rh antigens—D, C, c, E, and e— are responsible for the majority of clinically significant antibodies, but more than 50 Rh antigens have been characterized (Table 13-1).

The observation that ABO incompatibility between a mother and the fetus had a partial protective effect against immunization to Rh suggested the rationale for the development of Rh Immune Globulin (RhIG).[4] Although the hypothesis that maternal IgM antibodies were responsible for protection was incorrect (the use of IgM anti-D was not successful), IgG anti-D was found to be very effective.[5] By the 1960s, only 20 years after the discovery of Rh incompatibility, HDFN caused by anti-D could be prevented.

The extremely hydrophobic nature of the Rh proteins made biochemical studies difficult, as reflected in reports from the 1970s indicating the molecular weight was anywhere from 7000 kDa to >120,000 kDa. Key findings included those by Green,[6] who showed that Rh antigen activity depended on the presence of phospholipid, and studies by Gahmberg,[7] who demonstrated that the Rh proteins, unlike most membrane proteins, were not glycosylated and were not phosphorylated. The discovery that immune complexes of D with anti-D remained intact in the presence of membrane detergents led to the successful immunoprecipitation of a 30,000- to 32,000-kDa protein by several groups using anti-D, -c, or -E.[8-10] Large-scale isolation of the Rh proteins by chromatography, followed by N-terminal sequencing, was accomplished in the late 1980s.[11] These findings led to the cloning of the *RHCE* gene by Cartron and colleagues in 1990,[12] and cloning of *RHD* was successful in 1992.[13,14] The different *RHCE* alleles responsible for the C or c, and E or e antigens were clarified in 1994.[15]

The last decade has witnessed an abundance of information detailing the genetic diversity of the *RH* locus, which has exceeded all estimates predicted by serology. Well over 100 *RHD* and over 50 different *RHCE* alleles have been documented, and new alleles continue to be discovered. Population studies further demonstrate the ethnic and geographic variations in *RH* alleles, which have implications in transfusion and obstetric practices. A directory of *RHD* alleles is maintained on the Rhesus-Base website,[16] and *RHCE* alleles are found on the National Center for Biotechnology Information human blood group mutation website.[17] The International Society of Blood Transfusion (ISBT) Working Party on Red Cell Immunogenetics and Blood Group Terminology maintains and catalogs new alleles at http://ibgrl.blood. co.uk.

TERMINOLOGY

Early Rh nomenclature reflects the differences in opinion concerning the number of genes that encode DCE antigens. The terminology established by Fisher-Race in England was based on the premise that three closely linked genes, C/c, E/e, and D, were responsible, whereas the Wiener nomenclature (Rh-Hr) was based on the belief that a single gene encoded several blood group factors. Neither theory was correct. There are actually two genes, *RHD* and *RHCE*, as correctly proposed by Tippett.[18] The Fisher-Race CDE terminology is often preferred for written communication, but a modified version of Wiener's nomenclature allows one to convey the Rh antigens present on one chromosome, that is, a haplotype, in a single term (Table 13-2). A capital "R" is used to indicate that D is present, and subscripts are used to represent the C/c

TABLE 13-1. Numerical Terminology for Rh Antigens

Numerical Designation	Antigen or Symbol(s)	Prevalence	Numerical Designation	Antigen or Symbol(s)	Prevalence
Rh1	D	85% Whites 92% Blacks	Rh32[#]		1% Blacks R^N or others with DBT
Rh2	C	68% Whites 27% Blacks	Rh33	R_0^{Har}, D^{HAR}	0.01% Germans
Rh3	E	29% Whites 22% Blacks	Rh34[**]	Hr^B	High
Rh4	c	80% Whites 96% Blacks	Rh35		Low
Rh5	e	98%	Rh36	Be^a	Low
Rh6	ce or f	65% Whites 92% Blacks	Rh37	Evans	Low (several D/CE or CE/D hybrids)
Rh7	Ce or rh_i	68% Whites 27% Blacks	Rh39	C-like	High
Rh8	C^W	Low, 2% Whites	Rh40	Tar	Low (DVII)
Rh9	C^X	Low, 1.8% Finns	Rh41	Ce-like	70% Whites
Rh10	V	30% Blacks	Rh42	Ce^S, Cce^S	2% Blacks
Rh11	E^W	Low	Rh43	Crawford	0.1% Blacks
Rh12[*]	G	84% Whites 92% Blacks	Rh44	Nou	High
Rh17[†]	Hr_0	High	Rh45	Riv	Low
Rh18[‡]	Hr, Hr^S	High	Rh46	Sec	High
Rh19[§]	hr^s	98%	Rh47	Dav	High
Rh20	VS	32% Blacks	Rh48	JAL	Low
Rh21	C^G	68% Whites	Rh49[††]	STEM	6% Blacks
Rh22	CE	<1% (DCE, CE)	Rh 50	FPTT	Low (DFR, R_0^{Har})
Rh23[‖]	D^W	Low (DVa)	Rh51	MAR	High
Rh26	c-like	High (most c+)	Rh52[‖]	BARC	Low (DVI)
Rh27	cE	28% Whites 22% Blacks (DcE, cE)	Rh53	JAHK	Low
Rh28	hr^H	Low	Rh54[‖]	DAK	Low ($DIII^a$, DOL, R^N)
Rh29[¶]	total Rh	100%	Rh55	LOCR	Low

(Continued)

TABLE 13-1. Numerical Terminology for Rh Antigens (Continued)

Numerical Designation	Antigen or Symbol(s)	Prevalence	Numerical Designation	Antigen or Symbol(s)	Prevalence
Rh30[||]	Go^a	Low (DIVa)	Rh56	CENR	Low (Hybrid CE/D)
Rh31[§]	hr^B	98%	Rh57	CEST	High
			RH58	CELO	High

Note: Rh13 through Rh16, Rh24, Rh25, and Rh38 are obsolete.

*Present on red cells expressing C or D antigen.

†Antibody made by individuals with D-deletion phenotypes D––, Dc–, and DC^w–.

‡Antibody made by individuals with altered e and/or D phenotypes prevalent in African ethnic groups.

§Absent from red cells with DcE/DcE (R_2R_2) phenotype, or red cells with variant e found in African ethnic groups.

||Low-prevalence antigen associated with the partial D indicated.

¶Antibody made by individuals with Rh_{null} red cells.

#Low-prevalence antigen expressed by red cells with R^N or the partial DBT antigen.[44]

**Antibody made by individuals with altered C, E, and/or D phenotypes prevalent in African ethnic groups.

††Associated with 65% of hr^S– Hr– and 30% of hr^B– Hr^B– red cells.

and E/e antigens found with D: 1 for Ce (R_1), 2 for cE (R_2), 0 for ce (R_0), and "Z" for CE (R_z). A lowercase "r" ("little r") indicates the haplotype lacks D, and the C/c and E/e antigens present without D are represented by superscript symbols: "prime" for Ce (r), "double-prime" for cE (r), and y for CE (r^y) (Table 13-2).

A numerical nomenclature introduced in 1962 by Rosenfeld gave each Rh antigen a number based on the order of its discovery or assignment to the Rh system (Table 13-1). Although not in wide use, in addition to its historical contribution it is often applied when referring to high-prevalence antigens in the Rh system (eg, Rh17, Rh29, Rh32, etc).

With the goal of creating a uniform nomenclature, the ISBT Working Party on Terminology for Red Cell Surface Antigens adopted a

TABLE 13-2. Prevalence of the Principal Rh Haplotypes

Fisher-Race Haplotype	Modified Wiener Haplotype	Prevalence (%)		
		White	Black	Asian
Rh positive				
DCe	R_1	42	17	70
DcE	R_2	14	11	21
Dce	R_0	4	44	3
DCE	R_Z	<0.01	<0.01	1
Rh negative				
Ce	r	37	26	3
Ce	r′	2	2	2
cE	r″	1	<0.01	<0.01
CE	r^y	<0.01	<0.01	<0.01

six-digit number for each red cell antigen. The first three numbers represent the system, and the remaining three digits refer to the antigenic specificity; the Rh system was assigned the number 004. In 2008, the ISBT committee established Rh-associated glycoprotein (RHAG) as a new system (number 30).[19]

Contemporary Rh terminology distinguishes between the antigens, genes, and proteins. The antigens are referred to by the letter designations D, C, c, E, and e. The *RH* genes are indicated by capital letters, with or without italics, and include *RHD* and *RHCE.* Alleles of *RHCE* are designated *RHCE*ce, RHCE*Ce, RHCE*cE,* and *RHCE*CE,* according to which antigens they encode, and variant or partial *RHD* alleles are designated as *RHD*DVI, RHD*DFR,* etc. The proteins are indicated as RhD, or Rhce, RhCe, RhcE, and RhCE, according to the specific antigens they carry.

RH GENES AND Rh PROTEINS

Two genes (*RHD* and *RHCE*) in close proximity on chromosome 1 encode 416 amino acid Rh proteins; one encodes the D antigen, and the other encodes CE antigens in various combinations (ce, cE, Ce, or CE) [Fig 13-1(A)]. The genes each have ten exons, are 97% identical, and encode proteins that differ by 32 to 35 amino acids [Fig 13-1(B), shown as circles on RhD]. This contrasts with most blood group antigens that are encoded by single genes with alleles that differ by only one or a few amino acids.

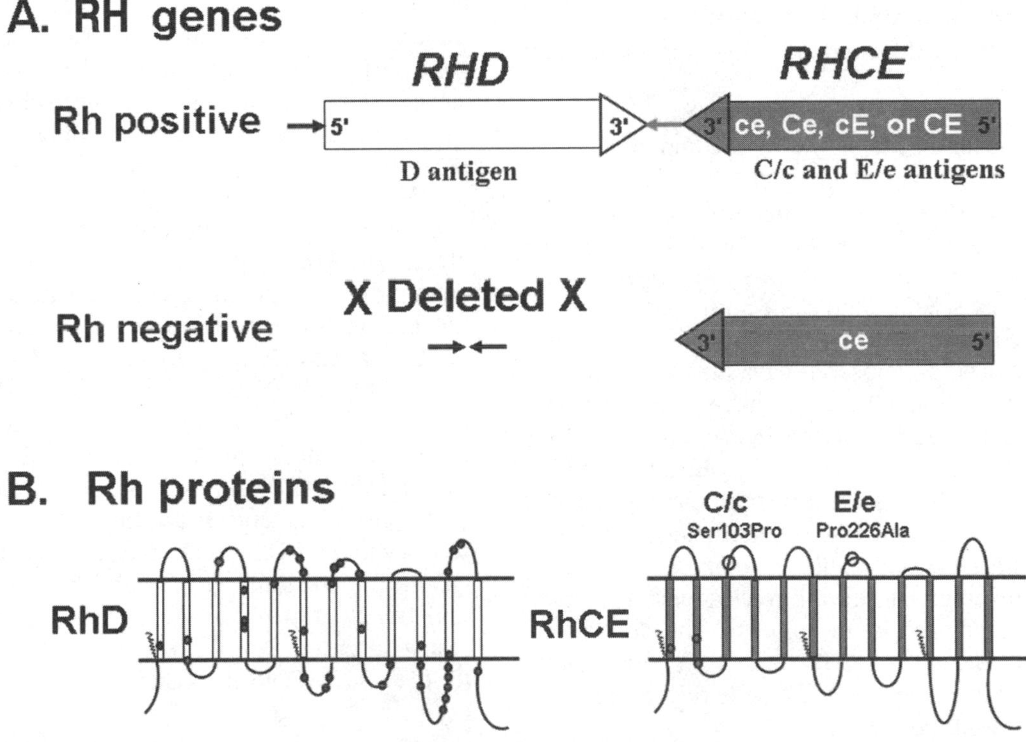

FIGURE 13-1. (A) Diagram of the RHD and RHCE genes. The inverted gene orientation, the antigens they encode, and the deletion of *RHD* that results in the D-negative red cell phenotype are shown. (B) Predicted 12-transmembrane domain model of the RhD and RhCE proteins. The amino acid differences between RhD and RhCE are shown as grey circles. The zigzag lines represent the location of possible palmitoylation sites. Positions 103 and 226 in RhCE critical for C or c and E or e expression are indicated as open circles.

Most D-negative (Rh-negative) phenotypes are the result of complete deletion of the *RHD* gene [Fig 13-1(A)]. Exposure to RhD in a D-negative individual often results in production of anti-D. The immunogenicity of a protein is correlated with the degree of foreignness to the host, and the large number of amino acid differences explains why exposure to RhD can result in a potent immune response.

RHCE (found in all but rare D–– individuals, where the dashes represent missing antigens) encodes both C/c and E/e antigens on a single protein. C and c antigens differ by four amino acids, but only the amino acid change Ser103Pro is extracellular [Fig 13-1(B)]. The E and e antigens differ by one amino acid, Pro226Ala, located on the fourth extracellular loop of the protein. The *RH* genes and proteins shown in the figure are typical for the majority of individuals, and commercial antibody reagents are available to detect expression of the principal Rh antigens—D, C, c, E, and e (Table 13-3).

The five principal antigens are responsible for the majority of Rh incompatibilities, although the system is more complex, and antigen numbers through Rh58 have been assigned (Table 13-1). New antigens may result from point mutations and gene rearrangements. For example, the numerous genetic exchanges between *RHD* and *RHCE* have created hybrid proteins that have RhD with a portion of RhCE, or vice versa. The rearrangements are facilitated by the inverted orientation of the *RH* genes where the 3′ ends are adjacent[20] [Fig 13-1(A)]. This structure promotes hairpin loop formation and subsequent genetic exchange via gene conversion; one member acts as a donor template during replication but remains unchanged in the process. The donated region can span several base pairs, single exons, or multiple exons. These hybrid proteins express unique epitopes.

ANTIGENS

D is the most immunogenic Rh antigen, followed by c and E. Routine donor and patient typing tests only for D. Testing for other common Rh antigens is performed primarily to resolve or confirm antibody identification, with the exception that some sickle cell transfusion programs perform Rh typing before transfusion to match patients and donors for D, C, and E (in addition to K) to reduce alloimmunization.

Rh Phenotypes

The results of testing red cells with the five principal Rh antisera are shown in Table 13-3, along with the Rh phenotype and the predicted *RH* genotype. Some genotypes are more common in a specific ethnic group (Table 13-2). For example, a person of European ancestry with the D, C, c, e phenotype would probably be DCe/ce (ie, R_1r). A person of African ancestry with this phenotype would probably be DCe/Dce (ie, R_1R_0). Prediction of the *RH* genotype in persons with mixed ethnicity is less certain. Serologic testing cannot determine whether the red cells are from a homozygote (D/D) or heterozygote (D/–), as anti-D seldom shows any difference in reactivity between red cells with a single or a double dose of D antigen. *RHD* zygosity can be determined by DNA molecular testing for the presence of a *RHD* deletion or an inactive *RHD*. Knowledge of paternal *RHD* zygosity is important in prenatal practice to predict the antigen status of the fetus to assess the risk of HDFN when the mother has anti-D.

The Rh haplotype influences the level of D antigen expression. Less D is expressed in the presence of C, and therefore the red cells from a DcE/DcE (R_2R_2) individual carry more D antigen sites and show higher titration scores with anti-D than red cells from a DCe/DCe (R_1R_1) individual. As measured by flow cytometry, D antigen strength decreases in the following order: DcE/DcE (R_2R_2) > DCe/DcE (R_1R_2) > DCe/DCe (R_1R_1) > DcE/ce (R_2r) > DCe/ce (R_1r).

D Antigen

The D antigen is composed of numerous epitopes (epD) that were originally defined by antibodies from D-positive people who made anti-D. Subsequent studies with monoclonal

TABLE 13-3. Results of Tests with Five Principal Rh Antisera with Phenotype and Predicted *RH* Genotype

Anti-D	Anti-C	Anti-E	Anti-c	Anti-e	Antigens Phenotype	Predicted Genotype	Alternative Genotype
					Rh positive*		
+	+	0	+	+	D, C, c, e	R^1r *DCe/ce*	R^1R^0 *DCe/Dce* $R^0\,r'$ *Dce/Ce*
+	+	0	0	+	D, C, e	R^1R^1 *DCe/DCe*	$R^1\,r'$ *DCe/Ce*
+	+	+	+	+	D, C, c, E, e	R^1R^2 *DCe/DcE*	$R^1\,r''$ *DCe/cE* $R^2\,r'$ *DcE/Ce* $R^Z\,r$ *DCE/ce* $R^0\,R^Z$ *Dce/DCE*
+	0	0	+	+	D, c, e	$R^0\,r$ *Dce/ce*	$R^0\,R^0$ *Dce/Dce*
+	0	+	+	+	D, c, E, e	$R^2\,r$ *DcE/ce*	$R^2\,R^0$ *DcE/Dce* $R^0\,r''$ *Dce/cE*
+	0	+	+	0	D, c, E	$R^2\,R^2$ *DcE/DcE*	$R^2\,r''$ *DcE/cE*
+	+	+	0	+	D, C, E, e	$R^1\,R^Z$ *DCe/DCE*	$R^Z\,r'$ *DCE/Ce*
+	+	+	+	0	D, C, c, E	$R^2\,R^Z$ *DcE/DCE*	$R^Z\,r''$ *DCE/cE*
+	+	+	0	0	D, C, E	$R^Z\,R^Z$ *DCE/DCE*	$R^Z\,r^y$ *DCE/CE*
					Rh negative†		
0	0	0	+	+	c, e	rr ce/ce	
0	+	0	+	+	C, c, e	$r'\,r$ Ce/ce	
0	0	+	+	+	c, E, e	$r''\,r$ cE/ce	
0	+	+	+	+	C, c, E, e	$r'\,r''$ Ce/cE	

*Not shown are rare genotypes (<0.01%) R^0r^y, R^1r^y, R^2r^y.

†Not shown are rare genotypes (<0.01%) rr^y, $r'\,r^y$, $r''\,r^y$, r^yr^y.

antibodies defined 30 or more epitopes,[21] designated epD1 to epD9 with further subdivisions of each (eg, epD6.1, etc). D epitopes are highly conformational and consist of more than simple linear amino acid residues. Many epitopes involve several of the extracellular loops, and amino acid changes in intracellular regions of the protein can also alter D epitopes. The availability of the crystal structure of the ancient homolog of Rh, the AmtB protein from *Escherichia coli*,[22] and the recent resolution of the crystal structure of the human kidney RhCG protein allow three-dimensional protein modeling, which has significantly advanced understanding of the structure of the Rh blood group proteins (Fig 13-2).

D Positive (Rh Positive)

Most D-positive red cell phenotypes have a conventional RhD protein [Fig 13-1(B)]. However, more than 100 different RHD alleles that encode proteins with amino acid changes have been reported. These can cause numerous variations in the expression of D and include weak D, partial D, and D_{el} phenotypes. Red cells with some form of altered D expression are not infrequently encountered in routine transfusion practice. An estimated 1% to 2% of individuals of European ethnicity carry RHD alleles that encode weak D or partial D antigens, and the incidence in individuals of African ethnicity is higher.

WEAK D (FORMERLY D^U^). Weak D red cells have historically been defined as having a reduced amount of D antigen, requiring an indirect antiglobulin test (IAT) for detection. The number of samples classified as weak D, however, depends on the characteristics of the typing reagents, which have changed over the years. Weak D expression results primarily from single nucleotide mutations in *RHD* that encode amino acid changes predicted to be located intracellularly, or in the transmembrane regions of RhD, rather than on the outer surface of the red cell[23] (Fig 13-2). The mutations affect insertion of the protein in the membrane, reflected in the reduced number of D antigen sites on the red cells. Many different mutations cause weak D expression, and they are designated Type 1 through Type 73.[16] The most common is Type 1, which has a Val270Gly amino acid mutation, and which, along with Types 2 and 3, represents approximately 90% of the weak D found in persons of European ethnicity.[23]

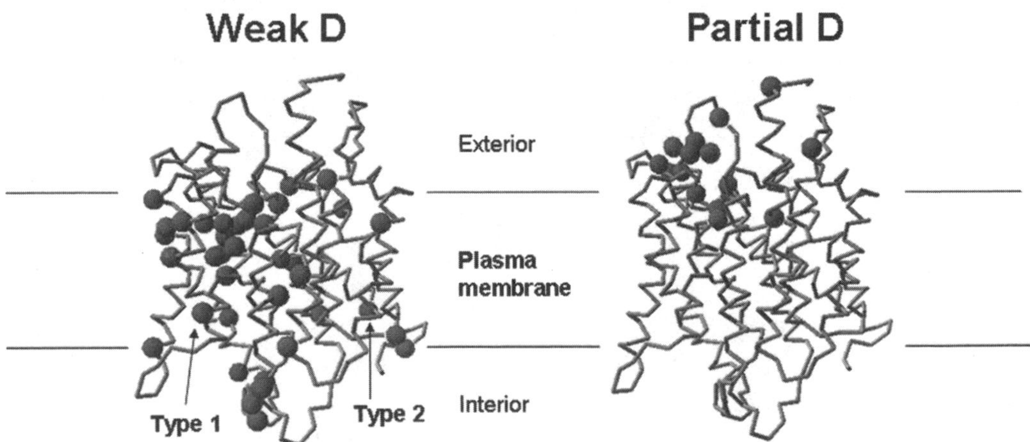

FIGURE 13-2. Homology model of weak D and partial D proteins. The predicted locations of amino acid mutations are shown as solid circles. The mutations associated with Type 1 and 2 (shown at the arrows) are found in approximately 80% of weak D phenotypes. The predicted extracellular locations of amino acid residues responsible for some partial D phenotypes encoded by single amino acid changes are shown.

WEAK D DUE TO C. A weak D phenotype can occur when Ce (r′) is present in *trans* to *RHD* (eg, R_0r'). In addition, the further depression of an already weak D (eg, *RHD*weak D)* by Ce can result in an apparent D-negative (r r′, r′ r′, or r″ r′) or D_{el} phenotype in a sample that is $R^{weak\ D}$ r′.

D_{EL}. D_{el} red cells express extremely low levels of D antigen that cannot be detected by routine serologic methods. However, these red cells can adsorb and subsequently elute anti-D. D_{el} cells are found in 10% to 30% of D-negative Asians and result from several different *RHD* mutations that severely reduce RhD expression in the membrane. D_{el} cells are much less common in individuals of European ancestry (0.027%) and carry a different mutation.[23-25] Because the red cells type serologically as D-negative or weak D-negative, D_{el} will usually be detected only by *RHD* genotyping.

PARTIAL D. Red cells with partial D have historically been classified as such based on the fact that the red cells type as D positive, but individuals make anti-D when exposed to conventional D antigen. These red cells were predicted to be missing portions of D, and indeed the majority of partial D phenotypes are due to hybrid genes in which portions of *RHD* are replaced by the corresponding portions of *RHCE* (Fig 13-3). The novel sequences of the hybrid protein resulting from regions of RhD joined to RhCE not only can result in the loss of D epitopes but also can generate new antigens. For example, DVI red cells carry the BARC antigen. A few partial D phenotypes, such as weak D discussed above, are the result of single amino acid changes. However, in contrast to weak D, the changes are predicted to be located on the exterior membrane surface (Fig 13-2).

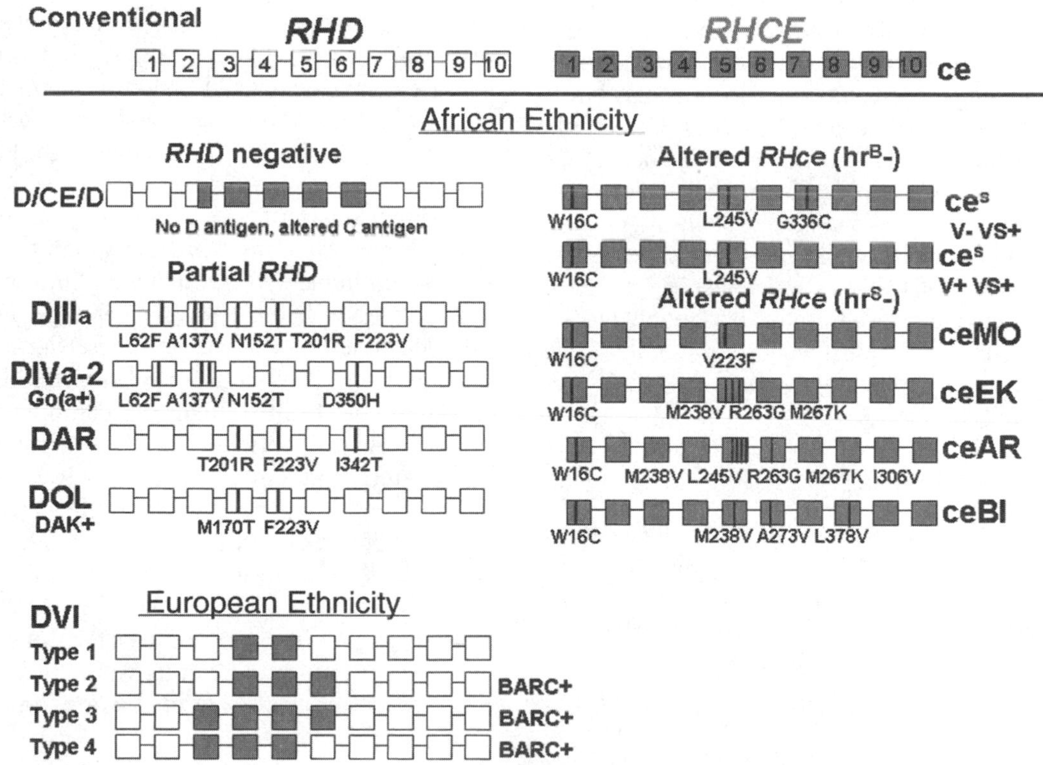

FIGURE 13-3. Diagram of the RHD and RHCE genes depicting the 10 exons as white and grey boxes, respectively. Also shown are some examples of *RHD* encoding partial D, and some examples of *RHCE* with mutations often found in those of African ethnicity that complicate transfusion in sickle cell patients.

ELEVATED D. Several rare deletion phenotypes, designated D––, Dc–, and DC^{w}–, have an enhanced expression of D antigen and no, weak, or altered C/c and E/e antigens.[26] These are the converse of partial D discussed above and result from replacement of portions of *RHCE* by *RHD*. The additional *RHD* sequences in *RHCE*, along with a normal *RHD*, explain the enhanced D antigen and account for the reduced or missing C/c and E/e antigens. People with CE-depleted phenotypes often make anti-Rh17 (Table 13-1).

D AND D-LIKE EPITOPES ON RHCE. Expression of D epitopes by the protein product of the *RHCE* gene, in the absence of *RHD*, further complicates serologic determination of the D status. Several Rhce proteins have D-specific amino acids that react with some monoclonal anti-D. They are more often found in a specific population group. Examples include D^{HAR}, found in individuals of German ancestry, and Crawford (ceCF), found in individuals of African ancestry. These two are notable because the red cells show strong reactivity with some monoclonal reagents but are nonreactive with others, including polyclonal anti-D reagents (Table 13-4). D^{HAR} and Crawford phenotypes can cause D typing discrepancies. Less dramatic are changes in Rhce proteins that mimic a D-epitope structure, encoded by alleles designated ceRT and ceSL.[27,28] The red cells are weakly reactive with some, but not all, monoclonal anti-D. Most importantly, individuals with these phenotypes lack RhD and can readily be sensitized.[29,30]

D Negative (Rh Negative)

The D-negative phenotype is prevalent in Whites (15%-17%), less likely in African Blacks (3%-5%), and rare in Asians (<0.1%).[1] The D-negative phenotype has arisen multiple times, as evidenced by the different mutations responsible for lack of D expression in various ethnic groups. In most Whites, it results from deletion of the entire *RHD* gene.[31] There are exceptions, however, and samples with uncommon haplotypes, r′ (Ce) or r″ (cE), are more likely to carry an inactive, rather than deleted, *RHD*.

In other ethnic groups, D-negative phenotypes are primarily caused by inactivating mutations in *RHD*. In individuals with African backgrounds, 66% have a 37-bp insertion in *RHD*, which results in a premature stop codon; 15% were reported to have a hybrid *RHD-CE-D*,[32] characterized by expression of weak C and no D antigen; and the remaining 19% have a deletion of the *RHD* (Fig 13-3). D-negative phenotypes in Asians result from mutations in *RHD* most often associated with a Ce (r′) haplotype, although 10% to 30% of Asians who type as D negative are actually D_{el}.

Testing for D

Reagents

Early reagents developed for D antigen testing exploited antibodies produced in women who were sensitized by pregnancy, or in hyperimmunized volunteers. These polyclonal antibodies are primarily IgG and recognize numerous epitopes of D. High-protein additives in these reagents enhance potency but can cause spontaneous agglutination of red cells and require that appropriate controls be performed (see "Technical Considerations for Rh Typing").

Monoclonal antibody technology, introduced in the 1980s, freed manufacturers from reliance on human source material; however, antibodies specific for a single D epitope did not detect all D-positive red cells. Consequently, many Food and Drug Aministration (FDA)-approved anti-D reagents combine a monoclonal IgM antibody, reactive at room temperature, and a monoclonal or polyclonal IgG antibody, reactive by an IAT, for the determination of weak D. Anti-D for column agglutination testing is an exception and contains only a monoclonal IgM. Three of five FDA-licensed reagents contain unique IgM clones, and these may react differently with red cells that have weak D, partial D, or D-like epitopes (Table 13-4).

Donors

The goal of D typing donors is to prevent anti-D immunization of recipients, which includes

TABLE 13-4. Reactivity of FDA-Licensed Anti-D Reagents with Some Rh Variant Red Cells

Reagent	IgM Monoclonal	IgG	DVI IS/AHG*	DBT IS/AHG*	D^{HAR} (Whites) IS/AHG*	Crawford (Blacks) IS/AHG*	ceRT	ceSL
Gammaclone	GAMA401	F8D8 monoclonal	Neg/Pos	Pos	Pos	Pos[†]		
Immucor Series 4	MS201	MS26 monoclonal	Neg/Pos	Pos	Pos	Neg	Weak pos	Neg
Immucor Series 5	Th28	MS26 monoclonal	Neg/Pos	Pos	Pos	Neg	Weak pos	Weak pos
Ortho BioClone	MAD2	Polyclonal	Neg/Pos	Neg/Pos	Neg/Neg	Neg		
Ortho Gel (ID-MTS)	MS201		Neg	Pos	Pos	Neg	Weak pos	Neg
Biotest RH1	BS226		Neg		Pos	Neg		
Biotest RH1 Blend	BS221	BS232 H41 11B7	Neg/Pos		Pos[†]	Neg		
Alba Bioscience alpha	LDM1		Neg		Pos	Neg		
Alba Bioscience beta	LDM3		Neg		Pos	Neg		
Alba Bioscience delta	LDM1 ESD1-M		Neg		Pos	Neg		
Alba blend	LDM3	ESD1	Neg/Pos		Pos	Neg		
Polyclonal			Neg/Pos	Neg/Pos	Neg/Neg	Neg/Neg	Weak pos[‡]	Neg

*Result following slash denotes anti-D test result by the indirect antiglobulin test (IAT).
[†]Test will be negative if IAT is performed.
[‡]Enzyme-treated cells.
IS = immediate spin; AHG = antihuman globulin.

identifying units with weak D or partial D antigens. Therefore, the AABB *Standards for Blood Banks and Transfusion Services* requires donor blood to be tested using a method designed to detect weak expression of D and to be labeled as "Rh positive" if the test is positive.[33(p29)] In addition, a unit labeled Rh negative (D negative) must be confirmed from an integrally attached segment before transfusion (confirmatory testing for weak D is not required), and discrepancies must be reported to the collecting facility and resolved before issue of blood for transfusion.[33(p33)] Most weak D or partial D antigen units are detected by these measures. Infrequently, however, some very weak D red cells are not detected, and D_{el} red cells are nonreactive with anti-D, even with IAT methods. Although red cells with weak D antigen are less immunogenic than normal D-positive red cells,[34] very weak D and D_{el} donor units have stimulated anti-D in some D-negative recipients.[35-38] Blood components labeled as Rh negative that may have stimulated anti-D in recipients should be investigated by serologic and genotyping methods to confirm the D antigen status. *RHD* genotyping can identify the presence of potentially immunogenic RhD expression not detected by serology.

Patients

When the D type of a patient is determined, a weak D test is not necessary except in testing the red cells of an infant of a mother at risk for D immunization. Historically, in the era of routine use of polyclonal IgG anti-D reagents, an IAT test for weak D was performed to conserve supplies of Rh-negative components and to prevent unnecessary RhIG administration. Current monoclonal IgM reagents type many samples as D positive in direct testing that would have previously been detected only by IAT, thereby eliminating some of the concerns regarding the unnecessary use of Rh-negative blood and RhIG. Additionally, current FDA-licensed monoclonal IgM reagents are specifically selected to be nonreactive with red cells from partial DVI in direct tests (Table 13-4). DVI is the most common partial D found in Whites, and anti-D produced by women with partial DVI has resulted in fatal hemolytic disease.[39] Performing only a direct test for female children and women of childbearing potential avoids the risk of sensitization by classifying DVI as D negative for transfusion and RhIG prophylaxis. These considerations, along with the cost savings realized by elimination of an IAT and potentially avoiding misinterpretation of the D type when the red cells are coated with immunoglobulin [positive direct antiglobulin test (DAT) causing a false-positive weak D test], prompt many transfusion services to perform only direct tests to determine the D status of a patient. However, as noted above, weak D testing must be performed on the red cells of the infant when determining if an Rh-negative mother is a candidate for RhIG.

D Typing Discrepancies

D typing discrepancies should always be investigated and resolved (see "Resolving D Typing Discrepancies"). Rh-negative blood is an appropriate option for patients needing immediate transfusion, but a thorough clerical and serologic investigation should be performed. *RHD* genotyping is also useful to resolve discrepancies. Because donor centers test for weak D, an individual who is appropriately Rh positive as a donor may be classified Rh negative as a recipient. This should not be considered problematic but rather should be communicated to the patient and health-care staff and become part of the patient's medical record.

Clinical Considerations

The long history of transfusing patients who have weak D red cells with D-positive blood suggests that weak D Types 1, 2, and 3, which represent the majority of Whites with weak D, are unlikely to make anti-D and can receive D-positive blood. The less common weak D Type 11 and Type 15 have been reported to make anti-D, suggesting they have altered D epitopes.[40] More data are needed to determine the risk for production of anti-D in other weak D types.

Patients with partial D red cells are at risk for production of anti-D and should receive D-negative blood and be considered candidates for RhIG. Unfortunately, serologic reagents cannot typically distinguish them from D-positive individuals. Many partial D red cells (eg, DIIIa, the most common partial D in Blacks) type strongly D-positive in direct tests and are recognized only after producing anti-D. Performing only a direct test with FDA-licensed anti-D reagents avoids the risk of sensitization for partial DVI, as discussed above.

Policies regarding D typing procedures and selection of blood components for transfusion should consider the patient population, the risk of immunization to D, and the limited supply of D-negative blood components. Anti-D is a clinically significant antibody, and it is important to prevent immunization in females of childbearing potential to avoid complications of HDFN. For other patients, the complications of anti-D are less serious and may include dependence on D-negative blood for future bleeding episodes and a possible increased risk of production of multiple blood group antibodies in addition to anti-D.[41] Not all D-negative patients make anti-D when exposed to D-positive red cells. The incidence of antibody production in volunteers undergoing repeat immunization was 80% to 90%, but the incidence in D-negative hospitalized patients switched to D-positive blood components was much lower, approximately 32%.[42] Transfusion services should have policies that address the administration of D-positive red cells to D-negative patients and the use of RhIG, which is a human blood product and not entirely without risk.

G Antigen

The G antigen is found on red cells possessing C or D and maps to the 103Ser residue present on RhD, RhCe, or RhCE (Fig 13-1). The antigen is of note because antibodies to G appear to be anti-D plus anti-C with serologic testing; they cannot be separated, but the antibody can be adsorbed by D–C+ or D+C– red cells. Anti-G can explain the D-negative person transfused with D– (C+) blood, or the D-negative woman who delivered a D– (C+) child, who subsequently appears to have made anti-D. Anti-D, -C, and -G can be distinguished by adsorption and elution studies.[43] This is not usually necessary in the pretransfusion setting, as patients with anti-G must receive D–C– blood. However, for obstetric patients it is important to provide RhIG prophylaxis to women with anti-G to prevent immunization to D when indicated (ie, the pregnant woman is D–C– and appears to have anti-D and anti-C, but because of anti-G she is stimulated by the C antigen, and the infant is potentially D+).

C/c and E/e Antigens

The common *RHCE* alleles encode the C or c and E or e antigens. However, more than 60 different alleles are known, and many are associated with altered or weak expression of the principal antigens and, in some cases, loss of high-prevalence antigens.[26,44] Partial C and many partial e antigens are well recognized, while fewer partial c antigens have been reported. The *RHCE* alleles encountered most frequently in transfusion practice are discussed below.

Compound Antigens (ce, Ce, cE, and CE)

Compound antigens define epitopes that depend on conformational changes that result from amino acids associated with *both* C/c and E/e. These were previously referred to as *cis* products, to indicate the antigens were expressed from the same haplotype, but it is now known that these are expressed on a single protein. These are shown in Table 13-5 and include ce or f, Ce or rh_i, cE or Rh27, and the uncommon CE or Rh22.

Altered or Variant C and e Antigens

Mutations in *RHCE* result in quantitative and qualitative changes in C/c or E/e antigen expression, with altered C and altered e encountered most frequently. In persons of European ancestry, altered C is associated with amino acid changes located on the first extracellular loop of RhCe and the expression of C^W (Gln41Arg) or C^X (Ala36Thr) antigens. Altered C is also associated with changes that result in expression of the novel antigens JAHK

TABLE 13-5. Compound Rh Antigens on Rh Proteins

Compound Antigen Designation	Rh Protein	Present on Red Cells with These Haplotypes
ce or f	Rhce	Dce (R_0) or ce (r)
Ce or rh_i, Rh7	RhCe	DCe (R_1) or Ce (r′)
cE or Rh27	RhcE	DcE (R_2) or cE (r″)
CE or Rh22	RhCE	DCE (R_z) or CE (r^y)

(Ser122Leu) and JAL (Arg114Trp). The red cells type as C-positive, but patients can make apparent anti-C or anti-Ce (rh_i) (Table 13-5) when stimulated.

In individuals of African ancestry, altered C expression most often results from the inheritance of a *RHDIIIa-CE(4-7)-D* hybrid, or less often a *RHD-CE(4-7)-D* hybrid. These do not encode D antigen, but encode C antigen on a hybrid background that differs from normal (Fig 13-3). The gene has an incidence of approximately 22% in those of African ancestry.[32] It is inherited with an *RHCE* allele designated ce^S, which encodes altered e antigen and a V–VS+ phenotype.[45] The hybrid *RHDIIIa-CE(4-7)-D* linked to *RHCE*ce*^{S} is referred to as the (C)ce^S or r'^S haplotype. Red cells with the r'^S haplotype often type strongly C-positive with monoclonal reagents, and the presence of the altered C goes undetected. These patients not infrequently make alloantibodies with C-like and e-like specificities that can appear to be autoantibodies. The red cells may also lack the high-prevalence hr^B antigen (hr^B–). Anti-hr^B can be clinically significant, and finding compatible blood can be difficult. Not all red cells designated hr^B– by serologic testing are compatible with antibodies produced by patients with different Rh genetic backgrounds.[46,47]

Altered or partial e expression is associated with many other *RHce* alleles that have multiple mutations.[48] These are also found primarily in African ethnic groups, and some examples are shown in Fig 13-3. The red cells type as e-positive, but individuals homozygous for these alleles make alloantibodies with e-like specificities that can appear to be autoantibodies. These red cells also lack the high-prevalence hr^S antigen (hr^S–). Anti-hr^S is a clinically significant antibody and has caused transfusion fatalities.[48] Not all red cells designated hr^S– by serologic testing are compatible with antibodies produced by patients with altered or partial e expression.

As an additional complication, altered *RHCE*ce* is often inherited with partial *RHD* (DIII, DAU, DAR, etc). As discussed above, patients with partial D red cells are at risk of producing anti-D. The inheritance of partial D with altered *RHCE*ce* can lead to production of anti-Hr^B (RH34) and anti-Hr (RH18).

Clinical Considerations

The prevalence of RH alleles that encode altered D, C, and e antigens in African ethnic groups often underlies the production of complex Rh alloantibody specificities in chronically transfused patients with sickle cell disease (SCD). It has long been recognized that alloimmunization represents a significant problem in this patient population, as 25% to 30% of chronically transfused SCD patients develop red cell antibodies. To address the problem, many programs determine the pretransfusion red cell phenotype and transfuse red cells that are antigen-matched for D, C, E, and K because these antigens are considered to be the most immunogenic. In addition, some programs also attempt to supply red cells from donors of African ancestry whenever possible. Although there is currently no consensus on the need to perform red cell phenotype-matching for all patients with SCD,[49] transfusion programs that have implemented transfusion of antigen-matched blood for D, C, E, and K have been successful in reducing the incidence of alloantibody production.[50] The implementation of this approach is limited by the donor phenotypes available and often requires major efforts to increase minority donor recruitment. Unfortunately, despite matching for D, C/c, and E/e, some patients still become sensitized to Rh antigens (D, C, e, and hr^B, Hr^B, hr^S, Hr^S) indicating they were not truly Rh antigen matched.

RH GENOTYPING

DNA molecular testing methods that use polymerase chain reaction (PCR) technology were introduced a decade ago, after the cloning of the genes made genetic testing for blood groups possible. Genotyping has been limited primarily to the reference laboratory setting, but the development of automated, high-throughput platforms expands testing and has the potential for cost-effective, rapid screening for all antigens of interest to potentially enable electronic selection of units antigen-matched at multiple blood group loci.

Assays that target allelic polymorphisms prevalent in all populations are reproducible and highly correlated with red cell phenotype. For some blood groups, assays that detect gene silencing mutations, such as those underlying Fy(a–b–) and S–s–(U–), are also required for accurate typing. ABO and Rh genotyping are challenging because numerous polymorphisms affect antigen expression, multiple regions of the genes must be sampled, and new polymorphisms are still being discovered.

Rh genotyping is a powerful adjunct to serologic testing for typing transfused patients, for *RHD* zygosity determination, for noninvasive fetal *D* typing, for resolution of D status, and for finding compatible blood for patients with SCD. Standardization of methods and FDA approval will be needed to move the technology into mainstream testing.

Typing Multitransfused Patients

In patients receiving chronic or massive transfusion, the presence of donor red cells in the peripheral blood often makes red cell phenotyping by agglutination difficult or inaccurate, especially for patients producing few reticulocytes. Genotyping overcomes this limitation, as reliable blood group determination can be obtained with DNA prepared from a blood sample collected after transfusion.[51] In transfusion-dependent patients who produce alloantibodies, an extended antigen profile allows the laboratory to determine additional blood group antigens to which the patient can become sensitized.

RHD Zygosity Testing

RHD zygosity can be determined by assaying for the presence of a recessive D-negative *RHD* allele. In prenatal practice, paternal *RHD* zygosity testing is important to predict the fetal D status when the mother has anti-D. Several different genetic events cause a D-negative phenotype, and multiple assays must be performed to accurately determine zygosity. If the father is *RHD* homozygous, the fetus will be D-positive, and monitoring of the pregnancy will be required. If the father is heterozygous, the D type of the fetus should be determined to prevent invasive and unnecessary testing during the pregnancy.

Fetal *RHD* Typing

To determine the D antigen status, fetal DNA can be isolated from cells obtained by amniocentesis or chorionic villus sampling. An alternative, noninvasive approach is to test the maternal plasma, which contains cell-free fetal-derived DNA at approximately 5 weeks' gestation.[52] Fetal DNA in the maternal plasma is derived from apoptotic syncytiotrophoblasts, increases in concentration with gestational age, and is rapidly cleared following delivery.[53] Testing requires several milliliters of maternal plasma, sensitive real-time PCR methods, and proper controls to appropriately amplify the small amounts of fetal DNA present. In the future, determination of fetal *RHD* status with this noninvasive procedure could become routine clinical practice to eliminate the unnecessary administration of antepartum RhIG to the approximately 40% of D-negative women who are carrying a D-negative fetus.[53]

Confirming D Status

RHD genotyping is useful to discriminate partial D and specific weak D or to resolve serologic D typing discrepancies. Although patients with an uncertain D status should be treated as D-negative for transfusion and RhIG administration, this may be unsatisfactory for females of childbearing potential facing unnecessary RhIG injections; *RHD* genotyping allows informed decisions to be made in this setting. For donors, D typing discrepancies must be resolved because errors in determining the D status may be reportable to the FDA and involve recall of blood components. Finally, screening of D-negative first-time donors for *RHD* to detect red cells with very weak D or D_{el} has been discussed in the literature and implemented in some European centers.[40,54,55] Additional data are needed to determine whether it would be prudent to eliminate these donors from the D-negative donor pool, but routine screening probably will not be considered until *RHD* genotyping methods become automated and readily available.

RH Genotyping for Sickle Cell Patients

Currently, extensive *RH* genotyping is time consuming and is limited to finding compatible donors in the American Rare Donor Program for patients with antibodies to high-prevalence Rh antigens.[47] The future availability of high-throughput *RH* genotyping platforms will enable patients who are homozygous for altered or variant *Rh* alleles prevalent in sickle cell patients to be recognized, and compatible donors to be identified by genetic matching.

RH_{NULL} SYNDROME AND RHAG BLOOD GROUP SYSTEM

Erythrocytes express a third Rh-protein termed RhAG, for Rh-associated glycoprotein. RhAG shares 38% identity with RhD/RhCE, has the same topology in the membrane, and is encoded by a single gene on chromosome 6. RhAG associates with the Rh blood group proteins in the membrane to form an Rh-core complex. Three red cell antigens resulting from single amino acid substitutions form the RHAG blood group system: Duclos is RHAG1, Ol(a) is RHAG2, and DSLK is provisionally RHAG3.[56] Several other proteins associate with the Rh complex and include CD47, or integrin-associated protein (IAP); LW (ICAM-4); and glycophorin B. Band 3 may also be associated with the complex (Chapter 14, Fig 14-1).

Red cells lacking all Rh antigens are designated Rh_{null}. Although uncommon, the phenotype most often results from mutations in *RHAG*, termed "regulator" mutations, indicating that RhAG protein plays a critical role in trafficking RhCE and RhD to the membrane. Less often, Rh_{null} individuals have *RHCE* mutations, along with the common deletion of *RHD*, and these are termed "amorph."[43] Rh_{null} red cells are stomatocytic and associated with mild anemia, suggesting that the Rh proteins have an important structural role in the erythrocyte membrane. The Rh complex is linked to the membrane skeleton through CD47-protein 4.2 interactions[57] and through Rh/RhAG-ankryin interactions.[58]

RH STRUCTURE AND FUNCTION

Hints to possible functions for the Rh/RhAG proteins initially came from structural predictions that suggested they were transport proteins. Phylogenetic analysis showed that Rh proteins share similarity to ammonia transporters from bacteria and yeast. The relationship of RhAG/Rh to the AMT/MEP family of ammonium transporters from other organisms has now been substantiated by functional transport data[56-59] and structural modeling.[60,61] These studies of Rh proteins reveal the power of comparative genomics and proteomics, in which sequence analysis and homology modeling can give important insight into mammalian protein function.

Nonerythroid Rh Glycoproteins: RhBG and RhCG

Nonerythroid Rh glycoproteins are present in many tissues, including kidney, liver, brain, and skin. These proteins have the same transmembrane structure as erythroid Rh proteins and mediate ammonia transport. In the kidney collecting segment and collecting duct, where large amounts of ammonium are excreted, RhBG and RhCG are found on the basolateral and apical membranes, respectively, of the intercalated cells where they mediate transepithelial movement of ammonium from the interstitium to the lumen of the collecting duct.[62] The mechanism of ammonia transport by Rh glycoproteins (RhAG, RhBG, RhCG) is an active area of investigation. Functional studies of the kidney, liver, and brain Rh-associated glycoproteins, along with the erythrocyte RhAG/Rh proteins, may lead to development of a unifying hypothesis of ammonium transport in mammals by the Rh family of proteins.[63]

Function of RhCE and RhD

The function of the more recently evolved erythrocyte blood group proteins, RhCE and RhD, has not been determined. RhCE and RhD lack the highly conserved histidine residues located in the membrane pore that are critical for ammonia transport, and functional studies suggest they do not transport ammonia.[61,64] An attractive alternative hypothesis is that the RhCE/RhD may mediate movement of the uncharged molecule CO_2; however, there is no direct evidence for this. Alternatively, these Rh proteins may contribute to the structural integrity of the red cell membrane.

Rh Antibodies

Most Rh antibodies are IgG, although some sera may have an IgM component. Typically, Rh antibodies do not activate complement, although rare exceptions have been reported. As a result, in transfusion reactions involving Rh antibodies, hemolysis is primarily extravascular rather than intravascular. Antibodies are almost always caused by red cell immunization from pregnancy or transfusion and usually persist for many years. Most Rh antibodies should be considered as having the potential to cause clinically significant HDFN and transfusion reactions. Anti-c, clinically the most important Rh antibody after anti-D, may cause severe HDFN. Anti-C, -E, and -e do not often cause HDFN, and when they do, it is usually mild. If serum antibody levels fall below detectable levels, subsequent exposure to the antigen characteristically produces a rapid secondary immune response. The reactivity of Rh antibodies is enhanced by enzyme treatment of the test red cells, and most react optimally at 37 C.

Concomitant Rh Antibodies

Some Rh antibodies are often found together. For example, a DCe/DCe (R_1R_1) patient with anti-E most certainly has been exposed to the c antigen as well. Anti-c may be present in addition to anti-E but may be weak and undetectable at the time of testing. Transfusion of seemingly compatible E-negative blood will most likely be c-positive and may elicit an immediate or delayed transfusion reaction; therefore, some advocate the avoidance of c-positive blood in this situation. In contrast, pursuing anti-E in serum containing anti-c is not warranted because the patient will likely have been exposed to c without being exposed to E; additionally, the vast majority of c-negative donor blood will be negative for E. (See Table 13-2.)

Antibodies to High-Prevalence Rh Antigens

Alloantibodies to high-prevalence Rh antigens include anti-Rh29, made by some Rh_{null} individuals who lack Rh antigens, and others that are most often encountered in transfused patients with SCD. These complex specificities, anti-hr^S, -hr^B, -Hr^B, and -Hr, can be difficult to identify, can be clinically significant, and have caused transfusion fatalities.[48] Autoantibodies to high-prevalence Rh antigens often occur in the sera of patients with warm autoimmune hemolytic anemia and in some cases of drug-induced autoimmune hemolytic anemia.[65]

Technical Considerations for Rh Typing

High-Protein Reagents and Controls

Some Rh reagents for use in slide, rapid tube, or microplate tests contain high concentrations of protein (20% to 24%) and other macromolecular additives. These reagents are prepared from pools of human sera and give reliable results; however, high-protein levels and macromolecular additives may cause false-positive reactions (See "Causes of False-Positive and False-Negative Rh Typing Results"). These reagents must be used according to manufacturers' directions and with the appropriate controls. False-positive results could cause a D-negative patient to receive D-positive blood and become immunized. If red cells exhibit aggregation in the control test, the results of the test are not valid.

Low-Protein Reagents and Controls

Most Rh reagents in routine use are low-protein reagents formulated predominantly with IgM monoclonal antibodies. These have a total protein concentration approximating that of human serum, and immunoglobulin-coated red cells can usually be successfully typed with these low-protein reagents in *direct* tests. Spontaneous agglutination causing a false-positive result can occur, although much less frequently than seen with high-protein reagents. A negative test result, performed concurrently in a similar manner, serves as a control. For example, for ABO and Rh typing, the absence of agglutination by anti-A or anti-B serves as a control for spontaneous aggregation. For red cells that show agglutination with all reagents (eg, group AB, D+), a control performed as described by the reagent manufacturer is required (with the exception of donor retyping). In most cases, a suitable control is a suspension of the patient's red cells with autologous serum or with 6% or 8% albumin. Most Rh typing reagents, with the exception of anti-D, are not intended for IAT testing and must not be used in this manner unless the manufacturer's instructions state otherwise. Indirect antiglobulin testing will not be valid on red cells with a positive DAT unless methods to remove the IgG antibody are used. Positive and negative controls should be tested, and the positive control cells should have a single dose of the antigen or be known to show weak reactivity.

Causes of False-Positive and False-Negative Rh Typing Results

False-positive typing can result from:

1. Warm or cold autoagglutinins causing immunoglobulin coating of the cells. IgM cold agglutinins can often be eliminated by washing the red cells several times with warm saline and retesting. Warm IgG autoagglutinins primarily cause false-positive results in the IAT phase of testing. Wash the red cells as above, and test with low-protein reagents by direct methods. If an IAT is required, IgG coating the red cells can be removed by treating with glycine/EDTA (Method 2-21) or chloroquine (Method 2-20) and retesting.
2. Serum factors that induce rouleaux and spontaneous red cell aggregation. Serum factors can be eliminated by thoroughly washing the red cells and retesting.
3. The wrong reagent being used inadvertently.
4. The reagent being contaminated with reagent from another vial.
5. Some component of the reagent other than the antibody (ie. a preservative, antibiotic, or dye) causing nonspecific aggregation of the red cells.
6. Polyagglutinable red cells being agglutinated with reagents that contain human serum.

False-negative typing can result from:

1. Failure to add the reagent. It is good practice to add typing reagent to all test tubes or wells before adding the red cells.
2. The wrong reagent being used.
3. A red cell suspension that is too heavy for the tube test or too weak for the slide test.
4. Undetected red cells with weak D antigen in direct tests on immediate centrifugation.
5. A specific reagent being unreactive with a variant or weak form of the antigen.
6. Agglutinates dispersed by aggressive resuspension of the red cell button.
7. Contamination, improper storage, or outdating of the reagent.

8. Red cells with a strongly positive DAT and with antigen sites blocked because of a large amount of bound antibody (primarily seen in severe HDFN caused by anti-D).

Rh Testing Considerations in Hemolytic Disease of the Fetus and Newborn

Red cells from an infant suffering from HDFN are coated with immunoglobulin, and a low-protein reagent is usually necessary for testing. Occasionally, red cells with a strongly positive DAT may be so heavily coated that they are not agglutinated by a reagent with the same specificity as the bound antibody. This "blocking" phenomenon probably results from steric hindrance and occupied antigen sites and can result in false-negative results. Heat elution of the antibody performed at 45 C permits red cell typing, but elution must be performed with caution to avoid denaturing the Rh antigens. Although detection of the antibody in an eluate confirms the presence of the antigen on the eluted red cells, *RHD* genotyping can be used for confirmation of D typing.

Resolving D Typing Discrepancies

Multiple variables contribute to D typing discrepancies. These include the use of different methods (ie, slide, tube, microplate, gel, and automated analyzers using enzyme-treated red cells), the phase of testing (direct or IAT), the different IgM clones in manufacturers' reagents, and the large number of *RHD* gene variations that affect the level of expression and epitopes of the D antigen.

It is important to know the characteristics of the D typing reagent being used and to always consult and follow the manufacturer's instructions. The FDA requires that manufacturers specify reactivity with partial DIV, DV, and DVI red cells. The IgM anti-D in all of the tube reagents reacts by direct testing (initial spin) with DIV and DV red cells but has been selected to be nonreactive with partial DVI red cells in direct testing. DVI donors will appropriately be classified as D-positive by IAT. Only limited studies have been performed to characterize the reactivity of reagents with other partial D or weak D red cells,[30,66] primarily because of the paucity of partial and weak D samples that have been confirmed by *RH* genotyping. Table 13-4 shows the reactivity of different reagents with some red cells that may be involved in D typing discrepancies.

To investigate D typing discrepancies, sample identification or clerical errors should be eliminated by obtaining and testing a new sample. Knowledge of the ethnic background of the donor or patient can be helpful in resolving the D discrepancy (Table 13-4). Discrepancies encountered when retyping donor units labeled as Rh negative must be reported to the collecting facility and resolved before issue of blood for transfusion. Key to assigning D antigen status should be whether the sample is from a blood donor or transfusion recipient. An individual with partial D should be considered D positive as a blood donor but D negative as a transfusion recipient.

KEY POINTS

1. The Rh system is highly immunogenic, complex, and polymorphic. More than 50 Rh antigens have been characterized, although the five principal antigens—D, C, c, E, and e—are responsible for the majority of clinically significant antibodies.
2. "Rh positive" and "Rh negative" refer to the presence or absence of the D antigen.
3. Contemporary Rh terminology distinguishes between antigens (letter designations such as D and C), genes (capital letters with or without italics, such as *RHD* and *RHCE*), alleles (*RHCE*ce* or *RHCE*Ce*), and proteins (RhD and Rhce).
4. Most D-negative (Rh-negative) phenotypes result from complete deletion of the *RHD* gene. Exposure of these individuals to RhD often results in anti-D.

5. *RHCE* encodes both C/c and E/e antigens on a single protein. C and c differ by four amino acids, while E and e differ by one amino acid.
6. Routine donor and patient Rh typing procedures test only for D. Testing for other common Rh antigens is used to resolve or confirm antibody identification, and for some sickle cell transfusion programs to match patients and donors for D, C, and E.
7. Weak D phenotypes are defined as having a reduced amount of D antigen, requiring an indirect antiglobulin test (IAT) for detection. Weak D usually results from single nucleotide mutations in *RHD* that impair insertion of the protein in the membrane. Many different mutations cause weak D expression.
8. Most anti-D reagents approved by the Food and Drug Administration combine a monoclonal IgM antibody (reactive at room temperature for routine testing) and a monoclonal or polyclonal IgG antibody (reactive by the IAT for the determination of weak D), except anti-D for column agglutination testing, which contains only IgM. These reagents may react differently with red cells that have weak D, partial D, or D-like epitopes.
9. When determining the D type of a patient, a weak D test is not necessary except when testing the red cells of an infant born to a mother at risk for D immunization. Rh-negative donors must be tested by a method that detects weak D.
10. Most Rh antibodies are IgG, although some may have an IgM component. With rare exceptions, Rh antibodies do not activate complement and thus cause primarily extravascular rather than intravascular hemolysis. Antibodies almost always result from red cell immunization through pregnancy or transfusion.

REFERENCES

1. Race RR, Sanger R. Blood groups in man. 6th ed. Oxford: Blackwell, 1975.
2. Levine P, Burnham L, Katzin WM, Vogel P. The role of isoimmunization in the pathogenesis of erythroblastosis fetalis. Am J Obstet Gynecol 1941;42:925-37.
3. Rosenfeld R. Who discovered Rh? A personal glimpse of the Levine-Wiener argument. Transfusion 1989;29:355-7.
4. Mollison PL, Hughes-Jones NC, Lindsay M, Wessely J. Suppression of primary RH immunization by passively-administered antibody. Experiments in volunteers. Vox Sang 1969;16: 421-39.
5. Freda V, Gorman J, Pollack W. Rh factor: Prevention of isoimmunization and clinical trials in mothers. Science 1966;151:828-30.
6. Green FA. Phospholipid requirement for Rh antigenic activity. J Biol Chem 1968;243:5519-21.
7. Gahmberg CG. Molecular characterization of the human red cell Rho(D) antigen. EMBO J 1983;2:223-7.
8. Gahmberg CG. Molecular identification of the human Rho (D) antigen. FEBS Lett 1982;140: 93-7.
9. Bloy C, Blanchard D, Lambin P, et al. Human monoclonal antibody against Rh(D) antigen: Partial characterization of the Rh(D) polypeptide from human erythrocytes. Blood 1987;69: 1491-7.
10. Moore S, Woodrow CF, McClelland DB. Isolation of membrane components associated with human red cell antigens Rh(D), (c), (E) and Fy. Nature 1982;295:529-31.
11. Saboori AM, Smith BL, Agre P. Polymorphism in the Mr 32,000 Rh protein purified from Rh(D)-positive and -negative erythrocytes. Proc Natl Acad Sci U S A 1988;85:4042-5.
12. Cherif-Zahar B, Bloy C, Le Van Kim C, et al. Molecular cloning and protein structure of a human blood group Rh polypeptide. Proc Natl Acad Sci U S A 1990;87:6243-7.
13. Le van Kim C, Mouro I, Cherif-Zahar B, et al. Molecular cloning and primary structure of the human blood group RhD polypeptide. Proc Natl Acad Sci U S A 1992;89:10925-9.
14. Arce MA, Thompson ES, Wagner S, et al. Molecular cloning of RhD cDNA derived from a gene present in RhD-positive, but not RhD-negative individuals. Blood 1993;82:651-5.
15. Simsek S, de Jong CAM, Cuijpers HTM, et al. Sequence analysis of cDNA derived from retic-

ulocyte mRNAs coding for Rh polypeptides and demonstration of E/e and C/c polymorphism. Vox Sang 1994;67:203-9.

16. Wagner FF, Flegel WA. The Rhesus site. Weak D types by number. [Available at http://www.uni-ulm.de/~fwagner/RH/RB/ (accessed October 15, 2010).]
17. Blumenfeld OO, Patnaik SK. Allelic genes of blood group antigens: A source of human mutations and cSNPs documented in the Blood Group Antigen Gene Mutation Database. Hum Mutat 2004;23:8-16. [Available at http://www.ncbi.nlm.nih.gov/gv/mhc/xslcgi.cgi?cmd=bgmut/home (accessed October 18, 2010).]
18. Tippett P. A speculative model for the Rh blood groups. Ann Hum Genet 1986;50(Pt 3):241-7.
19. Daniels G, Castilho L, Flegel WA, et al. International Society of Blood Transfusion Committee on terminology for red blood cell surface antigens: Macao report. Vox Sang 2009;96:153-6.
20. Wagner FF, Flegel WA. RHD gene deletion occurred in the Rhesus box. Blood 2000;95:3662-8.
21. Scott ML, Voak D, Liu W, et al. Epitopes on Rh proteins. Vox Sang 2000;78(Suppl 2):117-20.
22. Khademi S, O'Connell J 3rd, Remis J, et al. Mechanism of ammonia transport by Amt/MEP/Rh: Structure of AmtB at 1.35 A. Science 2004;305:1587-94.
23. Wagner FF, Gassner C, Muller TH, et al. Molecular basis of weak D phenotypes. Blood 1999;93:385-93.
24. Shao CP, Maas JH, Su YQ, et al. Molecular background of Rh D-positive, D-negative, D(el) and weak D phenotypes in Chinese. Vox Sang 2002;83:156-61.
25. Sun CF, Chou CS, Lai NC, Wang WT. RHD gene polymorphisms among RhD-negative Chinese in Taiwan. Vox Sang 1998;75:52-7.
26. Daniels G. Human blood groups. 2nd ed. Cambridge, MA: Blackwell Science, 2002.
27. Wagner FF, Ladewig B, Flegel WA. The RHCE allele ceRT: D epitope 6 expression does not require D-specific amino acids. Transfusion 2003;43:1248-54.
28. Chen Q, Hustinx H, Flegel WA. The RHCE allele ceSL: The second example for D antigen expression without D-specific amino acids. Transfusion 2006;46:766-72.
29. Beckers EA, Porcelijn L, Ligthart P, et al. The Ro^{Har} antigenic complex is associated with a limited number of D epitopes and alloanti-D production: A study of three unrelated persons and their families. Transfusion 1996;36:104-8.
30. Westhoff CM. Review: The Rh blood group D antigen . . . dominant, diverse, and difficult. Immunohematol 2005;21:155-63.
31. Colin Y, Cherif-Zahar B, Le Van Kim C, et al. Genetic basis of the RhD-positive and RhD-negative blood group polymorphism as determined by Southern analysis. Blood 1991;78:2747-52.
32. Singleton BK, Green CA, Avent ND, et al. The presence of an RHD pseudogene containing a 37 base pair duplication and a nonsense mutation in Africans with the Rh D-negative blood group phenotype. Blood 2000;95:12-18.
33. Carson TH, ed. Standards for blood banks and transfusion services. 27th ed. Bethesda, MD: AABB, 2011.
34. Schmidt PJ, Morrison EC, Shohl J. The antigenicity of the Rh_0 (D^u) blood factor. Blood 1962;20:196-202.
35. Wagner T, Kormoczi GF, Buchta C, et al. Anti-D immunization by DEL red blood cells. Transfusion 2005;45:520-6.
36. Yasuda H, Ohto H, Sakuma S, Ishikawa Y. Secondary anti-D immunization by Del red blood cells. Transfusion 2005;45:1581-4.
37. Flegel WA, Khull SR, Wagner FF. Primary anti-D immunization by weak D type 2 RBCs. Transfusion 2000;40:428-34.
38. Mota M, Fonseca NL, Rodrigues A, et al. Anti-D alloimmunization by weak D type 1 red blood cells with a very low antigen density. Vox Sang 2005;88:130-5.
39. Lacey PA, Caskey CR, Werner DJ, Moulds JJ. Fatal hemolytic disease of a newborn due to anti-D in an Rh-positive D_u variant mother. Transfusion 1983;23:91-4.
40. Flegel WA. Homing in on D antigen immunogenicity. Transfusion 2005;45:466-8.
41. Schonewille H, van de Watering LM, Brand A. Additional red blood cell alloantibodies after blood transfusions in a nonhematologic alloimmunized patient cohort: Is it time to take precautionary measures? Transfusion 2006;46:630-5.
42. Frohn C, Dumbgen L, Brand J-M, et al. Probability of anti-D development in D– patients receiving D+ RBCs. Transfusion 2003;43:893-8.
43. Issitt PD, Anstee DJ. Applied blood group serology. 4th ed. Durham, NC: Montgomery Scientific Publications, 1998.
44. Reid ME, Lomas-Francis C. The blood group antigen factsbook. 2nd ed. San Diego, CA: Academic Press, 2004.

45. Daniels GL, Faas BH, Green CA, et al. The VS and V blood group polymorphisms in Africans: A serologic and molecular analysis. Transfusion 1998;38:951-8.
46. Reid ME, Storry JR, Issitt PD, et al. Rh haplotypes that make e but not hr[B] usually make VS. Vox Sang 1997;72:41-4.
47. Vege S, Westhoff CM. Molecular characterization of GYPB and RH in donors in the American Rare Donor Program. Immunohematol 2006;22:143-7.
48. Noizat-Pirenne F, Lee K, Pennec PY, et al. Rare RHCE phenotypes in black individuals of Afro-Caribbean origin: Identification and transfusion safety. Blood 2002;100:4223-31.
49. Ness PM. To match or not to match: The question for chronically transfused patients with sickle cell anemia. Transfusion 1994;34:558-60.
50. Vichinsky EP, Luban NL, Wright E, et al. Prospective RBC phenotype matching in a stroke-prevention trial in sickle cell anemia: A multicenter transfusion trial. Transfusion 2001;41: 1086-92.
51. Reid ME, Rios M, Powell VI, et al. DNA from blood samples can be used to genotype patients who have recently received a transfusion. Transfusion 2000;40:48-53.
52. Lo YM, Corbetta N, Chamberlain PF, et al. Presence of fetal DNA in maternal plasma and serum. Lancet 1997;350:485-7.
53. Van der Schoot CE, Soussan AA, Koelewijn J, et al. Non-invasive antenatal RHD typing. Transfus Clin Biol 2006;13:53-7.
54. Gassner C, Doescher A, Drnovsek TD, et al. Presence of RHD in serologically D–, C/E+ individuals: A European multicenter study. Transfusion 2005;45:527-38.
55. Polin H, Danzer M, Hofer K, et al. Effective molecular RHD typing stategy for blood donations. Transfusion 2007;47:1350-5.
56. Tilley L, Green C, Poole J, et al. A new blood group system, RHAG: Three antigens resulting from amino acid substitutions in the Rh-associated glycoprotein. Vox Sang 2010;98:151-9.
57. Dahl KN, Parthasarathy R, Westhoff CM, et al. Protein 4.2 is critical to CD47-membrane skeleton attachment in human red cells. Blood 2004;103:1131-6.
58. Nicolas V, Le Van Kim C, Gane P, et al. Rh-RhAG/ankyrin-R, a new interaction site between the membrane bilayer and the red cell skeleton, is impaired by Rh(null)-associated mutation. J Biol Chem 2003;278:25526-33.
59. Ripoche P, Bertrand O, Gane P, et al. Human Rhesus-associated glycoprotein mediates facilitated transport of NH(3) into red blood cells. Proc Natl Acad Sci U S A 2004;101:17222-7.
60. Callebaut I, Dulin F, Bertrand O, et al. Hydrophobic cluster analysis and modeling of the human Rh protein three-dimensional structures. Transfus Clin Biol 2006;13:70-84.
61. Conroy MJ, Bullough PA, Merrick M, Avent ND. Modelling the human rhesus proteins: Implications for structure and function. Br J Haematol 2005;131:543-51.
62. Weiner ID, Miller RT, Verlander JW. Localization of the ammonium transporters, Rh B glycoprotein and Rh C glycoprotein, in the mouse liver. Gastroenterology 2003;124:1432-40.
63. Westhoff CM. The Rh blood group system in review: A new face for the next decade. Transfusion 2004;44:1663-73.
64. Westhoff CM, Wylie DE. Transport characteristics of mammalian Rh and Rh glycoproteins expressed in heterologous systems. Transfus Clin Biol 2006;13:132-8.
65. Petz LD, Garratty G. Immune hemolytic anemias. 2nd ed. Philadelphia: Churchill Livingstone/Elsevier Science, 2004.
66. Judd WJ, Moulds M, Schlanser G. Reactivity of FDA-approved anti-D reagents with partial D red blood cells. Immunohematol 2005;21:146-8.

SUGGESTED READING

1. Daniels G. Human blood groups. 2nd ed. Cambridge, MA: Blackwell Science, 2002.
2. Issitt PD, Anstee DJ. Applied blood group serology. 4th ed. Durham, NC: Montgomery Scientific Publications, 1998.
3. Westhoff CM. Review: The Rh blood group D antigen: Dominant, diverse, and difficult. Immunohematol 2005;21:155-63.
4. Westhoff CM. Structure and function of the Rh blood group antigens. Semin Hematol 2007; 44:42-50.
5. Reid ME, Lomas-Francis C. The blood group antigen factsbook. 2nd ed. San Diego, CA: Academic Press, 2004.

Chapter 14

Other Blood Groups

Geoff Daniels, PhD, FRCPath

THE INTERNATIONAL SOCIETY of Blood Transfusion (ISBT) recognizes 328 antigen specificities, 284 of which belong to one of 30 blood group systems.[1,2] Each system represents either a single gene or two or three closely linked homologous genes. The ABO and Rh systems are the best known and clinically most important systems and are described in detail in Chapters 12 and 13. The antigens of the H, Lewis, I, P1PK, and Globoside systems are carbohydrate structures that are biochemically closely related to ABO antigens and are included in Chapter 12. The remaining systems are described in this chapter; some, generally the most important in transfusion medicine, are described in some detail, others in a few lines. They are listed in ISBT order, as in Table 14-1.

In addition to the 30 systems, some groups of antigens that are serologically, biochemically, or genetically related but not eligible to join a system are classified together as collections. Other antigens that are not eligible to join a system or a collection are of either low or high prevalence in most major populations and make up the 700 and 901 series, respectively.[1] They are all mentioned at the end of this chapter.

The full ISBT classification can be found in Daniels et al[1,2]; on the website of the Bristol Institute for Transfusion Sciences and the International Blood Group Reference Laboratory, at http://blood.co.uk/ibgrl/; and in Appendix 6. Many more references to blood groups than can be provided here are available in various textbooks and reviews.[3-8]

The most important aspect of blood groups in transfusion medicine is whether their corresponding antibodies are hemolytic and therefore have the potential to cause hemolytic transfusion reactions (HTRs) and hemolytic disease of the fetus and newborn (HDFN).[3] A guide to the potential clinical significance of blood group antibodies is provided in Table 14-1.

THE MNS SYSTEM

MNS is a highly complex blood group system consisting of 46 antigens.[2-4(pp99-174)] As with the Rh system, much of the complexity arises from recombination between closely linked homologous genes.

Geoff Daniels, PhD, FRCPath, Senior Research Fellow, Bristol Institute for Transfusion Sciences, Bristol, United Kingdom

The author has disclosed no conflicts of interest.

TABLE 14-1. Clinical Significance of Antibodies to Blood Groups in the 30 Systems[3]

ISBT No.	System Symbol	No. of Antigens	Hemolytic Transfusion Reaction (HTR), Acute (AHTR) or Delayed (DHTR)	Hemolytic Disease of the Fetus and Newborn (HDFN)
001	ABO	4	See Chapter 12	See Chapter 12
002	MNS	46	Rare examples of anti-M and -N active at 37 C cause AHTRs and DHTRs; anti-S, -s, -U, and some other antibodies may cause AHTRs and DHTRs	Anti-S, -s, -U, and some other antibodies cause severe HDFN; anti-M, rarely
003	P1PK	2	Only very rare examples active at 37 C cause AHTRs and DHTRs	No
004	Rh	52	Cause severe AHTRs and DHTRs (see Chapter 13)	Cause severe HDFN (see Chapter 22)
005	Lutheran	20	Anti-Lu^a and -Lu^b have caused mild DHTRs; anti-Lu8, AHTRs	No
006	Kell	32	Cause severe AHTRs and DHTRs	Cause severe HDFN
007	Lewis	6	Not generally considered clinically significant	No
008	Duffy	5	Anti-Fy^a, -Fy^b, -Fy3 cause AHTRs and DHTRs; anti-Fy5, DHTRs	Anti-Fy^a and -Fy^b cause HDFN
009	Kidd	3	Common cause of DHTRs; anti-Jk^a and -Jk3 also cause AHTRs	Not usually
010	Diego	22	One anti-Di^a caused DHTR, but little evidence; anti-Di^b, DHTRs; anti-Wr^a, HTRs	Anti-Di^a, -Di^b, -Wr^a, and -Wr^b plus some others have caused severe HDFN
011	Yt	2	Anti-Yt^a very rarely caused HTR	No
012	Xg	2	No	No
013	Scianna	7	No	No
014	Dombrock	7	Anti-Do^a and -Do^b cause AHTRs and DHTRs	No

015	Colton	4	Anti-Co^a causes AHTRs and DHTRs; anti-Co^b and -Co3 have caused mild HTRs	Anti-Co^a has caused severe, and -Co3 mild, HDFN
016	LW	3	No	No
017	Ch/Rg	9	No	No
018	H	1	Anti-H in Bombay phenotype can cause severe intravascular HTRs; Anti-HI in para-Bombay is not usually clinically significant (see Chapter 12)	Anti-H in Bombay phenotype has potential to cause severe HDFN (see Chapter 12)
019	Kx	1	Anti-Kx and -Km in McLeod syndrome has caused severe HTRs	Antibodies found only in males
020	Gerbich	11	No	Three examples of anti-Ge3 causing HDFN
021	Cromer	16	No	No
022	Knops	9	No	No
023	Indian	4	One example of anti-In^b causing an HTR	No
024	Ok	3	Very rare and no HTR reported	No
025	Raph	1	No	No
026	JMH	6	1 example of anti-JMH reported to have caused AHTR	No
027	I	1	Anti-I in adult i phenotype has caused increased destruction of I+ red cells	No
028	Globoside	1	Intravascular HTRs	No, but high rate of spontaneous abortion
029	Gill	1	No	No
030	RHAG	3	No	No

ISBT = International Society of Blood Transfusion.

The MNS Glycoproteins and the Genes that Encode Them

The antigens of the MNS system are located on one or both of two glycoproteins: glycophorin A (GPA, CD235A) and glycophorin B (GPB, CD235B). Each crosses the membrane once, with an external N-terminal domain (GPA, 72 amino acids; GPB, 44 amino acids) and a C-terminal cytosolic domain (GPA, 36; GPB, 8). The extracellular domains of both molecules have many sialic acid-rich O-glycans; GPA is N-glycosylated at asparagine-45 (26 in native protein), whereas GPB is not N-glycosylated. The long cytosolic tail of GPA interacts with the cytoskeleton. GPA is very abundant with about 10^6 copies per red cell, but GPB has only about 200,000 copies per cell. GPA forms an association in the membrane with Band 3 (Diego antigen), and both GPA and GPB appear to be part of the Band 3/Rh ankyrin complex (Fig 14-1).[9,10]

GYPA and *GYPB*, the genes encoding GPA and GPB, comprise seven and five exons, respectively. A region of intron 3 of *GYPB* is homologous to exon 3 of *GYPA* but is not expressed because of a defective splice site (Fig 14-2).[11] Exon 1 of each gene encodes a 19-amino-acid signal peptide that is not present in the mature protein. A third gene, *GYPE*, probably produces a third glycoprotein, glycophorin E, but this plays little or no part in MNS antigen expression.

GPA is restricted to blood cells of erythroid origin and is often used as an erythroid marker. Both GPA and GPB are exploited by the malarial parasite *Plasmodium falciparum* as receptors for binding to red cells and may be critical to the invasion process.[12,13] A GPA-like molecule has been detected on renal endothelium.

M (MNS1), N (MNS2), S (MNS3), and s (MNS4)

M and N (as detected by most anti-N reagents) are antithetical antigens and polymorphic in all populations tested (Table 14-2). M and N are located at the N-terminus of GPA: M-active GPA has serine and glycine at the first and fifth positions of the native protein (positions 20 and 25); N-active GPA has leucine and glutamic acid at those positions.

S and s are another pair of polymorphic antithetical antigens of the MNS system (Table 14-2). Family studies showed tight linkage between *M/N* and *S/s*. S and s represent a Met48Thr (29 in native protein) polymorphism in GPB. The amino-terminal 26 amino acids of GPB mature protein are usually identical to those of the N form of GPA. Consequently, in almost all Whites and most people of other races, GPB expresses 'N'. However, because GPB is much less abundant than GPA, most anti-N reagents do not detect the 'N' antigen on GPB. The N-terminal region of GPA is cleaved from intact red cells by trypsin, whereas that of GPB is not. Consequently, M and N antigens on GPA are trypsin-sensitive, and S, s, and 'N' on GPB are trypsin-resistant. In contrast, with α-chymotrypsin treatment of red cells, M and N activity is only partially reduced, whereas S, s, and 'N' expression is completely destroyed. M, N, S, s, and 'N' are all destroyed by treatment of the red cells with papain, ficin, bromelin, or pronase, although this effect with S and s is variable.

TABLE 14-2. Frequencies of Some Phenotypes of the MNS system

Phenotype	Frequency (%)	
	Whites	Blacks
M+ N–	30	25
M+ N+	49	49
M– N+	21	26
S+ s–	10	6
S+ s+	42	24
S– s+	48	68
S– s–	0	2

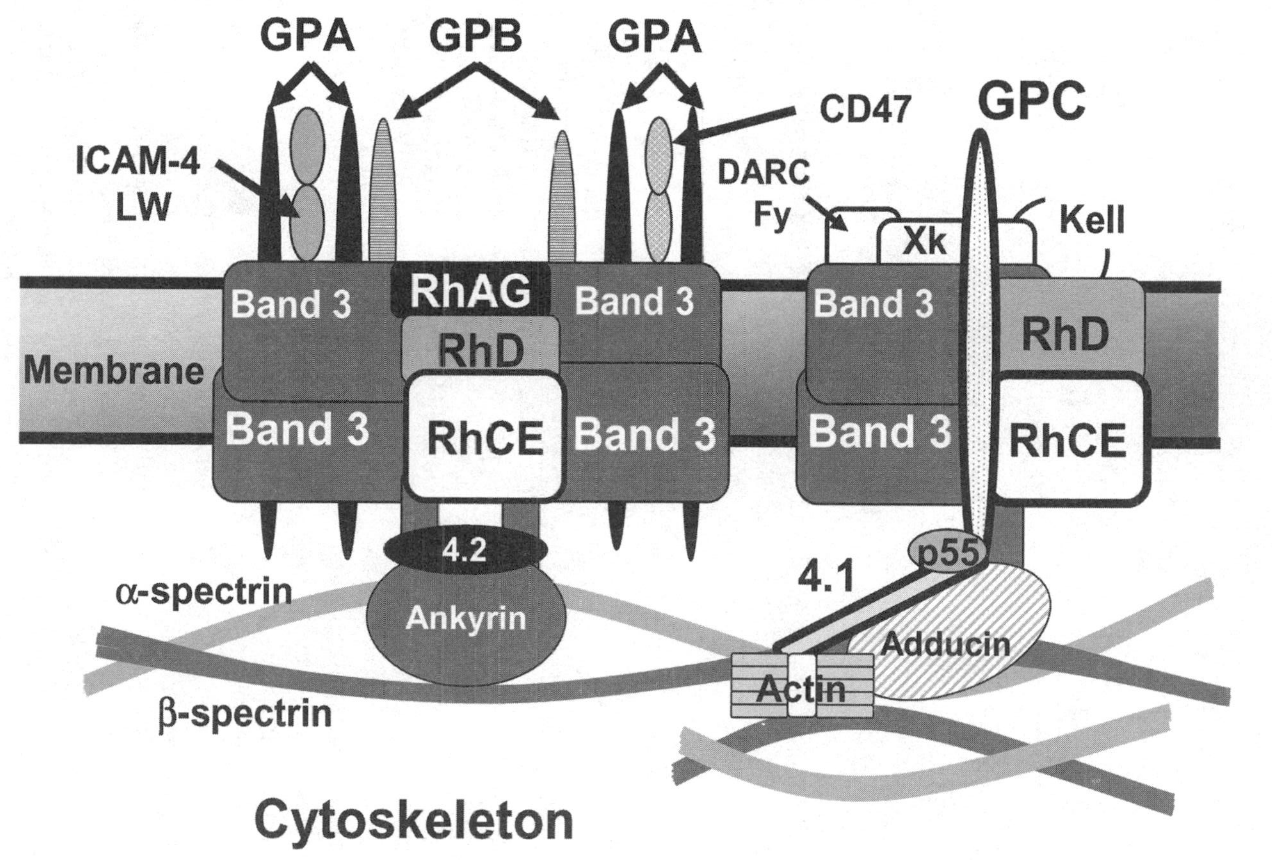

FIGURE 14-1. Model of two proposed membrane complexes containing Band 3 and Rh proteins: 1) containing tetramers of Band 3 and heterotrimers of RhD, RhCE, and RhAG, and linked to the spectrin matrix of the cytoskeleton through Band 3, protein 4.2, and ankyrin; and 2) containing Band 3, RhD, and RhCE, and linked to the spectrin/actin junction through glycophorin C (GPC), p55, and protein 4.1 and through Band 3 and adducin.

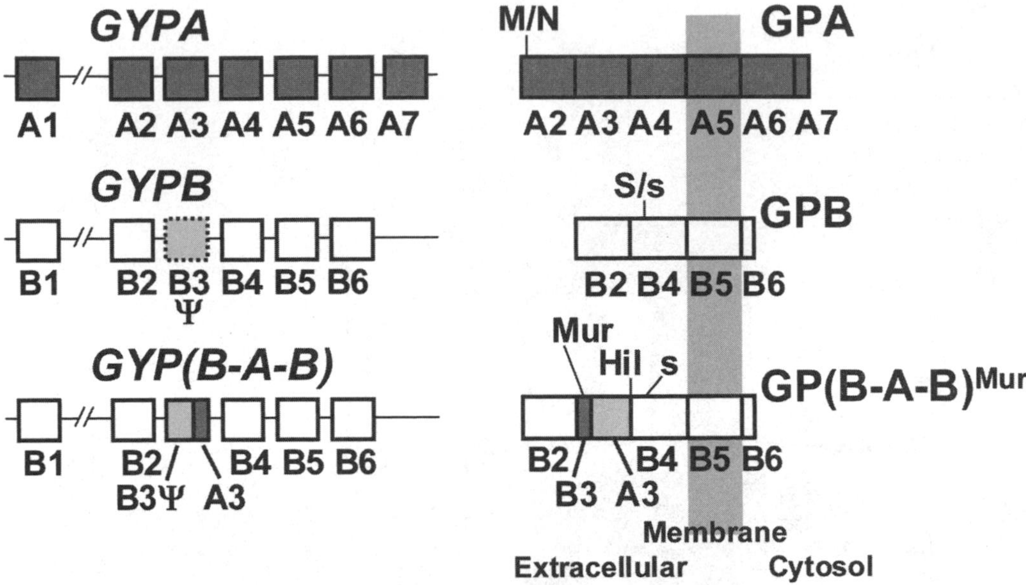

FIGURE 14-2. *GYPA, GYPB*, and the hybrid *GYPB–A–B* gene responsible for GP.Mur, and a representation of the proteins they encode, showing the regions of proteins encoded by the various exons.
Ψ= pseudoexon not represented in the mRNA or the encoded protein.

S–s–U– Phenotype

Red cells of about 2% of Americans of African descent and a higher proportion of Africans are S–s– and lack the high-prevalence antigen U (MNS5). The S–s–U– phenotype often results from homozygosity for a deletion of the coding region of *GYPB*, but other more complex molecular phenomena involving hybrid genes may also give rise to an S–s– phenotype, with expression of a variant U antigen. U is generally resistant to denaturation by proteases—papain, ficin, trypsin, α-chymotrypsin—although unusual examples of anti-U do not react with papain-treated red cells.

M, N, S, s, and U Antibodies and Their Clinical Significance

Anti-M is a relatively common "naturally occurring" antibody, whereas anti-N is quite rare. Most anti-M and -N are not active at 37 C and are not clinically significant.[5(pp220-223)] They can generally be ignored in transfusion practice, and if room-temperature incubation is eliminated from compatibility testing and screening for antibodies, they will not be detected. When M or N antibodies active at 37 C are encountered, antigen-negative or red cells compatible by an indirect antiglobulin test (IAT) should be provided.[3] Very occasionally anti-M and N have been implicated as the cause of acute and delayed HTRs, and anti-M has very rarely been responsible for severe HDFN.

A few cases of warm autoimmune hemolytic anemia (AIHA) caused by autoanti-N have been described, one of which had a fatal outcome. Autoanti-M responsible for warm AIHA has not been reported.

Anti-S and -s are generally IgG antibodies active at 37 C. They have been implicated in HTRs and have caused severe and fatal HDFN. Autoanti-S has caused AIHA.

If immunized, individuals with S–s–U– red cells may produce anti-U. Anti-U has been responsible for severe and fatal HTRs and HDFN. Autoanti-U has been implicated in AIHA.

Other MNS Antigens and Antibodies

The other MNS antigens are either of high or low prevalence in most populations. The similarity of sequence between certain regions of *GYPA* and *GYPB* may occasionally lead to *GYPA* pairing with *GYPB* during meiosis. If recombination then occurs, either by crossing over or by a less well-defined mechanism called gene conversion, then a hybrid gene can be formed consisting partly of *GYPA* and partly of *GYPB*. A large variety of these rare hybrid genes exists, and they give rise to low-prevalence antigens and, in the homozygous state, to phenotypes that lack high-prevalence antigens.[11] Red cells of some of the phenotypes resulting from hybrid genes react with an antibody called anti-Mi^a (MNS7), and the phenotypes were grouped together as the Miltenberger series, but this classification is now obsolete.[14]

One example, which is relatively common in Southeast Asia, is the hybrid gene that is responsible for the GP.Mur (previously Mi.III) phenotype. The hybrid gene is mostly *GYPB*, but a small region of *GYPB* encompassing the 3′ end of the pseudoexon and the 5′ end of the adjacent intron has been replaced by the equivalent region from *GYPA*. This means that the defective splice site in *GYPB* is now replaced by the functional splice site from *GYPA*, and the new, composite exon is expressed in the mRNA and represented in the protein.[11] This provides an unusual amino acid sequence that is immunogenic and represents the antigen Mur (MNS10), and the amino acid sequence that results from the junction of exons B3 and A3 gives rise to Hil (MNS20) and MINY (MNS34) (Fig 14-2).

Mur antigen is rare in people of European and African ethnicity but has a prevalence of about 7% in Chinese and 10% in Thais. Anti-Mur has the potential to cause severe HTRs and HDFN. In Hong Kong and Taiwan, anti-Mur is the most common blood group antibody after anti-A and -B. In Southeast Asia, it is important that red cells for antibody detection include a Mur+ sample.[15]

Antibodies to regions of GPA with the generic name En^a (MNS28), which may be made by very rare individuals who lack all or part of GPA, have caused severe HTRs and HDFN.

THE LUTHERAN SYSTEM

Lutheran is a complex system comprising 20 antigens, including four antithetical pairs: Lu^a/Lu^b (His77Arg); Lu6/Lu9 (Ser275Phe); Lu8/Lu14 (Met204Lys); and Au^a/Au^b (Thr529Ala).[16] The other Lutheran antigens are of high prevalence in all populations tested. Lu^a (LU1) has a prevalence of about 8% in people of European and African ethnicity but is rare elsewhere; its antithetical antigen, Lu^b (LU2), is common everywhere. In the other Lutheran polymorphism, Au^a (LU18) and Au^b (LU19) have a prevalence of around 80% and 50%, respectively, in Whites.

Lutheran antigens are destroyed by treatment of the red cells with trypsin or α-chymotrypsin, whereas papain and ficin have little effect. Most Lutheran antibodies do not react with red cells treated with the sulfhydryl reagents 2-aminoethylisothiouronium bromide (AET) or dithiothreitol (DTT), which reduce the disulfide bonds of the immunoglobulin superfamily (IgSF) domains (Method 3-10).

The Lutheran antigens are located on a pair of glycoproteins that span the membrane once, have five extracellular IgSF domains, and differ by the length of their cytoplasmic domains as a result of alternative RNA splicing. The isoform with the longer cytoplasmic domain interacts with spectrin of the membrane skeleton. The location of the Lutheran specificities on the IgSF domains is shown in Fig 14-3. The Lutheran glycoproteins are adhesion molecules that bind isoforms of laminin that contain α-5 chains. Laminin is a glycoprotein of the extracellular matrix, and Lutheran-laminin interactions may play a role in the migration of mature erythroid cells from the marrow to the peripheral blood at the latest stages of erythropoiesis. Up-regulation of Lutheran glycoproteins on red cells of patients with sickle cell disease could play a part in adhesion of these cells to the vascular endothelium and the resultant crises of vascular occlusion.[17]

The extremely rare Lu_{null} phenotype arises from homozygosity for inactive *LU* genes.[18]

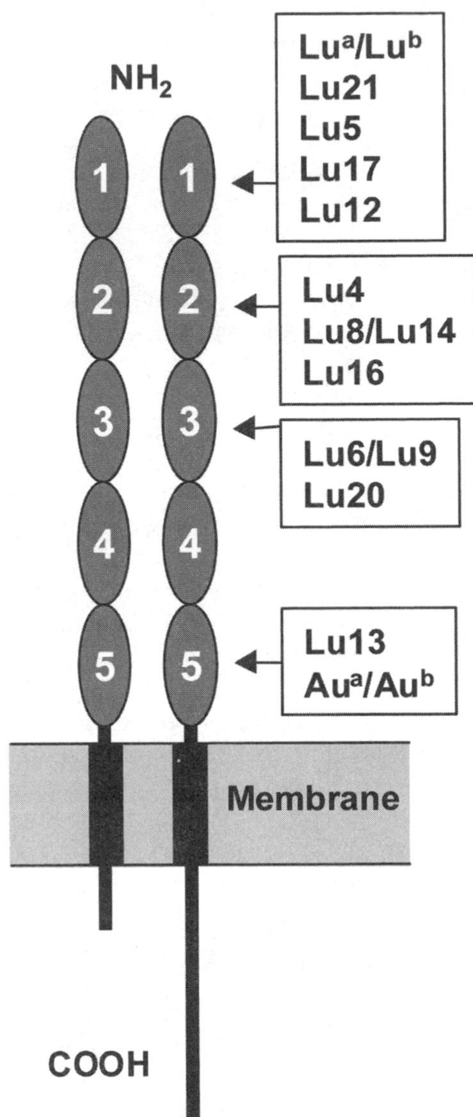

FIGURE 14-3. Diagram of the two isoforms of the Lutheran glycoprotein, showing the five extra-cellular immunoglobulin superfamily domains and the location of the Lutheran antigens on these domains, the single membrane-spanning domain, and the cytoplasmic domains.

The red cells completely lack any expression of Lutheran antigens, and individuals with this phenotype may produce an antibody to a high-prevalence antigen, anti-Lu3. Heterozygosity for inactivating mutations in the erythroid transcription factor EKLF is responsible for In(Lu), an Lu_{mod} phenotype with extremely weak expression of Lutheran antigens that are detectable only by adsorption/elution techniques, and also weakened expression of several other blood group antigens, including P1, In^b, and AnWj.[19] In(Lu) phenotype has a prevalence of around 0.03%. In one family, hemizygosity for a mutation in the X-linked gene for the major erythroid transcription factor GATA-1 resulted in an Lu_{mod} phenotype with an X-linked mode of inheritance.[20]

Lutheran antibodies have generally been implicated only in mild delayed HTRs and have not caused severe HDFN. Lu^a antibodies may be "naturally occurring" or immune, and they are often IgM but may also be IgG and IgA. They are usually reactive by direct agglutination of Lu(a+) red cells but often also react by an IAT. Antibodies to other Lutheran antigens are most often IgG and react best by IAT.

THE KELL AND Kx SYSTEMS

The antigen often referred to as Kell, but correctly named K or KEL1, is the original antigen of the Kell system and the first blood group antigen to be identified following the discovery of the antiglobulin test in 1946. Its antithetical antigen, k or KEL2, was identified 3 years later. The Kell system now consists of 32 antigens numbered from KEL1 to KEL35, with three obsolete.[4(pp295-323),21] They include five pairs (K/k, Js^a/Js^b, K11/K17, K14/K24, VLAN/VONG) and one triplet (Kp^a/Kp^b/Kp^c) of Kell antithetical antigens. Initially most antigens joined the Kell system through genetic associations observed by family studies. These associations have now been confirmed by DNA sequencing of the *KEL* gene.

The Kell Glycoprotein and the *KEL* Gene

The Kell antigens are located on a red cell membrane glycoprotein (CD238) with four or five N-glycans but no O-glycosylation. It is unique as a blood group antigen because it is a Type II membrane glycoprotein; it spans the membrane once and has a short N-terminal

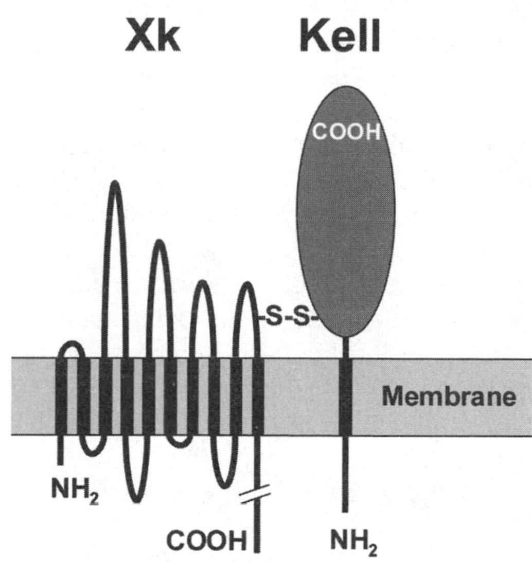

FIGURE 14-4. Diagram of the Kell and Xk proteins linked by a single disulfide bond. The Xk protein has cytoplasmic N- and C-terminal domains and 10 membrane-spanning domains. The Kell glycoprotein has a large, folded, extracellular, C-terminal domain and an intracellular N-terminal domain.

domain (47 amino acids) in the cytosol and a large C-terminal domain (665 amino acids) outside the membrane (Fig 14-4).[22] The extracellular domain has 15 cysteine residues and is extensively folded by disulfide bonding, although crystallographic studies are required to determine the three-dimensional structure of the molecule. Kell system antigens are dependent on the conformation of the glycoprotein and are sensitive to disulfide-bond-reducing agents such as DTT and AET.

The Kell glycoprotein is linked through a single disulfide bond to the Xk protein (Fig 14-4), an integral membrane protein that expresses the Kx blood group antigen (XK1). Absence of Xk protein from the red cell results in reduced expression of the Kell glycoprotein and weakened Kell antigens (McLeod phenotype, see below).

The *KEL* gene is located on chromosome 7q34. It is organized into 19 exons of coding sequence: exon 1 encodes the probable translation-initiating methionine; exon 2, the cytosolic domain; exon 3, the membrane-spanning domain; and exons 4 through 19, the large extracellular domain.

Kell Antigens

K (KEL1) has a prevalence of about 9% in people of European ethnicity and about 1.5% in people of African ethnicity, and it is rare in East Asia (Table 14-3). The k (KEL2) antigen is of high prevalence in all populations. K and k result from a single nucleotide polymorphism (SNP) in exon 6, which encodes Met193 in K and Thr193 in k. Asn191 is N-glycosylated in the product of the *k* allele but not the *K* allele.

Kp^a (KEL3) is found in about 2% of Whites and is not present in Blacks or in Japanese (Table 14-3); Kp^b (KEL4) is of high prevalence in all populations. Whereas 2.3% of Whites are Kp(a+), only 1.2% of K+ Whites are Kp(a+). Nine percent of Whites are K+, but only 2.7% of Kp(a+) people from the same population are K+. This strong allelic association was confirmed by family studies. Only one example of the KKp^a haplotype has been found.[23] Kp^c (KEL21), an antigen of very low prevalence, is

TABLE 14-3. Frequencies of Some Kell Phenotypes

Phenotype	Frequency (%)	
	Whites	Blacks
K– k+	91	98
K+ k+	8.8	2
K+ k–	0.2	Rare
Kp(a–b+)	97.7	100
Kp(a+b+)	2.3	Rare
Kp(a+b–)	Rare	0
Js(a–b+)	100	80
Js(a+b+)	Rare	19
Js(a+b–)	0	1

K, Kp^a, and Js^a are extremely rare in Asian populations.

the product of another allele of *Kp^a^* and *Kp^b^*. *KEL* alleles encoding the three Kp antigens differ by single base substitutions within codon 281 (exon 8): *Kp^a^*, TGG, Trp281; *Kp^b^*, CGG, Arg281; and *Kp^c^*, CAG, Gln281. The mutation associated with Kp^a expression appears to reduce the quantity of Kell glycoprotein in the red cell membranes, giving rise to a slight reduction in expression of Kell antigens in Kp^a/Kp^a homozygotes but a more obvious weakening of Kell antigens in individuals heterozygous for Kp^a and the null allele K^0.

Js^a (KEL6) is almost completely confined to people of African ethnicity. The prevalence of Js^a in African Americans is about 20% (Table 14-3). Js^b (KEL7) is of high prevalence in all populations, and Js(a+b–) has not been found in a person of non-African ethnicity. Js^a represents Pro597; Js^b, Leu597.

K17 (Wk^a) (Ala302) has a prevalence of 0.3% in English donors; K11 (Val302), its antithetical antigen, is of very high prevalence. K14 (Arg180) and K24 (Pro180) are very high- and very low-prevalence antigens, respectively. VLAN (KEL25) and VONG (KEL28) are low-prevalence antigens associated with Arg248Gln and Arg248Trp, respectively.

Presence of the low-prevalence antigens Ul^a, K23, and KYO and absence of the high-prevalence antigens K12, K13, K18, K19, K22, TOU, RAZ, KALT, KTIM, KUCI, KASH, KANT, and KELP all result from single amino acid substitutions in the Kell glycoprotein.

Kell antigens are resistant to papain, ficin, trypsin, and α-chymotrypsin but are destroyed by a mixture of trypsin and α-chymotrypsin. They are also destroyed by DTT and AET (see above) and by EDTA glycine.

Kell Antibodies and Their Clinical Significance

Kell antibodies are usually IgG and predominantly IgG1.[5(pp211-213)] They should be considered potentially clinically significant from the point of view of causing severe HDFN and HTRs. Patients with Kell antibodies should be transfused with antigen-negative blood whenever possible.

Anti-K is the most common immune red cell antibody outside the ABO and Rh systems; one-third of all non-Rh red cell immune antibodies are anti-K. An antiglobulin test is usually the method of choice for detection, although occasional examples may agglutinate red cells directly. Most anti-K appear to be induced by blood transfusion. Because anti-K can cause severe HDFN, it is usual practice in some countries for girls and women of childbearing potential to receive only K– red cells. Anti-K, -k, -Kp^a, -Kp^b, -Js^a, -Js^b, -Ku, -Ul^a, -K11, -K19, and -K22 are all reported to have caused severe HDFN. Anti-K, -k, -Kp^b, -Js^a, -Js^b, -Ku, and -K19 have all been implicated in acute or delayed HTRs.

The pathogenesis of HDFN caused by anti-K differs from that resulting from anti-D. Anti-K HDFN is associated with lower concentrations of amniotic fluid bilirubin than anti-D HDFN of comparable severity. Postnatal hyperbilirubinemia is not prominent in infants with anemia caused by anti-K. There is also reduced reticulocytosis and erythroblastosis in the anti-K disease compared with anti-D HDFN. These symptoms suggest that anti-K HDFN is associated with a lower degree of hemolysis and that fetal anemia in anti-K HDFN results predominantly from a suppression of erythropoiesis. The Kell glycoprotein appears on erythroid progenitors at a much earlier stage of erythropoiesis than do Rh antigens. Consequently, anti-K probably facilitates phagocytosis of K+ erythroid progenitors at an early stage of development by macrophages in the fetal liver, before the erythroid cells produce hemoglobin.[24]

Antibodies mimicking Kell specificities have been responsible for severe AIHA. Presence of the autoantibody is often associated with apparent depression of all Kell antigens.

Although most examples of anti-K are stimulated by pregnancy or transfusion, a few cases of apparently non-red-cell immune anti-K have been described. In some cases the antibodies were found in untransfused, healthy, male blood donors; in others microbial infection was implicated as an immunizing agent.

Null (K_0) and Mod Phenotypes

Like most blood group systems, Kell has a null phenotype (K_0), in which none of the Kell antigens is expressed and the Kell glycoprotein cannot be detected in the membrane. Immunized K_0 individuals may produce anti-Ku (anti-KEL5), an antibody that reacts with all cells except those of the K_0 phenotype. Homozygosity for a variety of nonsense mutations, missense mutations, and splice site mutations have been associated with K_0 phenotype.[25]

K_{mod} red cells have only very weak expression of Kell antigens, and individuals with this phenotype are homozygous (or doubly heterozygous) for missense mutations, resulting in single amino acid substitutions within the Kell glycoprotein.[26] Some K_{mod} individuals make an antibody that resembles anti-Ku but differs from anti-Ku by being nonreactive with K_{mod} cells.

Other phenotypes in which Kell antigens are substantially depressed in expression result from Kp^a/K^0 heterozygosity (see above), absence of Xk protein (see below), and absence of the Gerbich antigens Ge2 and Ge3, which are located on the glycophorins C and D. The reason for this phenotypic association between Kell and Gerbich is not known, although Kell glycoproteins, Xk, and glycophorins C and D could all be located within the same membrane protein complex (Fig 14-1).

Functional Aspects

The Kell protein has structural and sequence homology with a family of zinc-dependent endopeptidases that process a variety of peptide hormones. Although the function of the Kell glycoprotein is not known, it is enzymatically active and is able to cleave the biologically inactive peptide big-endothelin-3 to create the biologically active vasoconstrictor endothelin-3. Consequently, Kell might play a role in regulating vascular tone, but there is no direct evidence for this.[27] No obvious pathogenesis is associated with the K_0 phenotype.

In addition to erythroid cells, Kell antigens may be present on myeloid progenitor cells, and Kell glycoprotein has been detected in testis, lymphoid tissues, and with Xk protein in skeletal muscle.

Kx Antigen (XK1), McLeod Syndrome, and McLeod Phenotype

Kx is the only antigen of the Kx blood group system. It is located on a polytopic protein that spans the red cell membrane 10 times and is linked to the Kell glycoprotein by a single disulfide bond (Fig 14-4). Xk protein is encoded by the XK gene on chromosome Xp21.1.

McLeod syndrome is a very rare X-linked condition found almost exclusively in males and is associated with acanthocytosis and a variety of late-onset muscular, neurologic, and psychiatric symptoms. It results from hemizygosity for inactivating mutations and deletions of the XK gene.[28] McLeod syndrome is associated with McLeod phenotype, in which Kell antigens are expressed weakly and Km (KEL20) as well as Kx are absent. The function of the Xk-Kell complex is not known, but Xk has structural resemblance to a family of neurotransmitter transporters.

Deletion of part of the X chromosome that includes *XK* may also include *CYBB*, absence of which is responsible for X-linked chronic granulomatous disease (CGD). When transfused, CGD patients with McLeod syndrome usually produce anti-Kx plus anti-Km, making it almost impossible to find compatible donors. It is recommended, therefore, that transfusion of males with CGD and McLeod syndrome be avoided.

THE DUFFY SYSTEM

The Duffy system[4(pp324-341),21] officially comprises five antigens that reside on a glycoprotein encoded by the Duffy gene *(DARC)*, which consists of two exons, with exon 1 encoding only the first seven amino acids of the Duffy glycoprotein. *DARC* is on chromosome 1q23.2.

Fy^a (FY1) and Fy^b (FY2)

In Whites and Asians the Duffy polymorphism consists of two antigens, Fy^a and Fy^b, giving rise to three phenotypes, Fy(a+b–), Fy(a+b+),

TABLE 14-4. Duffy Phenotypes and Genotypes in Selected Populations

	Genotype		Frequency (%)		
Phenotype	European and Asian Ethnicity	African Ethnicity	Whites	African Americans	Japanese
Fy(a+b–)	*Fy^a/Fy^a*	*Fy^a/Fy^a* or *Fy^a/Fy*	20	10	81
Fy(a+b+)	*Fy^a/Fy^b*	*Fy^a/Fy^b*	48	3	15
Fy(a–b+)	*Fy^b/Fy^b*	*Fy^b/Fy^b* or *Fy^b/Fy*	32	20	4
Fy(a–b–)		*Fy/Fy*	0	67	0

and Fy(a–b+) (Table 14-4). The *Fy^a* and *Fy^b* alleles represent an SNP in exon 2 of *DARC*, encoding Gly42 and Asp42, respectively, in the N-terminal extracellular domain of the glycoprotein (Fig 14-5). Fy^a and Fy^b are very sensitive to most proteolytic enzymes, including papain, ficin, and bromelin, but are not destroyed by trypsin. In people of African ethnicity there is a third allele, *Fy*, more abundant than *Fy^a* and *Fy^b*. *Fy* produces no Duffy glycoprotein on red cells, and hence neither Fy^a nor Fy^b. Individuals homozygous for *Fy* have the red cell phenotype Fy(a–b–), the prevalence of which varies from about 70% in African Americans to 100% in Gambia (Table 14-4).

The coding region for the *Fy* allele in Africans is identical to that of the Fy^b allele, encoding Asp42. *Fy* produces no Duffy glycoprotein and no Fy^b antigen in red cells because of an SNP in the promoter region of *DARC*. This mutation disrupts the binding site for the erythroid-specific GATA-1 transcription factor and prevents expression of the gene in erythroid tissue.[29] Duffy glycoprotein is present on many cells throughout the body. Fy(a–b–) Africans lack Duffy glycoprotein on their red cells but not on cells from other tissues. This explains why they do not make anti-Fy^b and only very rarely make anti-Fy3 or anti-Fy5 (see below). Although in Africans the GATA-1 binding site mutation has been found only in Duffy genes with the *Fy^b* sequence, the mutation has been detected in silent *Fy^a* alleles in Papua New Guinea and in Brazil.

Fy^x is a weak form of Fy^b resulting from an *Fy^b* allele with a missense mutation encoding an Arg89Cys substitution in a cytosolic domain of the glycoprotein (Fig 14-5).

Fy3, Fy4, Fy5, and Fy6

Very rare non-Africans with Fy(a–b–) red cells are homozygous for inactivating mutations in their *DARC* genes. These individuals have no Duffy glycoprotein on their red cells and would not be expected to have it in any other tissues. All were found through the presence of

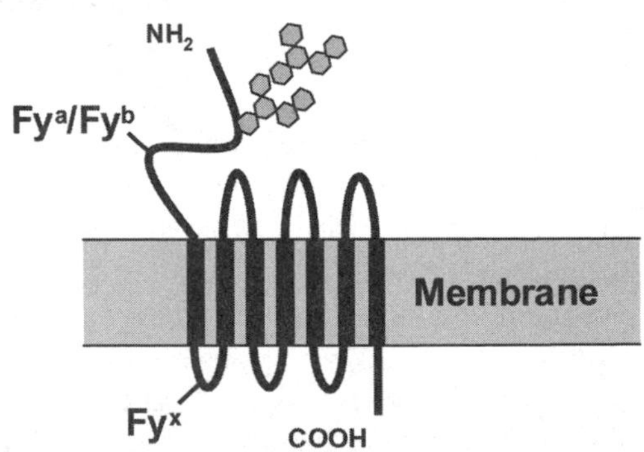

FIGURE 14-5. Diagram of the Duffy glycoprotein (DARC), with a glycosylated external N-terminal domain, seven membrane-spanning domains, and cytoplasmic C-terminus. The positions of the Fy^a/Fy^b polymorphism and of the amino acid substitution responsible for the Fy^x phenotype are shown.

anti-Fy3 in their sera, an antibody that reacts with all red cells except those of the Fy(a–b–) phenotype. Unlike Fy^a and Fy^b, Fy3 is protease resistant. Fy5 is also absent from cells of the Fy(a–b–) phenotype, but unlike Fy3, Fy5 is also absent from cells of the Rh_{null} phenotype. The Duffy glycoprotein may belong to the junctional membrane protein complex, which also contains Rh proteins (Fig 14-1).[10] Anti-Fy5 has been found only in multitransfused individuals of African ethnicity. Anti-Fy6 was the symbol given to a monoclonal antibody that gave serologic reactions very similar to those of anti-Fy3. Anti-Fy4 appeared to react with red cells of individuals with the silent *Fy* allele. However, the work could not be repeated, and the antibody is no longer available and Fy4 is now obsolete.

Duffy Antibodies and Their Clinical Significance

Anti-Fy^a is a relatively common antibody; anti-Fy^b is about 20 times less common.[5(p215)] IgG1 usually predominates, and these antibodies are generally detected by an antiglobulin test. Naturally occurring examples are very rare.

Anti-Fy^a and anti-Fy^b may cause acute or delayed HTRs. Although generally mild, some have proved fatal. These antibodies have also been responsible for HDFN, varying from mild to severe. Anti-Fy3 has been responsible for acute and delayed HTRs, and anti-Fy5 for delayed HTRs.

The Duffy Glycoprotein, a Receptor for Chemokines

The Duffy glycoprotein, also known as the Duffy antigen receptor for chemokines (DARC), is a red cell receptor for a variety of chemokines, including interleukin-8 (IL-8), monocyte chemotactic protein-1 (MCP-1), and melanoma growth stimulatory activity (MGSA).[30] It traverses the membrane seven times, with a 63-amino-acid extracellular N-terminal domain containing two potential N-glycosylation sites, and a cytoplasmic C-terminal domain (Fig 14-5). This arrangement is characteristic of the G protein-coupled superfamily of receptors, which includes chemokine receptors.

The function of the DARC on red cells is not known. It has been suggested that it might act as a clearance receptor for inflammatory mediators and that Duffy-positive red cells function as a "sink" or as scavengers for the removal of unwanted chemokines.[31] If so, this function must be of limited importance because Duffy is not present on the red cells of most individuals of African ancestry. It has been suggested that DARC on red cells reduces angiogenesis, and consequently the progression of prostate cancer, by clearing angiogenic chemokines from the tumor microenvironment. This potential effect of erythroid DARC could provide an explanation for the substantially higher levels of prostate cancer in men of African ancestry compared with those of European ancestry.[8]

DARC is present in many organs, where it is expressed on endothelial cells lining post-capillary venules.[32] Duffy glycoprotein on vascular endothelium may be involved in the inhibition of cancer-cell metastasis and induction of cellular senescence.[8] DARC may also function to facilitate movement of chemokines across the endothelium.

Duffy and Malaria

The Duffy glycoprotein is a receptor for merozoites of *Plasmodium vivax*, the parasite responsible for a form of malaria widely distributed in Africa but less severe than malaria resulting from *P. falciparum* infection. Red cells with the Fy(a–b–) phenotype are resistant to invasion by *P. vivax* merozoites. Consequently, the *Fy* allele confers a selective advantage in areas where *P. vivax* is endemic; this advantage probably balances with any potential disadvantage resulting from absence of the chemokine receptor on red cells.[33]

THE KIDD SYSTEM

Kidd comprises three antigens located on a glycoprotein with 10 membrane-spanning domains, cytoplasmic N- and C-termini, and one extracellular N-glycosylation site (Fig 14-6).[4(pp342-351),21] The Kidd gene (*SLC14A1*) contains 11 exons, with exons 4 through 11 encod-

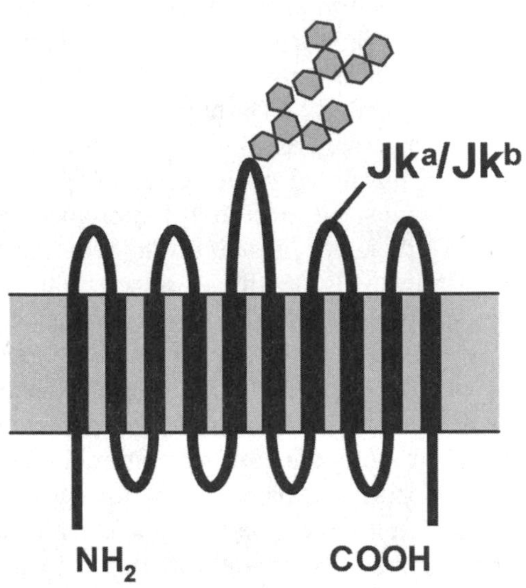

FIGURE 14-6. Diagram of the Kidd glycoprotein, a urea transporter, with cytoplasmic N- and C-terminal domains, 10 membrane-spanning domains, and an N-glycan on the third extracellular loop. The position of the Jk^a/Jk^b polymorphism is shown on the fourth external loop.

ing the mature protein, and is located on chromosome 18q12.3.

Jk^a (JK1) and Jk^b (JK2)

Jk^a and Jk^b are the products of alleles, representing Asp280 and Asn280 in the fourth external loop of the Kidd glycoprotein (Fig 14-6). They have similar prevalences to each other in White and Asian populations, but Jk^a is more abundant than Jk^b in Blacks (Table 14-5). Kidd antigens are resistant to proteolytic enzymes such as papain and ficin.

Jk(a–b–) and Jk3

The null phenotype, Jk(a–b–) Jk:–3, usually results from homozygosity for a silent gene at the *JK* locus. Although very rare in most populations, the null phenotype is relatively common in Polynesians, with a prevalence of around 1 in 400, but as high as 1.4% in Niueans. The Polynesian null allele contains a splice site mutation in intron 5, resulting in the loss of exon 6 from the mRNA. In Finns, where Jk(a–b–) is less rare than in other populations of European ethnicity, the mutation responsible encodes a Ser291Pro substitution. Immunized individuals with the Jk(a–b–) phenotype may produce anti-Jk3. An extremely rare form of Jk(a–b–) phenotype found in Japanese results from heterozygosity for a dominant inhibitor gene, named *In(Jk)* in analogy with the *In(Lu)* dominant inhibitor of Lutheran and other antigens. Very weak expression of Jk^a and/or Jk^b can be detected on In(Jk) red cells by adsorption/elution tests.

Kidd Antibodies and Their Clinical Significance

Anti-Jk^a and -Jk^b are not common antibodies and are generally found in antibody mixtures. They are usually IgG1 and IgG3, but some are partly IgG2, IgG4, or IgM. About 50% of anti-Jk^a and -Jk^b bind complement.[5(pp216-217)] Kidd antibodies are often difficult to detect. Some directly agglutinate antigen-positive cells, but the reactions are usually weak by this method. Generally, an antiglobulin test is required, and use of enzyme-treated cells may be necessary to detect weaker antibodies.

Kidd antibodies are dangerous, as they may cause severe acute HTRs. They are also a very common cause of delayed HTRs, probably because they are often not detected in pretransfusion testing because of their tendency to drop to low or undetectable levels in the plasma. Anti-Jk3 can also cause acute or de-

TABLE 14-5. Kidd Phenotypes in Three Populations

	Frequency (%)		
Phenotype	**Whites**	**Blacks**	**Asians**
Jk(a+b–)	26	52	23
Jk(a+b+)	50	40	50
Jk(a–b+)	24	8	27

layed HTRs. Despite their hemolytic potential, Kidd antibodies only very rarely cause severe HDFN.

Kidd antibodies have been implicated in acute renal transplant rejection, suggesting that Kidd antigens can behave as histocompatibility antigens.[34]

The Kidd Glycoprotein, a Urea Transporter

The Kidd antigens are located on a red cell urea transporter, also known as human urea transporter 11 (HUT11 or UT-B1).[35] When red cells approach the renal medulla, which contains a high concentration of urea, the urea transporter permits rapid uptake of urea and prevents the cells from shrinking in the hypertonic environment. As the red cells leave the renal medulla, urea is transported rapidly out of the cells, preventing the cells from swelling and carrying urea away from the kidney. HUT11 was detected on endothelial cells of the vasa recta, the vascular supply of the renal medulla, but it is not present in renal tubules.

Normal red cells are rapidly lysed by 2M urea because urea transported into the cells makes them hypertonic and they burst as a result of the osmotic influx of water. Because of the absence of the urea transporter, Jk(a–b–) cells are not hemolyzed by 2M urea, and this can be used as a method for screening for Jk(a–b–) donors.[36]

The Jk(a–b–) phenotype is not associated with any clinical defect, although two unrelated Jk(a–b–) individuals had a mild urine-concentrating defect.[37]

THE DIEGO SYSTEM

Band 3, the Red Cell Anion Exchanger

The 22 antigens of the Diego system are located on Band 3, the common name for the red cell anion exchanger or solute carrier family 4 A1 (*SLC4A1*).[38] Band 3 is a major red cell membrane glycoprotein with approximately 10^6 copies per red cell. In addition to a transmembrane domain that traverses the membrane about 14 times, with an N-glycan on the fourth extracellular loop, Band 3 has a long cytoplasmic N-terminal domain that interacts with the membrane skeleton proteins ankyrin, 4.1R, and protein 4.2 and also functions as a binding site for hemoglobin (Figs 14-1 and 14-7). The short, cytoplasmic C-terminal domain binds carbonic anhydrase II. Band 3 in red cells has at least two major functions: the rapid exchange of HCO_3^- and Cl^- ions, important in CO_2 transport, and attachment of the red cell membrane to the cytoskeleton.[10] Tetramers of Band 3 form the core of the Band 3/Rh ankyrin macrocomplex of red cell membrane proteins, which could function as a gas channel for O_2 and CO_2.[9] Band 3 is also a component of the junctional complex that links the red cell membrane to the membrane skeleton via glycophorin C (Fig 14-1).[10] The Band 3 gene (*SLC4A1*) consists of 20 exons of coding sequence and is on chromosome 17.

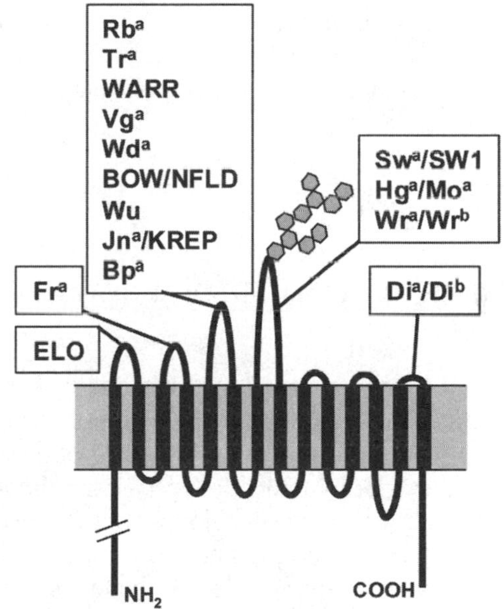

FIGURE 14-7. Diagram of Band 3, the Diego glycoprotein and anion exchanger, with cytoplasmic N- and C-terminal domains, 14 membrane-spanning domains, and an N-glycan on the fourth extracellular loop (although the precise conformation is still controversial). The locations of 21 antigens of Diego system on the extracellular loops are shown.

Di^a (DI1) and Di^b (DI2); Anti-Di^a and -Di^b

Di^a, the original Diego antigen, is very rare in people of European and African ancestry but has a prevalence of 5% in Chinese and Japanese and a higher prevalence in the native peoples of North and South America, reaching 54% in the Kainganges Indians of Brazil. Di^b is a high-prevalence antigen in almost all populations. Di^a and Di^b represent an amino acid substitution in the seventh extracellular loop of Band 3—Leu854 in Di^a and Pro854 in Di^b.

Anti-Di^a and -Di^b are usually IgG1 plus IgG3 and generally require an antiglobulin test for detection, although a few directly agglutinating examples have been found. Anti-Di^a occasionally binds complement and lyses untreated red cells. Anti-Di^a, which is present in 3.6% of multitransfused patients in Brazil, can cause severe HDFN. Anti-Di^b has, very rarely, been responsible for serious HDFN. Apart from one example of anti-Di^a causing a delayed reaction, neither anti-Di^a nor anti-Di^b has been reported to be responsible for an HTR.[4(p356),5(p226)]

Antigens of the Diego system are not destroyed by proteolytic enzymes such as papain, ficin, or trypsin.

Wr^a (DI3) and Wr^b (DI4); Anti-Wr^a and -Wr^b

The low-prevalence antigen Wr^a and its antithetical antigen of extremely high prevalence, Wr^b, represent an amino acid substitution in the fourth loop of Band 3—Lys658 in Wr^a and Glu658 in Wr^b. Wr^b expression, however, is also dependent on the presence of GPA. Despite homozygosity for the Glu658 codon in the Band 3 gene, Wr^b is not expressed in the rare phenotypes where there is complete absence of the MN glycoprotein GPA or absence of that part of GPA close to insertion into the red cell membrane. This provides strong evidence for an interaction between Band 3 and GPA within the red cell membrane.

Anti-Wr^a is a relatively common antibody, usually detected by an antiglobulin test but sometimes by direct agglutination of red cells. Wr^a antibodies are mostly IgG1 but sometimes IgM or IgM plus IgG. Anti-Wr^a has been responsible for severe HDFN and for HTRs. Alloanti-Wr^b is rare and little is known about its clinical significance, but autoanti-Wr^b is a relatively common autoantibody and may be implicated in AIHA.

Other Diego Antigens

Since 1996, 17 antigens of very low prevalence have been shown to represent amino acid substitutions in Band 3 and have joined the Diego system. These antigens are named Wd^a, Rb^a, WARR, ELO, Wu, Bp^a, Mo^a, Hg^a, Vg^a, Sw^a, BOW, NFLD, Jn^a, Krep, Tr^a, Fr^a, and SW1. Anti-DISK detects a high-prevalence antigen that is antithetical to Wu. Anti-ELO and anti-BOW have caused severe HDFN.

THE Yt SYSTEM

Yt^a (YT1, His353) and Yt^b (YT2, Asn353) are antithetical antigens on acetylcholinesterase, an enzyme important in neurotransmission but of unknown function on red cells. Yt^b has a prevalence of about 8% in people of European and African ancestry but has not been found in Japanese; Yt^a is of relatively high prevalence in all populations. Yt^a is not affected by trypsin but is destroyed by α-chymotrypsin treatment of the red cells; papain and ficin may also destroy the antigen, but this appears to depend on the anti-Yt^a used. Yt^a and Yt^b are sensitive to the disulfide-bond-reducing agents AET and DTT.

Yt antibodies are usually IgG and require an IAT for detection. They are not generally considered clinically significant, although anti-Yt^a may cause accelerated destruction of Yt(a+) transfused red cells and has been implicated in acute and delayed HTRs.[4(p371),38]

THE Xg SYSTEM

Xg^a (XG1) is the only polymorphic blood group antigen encoded by an X-linked gene.[38] Xg^a has a prevalence of about 66% in males and 89% in females. Part of the XG gene is within the X chromosome pseudoautosomal region, a section at the tip of the short arm that pairs with the Y chromosome. CD99 (XG2) is the second antigen of the Xg system. *CD99* gene is homologous to *XG* and is located on both X and Y chromosomes, with pairing occurring at meiosis. Both CD99 and Xg^a expression appear to be controlled by a common regulator gene, *XGR*. Although Xg^a antibodies occasionally agglutinate red cells directly, they are generally IgG and react by an IAT. They do not react with red cells treated with proteolytic enzymes. Anti-Xg^a is not clinically significant. CD99 antibodies in common use are mostly monoclonal of mouse origin; a few human alloanti-CD99 occur, although little is known of their characteristics.

THE SCIANNA SYSTEM

Scianna consists of seven antigens on erythrocyte membrane-associated protein (ERMAP), a member of the IgSF, with one IgSF domain.[38,39] SC1 (Gly57) and SC2 (Arg57) are antithetical antigens of high and low prevalence, respectively. Rd (SC4) is of very low prevalence; SC3, STAR (SC5), SCER (SC6), and SCAN (SC7) are all of very high prevalence. Anti-SC3 is produced by individuals with the very rare Scianna-null phenotype.

No Scianna antibody has been implicated in an HTR or in severe HDFN, although evidence is limited because of the scarcity of the antibodies. Although directly agglutinating SC1 antibodies are known, Scianna antibodies are generally reactive by an IAT. Treatment of red cells by proteolytic enzymes has little effect on their reactivity with Scianna antibodies, but disulfide-bond-reducing agents (AET and DTT) substantially reduce reactivity.

THE DOMBROCK SYSTEM

The Dombrock system consists of seven antigens: the polymorphic antithetical antigens Do^a (DO1, Asn265) and Do^b (DO2, Asp265), and the high-prevalence antigens Gy^a (DO3), Hy (DO4), Jo^a (DO5), DOYA (DO6), and DOMR.[2,40] Do^a and Do^b have a prevalence of 66% and 82%, respectively, in populations of European ancestry (Table 14-6). The prevalence of Do^a is somewhat lower in populations of African ancestry and substantially lower in people from the Far East. Anti-Gy^a is the antibody characteristically produced by immunized individuals with the Dombrock-null phenotype, which results from various inactivating mutations. Two uncommon phenotypes are found in individuals of African eth-

TABLE 14-6. Phenotypes of the Dombrock System and Their Approximate Frequencies

						Frequency (%)	
Phenotype	Do^a	Do^b	Gy^a	Hy	Jo^a	Whites	Blacks
Do(a+b–)	+	–	+	+	+	18	11
Do(a+b+)	+	+	+	+	+	49	44
Do(a–b+)	–	+	+	+	+	33	45
Gy(a–)	–	–	–	–	–	Rare	0
Hy–	–	$+^w$	$+^w$	–	–	0	Rare
Jo(a–)	$+^w$	–/$+^w$	+	$+^w$	–	0	Rare
DOYA–	–	–	$+^w$	$+^w$	$+^w$	Rare	Rare
DOMR–	–	+	–	$+^w$	$+^w$	Rare	Rare

$+^w$ = weakened expression of antigen.

nicity: Hy– Jo(a–) (Gly108Val) and Hy+^{w} Jo(a–) (Thr117Ile), usually associated with weak expression of Do^{b} and Do^{a}, respectively (Table 14-6). The Dombrock glycoprotein (CD297) has a structure characteristic of an ADP-ribosyltransferase, and the Dombrock gene has been given the symbol *ART4*.

Dombrock antigens are resistant to papain and ficin treatment of the red cells but are sensitive to trypsin, α-chymotrypsin, and pronase. They are also sensitive to the disulfide-bond-reducing agents AET and DTT.

Dombrock antibodies are usually IgG and reactive by an IAT. They are in short supply and are often of poor quality with very weak reactivity. Screening for Dombrock-compatible donors, therefore, is best performed by molecular genetics (SNP testing). Anti-Do^{a} and -Do^{b} have been responsible for acute and delayed HTRs. There is little information regarding the clinical significance of other Dombrock antibodies. No Dombrock antibody has caused HDFN.

THE COLTON SYSTEM

Co^{a} (Ala45) is a high-prevalence antigen; Co^{b} (Val45), its antithetical antigen, has a prevalence of about 8% in Whites, but lower in other ethnic groups.[38] Anti-Co3 reacts with all red cells except those of the extremely rare Colton-null phenotype, which results from various inactivating mutations. The Colton antigens are located on Aquaporin-1, a water channel (Fig 14-8).[41] Colton antibodies are usually IgG and reactive by an IAT, although agglutinating IgM

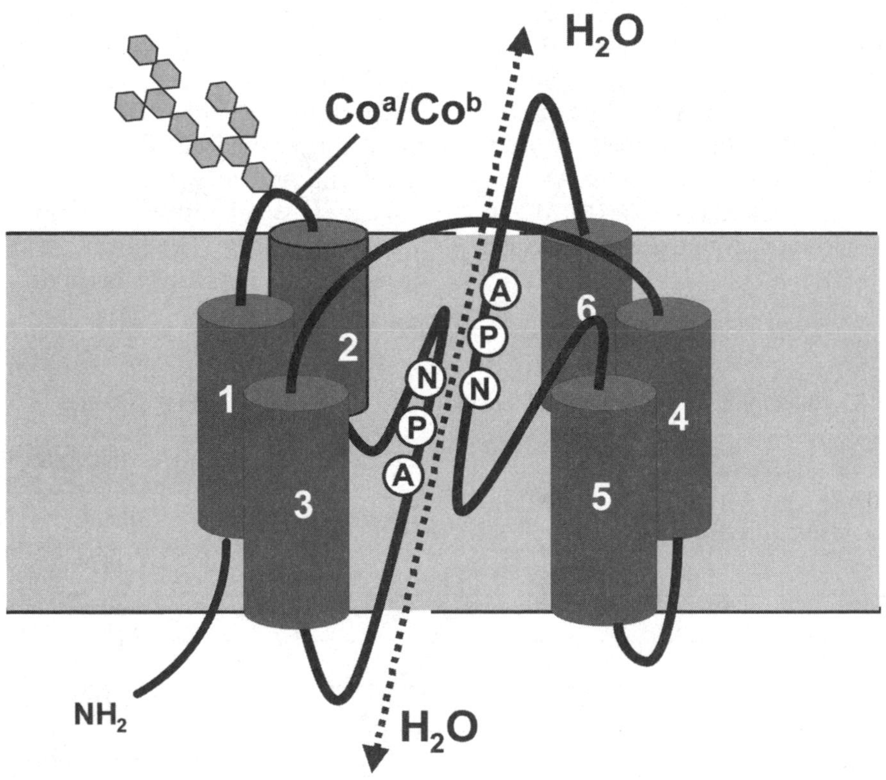

FIGURE 14-8. A three-dimensional model of aquaporin-1, showing the six membrane-spanning domains as cylinders. The first extracellular loop is glycosylated and contains the Co^{a}/Co^{b} polymorphism. The third extracellular loop and first intracellular loop contain alanine (A)-proline (P)-asparagine (N) motifs and form a channel in the membrane through which water molecules pass.

anti-Co^a has been found. Colton antibodies have been implicated in severe HDFN and in HTRs. Colton antigens are resistant to proteolytic enzymes.

THE LANDSTEINER-WIENER SYSTEM

LW^a and LW^b (Gln100Arg) are antithetical antigens of high and low prevalence, respectively.[38] Anti-LW^{ab} reacts with all red cells except those of the extremely rare LW-null phenotype and Rh_{null} cells, which are also LW(a–b–). LW antigens are expressed more strongly on D+ than D– red cells and more strongly on cord red cells than those of adults. They are unaffected by treatment of the red cells with papain, ficin, trypsin, or α-chymotrypsin but are destroyed by pronase. Disulfide-bond-reducing agents (AET and DTT) either destroy or greatly reduce LW^a or LW^{ab} on red cells.

The LW glycoprotein is intercellular adhesion molecule-4 (ICAM-4), an IgSF adhesion molecule. ICAM-4 binds integrins on macrophages and erythroblasts and is probably involved in the stabilization of erythroblastic islands in the marrow during the latter stages of erythropoiesis.[41] ICAM-4 is also part of the Band 3/Rh ankyrin macrocomplex (Fig 14-1) of red cell surface antigens and might function to maintain close contact between the red cell surface and the vascular endothelium.[9] Upregulation of ICAM-4 on red cells of patients with sickle cell disease could play a part in adhesion of these cells to the vascular endothelium and the resultant crises of vascular occlusion.[17]

Most LW antibodies are reactive by an IAT. They are not generally considered clinically significant and have not been implicated in HTRs or HDFN. Acquired and often temporary LW-negative phenotypes sometimes occur with production of anti-LW^a or anti-LW^{ab}, a phenomenon usually associated with pregnancy or hematologic malignancy. The transient antibodies behave like alloantibodies but strictly speaking should be considered autoantibodies.

THE CHIDO/RODGERS SYSTEM

The nine antigens of the Chido/Rodgers system are not true blood group antigens, as they are not produced by erythroid cells. They are located on a fragment of the fourth component of complement (C4d), which attaches to the red cells from the plasma. Ch1 to Ch6 (CH/RG1-CH/RG6), Rg1 (CH/RG11), and Rg2 (CH/RG12) have prevalences greater than 90%; WH (CH/RG7) has a prevalence of about 15%. A complex relationship exists between these nine determinants and SNPs in *C4A* and *C4B*, the genes encoding the C4α chains. Expression of Chido/Rodgers on red cells is destroyed by treatment of the cells with proteolytic enzymes such as papain or ficin.

No Chido/Rodgers antibodies are known to have caused HTRs or HDFN, and antigen-negative blood is not required for transfusion. Chido/Rodgers antibodies are generally IgG. Detection of these antibodies with native red cells usually requires an IAT, but they often directly agglutinate red cells coated artificially with C4d. Binding of Chido/Rodgers antibodies to red cells is readily inhibited by plasma from Ch/Rg+ individuals; this is useful as an aid to identification of these antibodies (Method 3-9).

THE GERBICH SYSTEM

The Gerbich system consists of six antigens of very high prevalence—Ge2, Ge3, Ge4, GEPL, GEAT, and GETI—and five antigens of very low prevalence—Wb (GE5), Ls^a (GE6), An^a (GE6), Dh^a (GE7), and GEIS (GE8). They are located on the sialoglycoproteins glycophorin C (GPC) or glycophorin D (GPD), or on both. These two glycoproteins are produced by the same gene, *GYPC*, by initiation of translation at two different sites on the mRNA. GPD lacks the N-terminal 21 amino acids of GPC. GPC and GPD are part of the junctional complex of membrane proteins. Their C-terminal cytoplasmic domains interact with the membrane skeleton through 4.1R, p55, and adducin and are important in functioning as a link between the membrane and its skeleton.[10,41] GPC appears to be exploited as a receptor by some strains of the malarial parasite *P. falciparum.*

There are three types of "Gerbich-negative" phenotypes (Table 14-7): Ge:–2,–3,–4, the true null in which both GPC and GPD are absent from the red cells, and Ge:–2,3,4 and Ge:–2,–3,4, in which GPD is absent and an abnormal form of GPC is present. Ge2, Ge3, and Ge4 are destroyed by trypsin treatment of red cells, but whereas Ge2 and Ge4 are also sensitive to papain, Ge3 is resistant to papain treatment. Consequently, papain-treated red cells can be used for distinguishing anti-Ge2 from anti-Ge3 in the absence of the very rare Ge:–2,3,4 phenotype red cells.

Gerbich antibodies may be IgM and directly agglutinating, but most are IgG and require an IAT for detection. They are not generally considered clinically significant and have not caused HTRs, but anti-Ge3 has caused HDFN that tends to manifest 2 to 4 weeks after birth. Some autoantibodies with specificities resembling anti-Ge2 or -Ge3 have been responsible for AIHA.

THE CROMER SYSTEM

The 16 Cromer antigens are located on the complement-regulatory glycoprotein, decay accelerating factor (DAF or CD55).[2,42] They include the antithetical antigens Tc^a (CROM2, Arg52), Tc^b (CROM3, Leu52), and Tc^c (CROM4, Pro52); and WES^a (CROM8, Arg82) and WES^b (CROM9, Leu82). Tc^a and WES^b are of high prevalence, and Tc^b, Tc^c, and WES^a, of low prevalence, although both Tc^b and WES^a have a prevalence of around 0.5% in Blacks, and WES^a was also found in 0.6% of Finns. Other antigens—Cr^a, Dr^a, Es^a, IFC, UMC, GUTI, SERF, ZENA, CROV, CRAM, and CROZ—are all of high prevalence. Anti-IFC (CROM7) is the antibody made by individuals with the very rare Cromer-null phenotype (Inab phenotype) and reacts with all red cells, apart from those of individuals with the Inab phenotype. Cromer antigens are readily destroyed by α-chymotrypsin treatment of red cells but not by papain, ficin, or trypsin treatment. Disulfide-bond-reducing agents, AET and DTT, cause only slight reduction of antigen expression.

CD55 helps to protect the red cells from lysis by autologous complement by inhibiting the action of C3-convertases. Inab phenotype red cells do not undergo undue hemolysis, however, because of the activity of another complement regulatory glycoprotein, CD59. CD55 and CD59 are both linked to the red cell membrane by a glycosylphosphatidylinositol (GPI) anchor. Pathological levels of hemolysis occur in paroxysmal nocturnal hemoglobinuria (PNH), where there is a clonal defect of GPI biosynthesis and both CD55 and CD59 are absent from affected red cells.

Cromer antibodies are not usually considered clinically significant because there is no firm evidence that any antibody has caused an HTR, and the evidence from functional cellular assays is equivocal. No Cromer antibodies have been implicated in HDFN, and they are probably sequestered by high levels of CD55 in the placenta. Cromer antibodies are usually IgG and require an IAT for detection. They are inhibited by serum or concentrated urine from antigen-positive individuals and are removed from serum by platelet concentrates.

TABLE 14-7. Phenotypes Lacking High-Frequency Gerbich Antigens, and the Antibodies That May Be Produced

Phenotype	Antibodies
Ge:–2,3,4 (Yus type)	Anti-Ge2
Ge:–2,–3,4 (Ge type)	Anti-Ge2 or -Ge3
Ge:–2,–3,–4 (Leach type)	Anti-Ge2 or -Ge3 or -Ge4

THE KNOPS SYSTEM

The nine antigens of the Knops system are located on the complement-regulatory glycoprotein, complement receptor-1 (CR1 or CD35).[2,43] All are polymorphic, although Kn^a (KN1), McC^a (KN3), Sl1 (KN4), and Yk^a (KN5) are of relatively high prevalence (Table 14-8).

TABLE 14-8. Approximate Frequencies of Knops Antigens in Two Populations

Antigen		Frequency	
		Whites	Blacks
Kn^a	KN1	99	100
Kn^b	KN2	6	0
McC^a	KN3	98	94
Sl1 (Sl^a)	KN4	98	60
Yk^a	KN5	92	98
McC^b	KN6	0	45
Sl2	KN7	0	80
Sl3	KN8	100	100
KCAM	KN9	98	20

Kn^a/Kn^b (KN1/KN2) represent Val 1561Met; McC^a/McC^b (KN3/KN6), Lys1590Glu; and Sl1/Sl2 (KN4/KN7), Arg1601Gly. Sl3 (KN8) requires the presence of Ser1610 and Arg1601 (Sl2) for expression. Absence of KCAM (KN9) results from an Ile1615Val substitution. An apparent null phenotype, the Helgeson phenotype, represents very low levels of red cell CR1 and very weak expression of Knops antigens. Knops antigens are generally resistant to papain and ficin, although this may depend on the antibodies used, and are destroyed by trypsin or α-chymotrypsin treatment. They are also destroyed, or at least weakened, by AET and DTT.

CR1 appears to be involved in the rosetting of red cells associated with severe *P. falciparum* malaria, and the *McC^b* and *Sl2* alleles, found almost exclusively in individuals of African ancestry, may confer a degree of protection from the parasite. This might explain the very obvious difference in prevalence of some antigens, especially Sl1, McC^b, Sl2, and KCAM, between populations of European and African ethnicity (Table 14-8).

Knops antibodies are not clinically significant and can be ignored when selecting blood for transfusion.[3] They are usually difficult to work with, often making it difficult to distinguish antigen-negative cells from those with weak expression. They are generally IgG and reactive only by an IAT.

THE INDIAN SYSTEM

The low-prevalence antigen In^a (IN1, Arg46) and its antithetical antigen In^b (IN2, Pro46),[38] plus two other high-prevalence antigens, INFI (IN3) and INJA (IN4), are located on CD44, the predominant cell surface receptor for the glycosaminoglycan hyaluronan, a component of the extracellular matrix. AnWj (901009), an antigen of very high prevalence, may also be located on or associated with CD44, but the evidence is incomplete. Indian antigens have reduced expression on red cells with the In(Lu) phenotype, and AnWj is virtually undetectable on In(Lu) cells. In^a and In^b are sensitive to treatment of red cells with proteolytic enzymes—papain, ficin, trypsin, α-chymotrypsin—and are also destroyed by the disulfide-bond-reducing agents AET and DTT. AnWj, however, is resistant to all these enzymes but shows variable effects with reducing agents.

Anti-In^a and -In^b often agglutinate red cells directly, but generally the reaction is enhanced by an IAT. Indian antibodies are not generally considered clinically significant, although there is one report of anti-In^b causing an HTR. AnWj, on the other hand, has caused severe HTRs, and In(Lu) red cells should be selected for transfusion.[3]

THE Ok SYSTEM

Ok^a (OK1), an antigen of very high prevalence, is located on the IgSF molecule CD147 or basigin, which has two IgSF domains. Ok^a is resistant to proteolytic enzymes and to disulfide-bond-reducing agents. Only two alloanti-Ok^a are known, both reactive by an IAT. In-vivo survival tests and cellular functional assays with one of them suggested that anti-Ok^a could be clinically significant, but no clinical information exists.

THE RAPH SYSTEM

MER2 (RAPH1), which is located on the tetraspanin CD151, was initially defined by mouse monoclonal antibodies that recognized a quantitative polymorphism, with about 8% of the population having undetectable levels of MER2 on their mature red cells. Alloanti-MER2 was found in three Israeli Jews originating from India, who had a RAPH-null phenotype resulting from a single nucleotide deletion leading to a premature stop codon. These three individuals were CD151-deficient and had end-stage renal failure, sensorineural deafness, and pretibial epidermolysis bullosa, suggesting that CD151 is essential for the proper assembly of basement membranes in kidney, inner ear, and skin.[44] MER2-negative individuals with anti-MER2 but with only single amino acid substitutions in CD151 do not have those symptoms.

MER2 antigen is resistant to treatment of red cells with papain but is destroyed by trypsin, α-chymotrypsin, and pronase and by AET and DTT. MER2 antibodies react by an IAT. There is no evidence that anti-MER2 is clinically significant.

THE JOHN MILTON HAGEN SYSTEM

This system comprises six antigens of very high prevalence on the semaphorin glycoprotein CD108 or Sema7A. Anti-JMH1 is typically produced by individuals with an acquired loss of CD108. This is most often found in elderly patients and is associated with a weakly positive direct antiglobulin test. Absence of JMH2 to JMH5 results from different missense mutations in *SEMA7A*.[45] JMH antigens are destroyed by proteolytic enzymes and by disulfide-bond-reducing agents. They are not detected on cord red cells.

JMH antibodies are usually reactive by an IAT. They are not generally considered to be clinically significant, although one example was implicated in an acute HTR.

THE GILL SYSTEM

GIL antibodies detect an antigen of very high prevalence (GIL1) located on Aquaporin 3 (AQP3), a member of the Aquaporin superfamily of water and glycerol channels (like the Colton antigen).[46] AQP3 enhances permeability of the red cell membrane to glycerol and water.

GIL antigen is resistant to proteolytic enzymes and to disulfide-bond-reducing agents. GIL antibodies are reactive by an IAT. Anti-GIL has not been implicated in HTRs or HDFN, although monocyte monolayer assays suggested a potential to cause accelerated destruction of GIL+ red cells.

THE RHAG SYSTEM

The three antigens of the RHAG system are located on the Rh-associated glycoprotein (RhAG),[47] which is also described in Chapter 13. RhAG is closely associated with the Rh protein in the membrane, as part of the Band 3/ Rh ankyrin macrocomplex (Fig 14-1). Ol^a (RHAG2) is very rare, and homozygosity for the allele encoding Ol^a is associated with an Rh_{mod} phenotype. Duclos (RHAG1) and DSLK (RHAG32) are of high prevalence, and absence of these antigens is associated with an aberrant U (MNS5) antigen.

ANTIGENS THAT DO NOT BELONG TO A BLOOD GROUP SYSTEM

Blood Group Collections

In addition to those antigens belonging to the 30 blood group systems, there are many antigens that have not been shown to belong to a system. These are mostly antigens of either very high or very low prevalence. Some of them are included in blood group collections, which contain two or more antigens that are related serologically, biochemically, or genetically but which do not fit the criteria for system status.[1]

The Cost collection contains Cs^a (COST1) and Cs^b (COST2), antithetical antigens of relatively high and low prevalence, respectively.

These antigens are serologically related to those of the Knops system but do not appear to be located on CR1. Cost antibodies are not clinically significant.

Er^a (ER1) and Er^b (ER2) are antithetical antigens of very high and low prevalence, respectively. Anti-Er3 is produced by individuals with Er(a–b–) red cells. There is no evidence that Er antibodies are clinically significant.

Vel (VEL1) and ABTI (VEL2) are serologically related antigens of high prevalence. Their strength of expression differs substantially between individuals, and they are generally expressed only weakly on cord red cells. They are resistant to treatment of the red cells with proteolytic enzymes or disulfide-bond-reducing agents. Vel antibodies are often IgM and complement activating. They can cause severe immediate HTRs but do not generally cause HDFN.

Carbohydrate antigens of the Ii and GLOB collections are described in Chapter 12.

High-Prevalence Antigens (901 Series)

The 901 series of the ISBT classification contains eight antigens (Table 14-9): seven have a prevalence well in excess of 99%; one, Sd^a, has a prevalence of about 91%. All are inherited, and none is eligible to join a system.[1] Of the eight antigens of very high prevalence, all are resistant to papain, trypsin, α-chymotrypsin, and AET treatment of the red cells, and all except AnWj and Sd^a are expressed strongly on cord cells.

Sd^a represents carbohydrate structures on red cells, and the product of the Sd^a gene is probably a β(1,4)N-acetylgalactosaminyltransferase. The strength of Sd^a on red cells is highly variable, and Sd^a is not detected on cord red cells. Agglutination of Sd(a+) red cells shows a characteristic "mixed-field" appearance of agglutinates and free red cells; when viewed microscopically, the agglutinates are refractile. Anti-Sd^a is inhibited by urine from Sd(a+) individuals (Method 3-11).

Low-Prevalence Antigens (700 Series)

Eighteen antigens of very low prevalence in all populations tested constitute the 700 series of the ISBT classification. All are inherited and do not fit any criteria for joining or forming a system.[1] They are as follows: By (700002); Chr^a (003); Bi (005); Bx^a (006); To^a (017); Pt^a (018); Re^a (019); Je^a (021); Li^a (028); Milne (039); RASM (040); JFV (044); Kg (045); JONES (047); HJK (049); HOFM (050); SARA (052); REIT (054).

Antibodies to low-prevalence antigens do not present transfusion problems because compatible blood is readily available. These

TABLE 14-9. Antigens of the 901 Series of High-Frequency Antigens, and Their Clinical Significance

Antigen		Clinical Significance
Lan	901002	One example caused AHTR
At^a	901003	Reported to have caused an HTR and mild HDFN
Jr^a	901005	Mild DHTRs and one case of AHTR reported
Emm	901008	No evidence of clinical significance
AnWj	901009	Severe AHTRs
Sd^a	901011	No evidence of clinical significance
PEL	901014	No evidence of clinical significance
MAM	901016	Severe HDFN

HTR = hemolytic transfusion reaction; AHTR = acute HTR; DHTR = delayed HTR; HDFN = hemolytic disease of the fetus and newborn.

antibodies will remain undetected if a serologic crossmatch is not employed. Anti-JFV, -Kg, -JONES, -HJK, and -REIT have all caused HDFN.

HLA Antigens on Red Cells

Bg is the name given to HLA Class I antigens expressed on mature red cells. Bg^a represents HLA-B7; Bg^b, HLA-B17 (B57 or B58); and Bg^c, HLA-A28 (A68 or A69) (crossreacting with HLA-A2). Many individuals, however, do not express Bg antigens on their red cells, despite having the corresponding HLA antigens on their lymphocytes. There are a few reports of Bg antibodies causing HTRs,[48] and they are sometimes present as contaminants in reagents. HLA antigens on red cells are not destroyed by papain, ficin, pronase, trypsin, α-chymotrypsin, AET, or DTT. They can be stripped from red cells with chloroquine (Method 2-20) or EDTA/glycine-HCl (Method 2-21).

KEY POINTS

1. Of 328 recognized antigen specificities, 284 belong to one of 30 blood group systems representing either a single gene or two or three closely linked homologous genes. Some groups of antigens that are not eligible to join a system are classified together as collections. Antigens not classified in a system or a collection are of either low or high prevalence and make up the 700 and 901 series, respectively.
2. M and N are antithetical, polymorphic antigens. M, N, S, s, and 'N' are all destroyed by treatment of the red cells with papain, ficin, bromelin, or pronase, although this effect with S and s is variable; M and N—but not S, s, or 'N'—are destroyed by trypsin treatment.
3. Anti-M is relatively common; anti-N, quite rare. Most anti-M and -N are not clinically significant. When M or N antibodies active at 37 C are encountered, antigen-negative or compatible red cells should be provided. Anti-S, -s, and -U are generally IgG antibodies active at 37 C. They have been implicated in hemolytic transfusion reactions (HTRs) and severe and fatal hemolytic disease of the fetus and newborn (HDFN).
4. The antigen often referred to as Kell is correctly named K or KEL1; its antithetical antigen is k or KEL2.
5. Because Kell antibodies can cause severe HDFN and HTRs, patients with Kell antibodies should be transfused with antigen-negative blood whenever possible. Anti-K is the most common immune red cell antibody outside the ABO and Rh systems.
6. In Whites and Asians, the Duffy polymorphism consists of two antigens, Fy^a and Fy^b, and three phenotypes: Fy(a+b–), Fy(a+b+), and Fy(a–b+). Fy^a and Fy^b are very sensitive to most proteolytic enzymes. In Blacks, a third allele, *Fy*, may result in neither Fy^a nor Fy^b. Individuals homozygous for *Fy* have the red cell phenotype Fy(a–b–).
7. Anti-Fy^a (common) and anti-Fy^b (rare) are generally detected by an antiglobulin test and may cause acute or delayed HTRs—generally mild, but some have proved fatal.
8. Kidd antigens are resistant to proteolytic enzymes such as papain and ficin.
9. Kidd antibodies anti-Jk^a and -Jk^b are not common, are generally found in antibody mixtures, and are often difficult to detect. An antiglobulin test is usually required, and use of enzyme-treated cells may be necessary to detect weaker antibodies. Kidd antibodies may cause severe acute HTRs and are a common cause of delayed HTRs.
10. The 22 antigens of the Diego system are located on Band 3, the red cell anion exchanger. Anti-Di^a and -Wr^a can cause severe HDFN. Anti-Wr^a can also cause HTRs.

REFERENCES

1. Daniels GL, Fletcher A, Garratty G, et al. Blood group terminology 2004. From the ISBT Committee on Terminology for Red Cell Surface Antigens. Vox Sang 2004;87:304-16.
2. Daniels G, Castilho L, Flegel WA, et al. International Society of Blood Transfusion Committee on Terminology for Red Cell Surface Antigens: Macao Report. Vox Sang 2009;96:153-6.
3. Poole J, Daniels G. Blood group antibodies and their significance in transfusion medicine. Transfus Med Rev 2007;21:58-71.
4. Daniels G. Human blood groups. 2nd ed. Oxford: Blackwell Science, 2002.
5. Klein HG, Anstee DJ. Mollison's blood transfusion in clinical medicine. 11th ed. Oxford: Blackwell Publishing, 2005.
6. Daniels G, Bromilow I. Essential guide to blood groups. 2nd ed. Oxford: Blackwell Publishing, 2010.
7. Reid ME, Lomas-Francis C. The blood group antigen factsbook. 2nd ed. London: Academic Press, 2004.
8. Daniels G. The molecular genetics of blood group polymorphism. Hum Genet 2009;126:729-42.
9. Bruce LJ, Beckmann R, Ribeiro ML, et al. A band 3-based macrocomplex of integral and peripheral proteins in the RBC membrane. Blood 2003;101:4180-8.
10. Mohandas N, Gallagher PG. Red cell membrane: Past, present, and future. Blood 2008;112:3939-48.
11. Huang C-H, Blumenfeld OO. MNS blood groups and major glycophorins. Molecular basis for allelic variation. In: Cartron J-P, Rouger P, eds. Blood cell biochemistry. Vol. 6. New York: Plenum, 1995:153-88.
12. Sim BKL, Chitnis CE, Wasniowska K, et al. Receptor and ligand domains for invasion of erythrocytes by *Plasmodium falciparum*. Science 1994;264:1941-4.
13. Mayer DCG, Cofie J, Jiang L, et al. Glycophorin B is the erythrocyte receptor of *Plasmodium falciparum* erythrocyte-binding ligand, EBL-1. Proc Natl Acad Sci U S A 2009;106:5348-52.
14. Tippett P, Reid ME, Poole J, et al. The Miltenberger subsystem: Is it obsolescent? Transfus Med Rev 1992;6:170-82.
15. Broadberry RE, Lin M. The incidence and significance of anti-"Mi^a" in Taiwan. Transfusion 1994;34:349-52.
16. Karamatic Crew V, Green C, Daniels G. Molecular bases of the antigens of the Lutheran blood group system. Transfusion 2003;43:1729-37.
17. Eyler CE, Telen MJ. The Lutheran glycoprotein: A multifunctional adhesion receptor. Transfusion 2006;46:668-77.
18. Karamatic Crew V, Mallinson G, Green C, et al. Different inactivating mutations in the *LU* genes of three individuals with the Lutheran-null phenotype. Transfusion 2007;47:492-8.
19. Singleton BK, Burton NM, Green C, et al. Mutations in *EKLF/KLF1* form the molecular basis of the rare blood group In(Lu) phenotype. Blood 2008;112:2081-8.
20. Singleton BK, Roxby D, Stirling J, et al. A novel GATA1 mutation (Ter414Arg) in a family with the rare X-linked blood group Lu(ab) phenotype (abstract). Blood 2009;114:1979.
21. Westhoff CM, Reid ME. The Kell, Duffy, and Kidd blood group systems. Immunohematology 2004;20:37-49.
22. Lee S, Zambas ED, Marsh WL, Redman CM. Molecular cloning and primary structure of Kell blood group protein. Proc Natl Acad Sci U S A 1991;88:6353-7.
23. Körmöczi G, Scharberg EA, Gassner C. A novel *KEL*1,3* allele with weak Kell antigen expression confirming the cis-modifier effect of KEL3. Transfusion 2009;49:733-9.
24. Daniels G, Hadley A, Green CA. Causes of fetal anemia in hemolytic disease due to anti-K. Transfusion 2003;43:115-16.
25. Lee S, Russo DCW, Reiner AP, et al. Molecular defects underlying the Kell null phenotype. J Biol Chem 2001;276:27281-9.
26. Lee S, Russo DCW, Reid ME, Redman CM. Mutations that diminish expression of Kell surface protein and lead to the K_{mod} RBC phenotype. Transfusion 2003;43:1121-5.
27. Lee S, Debnath AK, Redman CM. Active amino acids of the Kell blood group protein and model of the ectodomain based on the structure of neutral endopeptidase 24.11. Blood 2003;102:3028-34.
28. Danek A, Rubio JP, Rampoldi L, et al. McLeod neuroacanthocytosis: Genotype and phenotype. Ann Neurol 2001;50:755-64.
29. Tournamille C, Colin Y, Cartron JP, Le Van Kim C. Disruption of a GATA motif in the *Duffy* gene promoter abolishes erythroid gene ex-

pression in Duffy-negative individuals. Nat Genet 1995;10:224-8.
30. Hadley TJ, Peiper SC. From malaria to chemokine receptor: The emerging physiologic role of the Duffy blood group antigen. Blood 1997;89:3077-91.
31. Darbonne WC, Rice GC, Mohler MA, et al. Red blood cells are a sink for interleukin 8, a leukocyte chemotaxin. J Clin Invest 1991;88:1362-9.
32. Hadley TJ, Lu Z, Wasniowska K, et al. Postcapillary venule endothelial cells in kidney express a multispecific chemokine receptor that is structurally and functionally identical to the erythroid isoform, which is the Duffy blood group antigen. J Clin Invest 1994;94:985-91.
33. Horuk R, Chitnis CE, Darbonne WC, et al. A receptor for the malarial parasite *Plasmodium vivax*: The erythrocyte chemokine receptor. Science 1993;261:1182-4.
34. Holt S, Donaldson H, Hazlehurst G, et al. Acute transplant rejection induced by blood transfusion reaction to the Kidd blood group system. Nephrol Dial Transplant 2004;19:2403-6.
35. Sands JM. Molecular mechanisms of urea transport. J Membr Biol 2003;191:149-63.
36. Heaton DC, McLoughlin K. Jk(a–b–) red blood cells resist urea lysis. Transfusion 1982;22:70-1.
37. Sands JM, Gargus JJ, Fršhlich O, et al. Urinary concentrating ability in patients with Jk(a–b–) blood type who lack carrier-mediated urea transport. J Am Soc Nephrol 1992;2:1689-96.
38. Byrne KM, Byrne PC. Review: Other blood group systems—Diego, Yt, Xg, Scianna, Dombrock, Colton, Landsteiner-Wiener, and Indian. Immunohematology 2004;20:50-8.
39. Wagner FF, Poole J, Flegel WA. Scianna antigens including Rd are expressed by ERMAP. Blood 2003;101:752-7.
40. Reid ME. Complexities of the Dombrock blood group system revealed. Transfusion 2005;45 (Suppl 2):92S-9S.
41. Daniels G. Functions of red cell surface proteins. Vox Sang 2007;93:331-40.
42. Storry JR, Reid ME. The Cromer blood group system: A review. Immunohematology 2002; 18:95-103.
43. Moulds JM. Understanding the Knops blood group and its role in malaria. Vox Sang 2002;83 (Suppl 1):185-8.
44. Karamatic Crew V, Burton N, Kagan A, et al. CD151, the first member of the tetraspanin (TM4) superfamily detected on erythrocytes, is essential for the correct assembly of human basement membranes in kidney and skin. Blood 2004;104:2217-23.
45. Seltsam A, Strigens S, Levene C, et al. The molecular diversity of Sema7A that carries the JMH blood group antigens. Transfusion 2007; 47:133-46.
46. Roudier N, Ripoche P, Gane P, et al. AQP3 deficiency in humans and the molecular basis of a novel blood group system, GIL. J Biol Chem 2002;277:45854-9.
47. Tilley L, Green C, Poole J, et al. A new blood group system, RHAG: Three antigens resulting from amino acid substitutions in the Rh-associated glycoprotein. Vox Sang 2010;98:151-9.
48. Nance ST. Do HLA antibodies cause hemolytic transfusion reactions or decreased RBC survival? Transfusion 2004;43:687-90.

Chapter 15

Pretransfusion Testing

Katharine A. Downes, MD, and Ira A. Shulman, MD

PRETRANSFUSION TESTING IS performed in order to prevent transfusion of incompatible donor red cells that might result in an immune-mediated hemolytic transfusion reaction (HTR). Strategies to avoid the transfusion of incompatible platelets, plasma, and white cell components are discussed in other chapters. Table 15-1 shows the steps in pretransfusion testing and the associated AABB standards.[1]

The US federal government regulates pretransfusion testing by the authority of the Clinical Laboratory Improvement Amendments of 1988 (CLIA '88). Regulated pretransfusion tests include ABO group, Rh type, antibody detection, antibody identification, and compatibility testing.

REQUESTS FOR TRANSFUSION

Requests for blood and blood components may be submitted in an oral, electronic, or written format. Requests must contain sufficient information for accurate recipient identification (ID). Two independent patient identifiers are required, ideally including the patient's first and last names and an ID number that is unique to the patient. Other identifiers that may be used include the patient's birth date, driver's license number, photographic ID, or all three. The importance of accurate patient identification is fundamental in patient safety. The Joint Commission has listed improving the accuracy of patient identification and the elimination of transfusion errors related to patient misidentification during blood administration as part of its number one National Patient Safety Goal for hospitals, with the requirement of at least two patient identifiers for the provision of care, treatment, or other services.[2] Other information necessary to process a request for transfusion includes the specific component requested [eg, Red Blood Cells (RBCs)], the amount, any special requirements such as irradiation, the gender and age of the recipient, and the name of the authorized prescriber ordering the transfusion.[3] The recipient's diagnosis and a history of transfusion and pregnancy may provide useful information to guide testing, product/component

Katharine A. Downes, MD, Associate Medical Director, Blood Bank/Transfusion Medicine, University Hospitals-Case Medical Center, Medical Director of Coagulation Laboratories, University Hospitals-Case Medical Center, and Assistant Professor of Pathology, Department of Pathology, Case Western Reserve University, Cleveland, Ohio, and Ira A. Shulman, MD, Professor and Vice Chair of Pathology, Keck School of Medicine of the University of Southern California (USC), Director of the USC Transfusion Medicine Services Group, and Director of Laboratories and Pathology, Los Angeles County + USC Medical Center, Los Angeles, California
The authors have disclosed no conflicts of interest.

TABLE 15-1. Steps in Pretransfusion Testing and Associated AABB Standards

Steps in Pretransfusion Testing	Relevant AABB Standard(s)[1]
Request for transfusion	5.11.1 and 5.11.1.1
Identification of transfusion recipient and blood sample collected	5.11, 5.11.1, 5.11.2, 5.11.2.1, 5.11.2.2, 6.2.3.1, and 8.2
Testing of transfusion recipient's blood sample:	
◆ Blood sample acceptability	5.11.2.3 and 5.11.3
◆ ABO group and Rh type	5.13, 5.13.1, and 5.13.2
◆ Antibody detection testing	5.13.3, 5.13.3.1, 5.13.3.2, 5.13.3.3, and 5.13.3.4
◆ Antibody identification	5.13.3, 5.13.3.1, 5.13.3.2, 5.13.3.3, and 5.13.3.4
◆ Comparison of current and previous test results	5.13.5, 5.13.5.1, and 5.13.5.2
Donor RBC unit testing:	
◆ ABO group confirmation and Rh type confirmation for Rh-negative RBC units	5.12 and 5.12.1
Donor red cell unit selection:	
◆ Selection of components of ABO group and Rh type that are compatible with the transfusion recipient and with any unexpected allogeneic antibodies	5.14, 5.14.1, 5.14.2, 5.14.2.1, 5.14.3, 5.14.4, and 5.14.5
Compatibility testing (crossmatch):	
◆ Serologic	5.15, 5.15.1, and 5.15.1.1
◆ Computer or electronic	5.15.2, 5.15.2.1, 5.15.2.2, 5.15.2.3, 5.15.2.4, and 5.15.2.5
Labeling of blood or blood components with the recipient's identifying information and issue	5.1.6, 5.10, 5.20, 5.20.1, 5.21, 5.22, 5.23

selection, or both. Each institution should have a written policy defining the acceptance criteria for transfusion orders. Requests for blood or blood components that 1) lack the required information, 2) are inaccurate, or 3) are illegible should not be accepted. Verbal requests are acceptable in urgent situations but should be documented in accordance with local policies.

IDENTIFICATION OF RECIPIENTS AND LABELING OF BLOOD SAMPLES

Collection of a properly labeled pretransfusion blood sample from the intended recipient is critical to safe blood transfusion. The majority of HTRs arise from misidentification of patients or pretransfusion sample labeling errors.[4] Each institution must develop and implement policies and procedures for accurate patient identification and sample collection. At a minimum, the phlebotomist must identify the potential recipient before collecting a pretransfusion sample and must ensure that the correct patient information is placed on the label of the sample that is collected. Systems for patient identification and sample labeling may depend solely on eye-readable information, or they may be a combination of eye- and machine-readable information (bar codes or embedded radio-frequency-emitting chips).[5] Systems that use machine-readable labels and forms may be institutionally driven in their implementation by applications in various areas of the hospital or health-care facility, such as the pharmacy (for medication verification), patient registration, or both. "Positive" patient ID systems may perform and integrate many functions, including the initial identification of the patient, identification of general laboratory samples collected, blood unit identification, and linkage of blood components to their intended recipient(s).[6] Each system has its own method, device, or technology for identifying patients, sample tubes, and/or blood units.[7,8] (See Table 15-2.)

Patient Identification

Identification Wristband

Most institutions require hospitalized patients to wear an ID wristband, which ideally is placed on the patient before any samples are collected, and which remains on the patient until discharge. The phlebotomist is required to identify the patient by carefully examining the information on the wristband. It is important to realize, however, that a patient might be wearing the *wrong* wristband. If possible, the patient should be involved in verifying that he or she is wearing the correct ID band. For example, if a patient is wearing an ID band that displays his or her name, date of birth, and ID number, verification can be performed by asking the patient to spell the name and to state the date of birth. The phlebotomist can then compare the printed name and birth date as they appear on the ID band with verbal information provided by the patient. If the information does not match, the discrepancy must be resolved before a pretransfusion sample is collected or before a blood transfusion is given. One study found that patients were asked to verify the information on their ID bands less than 20% of the time before blood administration.[9]

Outpatient Setting and Preadmission Testing

The identification of samples used for preadmission testing must meet the same requirements as those used for inpatient transfusion. Because a patient's admission may occur on the same day as the patient's surgery, hospitals have developed different mechanisms to identify patients whose samples have been collected several days or weeks before surgery, including the following precautions:

- The requirement that patients wear ID wristbands.
- The use of a unique number on samples and on a patient ID form that the patient provides on the day of surgery so the preadmission sample can be valid for transfusion.
- The placement of the wristband used during sample collection on the patient's medical record. The wristband is attached to the patient on the day of surgery after *accurate* identification of the patient.

Alternative methods of patient identification are often used in the outpatient setting and might include identifying the patient by using his or her driver's license or other photographic identification. The patient's full name, ID number, birth date, or all three must be compared with the information on the test requisition; if there is any discrepancy in the information, a pretransfusion blood sample must not be collected until the patient's identity has been clarified.

Patient Identification When a Patient's Identity Is Unknown

An emergency ID method should be used when the patient's identity is unknown. A system should exist to assign temporary identification for an unidentified patient, such as an alias name and a medical record number. The temporary patient identification must be attached to the patient, must be affixed or reproduced on blood samples, and must be cross-referenced with the patient's name and

TABLE 15-2. Elements of Patient Identification Systems

Bar-code-based ID systems	◆ Bar-coded patients' wristbands and label printing at time of collection ◆ Bar-code enabled medication administration, sample collection, and blood administration ◆ Patients' wristbands with bar codes on medications and samples ◆ Bedside bar-code scanning: – Handheld computing device – Handheld bar-code reading wireless device
Non-bar-code ID systems	◆ Wristbands for patients ◆ Color-coded number linking wristband, collection tube, and unit ◆ Wristbands linked to embosser for label printing ◆ ID band with substitute or additional "blood bank number" as unique patient identifier ◆ Imprinted wristbands with patients' ID plate cards and software ◆ Biometrics fingerprint with wristband capability
Functions of ID systems	◆ Laboratory sample collection ◆ Patient and collection tube label matching before sample collection ◆ Patient and blood unit matching before blood transfusion ◆ Patient and medication matching before medication administration
Techniques to verify patient identification when creating a wristband	◆ ID card without a photograph ◆ ID card with a photograph ◆ Biometric identification: fingerprint, retinal scan, iris scan
Techniques to verify patient ID before intervention or sample collection	◆ ID card without a photograph ◆ ID card with a photograph ◆ Biometric identification: fingerprint ◆ One-dimensional, two-dimensional, bar-coded wristband, or both ◆ Passive, active radio-frequency identification, or both
Labels for sample identification at time of collection	◆ Peel-off label removed from wristband ◆ Bar-code label ◆ Radio frequency tag
Data elements that may be encoded on sample label	◆ Accession number; patient's location; container identification; date; sample type; tests ordered; patient's name; patient's account, admission, and medical record numbers; collector or staff identification
Location of performance of patient identification	◆ Handheld workstation ◆ Point-of-care workstation ◆ Handheld device
Interfaces	◆ Hospital information system ◆ Laboratory information system ◆ Pharmacy information system ◆ Order entry information system

Data from reference 8.

hospital ID number or code when that name and number become known. If a hospital permits the use of alias names, the hospital must have policies and procedures that govern their use.[10]

Sample Labeling

The phlebotomist must label each blood sample tube, in the presence of the patient, with two independent patient identifiers and the date of collection. Either handwritten or imprinted labels may be used provided that the information on the label is identical to that on the wristband and the transfusion request. All tubes must be indelibly labeled. There must be a mechanism to identify the phlebotomist and the date of sample collection.[1(p33)] The phlebotomist's identification may be placed on the label of the tube, placed on the requisition, or documented in a computer system. The identity of the phlebotomist must be traceable back to the collected sample.

Confirming Sample Linkage

When a pretransfusion sample is received in the laboratory, laboratory personnel must confirm that the information on the sample label and the information on the pretransfusion testing request are identical. If there is any doubt about the identity of the patient or about the labeling of the sample, a new sample must be obtained.[1(p33)]

It is extremely risky for anyone to correct identifying information on an incorrectly labeled sample. One study found that samples that failed to meet acceptability criteria were 40 times more likely to have a blood grouping discrepancy.[11] Thus, a strict policy of canceling the testing of incorrectly labeled samples should help avoid blood grouping errors and should decrease the likelihood of transfusing ABO-incompatible blood components. Each laboratory should establish policies and procedures that define sample identifying information, and describe how to document the receipt and management of mislabeled samples.

SAMPLE REQUIREMENTS

Pretransfusion red cell compatibility testing is performed on red cells and on either serum or plasma. Whereas both serum and plasma may be used for a variety of testing methods, plasma is often preferred. For example, incompletely clotted serum samples may contain small fibrin clots that trap red cells into aggregates and cause false-positive results with column agglutination technology. Additionally, clotting may be incomplete in anticoagulated serum samples, such as those from patients who have been treated with heparin. Adding thrombin or protamine sulphate to the sample may correct the problem. (See Method 1-2.)

At times it may be necessary to obtain a pretransfusion blood sample from the same extremity in which there is an intravenous infusion. If this is the case, steps should be taken to avoid dilution of the sample, which might cause failure to detect unexpected red cell antibodies.

Sample Hemolysis and Lipemia

The use of hemolyzed or lipemic samples may create difficulties in evaluating test results. Tests with a hemolyzed sample may mask antibody-induced hemolysis; therefore, whenever possible, a hemolyzed sample should be replaced with a new sample. If a hemolyzed sample is used, it should be noted in the patient's testing records to differentiate from hemolysis as a result of an antigen-antibody reaction. Each institution should have a procedure describing the indications, limitations, and exceptions for use of hemolyzed and lipemic samples.

Sample Age

When performing pretransfusion testing for a patient who has been pregnant or transfused within the previous 3 months, or if the pregnancy history and transfusion history are uncertain, the pretransfusion sample used for testing must be no more than 3 days old at the time of intended transfusion because recent transfusion or pregnancy may stimulate production of unexpected antibodies. The day of collection is counted as day zero; therefore, a sample collected on a Monday can be used for a transfusion given until 11:59 pm on Thursday of the same week.[1(p34)]

For patients without a recent history of transfusion or pregnancy, there is no requirement that a pretransfusion sample be less than 3 days old at the time of a transfusion. Although the selection of 3 days was arbitrary,[12] the 3-day requirement was created as a practical approach to ensure that the sample used for testing reflects the recipient's current immunologic status. If the histories of transfusion and pregnancy are certain and if no transfusion or pregnancy has occurred in the previous 3 months, the length of time that a pretransfusion sample is valid for testing should be determined based on the manufacturer's package or instructional insert recommendations for sample acceptability for the test being performed.[13]

Retention and Storage of Recipient and Donor Samples

The recipient's blood sample and a sample of the donor's red cells must be stored at refrigerator temperature for at least 7 days after each transfusion.[1(p33)] Retaining both the patient's sample and the donor's sample allows for repeat or additional testing if the patient has a transfusion reaction. Testing of stored samples should be based on the sample storage limitations in the reagent manufacturers' package inserts. Lack of appropriate storage space may also limit the length of time that samples are stored. Institutions that limit the use of a pretransfusion recipient's sample for no more than 3 days frequently store the pretransfusion sample of a transfused patient for 10 days (ie, 3 + 7). Institutions that permit the use of a pretransfusion sample beyond 3 days need to ensure that the pretransfusion sample is retained for at least an additional 7 days after the transfusion for which the sample was used for donor selection. For example, if an institution permits pretransfusion samples to be collected 14 days before a scheduled transfusion, the sample must be retained for at least 21 days if the patient is transfused on the 14th day after the sample was collected.

Donor red cells may be obtained from the remainder of the segment used in the crossmatch or from a segment removed before issuing the blood. If the opened crossmatch segment is saved, it should be placed in a tube labeled with the unit number and then sealed or stoppered.

SEROLOGIC TESTING PRINCIPLES

Pretransfusion serologic tests include ABO group and Rh type, antibody detection, antibody identification, and crossmatching. The purpose of these tests is to demonstrate in-vitro red cell antigen-antibody reactions. Antibody and red cell antigen combine in those laboratory tests and result in different observable results, often with a final endpoint of agglutination. Agglutination is a reversible chemical reaction thought to occur in two stages: 1) sensitization when the antibody attaches to the red cell antigen, and 2) agglutination when the sensitized red cells are bridged together to form the lattice that constitutes agglutination. Various factors may enhance or decrease sensitization and agglutination.

Sensitization

Antibody attachment requires both structural and chemical fit between antigen and antibody. The structural or spatial fit may be optimized by increasing the chance association between antigen and antibody through agitation, centrifugation of the sample, or both. Varying the relative concentrations of antibody and antigen is also effective; however, care should be exercised. Excess antigen in the test system should result in increased antibody uptake; however, excessive antigen also decreases the number of antibody molecules bound per cell and thus limits agglutination. Consequently, antibody excess is preferred in most pretransfusion tests. As with antigen excess, increasing the quantity of antibody can increase the test's sensitivity. However, occasionally significant antibody excess can, in contrast, inhibit direct agglutination in a phenomenon known as prozone. Although all antigen sites may be occupied by excess antibody, individual antibodies do not bind to two different cells. Thus, in the prozone effect, crosslinking does not occur, leading to false-negative results.

A ratio of 2 drops of serum to 1 drop of red cell suspension (2% to 5%) is most commonly used. As discussed above, sensitivity can be increased by increasing the ratio of serum to red cells. For example, decreasing the red cell concentration from 5% to between 2% and 3%, or adding 4 drops serum to 1 drop of a standard red cell suspension, doubles the ratio. When extra sensitivity is required, from 10 to as many as 20 drops of serum may be used. Caution must be exercised, however, because such changes affect the ionic strength if low-ionic-strength saline (LISS) is being used to reduce the dielectric constant. In those cases, modifications must be made to maintain the appropriate ratio of serum to LISS.

All chemical reactions are reversible. Antigen (Ag)-antibody (Ab) reactions may be expressed as

$$Ag + Ab \rightleftarrows AgAb$$

The reaction proceeds until a state of equilibrium is reached. This reaction is controlled by the rate constants of association (k_a) and dissociation (k_d).

$$Ag + Ab \underset{k_d}{\overset{k_a}{\rightleftarrows}} AgAb$$

By the law of mass action, the speed of the reaction is proportional to the concentrations of the reactants and their product. The equilibrium constant (K_o) is a function of these intrinsic association constants for the antibody being tested.

$$\frac{[AbAg]}{[Ab][Ag]} = \frac{k_a}{k_d} = K_o$$

FIGURE 15-1. The law of mass action and the equilibrium constant.

Chemical Bonds

Hydrogen bonds, hydrophobic bonds, electrostatic bonds, and van der Waals forces are responsible for the binding of antibody to antigen. The antigen-antibody interaction is reversible, with bond association and disassociation occurring until equilibrium occurs.

The relative rates of association and dissociation determine the equilibrium constant or affinity constant (K_0) of a reaction (see Fig 15-1). The K_0 reflects both the degree to which antibody and antigen bind to one another and the reaction speed; with a large K_0 value, the reaction occurs more readily and is more difficult to dissociate, while a small K_0 may require a higher ratio of antibody to antigen for detection. The reaction temperature, the pH, the ionic strength of the testing medium, the incubation time, and the relative antigen-to-antibody concentrations may affect the K_0. Alteration of those physical conditions may be used to increase or decrease the test's sensitivity. Most blood group antibodies with optimal reactivity in vitro fall into one of two categories, as follows: "cold-reactive antibodies" that are predominantly IgM and react optimally between 4 C and 25 C, and "warm-reactive antibodies" that are predominantly IgG and react between 30 C and 37 C. Antibodies that react at less than 30 C are considered clinically insignificant because they rarely destroy antigen-positive red cells. For most of the clinically significant blood group antibodies, optimal pH is assumed to approximate the physiologic pH range; thus, for most routine testing, a pH of around 7.0 should be used. In normal saline, clustering of Na^+ and Cl^- ions hinders antibody-antigen association; lowering the ionic strength of the reaction medium weakens the shielding effect of the ions and enhances the electrostatic attractions. Decreasing the salt concentration of the serum-cell system with the use of LISS increases the rate of antibody-antigen interactions and potentially the total amount of bound antibody. However, sensitivity may actually be decreased if incubation times are excessively prolonged.[14] Temperature, immunoglobulin class, and specific interactions between antigen configuration and the Fab site of the antibody all affect the incubation time necessary to reach equilibrium. If antihuman globulin (AHG) serum is used without enhancing media, a 30- to 60-minute incubation at 37 C is usually required to detect most clinically significant antibodies (see "The Antiglobulin Test"). If necessary, incubation can be extended past 60 minutes with no negative effects on sensitivity. Incubation time at 37 C may be shortened when LISS or polyethylene glycol (PEG) are used.

Agglutination

Following antibody attachment, the sensitized cells are linked into a lattice that allows for visualization of the reaction. Antibody size and physical properties, antigen concentration, and the distance between cells affect agglutination.[15] Although IgG molecules usually fail to bridge the distance between red cells, resulting in sensitization without lattice formation, larger multivalent IgM molecules readily cause agglutination. Antigen location and density also affect direct agglutination reactions. In fact, IgG antibodies against some relatively high-density antigens on the most external aspect of red cell glycoproteins, such as A, B, M, and N antigens, can directly agglutinate red cells. Red cells suspended in saline repel one another because of the net negative surface charge. To overcome or disrupt this repulsion and to promote agglutination, one can use a variety of strategies: sample centrifugation to force the red cells together; proteolytic enzyme treatment of red cells to reduce surface molecules' negative charge and cleave certain antigens; antiglobulin reagent to crosslink the reaction; albumin to reduce the hydration layer around the cells; or the addition of Polybrene, which is a positively charged macromolecule.

The Antiglobulin Test

Described in 1945 by Coombs, Mourant, and Race,[16] the antiglobulin test detects bound red cell antibodies that do not produce direct agglutination (sensitizing antibody). The antiglobulin test uses a secondary antibody, made in another species and directed against human globulins, that attaches and agglutinates sensitized red cells (see Fig 15-2). The antibody is produced by injecting animals with human globulins to stimulate antibody production against the foreign human protein and is called AHG serum. AHG sera may have different specificities, including anti-IgG as well as antibodies to several complement components. AHG reacts with human antibodies and with complement molecules that are bound to red cells. AHG can also bind to antibodies and complement that are unbound to cells, free in serum, which effectively neutralizes the AHG, making it unavailable to detect proteins that are bound to red cells. Neutralization of the AHG antibody may cause false-negative AHG test results. Therefore, to avoid neutralizing the AHG antibody, the red cells must be washed free of unbound proteins before the addition of AHG serum.

AHG sera may be used in performance of the direct antiglobulin test (DAT) and an indirect antiglobulin test (IAT). The DAT demonstrates in-vivo sensitization of red cells and is performed by directly testing a sample of a patient's washed red cells with AHG. An IAT dem-

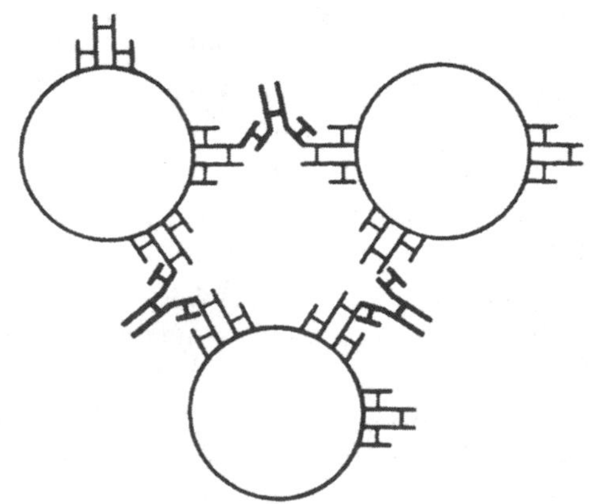

FIGURE 15-2. The antiglobulin reaction. Anti-human IgG molecules are shown reacting with the Fc portion of human IgG coating adjacent red cells (eg, anti-D coating D-positive red cells).

onstrates in-vitro reactions between red cells and antibodies. In an IAT, serum (or plasma) is incubated with red cells, which are then washed to remove unbound globulins. The presence of agglutination with the addition of AHG indicates antibody binding to a specific red cell antigen. An IAT is used in antibody detection, antibody identification, crossmatching, and blood group phenotyping. (See Tables 15-3[17,18] and 15-4[19,20] for sources of error in AHG testing.)

Reading and Interpreting Serologic Test Reactions

In serologic testing, hemolysis and/or agglutination that constitute the visible endpoint of a red cell antigen-antibody interaction must be observed accurately and consistently. The strength of agglutination (or adherence as seen in solid-phase methods) and the degree of hemolysis, or both, observed with each red cell sample should be recorded immediately after reading. All personnel in a laboratory should use the same interpretations and notations and should be consistent in grading (eg, 0 to 4+) reactions. Some laboratories prefer to use a numeric scoring system (eg, 0 to 12) to indicate reaction strength.[21] (Refer to Method 1-8 for grading and scoring.) An optical aid such as a concave mirror enhances visualization in reading tube tests. In automated methods such as column agglutination and solid phase, microcameras and computer algorithmic interpretations capture, record, and grade the reaction strength. If column agglutination technology or solid phase is used, the manufacturer's directions must be followed for reading and interpreting positive and negative reactions, as well as for possible interferences. Microscopic observation is not routinely recommended in manufacturers' inserts for enhancement media. A microscope can be useful in distinguishing rouleaux from true agglutination in tube methods and may also allow for the detection of specific patterns of agglutination that are characteristic of some antibodies. For example, anti-Sd^a typically produces small refractile agglutinates in a sea of free red cells, giving a mixed-field appearance.

PRETRANSFUSION TESTS

The patient's ABO group and Rh type must be determined in order to transfuse ABO- and Rh-compatible components. The red cells of the intended recipient must be typed for ABO and Rh, and the serum or plasma must be tested for expected and unexpected antibodies before components containing red cells are issued for transfusion.[1(pp33-34)] There should be written procedures for exceptions during emergencies. When only plasma, platelets, or Cryoprecipitated AHF are being infused, historical testing information in the patient's record may be used, although it is preferable that the results of testing from at least two different samples be available and that those historical results match. Table 15-5 lists the selection criteria of the ABO types for blood components when ABO-identical components are not available.

ABO Group and Rh Type of the Recipient

To determine the ABO group of the recipient, red cells must be tested with anti-A and anti-B, and the recipient's serum or plasma must be tested with A_1 and B red cells. The techniques used and interpretations of the results are described in Chapter 12 and in Methods Section 2. Any discrepant ABO group results should be resolved before blood is given. If transfusion is necessary before resolution, the patient should receive group O red cells.

The patient's red cells must also be tested with anti-D; routine testing for other Rh antigens (eg, C, c, E, e) is not required. The D test must be performed with suitable observations and/or controls to avoid a false-positive interpretation. Chapter 13 contains a more extensive discussion of Rh typing reagents, appropriate control techniques, and weak D types. If problems in D typing arise, especially if the patient is a female of childbearing potential, it is prudent to limit transfusion of red-cell-containing blood components to those that are D negative, at least until the problem is resolved.

As described in Chapter 13, the weak D test is used to detect forms of the D antigen

TABLE 15-3. Sources of False-Negative Results in Antiglobulin Testing

Neutralization of Antihuman Globulin (AHG) Reagent
◆ Failure to wash cells adequately to remove all serum or plasma. Fill tube at least ¾ full of saline for each wash. Check dispense volume of automated washers.
◆ If increased serum volumes are used, a routine wash may be inadequate. Wash additional times or remove serum before washing.
◆ Contamination of AHG by extraneous protein. Do not use finger or hand to cover tube. Contaminated droppers or wrong reagent dropper can neutralize entire bottle of AHG.
◆ High concentration of IgG paraproteins in test serum; protein may remain even after multiple washes.[17]
Interruption in Testing
◆ Bound IgG may dissociate from red cells and either leave too little IgG to detect or may neutralize AHG reagent.
◆ Agglutination of IgG-coated red cells will weaken. Centrifuge and read immediately.
Improper Reagent Storage
◆ AHG reagent may lose reactivity if frozen. Reagent may become bacterially contaminated.
◆ Excessive heat or repeated freezing or thawing may cause loss of reactivity of test serum.
◆ Reagent red cells may lose antigen strength on storage. Other subtle cell changes may cause loss of reactivity.
Improper Procedures
◆ Overcentrifugation may pack red cells so tightly that agitation required to resuspend red cells breaks up agglutinates. Undercentrifugation may not be optimal for agglutination.
◆ Failure to add test serum, enhancement medium, or AHG may cause negative test.
◆ Red cell suspensions that are too heavy may mask weak agglutination. Suspensions that are too light may be difficult to read.
◆ Improper or insufficient serum:cell ratios.
Complement
◆ Rare antibodies, notably some anti-Jk^a or anti-Jk^b, may be detected only when polyspecific AHG is used and when active complement is present.
Saline
◆ Low pH of saline solution can decrease sensitivity.[18] Optimal saline wash solution for most antibodies is pH 7.0 to 7.2.
◆ Some antibodies may require saline to be a specific temperature to retain antibody on the cell. Use 37 C or 4 C saline.

TABLE 15-4. Sources of False-Positive Results in Antiglobulin Testing

Cells Agglutinated Before Washing
◆ If potent agglutinins are present, agglutinates may not disperse during washing. Observe red cells before the addition of antihuman globulin (AHG) or use control tube substituting saline for AHG; reactivity before the addition of AHG or in the saline control invalidates AHG reading.
Particles of Contaminants
◆ Dust or dirt in glassware may cause clumping (not agglutination) of red cells. Fibrin or precipitates in test serum may produce red cell clumps that mimic agglutination.
Improper Procedures
◆ Overcentrifugation may pack cells so tightly that they do not easily disperse and appear positive.
◆ Centrifugation of test with polyethylene glycol or positively charged polymers before washing may create clumps that do not disperse.
Cells That Have Positive Direct Antiglobulin Test (DAT)
◆ Cells that are positive by DAT will be positive in any indirect antiglobulin test. Procedures for removing IgG from DAT-positive cells are given in Methods 2-20 and 2-21.
Complement
◆ Complement components, primarily C4, may bind to cells from clots or from CPDA-1 donor segments during storage at 4 C and occasionally at higher temperatures. For DATs, use red cells anticoagulated with EDTA, ACD, or CPD.
◆ Samples collected in tubes containing silicone gel may have spurious complement attachment.[19]
◆ Complement may attach to red cells in samples collected from infusion lines used to administer dextrose-containing solutions. Strongest reactions are seen when large-bore needles are used or when sample volume is less than 0.5 mL.[20]

that are not agglutinated directly by anti-D reagents but that require an IAT for detection. Weak D testing is required for typing of donated red cell components but not for pretransfusion testing on patients. Because many institutions do not perform weak D testing on transfusion recipients, weak D individuals are considered Rh negative and will receive Rh-negative RBC units without risk of D alloimmunization. Such a practice permits some partial D individuals who are capable of making alloanti-D to be called Rh negative. The

TABLE 15-5. Blood Component ABO Requirements

Whole Blood	Must be identical to that of the recipient.
Red Blood Cells	Must be compatible with the recipient's plasma.
Granulocytes	Must be compatible with the recipient's plasma.
Fresh Frozen Plasma	Must be compatible with the recipient's red cells.
Platelets	All ABO groups are acceptable. Although ABO-identical platelets are preferred, components compatible with the recipient's red cells are recommended.
Cryoprecipitated AHF	All ABO groups are acceptable.

practice also avoids errors in Rh interpretation resulting from a positive DAT or from mixed red cell populations (D-positive and D-negative) following red cell transfusion, causing a positive weak D test.

Nonetheless, some transfusion services prefer to test patients' pretransfusion samples for weak D. The services' objective is to discover weak D patients to whom the services will transfuse D-positive blood components, based on the reasoning that such individuals should not make alloanti-D. However, as discussed earlier, some of those individuals whose red cells react with anti-D only in the weak D test have a partial D antigen and may make anti-D when challenged with D-positive transfusions.[22]

Detection of Unexpected Antibodies

The goals of antibody detection testing are as follows:

- To detect as many clinically significant antibodies as possible.
- To detect as few clinically insignificant antibodies as possible.
- To complete the procedure in a timely manner.

In general, an antibody is considered potentially clinically significant if antibodies of its specificity have been previously associated with hemolytic disease of the fetus and newborn (HDFN), with an HTR, or with notably decreased survival of transfused red cells. Antibodies reactive at either 37 C or in the AHG test phase are more likely to be clinically significant than are cold-reactive antibodies.[23]

For transfusion recipients, tests for unexpected antibodies use unpooled reagent red cells and a method that detects clinically significant antibodies. Two, three, or four screening cells may be used. The procedure includes an antiglobulin test preceded by incubation at 37 C[1(p34)] or an equivalent test system.

The Food and Drug Administration (FDA) has licensed reagent red cells to detect specific antibodies that are considered potentially clinically significant. To this end, reagent red cells must express the following antigens: D, C, E, c, e, M, N, S, s, P1, Le^a, Le^b, K, k, Fy^a, Fy^b, Jk^a, and Jk^b.

Each negative AHG tube test must be followed by a control system of IgG-sensitized red cells (check cells) when called for by the manufacturer's instructional insert. If check cells are not used, the manufacturer's specified controls must be used.

It is imperative that antibody detection systems used by each laboratory be sufficiently sensitive because the failure to detect a weakly reactive red cell alloantibody can be followed by a rapid anamnestic production of antibody, and then by a delayed HTR. Data published by the College of American Pathologists (J-Surveys; JAT-Surveys) demonstrate the relative performance of various testing schemes (manual, semiautomated, and automated) to detect red cell antibodies when "challenge" samples are tested as part of an external proficiency testing program.[24]

Antibody detection tests may be performed in advance of, or together with, a crossmatch between the patient's serum or plasma and the donor red cells. Performing antibody detection tests before crossmatching permits early recognition and identification of clinically significant antibodies and thereby permits selection of the appropriate crossmatch procedure and RBC units.

Antibody Detection Methods

A variety of techniques are available for the detection and identification of antibodies, as described below.

Albumin Additives

Bovine serum albumin is available in 22% concentration. Addition of albumin during antibody detection may reduce repulsive forces between cells and thus may promote agglutination (see Method 3-2-2).

LISS

LISS, which has reduced ionic strength (approximately 0.03 M) compared to that of normal saline (approximately 0.17 M), markedly accelerates antibody binding to red cells. Popular formulations of LISS include glycine or other nonionic substances to prevent red cell lysis at low ionic strengths. LISS additives may also contain albumin. Nonetheless, because lysis remains a concern, most practitioners add LISS at the time the reactions are set up, rather than using LISS-suspended red cells. As discussed in the previous section on sensitization, increasing the ratio of serum to cells increases the ionic strength of the reaction, which must be taken into account when determining the volume of LISS to add (see Method 3-2-3).

Polyethylene Glycol

PEG is a water-soluble linear polymer that potentiates antigen-antibody reactions.[25] PEG appears to accelerate antibody-red-cell binding by steric exclusion of water molecules in the diluent. The acceleration raises the effective concentrations of antigen and antibody, brings them into closer proximity, and thus increases binding. Anti-IgG AHG is usually preferred, because some polyspecific AHG reagents may cause false-positive reactions. PEG promotes detection of potentially clinically significant antibodies and decreases detection of clinically insignificant antibodies.[23] However, PEG may enhance warm-reactive autoantibodies; in such cases, testing serum using LISS or saline IAT may be preferred in order to decrease the interference from autoantibodies in antibody detection and identification tests. Some described PEG reagents are prepared in LISS solution. Centrifugation of PEG with test serum and red cells after 37 C incubation and before washing should be avoided because centrifugation can lead to aggregates that are difficult to disperse and interpret. Following incubation with PEG, test cells should be washed immediately in saline for the AHG test (see Method 3-2-4).

Enzymes

Enzyme-treated red cells are not routinely used in antibody detection tests but rather play an adjunctive role in complex antibody identification. Enzyme treatment destroys some red cell antigens (eg, M, N, S, s, Fy[a], Fy[b]), and thus enzyme treatment cannot be the sole antibody detection method because some significant antibodies will not be detected (eg, anti-Fy[a]). The most commonly used enzymes are ficin and papain. By cleaving negatively charged sialic acid molecules from polysaccharide chains, the enzymes reduce the red cell surface charge and promote agglutination. Red cells are pretreated with the enzyme, and the patient's serum or plasma is then added to the test system for observation of agglutination (see Methods 3-5-5 and 3-5-6).

Autologous Control

An autologous control or DAT is not required or recommended as a part of routine pretransfusion testing. The DAT is of limited value as a screening test for unexpected antibodies, except for patients who have recently been transfused, where the test may permit early detection of newly emerging antibodies. An autologous control, however, is of value when performing antibody identification.[26] (See Chapter 16.)

TUBELESS METHODS FOR PRETRANSFUSION TESTING

In addition to tube tests, pretransfusion tests may be performed using column agglutination technology, microplate solid-phase technology, or hemagglutination-microplate technology. Several automated and semiautomated testing platforms have been developed for using these technologies.

Solid-Phase Red Cell Adherence Tests

Solid-phase tests are similar to enzyme-linked immunosorbent assay methods where red cell antigens or antibodies are immobilized in microplate wells in order to detect antibody-antigen interactions. In a typical configuration, intact red cells or red cell membranes, of known phenotype, are immobilized to microplate wells, and patient serum or plasma is added. Following incubation, unbound antibodies are washed off, and the remaining patient antibody bound to the immobilized red cell antigens is detected. A commonly used method to detect bound antibody is a suspension of anti-IgG-coated indicator red cells. Following brief centrifugation, the reaction is read as positive if the indicator cells adhere diffusely over the well, or as negative if the indicator cells pellet to the bottom.[27-30]

Column Agglutination Technology

Column agglutination uses gel or glass beads to trap agglutinated red cells. The commercially prepared systems use a card or strip of several microtubes of reactants that allows for performance of several tests simultaneously. Column agglutination can be used for detection of direct agglutination (eg, ABO and Rh tests, red cell phenotyping) and for the DAT or IAT. Red cells are typically allowed to interact with antibodies in chambers at the top of each column. The columns or microtubes are then centrifuged to force the red cells into the column medium. The column medium separates agglutinated red cells (which are too large to enter the gel matrix and thus remain at the top of the gel) from nonagglutinated cells that move through the pores in the gel to the bottom of the column. One advantage of this technology is that under appropriate centrifugation conditions, red cells enter the column, but serum or plasma remains on top, obviating the need for saline washing for antiglobulin tests.[31-33]

Automated Testing Systems

Automated testing systems have been developed for the detection of antigen-antibody reactions in immunohematologic testing. ABO, Rh, antibody detection and identification, and crossmatching may be performed on these systems. These systems perform multiple tests, using solid-phase, column agglutination, microtiter plate, and other technologies. Some or all steps in the testing process—from sample pipetting through results interpretation—may be performed under computerized control using bar-code technology to ensure "positive" sample identity. The test system's computer may be interfaced with a laboratory's information system for reporting results. Such systems should undergo validation before implementation and with any alteration in software functionality.

Molecular Methods

Molecular testing is not routinely performed as a part of pretransfusion testing. However, molecular red cell antigen typing may be employed in pretransfusion compatibility testing in certain clinical situations when serologic methodology may not be sufficient. Molecular methods may be useful for patients with the following:

- Recent transfusion without a known red cell phenotype.
- Autoimmune hemolytic anemia (for such patients, red cell phenotyping is required).
- HDFN.
- Rh typing discrepancies.

For additional discussion of molecular typing of red cell antigens, see Chapter 10.

COMPARISON OF CURRENT TESTING RESULTS WITH PREVIOUS RECORDS

Results of ABO and Rh tests on a current sample must be compared with previous transfusion service records if there has been prior testing during the past 12 months. The comparison must be documented.[1(p34)] Errors in identification or testing, or both, may be detected when discrepancies are found between previous and current ABO and Rh results. A potential problem can occur when a patient has no previous ABO and Rh results with which to compare current test results. If a sample collection or patient ID error were to occur, resulting in the wrong blood in tube (WBIT), it might not be detected by the blood bank because no previous ABO and Rh results are available for comparison. One approach that may detect such sample errors is to require a second, independently drawn sample on patients with no historical ABO group and Rh type available. Such an approach permits identification of WBIT sample errors and may prevent ABO-incompatible transfusions.[34,35]

Records should also be reviewed for the presence of clinically significant red cell antibodies, for difficulties in testing, for the occurrence of significant adverse reactions to transfusion, and for special transfusion requirements.[1(p34)] Clinically significant red cell alloantibodies may become undetectable in a recipient's serum over time. Between 30% and 35% of antibodies become undetectable within 1 year, and nearly 50% become undetectable after 10 or more years.[36]

DONOR RBC UNIT TESTING

A serologic test to confirm the ABO group of all RBC units and the Rh type of RBC units labeled as Rh negative must be performed at least once by the transfusing facility. Confirmatory testing for weak D is not required. Confirmatory testing is to be performed on a sample obtained from an attached segment. Any discrepancies are to be resolved before the unit is issued for transfusion and should be reported to the facility that collected the unit.[1(p33)]

DONOR RBC UNIT SELECTION

ABO Compatibility

Whenever possible, patients should receive ABO-identical blood; however, it may occasionally be necessary to make alternative selections. If the component to be transfused contains 2 mL or more of red cells, the donor's red cells must be ABO-compatible with the recipient's plasma.[1(p35)] Because plasma-containing components can also affect the recipient's red cells, the ABO antibodies in transfused plasma should be compatible with the recipient's red cells when feasible.[37] Requirements for components and acceptable alternative choices are summarized in Table 15-5.

Rh Type

D-positive blood components should routinely be selected for D-positive recipients. D-negative units will be compatible but should be reserved for D-negative recipients. D-negative patients (especially females of childbearing potential) should receive red-cell-containing components that are D negative to avoid immunization to the D antigen and possible HDFN. When ABO-compatible D-negative components are not available for a D-negative recipient, the blood bank physician and the patient's physician should weigh alternative courses of action. Depending on the childbearing potential of the patient and the volume of red cells transfused, it may be desirable to administer Rh Immune Globulin (RhIG) to a D-negative patient who is given D-positive blood.[38-41]

Other Blood Groups

Antigens other than ABO and D are not routinely considered in the selection of units of blood for nonalloimmunized patients. However, in certain medical conditions such as sickle cell disease, some institutions may elect to transfuse phenotypically matched RBCs to prevent alloimmunization in this frequently transfused population.[42] One study of North American hospital transfusion service laboratories showed that laboratories most commonly match for the C, E, and K antigens when phenotype-matched donor red cells are used to transfuse nonalloimmunized sickle cell patients.[43]

If the patient has a clinically significant unexpected antibody(ies), blood lacking the corresponding antigen(s) should be selected for crossmatching. If there is an adequate quantity of the patient's serum, or if another patient's serum with the same antibody specificity is available, and if that antibody reacts well with antigen-positive red cells, that serum may be used to screen for antigen-negative donor RBC units. Red cells found to be antigen negative must be confirmed with an FDA-licensed reagent, when available. When licensed reagents are not available (eg, anti-Lan or anti-Yt^a), expired reagents or stored serum samples from patients or donors may be used, provided that controls tested on the day of use are acceptable.[44,45]

When crossmatch-compatible units cannot be found, the transfusion service attending physician should be involved in the decision about how to manage the patient (see Chapter 20). Antigen-negative donor RBC units are not usually provided for patients whose antibodies are not clinically significant.

COMPATIBILITY TESTING OR CROSSMATCH (SEROLOGIC OR COMPUTER/ELECTRONIC)

Unless there is an urgent need for blood, a crossmatch must be performed before a red cell transfusion. When clinically significant antibodies are not detected in current antibody detection tests and there is no record of previous detection of such antibodies,[1(p35)] then a method is required that at least detects ABO incompatibility, such as an immediate-spin (IS) or computer/electronic crossmatch. If the patient's antibody detection test is negative, the risk of an overt hemolytic reaction is low.[46-48] The potential benefits of omitting a routine AHG crossmatch include reductions in turnaround time, in workload, and in reagent costs, as well as a more effective use of blood inventory. Omission of the AHG phase of the crossmatch for patients who meet the criteria must be in approved written standard operating procedures (SOPs).

Blood lacking relevant antigens should be selected for transfusion when a patient has a clinically significant antibody identified currently or historically, even if the antibody is presently nonreactive.[1(p35)] The crossmatch must include incubation at 37 C and the AHG test.[1(pp34-35)] The methods used for AHG crossmatches may be the same as those used for red cell antibody detection or identification, or the methods may be different. For example, column agglutination may be used for both antibody detection and identification, but the crossmatch may be performed using a tube test.

Immediate-Spin Crossmatch

The IS crossmatch and AHG phase crossmatch are both performed using the patient's serum or plasma and donor red cells, which must be obtained from a segment of tubing originally attached to the blood unit container.

The IS crossmatch method is designed to detect ABO incompatibilities between donor red cells and recipient serum. It can be used as the sole crossmatch method *only* if the patient has no present or previously detected clinically significant antibodies. In the IS saline technique, patient serum or plasma is mixed with saline-suspended red cells at room temperature, and the tube is centrifuged immediately and observed for the presence of agglutination. An IS crossmatch technique is described in Method 3-1.

The IS serologic crossmatch is considered the most efficacious serologic method to recognize ABO incompatibility.[47] Failure to properly perform the IS crossmatch test can cause *false-negative* results and the failure to detect ABO-incompatible donor RBC units.[49] It is imperative that when the IS crossmatch test is performed, no delay occurs when initiating the centrifugation step or reading the reaction upon completion of centrifugation.

Antiglobulin Crossmatch

The AHG crossmatch may be performed using tube, column agglutination, or solid-phase systems. Although tube AHG crossmatches will detect ABO incompatibility, the AHG crossmatch using solid-phase tests or column agglutination may not. The test manufacturer's package or instructional insert must be consulted to determine if any additional testing is required for the detection of ABO incompatibility.

For a routine tube AHG crossmatch, the donor red cells may be washed and resuspended to 2% to 5% in saline. Washing the donor's red cells removes small fibrin clots and some cold agglutinins that may interfere with interpretation of results. Because the ratio of serum to cells markedly affects the sensitivity of agglutination tests, it is important to stay within the 2% to 5% red cell suspension range or as specified by the manufacturer's instructions. If too many donor red cells are present, weak antibodies may be missed because too few antibody molecules bind to each cell. Many laboratorians find that a 2% to 3% concentration (tube testing) yields the best results. For tests using column agglutination or solid-phase systems, the manufacturer's directions should be followed.

Computer Crossmatch

When no clinically significant antibodies have been detected by the antibody detection test and history review, it is permissible to omit the IS and AHG phase of the crossmatch and to verify ABO compatibility by using the computerized/electronic crossmatch. Computerized crossmatching of blood can be used, provided that the following conditions have been met[1(p36)]:

- The computer system has been validated, on-site, to ensure that only ABO-compatible whole blood or red cells are selected for transfusion.
- Two determinations of the recipient's ABO group are made, as follows: one on a current sample, and a second one by one of the following methods: by retesting the same sample, by testing a second current sample, or by comparing with previous records.
- The computer system contains the unit number, component name, ABO group, and Rh type of the component; the confirmed donor unit ABO group; two unique recipient identifiers; the recipient's ABO group, Rh type, and antibody screen results; and interpretation of compatibility.
- A method exists to verify correct entry of data before the release of blood or components.
- The system contains logic to alert the user to discrepancies between the donor ABO group and Rh type on the unit label and the interpretation of the blood group confirmatory test, as well as to alert the user to ABO incompatibility between the recipient and donor unit.

Potential advantages of a computer crossmatch include decreased workload, reduced sample volume required for testing, reduced exposure of personnel to blood samples, and better use of blood inventory.[50-52]

Crossmatch/Transfusion Ratios

The crossmatch/transfusion ratio, or "C/T ratio," is the number of RBC units crossmatched divided by the number of RBC units transfused. Although the institution's average C/T ratio is not typically useful, determination of specialty-specific and individual physician C/T ratios may be helpful to identify which group of physicians is ordering a type and crossmatch for their patients when a type and screen preoperative transfusion order might be more appropriate.

INTERPRETATION OF ANTIBODY SCREENING AND CROSSMATCH RESULTS

Most samples tested have a negative antibody screen and will be crossmatch compatible with the donor RBC units selected. A negative antibody screen, however, does not guarantee that the serum or plasma does not have clinically significant red cell antibodies—only that it contains no detectable antibodies that react with the screening cells used or by the techniques used. Furthermore, a compatible crossmatch does not guarantee normal red cell survival. Table 15-6 reviews the possible causes of positive pretransfusion tests using tube testing. Spurious or unexpected reactions with other testing technologies may have the same causes as those seen in the tube tests, or other causes.[53] Depending on the antigen/antibody reaction strength and the testing conditions, not all of the scenarios will result in positive tests. The cause of the serologic problems should be identified before transfusion occurs. Chapter 16 reviews techniques for problem resolution and antibody identification. If the patient is found to have clinically significant antibodies, RBC units issued for transfusion should lack the antigens that cor-

TABLE 15-6. Causes of Positive Pretransfusion Tests*

Negative Antibody Screen, Incompatible Immediate-Spin Crossmatch
◆ Donor red cells are ABO-incompatible.
◆ Donor red cells are polyagglutinable.
◆ Anti-A1 is in the serum of an A_2 or A_2B individual.
◆ Other alloantibodies reactive at room temperature (eg, anti-M).
◆ Rouleaux formation.
◆ Cold autoantibodies (eg, anti-I).
◆ Passively acquired anti-A or anti-B.
Negative Antibody Screen, Incompatible Antiglobulin Crossmatch
◆ Donor red cells have a positive direct antiglobulin test.
◆ Antibody reacts only with red cells having strong expression of a particular antigen (eg, dosage) or variation in antigen strength (eg, P1).
◆ Antibody to a low-incidence antigen on the donor red cells.
◆ Passively acquired anti-A or anti-B.
Positive Antibody Screen, Compatible Crossmatches
◆ Autoanti-IH (-H) or anti-Le^{bH} and nongroup O units are selected.
◆ Antibodies dependent on reagent red cell diluent.
◆ Antibodies demonstrating dosage and donor red cells are from heterozygotes (ie, expressing a single dose of antigen).
◆ Donor unit is lacking corresponding antigen.
Positive Antibody Screen, Incompatible Crossmatches, Negative Auto Control
◆ Alloantibody(ies).
Positive Antibody Screen, Incompatible Crossmatches, Positive Auto Control, Negative Direct Antiglobulin Test
◆ Antibody to ingredient in enhancement media or enhancement dependent autoantibody.
◆ Rouleaux formation.
Positive Antibody Screen, Incompatible Crossmatches, Positive Auto Control, Positive DAT
◆ Alloantibody causing either a delayed serologic or hemolytic transfusion reaction.
◆ Passively acquired autoantibody (eg, intravenous immune globulin).
◆ Cold- or warm-reactive autoantibody.

*Causes depend on serologic methods used.

respond to those antibodies (see "Donor RBC Unit Selection," "Other Blood Groups"). When the antibody identified is considered clinically *insignificant* (eg, anti-A1, anti-M, anti-N, anti-P1, anti-Le^a, anti-Le^b) and is not reactive at 37 C, RBC units that are ABO and Rh-compatible (but that do not necessarily lack the corresponding antigen) may be selected for crossmatch.

PRETRANSFUSION ORDERS

A physician's order initiates the testing performed on a pretransfusion blood sample. The scope of pretransfusion testing might include merely "holding" the sample pending further instructions; performing an ABO and Rh test only, a type and screen, or a crossmatch; or using combinations of the aforementioned (see Table 15-7). Type and screen is a testing combination in which the patient's blood sample is tested for ABO group, for Rh type, and for unexpected antibodies, and then it is stored in the transfusion service laboratory for future crossmatching if a unit is needed for transfusion. The blood bank must have enough donor red cells available to meet the unexpected needs of patients undergoing operations under a type-and-screen policy. If transfusion becomes necessary, ABO- and Rh-compatible blood can be safely released after an IS or computer crossmatch if the antibody screen is negative and if there is no history of clinically significant antibodies.

However, if the antibody screen is positive, the cause of the positive screen must be determined, and any causative antibody(ies) must be identified following the type and screen. Depending on which antibodies are identified, RBC units lacking the corresponding antigen(s) must be available for use if needed. Each of these test combinations requires a certain amount of time to perform. If the antibody screen is positive, crossmatches should be performed to the extent that the worst-case bleeding scenario has been considered and covered. When a type and crossmatch is ordered, a sufficient number of units should be crossmatched to meet, on average, the transfusion demands for 90% of patients undergoing that procedure. (See Table 15-7.)

AVAILABILITY OF COMPATIBLE BLOOD

Certain steps may be taken to help ensure that sufficient compatible blood is available for each scheduled surgical procedure. The patient's blood sample should be received in the laboratory in advance of the scheduled procedure, with sufficient time allowed to complete all preoperative pretransfusion testing before surgery begins. Unfortunately, it is not uncommon for an initial pretransfusion sample to be received by the transfusion service laboratory on the morning of a "same-day admission" surgical procedure, which gives the laboratory only limited time to complete pretransfusion red cell compatibility testing.[54] Up to 7% of type and screen samples may not be tested completely until *after* the patient's surgery has begun. Such a sample may be the first and only opportunity that a laboratory has to determine a patient's ABO and Rh status. The risk of WBIT is about 1 in 2000 samples.[35] About 3% of samples received will have a serologic finding that requires further investigation.[55] Thus, discovery of either of these problems at the last minute may cause dangerous delays in blood availability for a patient. Collection of a type and screen sample days to weeks in advance of surgery, with a second sample collected the morning of a scheduled surgery, is an alternative approach that can mitigate the problem.[55]

LABELING OF BLOOD AND BLOOD COMPONENTS WITH THE RECIPIENT'S INFORMATION

The following activities are required at the time of issue[1(pp39-40)]:

- A tag or label indicating the recipient's two independent identifiers, the donor unit number, and the compatibility test inter-

TABLE 15-7. Pretransfusion Testing Schemes

Test Scheme	Tests Performed	Advantages	Limitations
No order	None		No sample has been collected. ABO, Rh, and antibody detection testing are *not* performed.
Hold clot	None	A sample has been collected.	ABO, Rh, and antibody detection testing are *not* performed.
Type (type and hold)	ABO, Rh	A sample has been collected; patient's ABO/Rh are known.	Antibody detection testing is *not* performed.
Type and screen	ABO, Rh, antibody detection test/identification	Most of the pretransfusion testing has been performed; compatible blood can be provided in most situations.	Does not include crossmatch.
Type and crossmatch	ABO, Rh, antibody detection test/identification, RBC unit selection or phenotyping, crossmatch	Routine pretransfusion testing has been performed; compatible blood can be provided in most situations.	Units are removed from inventory and may not be available for use by other patients in a timely manner.

pretation, if performed, must be attached securely to the blood container.

- A final check of records maintained in the blood bank for each unit of blood or component must include the following:

  1. Two independent identifiers, one of which is usually the patient's name.
  2. The recipient's ABO group and Rh type.
  3. The donor unit or pool ID number.
  4. The donor's ABO group and, if required, Rh type.
  5. The interpretation of the crossmatch tests (if performed).
  6. The date and time of issue.
  7. The expiration date (and time, as applicable).
  8. Special transfusion requirements (eg, cytomegalovirus reduced-risk, irradiated, or antigen-negative components).

- A process must exist to confirm that the identifying information, the request, the records, and the blood or component are all in agreement, and that any and all discrepancies have been resolved before issue.

Additional records that may be useful include those that identify the person issuing the blood, the person to whom the blood was issued, and the destination of the unit. After the transfusion, a record of the transfusion shall be made a part of the patient's medical record. That information may be part of a computer record or a paper form. Records must contain the identification of the person(s) performing the test and, if blood is issued before the resolution of compatibility problems, the final status of the serologic findings. Before issuing a unit of blood or component, personnel must inspect the blood or component to ensure that it is acceptable for use, that it does not have an abnormal color or appearance, that its container is not leaking, and that it is not outdated. Final identification of the transfusion recipient and the blood component rests with the transfusionist, who must identify the patient and donor unit and who must certify that identifying information on forms, tags, and labels is in agreement. The Joint Commission required in 2010 that hospitals use a two-person verification process before initiating a blood or blood component transfusion, and if two individuals are not available, an automated identification technology (ie, bar-coding) may be used in place of one of the individuals.[2]

SPECIAL CLINICAL SITUATIONS

Patients Less than 4 Months of Age

Requirements for compatibility testing for patients less than 4 months of age are discussed in Chapter 23. An initial pretransfusion sample must be obtained from the neonate/infant to determine the ABO group and Rh type. For determining ABO group, testing the red cells with anti-A and anti-B is the only test required. Serum or plasma from either the neonate/infant or the mother may be used to detect unexpected red cell antibodies and for crossmatching. The neonate/infant's serum does not need to be tested for ABO antibodies unless a non-group-O neonate/infant is to receive non-group-O cells that may be incompatible with passively acquired anti-A or anti-B. Such an antibody most often comes from the mother but can be found after transfusion of group O RBCs or out-of-group platelets. Tests in this case should include an AHG phase using either donor or reagent A_1 or B red cells.

If no clinically significant unexpected antibodies are present, it is unnecessary to crossmatch donor red cells for the initial or subsequent transfusions. Repeat testing may be omitted for patients less than 4 months of age during any one hospital admission[1(p37)] as long as they are receiving only group O RBCs. A crossmatch is not required if antibody of maternal origin is detected, as long as antigen-negative blood is transfused.

Blood Administered in Urgent Situations

When blood is urgently needed, the patient's physician must weigh the risk of transfusing uncrossmatched or partially crossmatched blood against the risk of delaying transfusion until compatibility testing is complete. Ideally, a transfusion service physician should provide consultation. (See Chapter 20.)

When blood is released before pretransfusion testing is complete, the records must contain a signed statement from the requesting physician indicating that the clinical situation was sufficiently urgent to require release of blood.[1(p41)] Such a statement does not need to be obtained before issuing lifesaving transfusions, nor does it absolve blood bank personnel from their responsibility to issue properly labeled donor blood that is ABO compatible with the patient. When urgent release is requested, blood bank personnel should take the following actions:

1. Issue uncrossmatched blood, which should be as follows:
   a. Group O RBCs if the patient's ABO group is unknown. It is preferable to give D-negative blood if the recipient's D type is unknown, especially if the patient is a female of childbearing potential.
   b. ABO and Rh compatible, if there has been time to test a current sample.
2. Indicate in a conspicuous fashion on the attached tag or label that compatibility testing was *not* completed at the time of issue.
3. Begin compatibility tests, and complete them promptly (for massive transfusion, see below). If incompatibility is detected at any stage of testing, the patient's physician and the transfusion service physician should be notified immediately.

Massive Transfusion

There are several different definitions of massive transfusion. In this chapter, massive transfusion is defined either as the administration of 8 to 10 RBC units to an adult patient in less than 24 hours, or as the acute administration of 4 to 5 RBC units in 1 hour. Exchange transfusion of an infant is also considered a massive transfusion.

Following massive transfusion, the pretransfusion sample no longer represents the blood currently in the patient's circulation. If possible, in the massive transfusion setting, an abbreviated crossmatch such as a computer crossmatch or an IS crossmatch should be performed to confirm ABO compatibility of units administered. If a more limited pretransfusion testing protocol is used in these situations, the protocol should be described in a written SOP.

Some facilities stop crossmatching RBC units (and routinely issue uncrossmatched RBCs) as soon as a patient has received 10 RBC units in less than 24 hours. These facilities justify the practice by stating that most of the circulating blood has been diluted with transfused blood and any antibodies capable of causing a hemolytic reaction have also been diluted. However, even if 99% of a patient's circulating red cells have been replaced with transfused red cells, massively transfused patients usually receive plasma-containing products, some of which may contain ABO antibodies incompatible with the RBC units selected for transfusion. The administration of RBCs incompatible with circulating anti-A or anti-B can still cause a significant reaction; thus, ABO incompatibility in such a situation will not be detected if the serologic crossmatch is eliminated after a patient receives massive RBC transfusion.

Blood Administration After Non-Group-Specific Transfusion

Transfusion services must sometimes release group O RBC units for transfusion during emergencies before a pretransfusion sample is received in the laboratory. Once a sample is received, the patient's ABO and Rh can be quickly determined and group specific products can begin to be released. Group O AS-1, AS-3, and AS-5 RBC units contain minimal residual plasma, which minimizes concerns regarding passive transfusion of anti-A and anti-B. In this case, switching to ABO-identical RBC components can be done safely, although an occasional patient may exhibit a transient positive DAT. In some cases, when large volumes of red cells are transfused, or when small children or infants receive transfusions, passively acquired ABO antibodies may be detected in the patient's serum/plasma.[56] If that should occur, transfusion with red cells that lack the corresponding ABO antigen should be continued. If a patient receives blood of an Rh type different from his or her own, it may become difficult to determine the patient's true Rh type. If there is any question about the patient's true Rh type, it may be prudent to administer D-negative blood, especially if the patient is female. The use of RhIG prophylaxis may be considered when D-positive components are transfused to D-negative patients. (See Chapter 20.)

KEY POINTS

1. Two independent patient identifiers are required for the pretransfusion samples, and ideally they include the patient's first and last names and an ID number that is unique to the patient.
2. The phlebotomist must label each blood sample tube, in the presence of the patient, with two independent patient identifiers and the date of collection.
3. When a pretransfusion sample is received in the laboratory, laboratory personnel must confirm that the information on the sample label and the information on the pretransfusion testing request are identical. If there is any doubt about the identity of the patient or about the labeling of the sample, a new sample must be obtained.
4. Pretransfusion serologic tests include ABO group and Rh type, antibody detection, and crossmatching. These tests, which demonstrate in-vitro red cell antigen/antibody reactions, are performed in order to prevent transfusion of incompatible red cells.
5. If the patient has been pregnant or transfused within the previous 3 months, or if the pregnancy history and transfusion history are uncertain, the pretransfusion sample used for testing must be no more than 3 days old at the time of intended transfusion, because recent transfusion or pregnancy may stimulate production of unexpected antibodies.
6. Any discrepant ABO group results should be resolved before blood is given. If transfusion is necessary before resolution of a discrepancy, the patient should receive group O red cells.
7. The goals of antibody detection testing are as follows:
   - To detect as many clinically significant antibodies as possible.
   - To detect as few clinically insignificant antibodies as possible.
   - To complete the procedure in a timely manner.
8. Results of ABO and Rh tests on a current sample must be compared with previous transfusion service records if there has been prior testing during the past 12 months. The comparison must be documented. Records are also reviewed for the presence of clinically significant red cell antibodies, for difficulties in testing, for the occurrence of significant adverse reactions, and for special transfusion requirements.
9. If the component to be transfused contains 2 mL or more of red cells, the donor's red cells must be ABO compatible with the recipient's plasma.
10. At the time of issue of a blood component, labeling information must be complete and be checked against blood bank records.

REFERENCES

1. Carson TH, ed. Standards for blood banks and transfusion services. 27th ed. Bethesda, MD: AABB, 2011.
2. National Patient Safety Goals. Oakbrook Terrace, IL: The Joint Commission, 2011. [Avail-

able at http://www.jointcommission.org (accessed March 6, 2011).]
3. Code of federal regulations. Title 42, CFR Part 493.1241. Washington, DC: US Government Printing Office, 2010 (revised annually).
4. Sazama K. Reports of 355 transfusion associated deaths: 1976 through 1985. Transfusion 1990; 30:583-90.
5. Turner CL, Casbard AC, Murphy MF. Barcode technology: Its role in increasing the safety of blood transfusion. Transfusion 2003;43: 1200-9.
6. Davies A, Staves J, Kay J, et al. End-to-end electronic control of the hospital transfusion process to increase the safety of blood transfusion: Strengths and weaknesses. Transfusion 2006;46:352-64.
7. Dzik WH. Technology for enhanced transfusion safety. Hematology Am Soc Hematol Educ Program 2005:476-82.
8. Positive patient identification systems and products. System review series. CAP Today, July 2006.
9. Murphy MF, Casbard AC, Ballard S, et al. Prevention of bedside errors in transfusion medicine (PROBE-TM) study: A cluster-randomized, matched-paired clinical areas trial of a simple intervention to reduce errors in the pre-transfusion bedside check. Transfusion 2007;47:771-80.
10. Wehrli G, Shulman IA. Transfusion therapy. In: Demetriades D, Asensio JA. Trauma management. Georgetown, TX: Landes Bioscience, 2000:636-45.
11. Lumadue JA, Boyd JS, Ness PM. Adherence to a strict specimen-labeling policy decreases the incidence of erroneous blood grouping of blood bank specimens. Transfusion 1997;37: 1169-72.
12. Shulman IA. When should antibody screening tests be done for recently transfused patients? Transfusion 1990;30:39-41.
13. What is the experience with using pretransfusion blood samples that are routinely used for up to 10 days (or longer) after their collection? California Blood Bank SocietyeNetwork Forum. [Available at http://www.cbbsweb.org/enf/2006/pretx_10dsample_all.html (accessed October 21, 2010).]
14. Jorgensen J, Nielsen M, Nielsen CB, Normark J. The influence of ionic strength, albumin and incubation time on the sensitivity of the indirect Coombs' test. Vox Sang 1979;36:186-91.
15. Van Oss CJ. Immunological and physio-chemical nature of antigen-antibody interactions. In: Garratty G, ed. Immunobiology of transfusion medicine. New York: Marcel Dekker, 1994: 327-64.
16. Coombs RRA, Mourant AE, Race RR. A new test for the detection of weak and "incomplete" Rh agglutinins. Br J Exp Pathol 1945;26:255-66.
17. Ylagen ES, Curtis BR, Wildgen ME, et al. Invalidation of antiglobulin tests by a high thermal amplitude cryoglobulin. Transfusion 1990;30: 154-7.
18. Rolih S, Thomas R, Fisher E, Talbot J. Antibody detection errors due to acidic or unbuffered saline. Immunohematology 1993;9:15-18.
19. Geisland JR, Milam JD. Spuriously positive direct antiglobulin tests caused by silicone gel. Transfusion 1980;20:711-13.
20. Grindon AJ, Wilson MJ. False-positive DAT caused by variables in sample procurement. Transfusion 1981;21:313-14.
21. Marsh WL. Scoring of hemagglutination reactions. Transfusion 1972;12:352-3.
22. Flegel WA. Homing in on D antigen immunogenicity. Transfusion 2005;45:466-8.
23. Issitt PD, Anstee DJ. Applied blood group serology. 4th ed. Durham, NC: Montgomery Scientific Publications, 1998:873-905.
24. Shulman IA, Maffei LM, Downes KA. North American pretransfusion testing practices, 2001-2004: Results from the College of American Pathologists Interlaboratory Comparison Program survey data, 2001-2004. Arch Pathol Lab Med 2005;129:984-9.
25. Nance SJ, Garratty G. Polyethylene glycol: A new potentiator of red blood cell antigen-antibody reactions. Am J Clin Pathol 1987;87:633-5.
26. Judd WJ, Barnes BA, Steiner EA, et al. The evaluation of a positive direct antiglobulin test (autocontrol) in pretransfusion testing revisited. Transfusion 1986;26:220-4.
27. Walker P. New technologies in transfusion medicine. Lab Med 1997;28:258-62.
28. Plapp FV, Sinor LT, Rachel JM, et al. A solid phase antibody screen. Am J Clin Pathol 1984; 82:719-21.
29. Rachel JM, Sinor LT, Beck ML, Plapp FV. A solid-phase antiglobulin test. Transfusion 1985;25:24-6.
30. Sinor L. Advances in solid-phase red cell adherence methods and transfusion serology. Transfus Med Rev 1992;6:26-31.

31. Malyska H, Weiland D. The gel test. Lab Med 1994;25:81-5.
32. Lapierre Y, Rigal D, Adam J, et al. The gel test: A new way to detect red cell antigen-antibody reactions. Transfusion 1990;30:109-13.
33. Reis KJ, Chachowski R, Cupido A, et al. Column agglutination technology: The antiglobulin test. Transfusion 1993;33:639-43.
34. Should pre-transfusion ABO/Rh testing be performed twice, and if so, on different samples or by different personnel? California Blood Bank Society eNetwork Forum. [Available at http://www.cbbsweb.org/enf/2002/pretxtesting_aborh.html (accessed October 21, 2010).]
35. Figueroa PI, Ziman A, Wheeler C, et al. Nearly two decades using the check-type to prevent ABO incompatible transfusions: One institution's experience. Am J Clin Pathol 2006;126: 422-6.
36. Ramsey G, Smietana SJ. Long-term follow-up testing of red cell alloantibodies. Transfusion 1994;34:122-4.
37. Fung M, Downes KA, Shulman IA. Transfusion of platelets containing ABO-incompatible plasma: A survey of 3,156 North American laboratories. Arch Pathol Lab Med 2007;131:909-16.
38. Pollack W, Ascari WQ, Crispen JF, et al. Studies on Rh prophylaxis II: Rh immune prophylaxis after transfusion with Rh-positive blood. Transfusion 1971;11:340-4.
39. Rh immune globulin (RHIG) administration after transfusion of Rh-pos platelets/plateletpheresis units to Rh-neg recipients. California Blood Bank Society eNetwork Forum. [Available at http://www.cbbsweb.org/enf/2001/rhig_incomptx.html (accessed October 21, 2010).]
40. How important is it to avoid Rh mismatched platelets for Rh-negative female neonates? California Blood Bank Society eNetwork Forum. [Available at http://www.cbbsweb.org/enf/2002/rhincomp_ plttx.html (accessed October 21, 2010).]
41. Is there evidence that girls and premenopausal women who need transfusion should receive donor RBC units that are phenotype tested and matched for CDE and K antigens, to reduce risk of alloimmunization and prevent future cases of hemolytic disease of the newborn? California Blood Bank Society eNetwork Forum. [Available at http://www.cbbsweb.org/enf/ 2006/phenomatch_females.html (accessed October 21, 2010).]
42. Afenyi-Annan A, Brecher ME. Pre-transfusion phenotype matching for sickle cell disease patients. Transfusion 2004;44:619-20.
43. Osby M, Shulman IA. Phenotype matching of donor red blood cell units for nonalloimmunized sickle cell disease patients: A survey of 1182 North American laboratories. Arch Pathol Lab Med 2005;129:190-3.
44. Food and Drug Administration. Compliance programs (CBER). 7342.001. Inspection of licensed and unlicensed blood banks, brokers, reference laboratories, and contractors. Rockville, MD: CBER Office of Compliance and Biologics Quality, 2010. [Available at http://www.fda.gov/BiologicsBloodVaccines/GuidanceComplianceRegulatoryInformation/ComplianceActivities/Enforcement/CompliancePrograms/ucm095226.htm (accessed April 4, 2011).]
45. Can expired panel cells be used in a manner that would be considered compliant? California Blood Bank Society eNetwork Forum. [Available at http://www.cbbsweb. org/enf/2004/reagentcells_exp2.html (accessed October 21, 2010).]
46. Oberman HA. The present and future crossmatch. Transfusion 1992;32:794-5.
47. Meyer EA, Shulman IA. The sensitivity and specificity of the immediate-spin crossmatch. Transfusion 1989;29:99-102.
48. Shulman IA, Odono V. The risk of overt acute hemolytic transfusion reaction following the use of an immediate-spin crossmatch. Transfusion 1994;34:87-8.
49. Shulman IA, Calderon C. Effect of delayed centrifugation or reading on the detection of ABO incompatibility by the immediate-spin crossmatch. Transfusion 1991;31:197-200.
50. Butch SH, Judd WJ, Steiner EA, et al. Electronic verification of donor-recipient compatibility: The computer crossmatch. Transfusion 1994; 34:105-9.
51. Butch SH, Judd WJ. Requirements for the computer crossmatch (letter). Transfusion 1994; 34:187.
52. Safwenberg J, Högman CF, Cassemar B. Computerized delivery control—a useful and safe complement to the type and screen compatibility testing. Vox Sang 1997;72:162-8.
53. Weisbach V, Kohnhauser T, Zimmermann R, et al. Comparison of the performance of microtube column systems and solid-phase systems

and the tube low-ionic-strength solution additive indirect antiglobulin test in the detection of red cell alloantibodies. Transfus Med 2006; 16:276-84.

54. Friedberg RC, Jones BA, Walsh MK. Type and screen completion for scheduled surgical procedures: A College of American Pathologists Q-Probes study of 8941 type and screen tests in 108 institutions. Arch Pathol Lab Med 2003; 127:533-40.

55. Saxena S, Nelson JM, Osby M, et al. Ensuring timely completion of type and screen testing and the verification of ABO/Rh status for elective surgical patients. Arch Pathol Lab Med 2007;131:576-81.

56. Garratty G. Problems associated with passively transfused blood group alloantibodies. Am J Clin Pathol 1998;109:169-77.

Chapter 16

Identification of Antibodies to Red Cell Antigens

Phyllis S. Walker, MS, MT(ASCP)SBB

NATURALLY OCCURRING anti-A and anti-B are the only red cell antibodies that are regularly found in normal human serum or plasma. All other antibodies are called unexpected red cell antibodies. This chapter discusses methods for detecting and identifying unexpected red cell antibodies.

There are two types of unexpected red cell antibodies: alloantibodies and autoantibodies. When someone produces an antibody to an antigen that he or she lacks, the antibody is called an alloantibody. When someone produces an antibody to an antigen that he or she possesses, the antibody is called an autoantibody. Therefore, by definition, alloantibodies react only with allogeneic red cells that express the corresponding antigens—not with the antibody producer's red cells. Conversely, autoantibodies do react with the red cells of the antibody producer. In fact, autoantibodies usually react with most reagent red cells as well as with the autologous red cells.

Depending on which group of patients or donors was studied and the sensitivity of the test methods used, alloantibodies were found in 0.3% to 38% of the population.[1] Immunization to red cell antigens may result from pregnancy, transfusion, transplantation, or injections of immunogenic material. In some instances, no specific immunizing event can be identified. In such a case, naturally occurring antibodies have presumably resulted from exposure to environmental, bacterial, or viral antigens that are similar to blood group antigens. Also, antibodies detected in serologic tests may be passively acquired. These antibodies may be acquired from injected immunoglobulin, donor plasma, passenger lymphocytes in transplanted organs, or hematopoietic progenitor cells (HPCs).

SIGNIFICANCE OF ALLOANTIBODIES

Alloantibodies to red cell antigens may be detected initially in any test that uses serum or plasma (eg, an ABO test, an antibody detection test, or a compatibility test) or in an eluate prepared from red cells coated with alloantibody. Serum and plasma are interchangeable for antibody testing unless complement is required for antibody detection. In such rare cases, only

Phyllis S. Walker, MS, MT(ASCP)SBB, Former Manager, Reference Laboratory, Blood Centers of the Pacific-Irwin Center, San Francisco, California (retired)

The author has disclosed no conflicts of interest.

serum provides complement. Throughout this chapter, serum can be considered to be interchangeable with plasma unless the text indicates otherwise.

After an antibody has been detected, its specificity should be determined and its clinical significance assessed. A clinically significant red cell antibody is defined as an antibody that is frequently associated with hemolytic disease of the fetus and newborn (HDFN), with hemolytic transfusion reactions, or with a notable decrease in the survival of transfused red cells. The degree of clinical significance varies among antibodies with the same specificity; some cause destruction of incompatible red cells within hours or even minutes, whereas others cause a decrease in the red cell survival by only a few days, and still others cause no discernible shortened red cell survival. Some antibodies are known to cause HDFN, whereas others may cause a positive direct antiglobulin test (DAT) in the fetus without clinical evidence of HDFN.

PREANALYTICAL CONSIDERATIONS

Before starting antibody identification testing, it may be helpful to consider the patient's medical history. Transfusion and pregnancy are the usual causes of red cell immunization. It is uncommon for patients who have never been transfused or pregnant to produce clinically significant alloantibodies, although "naturally occurring" antibodies may be present. If the patient has been transfused, it is critical to know when the most recent transfusion was given. If the patient was transfused during the past 3 months, the presence of circulating donor red cells may cause mixed-field results in antigen typing tests, and autologous adsorption techniques should not be used because alloantibodies could be adsorbed onto transfused donor red cells. In general, women who may have been sensitized by pregnancy are more likely to have alloantibodies than are men. Infants who are less than 6 months old usually do not produce alloantibodies, but newborns may have passive antibody of maternal origin.

Certain diseases have been associated with red cell antibodies; depending on the methods used, such antibodies may be detectable in antibody detection and identification tests. Cold agglutinin syndrome, Raynaud phenomenon, and infections with *Mycoplasma pneumoniae* are often associated with anti-I. Infectious mononucleosis is sometimes associated with anti-i. Patients with paroxysmal cold hemoglobinuria (PCH), which is associated with syphilis in adults and viral infections in children, may demonstrate autoantibodies with anti-P specificity. Warm autoantibodies often accompany diagnoses such as warm autoimmune hemolytic anemia (WAIHA), systemic lupus erythematosus (SLE), multiple myeloma, chronic lymphocytic leukemia, and lymphoma. Patients who have received solid organ or HPC transplants may demonstrate passive antibodies that originate from donor passenger lymphocytes.

Drugs are known to cause antibody identification problems. (See Chapter 17 for a discussion of drug-related mechanisms and a list of drugs that are associated with serologic problems.) Other sources of drug-related serologic problems include intravenous immune globulin (IVIG) and Rh Immune Globulin (RhIG) in antenatal and postnatal patients. Some lots of IVIG have been reported to contain unexpected antibodies, including anti-A and anti-B. Intravenous RhIG, which is sometimes used to treat thrombocytopenia, could explain the presence of anti-D in an Rh-positive patient.

Finally, when a patient is suspected of having an antibody to a high-prevalence antigen, the patient's ethnic origin may provide clues to the specificity of the antibody. Table 16-1 lists some rare blood types that are more commonly associated with certain ethnic groups.[2]

ANALYTICAL PHASE OF ANTIBODY IDENTIFICATION

Specimen Requirements

Either serum or plasma may be used for antibody detection and identification; however,

TABLE 16-1. Selected Rare Phenotypes in Certain Populations[2]

Antigen or Phenotype	Population
O_h (Bombay)	Indians > Japanese > any
Para-Bombay	Reunion Island > Indians > any
U	Blacks
En^a	Finns > Canadians > English > Japanese
M^kM^k	Swiss > Japanese
hr^S	Blacks
hr^B	Blacks
Lu20	Israelis (1)*
Lu21	Israelis (1)*
K	Whites > Blacks > any
Kp^b	Whites > Japanese
Js^b	Blacks
K12	Whites (4)*
K14	French-Cajuns (3)*
K22	Israelis (2)*
K_o (K_{null})	All
Fy(a–b–)	Blacks > Arabs/Jews > Mediterraneans > Whites
Lu(a–b–)	All
Jk(a–b–)	Polynesians > Finns > Japanese
Di^b	S. Americans > Native Americans > Japanese
LW^a	Baltic Sea region
LW(a–b–)	(Transient) > Canadians
Yt^a	Arabs > Jews
Gy^a	Eastern Europeans (Romany) > Japanese
Hy	Blacks
Jo^a	Blacks
Ge:–2,3,4 (Yus phenotype)	Mexicans > Israelis > Mediterraneans > any
Ge:–2, –3,4 (Gerbich phenotype)	Papua New Guinea > Melanesians > Whites > any
Ge:–2,–3,–4 (Leach phenotype)	All
Cr^a	Blacks

(Continued)

TABLE 16-1. Selected Rare Phenotypes in Certain Populations[2] (Continued)

Antigen or Phenotype	Population
Tc(a–b+c–)	Blacks
Tc(a–b–c+)	Whites
Dr^a	Jews from the Bukaran area of Uzbekistan > Japanese
WES^b	Finns > Blacks > any
IFC (Cr_{null}, Inab)	Japanese > any
UMC	Japanese
Es^a	Mexicans (1),* Blacks (1),* S. Americans (1)*
GUTI	Chileans
Kn^a	Whites > Blacks > any
McC^a	Blacks > Whites > any
Sl^a	Blacks > Whites > any
Yk^a	Whites > Blacks > any
In^b	Indians
Ok^a	Japanese
MER2	Indian Jews
At^a	Blacks
Jr^a	Japanese > Mexicans > any
Lan	Whites
AnWj	Israeli Arabs > (Transient in all)
PEL	French-Canadians (2)*

*Numbers in parentheses refer to probands.

Used with permission from Reid and Lomas-Francis.[2]

plasma may not be suitable for detecting complement-activating antibodies. A 5- to 10-mL aliquot of whole blood usually contains enough serum or plasma for identifying simple antibody specificities; more whole blood may be required for complex studies. When autologous red cells are studied, the use of samples anticoagulated with EDTA avoids problems associated with the in-vitro uptake of complement components by red cells, which may occur when clotted samples are used.

Reagents

Antibody Detection Red Cells

Group O red cells suitable for pretransfusion antibody screening are commercially available and are offered as sets of either two or three bottles of single-donor red cells. Pooled antibody detection red cells (usually obtained from two different donors) may be used only when testing donor serum.

Each laboratory should decide whether to use two or three red cell donor sets for antibody detection testing. Reagent red cells licensed by the Food and Drug Administration (FDA) for this purpose must express the following antigens: D, C, E, c, e, M, N, S, s, P1, Le^a, Le^b, K, k, Fy^a, Fy^b, Jk^a, and Jk^b. The red cell donor samples in both two-cell and three-cell sets express all of those antigens; however, the three-cell set usually offers red cells from presumed homozygous donors with double-dose expression for the following common antigens: D, C, E, c, e, M, N, S, s, Fy^a, Fy^b, Jk^a, and Jk^b. Some weakly reactive antibodies react only with red cells from donors who are homozygous for the genes encoding the antigens; the serologic phenomenon is known as dosage. Antibodies in the Rh, MNS, Duffy, and Kidd systems most commonly demonstrate dosage. Reagent red cells should be refrigerated when not in use, and they should not be used for antibody detection beyond their expiration date.

Antibody Identification Panels

Identification of an antibody to red cell antigen(s) requires testing the serum against a panel of selected red cell samples (typically 8-14 samples) with known antigenic composition for the major blood groups. Usually the red cell samples are obtained from commercial suppliers, but institutions may assemble their own panels using red cells from local sources. Except in special circumstances, panel cells are group O, thereby allowing the serum of any ABO group to be tested.

Each reagent red cell of the panel is from a different donor. The reagent red cells are selected so that if one takes all of the examples of red cells into account, a distinctive pattern of positive and negative reactions exists for each of many antigens. To be functional, a reagent red cell panel must make it possible to identify with confidence those clinically significant alloantibodies that are most commonly encountered, such as anti-D, -E, -K, and -Fy^a. The phenotypes of the reagent red cells should be distributed so that single specificities of the common alloantibodies can be clearly identified and most others can be excluded. Ideally, patterns of reactivity for most examples of single alloantibodies should not overlap with any other (eg, all of the K+ samples should not be the only ones that are also E+). Also, it is important to include reagent red cells with double-dose antigen expression to detect common antibodies that frequently show dosage. To lessen the possibility that chance alone has caused an apparently distinctive pattern, the panel must have an adequate number of reagent red cells that either express or lack most of the antigens listed in Table 16-2.

Commercially prepared panels are generally issued every 2 to 4 weeks. A sheet that lists the phenotypes of the reagent red cells accompanies each panel. The combination of reagent red cell samples varies from lot to lot, so it is essential to use the correct phenotype sheet when interpreting panel results. Commercial reagent red cells for tube testing are diluted to a 2% to 5% suspension in a preservative solution, which can be used directly from the bottle. Washing the red cells before use is usually unnecessary unless the preservative solution is suspected of interfering with antibody identification.

Panel cells should not be used beyond the expiration date; however, this restriction is not always practical. Most serologists use in-date reagent cells for initial antibody identification panels and, if necessary, use expired reagent red cells to exclude or confirm specificities. Each laboratory should establish a policy for using expired reagent red cells and validate any procedures associated with this practice.[3(p19)]

Antiglobulin Reagents

Most antibody detection and identification studies include an indirect antiglobulin test (IAT) phase. Either anti-IgG-specific antiglobulin reagent (AHG) or polyspecific reagent, which contains anti-IgG and anti-complement, may be used. Polyspecific reagent may detect—or may detect more readily—antibodies that bind complement. Complement binding occurs only when serum (not plasma) is tested, and it may be valuable in detecting and identifying certain Kidd antibodies.[4] Although

TABLE 16-2. Example of a Reagent Red Cell Panel for Antibody Identification

Cell	Rh-hr								MNS				Kell				P	Lewis		Duffy		Kidd		Others	Cell	Results	
	D	C	E	c	e	f	C^w	V	M	N	S	s	K	k	Kp^a	Js^a	P1	Le^a	Le^b	Fy^a	Fy^b	Jk^a	Jk^b			37 C	AHG
1	+	+	0	0	+	0	0	0	+	0	0	+	0	+	0	0	+	0	+	+	+	0	+	Bg(a+)	1		
2	+	+	0	0	+	0	+	0	+	+	+	0	0	+	0	0	+	0	0	0	0	+	0		2		
3	+	0	+	+	0	0	0	0	0	+	0	+	0	+	0	0	0	+	0	0	+	+	+		3		
4	0	+	0	+	+	+	0	0	+	0	+	+	0	+	0	0	+	0	+	+	0	+	0		4		
5	0	0	+	+	+	+	0	0	0	+	+	+	0	+	0	0	+	0	+	0	+	0	+		5		
6	0	0	0	+	+	+	0	0	+	0	+	0	+	+	0	0	+	0	+	+	0	0	+		6		
7	0	0	0	+	+	+	0	0	+	+	+	+	0	+	0	0	+	0	+	0	+	+	0		7		
8	+	0	0	+	+	+	0	+	0	+	0	0	0	+	0	0	+	0	0	0	0	0	+		8		
9	0	0	0	+	+	+	0	0	+	+	+	+	+	0	0	0	0	+	0	+	0	+	+		9		
10	0	0	0	+	+	+	0	0	+	0	0	+	+	+	+	0	+	0	0	0	+	+	+	Yt(b+)	10		
11	+	+	0	0	+	0	0	0	+	+	0	+	0	+	0	0	+	0	+	0	+	0	+		11		
AC																									AC		

+ indicates presence of antigen, 0 indicates absence of antigen, AC = autocontrol, AHG = antihuman globulin.

complement binding may be advantageous in some instances, many serologists prefer to use IgG-specific reagents to avoid unwanted reactivity resulting from in-vitro complement binding by cold-reactive antibodies.

Enhancement Media

Although the test system may consist solely of serum and red cells (either reagent red cells as provided by the manufacturer or saline-suspended red cells), most serologists use some type of enhancement medium. Many different techniques are available, including low-ionic-strength saline (LISS), polyethylene glycol (PEG), 22% bovine albumin, gel column agglutination, and solid-phase technology. Additional enhancement techniques may be used for complex studies. Enhancement techniques are discussed later in this chapter.

Basic Antibody Identification

Identification Panel

For initial panels, it is common to use the same methods and test phases used in the antibody detection test or crossmatch. Some serologists may choose to include an immediate centrifugation reading, a room-temperature incubation that is read before adding an enhancement medium, or both. Such an approach may enhance the detection of certain antibodies (anti-M, -N, -P1, -I, -Le^a, or -Le^b) and may help explain reactions detected in other phases. Many institutions omit these steps because most antibodies that react only at lower temperatures have little or no clinical significance.

Test observation after 37 C incubation may detect some antibodies (eg, potent anti-D, -E, or -K) that can cause direct agglutination of red cells. Other antibodies (eg, anti-Le^a, -Jk^a) may be detected by their lysis of antigen-positive red cells during the 37 C incubation if serum is tested. Some serologists believe that the reading at 37 C can be safely omitted because clinically significant antibodies will be detected with an IAT. The omission would lessen the detection of unwanted positive reactions caused by clinically insignificant cold-reactive autoantibodies and alloantibodies. However, in a study published in 1992, 103 potentially significant antibodies reactive at 37 C only (63-E, 27-K, 5-Jk^a, 4-D, 3-cE, and 1-C) were identified in a total of 87,480 samples.[5] An alternative strategy to avoid the uptake of cold antibodies during the centrifugation after the 37 C incubation includes setting up duplicate tests. One test is read after the 37 C incubation, and the other test is read only at the AHG phase.

If the patient has antibodies that were identified previously, the known antibodies may affect panel selection. For example, if the patient has known anti-e, it will not be helpful to test the patient's serum with a routine panel, in which 9 of 10 cell are e-positive. Testing a selected cell panel of e-negative red cells is a better approach to finding any newly formed antibodies. It is not necessary to test e-positive cells to reconfirm the previously identified anti-e.

If the patient's phenotype is known, a selected cell panel may be tested. For example, if a patient types D-negative and has known anti-D, an abbreviated panel or a selected cell panel of D-negative reagent cells may be tested to demonstrate the presence or absence of additional antibodies, thus minimizing the amount of testing required.[6]

INTERPRETING RESULTS. Antibody detection results are interpreted as positive or negative according to the presence or absence of reactivity (ie, agglutination or hemolysis). Interpretation of panel results can be a more complex process combining technique, knowledge, and intuitive skills. Panel results generally include both positive and negative results, which are sometimes at different phases of testing; each result should be explained by the final conclusion. The patient's phenotype and the probability of the antibody specificity are also taken into account in the final interpretation.

POSITIVE AND NEGATIVE REACTIONS. Both positive and negative reactions are important in antibody identification. The phase and strength of positive reactions can suggest certain specificities. (See Method 1-8 for grading agglutination.) Positive reactions can be compared to the antigen patterns of the panel cells to help assign specificity. A single alloantibody usually produces a clear pattern with antigen-positive and antigen-negative reagent red cells. For example, if a serum reacts only with red cell samples #3 and #5 of the reagent red cell panel shown in Table 16-2, anti-E is very likely present. Both reactive red cells express the antigen, and all nonreactive cells lack it. When there is no discernible pattern to explain the reactivity, possible explanations include multiple antibodies, dosage, and variations in antigen expression. Those factors are discussed in more detail later in this chapter.

Negative reactions are important in antibody identification because the reactions allow tentative exclusion of antibodies to antigens expressed on the nonreactive red cells. Exclusion of antibodies is an important step in the interpretation process and must be performed to ensure proper identification of all the antibodies present.

EXCLUSION, "RULE-OUT," OR "CROSS-OUT." A widely used first approach to the interpretation of panel results is to exclude specificities on the basis of nonreactivity of the patient's serum with red cells that express the antigen. Such a system is sometimes referred to as a "cross-out" or "rule-out" method. Once results have been recorded on the worksheet, the antigen profile of the first nonreactive red cell is examined. If an antigen is *present* on the red cell sample and the serum *did not react* with it, the presence of the corresponding antibody may be excluded, at least tentatively. Many technologists actually cross out such antigens from the list at the top of the panel sheet to facilitate the process. After all the antigens on that red cell have been crossed out, the same process is performed with the other nonreactive red cells; then additional specificities are excluded. In most cases, this process leaves a group of antibodies that have not been excluded.

Next, the red cells reactive with the serum are evaluated. The pattern of reactivity for each specificity that was not excluded is compared to the pattern of reactivity obtained with the test serum. If there is a pattern that matches the test serum pattern exactly, that is most likely the specificity of the antibody in the serum. If there are remaining specificities that were not excluded, additional testing is needed to eliminate remaining possibilities and to confirm the suspected specificity. This process requires testing the serum with selected red cells.

Although the exclusion (rule-out) approach often identifies simple antibodies, it should be considered only as a provisional step, particularly if the rule-out was based on the lack of reactivity with red cells that have weaker (eg, from heterozygous donors) expression of the antigen. (See "Variation in Antigen Expression," later in this chapter.)

SELECTED CELLS. Selected cells are red cells that have been chosen because they express certain specific antigens and lack others. Selected red cells with different antigen combinations can be used to confirm or rule out antibodies. For example, if a pattern of reactive red cells exactly fits anti-Jk^a, but anti-K and anti-S were not excluded, the serum should be tested with selected red cells. Ideally, red cells with the following phenotypes should be chosen: Jk(a–), K+, S–; Jk(a–), K–, S+; and Jk(a+), K–, S–. The reaction pattern with these red cells should both confirm the presence of anti-Jk^a and include or exclude anti-K and anti-S. Whenever possible, selected red cells should have a strong expression of the antigen being tested (ie, from homozygous donors or red cells with double-dose expression). Such red cells help to ensure that nonreactivity with the selected red cell indicates the absence of the antibody and does not indicate that the antibody was too weak to react with a selected red cell that had a weak expression of the antigen.

PROBABILITY. To ensure that an observed pattern of reactions is not the result of chance alone, conclusive antibody identification requires the serum to be tested against a sufficient number of reagent red cell samples that lack—and express—the antigen that corresponds with the apparent specificity of the antibody.

A standard approach (which is based on Fisher's exact method[7]) has been to require that three antigen-positive red cell samples react and that three antigen-negative red cell samples fail to react for each specificity identified. When that approach is not possible, a more liberal approach (which is derived from calculations by Harris and Hochman[8]) allows the minimum requirement for a probability (p) value of ≤0.05 to be met by having two reactive and three nonreactive red cell samples or by having one reactive and seven nonreactive red cell samples (or the reciprocal of either combination). Comparative p value calculations are shown in Table 16-3. The use of two reactive and two nonreactive red cell samples is also an acceptable approach for antibody confirmation.[3,9] Additional details on calculating probability may be found in the suggested readings by both Kanter and Menitove. The possibility of false-negative results with antigen-positive red cells must be considered, as well as that of unexpected positives (ie, positive results caused by the presence of an additional antibody or by an error in the presumptive antibody identification).

Autologous Control (Autocontrol)

The autologous control, in which serum and autologous red cells are tested under the same conditions as are serum and reagent red cells, is an important part of antibody identification. The autocontrol is not the same as a DAT (Method 3-6). Incubation and the presence of enhancement reagents may cause reactivity in the autologous control that is only an in-vitro phenomenon. If the autocontrol is positive in the antiglobulin phase, a DAT should be performed. If the DAT is negative, antibodies to an enhancement medium constituent or autoantibodies that react only in the enhancement

TABLE 16-3. Probability Values for Selected Antibody Identification Approaches

No. Tested	No. Positive	No. Negative	p (Fisher[7])	p (Harris and Hochman[8])
5	3	2	0.100	0.035
6	4	2	0.067	0.022
6	3	3	0.050	0.016
7	5	2	0.048	0.015
7	4	3	0.029	0.008
8	7	1	0.125	0.049
8	6	2	0.036	0.011
8	5	3	0.018	0.005
8	4	4	0.014	0.004
9	8	1	0.111	0.043
9	7	2	0.028	0.008
9	6	3	0.012	0.003
10	9	1	0.100	0.039
10	8	2	0.022	0.007
10	7	3	0.008	0.002
10	6	4	0.005	0.001
10	5	5	0.004	0.001

medium should be considered. Warm autoantibodies and cold autoantibodies, such as anti-I, -IH, or -Pr, may react by an IAT when certain enhancement media are used; therefore, testing should be repeated in another medium. If the DAT is positive, the result must be interpreted with careful attention to the transfusion history. Autoantibodies or drugs could explain a positive DAT; however, if the patient has an alloantibody and was recently transfused with blood that expressed the corresponding antigen, the circulating donor red cells could be coated with alloantibody, resulting in a positive DAT.

Phenotyping Autologous Red Cells

The phenotype of the autologous red cells is an important part of antibody identification. When an antibody has been tentatively identified in the serum, the corresponding antigen is expected to be absent from the autologous red cells. For example, if serum from an untransfused individual appears to contain anti-Fy^a but the autologous red cells have a negative DAT and type Fy(a+), the results are clearly in conflict and further testing is indicated. Thus, knowing the patient's phenotype can serve as a guide to exclusion testing.

It may be difficult to determine the patient's phenotype if the patient was transfused in the past 3 months. A pretransfusion specimen, if available, should be used to determine the phenotype. If a pretransfusion sample is not available, the patient's newly formed autologous red cells can be separated from the transfused red cells and then typed (Method 2-22). Separation of newly formed red cells by centrifugation is based on the difference in density of new red cells compared with mature red cells. Centrifugation is most successful when 3 or more days have elapsed since the last transfusion, which will provide time for new autologous red cell production. New autologous red cells must be isolated from the sample while the sample is fresh. The technique is ineffective if the sample is too old (>3 days), if the patient is not producing new red cells, or if the patient has sickle cell anemia.

Sickle cells are quite dense, and centrifugation is not an effective technique for separating the patient's autologous red cells from the transfused donor red cells. However, autologous sickle cells may be separated from donor red cells using washes with hypotonic saline (Method 2-23). Sickle cells containing hemoglobin SS are resistant to lysis by hypotonic saline, whereas the donor red cells containing hemoglobin AA are lysed.

The use of potent blood typing reagents, appropriate controls, and observation for mixed-field reactions often allow an unseparated specimen to be phenotyped. Phenotyping results on posttransfusion samples can be misleading, however, and should be interpreted with caution.[10] If the specificity of the antibody(ies) in the patient's plasma is clear, extensive efforts to separate and type the patient's own red cells are not necessary. A compatible AHG crossmatch using antigen-negative donor units provides additional confirmation of the antibody's specificity.[11(p35)] Definitive typing can be performed on the patient's red cells 3 months after the transfusion.

Additional problems that may complicate red cell typing include cold and warm autoantibodies. When red cells are coated with cold autoantibodies, it may be possible to remove the autoantibodies with warm (37 C) saline washes (Method 2-17). If the cold autoantibodies are very potent, it may be necessary to treat the red cells with dithiothreitol (DTT) to break the immunoglobulin M (IgM) molecules that cause spontaneous agglutination (Method 2-18). When red cells are coated with IgG autoantibodies, it is not possible to perform typing that requires an IAT. However, it is often possible to type antibody-coated red cells with direct-agglutinating antisera, such as IgM monoclonal reagents. With rare exceptions,[12] most direct-agglutinating monoclonal reagents will give valid phenotyping results despite a positive DAT. For antisera that require an IAT (eg, anti-Fy^a and anti-Fy^b), it will be necessary to strip the IgG antibodies from the test red cells before typing. Common techniques for removing IgG antibodies include gentle heat elution (Method 2-19), treatment with chloroquine diphosphate (Method 2-20), and treatment with acid glycine/EDTA (Method 2-21).

Molecular genotyping offers an alternative to serologic typing and is especially useful in situations where the patient has been recently transfused or where the patient's red cells are heavily coated with IgG. Molecular testing relies on the extraction of DNA from the nuclei of white cells. Because the life span of white cells in-vivo is short, the presence of transfused white cells from donors is not a limiting factor in determining the patient's genotype. There are situations, however, where the genotype of a person may not predict the red cell phenotype. Mutations that inactivate gene expression or rare new alleles may not be identified by these molecular assays. In addition, the genotype obtained from DNA isolated from leukocytes and other hematopoietic cells may differ from that of other tissues in people with a history of transplantation.

Complex Antibody Problems

Not all antibody identifications are simple. The exclusion procedure does not always lead directly to an answer, and additional testing may be required. When an antibody screen or incompatible crossmatch detects an unexpected antibody, the next step may be to determine whether the antibody is an autoantibody or an alloantibody. An autocontrol, which may not have been performed in the initial testing, can start the identification process. Figure 16-1 shows some approaches to identifying antibodies in a variety of situations when the autocontrol is negative, and Fig 16-2 shows some approaches to identifying antibodies when the autocontrol is positive.

Selected Serologic Procedures

Many techniques and methods are used in complex antibody identification. Some of the methods described in this chapter are used routinely by many laboratories; others are used selectively and may apply only in special circumstances. It is important to remember that no single method is optimal for detecting all antibodies. Any laboratory that performs antibody detection or identification should have routine methods as well as access to some alternative approaches.

When a pattern of weak reactions fails to indicate specificity, or when the presence of an antibody is suspected but cannot be confirmed, the use of enhancement techniques may be helpful. An autocontrol should always be included with each technique.

LISS and PEG

The rationale for LISS and PEG procedures and some technical details are discussed in Chapter 15 and in Methods 3-2-3 and 3-2-4. Both LISS and PEG techniques are used to enhance reactivity and to reduce incubation time. LISS may be used to suspend test red cells for use in tube or column agglutination tests, or as an additive medium for tube or solid phase tests. Care should be taken to adhere closely to the manufacturer's product insert to ensure that the appropriate proportion of serum to LISS is achieved. Commercially prepared LISS additives or PEG additives may contain additional enhancing agents. Because LISS and PEG enhance autoantibodies, their use may complicate alloantibody identification in samples that also contain autoantibodies.[13,14]

Enzymes

Ficin and papain are the most frequently used enzymes. They destroy or weaken antigens such as M, N, Fy^a, Fy^b, Xg^a, JMH, Ch, and Rg (Table 16-4). Antibodies to these antigens are expected to be nonreactive with treated red cells. Conversely, ficin-treated and papain-treated red cells show enhanced reactivity with other antibodies (eg, Rh, P, I, Kidd, and Lewis). Additional enzymes that are commonly used in immunohematology laboratories include trypsin, α-chymotrypsin, and pronase. Depending on the specific enzyme and method used, other antigens may be altered or destroyed. Antigens that are inactivated by one proteolytic enzyme may not be inactivated by other enzymes. The clinical significance of antibodies that react only with enzyme-treated cells is questionable; such "enzyme-only" antibodies may have no clinical significance.[16] In

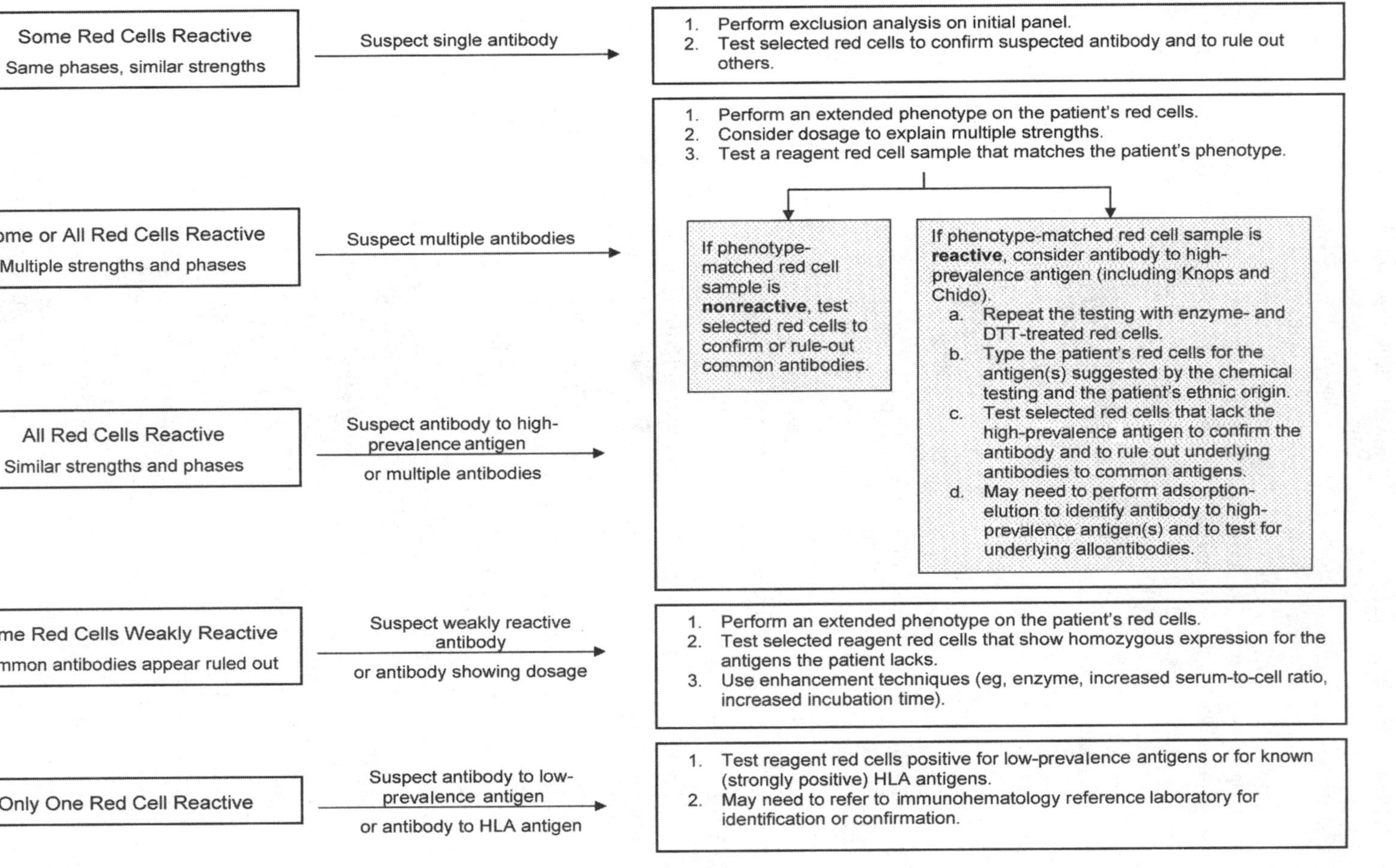

FIGURE 16-1. Antibody identification, with negative autocontrol.
DTT = dithiothreitol.

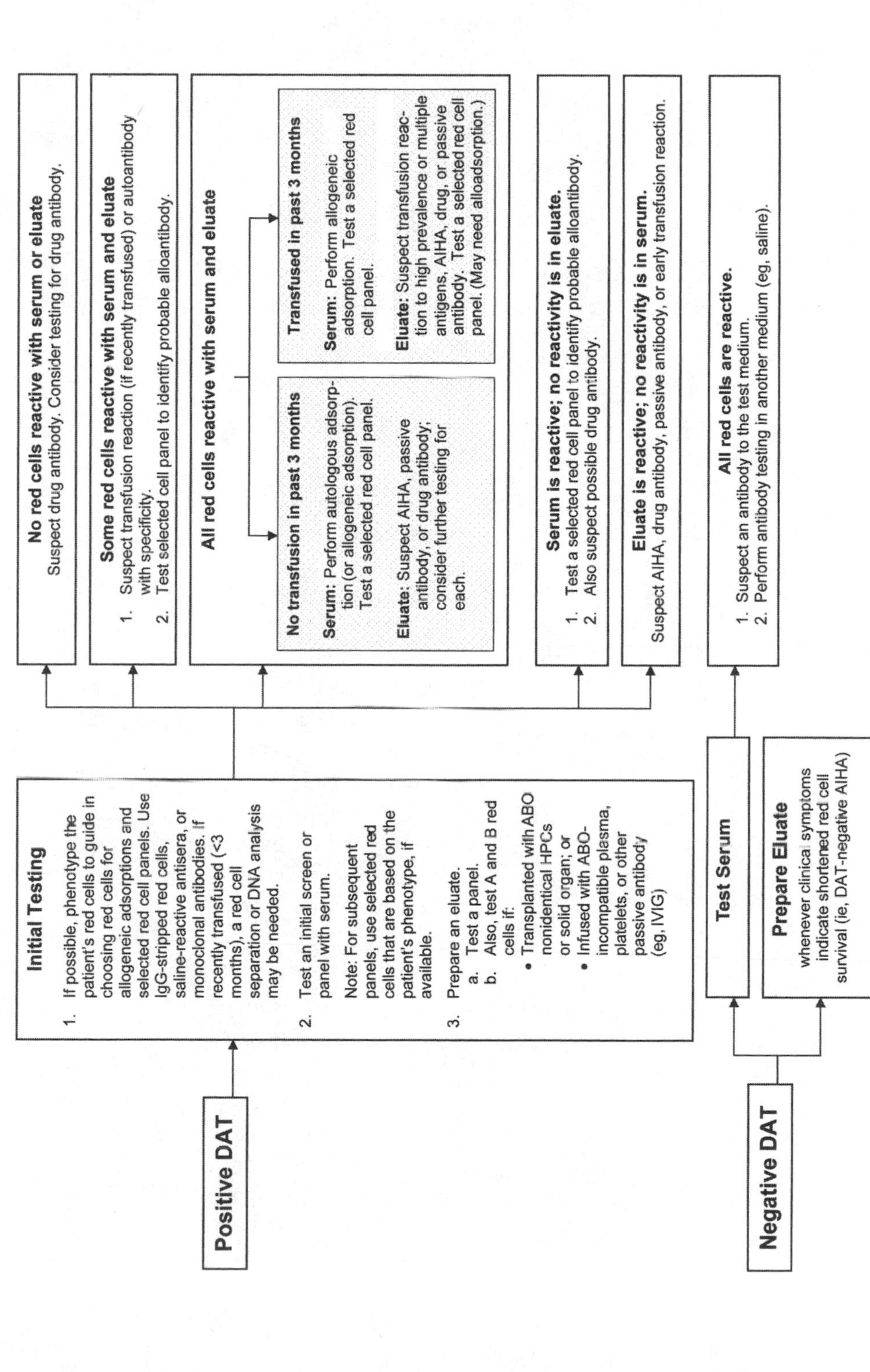

FIGURE 16-2. Antibody identification, with positive autocontrol.
HPCs = hematopoietic progenitor cells; IVIG = intravenous immune globulin.

TABLE 16-4. Alterations of Antigens by Various Agents*

Agent	Antigens Usually Denatured or Altered†
Proteolytic enzymes‡	M, N, S, Fy^a, Fy^b, Yt^a, Ch, Rg, Pr, Tn, Mg, Mi^a/Vw, Cl^a, Je^a, Ny^a, JMH, some Ge, In^b
Dithiothreitol (DTT) or 2-aminoethylisothiouronium bromide (AET)	Yt^a, JMH, Kn^a, McC^a, Yk^a, LW^a, LW^b, all Kell, Lutheran, Dombrock, and Cromer blood group antigens
ZZAP (a combination of DTT and proteolytic enzymes)	Alteration of all the antigens listed above

*Modified with permission from Wilkinson.[15]

†Some antigens listed may be weakened rather than completely denatured. Appropriate controls should be used with modified red cells.

‡Different proteolytic enzymes may have different effects on certain antigens.

addition to enhancing the reactivity of certain antibodies, enzyme techniques may be used to separate mixtures of antibodies. For example, if a serum contains anti-Fy^a and anti-Jk^a, many of the red cell samples on the initial panel would be reactive. Then, if a panel of enzyme-treated red cells were tested, the anti-Jk^a reactivity would be enhanced, whereas the anti-Fy^a reactivity would be destroyed. Procedures for the preparation and use of proteolytic enzymes are given in Method 3-5.

Temperature Reduction

Some antibodies react better at room temperature or below, and their specificity may be apparent only below 22 C (eg, anti-M, -N, -P1, -Le^a, -Le^b, -A1). An autocontrol is especially important for tests at cold temperatures because many sera also contain anti-I or other cold-reactive autoantibodies.

Increased Serum-to-Cell Ratio

Increasing the volume of serum incubated with a standard volume of red cells may enhance the reactivity of antibodies that are present in low concentrations. One acceptable procedure involves mixing 5 to 10 volumes of serum with one volume of a 2% to 5% saline suspension of red cells and incubating for 60 minutes at 37 C. Periodic mixing during the incubation promotes contact between the red cells and the antibodies. It is helpful to remove the serum before washing the cells for an IAT, because the standard three to four washes may be insufficient to remove all of the unbound immunoglobulin if increased amounts of serum are used. More than four washes are not recommended, because bound antibody molecules may dissociate. Increasing the serum-to-red-cell ratio is not appropriate for tests using LISS or commercial PEG, which may contain LISS. Tests performed in a low-ionic-strength medium require specific proportions of serum and additive.

Increased Incubation Time

For some antibodies, a 15-minute incubation period may not be sufficient to achieve equilibrium; therefore, the reactions may be weaker, particularly in saline or albumin media. Extending the incubation time to between 30 and 60 minutes might improve the reactivity and help clarify the pattern of reactions.

Extended incubation may be contraindicated when LISS or PEG is used. If the incubation exceeds the recommended times for those methods, the reactivity may diminish or be lost. Care must be taken to use all reagents according to the manufacturer's directions.

Alteration in pH

Altering the pH of the test system can change the reactivity of certain antibodies—enhancing some and decreasing others.

Some examples of anti-M are enhanced when the pH of the test system is lowered to pH 6.5.[17] If anti-M is suspected because the only reactive red cells are M+N–, a definitive pattern (ie, reactivity with M+N+ red cells also) may be seen if the serum is acidified. The addition of one volume of 0.1 N HCl to nine volumes of serum lowers the pH to approximately pH 6.5. The acidified serum should be tested with known M-negative cells to control for nonspecific agglutination.

Lowering the pH, however, significantly decreases the reactivity of other antibodies.[18] If unbuffered saline with a pH <6.0 is used to prepare red cell suspensions or for washing in an IAT, antibodies in the Rh, Duffy, Kidd, and MNS blood groups may lose reactivity. Phosphate-buffered saline (Method 1-7) can be used to control the pH and can enhance the detection of antibodies that react poorly at a lower pH.[19]

Inhibition Techniques

Soluble forms of some blood group antigens exist in body fluids such as saliva, urine, and plasma. These substances are also found in other natural sources, and they can be prepared synthetically. Soluble substance can be used to inhibit the reactivity of the corresponding antibody that could mask the presence of underlying nonneutralizable antibodies. Also, when an antibody is suspected, inhibition of the reactivity by soluble substance can help in the identification. For example, if a suspected anti-P1 does not produce a definitive pattern of agglutination, the loss of reactivity after the addition of soluble P1 substance strongly suggests that the specificity is anti-P1. A parallel dilution control with saline is essential when inhibition techniques are used. Inhibition results can be interpreted only when the test is nonreactive and when the dilution control that substitutes an equal volume of saline for the soluble substance is reactive.

Uses of soluble blood group substances include the following:

1. *Lewis substances.* Le^a or Le^b substances, or both, are present in the saliva of individuals who possess the Lewis gene (*FUT3*). Le^a substance is present in the saliva of Le(a+b–) individuals, and both Le^a and Le^b substances are present in the saliva of Le(a–b+) individuals (Method 2-8). Commercially prepared Lewis substance is also available.
2. *P1 substance.* Soluble P1 substance is present in hydatid cyst fluid and the ovalbumin of pigeon eggs. Commercially prepared P1 substance is also available.
3. *Sd^a substance.* Soluble Sd^a blood group substance is present in various body fluids, but urine has the highest concentration of Sd^a.[20] To confirm anti-Sd^a in a serum sample, urine from a known Sd(a+) individual (or a pool of urine specimens) can be used to inhibit the antibody reactivity. Urine known to lack Sd^a substance, or saline, should be used as a dilution control (Method 3-11).
4. *Chido and Rodgers substances.* Ch and Rg antigens are epitopes on the fourth component of human complement (C4).[21,22] Most normal red cells have a trace amount of C4 on their surface. Anti-Ch and anti-Rg react with this C4 by an IAT. If red cells are coated in vitro with excess C4, these antibodies may cause direct agglutination.[23] A useful test to identify anti-Ch and anti-Rg is inhibition of the antibodies with plasma from Ch+, Rg+ individuals (Method 3-9).

Inactivation of Blood Group Antigens

Certain blood group antigens can be destroyed or weakened by chemical treatment of the cells (Table 16-4). Modified red cells can be useful both in confirming the presence of suspected antibodies and in detecting additional antibodies. The use of modified red cells can be especially helpful if a sample contains an antibody to a high-prevalence antigen, because antigen-negative red cells are rare. Proteolytic enzymes, described above, are commonly used to alter red cell antigens. Sulfhydryl reagents such as 2-aminoethylisothiouronium bromide (AET), 2-mercaptoethanol (2-ME), or DTT can be used to weaken or destroy antigens in the Kell system and some other antigens (Method 3-10).[24,25] ZZAP reagent, which contains proteolytic enzyme and DTT, denatures antigens that are sensitive to DTT (eg, all Kell system antigens), as well as antigens that are sensitive to enzymes (Method 4-8).[26] Glycine-HCl/EDTA treatment of red cells destroys Bg and Kell system antigens as well as the Er^a antigen (Methods 2-21 and 4-2).[27] Chloroquine diphosphate can be used to weaken the expression of Class I HLA antigens (Bg antigens) on red cells.[28] Chloroquine treatment also weakens some other antigens, including Rh antigens (Method 2-20).

Sulfhydryl Reagents

Sulfhydryl reagents, such as DTT and 2-ME, can be used to cleave the disulfide bonds that join the monomeric subunits of the IgM immunoglobulin pentamer. Intact 19S IgM molecules are cleaved into 7S Ig subunits, which have altered serologic reactivity.[29] The interchain bonds of 7S Ig monomers are relatively resistant to such cleavage. Sulfhydryl reagents (DTT and 2-ME as well as AET) can also be used to cleave disulfide bonds that are responsible for the conformation of certain blood group antigens and, therefore, are used to destroy certain red cell antigens.

Uses of sulfhydryl reagents include the following:

1. Determining the immunoglobulin class of an antibody (Method 3-8).
2. Identifying antibodies in a mixture of IgM and IgG antibodies, particularly when an agglutinating IgM antibody masks the presence of IgG antibodies.
3. Determining the relative amounts of IgG and IgM components of a given specificity (eg, anti-A or -B).
4. Dissociating red cell agglutinates caused by IgM autoantibodies (Method 2-18).
5. Dissociating IgG antibodies from red cells using a mixture of DTT and proteolytic enzyme (ZZAP reagent); (Method 4-8).
6. Destroying selected red cell antigens for use in antibody investigations (eg, antigens in the Kell, Dombrock, Cartwright, LW, and Knops systems); (Method 3-10).

Adsorption

Antibody can be removed from a serum sample by adsorption onto red cells that express the corresponding antigen. After the antibody attaches to the membrane-bound antigens and the serum and cells are separated, the specific antibody remains attached to the red cells. It may be possible to harvest the bound antibody by elution or to examine the adsorbed serum for antibody(ies) remaining after the adsorption process.

Adsorption techniques are useful in the following situations:

1. Separating multiple antibodies present in a single serum.
2. Removing autoantibody to permit the detection or identification of underlying alloantibodies.
3. Removing unwanted antibody (often anti-A, anti-B, or both) from serum that contains an antibody that is suitable for reagent use.
4. Confirming the presence of specific antigens on red cells by their ability to remove antibody of corresponding specificity from previously characterized serum.
5. Confirming the specificity of an antibody by showing that it can be adsorbed onto red cells of only a particular blood group phenotype.

Adsorption serves different purposes in different situations; no single procedure is satisfactory for all purposes (Methods 4-5, 4-8, 4-9, and 4-10). A basic procedure for antibody adsorption can be found in Method 3-12. The usual serum-to-cell ratio is one volume of serum to an equal volume of washed, packed red cells. To enhance antibody uptake, a larger volume of red cells will increase the proportion of antigen. The incubation temperature should be the temperature at which the antibody reacts optimally. Pretreating red cells with a proteolytic enzyme may enhance antibody uptake and may reduce the number of adsorptions required to remove an antibody completely. Because enzymes destroy some antigens, antibodies directed against those antigens will not be removed by enzyme-treated red cells. To ensure that an adsorption process is complete (ie, that no unadsorbed antibody remains), it is essential to confirm that the adsorbed serum is nonreactive with a reserved sample of the adsorbing red cells that was not used for adsorption. Adsorption requires a substantial volume of red cells, and vials of reagent red cells are usually not sufficient. Blood samples from donor units or staff members are the most convenient sources.

When separating mixtures of antibodies, the selection of red cells of the appropriate phenotype is extremely important. If one or more antibodies have been previously identified, red cells that express the corresponding antigens can be used to remove the known antibodies and to leave the unknown antibody(ies) in the adsorbed serum. For example, if a person who types K+k–, Fy(a–b+) has produced anti-k, it may be necessary to adsorb the anti-k onto K–k+, Fy(a–b+) reagent red cells to remove the anti-k. Then, the adsorbed serum can be tested with common K–k+, Fy(a+b–) red cells to detect possible anti-Fy^a.

Elution

Elution dissociates antibodies from sensitized red cells. Bound antibody may be released by changing the thermodynamics of antigen-antibody reactions, by neutralizing or reversing forces of attraction that hold antigen-antibody complexes together, or by disturbing the structure of the antigen-antibody binding site. The usual objective is to recover bound antibody in a usable form.

Various elution methods have been described. Selected procedures are given in Methods 4-1 through 4-4. No single method is best for all situations. Heat or freeze-thaw elution techniques are usually restricted to the investigation of HDFN caused by ABO incompatibility because those elution procedures rarely work well for other antibodies. Acid or organic solvent methods are used for eluting warm-reactive auto- and alloantibodies. Commercial kits are also available for performing elutions. (See Table 17-2 for a list of elution methods and their uses, advantages, and disadvantages.)

Technical factors that influence the outcome of elution procedures include the following:

1. *Incomplete washing.* Sensitized red cells should be thoroughly washed before performing an elution, to prevent contamination of the eluate with unbound residual antibody. Six washes with saline are usually adequate, but more washes may be needed if the serum contains a high-titer antibody. To confirm the efficacy of the washing process, supernatant fluid from the final wash should be tested for antibody activity and found to be nonreactive.
2. *Binding of protein to glass surfaces.* If an eluate is prepared in the same test tube that was used during the sensitization or washing phases, antibody that nonspecifically binds to the test tube surface may dissociate during the elution. Similar binding can also occur from a whole blood sample when a patient has a positive DAT and has free antibody in the serum. To avoid such contamination, red cells used to prepare an eluate should be transferred to a clean test tube before washing and then again to a clean tube before beginning the elution procedure.
3. *Dissociation of antibody before elution.* IgM antibodies, such as anti-A or anti-M, may spontaneously dissociate from the red cells during the wash phase. To minimize the loss of bound antibody, cold (4 C) saline should be used for washing. Although this loss is not a concern with most IgG antibodies, some low-affinity IgG antibodies can also be lost during the wash phase. If such antibodies are suspected, washing with cold LISS instead of normal

saline may help maintain antibody association.

4. *Incorrect technique.* Such factors as incomplete removal of organic solvents or failure to correct the tonicity or pH of an eluate may cause the reagent red cells used to test the eluate to hemolyze or appear "sticky." The presence of stromal debris may interfere with the reading of tests. Careful technique and strict adherence to procedures should eliminate such problems.
5. *Instability of eluates.* Dilute protein solutions, such as those obtained by elution into saline, are unstable. Eluates should be tested as soon after preparation as possible. Alternatively, bovine albumin may be added to a final concentration of 6% w/v, and the preparation may be stored frozen. Eluates can also be prepared in antibody-free plasma, 6% albumin, or in a similar protein medium, instead of in saline.

Elution techniques are useful for the following:

1. Investigation of a positive DAT (Chapter 17).
2. Concentration and purification of antibodies, detection of weakly expressed antigens, and identification of multiple antibody specificities. Such studies are used in conjunction with an appropriate adsorption technique, as described below and in Method 2-7.
3. Preparation of antibody-free red cells for phenotyping or autologous adsorption studies. Procedures used to remove cold- and warm-reactive autoantibodies from red cells are discussed in Methods 4-5 and 4-8.

Combined Adsorption-Elution

Combined adsorption-elution tests can be used to separate a mixture of antibodies in a single serum, to detect weakly expressed antigens on red cells, or to help identify weakly reactive antibodies. The process consists of first incubating serum with selected red cells, then eluting antibody from the adsorbing red cells. Care must be taken when selecting the adsorbing cells to separate a mixture of antibodies. The cells should express only one of the antigens corresponding to an antibody in the mixture, so that the eluate from the cells will contain only that antibody. Both the eluate and adsorbed serum can be used for further testing. Unmodified red cells are generally used for adsorptions when subsequent elutions are being prepared. Eluates from enzyme- or ZZAP-treated red cells may create technical problems.

Titration

The titer of an antibody is usually determined by testing serial twofold dilutions of the serum with selected red cells. Results are expressed as the reciprocal of the highest serum dilution that shows macroscopic agglutination. Titration values can provide information about the relative amount of antibody present in a serum or about the relative strength of antigen expression on red cells.

Titration studies are useful in the following situations:

1. *Prenatal studies.* When the antibody has a specificity that is known to cause HDFN, or when the antibody's clinical significance is unknown, the results of titration studies may contribute to the decision about performing additional procedures (eg, Doppler sonography or amniocentesis). (See Chapter 22 and Method 5-3.)
2. *Antibody identification.* Some antibodies that agglutinate virtually all reagent red cells may give an indication of specificity by demonstrating reactivity of different strengths with different red cell samples in titration studies. For example, potent undiluted autoanti-I may react with both adult and cord blood red cells, but titration studies may reveal reactivity with adult I+ cells at a higher dilution than with cord blood I– red cells.

   The reactivity of most antibodies weakens progressively with serial dilutions (ie, a 2+ reaction becomes 1+ in the next dilution) and weak antibodies (<1+) may lose their reactivity when diluted. However, some antibodies that give weak reactions when undiluted continue to react at dilutions as high as 1 in 2048. Such antibodies include anti-Ch, -Rg, -Cs^a, -Yk^a, -Kn^a, -McC^a, -JMH, and others. When weak reactions are observed in an IAT, titration studies may be performed to determine whether the reactivity is consistent with the antibodies in this group; however, not all examples of these antibodies demonstrate such "high-titer, low-avidity" characteristics. Thus, the serologic characteristics may suggest certain specificities, but failure to do so does not eliminate those possibilities. The antibodies listed above are generally not expected to cause shortened red cell survival, although there are examples of other antibodies that may mimic these serologic characteristics and may cause shortened red cell survival (eg, anti-Lu^b, -Vel, and -Yt^a). Details about titration are given in Method 3-7.

3. *Separating multiple antibodies.* Titration results may suggest that one antibody reacts at higher dilutions than another antibody. That information can allow the serum to be diluted before testing with a red cell panel, effectively removing one antibody and allowing the other to be identified. For example, if a serum contains anti-c that reacts to a titer of 2 and anti-Jk^a that reacts to a titer of 16, it may be possible to eliminate the anti-c reactivity by diluting the serum to a titer of 8.

Other Methods

Methods other than traditional tube techniques may be used for antibody identification. Some methods are especially useful for testing small volumes of serum or reagents or for using automated equipment. Such methods include testing in capillary tubes, column agglutination microtubes, microplates, solid-phase systems, or enzyme-linked immunosorbent assays. Other methods that are useful in laboratories with specialized equipment include radioimmunoassay, immunofluorescence (including flow cytometric procedures), immunoblotting, and immunoelectrode biosensoring.

Factors Affecting Antibody Identification

Variation in Antigen Expression

For a variety of reasons, antibodies do not always react with all red cells that express the corresponding antigen. Basic interpretation by exclusion, as described previously, may result in an antibody being excluded because the serum was nonreactive with an antigen-positive red cell sample, despite the presence of the antibody. Technical error, weak antibody reactivity, and variant or weak antigenic expression are all possible causes. Therefore, whenever possible, antibody exclusions should be based only on red cells that strongly express the antigen. Enhancement techniques often help resolve problems associated with variation in antigen expression (Methods 3-2-2 through 3-5-6).

ZYGOSITY. Reaction strength of some antibodies may vary because of a phenomenon known as dosage, in which antibodies react more strongly (or only) with red cells that possess a "double-dose" expression of the antigen. Double-dose antigen expression occurs when an individual is homozygous for the gene that encodes the antigen. Red cells from individuals who are heterozygous for the gene may express fewer antigens and, therefore, may react weakly or be nonreactive with a weak example of the corresponding antibody. Alloantibodies vary in their tendency to demonstrate dosage. Many antibodies to antigens in the Rh, Duffy, MNS, and Kidd blood groups demonstrate dosage.

VARIATION IN ADULTS AND INFANTS. Some antigens (eg, I, P1, Le^a, and Sd^a) show variable expression on the red cells from different adult individuals. The antigenic differences can be demonstrated serologically; however, the variability is unrelated to zygosity. Certain antibodies (eg, anti-I, -Lu^b) demonstrate weaker reactivity with cord red cells than with red cells from adults (Table 16-5).

TABLE 16-5. Antigen Expression on Cord Red Blood Cells*

Expression	Antigens
Negative	Le^a, Le^b, Sd^a, Ch, Rg, AnWj
Weak	I, H, P1, Lu^a, Lu^b, Yt^a, Vel, Bg, McC^a, Yk^a, Sl^a, Cs^a, Hy, Gy, Jo^a, Do^a, Do^b, Fy3
Strong	i, LW^a, LW^b

*Modified with permission from Reid and Lomas-Francis.[2]

CHANGES WITH STORAGE. Blood group antibodies may react more weakly with stored red cells than with fresh red cells. Some antigens deteriorate more rapidly than others during storage (eg, Fy^a, Fy^b, M, P1, Kn^a/McC^a, Bg), and the rate varies among red cells from different individuals.[30] Because red cells from donors are often fresher than commercial reagent red cells, some antibodies give stronger reactions with donor red cells than with reagent red cells. Similarly, frozen storage of red cells may cause antigens to deteriorate, thus producing misleading antibody identification results.

The pH or other characteristics of the storage medium can affect the rate of antigen deterioration.[30,31] For example, Fy^a and Fy^b antigens may weaken when the red cells are stored in a medium with low pH and low ionic strength. Thus, certain antibodies may demonstrate differences in reactivity with red cells from different manufacturers if the suspending media are different.

The age and nature of the specimen must be considered when typing red cells. Antigens on red cells from clotted samples tend to deteriorate faster than antigens on red cells from donor units that are collected in citrate anticoagulants such as acid-citrate-dextrose (ACD) or citrate-phosphate-dextrose (CPD). Red cells in donor units collected in approved anticoagulants generally retain their antigens throughout the standard shelf life of the blood component. EDTA samples up to 14 days old are suitable for antigen typing[32]; however, the manufacturer's instructions should be consulted when using commercial typing reagents.

No Discernible Specificity

Factors other than variation in antigen expression may contribute to difficulty in interpreting results of antibody identification tests. If the reactivity with the serum is very weak, or if the pattern of reactivity and cross-out process have excluded all likely specificities, or both, alternative approaches to interpretation should be used.

ANTIGENS PRESENT IN COMMON. Instead of excluding antibodies to antigens on nonreactive red cells, it might be helpful to observe which antigens the reactive red cells have in common. For example, if all of the red cells reactive at room temperature are P1+, but the anti-P1 pattern is not complete, the antibody could be anti-P1 that is not reacting with red cells with a weaker expression of the antigen. (Sometimes such red cells are designated on the panel sheet as "+w.") In this case, it might be helpful to use a method that enhances anti-P1, such as testing at a colder temperature.

If all the reactive red cells are Jk(b+), but not all Jk(b+) red cells react, the reactive red cells might be Jk(a–b+), with a double-dose expression of the antigen. In this case, enhancement techniques, such as enzymes, LISS, or PEG, might help demonstrate reactivity with all of the Jk(b+) red cells. Typing the patient's red cells to confirm that they lack the corresponding antigen is also very helpful.

Finally, the presence of some antigens in common may suppress the expression of certain antigens. This suppression can cause weak antibodies to be missed or certain cells to be unexpectedly nonreactive when a suspected antibody fails to react with all antigen-positive cells. For example, *In(Lu)* is known to suppress the expression of Lutheran antigens, P1, In^b, and AnWj. Similarly, Kp^a is known to weaken the expression of Kell antigens. (See Chapter 14 for a more detailed discussion.)

INHERENT VARIABILITY. Nebulous reaction patterns that do not appear to fit any particular specificity are characteristic of certain antibodies, such as anti-Bg^a, -Kn^a, -McC^a, -Sl^a, -Yk^a, -Cs^a, and -JMH. Antigens corresponding to these antibodies vary markedly in their expression on red cells from different individuals. For example, the expression of Knops blood group antigens show marked differences between individuals of either African or European ethnicity, and this is caused by differences in the CR1 copy numbers on the red cells.[33] Rarely, a pattern of reactive and nonreactive red cells cannot be interpreted because the typing result for a reagent red cell is incorrect or the reagent red cell has a positive DAT. If the red cell sample is from a commercial source, the manufacturer should be notified immediately of the discrepancy.

UNLISTED ANTIGENS. Sometimes a serum reacts with an antigen that is not routinely listed on the antigen profile supplied by the reagent manufacturer—for example, Yt^b. Even though serum studies yield clearly reactive and nonreactive tests, anti-Yt^b may not be suspected. In such circumstances, it is useful to ask the manufacturer for additional phenotype information. If only one cell is unexpectedly reactive, the reaction is most likely caused by an antibody to a low-prevalence antigen. Antibodies to low-prevalence antigens are discussed in more detail later in this chapter.

ABO TYPE OF RED CELLS TESTED. A serum sample may react with many or all of the group O reagent red cells but not with red cells of the same ABO group as the autologous red cells. Such a reaction occurs most frequently with anti-H, anti-IH, or anti-Le^{bH}. Group O and A_2 red cells have larger amounts of H antigen than A_1 and A_1B red cells, which express very little H. (See Chapter 12 for more information.) Thus, sera containing anti-H or anti-IH will react strongly with group O reagent red cells, whereas autologous A_1 or A_1B red cells or donor red cells used for crossmatching may be weakly reactive or nonreactive. Anti-Le^{bH} reacts strongly with group O, Le(b+) red cells but reacts weakly or not at all with Le(b+) red cells from A_1 or A_1B individuals.

Multiple Antibodies

When a serum contains two or more alloantibodies, it may be difficult to interpret the results of testing performed with a single panel of reagent red cells. Perhaps the easiest way to identify multiple antibodies is to perform a phenotype on the patient's pretransfusion autologous red cells and then perform a selected-cell panel to identify or exclude all common antibodies to red cell antigens the patient lacks. (See the discussion on selected cells earlier in this chapter.) The presence of multiple antibodies may be suggested by a variety of test results, such as the following:

1. *The observed pattern of reactive and nonreactive red cells does not fit a single antibody.* When the exclusion approach fails to indicate a specific pattern, it is helpful to see if the pattern matches two combined specificities. For example, if the reactive red cells on the panel in Table 16-2 are numbers 3, 5, 6, 9, and 10, none of the specificities remaining after crossing-out exactly fits a pattern. However, if both E and K are considered together, a pattern is discerned, with cells 3 and 5 reacting because of anti-E, and cells 6, 9, and 10, because of anti-K. If the reaction pattern does not fit two combined specificities, the possibility of more than two antibodies must be considered. The more antibodies a serum contains, the more complex identification and exclusion become, but the basic process remains the same.
2. *Reactivity is present at different test phases.* When reactivity occurs at several phases, each phase should be analyzed separately. The pattern seen at room temperature may indicate a different specificity from the pattern at the AHG phase. It is also helpful to look for variations in the

strength of the reactions at each phase of testing. Table 16-6 provides information about the characteristic reactivity of several antibodies.

3. *Unexpected reactions are obtained when attempts are made to confirm the specificity of a suspected single antibody.* If a serum suspected of containing anti-e reacts with some e-negative cells, another antibody may be present, or the suspected antibody may not be anti-e. Testing a panel of selected e-negative red cells may help identify an additional specificity.
4. *No discernible pattern emerges.* When variable reaction strengths are observed, and dosage or other variations in antigen strength do not provide an explanation, additional approaches and methods of testing are needed. Some helpful steps include the following:
   - **a.** If strongly positive results are obtained, use the exclusion method with nonreactive cells to eliminate some specificities from initial consideration.
   - **b.** If weak or questionable positive results are obtained, test the serum against cells that show a strong expression of the antigen that corresponds with any suspected specificity, and combine this approach with methods to enhance the reactivity.
   - **c.** Type the patient's red cells for common red cell antigens, and eliminate from consideration specificities that correspond to antigens on the patient's autologous red cells. This step may not be possible if the patient has been transfused recently or has a positive DAT.
   - **d.** Use a method to inactivate certain antigens on the reagent cells. Enzyme treatment will render cells negative for such antigens as Fy^a and Fy^b (see Table 16-4).
   - **e.** Use adsorption or elution methods to separate antibodies (Methods 3-12, 4-1, and 4-2).
   - **f.** Enhance antibody reactivity by using a more sensitive method (eg, PEG, enzymes, increased incubation time, and increased serum-to-cell ratio; see Methods 3-2-4 and 3-5).

Antibodies to High-Prevalence Antigens

If all reagent red cells are reactive, but the autocontrol is nonreactive, an alloantibody to a high-prevalence antigen should be considered, especially if the strength and test phase of reactions are uniform for all the red cells tested. Antibodies to high-prevalence antigens can be identified by testing selected red cells of rare phenotypes and by typing the patient's autologous red cells with antisera to high-prevalence antigens. Knowing the race or ethnic origin of the antibody-producer can help in selecting additional tests to perform (Table 16-1). Red cells that lack all of the antigens in a blood group system (eg, Rh_{null} or K_o), or chemically modified red cells (eg, DTT-treated red cells), can help limit possible specificities (Table 16-4).

If red cells negative for a particular high-prevalence antigen are not available, red cells that are positive for the lower-prevalence antithetical antigen can sometimes be helpful. For example, if a serum contains anti-Co^a, which reacts with a high-prevalence antigen, weaker reactions may be observed with Co(a+b+) red cells than with Co(a+b–) red cells because of a dosage effect.

Antibodies to high-prevalence antigens may be accompanied by antibodies to common antigens, which can make identification much more difficult. In such cases, it may be necessary to determine the patient's phenotype for common antigens, to choose a phenotypically similar red cell sample (ie, lacking the same common antigens as the patient) that is incompatible with the patient's plasma, and to adsorb the antibody to the high-prevalence antigen onto that red cell sample. This approach leaves antibodies to common red cell antigens in the adsorbed plasma, where they can be identified with a routine selected red cell panel. Because the identification of antibodies to high-prevalence antigens is complicated, it may be necessary to refer such speci-

TABLE 16-6. Serologic Reactivity of Some Common Blood Group Antibodies

Antibody	Immunoglobulin Class	Reactivity				Papain/Ficin	DTT (200 mM)	Associated with	
		4 C	22 C	37 C	AHG			HDFN	HTR
Anti-M	IgG > IgM	Most	Most		Rare	Sensitive	Resistant	Rare	Rare
Anti-N	IgM > IgG	Most	Most		Rare	Sensitive	Resistant	No	Rare
Anti-S	IgG > IgM		Most		Most	Variable	Resistant	Yes	Yes
Anti-s	IgG > IgM				Most	Variable	Resistant	Yes	Yes
Anti-U	IgG				Most	Resistant	Resistant	Yes	Yes
Anti-P1	IgM (IgG rare)	Most	Most			Resistant	Resistant	No	Rare
Anti-D	IgG > IgM (IgA rare)		Some	Some	Most	Resistant	Resistant	Yes	Yes
Anti-C	IgG > IgM		Some	Some	Most	Resistant	Resistant	Yes	Yes
Anti-E	IgG > IgM		Some	Some	Most	Resistant	Resistant	Yes	Yes
Anti-c	IgG > IgM		Some	Some	Most	Resistant	Resistant	Yes	Yes
Anti-e	IgG > IgM		Some	Some	Most	Resistant	Resistant	Yes	Yes
Anti-Lu^a	IgM > IgG		Most		Most	Resistant or weakened	Variable	Rare	No
Anti-Lu^b	IgG > IgM		Some		Most	Resistant or weakened	Variable	Mild	Yes
Anti-K	IgG > IgM		Some		Most	Resistant	Sensitive	Yes	Yes
Anti-k	IgG > IgM				Most	Resistant	Sensitive	Yes	Yes
Anti-Kp^a	IgG				Most	Resistant	Sensitive	Yes	Yes
Anti-Kp^b	IgG > IgM				Most	Resistant	Sensitive	Yes	Yes
Anti-Js^a	IgG > IgM				Most	Resistant	Sensitive	Yes	Yes
Anti-Js^b	IgG				Most	Resistant	Sensitive	Yes	Yes
Anti-Le^a	IgM > IgG	Most	Most	Most	Most	Resistant	Resistant	No	Rare
Anti-Le^b	IgM > IgG	Most	Most	Most	Most	Resistant	Resistant	No	No
Anti-Fy^a	IgG > IgM				Most	Sensitive	Resistant	Yes	Yes
Anti-Fy^b	IgG > IgM				Most	Sensitive	Resistant	Yes	Yes
Anti-Jk^a	IgG > IgM				Most	Resistant	Resistant	Yes	Yes
Anti-Jk^b	IgG > IgM				Most	Resistant	Resistant	Yes	Yes
Anti-Di^a	IgG				Most	Resistant	Resistant	Yes	Yes
Anti-Di^b	IgG				Most	Resistant	Resistant	Yes	Yes

(Continued)

TABLE 16-6. Serologic Reactivity of Some Common Blood Group Antibodies (Continued)

Antibody	Immuno-globulin Class	Reactivity				Papain/Ficin	DTT (200 mM)	Associated with	
		4 C	22 C	37 C	AHG			HDFN	HTR
Anti-Yt[a]	IgG				Most	Variable	Sensitive or weak-ened	No	Yes
Anti-Yt[b]	IgG				Most	Variable	Sensitive or weak-ened	No	No
Anti-Xg[a]	IgG > IgM		Some		Most	Sensitive	Resistant	No	No
Anti-Sc1	IgG				Most	Resistant	Variable	No	No
Anti-Sc2	IgG				Most	Resistant	Variable	No	No
Anti-Do[a]	IgG				Most	Resistant	Variable	No	Yes
Anti-Do[b]	IgG				Most	Resistant	Variable	No	Yes
Anti-Co[a]	IgG > IgM				Most	Resistant	Resistant	Yes	Yes
Anti-Co[b]	IgG				Most	Resistant	Resistant	Yes	Yes

The reactivity shown in the table is based on the tube methods in common use. If tests are carried out by more sensitive test procedures (such as in capillary tubes, in microtiter plates, or by the albumin layering method), direct agglutination (before the antiglobulin phase) may be observed more often with some antibodies. Blank spaces indicate a lack of sufficient data for generalization about antibody behavior.

AHG = antihuman globulin; DTT = dithiothreitol; HDFN = hemolytic disease of the fetus and newborn; HTR = hemolytic transfusion reaction.

mens to an immunohematology reference laboratory (IRL).

SEROLOGIC CLUES. Knowing the serologic characteristics of particular antibodies to high-prevalence antigens and/or knowing the prevalence of such antigens in different populations may help in identification.

1. Reactivity in tests at room temperature suggests anti-H, -I, -IH, -P, -PP1P[k] (-Tj[a]), -En[a], -LW (some), -Ge (some), -Sd[a], or -Vel. Lysis of reagent red cells when testing with fresh serum is characteristic of anti-Vel, -P, -PP1P[k] (-Tj[a]), and -Jk3 and some examples of anti-H and -I.
2. Reduced or absent reactivity with enzyme-treated red cells occurs with anti-Ch, -Rg, -En[a], -In[b], -JMH, or -Ge2 and is seen with some examples of anti-Yt[a].
3. Weak nebulous reactions in the AHG phase are often associated with anti-Kn[a], -McC[a], -Yk[a], and -Cs[a]. Complement-binding autoantibodies such as anti-I and -IH, or alloantibodies such as anti-Lu[b], -Vel, and -Yt[a], may give similar results when polyspecific AHG reagent is used.

ETHNIC CLUES. Antibodies such as anti-U, -McC[a], -Sl[a], -Js[b], -Hy, -Jo[a], -Tc[a], -Cr[a], and -At[a] should be considered if the serum is from an individual of African ethnicity because the antigen-negative phenotypes occur almost exclusively in persons of African ethnicity. Individuals with anti-Kp[b] are almost always persons of European ethnicity. Anti-Di[b] is usually found among Asians, South American

Indians, and Native American populations (Table 16-1).

INTERPRETING A POSITIVE DAT. When a patient produces an antibody to a high-prevalence antigen after transfusion, the patient's posttransfusion red cells may have a positive DAT, and both serum and eluate may react with all red cells tested. Because that pattern of reactivity is identical to many warm-reacting autoantibodies that appear after transfusion, the two scenarios can be very difficult to differentiate. A posttransfusion alloantibody to a high-prevalence antigen would be expected to produce a DAT of mixed-field appearance (ie, some red cells agglutinated among many unagglutinated red cells) because only the transfused red cells would be coated with antibody. In practice, however, weak sensitization and mixed-field agglutination can be difficult to differentiate. If a pretransfusion specimen is not available, it may be helpful to use red cell separation procedures to isolate autologous red cells for testing or perform a DNA-based genotype, as described earlier in this chapter. Performing a DAT on autologous red cells or testing the posttransfusion serum with DAT-negative autologous red cells, or both, may help distinguish an autoantibody from an alloantibody. If a DAT on autologous red cells is negative, the reactivity is consistent with an alloantibody. If the posttransfusion serum reacts with DAT-negative autologous red cells, the reactivity is consistent with an autoantibody (Chapter 17 and Fig 16-2).

Antibodies to Low-Prevalence Antigens

If a serum reacts only with a single donor or reagent red cell sample, an antibody to a low-prevalence antigen should be suspected. To identify an antibody to a low-prevalence antigen, one can test the serum with a panel of reagent red cells that express low-prevalence antigens. Alternatively, the one reactive red cell sample could be tested with known antibodies to low-prevalence antigens. Unfortunately, sera that contain antibodies to low-prevalence antigens often contain multiple antibodies to low-prevalence antigens. Although, by definition, low-prevalence antigens are rare, antibodies that recognize some of them are much less rare. Many antibodies to low-prevalence antigens are reactive only at temperatures below 37 C and therefore have doubtful clinical significance. To confirm the suspected specificities, one may need the expertise and resources of an IRL.

If an antibody to a low-prevalence antigen is suspected, transfusion should not be delayed while identification studies are performed. Because antisera to type donor units for low-prevalence antigens are generally not available, it is usually necessary to rely on the crossmatch to avoid transfusion of antigen-positive units. When the serum reacts with only one donor unit or reagent red cell, the most likely cause is an antibody to a low-prevalence antigen; however, other possible explanations include the following: the red cells may be ABO incompatible, have a positive DAT, or be polyagglutinable.

If an antibody in the serum of a pregnant woman is suspected of reacting with a low-prevalence antigen, testing the father's red cells with maternal plasma (if ABO compatible) can predict the possibility of incompatibility with the fetus and can make identifying the antibody unnecessary. If a newborn has a positive DAT, testing the mother's serum or an eluate from the infant's red cells against the father's red cells can implicate an antibody to a low-prevalence antigen as the probable cause. That test can be done only if the mother's plasma is ABO compatible with the father's red cells or if the eluate from the infant's red cells does not contain anti-A or -B that would react with the father's red cells.

Some reference laboratories do not attempt to identify antibodies to low-prevalence antigens because the antibodies are often of academic interest only. Identification of antibodies may be made when time permits and when suitable reagents are available.

Antibodies to Reagent Components and Other Anomalous Serologic Reactions

Antibodies to a variety of drugs and additives can cause positive results in antibody detection and identification tests. The mechanisms are probably similar to those discussed in Chapter 17. Most of these anomalous reactions are in-vitro phenomena and have no clinical significance in transfusion therapy, other than causing laboratory problems that delay transfusions. The reactions rarely cause erroneous interpretations of ABO typing that could endanger the patient. For a more detailed discussion, see the suggested reading by Garratty.

ROULEAUX. Rouleaux are aggregates of red cells that give a "stack of coins" appearance when viewed microscopically. Rouleaux formation is an in-vitro phenomenon produced by abnormal serum protein concentrations. It may be difficult to detect antibodies by direct agglutination in a test serum that contains rouleaux-producing proteins; however, it is not a problem in an IAT, where the serum is washed away. The saline replacement technique can be used to detect direct-agglutinating antibodies in the presence of rouleaux (Method 3-4).

PRESERVATIVE SOLUTIONS. Antibodies that react with an ingredient in the solution used to preserve reagent red cells (eg, chloramphenicol, neomycin, tetracycline, hydrocortisone, EDTA, sodium caprylate, or various sugars) may agglutinate red cells suspended in that solution. The autologous control is often nonreactive, unless a suspension of autologous red cells is prepared with the manufacturer's red cell diluent or with a similar preservative. Such reactions can often be avoided by washing the reagent red cells with saline before testing. Adding the medium to the autologous control and converting a nonreactive test to a reactive test can often confirm the role of the preservative. In some cases, however, washing the reagent red cells will not circumvent the reactivity, and the resolution may be more complex.

ENHANCEMENT MEDIA. Antibodies that react with ingredients in other reagents, such as commercially prepared LISS additives or albumin, can cause agglutination in tests using reagent red cells, donor red cells, autologous red cells, or all three. Ingredients that have been implicated include parabens (in some LISS additives), sodium caprylate (in some albumins), and thimerosal (in some LISS/saline preparations). Antibody to ingredients in enhancement media may be suspected if the autologous control is positive but the DAT is negative. Omitting the enhancement medium will usually circumvent the reactivity.

In some cases, antibodies to reagent ingredients show blood group specificity (eg, paraben-dependent anti-Jk^a,[34] paraben-dependent antibody to Rh protein,[35] and caprylate-dependent autoanti-e).[36] The autocontrol may be reactive if the patient's own red cells express the antigen, but the DAT should be negative.

RED-CELL-RELATED ANOMALIES. The age of red cells can cause anomalous serologic reactions. Antibodies exist that react only with stored red cells. Such antibodies can cause agglutination of reagent red cells by all techniques, and the reactivity may be enhanced with enzyme-treated red cells. Such reactivity is not affected by washing the red cells, and the autocontrol is usually nonreactive. No reactivity will be seen when freshly collected red cells are tested (ie, from freshly drawn donor or autologous blood samples).

The Patient with a Positive Autocontrol

Reactivity of the patient's serum with the autologous cells may indicate the presence of warm or cold autoantibodies, antibodies to certain drugs, alloantibodies to transfused red cells if the patient was recently transfused, or antibodies to a constituent of the test medium. When the autocontrol is positive, a DAT should be performed (Chapter 17 and Fig 16-2).

NO RECENT TRANSFUSIONS. If the reactivity in the serum occurs at room temperature or below, the cause is often anti-I or another cold autoagglutinin. If the reactivity occurs in the AHG phase, the reactivity is usually associated with a positive DAT and possible autoantibodies. If, in addition, the serum reacts with all cells tested, autoadsorption or other special procedures may be necessary to determine whether there are underlying alloantibodies that are masked by the autoantibodies. If the serum is nonreactive or shows only weak reactivity, an eluate may demonstrate more potent autoantibody reactivity. (See both "Cold Autoantibodies" and "Warm Autoantibodies" later in this section, and Chapter 17 for a more detailed discussion.)

RECENT TRANSFUSIONS. If the autocontrol is positive in the AHG phase, there may be antibody-coated donor red cells in the patient's circulation, resulting in a positive DAT, which may show mixed-field reactivity. An elution should be performed, especially when tests on serum are inconclusive. For example, a recently transfused patient may have a positive autocontrol and serum that reacts weakly with most but not all Fy(a+) red cells. It may be possible to confirm anti-Fy[a] specificity in an eluate because often more antibody is bound to donor red cells than is free in the plasma. Furthermore the preparation of an eluate will concentrate the antibody. It is rare for transfused red cells to make the autocontrol positive at other test phases, but it can occur, especially with a newly developing or a cold-reacting alloantibody.

Some patients may form warm autoantibodies following red cell transfusion; therefore, if the positive DAT does not have a mixed-field appearance—and especially if the serum is reacting with all red cells—then the possibility of an autoantibody should be considered. Detection of masked alloantibodies may require allogeneic adsorptions (Method 3-12). If the patient's phenotype is known for the common red cell antigens, an allogeneic adsorption may require only one adsorption using a reagent cell that is matched for the antigens the patient lacks. If the patient's phenotype is unknown, it will be necessary to perform multiple allogeneic adsorptions using a combination of reagent cells, each of which lacks some of the common red cell antigens. Cells that are homozygous for the common red cell antigens, such as R_1 (DCe), R_2 (DcE), and r (dce), are frequently used. The adsorbed serum is tested with reagent cells to rule out the common antibodies that correspond with the antigens that are missing from the adsorbing cell. For example, if the adsorbing cell types R1 (DCe), K–, Fy(a+b–), Jk(a–b+), S–s+, the adsorbed plasma could be tested for possible anti-c, anti-E, anti-K, anti-Fy[b], anti-Jk[a], and anti-S. It is never possible, however, to rule out antibodies to high-prevalence antigens when allogeneic adsorption techniques are used.

If the DAT does have a mixed-field appearance and if the serum reacts with all cells tested, a transfusion reaction caused by an alloantibody to a high-prevalence antigen should be considered (Fig 16-2).

COLD AUTOANTIBODIES. Potent cold autoantibodies that react with all red cells, including the patient's own, can create special problems—especially when the reactivity persists at temperatures above room temperature. Cold autoantibodies may be benign or pathologic. (See Chapter 17 for a more detailed discussion.)

There are different approaches to testing sera with potent cold agglutinins. To detect underlying potentially clinically significant antibodies, methods that circumvent the cold autoantibody can be used. Procedures for the detection of alloantibodies in the presence of cold-reactive autoantibodies include the following:

1. Prewarming techniques, in which red cells and serum are prewarmed to 37 C separately before they are combined (Method 3-3).
2. The use of anti-IgG rather than polyspecific AHG reagent.
3. Cold autoadsorption of the patient's serum with autologous red cells to remove autoantibodies but not alloantibodies.
4. Adsorption with rabbit erythrocytes or rabbit erythrocyte stroma.

WARM AUTOANTIBODIES. Patients with warm-reactive autoantibodies in their serum create a special problem because the antibody reacts with virtually all red cells tested. The majority of warm autoantibodies are IgG immunoglobulins, although some warm autoantibodies are

IgM immunoglobulins. IgM warm autoantibodies are unusual, but they often cause severe autoimmune hemolytic anemia, with more fatalities than other types.[37] If patients with warm autoantibodies require transfusions, it is important to detect any underlying clinically significant alloantibodies that the autoantibodies may mask. (For more information, see Chapter 17 and Methods 4-8 through 4-10.)

Reactivity of most warm-reactive autoantibodies is greatly enhanced by methods such as PEG and enzymes, and to a lesser extent by LISS. It is often helpful to omit the enhancement media when testing sera that contain warm autoantibodies. If such tests are nonreactive, the same procedure can be used for compatibility testing, without the need for adsorptions.

Frequency of Antibody Testing

After a clinically significant antibody has been identified, antigen-negative RBC units must be selected for all future transfusions, even if the antibodies are no longer detectable.[11(p35)] In addition, an AHG crossmatch must be performed. It is rarely necessary to repeat identification of known antibodies. AABB *Standards for Blood Banks and Transfusion Services* states that in patients with previously identified antibodies, methods of testing shall be those that identify *additional* clinically significant antibodies.[11(p34)] Each laboratory should define and validate methods for the detection of additional antibodies in these patients.

In patients with previously identified antibodies, repeated testing of the patient's serum with routine antibody detection red cells is often not informative. It is more useful to test the patient's serum with red cells that are negative for the antigen(s) that corresponds to the patient's known antibody(ies). Ideally, if the patient's phenotype is known, a panel of red cells could be selected that is negative for the antigen that corresponds with the patient's antibody and is positive for other antigens the patient lacks. For example, if a routine commercial panel is tested with serum from a patient with anti-e, usually only one e-negative red cell is present; therefore, testing the entire panel would not be an effective way to detect additional antibody(ies). A better approach would be to test several known e-negative red cells that express other major antigens. Usually, appropriate red cells can be selected from available red cell panels. The selection of test red cells is simplified if the antigens expressed on the patient's cells are known.

Immunohematology Reference Laboratories

When antibody problems cannot be resolved or when rare blood is needed, an IRL can provide consultation and assistance through its access to the American Rare Donor Program (ARDP). (See Method 3-13.)

POSTANALYTICAL CONSIDERATIONS: SELECTING BLOOD FOR TRANSFUSION

After an antibody has been identified, it is important to determine its clinical significance. Antibodies that react at 37 C, by IAT, or both, are potentially clinically significant. Antibodies that react at room temperature and below are usually not clinically significant; however, there are many exceptions. For example, anti-Vel, -P, and -PP1P^k (-Tj^a) may react only at cold temperatures, yet may cause red cell destruction in vivo. Anti-Ch, anti-Rg, and many of the Knops and Cost antibodies have little or no clinical significance despite their reactivity by IAT. Reported experience with examples of antibodies with the same specificity can be used in assessing the clinical significance. Table 16-6 summarizes the expected reactivity and clinical significance of commonly encountered alloantibodies. Daniels et al have published a review of these and other specificities.[38] For some antibodies, little or no data exists, and the decision on clinical significance must be based on the premise that clinically significant antibodies are those active at 37 C, by an IAT, or both.

Certain laboratory tests have been used to predict the clinical significance of antibodies. The monocyte monolayer assay (MMA), which quantifies phagocytosis, adherence of antibody-coated red cells, or both, can be used to predict the in-vivo clinical significance of some antibodies. The test for antibody-dependent cellular cytotoxicity (ADCC), which measures lysis of antibody-coated red cells, and the chemiluminescence assay, which measures the respiratory release of oxygen radicals after phagocytosis of antibody-coated red cells, have been helpful in predicting in-vivo antibody reactivity—particularly for predicting the severity of HDFN. For cold-reactive antibodies, in-vitro thermal amplitude studies may predict the likelihood of in-vivo hemolysis.[39]

In-vivo tests may also be used to evaluate the significance of an antibody. The most common technique is a red cell survival study in which radiolabeled, antigen-positive red cells (usually labeled with ^{51}Cr) are infused into the patient. After a specified period has elapsed, a sample of blood from the patient is tested for radioactivity. With this technique, it is possible to measure the survival of 1 mL or less of infused cells. Another in-vivo technique, flow cytometry, can also be used to measure the survival of infused red cells, but a larger aliquot of red cells (about 10 mL) is generally required. Interpretation of in-vivo survival test results is complicated by the fact that small aliquots of incompatible red cells may have a faster rate of destruction than an entire transfused Red Blood Cell (RBC) unit. Comparison with documented cases in the literature and consultation with an IRL should provide guidance about previous examples of similar specificities.

Phenotyping Donor Units

Whenever possible, RBC units selected for transfusion to a patient with potentially clinically significant antibodies should be tested and found negative for the corresponding antigen(s). Even if the antibody is no longer detectable, all subsequent RBC transfusions to that patient should lack the antigen in order to prevent a secondary immune response. The transfusion service must maintain records of all patients in whom clinically significant antibodies have been previously identified, and an AHG crossmatch procedure is required if the serum contains—or has previously contained—a clinically significant antibody.[11(pp35,69)]

A potent example of the antibody should be used to identify antigen-negative blood. Often, the antibody is a commercial antiserum, but to save expensive or rare reagents, units can be tested first for compatibility with the patient's serum. Then, the absence of the antigen in compatible units can be confirmed with commercial reagents. If the antibody is unusual and if commercial antiserum is not available, a stored sample from the sensitized patient can be used to select units for transfusion at a later time, especially if the patient's later samples lose reactivity. If a patient's serum is used as a typing reagent, the antibody should be well characterized and should retain its reactivity after storage. Appropriate negative and weak-positive controls (eg, from heterozygous donors) should be used at the time of the testing. The following criteria, established by the FDA for licensing some reagents, should be used as guidelines for human-source reagents used in lieu of commercial reagents[40]:

1. Anti-K, -k, -Jk^a, -Fy^a, and -C^w: dilution of 1:8 must produce at least a 1+ reaction.
2. Anti-S, -s, -P1, -M, -I, -c (saline), -e (saline), and -A1: dilution of 1:4 must produce at least a 1+ reaction.
3. Most other specificities: undiluted must produce at least a 2+ reaction.

When selecting units for patients with clinically significant antibodies, some serologists recommend typing the units with antibodies from two different sources, but others consider it unnecessary—especially when potent reagents are available and when an AHG crossmatch will be performed. Different lots of antibody from the same manufacturer, and even reagents from different manufacturers, may have been prepared from the same source material because manufacturers often share the same resources.

If a donor unit is tested for selected antigens and labeled by the blood center, the use of licensed (commercial) reagents is preferred. If no licensed reagent is available, the unit may be labeled with appropriate wording (eg,

"Tested and found negative for XX antigen using unlicensed typing reagents").[41] Except for results of ABO and D typing, there is no requirement that results of antigen typing appear on the labels of donor units. The blood center may use a tag attached to the unit for indicating phenotype information.

Antigen-Negative Blood vs Crossmatch for Compatibility

For certain antibodies, typing the donor units may not be necessary, and the patient's serum can be used to select serologically compatible RBC units. This is especially true for antibodies that characteristically react below 37 C (eg, anti-M, -N, -P1, -Le^a, -Le^b, -A1) and that do not ordinarily produce a secondary immune response following the transfusion of antigen-positive RBC units.

It is rarely necessary to provide phenotypically matched antigen-negative RBC units as a prophylactic measure when the patient has no detectable antibody. However, special consideration is sometimes given to certain Rh antibodies. When a patient of the R_1R_1 phenotype produces anti-E, some serologists suggest that RBC units should be negative for both the E and c antigens. This is based on the assumption that the stimulus to produce anti-E may also have stimulated anti-c or anti-cE that remains undetected by routine tests.[42]

Similarly, for an R_2R_2 patient with demonstrable anti-C, the use of e-negative donor blood may be considered. When an antibody has not been specifically demonstrated but cannot be conclusively excluded, it may be prudent to select RBC units that lack the corresponding antigen.

When Rare Blood Is Needed

Rare blood includes units that are negative for high-prevalence antigens as well as units that are negative for a combination of common antigens. When a patient has multiple antibodies, it can be helpful to determine the prevalence of compatible donors. To calculate the prevalence, one must multiply the prevalence of donors negative for one antigen by the prevalence of donors negative for each of the other antigens. For example, if a serum contains anti-c, anti-Fy^a, and anti-S, and if the prevalence of antigen-negatives are c-negative = 18%, Fy(a–) = 34%, and S-negative = 45%, then the prevalence of compatible units is $0.18 \times 0.34 \times 0.45 = 0.028$, or 2.8%. If the patient is group O, the prevalence of group O donors (45%) is factored into the calculation, as follows: $0.028 \times 0.45 = 0.013$, or 1.3%. If any of these antibodies occurred alone, finding compatible blood would not be very difficult, but together the combination requires a large number of units to provide one compatible unit. The preceding calculation uses the prevalence in populations of European ethnicity. Prevalence may differ in populations of non-European ethnicity. In calculating the probability of compatible donors, one should use the prevalence that corresponds with the ethnic composition of the donor population, if available.

When units of rare (<1 in 5000) or uncommon (<1 in 1000) phenotypes are needed, the ARDP can be very helpful. That program, which can be accessed only by personnel from an accredited IRL, can identify blood suppliers that are known to have potentially compatible units (usually frozen RBC units) and donors who may be eligible to donate (Method 3-13).

Family members are another potential source of rare blood donors. Siblings are often the best source of serologically compatible blood. The absence of high-prevalence antigens is usually associated with the inheritance of the same rare recessive blood group gene from each heterozygous parent. Children from the same parents have one chance in four of inheriting the same two rare genes, making siblings much more likely than the general population to express the rare type. In most cases, blood from the patient's parents, children, and half of the patient's siblings will express only one rare gene. If transfusion is essential and if there is no alternative to transfusing incompatible blood, these heterozygous (single dose) donors would be preferable to random donors. For infants with HDFN resulting from multiple antibodies or an antibody to a high-prevalence antigen, the mother (if ABO compatible) is often the logical donor.

If the clinical situation allows, autologous RBC transfusions should be considered for patients with rare phenotypes who are expected to need rare blood in the future. For some patients with multiple antibodies who are not able to donate autologous units, it may be necessary to determine whether any of the antibodies is less likely to cause red cell destruction and, in a critical situation, to give blood that is incompatible for that particular antigen.

ACKNOWLEDGMENTS

The author wishes to acknowledge the contributions of members of the Technical Manual Committee who contributed anonymously to this chapter in previous editions of the *Technical Manual.* Also, thanks go to friends and coworkers who contributed their time and expertise, including Virginia Lew, MT(ASCP)SBB; Joseph L. Ong, MT(ASCP)SBB; Frances K. Sturtevant, MT(ASCP)SBB; and Debbie Warren, MT(ASCP)SBB.

KEY POINTS

1. It is important to consider the patient's medical history (transfusions, pregnancies, transplantations, diagnosis, drugs, and ethnic origin) before starting antibody identification testing.
2. An antibody may be tentatively excluded or "ruled out" if an antigen is present on a regent cell and the serum does not react with it.
3. Common clinically significant alloantibodies that should be excluded during antibody identification testing are anti-D, -C, -E, -c, -e, -K, -Fy^a, -Fy^b, -Jk^a, -Jk^b, -S, and -s.
4. Based on probability, the use of two reactive and two nonreactive red cell samples is an acceptable approach for antibody confirmation.
5. The autologous control, in which serum and autologous red cells are tested under the same conditions as the serum and reagent red cells, is an important part of antibody identification. The autologous control is not the same as a direct antiglobulin test (DAT).
6. The phenotype of the autologous red cells is an important part of antibody identification. When an antibody has been tentatively identified in the serum, the corresponding antigen is expected to be absent from the autologous red cells.
7. An antibody can be removed from a serum sample by adsorption onto red cells that express the corresponding antigen.
8. Elution dissociates antibodies from sensitized red cells. Bound antibody may be released by changing the thermodynamics of an antigen-antibody reaction, by neutralizing or reversing forces of attraction that hold antigen-antibody complexes together, or by disturbing the structures of the antigen-antibody binding site.
9. A clinically significant red cell antibody is an antibody that is frequently associated with hemolytic disease of the fetus and newborn (HDFN), with hemolytic transfusion reactions, or with a notable decrease in the survival of transfused red cells.
10. Whenever possible, red cell units selected for transfusion to a patient with a potentially clinically significant antibody should be tested and found negative for the corresponding antigen(s). Even if the antibody is no longer detectable, all subsequent red cell transfusions to the patient should lack the antigen in order to prevent a secondary immune response.

REFERENCES

1. Walker RH, Lin DT, Hartrick MB. Alloimmunization following blood transfusion. Arch Pathol Lab Med 1989;113:254-61.
2. Reid ME, Lomas-Francis C. The blood group antigens factsbook. 2nd ed. San Diego: Academic Press, 2004.

3. Michelle D, ed. Standards for immunohematology reference laboratories. 6th ed. Bethesda, MD: AABB, 2009.
4. Howard JE, Winn LC, Gottlieb CE, et al. Clinical significance of anti-complement component of antiglobulin antisera. Transfusion 1982;22:269-72.
5. Judd WJ, Steiner EA, Oberman HA, Nance S. Can the reading for serologic reactivity following 37 degrees C incubation be omitted? Transfusion 1992;32:304-8.
6. Shulman IA, Calderon C, Nelson JM, Nakayama R. The routine use of Rh-negative reagent red cells for the identification of anti-D and the detection of non-D red cell antibodies. Transfusion 1994;34:666-70.
7. Fisher RA. Statistical methods and scientific inference. 2nd ed. Edinburgh, Scotland: Oliver and Boyd, 1959.
8. Harris RE, Hochman HG. Revised p values in testing blood group antibodies: Fisher's exact test revisited. Transfusion 1986;26: 494-9.
9. Kanter MH, Poole G, Garratty G. Misinterpretation and misapplication of p values in antibody identification: The lack of value of a p value. Transfusion 1997;37:816-22.
10. Reid ME, Oyen R, Storry J, et al. Interpretation of RBC typing in multi-transfused patients can be unreliable (abstract). Transfusion 2000;40 (Suppl):123.
11. Carson TH, ed. Standards for blood banks and transfusion services. 27th ed. Bethesda, MD: AABB, 2011.
12. Rodberg K, Tsuneta R, Garratty G. Discrepant Rh phenotyping results when testing IgG-sensitized RBCs with monoclonal Rh reagents (abstract). Transfusion 1995;35(Suppl):67.
13. Reisner R, Butler G, Bundy K, Moore SB. Comparison of the polyethylene glycol antiglobulin test and the use of enzymes in antibody detection and identification. Transfusion 1996;36: 487-9.
14. Issitt PD, Combs MR, Bumgarner DJ, et al. Studies of antibodies in the sera of patients who have made red cell autoantibodies. Transfusion 1996;36:481-6.
15. Wilkinson SL. Serological approaches to transfusion of patients with allo- or autoantibodies. In: Nance SJ, ed. Immune destruction of red blood cells. Arlington, VA: AABB, 1989:227-61.
16. Issitt PD, Combs MR, Bredehoeft SJ, et al. Lack of clinical significance of "enzyme-only" red cell alloantibodies. Transfusion 1993;33:284-93.
17. Beattie KM, Zuelzer WW. The frequency and properties of pH-dependent anti-M. Transfusion 1965;5:322-6.
18. Bruce M, Watt AH, Hare W, et al. A serious source of error in antiglobulin testing. Transfusion 1986;26:177-81.
19. Rolih S, Thomas R, Fisher F, Talbot J. Antibody detection errors due to acidic or unbuffered saline. Immunohematol 1993;9:15-18.
20. Morton JA, Pickles MM, Terry AM. The Sd[a] blood group antigen in tissues and body fluids. Vox Sang 1970;19:472-82.
21. O'Neill GJ, Yang SY, Tegoli J, et al. Chido and Rodgers blood groups are distinct antigenic components of human complement C4. Nature 1978;273:668-70.
22. Tilley CA, Romans DG, Crookston MC. Localization of Chido and Rodgers determinants to the C4d fragment of human C4 (abstract). Transfusion 1978;18:622.
23. Judd WJ, Kraemer K, Moulds JJ. The rapid identification of Chido and Rodgers antibodies using C4d-coated red blood cells. Transfusion 1981;21:189-92.
24. Advani H, Zamor J, Judd WJ, et al. Inactivation of Kell blood group antigens by 2-aminoethylisothiouronium bromide. Br J Haematol 1982; 51:107-15.
25. Branch DR, Muensch HA, Sy Siok Hian AL, Petz LD. Disulfide bonds are a requirement for Kell and Cartwright (Yt[a]) blood group antigen integrity. Br J Haematol 1983;54:573-8.
26. Branch DR, Petz LD. A new reagent (ZZAP) having multiple applications in immunohematology. Am J Clin Pathol 1982;78:161-7.
27. Liew YW, Uchikawa M. Loss of Er[a] antigen in very low pH buffers. Transfusion 1987;27:442-3.
28. Swanson JL, Sastamoinen R. Chloroquine stripping of HLA A,B antigens from red cells. Transfusion 1985;25:439-40.
29. Freedman J, Masters CA, Newlands M, Mollison PL. Optimal conditions for use of sulphydryl compounds in dissociating red cell antibodies. Vox Sang 1976;30:231-9.
30. Issitt PD, Anstee DJ. Applied blood group serology. 4th ed. Durham, NC: Montgomery Scientific Publications, 1998.
31. Malyska H, Kleeman JE, Masouredis SP, Victoria EJ. Effects on blood group antigens from storage at low ionic strength in the presence of neomycin. Vox Sang 1983;44:375-84.

32. Westhoff CM, Sipherd BD, Toalson LD. Red cell antigen stability in K_3EDTA. Immunohematol 1993;9:109-11.
33. Moulds JM, Zimmerman PA, Doumbo OK, et al. Molecular identification of Knops blood group polymorphisms found in long homologous region D of complement receptor 1. Blood 2001;97:2879-85.
34. Judd WJ, Steiner EA, Cochran RK. Paraben-associated autoanti-Jk[a] antibodies: Three examples detected using commercially prepared low-ionic strength saline containing parabens. Transfusion 1982;22:31-5.
35. Judd WJ, Storry JR, Amnesley TD, et al. The first example of a paraben-dependent antibody to an Rh protein. Transfusion 2001;41: 371-4.
36. Dube VE, Zoes C, Adesman P. Caprylate-dependent auto-anti-e. Vox Sang 1977;33:359-63.
37. Arndt PA, Leger RM, Garratty G. Serologic findings in autoimmune hemolytic anemia associated with immunoglobulin M warm autoantibodies. Transfusion 2009;49:235-42.
38. Daniels G, Poole J, deSilva M, et al. The clinical significance of blood group antibodies. Transfus Med 2002;12:287-95.
39. Petz LD, Garratty G. Immune hemolytic anemias. 2nd ed. Philadelphia: Churchill Livingstone, 2004.
40. Code of federal regulations. Title 21, CFR Part 660.25. Washington, DC: US Government Printing Office, 2010 (revised annually).
41. Food and Drug Administration. Compliance programs (CBER). 7342.001: Inspection of licensed and unlicensed blood banks, brokers, reference laboratories, and contractors. Attachment C—Product testing system, infectious disease testing including invalidation of test results, blood grouping and typing (ABO and Rh), and crossmatching. Rockville, MD: CBER Office of Compliance and Biologics Quality, 2010. [Available at http://www.fda.gov/BiologicsBloodVacines/GuidanceComplianceRegulatoryInformation/ComplianceActivities/Enforcement/CompliancePrograms/ucm095226.htm (accessed October 21, 2010).]
42. Shirey RS, Edwards RE, Ness PM. The risk of alloimmunization to c (Rh4) in R_1R_1 patients who present with anti-E. Transfusion 1994;34: 756-8.

SUGGESTED READINGS

Carson TH, ed. Standards for blood banks and transfusion services. 27th ed. Bethesda, MD: AABB, 2011.

Daniels G. Human blood groups. 2nd ed. Oxford: Blackwell Science, 2002.

Engelfriet CP, Overbeeke MA, Dooren MC, et al. Bioassays to determine the clinical significance of red cell antibodies based on Fc receptor-induced destruction of red cells sensitized with IgG. Transfusion 1994;34:617-26.

Garratty G. In-vitro reactions with red blood cells that are not due to blood group antibodies: A review. Immunohematology 1998;14:1-11.

Harmening DM. Modern blood banking and transfusion practices. 5th ed. Philadelphia: FA Davis, 2005.

Issitt PD, Anstee DJ. Applied blood group serology. 4th ed. Durham, NC: Montgomery Scientific Publications, 1998.

Judd WJ. Elution of antibody from red cells. In: Bell CA, ed. A seminar on antigen-antibody reactions revisited. Washington, DC: AABB, 1982: 175-221.

Judd WJ, Johnson S, Storry J. Judd's methods in immunohematology. 3rd ed. Bethesda, MD: AABB Press, 2008.

Kanter MH. Statistical analysis. In: Busch MP, Brecher ME, eds. Research design and analysis. Bethesda, MD: AABB, 1998:63-104.

Klein HG, Anstee DJ. Mollison's blood transfusion in clinical medicine. 11th ed. Oxford: Blackwell Publishing, 2005.

Mallory D, ed. Immunohematology methods and procedures. Rockville, MD: American Red Cross, 1993.

Menitove JE. The Hardy-Weinberger principle: Selection of compatible blood based on mathematic principles. In: Fridey JL, Kasprisin CA, Chambers LA, Rudmann SV, eds. Numbers for blood bankers. Bethesda, MD: AABB, 1995:1-11.

Michelle D, ed. Standards for immunohematology reference laboratories. 6th ed. Bethesda, MD: AABB, 2009.

Reid ME, Lomas-Francis C. The blood group antigen factsbook. 2nd ed. London: Elsevier Academic Press, 2004.

Rolih S. A review: Antibodies with high-titer, low-avidity characteristics. Immunohematology 1990;6:59-67.

Rudmann SV, ed. Serologic problem-solving: A systematic approach for improved practice. Bethesda, MD: AABB Press, 2005.

Telen MJ. New and evolving techniques for antibody and antigen identification. In: Nance ST, ed. Alloimmunity: 1993 and beyond. Bethesda, MD: AABB, 1993:117-39.

Weisbach V, Kohnhauser T, Zimmermann R, et al. Comparison of the performance of microtube column systems and solid-phase systems and the tube low-ionic-strength solution additive indirect antiglobulin test in the detection of red cell alloantibodies. Transfus Med 2006;16: 276-84.

Wilkinson SL. Serological approaches to transfusion of patients with allo- or autoantibodies. In: Nance SJ, ed. Immune destruction of red blood cells. Arlington, VA: AABB, 1989:227-61.

Chapter 17

The Positive Direct Antiglobulin Test and Immune-Mediated Hemolysis

◆

Regina M. Leger, MSQA, MT(ASCP)SBB, CMQ/OE(ASQ)

THE DIRECT ANTIGLOBULIN test (DAT) is a simple test used to determine if red cells have been coated in vivo with immunoglobulin, complement, or both. A positive DAT may or may not be associated with immune-mediated hemolysis. As shown in Table 17-1, there are many causes of a positive DAT. The DAT is used primarily for the investigation of hemolytic transfusion reactions, hemolytic disease of the fetus and newborn (HDFN), autoimmune hemolytic anemia (AIHA), and drug-induced immune hemolysis.

THE DIRECT ANTIGLOBULIN TEST

The DAT should be performed on every patient in whom the presence of hemolysis has been established to distinguish immune from nonimmune hemolytic anemia. The predictive value of a positive DAT is 83% in a patient with hemolytic anemia, but only 1.4% in a patient without hemolytic anemia.[1] Small amounts of IgG and complement appear to be present on all red cells. Healthy individuals can have 5 to 90 IgG molecules/red cell[2] and 5 to 40 C3d molecules/red cell[3]; these levels are below the threshold of detection in routine testing. Depending on the technique and reagents used, the DAT can detect 100 to 500 molecules of IgG/red cell and 400 to 1100 molecules of C3d/red cell. Positive DATs are reported in 1:1000 up to 1:14,000 blood donors and 1% to 15% of hospital patients.[4] These large differences in incidence probably relate to different techniques (eg, tube vs tile) used. Most blood donors with positive DATs appear to be perfectly healthy, and most patients with positive DATs have no obvious signs of hemolytic anemia, although after careful evaluation some may show slight evidence of increased red cell destruction.

Although a positive DAT in a patient with hemolytic anemia indicates the most likely diagnosis is one of the immune hemolytic anemias, the DAT can be positive, coincidentally, in patients with hemolytic anemia that is not immune mediated. Conversely, some patients

Regina M. Leger, MSQA, MT(ASCP)SBB, CMQ/OE(ASQ), Research Associate, American Red Cross Blood Services, Southern California Region, Pomona, California
The author has disclosed no conflicts of interest.

◆17

TABLE 17-1. Some Causes of a Positive DAT

Autoantibodies to intrinsic red cell antigens
Hemolytic transfusion reactions
Hemolytic disease of the fetus and newborn
Drug-induced antibodies
Passively acquired alloantibodies (eg, donor plasma, derivatives, immunoglobulin)
Nonspecifically adsorbed proteins (eg, hypergammaglobulinemia, high-dose intravenous immune globulin, modification of red cell membrane by some drugs)
Complement activation due to bacterial infection, autoantibodies, or alloantibodies
Antibodies produced by passenger lymphocytes (eg, in transplanted organs or hematopoietic components)

with immune hemolytic anemia have a negative DAT (see "DAT-Negative AIHA" below).

Positive DATs caused by elevated levels of IgG or complement, with no clear correlation with anemia, have been noted with the red cells of patients with sickle cell disease, β-thalassemia, renal disease, multiple myeloma, autoimmune disorders, AIDS, and other diseases associated with elevated serum globulin or blood urea nitrogen (BUN) levels.[5-7] Interpretation of positive DATs should include the patient's history, clinical data, and the results of other laboratory tests.

When investigating a transfusion reaction, performance of the DAT on postreaction specimens is part of the initial transfusion reaction investigation. In the presence of immune-mediated hemolysis, the DAT may be positive if sensitized red cells have not been destroyed, or negative if hemolysis and rapid clearance have occurred.

The Principles of the DAT

The DAT is based on the test developed by Coombs, Mourant, and Race[8] for the detection of antibodies attached to red cells that do not produce direct agglutination. Initially, this test (the antiglobulin test) was used to demonstrate antibody in serum, but it was later applied to demonstrate the in-vivo coating of red cells with antibody or complement components. The two Fab sites on the antiglobulin molecule bind to the Fc portion of the sensitizing antibody (or to the complement component), thus bridging the gap between adjacent red cells to produce visible agglutination. The strength of the observed agglutination is usually proportional to the amount of bound protein.

The DAT is performed by testing freshly washed red cells directly with antiglobulin reagents containing anti-IgG and anti-C3d. The red cells need to be washed to remove globulins and complement that are present in the surrounding plasma; otherwise the antiglobulin reagent can be neutralized, resulting in a false-negative test. The red cells should be tested immediately after washing to prevent false-negative results due to the potential elution of IgG. Although any red cells may be tested, EDTA-anticoagulated blood samples are preferred; the EDTA prevents in-vitro fixation of complement by chelating the calcium that is needed for C1 activation. If red cells from a clotted blood sample have a positive DAT due to complement, the results should be confirmed on cells from freshly collected blood kept at 37 C or an EDTA-anticoagulated specimen if those results are to be used for diagnostic purposes.

The DAT can initially be performed with a polyspecific antihuman globulin (AHG) reagent capable of detecting both IgG and C3d (see Method 3-6). If positive, tests with monospecific reagents (anti-IgG and anticomplement) need to be performed for appropriate characterization of the immune process involved and to determine the diagnosis. Because polyspecific reagents are commonly blended reagents, and testing conditions for optimally detecting IgG and C3d on red cells may differ, some laboratories elect to perform the DAT initially with the specific anti-IgG and anti-C3d reagents separately. If the polyspecific reagent is polyclonal, proteins other than IgG or C3d (eg, IgM, IgA, or other complement components) can occasionally be detected; however, specific reagents to distinguish these other proteins by serologic techniques are not readily available. If cord blood samples are to be tested, it is appropriate to use anti-IgG only, because HDFN results from fetal red cell sensitization with maternally derived IgG antibody, and complement activation rarely occurs.[4]

It is important to follow the antiglobulin reagent manufacturer's instructions and recognize any stated product limitations. False-negative or weaker results can be obtained if the washed red cells are allowed to sit before testing with anti-IgG, or if the reading is delayed. Some anticomplement reagents, on the other hand, demonstrate stronger reactivity if centrifugation is delayed for a short time after the reagent has been added. When the DAT is positive with both anti-IgG and anti-C3, the red cells should be tested with an inert control reagent (eg, 6% albumin or saline). Lack of agglutination of the red cells in the control reagent will provide some assurance that the test results are accurately interpreted. If the control is reactive, the DAT result is invalid (see sections below on warm AIHA and cold agglutinin syndrome, respectively). Reactivity with this control reagent can indicate spontaneous agglutination caused by heavy coating of IgG or rare warm-reactive IgM, or IgM cold autoagglutinins that were not dissociated during routine washing.

Evaluation of a Positive DAT

A positive DAT alone is not diagnostic. The interpretation of the significance of this positive result requires knowledge of the patient's diagnosis; recent drug, pregnancy, and transfusion history; and information on the presence of acquired or unexplained hemolytic anemia. Dialogue with the attending physician is important. Clinical considerations together with laboratory data should dictate the extent to which a positive DAT is evaluated.

Patient History

The following situations may warrant further investigation of a positive DAT.

1. *Evidence of in-vivo red cell destruction.* If an anemic patient with a positive DAT does show evidence of hemolysis, testing to evaluate a possible immune etiology is appropriate. Reticulocytosis, spherocytes observed on the peripheral blood film, hemoglobinemia, hemoglobinuria, decreased serum haptoglobin, and elevated levels of serum unconjugated bilirubin or lactate dehydrogenase (LDH), especially LDH1, may be associated with increased red cell destruction. *If there is no evidence of immune hemolysis, no further studies are necessary* unless the patient requires red cell transfusion and the serum contains incompletely identified unexpected antibodies to red cell antigens; an eluate may be helpful with antibody identification (see "Elution" below).
2. *History of recent transfusion.* When a patient has recently been transfused, a positive DAT may be the first indication of a developing immune response. The developing antibody sensitizes the transfused red cells that have the corresponding antigen and the DAT becomes positive; the antibody may not be of sufficient quantity to be detected in the serum. Antibody may appear as early as 7 to 10 days after transfusion in primary immunization or as early as 1 to 2 days in a secondary response[4,9]; these alloantibodies could shorten the survival of red cells already transfused or given in subsequent transfusions. A mixed-field appearance in the posttransfusion DAT (ie, agglutination of donor red cells and no agglutination of the patient's red cells) may or may not be observed.

3. *Administration of drugs previously associated with immune-mediated hemolysis.* Many drugs have been reported to cause a positive DAT and/or immune-mediated hemolysis, but the occurrence is rare.[10] (See "Drug-Induced Immune Hemolytic Anemia" below.)
4. *History of hematopoietic progenitor cell or organ transplantation.* Passenger lymphocytes of donor origin produce antibodies directed against ABO or other blood group antigens on the recipient's cells, causing a positive DAT.[4]
5. *Administration of intravenous immunoglobulin (IVIG) or IV anti-D.* IVIG may contain ABO antibodies, anti-D, or sometimes other antibodies. Intravenous anti-D used to treat immune thrombocytopenia (ITP, previously known as immune thrombocytopenic purpura) causes Rh-positive patients to develop a positive DAT[11]; IV anti-D may also contain other antibodies.

Serologic Investigation

Three investigative approaches are helpful in the evaluation of a positive DAT:

1. Test the DAT-positive red cells with anti-IgG and anti-C3d reagents to characterize the type of protein(s) coating the red cells.
2. Test the serum/plasma to detect and identify clinically significant antibodies to red cell antigens. Additional tests useful in classifying the hemolytic anemias and procedures for detecting alloantibodies in the presence of autoantibodies are described later in this chapter.
3. Test an eluate prepared from the DAT-positive red cells with reagent red cells to define whether the coating protein has red cell antibody activity. When the only coating protein is complement, eluates are frequently nonreactive. However, an eluate from the patient's red cells coated only with complement should be tested if there is clinical evidence of antibody-mediated hemolysis, for example, after transfusion. The eluate preparation can concentrate small amounts of IgG that may not be detectable in routine testing of the patient's plasma.

Results of these tests combined with the patient's history and clinical data should assist in classification of the problem involved.

Elution

Elution frees antibody from sensitized red cells and recovers antibody in a usable form. Multiple elution methods have been described and reviewed.[12] Many laboratories use the commercial acid elution kits, primarily for ease of use and decreased exposure to potentially harmful chemicals; these kits are suitable to recover antibody in most cases. Because no single elution method is ideal in all situations, use of an alternative elution method (eg, organic solvents)[13] may be indicated when a nonreactive eluate is not in agreement with clinical data. Table 17-2 lists the uses of some common elution methods.

Very thorough washing of the red cells before elution is essential to ensure that antibody detected in the eluate is only red-cell-bound antibody and does not represent free antibody from the plasma. A control to show that all free antibody has been removed by washing can be obtained by saving the saline from the last wash and testing it in parallel with the eluate. Also, transferring the red cells to a clean tube before the elution step eliminates the possibility of dissociating any plasma antibody that may have nonspecifically bound to the test tube during preparation.

In cases of HDFN or hemolytic transfusion reactions, specific antibody (or antibodies) is usually detected in the eluate that may or may not be detectable in the serum. In the case of transfusion reactions, newly developed antibodies initially detectable only in the eluate are usually detectable in the serum after about 14 to 21 days.[15] Eluate preparation from the patient's posttransfusion red cell sample may concentrate antibody activity and facilitate identification of weakly reactive serum antibodies.

When the eluate reacts with all cells tested, autoantibody is the most likely explanation, especially if the patient has not been transfused recently. When no unexpected antibodies are present in the serum, and if the patient has not been transfused recently, no further serologic testing of an autoantibody is necessary.

A nonreactive eluate prepared from IgG-coated red cells may have several causes. One cause may be that the eluate was not tested against cells positive for the corresponding antigen, notably group A or group B cells, or antigens of low prevalence, which are absent from most reagent red cells. If a non-group-O patient has received plasma containing anti-A or anti-B (as in transfusion of group O platelets), and the recipient appears to have immune hemolysis, the eluate should be tested against A_1 and/or B cells. If the expected ABO antibodies are not detected, other causes of the positive DAT should be sought. It may be appropriate to test the eluate against red cells from recently transfused donor units, which could have caused immunization to a rare antigen, or, in HDFN, against cells from the father, from whom the infant may have inherited a rare gene encoding a low-prevalence antigen. Pursuing the cause of a nonreactive eluate for patients with no evidence of hemolysis is usually not indicated. Toy et al[5] showed that 79% of pretransfusion patients with a positive DAT have a nonreactive eluate.

Reactivity of eluates can be enhanced by testing them against enzyme-treated cells or by the use of enhancement techniques such as polyethylene glycol (PEG). Washing the red cells with low-ionic-strength saline (LISS) or cold wash solutions (eg, saline) may prevent the loss of antibody while the cells are being prepared for elution.

If both the serum and eluate are nonreactive, there is evidence of immune hemolysis, and the patient has received a drug previously reported to have caused hemolysis, testing to demonstrate drug-related antibodies should be considered (see later section on laboratory investigation of drug-induced immune hemolysis).

AUTOIMMUNE HEMOLYTIC ANEMIA

Immune-mediated hemolysis is the shortening of red cell survival as a result of an immune response. If the marrow is able to adequately compensate, the reduced red cell survival may not result in anemia. Immune-mediated hemolysis is only one cause of hemolytic anemia, and many causes of hemolysis are unrelated to immune reactions. The serologic investigations carried out in the blood bank do not determine whether a patient has a "hemolytic" anemia. The diagnosis of hemolytic anemia

TABLE 17-2. Antibody Elution Methods

Method	Use	Comments
Lui freeze-thaw	ABO HDFN	Quick; small volume of red cells needed; poor recovery of other antibodies
Heat (56 C)	ABO HDFN; IgM agglutinating antibodies	Easy; poor recovery of IgG allo- and autoantibodies
Acid elution kits (commercial)	Warm auto- and alloantibodies	Easy; possible false-positive eluates when high-titer antibody present[14]
Digitonin acid	Warm auto- and alloantibodies	Time-consuming washing of stroma

HDFN = hemolytic disease of the fetus and newborn.

rests on clinical findings and laboratory data such as hemoglobin or hematocrit values; reticulocyte count; red cell morphology; bilirubin, haptoglobin, and LDH levels; and sometimes red cell survival studies. The serologic findings help determine whether the hemolysis has an immune basis and, if so, what type of immune hemolytic anemia is present. This is important because the treatment for each type is different.

In some cases, the destruction of red cells takes place in the intravascular space, with release of free hemoglobin into the plasma. The red cells are ruptured following activation of the classical complement cascade. The characteristic features of this rare type of hemolysis are hemoglobinemia and, when the plasma hemoglobin exceeds the renal threshold, hemoglobinuria. Conversely, extravascular hemolysis results when macrophages in the spleen and liver phagocytose red cells completely or partially (producing spherocytes) or destroy red cells by cytotoxic events, with a subsequent increase in serum bilirubin. Such a distinction is a simplification, however, because hemoglobin can also be released into the plasma following extravascular destruction if hemolysis is brisk.

Immune hemolytic anemias can be classified in various ways. One classification system is shown in Table 17-3. The AIHAs are subdivided into the major types: warm AIHA (WAIHA), cold agglutinin syndrome (CAS), mixed- or combined-type AIHA, and paroxysmal cold hemoglobinuria (PCH). Not all cases fit neatly into these categories. Table 17-4 shows the typical serologic characteristics of the AIHAs. Drugs (discussed in a later section of this chapter) may also induce immune hemolysis; effects of drug-induced *auto*antibodies are serologically indistinguishable from WAIHA.

TABLE 17-3. Classification of Immune Hemolytic Anemias

Autoimmune Hemolytic Anemia (AIHA)
Warm AIHA
Cold agglutinin syndrome
Mixed-type AIHA
Paroxysmal cold hemoglobinuria
Alloimmune Hemolytic Anemia
Hemolytic transfusion reaction
Hemolytic disease of the fetus and newborn
Drug-Induced Immune Hemolytic Anemia

Warm Autoimmune Hemolytic Anemia

The majority of AIHA cases are caused by warm-reactive autoantibodies, optimally reactive with red cells at 37 C. The autoantibody is usually IgG (but can be IgM or IgA).

Serologic Characteristics

The DAT may be positive due to IgG plus complement (67%), IgG only (20%), or complement only (13%).[4] The presence of an IgG autoantibody on the red cells may be confirmed by elution upon initial diagnosis and/or at pretransfusion testing. Typically, the eluate reacts with virtually all cells tested, with reactivity enhanced in tests against enzyme-treated cells or when enhancement such as PEG is used. The eluate will usually have no serologic activity if the only protein coating the red cells is complement.

If the autoantibody has been adsorbed by the patient's red cells in vivo, the serum may not contain detectable free antibody. The serum will contain antibody after all the specific antigen sites on the red cells have been occupied and no more antibody can be bound in vivo. The DAT in such cases is usually strongly positive. Autoantibody in the serum typically reacts by indirect antiglobulin testing against all cells tested. Approximately 60% of patients with WAIHA have serum antibodies that react with untreated saline-suspended red cells. When testing with PEG, enzyme-treated red cells, or solid-phase methods, over 90% of these sera can be shown to contain autoantibody. Agglutination at room temperature can

TABLE 17-4. Typical Serologic Findings in Autoimmune Hemolytic Anemia

	WAIHA	CAS	Mixed-type AIHA	PCH
DAT (routine)	IgG IgG + C3 C3	C3 only	IgG + C3 C3	C3 only
Immunoglobulin type	IgG	IgM	IgG, IgM	IgG
Eluate	IgG antibody	Nonreactive	IgG antibody	Nonreactive
Serum	IAT; 35% agglutinate untreated red cells at 20 C	IgM agglutinating antibody; titer ≥1000 (60%) at 4 C; react at ≥30 C	IgG IAT-reactive antibody plus IgM agglutinating antibody react at ≥30 C	Routine IAT negative; IgG biphasic hemolysin in Donath-Landsteiner test
Specificity	Broadly reactive; multiple specificities reported	Usually anti-I	Usually unclear	Anti-P

AIHA = autoimmune hemolytic anemia; WAIHA = warm AIHA; CAS = cold agglutinin syndrome; PCH = paroxysmal cold hemoglobinuria; DAT = direct antiglobulin test; IAT = indirect antiglobulin test.

be seen in about one-third of patients with WAIHA, but the cold agglutinins have normal titers at 4 C and are nonreactive at 30 C and 37 C. Thus, these cold agglutinins are nonpathogenic and the patient would not have CAS in addition to WAIHA.[4]

An unusual subcategory of WAIHA is associated with IgM agglutinins that react at 37 C.[4,16] This type of WAIHA is characterized by severe hemolysis, and the prognosis for these patients is poor. The patient's red cells are typically spontaneously agglutinated in the DAT; that is, the red cells are reactive with all reagents tested, including a control such as 6% albumin (see "Serologic Problems" below). Complement is usually detected on the red cells; IgG or IgM may or may not be detected. IgM agglutinins are often detected in an eluate (eg, acid) when inspected for agglutination after the 37 C incubation and before proceeding to the antiglobulin test. Serum IgM warm autoagglutinins are typically weak and may be difficult to detect; some are enhanced in the presence of albumin or at low pH. Optimal reactivity is sometimes seen between 20 C and 30 C rather than at 37 C. These antibodies have low antibody titers; a 4 C titer of <64 easily differentiates this IgM warm antibody from those seen in CAS. To prevent misinterpretation of titration results, titrations at different temperatures need to be carried out with separate sets of tubes to avoid carryover agglutination.[4]

Serologic Problems

Warm autoantibodies can cause technical difficulties during red cell testing. Spontaneous agglutination can occur if the red cells are heavily coated with IgG and the reagent contains a potentiator such as albumin. This has been observed when high-protein Rh typing sera are used; if the control reagent provided by the manufacturer for these antisera reacts, the typing is invalid. IgG can less commonly cause spontaneous agglutination in lower protein reagents—eg, monoclonal typing sera; this reactivity is often weaker or fragile in comparison to true agglutination and may not be detected by a 6% albumin control.[17]

Warm-reactive IgM agglutinins can also cause spontaneous agglutination, resulting in ABO and Rh typing problems and/or reactivity with the negative control reagent for the DAT.[16] In these cases, treatment with dithiothreitol (DTT) or 2-mercaptoethanol (2-ME) (Method 2-18) to disrupt the IgM agglutinin is required to accurately interpret typing and DAT results. When the spontaneous agglutination is disrupted, the control reagent will be nonreactive.

When the DAT is positive due to IgG, antiglobulin-reactive typing reagents cannot be used unless the red-cell-bound IgG is first removed (see Methods 2-20 and 2-21). An alternative is to use low-protein antisera (eg, monoclonal reagents) that do not require an antiglobulin test (refer to the manufacturer's instructions for detection of spontaneous agglutination).

The presence of autoantibody in the serum increases the complexity of the serologic evaluation and increases the time needed to complete pretransfusion testing, which often requires some hours. If a patient who has warm-reactive autoantibodies in the serum needs transfusion, it is important to determine if alloantibodies are also present. Some alloantibodies may make their presence known by reacting more strongly or at different phases than the autoantibody, but quite often studies may not suggest the existence of masked alloantibodies.[18,19]

Methods to detect alloantibodies in the presence of warm-reactive autoantibodies attempt to remove, reduce, or circumvent the autoantibody. Antibody detection methods that use PEG, enzymes, column agglutination, or solid-phase red cell adherence generally enhance autoantibodies. Antibody detection tests using LISS or saline tube methods may not detect autoantibodies, but most significant alloantibodies will be detected. Other procedures involve adsorption; two widely used approaches are discussed below.

It is helpful to know which of the common red cell antigens are lacking on the patient's red cells to predict which clinically significant alloantibodies the patient may have produced or may produce. Antigens absent from autologous cells could well be the target of present or future alloantibodies.

Adsorption with Autologous Red Cells

In a patient who has not been transfused recently, adsorption with autologous red cells (autologous adsorption; see Method 4-8) is the best way to detect alloantibodies in the presence of warm-reactive autoantibodies. Only autoantibodies will be removed, and alloantibodies, if present, will remain in the serum.

Autologous adsorption generally requires some initial preparation of the patient's red cells. At 37 C, in-vivo adsorption will have occurred, and all antigen sites on the patient's own red cells may be blocked. A gentle heat elution at 56 C for 5 minutes can dissociate some of the bound IgG. This can be followed by treatment of the autologous red cells with proteolytic enzymes to increase their capacity to adsorb autoantibody. Treatment of the red cells with ZZAP, a mixture of papain or ficin and DTT, accomplishes both of these actions in one step; it is proposed that the sulfhydryl component makes the IgG molecules more susceptible to the protease and dissociates the antibody molecules from the cell.[20] Multiple sequential autologous adsorptions with new aliquots of red cells may be necessary if the serum contains high levels of autoantibody. Once autoantibody has been removed, the adsorbed serum is tested for alloantibody reactivity.

Autologous adsorption is not recommended for patients who have been transfused within the last 3 months because a blood sample may contain some of the transfused red cells that might adsorb alloantibody. Red cells normally survive for about 110 to 120 days. In patients with AIHA, autologous and transfused red cells can be expected to have shortened survival. However, determining how long transfused red cells remain in circulation in patients who need repeated transfusions is not feasible. It has been demonstrated that very small amounts (<10%) of antigen-positive red cells are capable of removing alloantibody reactivity in in-vitro studies[21]; therefore, it is recommended to wait for 3 months after transfusion before autologous adsorptions are performed.

Adsorption with Allogeneic Red Cells

The use of allogeneic red cells for adsorption (allogeneic adsorption) may be helpful when the patient has been recently transfused or when insufficient autologous red cells are available. The goal is to remove autoantibody and leave the alloantibody in the adsorbed serum. The adsorbing red cells must not have the antigens against which the alloantibodies react. Because alloantibody specificity is unknown, red cells of different phenotypes will usually be used to adsorb several aliquots of the patient's serum.

Given the number of potential alloantibodies, the task of selecting the red cells may appear formidable. However, red cell selection is based only on those few antigens for which alloantibodies of clinical significance are likely to be present. These include the common Rh antigens (D, C, E, c, and e), K, Fy^a and Fy^b, Jk^a and Jk^b, and S and s. Red cell selection is made easier by the fact that some of these antigens can be destroyed by appropriate treatment (eg, with enzymes or ZZAP) before use in adsorption procedures (see Table 16-4). Antibodies to high-prevalence antigens cannot be excluded by allogeneic adsorptions because the adsorbing red cells will be expected to express the antigen and adsorb the alloantibody along with autoantibody.

When the patient's phenotype is not known, group O red cell samples of three different Rh phenotypes (R_1R_1, R_2R_2, and rr) should be selected (see Method 4-9). One should lack Jk^a, and another, Jk^b. As shown in Table 17-5, ZZAP or enzyme pretreatment of the adsorbing red cells reduces the phenotype requirements. Untreated red cells may be used, but antibody may be more difficult to remove, and the adsorbing red cells must include, at a minimum, at least one negative for the S, s, Fy^a, Fy^b, and K antigens in addition to the Rh and Kidd requirements stated above.

If the patient's phenotype is known or can be determined, adsorption with a single sample of red cells may be possible. Red cells can

TABLE 17-5. Selection of Red Cells for Allogeneic Adsorption

Step 1. Select red cells for each Rh phenotype.

R_1R_1
R_2R_2
rr

Step 2. On the basis of the red cell treatment, or lack of treatment (below), at least one of the Rh-phenotyped cells should be negative for the antigens listed below.

ZZAP-Treated Red Cells	Enzyme-Treated Red Cells	Untreated Red Cells
Jk(a–)	Jk(a–)	Jk(a–)
Jk(b–)	Jk(b–)	Jk(b–)
	K–	K–
		Fy(a–)
		Fy(b–)
		S–
		s–

be selected that match the patient's phenotype, or at least match the Rh and Kidd phenotypes if ZZAP treatment is used.

Testing of Adsorbed Serum

Each aliquot of serum may need to be adsorbed two or three times. The fully adsorbed aliquots are then tested against reagent red cells known either to lack or to carry common antigens of the Rh, MNS, Kidd, Kell, and Duffy blood group systems (eg, antibody detection cells). If an adsorbed aliquot is reactive, the aliquot should be tested to identify the antibody. Adsorbing several aliquots with different red cell samples provides a battery of potentially informative specimens. For example, if the aliquot adsorbed with Jk(a–) red cells subsequently reacts only with Jk(a+) red cells, the presence of alloanti-Jk^a can be inferred confidently.

Occasionally, autoantibody will not be removed by three sequential adsorptions. Further adsorptions can be performed, but multiple adsorptions have the potential to dilute the serum. If the adsorbing cells do not appear to remove the antibody, the autoantibody may have an unusual specificity that does not react with the red cells used for adsorption. For example, autoantibodies with Kell, LW, or En^aFS specificity would not be removed by ZZAP-treated red cells (see Table 16-4 for a list of antigens altered by various agents).

Autoantibodies sometimes have patterns of reactivity that suggest the presence of alloantibody. For example, the serum of a D– patient may have apparent anti-C reactivity. The anti-C reactivity may reflect warm-reactive autoantibody even if the patient's red cells lack C. The autoantibody nature of the reactivity can be demonstrated by autologous and allogeneic adsorption studies. The apparent alloanti-C would, in this case, be adsorbed by C– red cells, both autologous and allogeneic. This is quite unlike the behavior of a true alloanti-C, which would be adsorbed only by C+ red cells. In one study,[22] the serum prepared from an initial autologous adsorption would often retain autoantibodies that mimicked alloantibodies in addition to the true alloantibody(ies) present. Serum prepared from an initial allogeneic adsorption most often contains only alloantibodies. The differences in the auto- or alloantibody nature of specificities detected in the autoadsorbed serum as compared to the alloadsorbed serum reflect an inefficiency of autologous adsorption. This is primarily caused by limited volumes of autologous red cells available for removing all of the autoantibody reactivity from the serum.[22]

Specificity of Autoantibody

In many cases of WAIHA, no autoantibody specificity is apparent. The patient's serum reacts with all red cell samples tested. If testing is performed with cells of rare Rh phenotypes, such as D–– or Rh_{null}, some autoantibodies will react weaker or be nonreactive, and the autoantibody would appear to have broad specificity in the Rh system. Apparent specificity for simple Rh antigens (D, C, E, c, e) is occasionally seen, especially in saline or LISS indirect antiglobulin tests. A "relative" specificity may also be seen, based on stronger reactivity with cells of certain phenotypes. Autoantibody specificities are clearer in the serum than in the eluate.

Apart from Rh specificity, warm autoantibodies with many other specificities have been reported (eg, specificities in the LW, Kell, Kidd, Duffy, and Diego systems).[23,24] Patients with autoantibodies of Kell, Rh, LW, Ge, Sc, Lu, and Lan specificities may have depressed expression of the respective antigen, and the DAT may be negative or very weakly positive[24]; in these cases, the autoantibody may initially appear to be alloantibody.

Tests against red cells of rare phenotype and by special techniques have limited clinical or practical application. If apparent specificity is directed to a high-prevalence antigen (eg, anti-U), or when the autoantibody reacts with all red cells except those of a rare Rh phenotype (eg, D––, Rh_{null}), compatible donor blood is unlikely to be available and there is little point in determining specificity. Such blood, if available, should be reserved for alloimmunized patients of that uncommon phenotype.

Selection of Blood for Transfusion

The most important consideration is to exclude the presence of potentially clinically significant alloantibodies *before* selecting red cells for transfusion. There are multiple reports in the literature demonstrating that patients who have warm autoantibodies in their sera have a higher rate of alloimmunization (eg, 12% to 40%, with a mean of 32%).[18,25-28] Although these patients present a serologic challenge, they deserve the same protection from hemolytic transfusion reactions as any other patient. Autoantibodies that react with all reagent red cells, even weakly, are capable of masking alloantibody reactivity (ie, reactivity of red cells with both alloantibody and autoantibody may not be any stronger than reactivity observed with autoantibody alone).[18,19] It is the exclusion of newly formed alloantibodies that is of concern. Because of the presence of autoantibodies, all crossmatches will be incompatible. This is unlike the case of clinically significant alloantibodies without autoantibodies, where a compatible crossmatch with antigen-negative red cells can be obtained. Monitoring for evidence of red cell destruction caused by *alloantibodies* is difficult in patients who already have AIHA; the patient's own red cells and transfused red cells will have shortened survival.

If no alloantibodies are detected in adsorbed serum, random units of the appropriate ABO group and Rh type may be selected for transfusion. If clinically significant alloantibodies are present, the transfused cells should lack the corresponding antigen(s).

If the autoantibody has clear-cut specificity for a single antigen (eg, anti-e) and there is active ongoing hemolysis, blood lacking that antigen may be selected. There is evidence that such red cells survive better than the patient's own red cells.[4] In the absence of hemolysis, autoantibody specificity is not important, although donor units negative for the antigen may be chosen because this is a simple way to circumvent the autoantibody and detect potential alloantibodies. If the autoantibody shows broader reactivity, reacting with all cells but showing some relative specificity (eg, it reacts preferentially with e+ red cells), the use of blood lacking the corresponding antigen is debatable. It may be undesirable to expose the patient to Rh antigens absent from autologous cells, especially D and especially in females of childbearing potential, merely to improve serologic compatibility testing with the autoantibody. (For example, when a D– patient has autoanti-e, available e– units will be D+; D–e– units are extremely rare.)

Some laboratories will use the adsorbed serum to screen and select nonreactive units for transfusion (antigen-negative for clinically significant alloantibodies, if detected). Other laboratories do not perform a crossmatch with the adsorbed serum because all units will be incompatible in vivo because of the autoantibody. Issuing a unit that is serologically compatible with adsorbed serum may provide some assurance that the correct unit is selected and avoid incompatibility because of additional antibodies (eg, anti-Wr[a]), but this practice can also provide a false sense of security for the transfusion of these patients.

A transfusion management protocol proposed by one group uses prophylactic antigen-matched units for patients with warm autoantibodies where feasible, in combination with streamlined adsorption procedures.[29] Such a protocol depends on the ability of the transfusion service and/or blood supplier to consistently maintain an adequate inventory of fully phenotyped units (eg, C, E, c, e, K, S, s, Fy[a], Fy[b], Jk[a], and Jk[b]) whenever needed.

Others propose that an electronic crossmatch can be safely used for patients with autoantibodies when presence of the common clinically significant alloantibodies has been excluded.[30,31] This approach circumvents issuing units that are labeled "incompatible"; however, as discussed above, this practice can also lead to a false sense of security.

Although resolving these serologic problems is important, delaying transfusion in the hope of finding serologically compatible blood may, in some cases, cause greater danger to the patient. Only clinical judgment can resolve this dilemma; therefore, dialogue with the patient's physician is important.

Transfusion of Patients with Warm-Reactive Autoantibodies

Patients with warm-reactive autoantibodies may have no apparent hemolysis or may have life-threatening anemia. Patients with little or no evidence of significant hemolysis tolerate transfusion quite well. The risk of transfusion is somewhat increased in these patients because of the difficulties encountered in pretransfusion testing. Survival of the transfused red cells is about the same as the survival of the patient's own red cells.

In patients with active hemolysis, transfusion may increase hemolysis, and the transfused red cells may be destroyed more rapidly than the patient's own red cells. This is related to the increased red cell mass available from the transfusion and the kinetics of red cell destruction.[4] Destruction of transfused cells may increase hemoglobinemia and hemoglobinuria. Disseminated intravascular coagulation can develop in patients with severe posttransfusion hemolysis.[4]

Transfusion of patients with AIHA is a clinical decision, balancing the risks and clinical need. Transfusion should not be withheld solely because of serologic incompatibility. The volume transfused should usually be the smallest amount required to maintain adequate oxygen delivery, not necessarily to reach an arbitrary hemoglobin level.[4] The patient should be carefully monitored throughout the transfusion.

DAT-Negative AIHA

Clinical and hematologic evidence of WAIHA is present in some patients whose DAT is nonreactive. The most common causes for AIHA associated with a negative DAT are red-cell-bound IgG below the threshold of the antiglobulin test, red-cell-bound IgM and IgA that are not detectable by routine AHG reagents, and low-affinity IgG that is washed off the red cells during the washing phase for the DAT.[4,32] Nonroutine tests can be applied in these situations. Unfortunately, these assays require standardization and many have a low predictive value. One of the easier tests is for low-affinity antibodies. Washing with ice-cold saline (eg, 4 C) or LISS may help retain antibody on the cells; a control (eg, 6% albumin) is necessary to confirm that cold autoagglutinins are not causing the positive results.[4] Complement fixation antibody consumption assay, enzyme-linked antiglobulin test, radiolabeled anti-IgG, flow cytometry, solid phase, direct PEG test, direct Polybrene test, column agglutination, and concentrated eluate are all methods that have been used to detect lower levels of red-cell-bound IgG.[32] Anti-IgG, anti-C3d, and the combined anti-C3b, -C3d reagents are the only licensed products available in the United States for use with human red cells. AHG reagents that react with IgA or IgM are available commercially but probably have not been standardized for use with red cells in agglutination tests. They must be used cautiously, and their hemagglutinating reactivity carefully standardized by the user.[4] In other countries, AHG reagents for the detection of IgM and IgA in tube tests or column agglutination tests may be available.

Cold Agglutinin Syndrome

CAS is less common than WAIHA and is the hemolytic anemia most commonly associated with autoantibodies that react preferentially in the cold. It occurs as an acute or chronic condition. The acute form is often secondary to *Mycoplasma pneumoniae* infection. The chronic form is often seen in elderly patients, sometimes associated with lymphoma, chronic lymphocytic leukemia, or Waldenström macroglobulinemia. Acrocyanosis and hemoglobinuria may occur in cold weather. CAS is often characterized by agglutination, at room temperature, of red cells in an EDTA specimen, sometimes to the degree that it appears that the red cells are clotted.

Serologic Characteristics

Complement is the only protein detected on the red cells in almost all cases of CAS. If the red cells have been collected properly and washed at 37 C, there will be no immunoglobulin on the cells and no reactivity will be found in the eluate. If other proteins are detected, a negative control for the DAT (eg, 6% albumin or saline), should be tested to ensure that the cold autoagglutinin is not causing a false-positive result. The cold-reactive autoagglutinin is usually IgM, which binds to red cells in the lower temperature of the peripheral circulation and causes complement components to attach to the red cells. As the red cells circulate to warmer areas, the IgM dissociates but the complement remains.

IgM cold-reactive autoagglutinins associated with immune hemolysis usually react at ≥30 C, and 60% have a titer of ≥1000 when tested at 4 C.[4] If 22% to 30% bovine albumin is included in the test system, pathologic cold agglutinins will react at 30 C or 37 C.[4] Occasionally, pathologic cold agglutinins will have a lower titer (ie, <1000), but they will have a high thermal amplitude (ie, reactive at 30 C with or without the addition of albumin). Hemolytic activity against untreated red cells can sometimes be demonstrated at 20 C to 25 C, and except in rare cases with Pr specificity, enzyme-treated red cells are hemolyzed in the presence of adequate complement.

To determine the true thermal amplitude or titer of the cold autoagglutinin, the specimen is collected and maintained strictly at 37 C until the serum and red cells are separated, to avoid in-vitro autoadsorption. Alternatively, plasma can be used from an EDTA-anticoagulated specimen that has been warmed for 10 to 15 minutes at 37 C (with repeated mixing) and then separated from the cells, ideally at 37 C. This should release autoadsorbed antibody back into the plasma.

In chronic CAS, the IgM autoagglutinin is usually a monoclonal protein with kappa light chains. In the acute form induced by *Mycoplasma* or viral infections, the antibody is polyclonal IgM with normal kappa and lambda light-chain distribution. Rare examples of IgA and IgG cold-reactive autoagglutinins have also been described.[4]

Serologic Problems

Problems with ABO and Rh typing and other tests are not uncommon. Often, it is only necessary to maintain the blood sample at 37 C immediately after collection and to wash the red cells with warm (37 C) saline before testing. Alternatively, an EDTA sample can be warmed to 37 C for about 10 minutes, followed by washing the red cells with warm saline. It is helpful to perform a parallel control test with 6% bovine albumin to determine if autoagglutination persists. If the control test is nonreactive, the results obtained with anti-A and anti-B are usually valid. If autoagglutination still occurs, it may be necessary to treat the red cells with sulfhydryl reagents.

Because cold-reactive autoagglutinins are almost always IgM, and sulfhydryl reagents denature IgM molecules, reagents such as 2-ME or DTT can be used to abolish autoagglutination (see Method 2-18). Treating the red cells with ZZAP reagent, as in the preparation for adsorptions, can also be used (see Method 4-8).

When the serum agglutinates group O reagent red cells, ABO serum tests are invalid. Repeating the tests using prewarmed serum and group A_1, B, and O red cells and allowing the red cells to "settle" after incubation at 37 C for 1 hour (instead of centrifuging the test) will often resolve any discrepancy (see Method 2-11). By eliminating the centrifugation step, interference by cold-reactive autoantibodies might be avoided. Weak anti-A and/or -B in some patients' sera may not react at 37 C. Alternatively, adsorbed serum (either autoadsorbed or adsorbed with allogeneic group O red cells) can be used. Rabbit erythrocyte stroma should not be used for ABO serum tests because the adsorbed sera may not contain anti-B or anti-A1.[33,34]

Detection of Alloantibodies in the Presence of Cold-Reactive Autoantibodies

Cold-reactive autoagglutinins rarely mask clinically significant alloantibodies if serum tests are conducted at 37 C and if IgG-specific reagents are used for the antiglobulin phase. The use of potentiators (eg, albumin, PEG) is not recommended because they may increase the reactivity of the autoantibodies. In rare instances, it may be necessary to perform autologous adsorption at 4 C (see Method 4-5). Achieving the complete removal of potent cold-reactive autoagglutinins is very time consuming and is usually unnecessary. Removal of sufficient cold autoagglutinins may be facilitated by treating the patient's cells with enzymes or ZZAP before adsorption. One or two cold autologous adsorptions should remove enough autoantibody to make it possible to detect alloantibodies at 37 C that were otherwise masked by the cold-reactive autoantibody. Alternatively, allogeneic adsorption as for WAIHA can be performed at 4 C. Rabbit erythrocyte stroma, used to remove autoanti-I and -IH from sera, should be used with caution because clinically significant alloantibodies—notably anti-D, -E, -Vel, and IgM antibodies regardless of blood group specificity—have been removed by this method.[35,36]

Specificity of Autoantibody

The autoantibody specificity in CAS is most often anti-I but is usually of academic interest only. Less commonly, anti-i is found, usually associated with infectious mononucleosis. On rare occasions, other specificities are seen.

Autoantibody specificity is not diagnostic for CAS. Autoanti-I may be seen in healthy individuals as well as in patients with CAS. The nonpathologic forms of autoanti-I, however, rarely react to titers above 64 at 4 C and are usually nonreactive with I– (cord i and adult i) red cells at room temperature. In contrast, the autoanti-I of CAS may react quite strongly with I– red cells in tests at room temperature, and equal or even stronger reactions are observed with I+ red cells. Autoanti-i reacts in the opposite manner, demonstrating stronger reactions with I– red cells than with red cells that are I+. Anti-I^T, originally thought to recognize a transition state of i to I (thus the designation I^T), reacts strongly with cord red cells, weakly with normal adult I red cells, and most weakly with the rare adult i red cells. Rarely, the cold agglutinin specificity may be anti-Pr, which reacts equally well with untreated red cells of I or i phenotypes but does not react with enzyme-treated red cells. Procedures to determine the titer and specificity of cold-reactive autoantibodies are given in Methods 4-6 and 4-7. Typical reactivity patterns of cold autoantibodies are shown in Methods Table 4-6-1.

Mixed-Type AIHA

Although about one-third of patients with WAIHA have nonpathologic IgM antibodies that agglutinate at room temperature, another group of patients with WAIHA have cold agglutinins that react at or above 30 C. This latter group is referred to as having "mixed"[37] or "combined warm and cold"[38] AIHA and can be subdivided: patients with high-titer, high-thermal-amplitude IgM cold antibodies (the rare WAIHA plus classic CAS), and patients with normal-titer (<64 at 4 C), high-thermal-amplitude cold antibodies.[37-39] Patients with mixed-type AIHA often present with hemolysis and complex serum reactivity present in all phases of testing.

Serologic Characteristics

In mixed-type AIHA, both IgG and C3 are usually detectable on patients' red cells; however, C3, IgG, or IgA alone may be detectable on the red cells.[4] An eluate will contain a warm-reactive IgG autoantibody.

Both warm-reactive IgG autoantibodies and cold-reactive, agglutinating IgM autoantibodies are present in the serum. These usually result in reactivity at all phases of testing, with virtually all cells tested. The IgM agglutinating autoantibody reacts at 30 C or above. If adsorptions are performed to detect alloantibodies, it may be necessary to perform adsorptions at both 37 C and 4 C.

Specificity of Autoantibodies

The unusual cold-reactive IgM agglutinating autoantibody can have specificities typical of CAS (ie, anti-I or -i) but often has no apparent specificity.[37,38] The warm-reactive IgG autoantibody often appears serologically indistinguishable from autoantibodies encountered in typical WAIHA.

Transfusion of Patients with Mixed-Type AIHA

If blood transfusions are necessary, the considerations for the exclusion of alloantibodies and the selection of blood for transfusion are identical to those described for patients with acute hemolysis caused by WAIHA and CAS (see above).

Paroxysmal Cold Hemoglobinuria

PCH is the rarest form of DAT-positive AIHA. Historically, PCH was associated with syphilis, but this association is now unusual.[40] More commonly, PCH presents as an acute transient condition secondary to viral infections, particularly in young children. In such cases, the biphasic hemolysin may be only transiently detectable. PCH can also occur as an idiopathic chronic disease in older people.

Serologic Characteristics

PCH is caused by a cold-reactive IgG complement-binding antibody. As with IgM cold-reactive autoagglutinins, it reacts with red cells in colder areas of the body (usually the extremities), causes C3 to bind irreversibly to red cells, and then the antibody dissociates from the red cells as the blood circulates to warmer parts of the body. Red cells washed in a routine manner for the DAT are usually coated only with complement, but IgG may be detectable on cells that have been washed with cold saline and tested with cold anti-IgG reagent.[4] Keeping the test system nearer its optimal binding temperature allows the cold-reactive IgG autoantibody to remain attached to its antigen. Because complement components are usually the only globulins present on circulating red cells, eluates prepared from red cells of patients with PCH are almost always nonreactive.

The IgG autoantibody in PCH is classically described as a biphasic hemolysin, because binding to red cells occurs at low temperatures, but hemolysis does not occur until the complement-coated red cells are warmed to 37 C. This is the basis of the diagnostic test for the disease, the Donath-Landsteiner test (see Method 4-11). The autoantibody may agglutinate normal red cells at 4 C but rarely to titers greater than 64. Because the antibody rarely reacts above 4 C, pretransfusion antibody detection tests are usually nonreactive and the serum is usually compatible with random donor cells by routine crossmatch procedures.

Specificity of Autoantibody

The autoantibody of PCH has most frequently been shown to have P specificity, reacting with all red cells by the Donath-Landsteiner test (including the patient's own red cells) except those of the very rare p or P^k phenotypes. Exceptional examples with other specificities have been described.[23]

Transfusion of Patients with PCH

Transfusion is rarely necessary for adult patients with PCH, unless their hemolysis is severe. In young children, the thermal amplitude of the antibody tends to be much wider than in adults and hemolysis more brisk, so transfusion may be required as a lifesaving measure. Although there is some evidence that p red cells survive better than P+ (P1+ or P1–) red cells, the prevalence of p blood is approximately 1 in 200,000, and the urgent need for transfusion usually precludes attempts to obtain this rare blood. Transfusion of donor blood should not be withheld from PCH patients whose need is urgent. Red cells negative for the P antigen should be considered only for those patients who do not respond adequately to randomly selected units of donor blood.[4]

DRUG-INDUCED IMMUNE HEMOLYTIC ANEMIA

Drugs rarely cause immune hemolytic anemia; the estimated incidence is 1 in 1 million of the population.[10] Many drugs have been implicated over the years, as can be seen in the list provided in Appendix 17-1 and reviewed elsewhere.[41] The most recent additions to this list are hydrocortisone[42] and cimetidine.[43]

Drugs sometimes induce the formation of antibodies—against the drug itself, against red cell membrane components, or against an antigen formed by the drug and the red cell membrane. These antibodies may result in a positive DAT, immune red cell destruction, or both.[41] In some instances, a positive DAT can result from nonimmunologic protein adsorption (NIPA) onto the red cell, caused by the drug.

Theoretical Mechanisms of Drug-Induced Antibodies

Numerous theories have been suggested to explain how drugs induce immune responses and what relation such responses may have to the positive DAT and immune-mediated cell destruction observed in some patients.[4] For many years, drug-associated positive DATs were classified into four mechanisms: drug adsorption (penicillin-type), immune complex formation, autoantibody production, and nonspecific protein adsorption. Such classification has been useful serologically, but many aspects lack definitive proof. In addition, some drugs demonstrate serologic reactivity that appears to involve more than one mechanism. A more comprehensive approach, termed a "unifying hypothesis," is shown in Fig 17-1. One or more populations of antibodies may be present. In addition, NIPA, which is independent of antibody production, appears to play a role in drug-induced immune hemolytic anemia.[10]

Serologic and Clinical Classification

Drug-induced antibodies can be classified into two groups: drug-dependent antibodies (those that require the presence of the drug in the test system to be detected) and drug-independent antibodies (those that do not require the in-vitro addition of the drug for detection).[4] Drug-dependent antibodies are subdivided into those that react with drug-treated red cells (eg, antibodies to penicillin), and those that react with untreated red cells in the presence of a solution of the drug (eg, antibodies to quinidine and ceftriaxone). Drug-independent antibodies (eg, antibodies induced by methyldopa, procainamide, and fludarabine) have serologic reactivity that is independent of the drug, despite the fact that it was the drug that originally induced the immune response. Serologically, because the drug does not need to be added to the test system, these antibod-

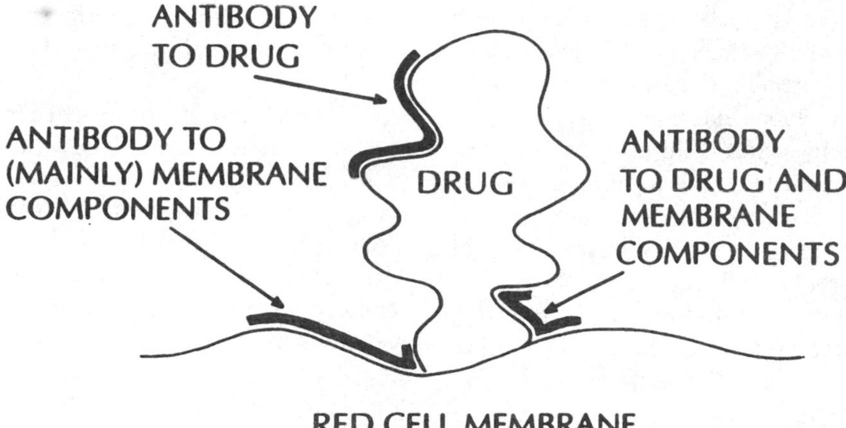

FIGURE 17-1. Proposed unifying theory of drug-induced antibody reactions (based on a cartoon by Habibi as cited by Garratty[23]). The thicker, darker lines represent antigen-binding sites for the Fab region of the drug-induced antibody. Drugs (haptens) bind loosely or firmly to cell membranes, and antibodies may be made to 1) the drug [producing in-vitro reactions typical of a drug adsorption (penicillin-type) reaction]; 2) membrane components, or mainly membrane components (producing in-vitro reactions typical of autoantibody); or 3) part-drug, part-membrane components (producing an in-vitro reaction typical of the so-called immune complex mechanism).[23(p55)]

ies behave as autoantibodies that are serologically indistinguishable from idiopathic warm autoantibodies.

Drug-Dependent Antibodies Reactive with Drug-Treated Red Cells

The clinical and laboratory features of drug-induced immune hemolytic anemia detected in this manner are as follows:

1. The DAT is strongly positive because of IgG coating. Complement coating may also be present.
2. Antibody eluted from the patient's red cells reacts with drug-treated red cells but not with untreated red cells.
3. The serum contains a high-titer IgG antibody (especially when the target is penicillin) reactive with the drug-treated red cells but not with the untreated red cells unless the patient also has alloantibodies to red cell antigens.
4. For penicillin, the hemolysis-inducing dose is millions of units daily for a week or more.
5. Hemolysis develops gradually but may be life threatening if the etiology is unrecognized and drug administration is continued.
6. Discontinuation of the drug is usually followed by increased cell survival, although hemolysis of decreasing severity may persist for several weeks.

Although not commonly seen anymore, approximately 3% of patients receiving large doses of penicillin intravenously (ie, millions of units per day) will develop a positive DAT; only occasionally will these patients develop hemolytic anemia.[4] The penicillin becomes covalently linked to the red cells in vivo. If the patient has antibodies to penicillin, they bind to the penicillin bound to the red cells. The result is that the penicillin-coated red cells become coated with IgG. If cell destruction occurs, it takes place extravascularly, probably in the same way that red cells coated with IgG alloantibodies are destroyed. Intravascular hemolysis is rare. Antibodies to a semisynthetic penicillin, piperacillin, have been shown to have different serologic and clinical characteristics than those in classic penicillin-induced immune hemolytic anemia.[44] Rather than testing with piperacillin-coated red cells, investigations for piperacillin antibodies should be performed by testing in the presence of a solution of piperacillin. This is because an antibody that reacts with piperacillin-coated red cells has been detected in a high percentage of blood donors' and patients' plasma.[44]

Many cephalosporins, which are related to penicillins, bind well to red cells. The cephalosporins are generally classified by "generations," based on their effectiveness against gram-negative organisms. Dramatically reduced red cell survival has been associated with second- and third-generation cephalosporins.[10]

Drug-Dependent Antibodies Reacting with Untreated Red Cells in the Presence of Drug

Antibodies to many drugs that have been reported as causing hemolytic anemia are detected by testing untreated red cells in the presence of the drug. Piperacillin and some of the second- and third-generation cephalosporins react by this method; anti-ceftriaxone has been detected only by testing in the presence of drug.[10] The following observations are characteristic:

1. Complement may be the only protein easily detected on the red cells, but IgG may be present.
2. The serum antibody can be IgM, IgG, or IgM with IgG.
3. A drug (or metabolite) must be present in vitro for demonstration of the antibody in the patient's serum. Antibodies may cause hemolysis, agglutination, and/or sensitization of red cells in the presence of the drug.
4. The patient need only take a small amount of the drug (eg, a single dose).
5. Acute intravascular hemolysis with hemoglobinemia and hemoglobinuria is the usual presentation. Renal failure is quite common.
6. Once antibody has been formed, severe hemolytic episodes may recur after exposure to very small quantities of the drug.

On occasion, it appears that a patient's serum contains an "autoantibody" in addition to a drug antibody reacting in the presence of the drug. Rather than a true autoantibody, it is believed that this reactivity may be due to the presence of circulating drug or drug plus antibody complexes.[45] In these cases, an eluate is generally nonreactive without drug present in the system, and a sample collected several days after the drug has been discontinued will be nonreactive. A true warm autoantibody would be expected to be reactive in an eluate prepared from the patient's red cells, and free autoantibody would not disappear a few days later. Differentiation of warm-reactive autoantibody from drug-induced immune hemolytic anemia is important for clinical management of the patient.[45]

Drug-Independent Antibodies: Autoantibody Production

Some drugs induce autoantibodies that appear serologically indistinguishable from those of WAIHA. Red cells are coated with IgG, and the eluate as well as the serum react with virtually all cells tested in the absence of the drug. Blood group specificity has been demonstrated at times, similar to that seen in AIHA. The antibody has no in-vitro interaction with the drug, directly or indirectly.

The best studied of such cases are those induced by α-methyldopa. A closely related drug, L-dopa, has been implicated, as have several drugs unrelated to α-methyldopa, including procainamide, nonsteroidal anti-inflammatory drugs (eg, mefenamic acid), second- and third-generation cephalosporins, fiudarabine, and cladribine. In some cases, drug-dependent antibodies are also present.

Proof that a drug causes autoantibody production is difficult to obtain. Sufficient evidence would include demonstration that autoantibody production began after drug administration; resolution of the immune process after withdrawal of the drug; *and* recurrence of hemolytic anemia or autoantibodies if the drug is readministered.

Nonimmunologic Protein Adsorption

The positive DAT associated with some drugs is caused by a mechanism independent of antibody production. Hemolytic anemia associated with this mechanism occurs rarely.

Cephalosporins (primarily cephalothin) are the drugs with which positive DATs and NIPA were originally associated. In vitro, red cells coated with cephalothin (Keflin) in pH 9.8 buffer and incubated with normal plasma will adsorb albumin, IgA, IgG, IgM, and C3 in a nonimmunologic manner. As a result, the indirect antiglobulin test with these plasmas will be positive. Other drugs that may cause NIPA and a positive DAT include diglycoaldehyde, cisplatin, oxaliplatin, clavulanate (in Timentin and Augmentin), sulbactam (in Unasyn), and tazobactam (in Tazocin and Zosyn).[44,46] NIPA should be suspected when a patient's plasma/serum and most normal plasma/sera react in an indirect antiglobulin test with drug-treated red cells, but the eluate from the patient's red cells is nonreactive with the drug-treated cells.

Laboratory Investigation of Drug-Induced Immune Hemolysis

The drug-related problems most commonly encountered in the blood bank are those associated with a positive DAT and a nonreactive eluate. Recent red cell transfusions and/or dramatic hemolysis may result in a weak DAT by the time hemolysis is suspected. When other more common causes of immune-mediated hemolysis have been excluded *and* a temporal relationship exists between the administration of a drug and the hemolytic anemia, a drug antibody investigation should be pursued.

The patient's serum should be tested for unexpected antibodies by routine procedures. If the serum does not react with untreated red cells, the tests should be repeated with the drug(s) suspected of causing the problem. Some drug formulations contain inert ingredients (eg, oral medications such as Augmentin), and other drugs are combinations of two drugs (eg, piperacillin plus tazobactam). Although it would seem logical to test with the actual drug the patient received, inert ingredients or drug combinations can make preparation of drug-treated red cells difficult or confuse results. It is preferable to test using pure drug formulations as well as separate components of combination drugs.

If the drug has already been reported as causing hemolytic anemia, testing methods may be available in the case reports. Far more drug antibodies are detected by testing in the presence of drug; therefore, when a previous report is not available, an initial screening test can be performed with a solution of the drug at a concentration of approximately 1 mg/mL in phosphate-buffered saline (see Method 4-13). Serum, rather than plasma, is the preferred specimen for this testing for the observation for hemolysis; this also allows fresh normal serum as a source of complement to be added to the test system. The addition of the fresh complement increases the sensitivity of the test for the detection of in-vitro hemolysis resulting from complement activation.

If these tests are not informative, attempts can be made to coat normal red cells with the drug, and the patient's serum, and an eluate from the patient's red cells can be tested against the drug-treated red cells (see Method 4-12). This is the method of choice when penicillin or cephalosporins are thought to be implicated. Results definitive for a penicillin-induced positive DAT are reactivity of the eluate against penicillin-treated red cells and absence of reactivity between the eluate and untreated red cells.

Drug-treated red cells should always be tested with saline and normal serum (or plasma) as negative controls. This ensures that reactivity observed with the patient's serum/plasma is appropriately interpreted. Drugs present in the environment (eg, piperacillin or a chemically related structure) can result in a proportion of normal blood donors and patients without hemolytic anemia demonstrating an antibody reactive with drug-treated red cells, and thus in a possible misinterpretation of reactivity found in a patient's serum.[44]

Whenever possible, a positive control should also be tested with drug-treated red cells. Negative results of a patient's serum and eluate without a positive control can only be interpreted that antibodies to that drug were not detected; drug may or may not be bound to the test red cells.

If the drug in question is known to cause NIPA, the patient's serum and the controls (negative and positive) should also be tested at a dilution of 1 in 20. Normal sera diluted 1 in 20 generally do not react nonspecifically.

The immune response may be caused by a metabolite of a drug rather than the drug itself. If the clinical picture is consistent with immune-mediated hemolysis and the above tests are noninformative, it may be helpful to test drug metabolites in the place of the parent drug (ie, serum or urine from an individual taking the drug in question). Antibodies to some nonsteroidal anti-inflammatory drugs have been detected only by testing in the presence of a urine metabolite of the drug.[47] The metabolism and half-life of the specific drug will determine when the drug metabolite should be collected; reference should be made to information about the metabolite(s) detectable in serum or urine and previous reports for the drug under investigation.

KEY POINTS

1. The direct antiglobulin test (DAT) is used to determine if red cells have been coated in vivo with immunoglobulin, complement, or both. The DAT is used primarily for the investigation of hemolytic transfusion reactions, hemolytic disease of the fetus and newborn (HDFN), autoimmune hemolytic anemia (AIHA), and drug-induced immune hemolysis.
2. A positive DAT may or may not be associated with immune-mediated hemolysis.
3. When investigating a transfusion reaction, performance of the DAT on postreaction specimens is part of the initial investigation. The DAT may be positive if sensitized red cells have not been destroyed, or negative if hemolysis and rapid clearance have occurred.
4. The DAT is performed by testing freshly washed red cells directly with antiglobulin reagents containing anti-IgG and anti-C3d. False-negative or weaker results can be obtained if the washed red cells are allowed to sit before testing with anti-IgG or if the reading is delayed.
5. When the DAT is positive with both anti-IgG and anti-C3, the red cells should be tested with an inert control reagent (eg, 6% albumin or saline). If the control is reactive, the DAT result is invalid, possibly indicating spontaneous agglutination from heavy coating of IgG or rare warm-reactive IgM, or IgM cold autoagglutinins that were not dissociated during routine washing.
6. A positive DAT alone is not diagnostic. The interpretation of the significance of this positive result requires additional patient-specific information. Dialogue with the attending physician is important. Clinical considerations together with laboratory data should dictate the extent to which a positive DAT is evaluated.
7. The following situations may warrant further investigation of a positive DAT:
   - **a.** Evidence of in-vivo red cell destruction.
   - **b.** History of recent transfusion.
   - **c.** Administration of drugs previously associated with immune-mediated hemolysis.
   - **d.** History of hematopoietic progenitor cell or organ transplantation.
   - **e.** Administration of intravenous immune globulin or intravenous anti-D.
8. Elution frees antibody from sensitized red cells and recovers antibody in a usable form. Elution is useful in certain situations for implicating an autoantibody, detecting specific antibodies that may not be detectable in the serum, and deciding to test for drug-related antibodies.

9. Immune-mediated hemolysis is the shortening of red cell survival caused by an immune response.

10. AIHAs are subdivided into the major types: warm AIHA (WAIHA), cold agglutinin syndrome (CAS), mixed- or combined-type AIHA, and paroxysmal cold hemoglobinuria (PCH). Drugs may also induce immune hemolysis.

REFERENCES

1. Kaplan HS, Garratty G. Predictive value of direct antiglobulin test results. Diagnostic Med 1985;8:29-32.
2. Garratty G. The significance of IgG on the red cell surface. Transfus Med Rev 1987;1: 47-57.
3. Freedman J. The significance of complement on the red cell surface. Transfus Med Rev 1987; 1:58-70.
4. Petz LD, Garratty G. Immune hemolytic anemias. 2nd ed. Philadelphia: Churchill-Livingstone, 2004.
5. Toy PT, Chin CA, Reid ME, Burns MA. Factors associated with positive direct antiglobulin tests in pretransfusion patients: A case control study. Vox Sang 1985;49:215-20.
6. Heddle NM, Kelton JG, Turchyn KL, Ali MAM. Hypergammaglobulinemia can be associated with a positive direct antiglobulin test, a nonreactive eluate, and no evidence of hemolysis. Transfusion 1988;28:29-33.
7. Clark JA, Tanley PC, Wallas CH. Evaluation of patients with positive direct antiglobulin tests and nonreactive eluates discovered during pretransfusion testing. Immunohematology 1992;8:9-12.
8. Coombs RRA, Mourant AE, Race RR. A new test for the detection of weak and "incomplete" Rh agglutinins. Br J Exp Pathol 1945;26:255-66.
9. Heddle NM, Soutar RL, O'Hoski PL, et al. A prospective study to determine the frequency and clinical significance of alloimmunization post-transfusion. Br J Haematol 1995;91:1000-5.
10. Arndt PA, Garratty G. The changing spectrum of drug-induced immune hemolytic anemia. Semin Hematol 2005;42:137-44.
11. Garratty G. Problems associated with passively transfused blood group alloantibodies. Am J Clin Pathol 1998;109:769-77.
12. Judd WJ. Elution—dissociation of antibody from red blood cells: Theoretical and practical considerations. Transfus Med Rev 1999;13: 297-310.
13. Judd WJ, Johnson ST, Storry JR. Judd's methods in immunohematology. 3rd ed. Bethesda, MD: AABB Press, 2008.
14. Leger RM, Arndt PA, Ciesielski DJ, Garratty G. False-positive eluate reactivity due to the low-ionic wash solution used with commercial acid-elution kits. Transfusion 1998;38:565-72.
15. Judd WJ, Barnes BA, Steiner EA, et al. The evaluation of a positive direct antiglobulin test (autocontrol) in pretransfusion testing revisited. Transfusion 1986;26:220-4.
16. Arndt PA, Leger RM, Garratty G. Serologic findings in autoimmune hemolytic anemia associated with immunoglobulin M warm autoantibodies. Transfusion 2009; 49:235-42.
17. Rodberg K, Tsuneta R, Garratty G. Discrepant Rh phenotyping results when testing IgG-sensitized RBCs with monoclonal Rh reagents (abstract). Transfusion 1995;35 (Suppl):67S.
18. Leger RM, Garratty G. Evaluation of methods for detecting alloantibodies underlying warm autoantibodies. Transfusion 1999;39:11-16.
19. Church AT, Nance SJ, Kavitsky DM. Predicting the presence of a new alloantibody underlying a warm autoantibody (abstract). Transfusion 2000;40(Suppl): 121S.
20. Branch DR, Petz LD. A new reagent (ZZAP) having multiple applications in immunohematology. Am J Clin Pathol 1982;78:161-7.
21. Laine EP, Leger RM, Arndt PA, et al. In vitro studies of the impact of transfusion on the detection of alloantibodies after autoadsorption. Transfusion 2000;40:1384-7.
22. Issitt PD, Combs MR, Bumgarner DJ, et al. Studies of antibodies in the sera of patients who have made red cell autoantibodies. Transfusion 1996;36:481-6.
23. Garratty G. Target antigens for red-cell-bound autoantibodies. In: Nance SJ, ed. Clinical and basic science aspects of immunohematology. Arlington, VA: AABB, 1991:33-72.
24. Garratty G. Specificity of autoantibodies reacting optimally at 37° C. Immunohematology 1999;15:24-40.

25. Branch DR, Petz LD. Detecting alloantibodies in patients with autoantibodies (editorial). Transfusion 1999;39:6-10.
26. Young PP, Uzieblo A, Trulock E, et al. Autoantibody formation after alloimmunization: Are blood transfusions a risk factor for autoimmune hemolytic anemia? Transfusion 2004;44: 67-72.
27. Maley M, Bruce DG, Babb RG, et al. The incidence of red cell alloantibodies underlying panreactive warm autoantibodies. Immunohematology 2005;21:122-5.
28. Ahrens N, Pruss A, Kähne A, et al. Coexistence of autoantibodies and alloantibodies to red blood cells due to blood transfusion. Transfusion 2007;47:813-16.
29. Shirey RS, Boyd JS, Parwani AV, et al. Prophylactic antigen-matched donor blood for patients with warm autoantibodies: An algorithm for transfusion management. Transfusion 2002;42:1435-41.
30. Lee E, Redman M, Burgess G, Win N. Do patients with autoantibodies or clinically insignificant alloantibodies require an indirect antiglobulin test crossmatch? Transfusion 2007; 47:1290-5.
31. Richa EM, Stowers RE, Tauscher CD, et al. The safety of electronic crossmatch in patients with warm autoantibodies (letter). Vox Sang 2007;93:92.
32. Garratty G. Immune hemolytic anemia associated with negative routine serology. Semin Hematol 2005;42:156-64.
33. Waligora SK, Edwards JM. Use of rabbit red cells for adsorption of cold autoagglutinins. Transfusion 1983;23:328-30.
34. Dzik WH, Yang R, Blank J. Rabbit erythrocyte stroma treatment of serum interferes with recognition of delayed hemolytic transfusion reaction (letter). Transfusion 1986;26:303-4.
35. Mechanic SA, Maurer JL, Igoe MJ, et al. Anti-Vel reactivity diminished by adsorption with rabbit RBC stroma. Transfusion 2002;42:1180-3.
36. Storry JR, Olsson ML, Moulds JJ. Rabbit red blood cell stroma bind immunoglobulin M antibodies regardless of blood group specificity (letter). Transfusion 2006;46:1260-1.
37. Sokol RJ, Hewitt S, Stamps BK. Autoimmune haemolysis: An 18-year study of 865 cases referred to a regional transfusion centre. Br Med J 1981;282:2023-7.
38. Shulman IA, Branch DR, Nelson JM, et al. Autoimmune hemolytic anemia with both cold and warm autoantibodies. JAMA 1985;253: 1746-8.
39. Garratty G, Arndt PA, Leger RM. Serological findings in autoimmune hemolytic anemia (AIHA) associated with both warm and cold autoantibodies (abstract). Blood 2003;102: 563a.
40. Eder AF. Review: Acute Donath-Landsteiner hemolytic anemia. Immunohematology 2005; 21:56-62.
41. Garratty G, Arndt PA. An update on drug-induced immune hemolytic anemia. Immunohematology 2007;23:105-19.
42. Martinengo M, Ardenghi DF, Tripodi G, Reali G. The first case of drug-induced immune hemolytic anemia due to hydrocortisone. Transfusion 2008;48:1925-9.
43. Arndt PA, Garratty G, Brasfield FM, et al. Immune hemolytic anemia due to cimetidine: The first example of a cimetidine antibody. Transfusion 2010;50:302-7.
44. Leger RM, Arndt PA, Garratty G. Serological studies of piperacillin antibodies. Transfusion 2008;48:2429-34.
45. Bandara M, Seder DB, Garratty G, et al. Piperacillin-induced immune hemolytic anemia in an adult with cystic fibrosis. Case Report Med 2010;2010:161454.
46. Arndt P, Garratty F, Isaak E, et al. Positive direct and indirect antiglobulin tests associated with oxaliplatin can be due to drug antibody and/or drug-induced nonimmunologic protein adsorption. Transfusion 2009;49:711-18.
47. Johnson ST, Fueger JT, Gottschall JL. One center's experience: The serology and drugs associated with drug-induced immune hemolytic anemia—a new paradigm. Transfusion 2007; 47:697-702.

◆ APPENDIX 17-1
Drugs Associated with a Positive DAT and/or Immune Hemolytic Anemia

Drug		Method of Detection		
Aceclofenac			+Drug	
Acetaminophen			+Drug	
Acyclovir		DT		
Aminopyrine		DT		
Amoxicillin		DT		
Amphotericin B			+Drug	
Ampicillin		DT	+Drug	
Antazoline			+Drug	
Azapropazone	AA	DT		
Butizide			+Drug	
Carbimazole	AA	DT	+Drug	
Carboplatin	AA	DT	+Drug	
Carbromal		DT		
Cefamandole		DT		
Cefazolin		DT		
Cefixime		DT	+Drug	
Cefotaxime		DT	+Drug	
Cefotetan	AA	DT	+Drug	NIPA
Cefoxitin	AA	DT	+Drug	
Ceftazidime	AA	DT	+Drug	
Ceftizoxime		DT	+Drug	
Ceftriaxone			+Drug	
Cefuroxime		DT		
Cephalexin		DT		
Cephalothin		DT	+Drug	NIPA
Chloramphenicol	AA	DT		
Chlorinated hydrocarbons	AA	DT	+Drug	
Chlorpromazine	AA		+Drug	
Chlorpropamide			+Drug	

(Continued)

◆ APPENDIX 17-1
Drugs Associated with a Positive DAT and/or Immune Hemolytic Anemia (Continued)

Drug	Method of Detection			
Cimetidine		DT	+Drug	
Ciprofloxacin			+Drug	
Cisplatin		DT		NIPA
Cladribine	AA			
Clavulanate				NIPA
Cyanidanol	AA	DT	+ Drug	
Cyclofenil	AA		+ Drug	
Cyclosporin		DT		
Diclofenac	AA	DT	+ Drug	
Diethylstilbestrol			+ Drug	
Diglycoaldehyde				NIPA
Dipyrone		DT	+ Drug	
Erythromycin		DT		
Etodolac			+ Drug	
Fenoprofen	AA		+ Drug	
Fluconazole		DT	+ Drug	
Fludarabine	AA			
Fluorescein		DT	+ Drug	
Fluorouracil			+ Drug	
Furosemide			+ Drug	
Hydralizine		DT		
Hydrochlorothiazide		DT	+ Drug	
Hydrocortisone		DT	+ Drug	
9-Hydroxy-methyl-ellipticinium			+ Drug	
Ibuprofen			+Drug	
Imatinib mesylate		DT		
Insulin		DT		
Isoniazid		DT	+ Drug	
Levodopa	AA			
Levofloxacin		DT	+Drug	
Mefenamic acid	AA			

◆ APPENDIX 17-1

Drugs Associated with a Positive DAT and/or Immune Hemolytic Anemia (Continued)

Drug	Method of Detection			
Mefloquine		DT	+ Drug	
Melphalan			+ Drug	
6-Mercaptopurine		DT		
Methadone		DT		
Methotrexate	AA	DT	+ Drug	
Methyldopa	AA			
Nabumetone			+Drug	
Nafcillin		DT		
Naproxen			+ Drug	
Oxaliplatin		DT	+ Drug	NIPA
p-Aminosalicylic acid			+ Drug	
Penicillin G		DT		
Phenacetin			+ Drug	
Phenytoin		DT		
Piperacillin		DT	+ Drug	
Probenicid			+ Drug	
Procainamide	AA			
Propyphenazone			+ Drug	
Pyrazinamide		DT	+ Drug	
Pyrimethamine		DT		
Quinidine		DT	+ Drug	
Quinine			+ Drug	
Ranitidine		DT	+ Drug	
Rifabutin			+ Drug	
Rifampicin		DT	+ Drug	
Sodium pentothal/thiopental			+ Drug	
Stibophen			+ Drug	
Streptomycin	AA	DT	+ Drug	
Sulbactam				NIPA

(Continued)

♦ APPENDIX 17-1
Drugs Associated with a Positive DAT and/or Immune Hemolytic Anemia (Continued)

Drug	Method of Detection			
Sulfamethoxazole			+Drug	
Sulfasalazine			+Drug	
Sulfisoxazole			+Drug	
Sulindac	AA	DT	+Drug	
Suprofen	AA		+Drug	
Tazobactam				NIPA
Teicoplanin	AA		+Drug	
Teniposide	AA		+Drug	
Tetracycline		DT		
Ticarcillin	AA	DT		
Tolbutamide		DT		
Tolmetin	AA		+Drug	
Triamterene		DT	+Drug	
Trimethoprim			+Drug	
Vancomycin			+Drug	
Zomepirac	AA		+Drug	

AA = drug-independent autoantibody; DT = testing with drug-treated red cells; + Drug = testing in the presence of drug; NIPA = nonimmunologic protein adsorption.

Chapter 18

Platelet and Granulocyte Antigens and Antibodies

Janice G. McFarland, MD

THIS CHAPTER DISCUSSES antigens expressed on platelets and granulocytes, together with antibodies that arise when individuals are sensitized to these markers. These antigens and the immune responses to them are of importance in alloimmune, autoimmune, and drug-induced immune syndromes involving platelets and granulocytes.

PLATELET ANTIGENS AND ANTIBODIES

Platelets express a variety of antigenic markers on their surface. Some of these antigens are shared with other cells, as in the case of ABO antigens and HLA antigens, while others are essentially platelet specific.

ABO Antigens on Platelets

The ABO antigens expressed on platelets are a combination of material both intrinsic to the platelet surface membrane and adsorbed from the plasma. The amount of ABO antigen present on platelets is quite variable from individual to individual, with from 5% to 10% of non-group-O individuals expressing extremely high levels of A or B substance on their platelets. These people appear to have a "high-expresser" form of glycosyltransferase in their sera.[1,2]

Although platelets are often transfused without regard to ABO compatibility, using mismatched platelets frequently results in lower posttransfusion recoveries.[3,4] In some cases, high-titer IgG ABO antibodies in blood group O recipients may react with platelets carrying large amounts of A or B antigens, resulting in platelet transfusion refractoriness. High-expresser platelets are particularly vulnerable to this type of immune destruction. Studies by Heal et al suggest that recovery of transfused platelets can also be influenced by *indirect* incompatibility between donor and recipient; for example, transfusion of group O platelets to a group A recipient.[5] A possible explanation is that anti-A and/or anti-B in the donor plasma transfused with the platelets might react with soluble A or B substance in recipient plasma to form immune complexes that bind to transfused (and autologous) platelets via Fc receptors (FcγRII), thereby influenc-

Janice G. McFarland, MD, Medical Director, Platelet/Neutrophil Immunology Laboratory, BloodCenter of Wisconsin, Inc., Milwaukee, Wisconsin

The author has disclosed no conflicts of interest.

ing their survival. Clinical trials in oncology patients requiring multiple platelet transfusions, comparing ABO-identical platelets to those that are unmatched, suggest that rates of refractoriness are significantly increased when unmatched components are used.[6] Although other red cell antigens (Le^a, Le^b, I, i, P, P^k, and Cromer antigens associated with decay accelerating factor)[7,8] are also found on platelets, there is no evidence that antibodies to these antigens significantly reduce platelet survival in vivo.

HLA Antigens on Platelets

HLA antigens are found on the surfaces of both platelets and white cells as well as on other nucleated cells of the body (see Chapter 19). HLA antigens associated with platelets are recognized as the main source of Class I HLA antigen in whole blood.[9] Most of the Class I HLA molecules on platelets are integral membrane proteins, while smaller amounts may be adsorbed from surrounding plasma.[10] With rare exceptions,[11] Class II HLA molecules are not present on the platelet membrane, and until recently it was thought that of the Class I molecules, only the HLA-A and -B locus antigens were significantly represented. A report from Japan, however, suggests that HLA-C antibodies might mediate between 5% and 10% of alloimmune refractoriness. This study, using careful absorption and elution techniques, showed that patients refractory to HLA-A-and-B-matched and -C-mismatched platelets but responsive to platelets matched for all three Class I antigens had antibodies reactive with HLA-C antigens on the HLA-C-mismatched platelets.[12]

Several factors influence the likelihood that HLA antibodies will develop after transfusions, and such sensitization may be clinically important in patients receiving multiple platelet transfusions. Studies of HLA alloimmunization in patients transfused with platelets, before the now widespread use of leukocyte-reduced (LR) blood components, documented the development of antibodies as early as 10 days (but generally 21-28 days) after primary exposure and 4 days after secondary exposure in patients previously transfused or pregnant.[13] The development of HLA alloimmunization in patients not previously sensitized was variable, ranging from 18%[13] to 50%[14] when non-LR components were used.

A dose-response relationship between donor exposures and the rate of HLA alloimmunization is not always evident. One group failed to detect such a relationship in patients with acute myelogenous leukemia receiving induction therapy,[15] while others have demonstrated a dose-response relationship in animal studies.[16] More recently, a large-scale study of patients receiving multiple platelet transfusions found that exposure to 13 or more apheresis platelet transfusions was among the few factors significantly associated with higher rates of HLA alloimmunization; the others were prior pregnancy or transfusion and receipt of non-LR components.[17] Transfusion-associated HLA alloimmunization appears to be influenced by the underlying disease, immunosuppressive effects of treatment regimens, and whether or not the blood components contain significant leukocyte content.

The white cells in blood components appear to be most responsible for primary HLA alloimmunization that occurs with transfusion. A number of studies in animals and humans demonstrate that when platelets devoid of white cells are transfused, primary immunization to HLA is very much delayed or does not occur at all, whereas unmodified platelet concentrates are associated with high rates of HLA immunization.[18,19] These observations implicate leukocytes in both platelet and red cell transfusions as the source of primary alloimmunization.

Sensitization to HLA antigens becomes important in managing patients receiving platelet transfusions when HLA antibodies cause destruction of transfused platelets.

Platelet Transfusion Refractoriness

A less-than-expected increase in platelet count occurs in about 20% to 70% of multitransfused thrombocytopenic patients.[20] Those treated for malignant hematopoietic disorders are particularly likely to become refractory to platelet transfusions. Responses to platelet transfusions are often determined 10 and 60 minutes after transfusion by calculating either a corrected platelet count increment (CCI) or a posttransfusion platelet recovery (PPR), both of which normalize transfusion responses for patient blood volume and platelet dose (see Table 18-1). Most would agree that a 1-hour posttransfusion CCI of less than 5000 to 7500 after two consecutive transfusions adequately defines the refractory state.

Although the CCI and PPR measurements are commonly used to assess the success of platelet transfusions, these calculations may be misleading, particularly when smaller doses of platelets are administered. In a recent reevaluation of data from a large clinical trial of platelet transfusions,[3] the authors argue that absolute posttransfusion platelet count increments are more useful in assessing the impact of different manipulations of platelet components, such as leukocyte reduction by filtration, particularly if these manipulations result in lower doses of platelets in the final product transfused. In the setting of large transfusion studies, where sufficient numbers of patients and transfusions can be analyzed, the posttransfusion platelet count increment along with multiple immune and nonimmune factors, blood volume, and platelet dose can be analyzed by multiple regression analysis to better assess the impact of different manipulations of the platelet components on transfusion response.[3]

Diagnosis of Alloimmune Refractoriness Caused by HLA Antibodies

HLA sensitization is the most common immune cause of platelet refractoriness and can be diagnosed by demonstration of significant levels of HLA Class I antibodies in the refractory patient's serum. In the standard microlymphocytotoxicity assay, the percent of the panel cells to which the recipient has formed cyto-

TABLE 18-1. Determination of Response to Transfused Platelets

Calculation of Corrected Count Increment (CCI)

$$\text{CCI} = \frac{\text{Body Surface Area } (\text{m}^2) \times \text{Platelet Count Increment} \times 10^{11}}{\text{Number of Platelets Transfused}}$$

EXAMPLE: If 4×10^{11} platelets are transfused to a patient whose body surface area is 1.8 m^2, and the increase in posttransfusion platelet count is 25,000/µL, then:

$$\text{CCI} = \frac{1.8\ \text{m}^2 \times 25{,}000/\mu\text{L} \times 10^{11}}{4 \times 10^{11}} = 11{,}250$$

Calculation of Posttransfusion Platelet Recovery

$$\text{PPR}(\%) = \frac{\text{Estimated Total Blood Volume}^* \times \text{Platelet Count Increment} \times 10^3}{\text{Number of Platelets Transfused}}$$

*Total blood volume can be estimated in adult patients as 75 mL/kg.

EXAMPLE: If 4×10^{11} platelets are transfused to a 70-kg patient and the increase in posttransfusion platelet count is 25,000/µL, then

$$\text{PPR} = \frac{(70\ \text{kg} \times 75\ \text{mL/kg}) \times 25{,}000\ \text{platelets}/\mu\text{L} \times 10^3}{4 \times 10^{11}\ \text{platelets}} = 0.328 = 32.8\%$$

toxic antibodies is referred to as the panel-reactive antibody (PRA) level. A commonly accepted level of alloimmunization to explain refractory responses to randomly selected platelet components is a PRA of 20%.[21] (See Chapter 19 for additional information on detecting HLA antibodies.)

Although platelet alloimmunization is one cause of refractoriness, there are multiple, nonimmune-related reasons that transfused platelets may not yield the expected increase in platelet count, such as sepsis, disseminated intravascular coagulation (DIC), or the administration of certain drugs. In fact these nonimmune factors are more often implicated in transfusion refractoriness than is alloimmunization.[22,23] Some of the most commonly cited nonimmune factors are listed in Table 18-2. A study of patients undergoing hematopoietic progenitor cell (HPC) transplant procedures suggested that patient-related variables such as treatment regimen (total body irradiation), disease status (advanced), and liver dysfunction are important predictors of poor platelet count increments as well.[24] Even when possible immune causes of refractoriness are identified, nonimmune factors are often simultaneously present.

TABLE 18-2. Some Nonimmune Causes of Platelet Refractoriness

◆ Massive bleeding
◆ Fever
◆ Sepsis
◆ Splenomegaly (splenic sequestration)
◆ Disseminated intravascular coagulation
◆ Allogeneic transplantation
◆ Poor storage of platelets before transfusion
◆ Effects of drugs (may include immune mechanisms)
◆ Intravenous amphotericin B
◆ Thrombotic thrombocytopenic purpura

Selection of Platelets for Transfusion in Alloimmune Refractoriness

Several strategies may be considered when selecting platelets for transfusion to patients with alloimmune refractoriness. When antibodies to HLA antigens are demonstrated, a widely used approach is to supply apheresis platelets from donors whose Class I HLA antigens are similar to those of the patient. Class I HLA typing can be performed on donors using serologic methods such as microlymphocytotoxicity or, more recently, by molecular methods (see Chapter 19). A disadvantage of relying on HLA-matched platelets is that a pool of 1000 to 3000 or more random, HLA-typed, potential apheresis donors is generally necessary to find sufficient HLA-compatible matches to support a typical patient.[25] Moreover, donor selection on the basis of HLA type can lead to the exclusion of donors whose HLA types, although different from that of the recipient, may still be effective.[26] For patients likely to require multiple platelet transfusions, HLA typing should be performed in advance of a planned course of treatment when white cell counts are sufficient to perform either serologic or DNA-based HLA typing.

An additional concern when using HLA-selected platelets is that requesting "HLA-matched" platelets does not necessarily lead to receiving HLA-identical or even well-matched platelets. It is important to understand the degree of match that may be provided (Table 18-3). Platelets received following an "HLA-matched" request are typically the closest match obtainable within the constraints of time and donor availability. In one study, 43% of platelets provided as HLA matched were relatively poor grade B or C matches.[27] In alloimmune refractory patients, the best increases in CCI occur with the subset of grade A and B1U or B2U HLA-matched platelets, but platelets mismatched for some antigens (eg, B44, 45) that are poorly expressed on platelets can also be successful.[26]

According to AABB *Standards for Blood Banks and Transfusion Services*, HLA-matched platelets should be irradiated to prevent transfusion-associated graft-vs-host disease

TABLE 18-3. Degree of Matching for HLA-Matched Platelets

Match Grade	Description	Examples of Donor Phenotypes for a Recipient Who Is A1, 3; B8, 27
A	4-antigen match	A1, 3; B8, 27
B1U	1 antigen unknown or blank	A1, –; B8, 27
B1X	1 cross-reactive group	A1, 3; B8, 7
B2UX	1 antigen blank and 1 cross-reactive	A1, –; B8, 7
C	1 mismatched antigen present	A1, 3; B8, 35
D	2 or more mismatched antigens present	A1, 32; B8, 35
R	Random	A2, 28; B7, 35

(GVHD).[28(p38)] This complication may arise when a recipient's immune system fails to recognize and destroy donor T lymphocytes because no Class I HLA antigens are present on donor cells that are mismatched to the recipient. In contrast, the immune-competent *donor* lymphocytes may recognize foreign HLA antigens on the *recipient's* tissue and mount an immune attack (ie, GVHD). A typical scenario for this process to occur is when a donor is homozygous for a Class I HLA haplotype shared with the recipient who has an additional haplotype not found in the donor. Because HLA-matched platelets are deliberately selected to minimize incompatible Class I HLA antigens that the recipient may react to in the transfusion, those components are more likely to cause GVHD than randomly selected platelets. Treating the component with gamma irradiation effectively eliminates this risk by inactivating the donor lymphocytes so that they cannot proliferate in response to foreign (recipient) tissue.

An alternative approach for supplying HLA-compatible transfusions is to determine the specificity of the patient's HLA antibodies and select donors whose platelets lack the antigens with which the antibodies react. This is termed the antibody specificity prediction (ASP) method.[29] One study compared the effectiveness of transfused platelets selected by the ASP method with those selected on the basis of HLA matching, platelet crossmatching, or on a random basis.[29] Platelets selected by the ASP method were equally effective to those selected by HLA matching or by crossmatching, and superior to randomly selected platelets. Further, in a file of HLA-typed donors, many more potential donors were identified by the ASP method than were available using traditional HLA matching criteria.

A variation of the ASP method involves analysis of patient antibody specificities detected in sensitive assays (either of flow cytometry[30] or Luminex-based[31,32] platforms) where single HLA antigens are represented on discrete and identifiable populations of beads. Reactivity of the patient's serum with the specific bead populations yields both the specificity and the relative strength of antibody binding to specific HLA antigens represented on the beads. Bead populations that lack reactivity with patient serum identify HLA antigens that could be used in donor selection even though they may not be matched to the patient's HLA type using more classic criteria for HLA matching. The identification of so-called permissive HLA antigens is modeled on a strategy used for identifying potentially compatible deceased donor kidney grafts for HLA-sensitized renal graft recipients.[33,34] This is yet another way to expand the donor pool to provide platelets that are compatible with the patient's HLA antibodies.

Pretransfusion platelet crossmatching is an additional approach to providing effective platelet transfusions to patients who are alloimmune refractory. Crossmatching can be used to predict, and therefore avoid, subsequent platelet transfusion failures.[35] Each platelet product intended for such patients needs to be tested in the crossmatch assay with a current sample of the patient's serum. The solid-phase red cell adherence (SPRCA) test is the most widely used method for this purpose. Good correlation between test results and posttransfusion platelet counts has been achieved.[35-37] Compared with HLA matching, crossmatching can prove to be both more convenient and cost effective. It avoids exclusion of HLA-mismatched but compatible donors and has the added advantage of facilitating the selection of platelets when the antibodies involved are directed at platelet-specific rather than HLA antigens. Platelet crossmatching, however, will not always be successful, particularly when patients are highly alloimmunized (PRA >50%). In these instances, finding sufficient compatible units may be problematic, and the use of HLA-matched platelets may be more practical.

Although the incidence of platelet-specific antibodies causing patients to be refractory to most or all attempted platelet transfusions is very small, this possibility should be investigated when most of the attempted crossmatches are positive or when HLA-matched transfusions fail. If platelet-specific antibodies are present, donors of known platelet antigen phenotype or family members, who may be more likely to share the patient's phenotype, should be tested.

Prevention of Alloimmunization

Once refractoriness caused by platelet alloimmunization is established, it is very difficult, if not impossible, to reverse. Therefore, in addition to developing methods of selecting compatible platelet donors for the refractory patient, several strategies have been evaluated to *prevent* alloimmunization in the first place. These include reduction of leukocytes in the platelet components and treating platelets with ultraviolet B (UVB) irradiation. In the Trial to Reduce Alloimmunization to Platelets (TRAP),[18] patients were randomly assigned to receive whole-blood-derived platelets that were filtered (LR) and pooled, that were UVB irradiated, or that were unfiltered and pooled, or apheresis platelets that were filtered. Use of either the LR or the UVB-irradiated platelets significantly reduced the incidence of HLA antibody generation from 45% to between 17% and 21%. The prevalence of platelet refractoriness was also reduced from 16% to between 7% and 10%. These treatments had no effects on the incidence of alloimmunization to platelet-specific glycoprotein antigens.

Thus, LR pooled platelets may be clinically equivalent to LR apheresis platelets, at least in terms of reducing primary HLA alloimmunization. UVB irradiation of pooled components is similarly effective, but this technology is not approved for use in patients in the United States. Although the TRAP study was limited to acute leukemia patients, its conclusions have been widely extrapolated to other patient groups receiving repeated platelet transfusions.

Platelet-Specific Antigens

Of the dozens of recognized platelet membrane glycoproteins, at least five [GPIa, -Ib (alpha and beta), -IIb, and -IIIa, and CD109] are polymorphic and demonstrated to be alloimmunogenic.[38] To date, 24 platelet-specific antigens have been characterized, including their localization to platelet surface glycoprotein structures, quantification of their density on the platelet surface, and determination of DNA polymorphisms in the genes encoding them (see Fig 18-1 and Table 18-4). Several others have been described serologically, but genetic polymorphisms underlying these have not yet been determined. The term "platelet-specific" is a misnomer for some of these markers, as they may be found on other types of cells as well (especially endothelial cells), although their chief clinical importance appears to be linked to their presence on platelets.

In addition to sensitization to polymorphic platelet glycoproteins, isoimmunization to a sixth membrane glycoprotein, GPIV (CD36), may occur in individuals who lack this

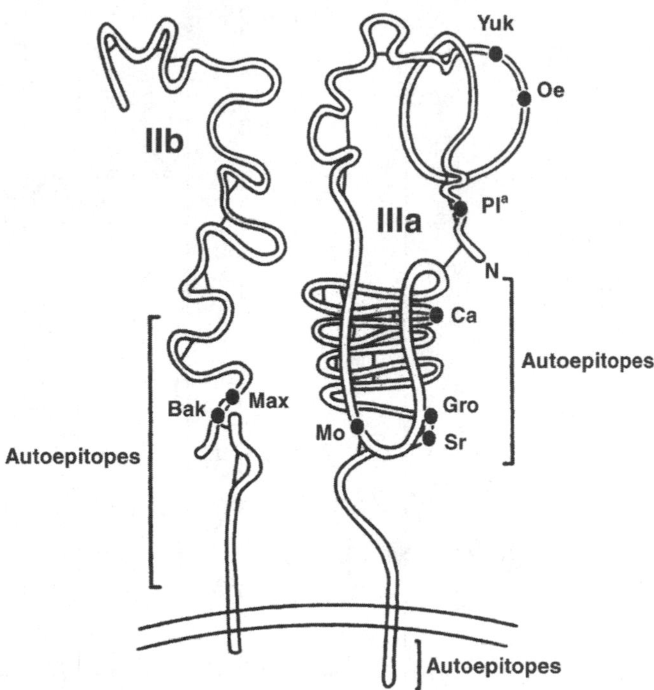

FIGURE 18-1. Schematic diagram of platelet glycoprotein complex IIb/IIIa. Dots and letters (Yuk, Oe, Pl^a, Ca, Gro, Sr, Mo, Bak, Max) designate positions and names of recognized allotypic epitopes. The molecular regions where autoepitopes have been recognized are indicated by brackets.[39]

structure on their platelets. Approximately 3% to 5% of Asians and Blacks lack GPIV on their platelets and can become sensitized to GPIV by transfusion or pregnancy.[38]

Several antigen "systems" on platelets are now recognized (Table 18-4). The nomenclature adopted by the International Society of Blood Transfusion (ISBT) classifies the systems numerically according to the date of publication and alphabetically to reflect their prevalence in the population.[40] As with red cells, different terminologies for platelet antigens often coexist. The first recognized antigen, Zw^a,[41] is now designated as human platelet antigen (HPA)-1a of the HPA-1 system. The HPA-1a antigen is often known as Pl^{A1}. HPA-1a is present on the platelets of about 98% of Whites, and anti-HPA-1a (anti-Pl^{A1}) is the most frequently encountered clinically significant platelet-specific antibody in the White population. Its antithetical antigen, HPA-1b (Pl^{A2}), occurs in 27% of Whites.

The HPA-1a and HPA-1b antigens reside on the platelet membrane glycoprotein GPIIIa. Patients with Glanzmann thrombasthenia Type I, who lack this glycoprotein, do not express HPA-1 antigens. The HPA-1 polymorphism arises by the substitution of a single DNA base pair, leading to an amino acid change (leucine in HPA-1a and proline in HPA-1b) at position 33 of the protein. Additional single nucleotide substitutions lead to other polymorphisms of GPIIIa, including HPA-4, -6, -7, -8, -10, -11, -14, -16, and -17. The HPA-2 and -12 antigen systems are situated on GPIb-alpha and -beta, respectively; the HPA-3 and -9 systems, on GPIIb; and the HPA-5 and 13 systems, on GPIa.[38]

On the platelet membrane, most of the glycoproteins that carry these platelet-specific antigens are present as heterodimeric compounds, that is, each consisting of two different glycoprotein molecules. Therefore, platelet glycoprotein names are often paired (eg, Ia/

TABLE 18-4. Alloantigenic Polymorphisms of Platelet Glycoproteins

HPA System Name	Other Names	Phenotypic Frequencies	GP Location	Amino Acid Change	Alloimmune Syndromes
Polymorphisms of Glycoprotein IIIa					
HPA-1a	Pl^{A1}, Zw^{a}	98%	IIIa	LeuPro33	NAIT, PTP, multiple transfusions
HPA-1b	Pl^{A2}, Zw^{b}	27%	IIIa		NAIT, PTP, multiple transfusions
HPA-1c		<1%	IIIa	$LeuVa_{l33}$	
HPA-4a	Pen^{a}, Yuk^{b}	99.9%	IIIa	$ArgGln_{143}$	NAIT, PTP
HPA-4b	Pen^{b}, Yuk^{a}	<1%	IIIa		NAIT, PTP
HPA-6(b)w	Ca, Tu	<1%	IIIa	$ArgGln_{489}$	NAIT
HPA-7(b)w	Mo	<1%	IIIa	$ProAla_{407}$	NAIT
HPA-8(b)w	Sr-a	<1%	IIIa	$ArgCys_{636}$	NAIT
HPA-10(b)w	La(a)	<1%	IIIa	$ArgGln_{62}$	NAIT
HPA 11(b)w	Gro (a)	<1%	IIIa	$ArgHis_{633}$	NAIT
HPA-14(b)w	Oe(a)	<1%	IIIa	Lys_{611} deleted	NAIT
HPA-16(b)w	Duv (a)	<1%	IIIa	$IleThr_{140}$	NAIT
HPA-17(b)w	Va (a)	<1%	IIb/IIIa	$ThrMet_{622}$	

Polymorphisms of Glycoprotein IIb					
HPA-3a	Bak^a, Lek	85%	IIb	$IleSer_{843}$	NAIT, PTP
HPA-3b	Bak^b	63%	IIb		NAIT, PTP
HPA-9(b)w	Max^a	0.6%	IIb	$ValMet_{837}$	NAIT
Polymorphisms of Glycoprotein Ia					
HPA-5a	Br^b, Zav^b	99%	Ia	$LysGlu_{505}$	NAIT, PTP
HPA-5b	Br^a, Zav^a	20%			NAIT, PTP
HPA-13(b)w	Sit(a)	<0.2%	Ia	$ThrMet_{799}$	NAIT
Polymorphisms of Glycoprotein Ib					
HPA-2a	Ko^b, Sib-b	99%	Ib alpha	$ThrMet_{145}$	Multiple transfusions
HPA-2b	Ko^a, Sib-a	15%			NAIT
HPA-12(b)w	Iy(a)	0.3%	Ib beta	$GlyGlu_{15}$	NAIT
Polymorphisms of CD109					
HPA-15a	Gov-b	80%	CD109	$TyrSer_{703}$	NAIT, PTP
HPA-15b	Gov-a	60%	CD109		NAIT, PTP

NAIT = neonatal alloimmune thrombocytopenia; PTP = posttransfusion purpura.

IIa, IIb/IIIa, or Ib/IX), referring to the alpha and beta chains in each complex. GPIb/IX is a leucine-rich membrane glycoprotein that serves as a receptor for von Willebrand factor on platelets. The Ia/IIa and IIb/IIIa complexes are members of a broadly distributed family of adhesion molecules called integrins. Integrins are essential for platelet adhesion and aggregation because the molecules serve as receptors for ligands such as fibrinogen (GPIIb/IIIa), von Willebrand factor (GPIb/IX), and collagen (GPIa/IIa). When present on other cells, the glycoprotein pairings may differ. For example, on platelets, GPIIIa is normally paired with GPIIb, but on endothelial cells, fibroblasts, and smooth muscle, GPIIIa is paired with a different glycoprotein. Thus, these cells share the HPA antigens found on the GPIIIa molecule but not those found on the GPIIb molecule.

CD109 is an exception to the heterodimeric rule because it occurs as a monomeric structure on the platelet membrane. This GPI-linked protein is also found on activated T cells, cultured endothelial cells, and several tumor cell lines as well as platelets.[42] The antigens HPA-15a (Gov[b]) and HPA-15b (Gov[a]) have been localized to platelet CD109, and unlike most platelet-specific antigens, both have a fairly high prevalence, with frequencies of 80% and 60%, respectively, in Whites. Sensitization to HPA-15 antigens has been associated with platelet refractoriness, neonatal alloimmune thrombocytopenia (NAIT), and posttransfusion purpura (PTP), albeit usually along with alloantibodies to other platelet antigens.[38]

Although antibodies to these various membrane glycoproteins may in rare instances cause refractoriness to platelet transfusions, they are more often associated with the alloimmune syndromes NAIT and PTP.

Neonatal Alloimmune Thrombocytopenia

Neonatal alloimmune thrombocytopenia (variously abbreviated as NAIT, NATP, NAT, or NIT) is a syndrome involving immune destruction of fetal platelets by maternal antibody, analogous to red cell destruction in hemolytic disease of the fetus and newborn. During pregnancy, a mother may become sensitized to an incompatible fetal platelet antigen inherited from the father. IgG specific for the platelet antigen is formed and crosses the placenta, causing fetal and neonatal thrombocytopenia. NAIT is the single most common cause of severe fetal/neonatal thrombocytopenia, and affected infants are at risk of major bleeding complications, especially intracranial hemorrhage. The most commonly implicated platelet antigen incompatibility in NAIT is for HPA-1a, but a large number of other antigens have been implicated as well.[43] A serologic diagnosis for NAIT may be made 1) by testing maternal serum for platelet antibodies using assays that can differentiate platelet-specific from non-platelet-specific reactivity and 2) by performing platelet antigen genotyping on parental DNA. Demonstration of both a platelet-specific antibody in the maternal serum and the corresponding incompatibility for the antigen in the parental platelet types confirm the diagnosis. Treatment of acutely thrombocytopenic newborns includes intravenous immune globulin (IVIG) with or without antigen-compatible platelet transfusions. Once the diagnosis of NAIT has been made in a family, subsequent fetuses are at risk. Antenatal treatment with IVIG with or without steroids has been proven to be an effective means of ameliorating fetal thrombocytopenia and preventing intracranial hemorrhage.[44] (For a more in-depth discussion of NAIT, see Chapter 22.)

Posttransfusion Purpura

PTP is characterized by the development of dramatic, sudden, and self-limiting thrombocytopenia 5 to 10 days after a blood transfusion in a patient with a previous history of sensitization by pregnancy or transfusion. Coincident with the thrombocytopenia is the development of a potent platelet-specific alloantibody in the patient's serum, usually anti-HPA-1a. Other specificities have been implicated, almost always associated with antigens on GPIIb/IIIa.[45] PTP differs from transfusion reactions caused by red cell antibodies, because the patient's own antigen-negative platelets (usually HPA-1a negative) as well as any transfused antigen-positive platelets are destroyed. The pathogenesis of autologous platelet destruction in PTP is not fully understood; however, mounting evidence suggests that either 1) the alloantibodies produced also have autoreactivity or 2) distinct platelet autoantibodies transiently arise along with the alloantibodies and cause both autologous and transfused antigen-negative platelet destruction.[45]

Plasma exchange—once the treatment of choice for PTP—has now largely been supplanted by IVIG as first-line therapy. Transfusion of antigen-negative platelets may be of value during the acute phase of PTP; however, such platelets have a reduced in-vivo survival.[46] Platelet antibody assays usually reveal an antibody in the serum with HPA-1a specificity. Genotyping will document the absence of HPA-1a or analogous markers for other platelet-specific antigen systems.[47]

Following recovery, future red cell transfusions should be from HPA-1a-negative donors if possible. Washed red cells may offer some protection against recurrence, although there is at least one report of PTP being precipitated by a washed red cell transfusion.[48]

Testing for Platelet-Specific Antigens and Antibodies

Three types of platelet antibody detection methods have been developed.[49] The earliest were Phase I assays that involved mixing patients' sera with normal platelets and used platelet function-dependent endpoints such as alpha granule release, aggregation, or agglutination. Phase I assays were succeeded by Phase II tests that measured either surface or total platelet-associated immunoglobulin (PAIG) on patients' platelets or on normal platelets after sensitization with patients' sera. Most recently, Phase III solid-phase assays were developed in which the binding of antibodies to isolated platelet surface glycoproteins is detected. The test methods that follow are examples of Phase II and III assays. (See "Heparin-Induced Thrombocytopenia" later in this chapter for an example of a Phase I assay.)

MIXED PASSIVE HEMAGGLUTINATION ASSAY (MPHA). A widely used Phase II assay for the detection of platelet-specific antibodies as well as for platelet crossmatching is the MPHA, also called the SPRCA assay.[35] Shibata et al were first to use this method to detect and identify clinically significant platelet alloantibodies.[50] In the assay, intact platelets are immobilized in round-bottom wells of a microtiter tray and are then incubated with the patient's serum. After washing, detector red cells previously coated with an antibody specific for human immunoglobulin are added. After incubation the tray is centrifuged and examined visually. The method's main limitation is that it fails to distinguish platelet-specific from non-platelet-specific antibodies. A modification of the MPHA is available as a commercial kit and is most often marketed for platelet crossmatching. Treatment of target platelets with chloroquine or acid disrupts the Class I HLA heavy-chain-peptide-β_2-microglobulin tri-molecular complex, which modifies antigenic epitopes, reducing the binding of antibodies directed at HLA on platelets.[51,52] Residual reactivity in the MPHA, when performed using chloroquine-treated platelets, can signal the presence of platelet-specific antibody.

FLOW CYTOMETRY. Another example of a Phase II assay is platelet antibody detection using immunofluorescence. The original slide-based method has given way to the flow cytometer to measure fluorescence of platelet-bound immunoglobulins. The latter method is used to detect platelet antibodies in patient sera that bind to intact platelets.[53] In the assay, washed platelets are sensitized with patient or control serum. The platelets are washed and platelet-bound antibodies are detected with a fluorescent-labeled (usually fluorescein isothiocyanate, or FITC) polyclonal or monoclonal antibody specific for human immunoglobulin (eg, IgG). The platelets are analyzed in the flow cytometer, and results can be expressed as a ratio of the median or peak channel fluorescence of normal platelets sensitized with patient serum over that of normal platelets incubated in normal serum. A second fluorescent label (eg, phycoerythrin, or PE) can be attached to an antihuman IgM probe to detect IgM platelet antibodies. Using two labels, IgG and IgM platelet antibodies can be detected simultaneously in the same reaction mixture.

Flow cytometry has proven to be a very sensitive method for detection of alloantibodies. The assay is capable of detecting very small numbers of antibody molecules bound to platelets, as is the case with alloantibodies specific for antigens of the HPA-5 (Br) system having only 1000 to 2000 sites per platelet. Moreover, some alloantibodies that are specific for labile epitopes that are unreliably detected in Phase III assays can be detected on intact platelets using immunofluorescence-based methods such as flow cytometry.[54]

Because the target platelets used in the assay are intact, flow cytometry does not differentiate between platelet-specific (ie, platelet-glycoprotein-directed) and non-platelet-specific antibodies. This is an advantage when the method is used to detect antibodies that will affect the success of a platelet transfusion; for this reason, flow cytometry has been advocated as a platelet crossmatching method. However, when the method is used to investigate cases of suspected NAIT or PTP, it is a potential drawback because the more relevant platelet-specific antibodies characteristic in these syndromes can be obscured by non-platelet-specific reactivity.

MONOCLONAL ANTIBODY-SPECIFIC IMMOBILIZATION OF PLATELET ANTIGEN (MAIPA) ASSAY. An example of a Phase III assay is the MAIPA,[55] perhaps the most widely used assay to detect platelet-specific antibodies. The assay requires the use of murine monoclonal antibodies (MoAbs) that recognize the target antigens of interest but do not compete with the human antibody being detected. In the assay, target platelets are simultaneously sensitized with patient serum and a murine MoAb recognizing the desired target molecule on the platelet surface. After the initial sensitization step, platelets are washed and solubilized in a nonionic detergent. An aliquot of the supernatant lysate is added to wells of a microtiter tray containing immobilized goat antibody specific for mouse IgG. The MoAb is thereby captured, and the platelet surface GP with its bound human antibody, immobilized. After a wash step, the human antibody is detected with an enzyme-labeled goat antihuman immunoglobulin probe.

There are several other versions of Phase III assays in use today, including the antigen capture enzyme-linked immunosorbent assay (ELISA), or ACE; the modified antigen capture ELISA, or MACE[43,56]; and a commercially available kit (PAKPLUS, GTI Diagnostics, Wakesha, WI). Each relies on MoAbs to immobilize only the glycoproteins of interest, thereby reducing or eliminating interfering reactions from non-platelet-specific antibodies, especially anti-HLA.

PLATELET TYPING USING MOLECULAR METHODS. Molecular typing is available for many platelet antigens. Because serologic phenotyping is limited by the shortage of well-characterized typing antisera and by low platelet counts, several DNA-based HPA typing techniques have been developed, such as restriction fragment length polymorphism (RFLP) analysis and sequence-specific oligonucleotide hybridization.[57,58] All of these techniques are reliable, but they are also laborious and time consuming. For this reason, polymerase chain reaction (PCR) genotyping with sequence-specific primers (SSP) appears to be much more practical. In an international workshop, SSP-PCR was the most common and reliable method of determining platelet genotypes,[59] making it feasible for genotyping HPAs independent of the patient's platelet count and the availability of rare typing sera.

Platelet Autoantibodies

Autoantibodies directed against platelet antigens may result in immune thrombocytopenia (ITP), also known as immune thrombocytopenic purpura. Chronic ITP, most often a disease in adults, is characterized by an insidious onset and moderate thrombocytopenia that may exist for months to years before diagnosis. Females are twice as likely to be affected as males. Spontaneous remissions are rare, and treatment is usually required to raise the platelet count. First-line therapy consists of steroids or IVIG, followed by more potent immunosuppressive agents or splenectomy in nonresponders. Many other therapies have been used in patients who fail splenectomy, with variable results. Chronic autoimmune thrombocytopenia may be idiopathic or associated with other conditions such as human immunodeficiency virus infection, malignancy, or other autoimmune diseases.

Acute ITP is mainly a childhood disease characterized by abrupt onset of severe thrombocytopenia and bleeding symptoms, often after a viral infection. The majority of cases resolve spontaneously over a 2- to 6-month period. If treatment is required, IVIG or anti-D immunoglobulin infusions given to D-positive patients are usually effective in raising the platelet count. Steroids are used less often because of serious side effects of this therapy in children. Splenectomy, if used, is reserved for children whose disease is severe and lasts longer than 6 months, similar to chronic ITP in adults.

Studies of both sera and washed platelets from patients with ITP have identified autoantibodies of IgG, IgM, and IgA classes reactive with a number of platelet surface membrane structures, including GP complexes IIb/IIIa, Ia/IIa, and Ib/IX and GPs IV and V.[60,61] In the majority of cases studied, platelet-associated autoantibodies reacted with two or more of these platelet glycoproteins.[61] There is no compelling evidence to date suggesting that a patient's particular profile of autoantibody specificities correlates with severity of disease or predicts response to therapy.[62]

Numerous Phase I, II, and III platelet antibody assays have been developed to detect relevant autoantibodies in ITP patients. Although many tests are quite sensitive, particularly in detecting total or cell surface platelet-associated immunoglobulins (Phase II assays),[63] none has been sufficiently specific to be particularly useful in either the diagnosis or management of ITP. The American Society of Hematology practice guidelines for ITP state that serologic testing is unnecessary, assuming the clinical findings are compatible with the diagnosis.[64] However, platelet antibody tests may be helpful in evaluation of patients suspected of having ITP when other, nonimmune causes may be present.

The goal of serologic testing in ITP is to detect autoantibody bound to the patient's own platelets with or without demonstration of similar reactivity in the patient's plasma. Most of the newer assays offered for evaluation of patients suspected of having ITP are Phase III assays, designed to detect immunoglobulin binding to platelet-specific epitopes found on platelet glycoprotein complexes IIb/IIIa, Ia/IIa, and/or Ib/IX. These solid-phase GP-specific assays appear to have improved specificity in distinguishing ITP from nonimmune thrombocytopenia when compared to Phase II assays, but this is often balanced by a decrease in sensitivity.[61,65] Moreover, all of these methods have limited utility in patients who have very low platelet counts preventing adequate numbers of platelets to be collected for use in the tests.

One commercially available Phase III test uses eluates prepared from washed patient platelets.[66] The eluates are tested against a panel of MoAb-immobilized platelet glycoprotein complexes, and antibody binding is detected using an enzyme-linked antihuman immunoglobulin probe. In the indirect phase of the assay, patient plasma is tested against the same glycoprotein panel. In general, plasma antibodies are detected less often than antibodies in the eluates. ITP patients may have antibodies reactive with one or several GP targets.[61]

Drug-Induced Platelet Antibodies

Thrombocytopenia caused by drug-induced platelet antibodies is a recognized complication of drug therapy. Drugs commonly implicated include quinine/quinidine, sulfa drugs, heparin, and colloidal gold. Both drug-dependent and drug-independent antibodies may be produced. Drug-independent antibodies, although stimulated by drugs, do not require the continued presence of the drug to react with platelets and are serologically indistinguishable from other platelet autoantibodies. However, unlike antibodies associated with typical autoimmune thrombocytopenia, drug-induced antibodies are transient except when caused by gold compounds, which are excreted very slowly. Recent evidence suggests that clinically relevant drug-dependent platelet antibodies may result when a drug interacts with certain platelet membrane epitopes. Alternatively, the drug may bind to preexisting low-affinity antibodies that recognize self-epitopes in such a way that the binding of antibody to platelet antigen is increased, leading to platelet destruction only in the presence of the drug molecules.[67] These antibodies can cause a thrombocytopenia of sudden and rapid onset, usually resolving when the drug is discontinued.

Testing for Drug-Dependent Platelet Antibodies

A number of assays for the detection of platelet antibodies have been adapted for the detection of drug-dependent platelet antibodies.[56,68] Among these are flow cytometry, the SPRCA assay, and assays designed to identify specific platelet membrane GPs with which drugs react before binding of drug-dependent antibody. In some cases, determination of the specific GP to which antibody is directed may provide useful clinical information. For example, drug-dependent antibody to GPIb/IX was associated with a more acute but reversible quinine-induced thrombocytopenia, whereas antibody to GPIIb/IIIa was associated with a more prolonged course.[68]

Virtually any platelet serology test that is used to detect platelet-bound immunoglobulin can be modified for use in the detection of drug-dependent platelet antibodies. In performing drug-dependent antibody testing, it is essential to establish the proper positive and negative controls for the assay. Each serum or plasma suspected of containing drug-dependent antibody must be tested against normal target platelets in the presence and absence of drug. Moreover, at least one normal serum should be tested with and without drug to control for nonspecific antibody binding that might be induced by the presence of the drug. Finally, a positive control serum known to be reactive with the drug being assayed should be tested with and without drug to complete the evaluation. A positive result must show that the serum is positive (or more positive) against normal target platelets in the presence of drug vs without drug, and that the drug did not nonspecifically cause a positive result in the target platelets. The positive control must likewise be positive with the drug and negative without it.

The flow cytometry test can be readily adapted to detect both IgG and IgM drug-dependent platelet antibodies.[56,69] In this modification, fluorescence of normal platelets sensitized with the patient's serum in the presence of drug can be compared with that of the patient's sample without drug or to a normal serum with drug to determine relative intensity of labeling. Flow cytometry has proven to have superior sensitivity to other assays for detection of quinine-, quinidine-, and sulfonamide-dependent platelet antibodies.[56] Other agents for which drug-dependent platelet antibodies have been detected and confirmed by flow cytometry in a large platelet immunology reference laboratory are shown in Table 18-5.

There are limitations of flow cytometry, or indeed any other antibody detection method, in detecting drug-dependent antibodies. For many drugs, the optimal concentration to demonstrate in-vitro binding of antibody has not been determined. Probably the most extensively studied drugs in this regard are quinine and quinidine.[71] Another cause of poor sensitivity is the weak binding of drug to platelets, leading to rapidly declining numbers of drug molecules on the platelet surface once drug is removed from the environment of the platelet. It is therefore important to maintain a critical concentration of drug in all washing buffers before addition of probe at the end of an assay.[69] Yet another potential reason for insensitivity is that a patient may not be sensitized to the native drug but rather to a metabolite of the drug. Antibodies dependent on metabolites of acetaminophen and sulfamethoxazole have been reported.[67]

Heparin-Induced Thrombocytopenia

Among the drug-induced immune responses to platelets, those triggered by exposure to he-

TABLE 18-5. Drugs Confirmed to Elicit Drug-Dependent Platelet-Reactive Antibodies In Vitro Using Flow Cytometry Testing[70]

Drug Category	Individual Drug
ACE inhibitor	Lisinopril
Analgesic	Acetaminophen,* propoxyphene
Antibiotic, antifungal	Sulfamethoxazole, vancomycin
	Ceftriaxone, levofloxacin, nafcillin, piperacillin, rifampin, trimethoprim
	Ampicillin, amoxicillin, cefazolin, cefadroxil, cefepime, cefpodoxime, ceftazidime, ceftizoxime, cefpodoxime, ciprofloxacin, ethambutol, lisinopril, loracarbef, metronidazole, nitrofurantoin, sulfisoxazole
Anticonvulsant	Carbamazepine
	Phenytoin
	Lorazepam, valproic acid
Antidepressant, antipsychotic	Amitriptylene, bupropion, haldol, olanzepine, sertraline
Beta blocker	Atenolol, propranolol
Cardiac	Amiodarone
	Dobutamine
Chemotherapeutic agent	Oxaliplatin
	Geldanamycin, irinotecan, suramin
Cinchona alkaloid	Quinine, quinindine
Diuretic	Furosemlde
GPIIb/IIIa inhibitor	Abciximab, eptifibatide, tirofiban
	Orbofiban, xemolifiban
Histamine receptor antagonist	Fexofenadine, ranitidine
Narcotic	Fentanyl
Nonsteroidal anti-inflammatory	Naproxen*
	Celecoxib, ibuprofen, oxaprozin
Proton pump inhibitor	Esomeprozole, lansoprazole, pantoprazole
Thrombin inhibitor	Argatroban
Vasodilator	Papaverine

*Drug-dependent antibodies that were specific for drug metabolites only.
ACE = angiotensin-converting enzyme; GP = glycoprotein.

parin have particular clinical importance, both because of the widespread use of this anticoagulant and because of the devastating thrombotic complications associated with the syndrome of heparin-induced thrombocytopenia (HIT).

The exact incidence of HIT is unknown, but it may develop in up to 4% of patients treated with unfractionated heparin. Low-molecular-weight heparin is less likely to be associated with HIT.[72,73] Bovine heparin appears somewhat more likely to cause the syndrome than porcine heparin.[73] A reduction in baseline platelet count by 30% to 50% occurs generally within 5 to 14 days after primary exposure, and sooner if the patient has been exposed to heparin within the last 3 months. The platelet count is often less than 100,000/µL but usually recovers within 5 to 7 days upon discontinuation of heparin.

More than 50% of patients with HIT develop thrombosis, which can occur in the arterial or venous systems, or both.[74] Patients may develop stroke, myocardial infarction, limb ischemia, deep venous thrombosis, or ischemia of other organs. The thrombotic complications may force limb amputation or may prove fatal. Because the rate of HIT-associated thrombosis is so significant, it is of critical importance to discontinue heparin therapy when the diagnosis of HIT is suspected. Moreover, strong consideration should be given to using an alternative (nonheparin) anticoagulant (eg, a direct thrombin inhibitor) to prevent thrombosis.[74]

The mechanism of HIT has become more completely understood in recent years. Heparin forms a complex with platelet factor 4 (PF4), a tetrameric protein released from platelet alpha granules. Antibodies (IgG, IgM, and some IgA) form against various epitopes on this complex and bind. HIT antibodies, IgG in particular, then attach secondarily to platelet FcγRIIa via their Fc portions, resulting in platelet activation with subsequent thrombin generation. The antibody may also bind to the complexes at other sites, notably on endothelial cells. Thus, HIT might involve activation and damage not only of platelets but also of endothelium, causing increased susceptibility to thrombosis. This understanding of the mechanism of HIT antibodies is exploited by ELISA tests in which microtiter wells are coated with the complexes of PF4 and heparin (or heparin-like molecules) rather than with the platelets themselves.[75,76]

The PF4 ELISA is an example of a Phase III assay for HIT. Target complexes of PF4 and heparin or heparin-like molecules are immobilized on a solid phase. To perform the test, the patient's serum is added to pre-made complexes of PF4 and heparin or heparin-like molecules (eg, polyvinyl sulfate, or PVS) alone and in the presence of high-dose (100 U/mL) heparin. Heparin-dependent antibody binds to the complexes and is detected via enzyme-conjugated antihuman immunoglobulin. An optical density value above 0.4 in the PF4-PVS well that can be inhibited by high-dose heparin confirms the presence of a heparin-dependent antibody in the patient's sample. Although IgG antibodies are the most clinically relevant antibodies causing this syndrome,[77] occasional patients with HIT appear to have only non-IgG (IgM or IgA) antibodies.[78] PF4 ELISA assays are available in two forms: those that detect but do not differentiate IgG, IgM, and IgA heparin-dependent antibodies, and those that detect only IgG.

The ^{14}C-serotonin release assay (SRA) is an example of a Phase I assay for detection of heparin-dependent antibodies. Normal, fresh target platelets are incubated with ^{14}C-serotonin, which is taken up into the dense granules of the platelets. The target platelets are then exposed to the patient's serum in the presence of low and high concentrations of heparin. Release of at least 20% of the radioactive label at the low dose of heparin and inhibition of this release at the high dose confirms the presence of heparin-dependent antibodies. Other functional tests used to detect heparin-dependent antibodies include the heparin-induced platelet aggregation test and the heparin-induced platelet activation test.

The PF4 ELISA and the SRA are both more sensitive and specific than the platelet aggregation test for the detection of heparin-dependent platelet antibodies in patients for whom there is clinical suspicion. However, in asymptomatic patients receiving heparin or in those who have not yet received the drug, neither test is sufficiently predictive of HIT to warrant its use in screening.[74]

GRANULOCYTE ANTIGENS AND ANTIBODIES

Antibodies against granulocyte (neutrophil) antigens are implicated in the following clinical syndromes: neonatal alloimmune neutropenia (NAN), transfusion-related acute lung injury (TRALI), immune neutropenia after HPC transplantation, refractoriness to granulocyte transfusion, and chronic benign autoimmune neutropenia of infancy. To date, seven neutrophil antigens carried on five different glycoproteins have been characterized and given human neutrophil antigen (HNA) designations by the Granulocyte Antigen Working Party of the ISBT[79] (Table 18-6).

The first granulocyte-specific antigen, NA1 (HNA-1a), was demonstrated in 1966 by Lalezari and Bernard.[80] HNA-1a and its antithetical antigen HNA-1b are located on a receptor protein for IgG, FcγRIIIb, which is present on the surface of granulocytes. Antibodies to HNA-1a and -1b have been implicated in TRALI, NAN, and autoimmune neutropenia of infancy. About 0.1% of Whites have neutrophils with no detectable FcγRIIIb (NA_{null}). The FcγRIII protein also carries the neutrophil antigen SH (HNA-1c).[81] NB1 (HNA-2a) is found on another granulocyte surface glycoprotein, CD177, the function of which is as yet undetermined. HNA-2a has been reported to have an allele, NB2, but the product of this gene cannot be reliably identified with human antisera, and no monoclonal antibody specific for NB2 has been identified, leaving the existence of an allele to HNA-2a unproven.[82] HNA-2a has been associated with TRALI and NAN. The DNA sequence of the *HNA-2a* gene has been determined, as have the molecular polymorphisms associated with HNA-1a, HNA-1b, and HNA-1c on the gene for FcγRIII. Genotyping for these specificities can therefore be performed on genomic DNA using PCR-SSP.[83]

Additional antigens on granulocytes are shared with other cells and are not granulocyte specific. These include 5b (HNA-3a), MART[a] (HNA-4a), and OND[a] (HNA-5a). The protein carrying HNA-3a has recently been identified as the choline transporter-like protein 2 (CTL2), and a single nucleotide polymorphism (SNP) in the gene encoding for the protein accounts for the HNA-3a and -3b alleles (Table 18-6).[84] This antigen is also expressed on the surface of lymphocytes. HNA-3a antibodies

TABLE 18-6. Granulocyte (Neutrophil) Alloantigens

Antigen System	Allele	HNA Designation	Antigen Prevalence (%) Whites	Antigen Prevalence (%) Blacks	Glycoprotein Location
Neutrophil-specific:					
NA	*NA1*	HNA-1a	46	46	FcγRIIIb (CD16)
NA	*NA2*	HNA-1b	88	84	FcγRIIIb (CD16)
SH	*SH*	HNA-1c	5	22	FcγRIIIb (CD16)
NB	*NB1*	HNA-2a	97	—	CD177
Neutrophil-nonspecific:					
—	*5b*	HNA-3a	97	—	CTL2
MART	*MART[a]*	HNA-4a	99	—	CD11b
OND	*OND[a]*	HNA-5a	99	—	CD11a

are usually agglutinins; they occasionally occur in women after pregnancy and may be associated with febrile transfusion reactions. Potent anti-HNA-3a agglutinins in transfused plasma have been responsible for fatal TRALI. HNA-4a and HNA-5a, both high-prevalence antigens, are also present on monocytes and lymphocytes as well as granulocytes. HNA-4a has been localized to the alpha M chain (CD11b) of the C3bi receptor (CR3) and results from a SNP. Sensitization to HNA-4a has been reported to cause NAN.[85] HNA-5a is expressed on the alpha L integrin unit, leukocyte function antigen-1 (CD11a), and also results from a SNP. Antibodies reactive with this marker, found in a chronically transfused aplastic anemia patient, have not been reported to be associated with clinical disease.

Neonatal Alloimmune Neutropenia

NAN is caused by maternal antibodies against antigens on fetal neutrophils; the most frequent specificities seen are against HNA-1a, HNA-1b, and HNA-2a antigens. NAN occurs most often in the newborns of women with HNA-1a/a and HNA-1b/b phenotypes; it may also occur in children of women with the rare HNA-1_{null} phenotype who lack the FcγRIII protein. The severity of neutropenia in NAN can occasionally be life-threatening because of increased susceptibility to infection. Management with antibiotics, IVIG, granulocyte colony-stimulating growth factor, and/or plasma exchange may be helpful.

Transfusion-Related Acute Lung Injury

TRALI is an acute, often life-threatening reaction characterized by respiratory distress, hypo- or hypertension, and noncardiogenic pulmonary edema that generally occurs within 2 hours of a transfusion of a plasma-containing blood component. TRALI has been reported to be induced by antibodies directed at granulocyte-specific antigens, although recent reports more commonly implicate antibodies to HLA antigens.[86] In TRALI, the causative antibodies are most often found in the plasma of the blood donor, although in about 10% of cases the granulocyte antibodies are of recipient, not donor, origin. (For a more in-depth discussion of TRALI, see Chapter 27).

Autoimmune Neutropenia

Autoimmune neutropenia may occur in adults or in infants. When present in adults, it may be idiopathic or may occur secondary to such diseases as rheumatoid arthritis, systemic lupus erythematosus, or bacterial infections. In autoimmune neutropenia of infancy, usually occurring in children between the ages of 6 months to 2 years, the autoantibody has neutrophil antigen specificity (usually HNA-1a or -1b) in about half the cases. The condition is generally self-limiting, with recovery usually in 7 to 24 months, and is relatively benign and manageable with antibiotics.[87]

Testing for Granulocyte Antibodies

Tests for granulocyte antibodies are not widely performed, although the implication of neutrophil antibodies as a cause of TRALI has increased the demand for this laboratory resource. Agglutination tests, performed in tube, capillary, or microplate formats, use heat-inactivated serum in the presence of EDTA and require fresh granulocytes. Immunofluorescence tests, also requiring fresh target cells, are read with either a fluorescence microscope or a flow cytometer and are capable of detecting granulocyte-bound immunoglobulins IgG and IgM. A combination of agglutination and immunofluorescence tests is beneficial.[79,88] Other methods include chemiluminescence and a MoAb immobilization of granulocyte antigens (MAIGA) assay, similar to the MAIPA assay. As with the latter, an advantage of the MAIGA assay is its ability to differentiate between HLA and granulocyte-specific antibodies.

KEY POINTS

1. Platelets express a variety of antigenic markers on their surface. Some of these antigens are shared with other cells, as in the case of ABO antigens and HLA, while others are essentially platelet specific.
2. HLA sensitization is the most common immune cause of platelet refractoriness and can be diagnosed by demonstration of significant levels of HLA Class I antibodies in the refractory patient's serum. When antibodies to HLA antigens are demonstrated, a widely used approach is to supply apheresis platelets from donors whose Class I HLA antigens are similar to those of the patient. HLA-matched platelets should be irradiated to prevent transfusion-associated graft-vs-host disease (GVHD).
3. Compared with HLA matching, crossmatching can prove to be both more convenient and cost effective. It avoids exclusion of HLA-mismatched but compatible donors and has the added advantage of selecting platelets when the antibodies involved are directed at platelet-specific rather than HLA antigens.
4. Although blood group antibodies (anti-A, -B) and platelet-specific antibodies can be responsible for refractory responses to platelet transfusion, they are less commonly implicated in this complication, compared to HLA antibodies.
5. Sensitization to platelet-specific antigens is the most common cause of neonatal alloimmune thrombocytopenia (NAIT), a syndrome involving immune destruction of fetal platelets by maternal antibody, analogous to red cell destruction in hemolytic disease of the fetus and newborn. Platelet-specific antibodies are also involved in posttransfusion purpura (PTP), a syndrome characterized by severe thrombocytopenia occurring 5 to 10 days after a blood transfusion. The most commonly implicated antibody in both conditions is anti-HPA-1a. Serologic testing using Phase III assays and molecular typing for platelet-specific antigens is useful in confirming both of these diagnoses.
6. Autoantibodies directed against platelet antigens may result in immune thrombocytopenia, or ITP. Chronic ITP, most often a disease in adults, is characterized by an insidious onset and moderate thrombocytopenia that may exist for months to years before diagnosis. Females are twice as likely to be affected as males. The goal of serologic testing in ITP is to detect autoantibody bound to the patient's own platelets with or without demonstration of similar reactivity in the patient's plasma.
7. Granulocyte (neutrophil) antigens are implicated in the clinical syndromes neonatal alloimmune neutropenia (NAN), transfusion-related acute lung injury (TRALI), immune neutropenia after hematopoietic progenitor cell transplantation, refractoriness to granulocyte transfusion, and chronic benign autoimmune neutropenia of infancy.

REFERENCES

1. Ogasawara K, Ueki J, Takenaka M, Furihata K. Study on the expression of ABH antigens on platelets. Blood 1993;82:993-9.
2. Curtis BR, Edwards JT, Hessner MJ, et al. Blood group A and B antigens are strongly expressed on platelets of some individuals. Blood 2000; 96:1574-81.
3. Slichter SJ, Davis K, Enright H, et al. Factors affecting posttransfusion platelet increments, platelet refractoriness, and platelet transfusion intervals in thrombocytopenic patients. Blood 2005;105:4106-14.
4. Julmy F, Ammann RA, Taleghani BM, et al. Transfusion efficacy of ABO major-mismatched platelets (PLTs) in children is inferior to that of ABO-identical PLTs. Transfusion 2009;49:21-33.
5. Heal JM, Masel D, Blumberg N. Interaction of platelet fc and complement receptors with cir-

culating immune complexes involving the ABO system. Vox Sang 1996; 71:205-11.

6. Heal JM, Rowe JM, McMican A, et al. The role of ABO matching in platelet transfusion. Eur J Haematol 1993;50:110-17.
7. Dunstan RA, Simpson MB. Heterogeneous distribution of antigens on human platelets demonstrated by fluorescence flow cytometry. Br J Haematol 1985;61:603-9.
8. Spring FA, Judson PA, Daniels GL, et al. A human cell-surface glycoprotein that carries Cromer-related blood group antigens on erythrocytes and is also expressed on leucocytes and platelets. Immunology 1987;62:307-13.
9. Bialek JW, Bodmer W, Bodmer J, Payne R. Distribution and quantity of leukocyte antigens in the formed elements of blood. Transfusion 1966;6:193-204.
10. Feuerstein N, Monos DS, Cooper HL. Phorbol ester effect in platelets, lymphocytes, and leukemic cells (HL-60) is associated with enhanced phosphorylation of class I HLA antigens. Coprecipitation of myosin light chain. Biochem Biophys Res Commun 1985;126:206-13.
11. Boshkov LK, Kelton JG, Halloran PF. HLA-DR expression by platelets in acute idiopathic thrombocytopenic purpura. Br J Haematol 1992;81:552-7.
12. Saito S, Ota S, Seshimo H, et al. Platelet transfusion refractoriness caused by a mismatch in HLA-C antigens. Transfusion 2002;42:302-8.
13. Howard JE, Perkins HA. The natural history of alloimmunization to platelets. Transfusion 1978;18:496-503.
14. Godeau B, Fromont P, Seror T, et al. Platelet alloimmunization after multiple transfusions: A prospective study of 50 patients. Br J Haematol 1992;81:395-400.
15. Dutcher JP, Schiffer CA, Aisner J, Wiernik PH. Alloimmunization following platelet transfusion: The absence of a dose-response relationship. Blood 1981;57:395-8.
16. Slichter SJ, O'Donnell MR, Weiden PL, et al. Canine platelet alloimmunization: The role of donor selection. Br J Haematol 1986;63:713-27.
17. Seftel MD, Growe GH, Petraszko T, et al. Universal prestorage leukoreduction in Canada decreases platelet alloimmunization and refractoriness. Blood 2004;103:333-9.
18. Leukocyte reduction and ultraviolet B irradiation of platelets to prevent alloimmunization and refractoriness to platelet transfusions. The Trial to Reduce Alloimmunization to Platelets Study Group. N Engl J Med 1997;337:1861-9.
19. Eernisse JG, Brand A. Prevention of platelet refractoriness due to HLA antibodies by administration of leukocyte-poor blood components. Exp Hematol 1981;9:77-83.
20. Triulzi DJ, Dzik WH. Leukocyte-reduced blood components: Laboratory and clinical aspects. In: Simon TL, Snyder EL, Solheim BG, et al, eds. Rossi's principles of transfusion medicine. 4th ed. Bethesda, MD: AABB Press, 2009:228-46.
21. Hogge DE, Dutcher JP, Aisner J, Schiffer CA. Lymphocytotoxic antibody is a predictor of response to random donor platelet transfusion. Am J Hematol 1983;14:363-9.
22. Hod E, Schwartz J. Platelet transfusion refractoriness. Br J Haematol 2008;142:348-60.
23. Alcorta I, Pereira A, Ordinas A. Clinical and laboratory factors associated with platelet transfusion refractoriness: A case-control study. Br J Haematol 1996;93:220-4.
24. Ishida A, Handa M, Wakui M, et al. Clinical factors influencing posttransfusion platelet increment in patients undergoing hematopoietic progenitor cell transplantation—a prospective analysis. Transfusion 1998;38:839-47.
25. Bolgiano DC, Larson EB, Slichter SJ. A model to determine required pool size for HLA-typed community donor apheresis programs. Transfusion 1989;29:306-10.
26. Schiffer CA, O'Connell B, Lee EJ. Platelet transfusion therapy for alloimmunized patients: Selective mismatching for HLA B12, an antigen with variable expression on platelets. Blood 1989;74:1172-6.
27. Dahlke MB, Weiss KL. Platelet transfusion from donors mismatched for crossreactive HLA antigens. Transfusion 1984;24:299-302.
28. Carson TH, ed. Standards for blood banks and transfusion services. 27th ed. Bethesda, MD: AABB, 2011.
29. Petz LD, Garratty G, Calhoun L, et al. Selecting donors of platelets for refractory patients on the basis of HLA antibody specificity. Transfusion 2000;40:1446-56.
30. Gebel HM, Bray RA. Sensitization and sensitivity: Defining the unsensitized patient. Transplantation 2000;69:1370-4.
31. Tait BD. Solid phase assays for HLA antibody detection in clinical transplantation. Curr Opin Immunol 2009;21:573-7.

32. Tait BD, Hudson F, Cantwell L, et al. Review article: Luminex technology for HLA antibody detection in organ transplantation. Nephrology (Carlton) 2009;14:247-54.
33. Bray RA, Nolen JD, Larsen C, et al. Transplanting the highly sensitized patient: The emory algorithm. Am J Transplant 2006;6:2307-15.
34. Tambur AR, Ramon DS, Kaufman DB, et al. Perception versus reality?: Virtual crossmatch—how to overcome some of the technical and logistic limitations. Am J Transplant 2009;9:1886-93.
35. Rachel JM, Summers TC, Sinor LT, Plapp FV. Use of a solid phase red blood cell adherence method for pretransfusion platelet compatibility testing. Am J Clin Pathol 1988;90:63-8.
36. O'Connell BA, Schiffer CA. Donor selection for alloimmunized patients by platelet crossmatching of random-donor platelet concentrates. Transfusion 1990;30:314-17.
37. Friedberg RC, Donnelly SF, Mintz PD. Independent roles for platelet crossmatching and HLA in the selection of platelets for alloimmunized patients. Transfusion 1994;34:215-20.
38. Curtis BR, McFarland JG. Platelet immunology and alloimmunization. In: Simon TL, Snyder EL, Solheim BG, et al, eds. Rossi's principles of transfusion medicine. Bethesda, MD: AABB Press, 2009:168-86.
39. Müeller-Eckhardt C. Platelet autoimmunity. In: Silberstein LE, ed. Autoimmune disorders of blood. Bethesda, MD: AABB, 1996:115-50.
40. Metcalfe P, Watkins NA, Ouwehand WH, et al. Nomenclature of human platelet antigens. Vox Sang 2003;85:240-5.
41. Van Loghem Jj J, Dorfmeijer H, Van Hart M, Schreuder F. Serological and genetical studies on a platelet antigen (Zw). Vox Sang 1959;4:161-9.
42. Smith JW, Hayward CP, Horsewood P, et al. Characterization and localization of the Gova/b alloantigens to the glycosylphosphatidylinositol-anchored protein CDw109 on human platelets. Blood 1995;86:2807-14.
43. Davoren A, Curtis BR, Aster RH, McFarland JG. Human platelet antigen-specific alloantibodies implicated in 1162 cases of neonatal alloimmune thrombocytopenia. Transfusion 2004;44:1220-5.
44. Bussel JB, Zabusky MR, Berkowitz RL, McFarland JG. Fetal alloimmune thrombocytopenia. N Engl J Med 1997;337:22-6.
45. McFarland JG. Posttransfusion purpura. In: Popovsky M, ed. Transfusion reactions. 3rd ed. Bethesda, MD: AABB Press, 2007.
46. Brecher ME, Moore SB, Letendre L. Posttransfusion purpura: The therapeutic value of PlA1-negative platelets. Transfusion 1990;30:433-5.
47. Skogen B, Bellissimo DB, Hessner MJ, et al. Rapid determination of platelet alloantigen genotypes by polymerase chain reaction using allele-specific primers. Transfusion 1994;34:955-60.
48. Christie DJ, Pulkrabek S, Putnam JL, et al. Posttransfusion purpura due to an alloantibody reactive with glycoprotein Ia/IIa (anti-HPA-5b). Blood 1991;77:2785-9.
49. Warner M, Kelton JG. Laboratory investigation of immune thrombocytopenia. J Clin Pathol 1997;50:5-12.
50. Shibata Y, Juji T, Nishizawa Y, et al. Detection of platelet antibodies by a newly developed mixed agglutination with platelets. Vox Sang 1981;41:25-31.
51. Neumuller J, Tohidast-Akrad M, Fischer M, Mayr WR. Influence of chloroquine or acid treatment of human platelets on the antigenicity of HLA and the 'thrombocyte-specific' glycoproteins Ia/IIa, IIb, and IIb/IIIa. Vox Sang 1993;65:223-31.
52. Gouttefangeas C, Diehl M, Keilholz W, et al. Thrombocyte HLA molecules retain nonrenewable endogenous peptides of megakaryocyte lineage and do not stimulate direct allocytotoxicity in vitro. Blood 2000;95:3168-75.
53. Garratty G, Arndt P. Applications of flow cytofluorometry to transfusion science. Transfusion 1995;35:157-78.
54. Lin M, Shieh SH, Liang DC, et al. Neonatal alloimmune thrombocytopenia in Taiwan due to an antibody against a labile component of HPA-3a (Baka). Vox Sang 1995;69:336-40.
55. Kiefel V, Santoso S, Weisheit M, Müeller-Eckhardt C. Monoclonal antibody—specific immobilization of platelet antigens (MAIPA): A new tool for the identification of platelet-reactive antibodies. Blood 1987;70:1722-6.
56. Visentin GP, Wolfmeyer K, Newman PJ, Aster RH. Detection of drug-dependent, platelet-reactive antibodies by antigen-capture ELISA and flow cytometry. Transfusion 1990;30:694-700.
57. McFarland JG, Aster RH, Bussel JB, et al. Prenatal diagnosis of neonatal alloimmune thrombocytopenia using allele-specific oligonucleotide probes. Blood 1991;78:2276-82.

58. Simsek S, Faber NM, Bleeker PM, et al. Determination of human platelet antigen frequencies in the Dutch population by immunophenotyping and DNA (allele-specific restriction enzyme) analysis. Blood 1993;81:835-40.
59. Panzer S. Report on the Tenth International Platelet Genotyping and Serology Workshop on behalf of the International Society of Blood Transfusion. Vox Sang 2001;80:72-8.
60. McMillan R. Antiplatelet antibodies in chronic adult immune thrombocytopenic purpura: Assays and epitopes. J Pediatr Hematol Oncol 2003;25(Suppl 1):S57-61.
61. Davoren A, Bussel J, Curtis BR, et al. Prospective evaluation of a new platelet glycoprotein (GP)-specific assay (PakAuto) in the diagnosis of autoimmune thrombocytopenia (AITP). Am J Hematol 2005;78:193-7.
62. Kiefel V, Santoso S, Kaufmann E, Müeller-Eckhardt C. Autoantibodies against platelet glycoprotein Ib/IX: A frequent finding in autoimmune thrombocytopenic purpura. Br J Haematol 1991;79:256-62.
63. George JN. Platelet immunoglobulin G: Its significance for the evaluation of thrombocytopenia and for understanding the origin of alpha-granule proteins. Blood 1990;76:859-70.
64. George JN, Woolf SH, Raskob GE, et al. Idiopathic thrombocytopenic purpura: A practice guideline developed by explicit methods for the American Society of Hematology. Blood 1996;88:3-40.
65. Warner MN, Moore JC, Warkentin TE, et al. A prospective study of protein-specific assays used to investigate idiopathic thrombocytopenic purpura. Br J Haematol 1999;104:442-7.
66. GTI PAKAUTO™ ELISA screening test for autoantibodies to platelet glycoproteins IIb/IIIa, Ib/IX and Ia/IIa (package insert). Brookfield, WI: GTI Diagnostics, 2004.
67. Aster RH, Bougie DW. Drug-induced immune thrombocytopenia. N Engl J Med 2007;357:580-7.
68. Nieminen U, Kekomaki R. Quinidine-induced thrombocytopenic purpura: Clinical presentation in relation to drug-dependent and drug-independent platelet antibodies. Br J Haematol 1992;80:77-82.
69. Curtis BR, McFarland JG, Wu GG, et al. Antibodies in sulfonamide-induced immune thrombocytopenia recognize calcium-dependent epitopes on the glycoprotein IIb/IIIa complex. Blood 1994;84:176-83.
70. Aster RH, Curtis BR, McFarland JG, Bougie DW. Drug-induced immune thrombocytopenia: Pathogenesis, diagnosis, and management. J Thromb Haemost 2009;7:911-18.
71. Christie DJ, Aster RH. Drug-antibody-platelet interaction in quinine- and quinidine-induced thrombocytopenia. J Clin Invest 1982;70:989-98.
72. Warkentin TE, Levine MN, Hirsh J, et al. Heparin-induced thrombocytopenia in patients treated with low-molecular-weight heparin or unfractionated heparin. N Engl J Med 1995;332:1330-5.
73. Warkentin TE. Pork or beef? Ann Thorac Surg 2003;75:15-16.
74. Warkentin TE, Greinacher A, Koster A, Lincoff AM. Treatment and prevention of heparin-induced thrombocytopenia: American College of Chest Physicians Evidence-Based Clinical Practice Guidelines (8th Edition). Chest 2008;133:340S-80S.
75. GTI-HAT™ for the detection of heparin associated antibodies (package insert). Brookfield, WI: GTI Diagnostics, 1997.
76. Suh JS, Malik MI, Aster RH, Visentin GP. Characterization of the humoral immune response in heparin-induced thrombocytopenia. Am J Hematol 1997;54:196-201.
77. Warkentin TE, Sheppard JA, Moore JC, et al. Laboratory testing for the antibodies that cause heparin-induced thrombocytopenia: How much class do we need? J Lab Clin Med 2005;146:341-6.
78. Amiral J, Wolf M, Fischer A, et al. Pathogenicity of IgA and/or IgM antibodies to heparin-PF4 complexes in patients with heparin-induced thrombocytopenia. Br J Haematol 1996;92:954-9.
79. Bux J. Human neutrophil alloantigens. Vox Sang 2008;94:277-85.
80. Lalezari P, Bernard GE. An isologous antigen-antibody reaction with human neutrophiles, related to neonatal neutropenia. J Clin Invest 1966;45:1741-50.
81. Steffensen R, Gulen T, Varming K, Jersild C. Fcγ RIIIB polymorphism: Evidence that NA1/NA2 and SH are located in two closely linked loci and that the SH allele is linked to the NA1 allele in the Danish population. Transfusion 1999;39:593-8.
82. Stroncek D. Neutrophil alloantigens. Transfus Med Rev 2002;16:67-75.
83. Hessner MJ, Curtis BR, Endean DJ, Aster RH. Determination of neutrophil antigen gene fre-

quencies in five ethnic groups by polymerase chain reaction with sequence-specific primers. Transfusion 1996;36:895-9.

84. Curtis BR, Cox NJ, Sulliman MJ, et al. The neutrophil alloantigen HNA-3a (5b) is located on choline transporter-like protein 2 and appears to be encoded by an R>Q154 amino acid substitution. Blood 2010;115:2073-6.
85. Fung YL, Pitcher LA, Willett JE, et al. Alloimmune neonatal neutropenia linked to anti-HNA-4a. Transfus Med 2003;13:49-52.
86. Curtis BR, McFarland JG. Mechanisms of transfusion-related acute lung injury (TRALI): Anti-leukocyte antibodies. Crit Care Med 2006; 34:S118-23.
87. Bux J, Behrens G, Jaeger G, Welte K. Diagnosis and clinical course of autoimmune neutropenia in infancy: Analysis of 240 cases. Blood 1998;91:181-6.
88. Bierling P, Bux J, Curtis B, et al. Recommendations of the ISBT Working Party on Granulocyte Immunobiology for leucocyte antibody screening in the investigation and prevention of antibody-mediated transfusion-related acute lung injury. Vox Sang 2009;96:266-9.

Chapter 19

The HLA System

Howard M. Gebel, PhD; Marilyn S. Pollack, PhD; and Robert A. Bray, PhD

THE HLA SYSTEM is composed of a complex array of genes and their protein products located within the human major histocompatibility complex (MHC) on the short arm of chromosome 6. HLA antigens contribute to the recognition of self and nonself, to the immune responses to antigenic stimuli, and to the coordination of cellular and humoral immunity. The HLA antigens are cell-surface glycoproteins that are divided into two groups (Class I and Class II) according to their coding gene locus, their function, tissue distribution, and biochemistry. HLA Class I molecules contain one copy each of two polypeptides: a heavy chain that is an integral cell membrane protein, and a noncovalently associated light chain that is called β_2-microglobulin (β_2-microglobulin is not encoded by a chromosome 6 "HLA gene" but by a gene that resides on chromosome 15). The HLA Class II molecules are composed of one copy each of an alpha-chain and a beta-chain, both of which are integral membrane proteins and coded for by "HLA genes." Class I molecules are found on the surface of platelets and, with a few exceptions, all nucleated cells of the body. Mature red cells usually lack HLA antigens that are demonstrable by conventional methods, whereas nucleated immature erythroid cells do express HLA antigens. MHC Class II antigens are typically restricted to a few cell types, including B lymphocytes, monocytes, macrophages, dendritic cells, and activated T lymphocytes. Other terms that have been applied to antigens of the HLA system include major histocompatibility locus antigens, transplantation antigens, and tissue antigens.

HLA molecules play a key role in antigen presentation. Immunologic recognition of differences in HLA antigens is probably the first step in the rejection of transplanted tissue. The HLA system is generally viewed as second in importance only to the ABO antigens in influencing the survival of transplanted solid or-

Howard M. Gebel, PhD, Professor of Pathology, and Codirector, Histocompatibility and Molecular Immunogenetics Laboratory, Department of Pathology, Emory University, Atlanta, Georgia; Marilyn S. Pollack, PhD, Professor of Pathology, University of Texas Health Science Center, and Director, University Health System Histocompatibility and Immunogenetics Laboratory, San Antonio, Texas; and Robert A. Bray, PhD, Professor of Pathology, and Codirector, Histocompatibility and Molecular Immunogenetics Laboratory, Department of Pathology, Emory University, Atlanta, Georgia

The authors have disclosed no conflicts of interest.

gans in the immediate posttransplant period. In hematopoietic progenitor cell (HPC) transplantation, the HLA system is paramount with regard to graft rejection and graft-vs-host disease (GVHD). HLA antigens and antibodies are also important in complications of transfusion therapy such as platelet refractoriness, febrile nonhemolytic transfusion reactions (FNHTRs), transfusion-related acute lung injury (TRALI), and transfusion-associated GVHD (TA-GVHD).

Interest in HLA polymorphisms has extended beyond their role as transplantation antigens. Studies correlating them with disease susceptibility and disease resistance began soon after serologic techniques for HLA Class I typing were developed. Historically, HLA antigen typing had been of value in relationship assessments and forensic investigations. With the development of DNA typing, molecular methods replaced the mixed lymphocyte culture (MLC) as the preferred method for selecting matched donor-recipient pairs for HPC transplantation. Molecular HLA testing also fostered resurgence in the investigation of disease associations, permitted the analysis of peptide-binding restriction parameters needed for effective vaccine development, and provided a more accurate tool for anthropologic population studies. Because of the polymorphic nature of the HLA genes, a complex nomenclature was developed (and is continually evolving) to define unique allele sequences based on the relationship of each allele's protein sequence to the serologic specificity of the corresponding antigen.[1,2]

GENETICS OF THE MAJOR HISTOCOMPATIBILITY COMPLEX

Class I and II HLA antigens are cell-surface glycoproteins that are products of closely linked genes mapped to the p21.3 band on the short arm of chromosome 6 (Fig 19-1). That genomic region is called the MHC and is usually inherited en bloc as a haplotype. Each of the several loci has multiple alleles with codominant expression of the products from each chromosome. With the exception of immunoglobulin idiotypes, the HLA system is the most polymorphic genetic system described in humans.

The genes *HLA-A*, *HLA-B*, and *HLA-C* encode the corresponding Class I A, B, and C antigens. The gene cluster *HLA-DR*, *HLA-DQ*, and *HLA-DP* encodes for the synthesis of the correspondingly named Class II antigens. Located between the Class I and Class II genes is a group of non-HLA genes that code for molecules that include the complement proteins C2, Bf, C4A, and C4B; a steroid enzyme (21-hydroxylase); and a cytokine (tumor necrosis factor). The non-HLA region is often referred to as MHC Class III even though it does not contain any HLA genes.

Organization of HLA Genetic Regions

The HLA Class I region contains (in addition to the classical genes *HLA-A*, *HLA-B*, and *HLA-C*) other gene loci designated *HLA-E*, *HLA-F*, *HLA-G*, *HLA-H*, *HFE*, *HLA-J*, *HLA-K*, *HLA-L*, *MICA*, and *MICB*. The latter genes encode nonclassical, or Class Ib, HLA proteins, and they frequently have limited polymorphism and low levels of expression.[4] Some Class Ib genes express nonfunctional proteins or no protein whatsoever. Genes that are unable to express a functional protein product are termed pseudogenes and presumably represent an evolutionary dead end. Other nonclassical HLA proteins have been associated with a variety of functions. For example, HLA-E is associated with the surveillance system of natural killer cells. HLA-G is expressed by the trophoblast and may be involved in the development of maternal immune tolerance of the fetus. Hereditary hemochromatosis (HH), an iron overload disorder with a 10% carrier frequency in Northern Europeans, is associated with two missense mutations in a Class I-like gene.[5] The gene conferring HH was initially named *HLA-H*; however, the *HLA-H* designation had already been assigned to an HLA Class I pseudogene by the World Health Organization (WHO) Nomenclature Committee.[6] The gene conferring HH is now called *HFE*. Additional Class I-like molecules are also located outside the MHC, such as CD1. These

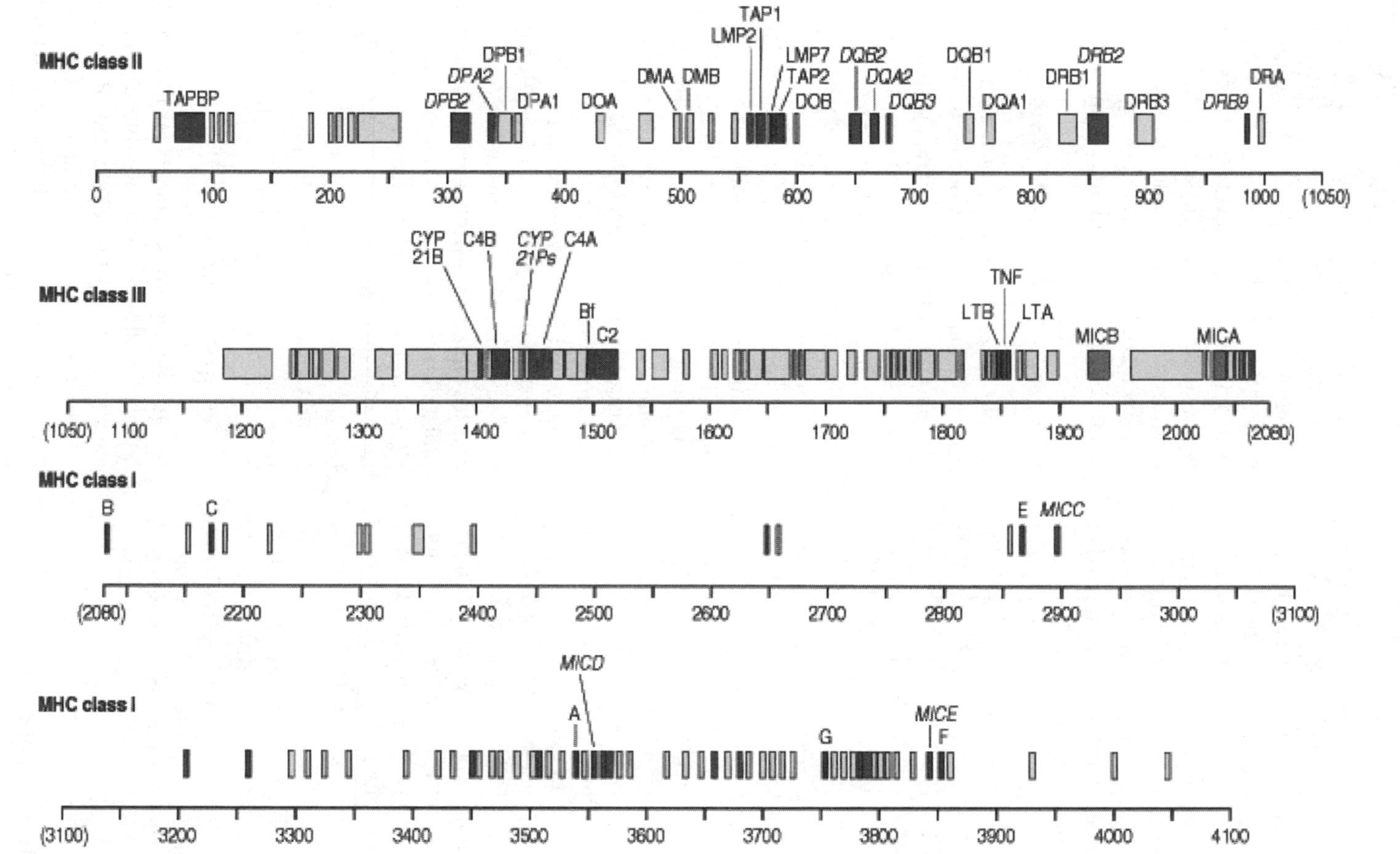

FIGURE 19-1. The HLA complex is located on the short arm of chromosome 6. The centromere is to the top left of the figure, the telomere to the bottom right. The organization of the Class I, II, and III regions is shown.[3]

molecules present nonprotein antigens (such as lipids) to T cells.

The genomic organization of the MHC Class II region (*HLA-D* region) is more complex. An MHC Class II molecule consists of a noncovalent complex of two structurally similar chains: the alpha-chain and the beta-chain. Both of those chains are encoded within the MHC. The polymorphism of HLA Class II molecules results from differences in both the alpha-chain and the beta-chain; this polymorphism depends on the Class II isoform. For example, with HLA-DR, the alpha-chain is essentially monomorphic, but the beta-chain is very polymorphic. Multiple loci code for the alpha- and beta-chains of the Class II MHC proteins. Different haplotypes have different numbers of Class II genes and pseudogenes. The proteins coded by *DRA* and *DRB1* result in HLA-DR1 through HLA-DR18. The products of *A* and *B3* (if present) express HLA-DR52; those of *A* and *B4* (if present) express HLA-DR53; and those of *A* and *B5* (if present) express HLA-DR51. The HLA-DQ1 through DQ9 antigens are expressed on the glycoproteins coded by *DQA1* and *DQB1* in the DQ cluster genes. Many of the other genes of the DQ cluster are probably pseudogenes. A similar organization is found in the HLA-DP gene cluster.

Although not generally considered part of the HLA system, the MHC Class III region contains four complement genes, whose alleles are generally inherited together as a unit, termed a complotype. More than 10 different complotypes are inherited in humans. Two of the Class III genes, *C4A* and *C4B*, encode for variants of the C4 molecule and antigens of the Chido/Rodgers blood group system. These variants have distinct protein structures and functions; the C4A molecule (if present) carries the Rg antigen, and the C4B molecule (if present) carries the Ch antigen, both of which are adsorbed onto the red cells of individuals who possess the gene(s).

Patterns of Inheritance

Although MHC organization is complicated, its inheritance follows the established principles of genetics. Every person has two different copies of chromosome 6 and possesses two HLA haplotypes, one from each parent. The expressed gene products constitute the phenotype, which can be determined by typing for HLA antigens or alleles. Because HLA genes are autosomal and codominant, the phenotype represents the combined expression of both haplotypes. However, to define haplotypes, parents (and possibly other family members) must also be phenotyped to determine which alleles are inherited together. Figure 19-2 illustrates inheritance of haplotypes.

Finding HLA-Identical Siblings

A child inherits one copy of chromosome 6 from each parent; hence, one MHC haplotype is inherited from each parent. Because each parent has two different copies of chromosome 6, four different combinations of haplotypes are possible in the offspring (assuming no recombination). The inheritance pattern is important in predicting whether family members will be compatible donors for transplantation. The chance that two siblings will be genotypically HLA identical is 25%. The chance that any one patient with "n" siblings will have at least one HLA-identical sibling is $1 - (3/4)^n$. Having two siblings provides, a priori, a 44% chance, and having three siblings provides a 58% chance that one sibling will be HLA identical. No matter how many siblings are available for typing (aside from identical twins), the probability will never be 100% for finding an HLA-identical sibling. Moreover, each time a new sibling is tested, that new sibling has (only) a 25% chance of being a match, no matter how many siblings have previously been tested.

Absence of Antigens

Before the advent of molecular-based HLA typing, the absence of an antigen upon serologic phenotyping was attributed to homozygosity at a locus (eg, inheritance of A1 from both parents, which in reality represented only an apparent absence of the antigen as a result of limitations of phenotyping methods) or to a null allele. With DNA sequencing and other molecular methods, homozygosity can now be

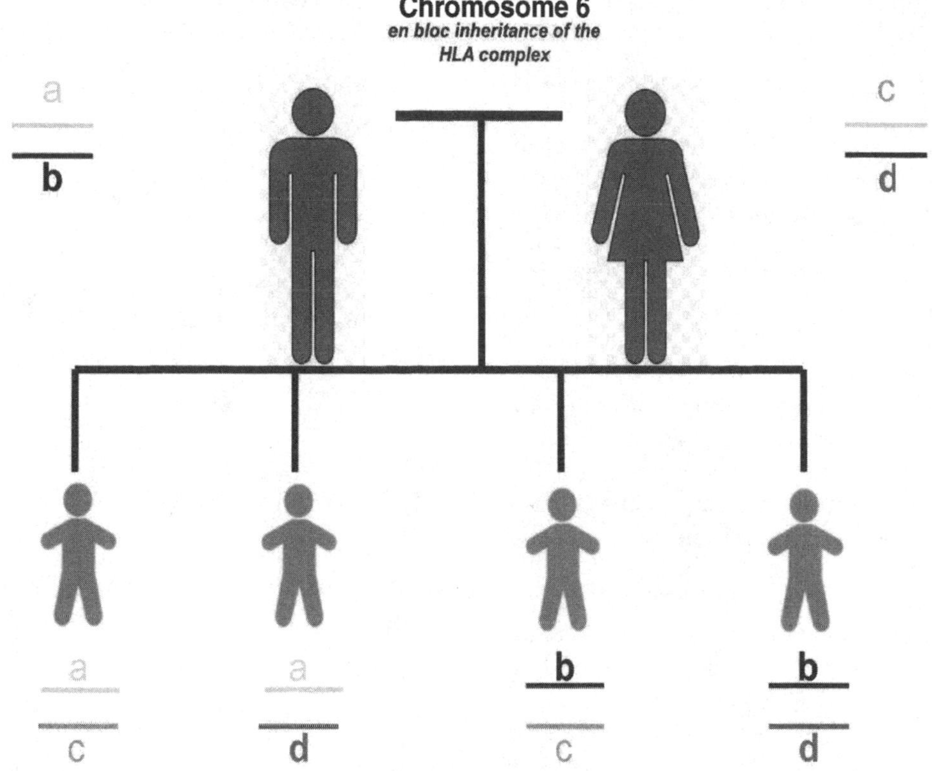

FIGURE 19-2. The designations a/b and c/d represent maternal and paternal HLA haplotypes, respectively. Except for crossovers, the HLA complex is transmitted en bloc from parent to offspring.

presumed with a higher degree of confidence, although homozygosity still can be proven only through family studies or methods permitting hemizygous typing (ie, typing of individual haplotypes). A null allele is characterized by one or more substitutions that are within or outside the coding region of the gene and that prevent expression of a functional protein at the cell surface. Such inactivation of a gene may be caused by nucleotide substitutions, deletions, or insertions, which lead to a premature cessation in the antigen's synthesis. When one refers to phenotypes, in the absence of a family study, a single allele at any locus is only presumptive evidence for homozygosity and should be listed only once because it is unknown whether that allele is present twice (a true homozygote) or whether there is another allele not detected by the available method.

Crossing Over

The genes of the HLA region occasionally demonstrate chromosome crossover in which segments containing linked genetic material are exchanged between the two chromosomes during meiosis or gametogenesis. The recombinant chromosomes are then transmitted as new haplotypes to the offspring. Crossover frequency is in part related to the physical distance between the genes and their resistance or susceptibility to recombination. For example, the *HLA-A*, *HLA-B*, and *HLA-DR* loci are close together, with 0.8% crossover between the *A* and *B* loci and 0.5% between the *B* and *DR* loci. Crossovers between the *HLA-B* and *HLA-C* loci or between the *HLA-DR* and the *HLA-DQ* loci are extremely rare, whereas crossovers between the *DQ* and *DP* loci are relatively common.[7,8] In family studies and in relationship evaluation, the possibility of recombination should always be considered.

Linkage Disequilibrium

The MHC system is so polymorphic that the number of possible unique HLA phenotypes is theoretically greater than that of the global human population. Moreover, new HLA alleles are constantly being discovered and characterized. As of July 2010, 1193 *HLA-A* alleles, 1800 *HLA-B* alleles, and 902 *DRB1* alleles[9] had been identified. In reality, many HLA haplotypes are overrepresented compared with what would be expected if the distribution of HLA genes were random. The phenomenon of linkage disequilibrium accounts for the discrepancy between expected and observed HLA haplotype frequencies.

Expected frequencies for HLA haplotypes are derived by multiplication of the frequencies of each allele. For example, in individuals of European ancestry, the overall frequency of the gene coding for HLA-A1 is 0.15 and that for HLA-B8 is 0.10; therefore, 1.5% (0.15 × 0.10) of all HLA haplotypes in the European population would be expected to contain genes coding for both HLA-A1 and HLA-B8 if the haplotypes were randomly distributed. The actual haplotype frequency of the A1 and B8 combination, however, is 7% to 8% in that population. Certain allelic combinations occur with increased frequency in different racial groups and constitute common haplotypes in those populations. The common haplotypes are called ancestral haplotypes because they appear to be inherited from a single common ancestor or to be conserved within the population because of resistance to recombination or survival advantage. The most common ancestral haplotype in Northern Europeans—the *A1, B8, DR17 (DRB1*03:01), DQ2* haplotype—includes both Class I and Class II regions. Some haplotypes in apparent linkage disequilibrium may represent relatively young haplotypes that have not had sufficient time to undergo recombination, whereas some old haplotypes are resistant to recombination because of selection or physical limitations. For example, the *A1, B8, DRB1*03:01* haplotype appears to be resistant to recombination because that sequence of DNA has a different length than that of most other comparable sequences due to the deletion of the complement gene *C4A*. Linkage disequilibrium in the HLA system is important in studies of relationship because haplotype frequencies in the relevant population make the transmission of certain gene combinations more likely than others. Linkage disequilibrium also affects the likelihood of finding suitable unrelated donors for HLA-matched platelet transfusions and for HPC transplantation.

BIOCHEMISTRY, TISSUE DISTRIBUTION, AND STRUCTURE

Characteristics of Class I and Class II Antigens

Class I antigens (HLA-A, -B, and -C) have a molecular weight around 57,000 Daltons and consist of two chains: a glycoprotein heavy chain (45,000 Daltons) encoded on the short arm of chromosome 6 and, as a light chain, the β_2-microglobulin molecule (12,000 Daltons) encoded by a gene on chromosome 15. The heavy chain penetrates the cell membrane. β_2-microglobulin is not attached to the cell membrane; $\beta_2$micro-globulin associates with the heavy chain through the latter's nonvariable (α3) domain but is not covalently bound to it (see Fig 19-3). The external portion of the heavy chain consists of three amino acid domains (α1, α2, and α3), of which the outermost α1 and α2 domains contain the majority of polymorphic regions conferring HLA antigen specificity.

Class I molecules are found on platelets and on most nucleated cells in the body, with some exceptions including neurons, corneal epithelium, trophoblasts, and germinal cells. Only vestigial amounts remain on mature red cells, with certain allotypes better expressed than others. Those Class I polymorphisms were independently recognized as red cell antigens by serologists and were designated as Bennett-Goodspeed (Bg) antigens. The specificities called Bg^a, Bg^b, and Bg^c are actually

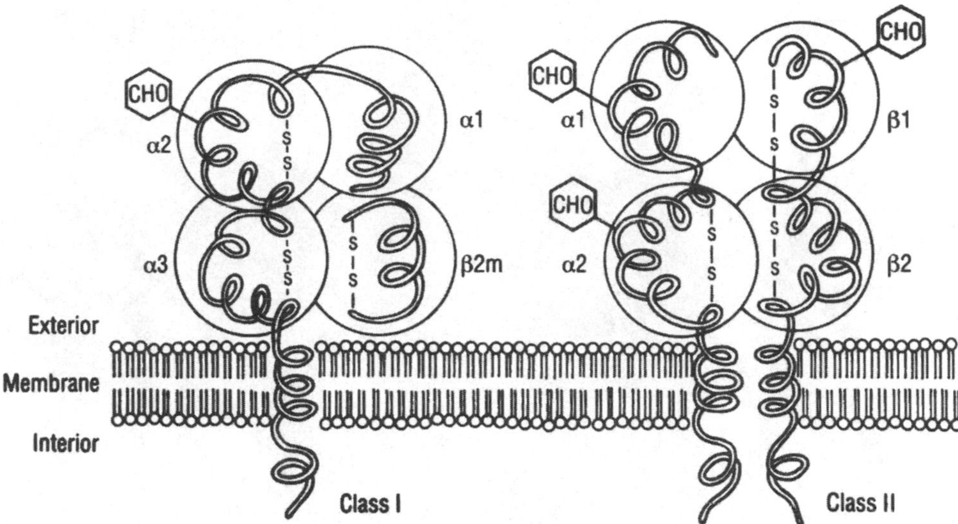

FIGURE 19-3. Stylized diagram of Class I and Class II MHC molecules showing α and β polypeptide chains, their structural domains, and attached carbohydrate units.

HLA-B7, HLA-B17 (B57 or B58), and HLA-A28 (A68 or A69), respectively. Platelets express primarily HLA-A and HLA-B antigens. HLA-C antigens are present at very low levels, and Class II antigens are generally not expressed at all on platelets.

Class II antigens (HLA-DR, -DQ, and -DP) have a molecular weight of approximately 63,000 Daltons and consist of two structurally similar glycoprotein chains (α and β), both of which traverse the membrane (see Fig 19-3). The extramembranous portion of each chain has two amino acid domains, of which the outermost contains the variable regions of the Class II alleles. The expression of Class II antigens is more restricted than that of Class I. Class II antigens are expressed constitutively on B lymphocytes, monocytes, macrophages, dendritic cells, intestinal epithelium, and early hematopoietic cells. There is also constitutive expression of Class II antigens on some endothelial cells, especially those lining the microvasculature. However, in general, endothelium, particularly that of larger blood vessels, is negative for Class II antigen expression, although it can be induced (for instance, by interferon-gamma during immune activation). T lymphocytes are negative for Class II antigen expression but can become positive when activated. Class II antigens are expressed abnormally in autoimmune diseases and on some tumor cells.

Soluble HLA Class I and Class II antigens shed from cells are found in blood and body fluids and may play a role in modulating immune reactivity.[10] Levels of soluble HLA increase with infection [including human immunodeficiency virus (HIV)], inflammatory disease, and transplant rejection, but HLA levels decline with progression of malignancy. Levels of soluble HLA in blood components are proportional to the number of residual donor leukocytes and to the length of storage.[11] Soluble HLA in blood components may be involved in the immunomodulatory effect of blood transfusion.

Configuration

A representative three-dimensional structure of Class I and Class II molecules can be obtained by x-ray crystallographic analysis of purified HLA antigens (see Fig 19-4). The outer domains, which contain the regions of amino acid variability and the antigenic epitopes of the molecules, form a structure known as the "peptide-binding groove." Alleles that are defined by polymorphisms in the HLA gene se-

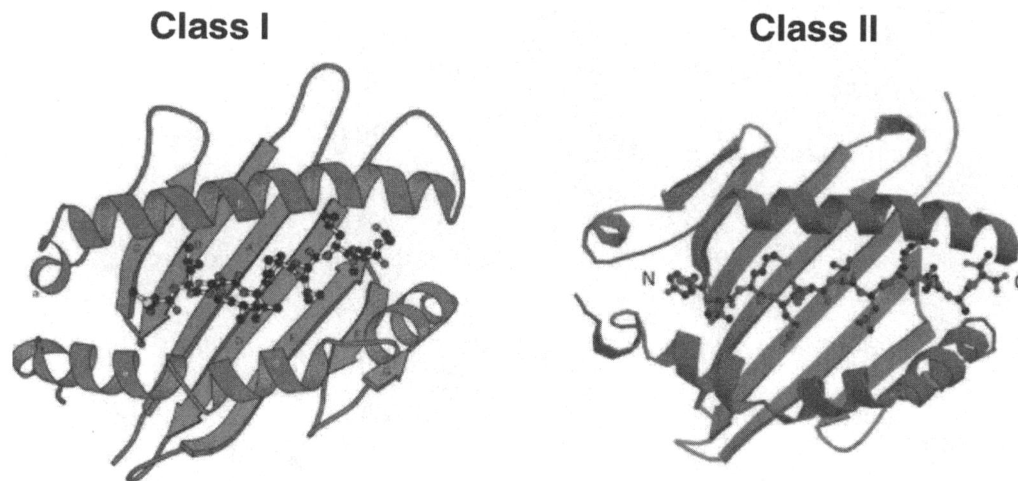

FIGURE 19-4. Ribbon diagram of HLA Class I and Class II molecule. Note the peptide in the groove of each molecule.

quences encode unique amino acid sequences and therefore form unique binding grooves, each being able to bind peptides of different sequences. The peptide-binding groove is critical for the functional aspects of HLA molecules (see section on biologic function).

Nomenclature for HLA Antigens

An international committee sponsored by the WHO establishes the nomenclature of the HLA system. It is updated regularly to incorporate new HLA alleles.[2] HLA antigens are designated by a number following the letter that denotes the HLA series (eg, HLA-A1 or HLA-B8). Previously, antigenic specificities that were not fully confirmed carried the prefix "w" (eg, HLA-Aw33) for "workshop." When identification of the antigen became definitive, the WHO Nomenclature Committee dropped the "w" from the designation. (The Committee meets regularly to update nomenclature by recognizing new specificities or genetic loci.) The "w" prefix is no longer applied in this manner and is now used only for the following: 1) Bw4 and Bw6, to distinguish such "public" antigens (see below) from other B locus alleles; 2) all serologically defined C locus specificities, to avoid confusion with members of the complement system; and 3) Dw specificities that were defined by mixed leukocyte reactions but are now known to be caused by *HLA-DR, HLA-DQ,* and *HLA-DP* polymorphisms. The numeric designations for the HLA-A and HLA-B specificities were assigned according to the order of their discovery.

"Splits"

Refinement of serologic methods permitted antigens that were previously believed to represent a single specificity to be "split" into specificities that were serologically (and, later, genetically) distinct. The designation for an individual antigen that is a split of an earlier recognized antigen often includes the number of the parent antigen in parentheses [eg, HLA-B44 (12)].

Cross-Reactive Groups

In addition to "splits," HLA antigens and antigen groups may have other epitopes in common. Antibodies that react with the shared determinants often cause cross-reactions in serologic testing. The collective term for a group of HLA antigens that exhibits such cross-reactivity is cross-reactive group (CREG).

"Public" Antigens

In addition to splits and CREGs, HLA proteins have reactivity that is common to many different HLA specificities. Called "public" antigens, those common amino acid sequences appear to represent the less variable portion of the HLA molecule. Two well-characterized public antigens, HLA-Bw4 and HLA-Bw6, are found in all HLA-B molecules except B*18:06, B*46:01, B*55:03, and B*73:01.[12] The *HLA-A* locus molecules A23, A24, A25, and A32 also have a Bw4-like epitope. Public antigens are clinically important because patients exposed to public HLA antigens through pregnancy, transfusion, or transplantation can make antibodies to those antigens if the patients do not express the epitopes themselves. A single antibody, when directed against a public antigen, can resemble multiple discrete alloantibodies and has significant consequences for identifying compatible donors for transplantation and platelet transfusion.

Nomenclature for HLA Alleles

Because nucleotide sequencing is used to investigate the HLA system, increasing numbers of HLA alleles are being identified, many of which share a common serologic phenotype. The minimum requirement for designation of a new allele is the sequence of exons two and three for HLA Class I and exon two for HLA Class II (*DRB1*). These exons encode the variable amino acids that confer HLA antigen specificity. A uniform nomenclature has been adopted that takes into account the locus, the major serologic specificity, and the allele group determined by molecular typing techniques. For example, nucleotide sequencing has identified at least 90 unique exon 2 amino acid sequence variants (alleles) of HLA-DR4.[2] The first HLA-DR4 variant is designated *DRB1*04:01*, indicating the locus (DR), the protein (β1 chain), an asterisk to denote that an allele name follows (and that the typing was determined by molecular techniques), the major serologic specificity (04 for HLA-DR4), and the sequence 2 variation allele number (variant 01). A similar system is used for naming Class I alleles. The name of the locus—for example, HLA-B—is followed by an asterisk and then by a number of digits separated by colons. The first two digits correspond to the serologic specificity of the antigen in most cases. The next group of digits is used to indicate coding for a unique amino acid sequence in exons 2 and 3, with numbers being assigned in the order in which the DNA sequences have been determined. Therefore, *B*27:04* represents the HLA-B locus, with a serologic specificity of B27, and was the fourth unique sequence 2 and 3 allele described in this family (see Table 19-1). A third "place" in the allele name is added for alleles that differ only by

TABLE 19-1. HLA Nomenclature 2010

Species	Locus	Antigen Equivalent	Allele	Silent Mutation	Outside Exon	Expression Modifier
HLA	DRB1 *	04 :	01 :	01 :	01:02	N,L,S,Q

Examples:

DR4 - Serology
DRB1*04:xx - Serologic Equivalent
DRB1*04:02 - Allele
DRB1*04:01:01; DRB1*04:01:02 - Silent Mutation
A*02:15N; DRB4*01:03:01:02N - Null Alleles (exon, intron)
A*24:02:01:02L
B*44:02:01:02S
A*32:11Q
(A*24:02:01:02L, B*44:02:01:02S, A*32:11Q) - Expression Modifiers

synonymous ("silent") nucleotide substitutions in exons 2 and 3 for Class I or in exon 2 for Class II. For example, A*01:01:02 differs from A*01:01:01 only in that the codon for isoleucine in position 142 is ATT instead of ATC. A fourth "place" in the allele name can be added for alleles that differ only in sequences within introns or in 3′ or 5′ untranslated regions. Finally, the nomenclature accommodates alleles with null or low expression or other characteristics by the addition of an "N" or "L," respectively, or another letter as appropriate, to the end of the allele name. The other official expression modifiers are as follows: S (secreted, not on cell surface), Q (expression level questionable), A (unknown but aberrant expression, perhaps null), and C (cytoplasmic expression only). The last two have not been used to date.

Biologic Function

The essential function of the HLA system is self/nonself discrimination. Discrimination of self from nonself is accomplished by the interaction of T lymphocytes with peptide antigens. T lymphocytes interact with peptide antigens only when the T-cell receptor (TCR) for antigen engages both an HLA molecule and the antigenic peptide contained with the TCR's peptide-binding groove. That limitation is referred to as "MHC restriction."[13]

In the thymus, T lymphocytes with TCRs that bind to a self HLA molecule are selected (positive selection), with the exception of those with TCRs that also bind to a peptide derived from a self-antigen, in which case the T lymphocytes are deleted (negative selection). Some self-reactive T cells escape negative selection. If not functionally inactivated (for instance, by the mechanism of anergy), such self-reactive T cells may become involved in an autoimmune process.

Role of Class I

Class I molecules are synthesized, and peptide antigens are inserted into the peptide-binding groove, in the endoplasmic reticulum. Peptide antigens that fit into the Class I peptide-binding groove are typically eight or nine amino acids in length and are derived from proteins made by the cell (endogenous proteins). Such endogenous proteins—which may be normal self-proteins, altered self-proteins such as those found in cancer cells, or viral proteins such as those found in virus-infected cells—are degraded in the cytosol by a large multifunctional protease (LMP) and are transported to the endoplasmic reticulum by a transporter associated with antigen processing (TAP). The LMP and TAP genes are both localized to the MHC.

Class I molecules are transported to the cell surface, where the molecules are available to interact with CD8-positive T lymphocytes. If the TCR of a CD8 cell can bind the antigenic peptide in the context of the specific Class I molecule displaying it, then TCR binding activates the cytotoxic properties of the T cell, which will attack the cell, characteristically eliciting an inflammatory response. The presentation of antigen by Class I molecules is especially important in host defense against viral pathogens and against malignant transformation. Tumor cells that do not express Class I escape this immune surveillance.

Role of Class II

Like Class I molecules, Class II molecules are synthesized in the endoplasmic reticulum, but peptide antigens are not inserted into the peptide-binding groove there. Instead, an invariant chain (Ii) is inserted. The Class II-invariant chain moiety is transported to an endosome where the invariant chain is removed by a specialized Class II molecule called DM. The DM locus is also localized to the MHC. A Class II antigenic peptide is then inserted into the peptide-binding groove. Peptide antigens that fit into the Class II peptide-binding groove are typically 12 to 25 amino acids in length and are derived from proteins that are taken up by the cell by endocytosis (exogenous proteins). Exogenous proteins, which may be normal self-proteins or proteins derived from pathogens such as bacteria, are degraded to peptides by enzymes in the endosomal pathway. Class II molecules are then transported to the cell surface where the molecules are available to interact with CD4-positive T lymphocytes, which secrete immunostimulatory cytokines in response. That mechanism is especially important for the production of antibodies.

DETECTION OF HLA ANTIGENS AND ALLELES

Methods for the identification of HLA antigens and alleles fall into three groups: molecular (DNA-based), serologic, and cellular assays. Detailed procedures for commonly used assays are provided in the *ASHI Laboratory Manual*, from the American Society for Histocompatibility and Immunogenetics.[14] Depending on the clinical situation, a particular HLA antigen/allele detection or typing method may be preferable (see Table 19-2).

DNA-Based Assays

DNA-based typing has several advantages over serologic and cellular assays: high sensitivity and specificity, small sample volumes, decreased turnaround time in comparison with cellular assays, and absence of the need for cell surface antigen expression or cell viability. Although serologic methods can distinguish a limited number of HLA specificities, high-resolution DNA-based methods have the capability to identify all known alleles.

Polymerase Chain Reaction Testing

Polymerase chain reaction (PCR) technology allows amplification of large quantities of a particular target segment of genomic DNA. Low- to intermediate-resolution typing detects the HLA serologic equivalents with great accuracy (eg, it distinguishes DR15 from DR16), whereas high-resolution typing distinguishes individual alleles (eg, DRB1*01:01 from DRB1*01:02). Several PCR-based methods have been developed; three general approaches are described below.

OLIGONUCLEOTIDE PROBES. This method for establishing HLA genotypes features arrays of oligonucleotide probes on a solid-phase matrix—for example, microbeads or an enzyme-linked immunosorbent assay (ELISA) plate. The microbead array assay is a sequence-specific oligonucleotide probe (SSOP) method for

TABLE 19-2. HLA Typing Methods and Appropriate Applications

Method	Clinical Application	Resolution
SSP (PCR)	Solid organ, related and unrelated HPC transplantation	Serologic to allele level, higher resolution with large number of primers
DNA sequencing	Unrelated HPC transplantation, resolution of typing problems with other methods, characterization of new alleles	Allele level
Forward SSOP hybridization	Solid organ and HPC transplantation (can accommodate high-volume testing)	Serologic to allele level
Reverse SSOP hybridization	Solid organ, related and unrelated HPC transplantation	Serologic, higher resolution with larger number of probes
Microlymphocytotoxicity	Solid organ transplantation, evaluation of platelet refractoriness, HLA typing (Class I only) of platelet recipients and platelet donors	Serologic specificity

HLA Class I and Class II low-to-high-resolution DNA-based tissue typing, with a reduction in sample processing time.[15]

SEQUENCE-SPECIFIC PRIMERS. A second major technique uses sequence-specific primer (SSP) pairs that target and amplify a particular DNA sequence.[16] The sequence-specific method requires the performance of multiple PCR assays in which each reaction is specific for a particular allele or group of alleles. Direct visualization of the amplified alleles is seen after agarose gel electrophoresis. Because SSPs have such specific targets, presence of the amplified material indicates presence of the corresponding allele(s). The pattern of positive and negative PCR amplifications is examined to determine the HLA alleles present. Primer pair sets are commercially available that can determine a complete HLA-A, -B, -C, -DR, -DQ, and -DP allele-level phenotype.

SEQUENCE-BASED TYPING. High-resolution nucleic acid sequencing of HLA alleles generates allele-level sequences. Sequence-based typing (SBT) can be used to characterize new allele(s). Although SBT is considered the "gold standard" for HLA typing, ambiguities do result from *cis/trans* polymorphisms (ie, two different base pairs at the same position). These ambiguities occur because SBT evaluates both maternal and paternal HLA genes (haplotypes) simultaneously. In contrast, new techniques for high-resolution SBT allow separation of HLA haplotypes before sequencing, thereby avoiding ambiguities.

Serologic (Lymphocytotoxicity) Assays

The microlymphocytotoxicity test can be used to detect HLA-A, -B, -C, -DR, and -DQ antigens. Lymphocytes are used for testing because they are readily obtained from anticoagulated peripheral blood and are a more reliable target than granulocytes. Lymphocytes obtained from lymph nodes or spleen may also be used. HLA typing sera are obtained primarily from multiparous women. Some mouse monoclonal antisera are also available.

HLA sera of known specificities are placed in wells of a microdroplet test plate. A suspension of lymphocytes is added to each well. Rabbit complement is then added; if sufficient antibody has bound to the lymphocyte membranes, the complement cascade will be activated through the membrane attack complex, leading to lymphocytotoxicity. Damage to the cell membrane can be detected by the addition of dye. Cells that have no attached antibody, no activated complement, and no damage to the membrane keep the vital dyes from penetrating; cells with damaged membranes allow the dye to enter. The cells are examined for dye exclusion or uptake under phase contrast microscopy. If a fluorescent microscope is available, fluorescent vital dyes can also be used.

Because HLA-DR and HLA-DQ antigens are expressed on B cells and not on resting T cells, typing for those antigens usually requires that the initial lymphocyte preparation be manipulated to yield an enriched B-cell population before testing. The manipulation is typically accomplished by the use of magnetic beads, to which monoclonal antibodies to B cells have been bound.

The interpretation of serologic reactions requires skill and experience. Control wells of known reactivity and careful quality control (QC) of reagents are required, especially for the activity of the complement used to induce lymphocytotoxicity. In addition, antigen assignments can be made only on the basis of results obtained with multiple antisera because few reagent antisera have sufficient monospecific reliability to be used alone. The extreme polymorphism of the HLA system; the variation in antigen frequencies among different racial groups; the reliance on biologic antisera and living target cells; and the complexities introduced by splits, CREGs, and "public" antigens all contribute to difficulties in accurate serologic HLA typing. Given these problems, most US laboratories now rely primarily on DNA-based methods for HLA typing. However, it should be noted that although the more common "null alleles" such as *DRB4*01:03:01:02N* and *Cw*04:09N* can be identified by routine molecular typing methods, rare null alleles may not be as easily identified. It is important to stay current with the ever-changing array of expressed and nonexpressed HLA polymorphisms. A very useful resource is the International Immunogenetics Project (IMGT)/ HLA database.[2,9]

Cellular Assays

Historically, the MLC (also called mixed lymphocyte reaction, or MLR) and primed lymphocyte typing (PLT) assays were used to detect genetic differences in the Class II region. In the MLC, mononuclear cells from different individuals are cultured together; the ability of one population (the responder) to recognize the HLA-D (combined DR, DQ, and DP) antigens of the other (the target) as foreign can be detected by measuring the proliferation of the responders. In PLT, reagent cells previously stimulated by specific Class II mismatched types allow the identification of those types by their accelerated proliferative responses to stimulator cells sharing the original mismatches. These classical cellular assays have been largely replaced by molecular typing methods for HLA antigens. However, these assays are still used as monitors of immune function or relative functional compatibility in some laboratories.

CROSSMATCHING AND DETECTION OF HLA ANTIBODIES

Serologic Assays

The same type of microlymphocytotoxicity testing used for serologic HLA typing can be used to test serum specimens for antibodies against selected target cells. This type of testing is referred to as lymphocyte crossmatching. Crossmatching consists of incubating serum from a potential recipient with lymphocytes (unfractioned or separated into T and B lymphocytes) from prospective donors. A variation of the microlymphocytotoxicity test uses an antiglobulin reagent, which increases assay sensitivity. Flow cytometry is yet another crossmatch method with even greater sensitivity than the antiglobulin-enhanced crossmatch.

Testing the patient's serum against a panel of 30 to 60 (or more) different target cells was historically used to assess the extent of HLA alloimmunization. A positive result was target cell death. The percentage of panel cells that died after reacting with the cytotoxic antibodies in patient serum was referred to as the panel-reactive antibody (PRA) level in that patient. Determination of cytotoxic PRA was (and may still be) useful in following patients awaiting deceased-donor solid organ transplantation, in the workup of patients for platelet refractoriness, and in the investigation of FNHTR or TRALI cases. The PRA "HLA antibody screen" not only detects the presence of cytotoxic HLA antibodies but can also identify the specificity of those antibodies. Although they have long been the gold standard for antibody identification, complement-dependent cytotoxic assays are not optimal tests. Sensitivity and specificity are marginal, but more importantly, most cytotoxic assays cannot identify specific antibodies in highly sensitized patients reactive with 80% or more of test panel cells.

Solid-Phase Assays

The current approach to identify HLA antibodies (especially for highly sensitized solid organ transplant candidates) relies on the use of beads or microparticles coated either with clusters of HLA Class I or Class II antigens or with single purified HLA antigens (solid-phase methodology).[17] Antibody binding is detected by staining with a fluorescent-labeled antihuman globulin (AHG). Flow cytometry and microarray methods are more sensitive than lymphocytotoxicity testing and focus on the detection of IgG antibodies. Newer adaptations of this technology include the ability to determine if those antibodies do or do not fix complement. The clinical significance of the low level of antibodies detectable by solid-phase assays, and which may not cause a positive cytotoxicity or flow-cytometric crossmatch, is controversial.

THE HLA SYSTEM AND TRANSFUSION

HLA system antigens and antibodies play important roles in a number of transfusion-related events, including platelet refractoriness, FNHTRs, TRALI, and TA-GVHD. HLA antigens are highly immunogenic. In response to pregnancy, transfusion, or transplantation, immunologically normal individuals are more likely to form antibodies to HLA antigens than to any other antigens.

Platelet Refractoriness

The incidence of HLA alloimmunization and platelet refractoriness among patients receiving repeated transfusions of cellular blood components ranges from 20% to 71%.[18] The refractory state exists when transfusion of suitably preserved platelets fails to increase the recipient's platelet count. Platelet refractoriness may be caused by clinical factors such as sepsis, high fever, disseminated intravascular coagulopathy, medications, hypersplenism, complement-mediated destruction, or a combination of those factors, or it may have an immune basis.

Antibody Development

Antibodies against HLA antigens are a common cause of immune-mediated platelet refractoriness, but antibodies to platelet-specific or ABH antigens may also be involved. HLA alloimmunization can follow pregnancy, transfusion, or organ transplantation because the foreign antigens are the donor MHC antigens themselves. A common example is the development of HLA antibodies directed against Class I and Class II antigens that occurs with transfusion of platelets, even though platelets express only Class I antigens. It is likely that the presence of donor leukocytes (bearing Class I and II antigens) elicits alloimmunization. The likelihood of HLA immunization can be lessened (but not eliminated) with leukocyte-reduced blood components or by treatment with ultraviolet light, which alters costimulatory molecules or impairs antigen-presenting cell activity. The threshold level of leukocytes required to provoke a primary HLA alloimmune response is unclear and probably varies among different recipients. Some studies have suggested that 5×10^6 leukocytes per transfusion may represent an immunizing dose. In patients who have been sensitized by prior transplantation, pregnancy, or transfusion, exposure to even lower numbers of allogeneic cells is likely to provoke an anamnestic antibody response.

Identifying Compatible Donors

The HLA antibody response of transfused individuals may be directed against individual specificities present on donor cells or against public alloantigens. Precise characterization may be difficult. An overall assessment of the degree of HLA alloimmunization can be obtained by measuring the PRA of the recipient's serum. Platelet-refractory patients with a high PRA are broadly alloimmunized and may be difficult to support with platelet transfusions. HLA-matched platelets, obtained by plateletpheresis, benefit some, but not all, of those refractory patients. Donors who are phenotypically matched with the immunized recipient for four Class I antigens (two alleles each at the *HLA-A* and *HLA-B* loci) are difficult to find, and strategies to obtain HLA-compatible platelets vary. Although selection of partially mismatched donors (based on serologic CREGs) has been emphasized, such donations may fail to provide an adequate transfusion response in vivo. An alternative approach to the selection of donors is based on matching for immunogenic epitopes as described by the "HLA Matchmaker" program developed at the University of Pittsburgh. HLA Matchmaker considers epitopes present on all the HLA Class I (and if indicated, Class II) molecules of the patient regardless of which allele encodes them. HLA Matchmaker is an excellent tool to predict compatibility between a specific donor-recipient pair, but unfortunately the tool does not accurately predict 100% of the time. Use of single-antigen beads or microarrays to identify HLA antibody specificities can also help to allow a better selection of donors with acceptable mismatched antigens.[19] Approaches such as HLA Matchmaker can be referred to as "pull" approaches, wherein donors are selected (or pulled into) the process. In contrast, antibody specificity identification can be considered "push" approaches that exclude (push away) inappropriate donors. Either approach has a similar net effect: identification of donors who will have the greatest likelihood for a negative crossmatch with the recipient, thus optimizing posttransfusion platelet counts.

As an alternative approach, HLA-alloimmunized patients often respond to crossmatch-compatible platelets selected by using patient serum and samples of apheresis platelets in a platelet antibody assay. Crossmatching techniques may assess compatibility for both HLA and platelet-specific antibodies.[20] Histocompatible platelet components are discussed further in Chapter 18.

Febrile Nonhemolytic Transfusion Reactions

HLA antibodies, as well as granulocyte and platelet-specific antibodies, have been implicated in the pathogenesis of FNHTRs. The recipient's antibodies, reacting with transfused antigens, elicit the release of cytokines (eg, interleukin-1) that are capable of causing fever. Serologic investigation, if undertaken, may require multiple techniques and target cells from a number of different donors (see Chapter 27).

Transfusion-Related Acute Lung Injury

In TRALI (a potentially fatal transfusion reaction that is being recognized with increasing frequency), acute noncardiogenic pulmonary edema develops in response to transfusion (see Chapter 27). Pathogenesis appears to reflect the presence of HLA antibodies in donor blood, which react with and fix complement to the granulocytes of the recipient, leading to severe capillary leakage and pulmonary edema. Rarely, HLA antibodies of the recipient react with transfused leukocytes from the donor. Cases of TRALI have been reported that appear to be caused by donor antibodies against Class I or Class II antigens in recipients. Because Class II antigens are not expressed on neutrophils, an alternate explanation for activation of neutrophils is required in these instances. One hypothesis is that Class II antigens on the recipient's pulmonary macrophages are targeted by the complement-activating antibodies. Subsequent release of cytokines and chemokines results in the recruitment and activation of neutrophils in the lungs.[21]

Chimerism and Transfusion-Associated Graft-vs-Host Disease

Chimerism refers to the presence of two cell populations in an individual, such as transfused or transplanted donor cells in a recipient. Persistent chimerism after blood transfusion may lead to the development of GVHD in the recipient. The development of TA-GVHD depends on the following factors: the degree to which the recipient is immunocompromised, the number and viability of lymphocytes in the transfused component, and the degree of HLA similarity between donor and recipient. The observation of TA-GVHD with the use of fresh blood components from blood relatives has highlighted the pathogenic role of the HLA system.

Figure 19-5 illustrates the conditions for increased risk for TA-GVHD. The parents have one HLA haplotype in common. Each child, therefore, has one chance in four of inheriting the same haplotype from each parent, and child 1 is homozygous for the shared parental HLA haplotype. Transfusion of blood from this person to an unrelated recipient with different haplotypes would have no untoward consequences. If, however, child 1 were a directed donor for a relative who was heterozygous for that haplotype (eg, either parent or child 3), the recipient would fail to recognize the antigens on the transfused lymphocytes as foreign and would not eliminate them. The donor cells would recognize the recipient's other haplotype as foreign and would become activated, proliferate, and attack the host. If one is to avoid this situation, it is recommended that all cellular components from blood relatives be irradiated before transfusion. Other specially

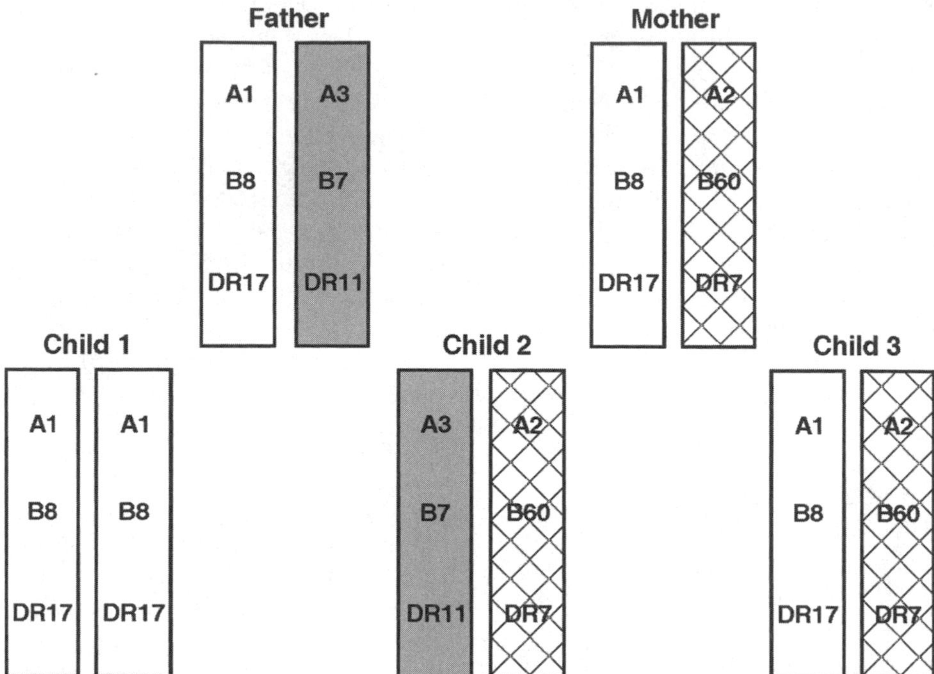

FIGURE 19-5. HLA haplotypes in a family at risk for transfusion-associated GVHD. In contrast to the family shown in Fig 19-2, each parent shares a common HLA haplotype, *HLA-A1,B8,DR17*. Child 1 is homozygous for the haplotype shared by the parents and by child 3. The lymphocytes of child 1 are capable of producing posttransfusion GVHD if transfused to either parent or to child 3.

chosen donor units, including HLA-matched platelets, may also present an increased risk for TA-GVHD. Rarely, TA-GVHD has occurred after the transfusion of blood from an unrelated donor, usually within populations with relatively limited genetic diversity such as in Japan.[22]

Chimerism is proposed to be responsible for the maintenance of tolerance in some organ transplant recipients[23] as well as for the maintenance of HLA sensitization.[24] It has been postulated that scleroderma is a form of GVHD resulting from chimeric cells derived from fetal cells transferred across the placenta during pregnancy.[25] Furthermore, the persistence of donor lymphocytes originally present in and transplanted with a solid organ allograft has been documented to cause fatal GVHD[26] in recipients of those organs.

Hemolytic Transfusion Reactions

HLA incompatibility has rarely been implicated as a cause of shortened red cell survival in patients with antibodies to HLA antigens such as Bg^a (B7), Bg^b (B17-B57 or B58), and Bg^c (A28-A68 or A69) that are expressed, although weakly, on red cells. Such an incompatibility may not be detected with conventional pretransfusion testing.

HLA TESTING AND TRANSPLANTATION

HLA testing is an integral part of solid organ and HPC transplantation. The extent of testing differs for different types of transplantation (see Chapters 29-32).

Hematopoietic Progenitor Cell Transplants

It has long been recognized that disparity within the HLA system represents an important barrier to successful HPC transplantation.[27] HLA similarity and compatibility between the donor and the recipient are required for engraftment and to help prevent GVHD, but some degree of rejection or GVHD remain as common problems for recipients of allogeneic HPCs, despite immunosuppressive conditioning.

Candidate donors and recipients are typed for their HLA-A, -B, -C, -DR, and -DQ alleles and, in some cases, for their HLA-DP alleles. The goal is to match the alleles of the prospective donor and recipient at the *HLA-A, -B, -C,* and *-DRB1* loci, with the optimal match being an allele-level match.[28] Some transplant programs additionally attempt to match for HLA-DQ or -DP alleles, or both. Molecular HLA typing is performed on samples from both the donor and recipient for optimal assessment of Class I and Class II region compatibility. Although HLA-identical sibling donors remain the best choice for HPC transplantation, there is increasing use of unrelated donors identified by searching the files of more than 7 million HPC donors listed in the National Marrow Donor Program's registry of volunteer donors or other international registries. The use of umbilical cord HPCs and HPC grafts from mismatched donors that have undergone T-cell depletion may allow greater donor-recipient mismatches.[29,30]

Kidney Transplants

ABO compatibility is considered the most important factor determining the immediate fate of kidney transplants. Because ABH antigens are expressed in varying amounts on all cells of the body, transplanted ABO-incompatible tissue comes into continuous contact with the recipient's ABO antibodies. Of particular importance is the expression of ABH antigens on vascular endothelial cells because the vascular supply in the transplant is a common site for rejection. Currently, the use of A_2 blood group organs for group B and group O recipients with low anti-A blood group titers has become an acceptable procedure.[31,32] In fact, several transplantation programs have used ABO-incompatible donors with higher anti-A titers following protocols that include various combinations of rituximab, splenectomy, plasmapheresis with intravenous immune globulin, and other treatments to remove preexisting antibodies and to promote accommodation of the transplanted organ.

Both the recipient and the donor are routinely typed for ABO, HLA-A, -B, and -DR antigens. HLA-C and -DQ typing is usually also performed. Before surgery, a crossmatch between recipient serum and donor lymphocytes is required. ASHI *Standards for Accredited Laboratories*[33] requires that the crossmatch be performed using a method more sensitive than routine microlymphocytotoxicity testing, such as prolonged incubation, washing, augmentation with AHG reagents, or flow cytometry. Flow cytometry is the most sensitive method and has been credited with predicting early acute rejection and delayed graft function, both of which are strong predictors of chronic rejection (if results are positive) and long-term allograft survival (if results are negative).[34] In patients undergoing deceased-donor kidney retransplantation, the 7-year graft survival rate using a negative T-cell flow crossmatch to select the donor kidney was comparable to that of patients undergoing primary deceased-donor transplantation (68% vs 72%) and was significantly better than that of regraft patients for whom only the antiglobulin lymphocytotoxicity crossmatch was used (45%).[35] Because HLA antibody responses are dynamic, the serum used for the crossmatch is often obtained within 48 hours of surgery for sensitized potential recipients and is retained in the frozen state for any required subsequent testing. An incompatible crossmatch with unfractionated or T lymphocytes is typically a contraindication to kidney transplantation. A positive B-cell crossmatch is significant when caused by donor-specific HLA Class I or Class II antibodies.

Serum from a patient awaiting deceased-donor kidney transplant surgery is tested at regular intervals for the degree of alloimmunization by determining the percent PRA as well as the specificities of the detected antibodies. If an antibody with a defined HLA specificity is identified in a recipient, common practice is to avoid donors who express the corresponding HLA antigen(s). Such antigens are deemed "unacceptable." More recently, using solid-phase assays to identify HLA antibodies and unacceptable antigens, a patient's "PRA" is calculated (cPRA) using a database of over 12,000 HLA typed donors.[36] The serum samples used for periodic PRA testing are often stored frozen so that "historic" samples with the highest PRA can be used in addition to the preoperative sample for pretransplantation crossmatching. Prospective crossmatching is not typically performed for recipients who are conclusively devoid of HLA antibodies (ie, cPRA = 0%). Prompt transplantation with reduced cold ischemia time for the renal allograft may provide greater benefit to the patient than prospective crossmatching, provided that 1) a very sensitive method for antibody detection, such as flow cytometry or microarrays, has been used,[37] and 2) it is certain that the patient has had no additional sensitizing event (ie, immunization or transfusions within 2 weeks before or at any time since that serum was screened).

The approach to kidney transplants with living donors is different. In the past, when several prospective living donors were being considered, MLC testing between the recipient and the donors was sometimes performed, but that is rarely (if ever) the situation today. HLA matching of recipients with kidney donors (both living and deceased donors) contributes to long-term allograft survival by decreasing the likelihood of chronic rejection. According to the Scientific Registry for Transplant Recipients (SRTR: www.ustransplant.org), recent 1-year graft survival rates from living and deceased renal donors were 96.5% and 91.7%, respectively, and the half-lives of living-donor and deceased-donor renal allografts were 21.6 years and 13.8 years, respectively.

The significantly better graft survival for recipients of living vs deceased donor renal allografts, even when donors are completely unrelated,[38] coupled with inadequate numbers of deceased organ donors has led to a relatively new practice, namely, paired donor exchange (PDE). Recently, PDEs have been facilitated through local and national registries, permitting patients with ABO- or HLA-incompatible potential living donors to exchange those donors with the donors of other patients in the same situation. As a simple example, a blood group A transplant candidate with an incompatible blood group B potential living kidney donor could exchange donors with a blood group B transplant candidate with an incompatible blood group A potential living kidney donor. Patients with HLA-incompatible potential donors have similar possibilities for donor exchange, and multiple "pairs" can be involved in one continuous exchange (chain) process. The introduction of altruistic donors (ie, individuals who choose to donate a kidney without having a specific recipient) can significantly expand the PDE process. Briefly described, the altruistic donor donates a kidney to a patient with an incompatible potential living donor who then donates to a different recipient with an incompatible donor, starting a "chain" with the possibility for a large number of living donor transplants. One chain of 10 transplants was recently reported.[39]

Other Solid Organ Transplants

For liver, heart, lung, and heart/lung transplants, ABO compatibility remains the primary immunologic system for donor selection, and determining pretransplant ABO compatibility between donor and recipient is mandatory. However, it has been shown that young pediatric heart or liver transplant recipients, who have low levels of ABO isoagglutinins, have successful outcomes with ABO-incompatible hearts[40] or livers.[41] Although it is not a requirement, HLA typing of potential recipients of the above organs is recommended. Furthermore, a crossmatch should be available before transplantation when the recipient has demonstrated presensitization, except for emergency situations. Although a degree of HLA compatibility correlates with graft survival after heart, lung, small intestine, and liver transplantations, prospective HLA matching is generally not performed.[42]

Relationship and Other Forensic Testing

HLA typing (particularly DNA-based HLA typing) has proven useful in forensic testing. Although rarely used now for relationship testing, DNA-based HLA typing alone can exclude greater than 90% of falsely accused males. Haplotype frequencies, rather than gene frequencies, are used in such calculations because linkage disequilibrium is very common in the HLA system. It is important, however, to consider the racial differences that exist in HLA haplotype frequencies in the calculations used; the possibility for recombination events should also be considered.

Other useful DNA-based assays for forensic detection of polymorphisms between individuals are the variation in the number of short tandem repeats (STRs), which assess other polymorphic, non-HLA genetic regions, and single nucleotide polymorphisms (SNPs). DNA-based assays, including HLA typing, allow identification of individuals on the basis of extremely small samples of fluid or tissue, such as hair, epithelial cells, or semen.

OTHER CLINICALLY SIGNIFICANT ASPECTS OF HLA

For some conditions, especially those believed to have an autoimmune etiology, an association exists between HLA phenotype and the occurrence of, or resistance to, clinical disease (see Table 19-3).[42-45] HLA-associated disease susceptibilities have several features in common. The susceptibilities are known or suspected to be inherited, display a clinical course with acute exacerbations and remissions, and usually have characteristics of autoimmune disorders; also, often their exact cause is unknown. Evidence has been accumulating that implicates the HLA molecules themselves, rather than linked genes, in most cases of disease susceptibility. One mechanism that could lead to the association of HLA phenotype and disease is the presence of a Class I or Class II heterodimer encoded by a specific allele that preferentially presents autoantigens to the TCR.

The ancestral haplotype *A1, B8, DR17 (DRB1*03:01), DQ2* discussed previously (under "Linkage Disequilibrium") is associated with susceptibility to Type I diabetes, systemic lupus erythematosus, celiac disease, common variable immunodeficiency, IgA deficiency, and myasthenia gravis, and also to an acceler-

TABLE 19-3. HLA-Associated Diseases

Disease	HLA	RR[42-44]
Celiac disease	DQ2	>250
Ankylosing spondylitis	B27	>150
Narcolepsy	DQ6	>38
Subacute thyroiditis	B35	14
Type 1 diabetes	DQ8	14
Multiple sclerosis	DR15, DQ6	12
Rheumatoid arthritis	DR4	9
Juvenile rheumatoid arthritis	DR8	8
Grave disease	DR17	4

RR = relative risk.

ated course of HIV infection, which is likely caused by the presence of multiple genes.[46] However, HLA typing has only limited value in assessing risk for most diseases because the association is incomplete. The association of HLA-B27 and ankylosing spondylitis in patients of European ancestry is instructive. The test is highly sensitive; more than 90% of patients with ankylosing spondylitis possess the HLA-B27 antigen. Conversely, specificity is low; only 20% of individuals with the B27 antigen will develop ankylosing spondylitis. A second condition, narcolepsy, is strongly associated with the HLA allele *DQB1*06:02*.[47] As with the case of HLA-B27 and ankylosing spondylitis, more than 90% of individuals with narcolepsy are positive for *HLA-DQB1*06:02*, but only a minority of individuals with that HLA allele develop the disease. For some autoimmune diseases, the specific peptide that might trigger the autoimmune response is at least tentatively identified: a gluten peptide, gliadin, for celiac disease[48]; cyclic citrullinated peptides for rheumatoid arthritis[49]; and a peptide from glutamic acid decarboxylase for Type I diabetes.[50]

In relation to disease resistance, resistance to cerebral malaria seems to result from a strong cytotoxic T-cell response to particular malarial peptides that are restricted by (ie, fit into the peptide-binding grooves of) two specific HLA molecules.[51]

A similar peptide binding specificity is important in consideration of the development of vaccines—for example, a vaccine to enhance immune responses to melanoma using a melanoma-specific peptide that binds only to the cells of individuals with the HLA type HLA-A*0201.[52]

HLA is also important in pharmacogenomic applications. For example, the presence of certain HLA phenotypes confers an increased sensitivity to some specific drugs: *HLA-B*57:01* confers sensitivity to the drug abacavir; *HLA-B*15:02*, to the drug carbamazepine; and *HLA-B*58:01*, to the drug allopurinol.[53,54]

The degree of association between a given HLA type and a disease is often described in terms of relative risk (RR), which is a measure of how much more frequently a disease occurs in individuals with a specific HLA type than in individuals not having that HLA type. Calculation of RR is usually based on the cross-product ratio of a 2 × 2 contingency table. However, because the HLA system is so polymorphic, there is an increased possibility of finding an association between an HLA antigen and a disease by chance alone. Therefore, calculation of RR for HLA disease associations is more complex and is typically accomplished by use of Haldane's modification of Woolf's formula.[55,56] The RR values for some diseases associated with HLA are shown in Table 19-3.

SUMMARY

In conclusion, the HLA system represents a complex and highly polymorphic set of genes that collectively are involved in all aspects of the immune response. The recent development of molecular tools to explore this genetic oasis is providing additional information such as the elucidation of unrecognized polymorphisms within the HLA complex (ie, SNPs). In the future, perhaps the translation of this basic information will lead to novel clinical applications in organ transplantation, autoimmunity, and infectious diseases.

KEY POINTS

1. Genes encoded by the major histocompatibility complex (or HLA complex in humans) are critical components of the immune system, distinguishing self from non-self.
2. HLA genes are located within multiple loci on chromosone 6. Each locus is extremely polymorphic.
3. HLA genes encode multiple Class I (eg, HLA-A, HLA-B, HLA-C) and Class II (eg, HLA-DR, HLA-DQ, and HLA-DP) cell surface proteins.

4. Class I proteins are expressed ubiquitously, while Class II proteins have a restricted tissue distribution.
5. Every individual inherits a set of HLA genes from his or her mother and father referred to as a maternal and paternal haplotype, respectively.
6. Together, the maternal and paternal haplotypes are referred to as a genotype. The cell surface expression of proteins encoded by those HLA genes is referred to as a phenotype.
7. Class I and Class II HLA proteins are strongly immunogenic and can induce an immune response, eg, HLA antibodies.
8. Donor-directed HLA antibodies are associated with graft dysfunction and/or survival.
9. Solid-phase assays (eg, flow cytometry, Luminex) have become the gold standard to detect and identify HLA antibodies.
10. Identification of donor directed HLA antibodies can be used to perform a virtual (in silico) crossmatch.

REFERENCES

1. Holdsworth R, Hurley CK, Marsh SG, et al. The HLA dictionary 2008: A summary of HLA-A, -B, -C, -DRB1/3/4/5, and -DQB1 alleles and their association with serologically defined HLA-A, -B, -C, -DR, and -DQ antigens. Tissue Antigens 2009;73:95-170.
2. Marsh SG, Albert ED, Bodmer WF, et al. Nomenclature for factors of the HLA system, 2010. Tissue Antigens 2010;75:291-455.
3. Janeway CA, Travers P, Walport M, et al. The immune system in health and disease. 5th ed. New York: Garland Science, 2001.
4. Braud VM, Allan DSJ, McMichael AJ. Functions of nonclassical MHC and non-MHC-encoded class I molecules. Curr Opin Immunol 1999;11:100-8.
5. Feder JN, Gnirke A, Thomas W, et al. A novel MHC class I-like gene is mutated in patients with hereditary haemochromatosis. Nat Genet 1996;13:399-408.
6. Bodmer JG, Parham P, Albert ED, Marsh SG. Putting a hold on "HLA-H." Nat Genet 1997;15:234-5.
7. Termijtelen A, Meera Khan P, Shaw S, van Rood JJ. Mapping SB in relation to HLA and GLO1 using cells from first-cousin marriage offspring. Immunogenetics 1983;18:503-12.
8. Buchler T, Gallardo D, Rodriguez-Luaces M, et al. Frequency of HLA-DPB1 disparities detected by reference strand-mediated conformation analysis in HLA-A, -B, and -DRB1 matched siblings. Hum Immunol 2002;63:139-42.
9. International Immunogenetics Project, IMGT/HLA database. Release 3.2.0, 15 October 2010. Cambridge, UK: European Bioinformatics Institute, 2010. [Available at http://www.ebi.ac.uk/imgt/hla (accessed December 10, 2010).]
10. McDonald JC, Adamashvili I. Soluble HLA: A review of the literature. Hum Immunol 1998;59:387-403.
11. Ghio M, Contini P, Mazzei C, et al. Soluble HLA class 1, HLA class II, and Fas ligand in blood components: A possible key to explain the immunomodulatory effects of allogeneic blood transfusion. Blood 1999;93:1770-7.
12. Voorter CE, van der Vlies S, Kik M, van den Berg-Loonen EM. Unexpected Bw4 and Bw6 reactivity patterns in new alleles. Tissue Antigens 2000;56:363-70.
13. Zinkernagel RM, Doherty PC. The discovery of MHC restriction. Immunol Today 1997;18:14-17.
14. Phelan DL, Mickelson EM, Noreen HS, et al, eds. ASHI laboratory manual. 4th ed. Mt. Laurel, NJ: American Society for Histocompatibility and Immunogenetics, 2001.
15. Petrik J. Microarray technology: The future of blood testing? Vox Sang 2001;80:1-11.
16. Welsh K, Bunce M. Molecular typing for the MHC with PCR-SSP. Rev Immunogenet 1999;1:157-76.
17. Bray RA, Gebel HM. Strategies for human leukocyte antigen antibody detection. Curr Opin Organ Transplant 2009;14:392-7.
18. Triulzi DJ, Dzik WH. Leukocyte-reduced blood components: Laboratory and clinical aspects. In: Simon TL, Snyder EL, Solheim BG, et al, eds. Rossi's principles of transfusion medicine. 4th ed. Bethesda, MD: AABB Press, 2009:228-46.

19. Duquesnoy R. Structural epitope matching for HLA-alloimmunized thrombocytopenic patients: A new strategy to provide more effective platelet transfusion support. Transfusion 2008; 48:221-7.
20. Friedberg RC. Independent roles for platelet crossmatching and HLA in the selection of platelets for alloimmunized patients. Transfusion 1994;34:215-20.
21. Kopko PM, Popovsky MA, MacKenzie MR, et al. HLA class II antibodies in transfusion-related acute lung injury. Transfusion 2001;41: 1244-8.
22. Gorman TE, Julius CJ, Barth RF, et al. Transfusion-associated graft-vs-host disease. A fatal case caused by blood from an unrelated HLA homozygous donor. Am J Clin Pathol 2000; 113:732-7.
23. Starzl TE, Demetris AJ, Murase N, et al. Chimerism after organ transplantation. Curr Opin Nephrol Hypertens 1997;6:292-8.
24. Sivasai KSR, Jendrisak M, Duffy BF, et al. Chimerism in peripheral blood of sensitized patients waiting for renal transplantation. Transplantation 2000;69:538-44.
25. Artlett CM, Smith JB, Jimenez SA. Identification of fetal DNA and cells in skin lesions from women with system sclerosis. N Engl J Med 1998;338:1186-91.
26. Pollack MS, Speeg KV, Callander NS, et al. Severe, late-onset graft vs. host disease in a liver transplant recipient documented by chimerism analysis. Hum Immunol 2005;66:28-31.
27. Thomas ED. Bone marrow transplantation: A review. Semin Hematol 1999;36:95-103.
28. Mickelson EM, Petersdorf E, Anasetti PM, et al. HLA matching in hematopoietic cell transplantation. Hum Immunol 2000;61:92-100.
29. Kurtzberg J, Laughlin M, Graham ML, et al. Placental blood as a source of hematopoietic stem cells for transplantation into unrelated recipients. N Engl J Med 1996;335:157-66.
30. Aversa F, Tabilio A, Velardi A. Treatment of high-risk acute leukemia with T cell depleted stem cells from related donors with one fully mismatched HLA haplotype. N Engl J Med 1998;339:1186-93.
31. Bryan CF, Winklhofer FT, Murillo D, et al. Improving access to kidney transplantation without decreasing graft survival: Long-term outcomes of blood group A2/A2B deceased donor kidneys in B recipients. Transplantation 2005; 80:75-80.
32. Tyden G, Donauer J, Wadstrom J, et al. Implementation of a protocol for ABO-incompatible kidney transplantation—a three-center experience with 60 consecutive transplantations. Transplantation 2007; 83:1153-5.
33. Standards for accredited laboratories. Mt. Laurel, NJ: American Society for Histocompatibility and Immunogenetics, 2009.
34. Bryan CF, Baier KA, Nelson PW, et al. Long-term graft survival is improved in cadaveric renal retransplantation by flow cytometric crossmatching. Transplantation 2000;66: 1827-32.
35. Taylor CJ, Smith SI, Morgan CH, et al. Selective omission of the donor crossmatch before renal transplantation: Efficacy, safety, and effects of cold storage time. Transplantation 2000;69: 719-23.
36. Cecka JM. Calculated PRA (CPRA): The new measure of sensitization for transplant candidates. Am J Transplant 2010;10:26-9.
37. Gebel HM, Bray RA. Sensitization and sensitivity: Defining the unsensitized patient. Transplantation 2000;69:1370-4.
38. Terasaki PI, Cecka JM, Gjertson DW, Takemoto S. High survival rates of kidney transplants from spousal and living unrelated donors. N Engl J Med 1995;333:333-6.
39. Rees MA, Kopke JE, Pelletier RP, et al. A nonsimultaneous, extended, altruistic-donor chain. N Engl J Med 2009;360:1096-101.
40. Daebritz SH, Schmoeckel M, Mair H, et al. Blood type incompatible cardiac transplantation in young infants. Eur J Cardiothorac Surg 2007;31:339-43. [See comment in Eur J Cardiothorac Surg 2007;31:343.]
41. Heffron T, Welch D, Pillen T, et al. Successful ABO-incompatible pediatric liver transplantation utilizing standard immunosuppression with selective postoperative plasmapheresis. Liver Transpl 2006;12:972-8.
42. Ketheesan N, Tay GK, Witt CS, et al. The significance of HLA matching in cardiac transplantation. J Heart Lung Transplant 1999;18:226-30.
43. Thorsby E. Invited anniversary review: HLA associated diseases. Hum Immunol 1997;53:1-11.
44. Pile KS. HLA and disease associations. Pathology 1999;31:202-12.
45. Howell WM, Jones DB. The role of human leukocyte antigen genes in the development of malignant disease. J Clin Pathol Mol Pathol 1995;48:302-6.

46. Price P, Witt C, Allcock R, et al. The genetic basis for the association of the 8.1 ancestral haplotype (A1, B8, DR3) with multiple immunopathological diseases. Immunol Rev 1999;167: 257-74.
47. Pelin Z, Guilleminault C, Risch N, et al. HLA-DQB1*0602 homozygosity increases relative risk for narcolepsy but not for disease severity in two ethnic groups. US Modafinil in Narcolepsy Multicenter Study Group. Tissue Antigens 1998;51:96-100.
48. Cinova J, Palova-Jelinkova L, Smythies LE, et al. Gliadin peptides activate blood monocytes from patients with celiac disease. J Clin Immunol 2007;27:201-9.
49. Van Gaalen FA, van Aken J, Huizinga TW, et al. Association between HLA class II genes and autoantibodies to cyclic citrullinated peptides (CCPs) influences the severity of rheumatoid arthritis. Arthritis Rheum 2004;50:2113-21.
50. Mayr A, Schlosser M, Grober N, et al. GAD autoantibody affinity and epitope specificity identify distinct immunization profiles in children at risk for type 1 diabetes. Diabetes 2007; 56:1527-33.
51. Hill AV. The immunogenetics of resistance to malaria. Proc Assoc Am Physicians 1999;111: 272-7.
52. Slingluff CL Jr, Yamshchikov G, Neese P, et al. Phase I trial of a melanoma vaccine with gp100(280-288) peptide and tetanus helper peptide in adjuvant: Immunologic and clinical outcomes. Clin Cancer Res 2001;7:3012-24.
53. Hughes DA, Vilar FJ, Ward CC, et al. Cost-effectiveness analysis of HLA B*5701 genotyping in preventing abacavir hypersensitivity. Pharmacogenetics 2004;14:335-42.
54. Chung W-H, Hung S-I, Chen YT. Human leukocyte antigens and drug hypersensitivity. Curr Opin Allergy Clin Immunol 2007;7:317-23.
55. Haldane JBS. The estimation and significance of the logarithm of a ratio of frequencies. Ann Hum Genet 1955;20:309-11.
56. Woolf B. On estimating the relation between blood groups and disease. Ann Hum Genet 1955;19:251-3.

Chapter 20

Hemotherapy Decisions and Their Outcomes

Theresa Nester, MD, and James P. AuBuchon, MD

TRANSFUSION, LIKE ANY other medical intervention, carries with it both benefits and risks that must be balanced for each patient. Although myriad situations in which transfusion might be considered prevent the promulgation of "one size fits all" transfusion guidelines, the growing accumulation of data in the medical literature can certainly help inform hemotherapy decisions so that patient therapy is based on increasingly sound evidence.

This chapter provides a review of the current literature regarding the indications for and outcomes of transfusion of blood components. When used in combination with information presented elsewhere in the *Technical Manual* regarding the content of blood components and the risks they pose, this chapter provides physicians with sufficient data to make evidence-based decisions in hemotherapy.

RED CELL TRANSFUSION

It is axiomatic that the impetus for red cell transfusion is predicated on the need to increase oxygen delivery to key tissues. However, assessing whether an oxygen delivery deficiency exists and whether it is best remedied by transfusion are difficult decisions, too complex to be based, for example, on a single hemoglobin concentration determination.

Resuscitation in Acute Anemia

With 50% to 65% of red cell transfusions occurring in surgery, and about 30% occurring in intensive care units, clearly the vast majority of transfusion decisions are made in "acute" settings. Acutely bleeding patients have not had sufficient time to engage all compensatory mechanisms, such as increased 2,3-diphosphoglycerate (2,3-DPG) synthesis. Furthermore, they may also be suffering from concomitant hypovolemia and may have multiple organ system dysfunction. At the same time, estimation of the amount of blood lost (except in surgical settings) is fraught with inexactitude. The symptoms and signs of anemia—including weakness, headache, dizziness, disorientation, dyspnea, palpitations, tachycardia,

Theresa Nester, MD, Associate Medical Director, Puget Sound Blood Center, and Associate Professor of Laboratory Medicine, University of Washington, and James P. AuBuchon, MD, President and Chief Executive Officer, Puget Sound Blood Center, and Professor of Medicine and of Laboratory Medicine, University of Washington, Seattle, Washington

The authors have disclosed no conflicts of interest.

angina, and pallor—must be distinguished from a similar set related to hypovolemia (Table 20-1). Hypotension, with both reduced arterial and central venous pressure; acidosis; and decreased urinary output are often the primary distinguishing features of acute blood loss. Even in a healthy patient, the loss of 30% of one's blood volume acutely overwhelms the compensatory mechanisms, and shock sets in.

The primary goal of acute treatment is the restoration of blood volume through control of hemorrhage and replacement of intravascular volume. Given the hemoglobin reserve of approximately 50% that is available in most patients, and the more ready availability, lower cost, and greater safety of nonblood solutions, resuscitation is usually performed first with crystalloids. Although crystalloids redistribute rapidly outside the vascular space, many regard them as the best first line of correction for hypovolemia. Ultimately, colloids such as hydroxyethyl starch, dextran solutions, or albumin, all of similar safety and efficacy, may be needed to maintain sufficient intravascular volume. Of course, the patient may well need plasma for procoagulant replenishment by this point. The slow pace of "natural" reconstitution of blood volume after acute blood loss should be recognized so as not to underestimate the extent of the blood loss.[1] For example, loss of 1000 mL may require more than 72 hours for complete compensation,[2,3] and thus the hematocrit (or hemoglobin) cannot be followed as an indicator of the patient's status. Furthermore, partial compensation and return of the systolic blood pressure to near normal levels (100 mm Hg) may not reflect the limited reserve that has been reestablished, and quick decompensation of the patient is possible on standing or further blood loss.[4] The effect of

TABLE 20-1. Signs and Symptoms of Anemia vs Acute Blood Loss

Symptom	Anemia	Hypovolemia
Tachycardia	X	X
Palpitations	X	X
Cooling of extremities		X
Pallor	X	X
Hypotension		X
Reduced arterial pressure		X
Reduced central venous (jugular) pressure		X
Acidosis		X
Increased respirations		X
Decline in urinary output		X
Mental status changes		X
Weakness	X	
Headache	X	
Dizziness	X	X
Disorientation	X	X
Dyspnea	X	
Angina	X	

transfusion on hemoglobin concentration, however, can be estimated accurately by measurement in as little as 15 minutes after transfusion.[5]

Once something close to normovolemia has been reestablished, the extent of the acute blood loss can be better understood, and the ability of the patient to withstand the anemia is more evident. [This is not to say that Red Blood Cells (RBCs) should not be transfused during rapid blood loss, but estimation of the amount that will be needed would require a projection of 1) the amount already lost, 2) the amount that will be lost before bringing the situation under control, and 3) the patient's ability to tolerate this level of anemia, separate from the hypovolemia.] Induction of normovolemic anemia in normal subjects (without known cardiovascular disease) has shown that a hemoglobin reduction to around 6 g/dL is well tolerated before oxygen delivery suffers (from limitations in cardiac output) and venous oxygen drops. An increase in cardiac output, the principal compensatory mechanism, is achieved primarily through increases in heart rate in healthy individuals,[6] as opposed to increased stroke volume in anesthetized patients.[7] By challenging normovolemic anemic subjects with arithmetic problems or reaction time tests or by measuring parameters of cardiovascular/cardiorespiratory function, the effects of oxygen deprivation become evident at hemoglobin between 5 and 6 g/dL. These deficits are recoverable on reinfusion of the red cells.[8-12] These studies parallel the observation that patients refusing transfusion on religious grounds and undergoing elective surgery without evidence of cardiovascular disease tolerate hemoglobin reductions to 6 to 7 g/dL with only a minimal rise in perioperative mortality risk.[13] Although many otherwise healthy adults can tolerate significant anemia equivalent to a halving of their red cell mass, co-morbidities in many patients may limit their reserve.

Thus, what should be the indication for red cell transfusion in the setting of acute anemia?

Patients studied immediately after surgical "correction" of their arteriosclerotic disease (that is, after revascularizing coronary artery bypass grafting, or CABG) appear to do well with a transfusion goal in the range of approximately 25% hematocrit (8 g/dL hemoglobin), with recovery times, exercise capacity, and fatigue assessment equivalent to those maintained at a higher hematocrits.[14] In fact, patients reaching the intensive care unit after CABG with hematocrits above 24% have been reported to have an increasing probability of Q-wave myocardial infarcts and evidence of left ventricular dysfunction, possibly because the optimal point in oxygen delivery (vs the work of moving the increasingly viscous blood) has been reached or surpassed.[15-16] A similar phenomenon was noted in end-stage renal disease patients whose anemia was being treated with erythropoietin to target hematocrits of either 30% or 42%; the latter group was trending toward an increased rate of death or myocardial infarction that prompted cessation of the trial.[17] However, the question of appropriate handling of patients with real or presumed coronary artery disease is less clear. An observational study of peripheral vascular disease patients[18] suggested that "morbid cardiac events" were confined to those with hematocrits ≤28%, but those patients also more frequently had evidence of anemia *and* ischemia before their peripheral vascular surgery, thus limiting the impact of the observation. In patients undergoing elective orthopedic surgery, the use of a transfusion threshold of 8 g/dL or the presence of symptomatic anemia obviated transfusion for 45% of patients and was not related to increased morbidity as compared to a threshold of 10 g/dL.[19] In fact, a similar group of patients had *longer* periods of ischemia when a transfusion threshold of 10 g/dL was applied as opposed to 8 g/dL.[20] Similarly, trauma patients were found to tolerate a hematocrit of 30% as well as 40%, apparently through increased oxygen extraction.[21] A randomized controlled trial of 7 vs 10 g/dL hemoglobin thresholds in critically ill patients, including those with atherosclerotic disease (but not acute, unstable myocardial situations), showed that the lower threshold reduced morbidity and mortality significantly overall; it was not associated with increased length of stay or morbidity in patients with heart disease nor prolonged ventilation time for those requiring a respirator.[22-24] These authors concluded that a threshold of 7 g/dL hemoglobin was appropriate across all critically ill patients, except perhaps those with unstable cardiac situations in whom there was a statistically nonsignificant trend toward increased mortality with the more restrictive threshold. Indeed, mortality in patients refusing transfusion on religious grounds who had evidence of arteriosclerotic vascular disease increased dramatically when preoperative anemia was present.[25] Below 8 g/dL, the mortality rate increased 2.5-fold for every decrease in hemoglobin of 1 g/dL. (However, these findings in adults may not be applicable to neonates, where use of a more restrictive threshold was associated with increased risk of intraventricular hemorrhage.[26])

Unfortunately, two large retrospective analyses of patients with acute coronary syndromes have not clarified the matter further. An analysis of a Medicare database indicated that lower hematocrits were associated in a stepwise fashion with increased mortality during admission for acute myocardial infarction.[27] Furthermore, transfusion when the admission hematocrit was below 30% was associated with an improvement in outcome even with adjustment for common comorbidities. However, the reanalysis of three studies involving such patients failed to identify any hematocrit, even to 20%, below which transfusion was associated with an improved outcome.[28,29] In fact, transfusion at 30% hematocrit was associated with a 169-fold *increase* in mortality. The patients who were transfused were older and had more comorbidities, indicative of the difficulties associated with retrospective analysis of complex medical situations.

Clearly, the requirement of achieving a hemoglobin ≥10 g/dL before general anesthesia that was previously promulgated has passed into antiquity (a passage endorsed by a National Institutes of Health consensus conference).[30] Gone also is the assumption that anemia slows healing [whereas oxygen partial pressure (pO_2) is a more important determinant than hemoglobin]. The most appropriate hemoglobin is understood to be a patient-specific (and even situation-specific) parameter. A hemoglobin <6 g/dL almost always requires transfusion, and a hemogloblin >10 g/dL rarely (but occasionally) requires intervention. Of course, most patients have a hemoglobin between these limits and may have one or more co-morbidities to cloud the issue of their tolerance of the situation. This is where the assemblage of experience and knowledge must still be blended as the "art of medicine." However, the fact that 21% of perioperative red cell transfusions in one study were given to patients with hemoglobin >10 g/dL, and a third of medical transfusions were given to patients with a hemoglobin >8 g/dL, demonstrates that there is substantial opportunity for integrating objective information into the hemotherapy decision-making process of many physicians.[31]

Transfusion in Chronic Anemia

Transfusion is much less commonly indicated when anemia has persisted for weeks or months, because compensatory mechanisms have had time to work. These anemias are usually best treated through addressing their etiologies, such as replacing a nutritional deficiency (eg, iron) or by reducing the rate of autoimmune hemolysis. Congenital hemoglobinopathies, such as sickle cell disease, are treated according to specific disease-related protocols for reasons not necessarily directly related to oxygen delivery. Hypoproliferative anemias secondary to chemotherapy or end-stage renal disease are often addressed through marrow stimulants such as recombinant erythropoietin. Any of these situations could conceivably necessitate a transfusion intervention if patient symptomatology requires more rapid reversal than can be effected by means directed at underlying mechanisms, but transfusion is usually considered only as a last resort. Some patients become transfusion-dependent because of their inability to create and maintain an adequate red cell mass, and these patients often "declare" the hemoglobin at which their symptoms are best controlled. The symptomatology reported by chronic anemia patients does not generally correlate well with laboratory values between patients but often corresponds well in an individual over time.

Selected Clinical Issues

Use of Whole Blood

Whole Blood provides oxygen-carrying capacity, stable coagulation factors (the concentrations of Factors V and VIII decrease during storage), and blood volume expansion. Thus, it is potentially useful for patients with concomitant red cell and volume deficits, such as actively bleeding patients, and will help support coagulation in appropriate clinical settings such as liver transplantation.[32] However, Whole Blood is rarely available for allogeneic transfusion; RBCs and asanguinous solutions have become the standard for most cases of active bleeding in trauma and surgery, with supplementation of hemostatic elements as needed. The major use of Whole Blood in the United States today is for autologous transfusion. Whole Blood must be ABO identical to the recipient.

Length of Storage

With the rapid disappearance of 2,3-DPG from stored red cells and the concomitant increase in hemoglobin's affinity for O_2, some have expressed concern that units stored for more than 1 to 2 weeks may not provide the intended increased availability of O_2 at the tissue level, at least for the first 12 to 24 hours after transfusion.[33,34] (Beyond 7-10 days of storage, the P_{50} of hemoglobin drops from 27 to 16 mm Hg, markedly shifting the dissociation curve to the left.) There are other known changes to red cells that occur with storage over time, sometimes referred to collectively as the "storage lesion." These include shape changes, decreased deformability of the red cell, and decreased adenosine triphosphate. Additionally, a loss of nitric oxide occurs within a few hours after collection.[35] Whether these changes are clinically important is unclear. A series of retrospective data exists, and the results show conflicting findings. In a rat model, exchange transfusion with DPG-depleted blood resulted in the supply dependency point of the oxygen utilization curve occurring at a higher hematocrit.[36] Subsequent retrospective observational studies suggested an increased rate of untoward outcomes in patients receiving older units, although this was attributable to increased comorbidities in this group in several studies.[37-40] A well-publicized retrospective analysis in cardiac surgery was difficult to interpret because of clinical differences in the two groups of patients.[40] A prospective, randomized, blinded study in critically ill patients failed to show any difference in key clinical outcomes associated with the transfusion of older vs "fresh" RBC units.[41] A small pilot study in critically ill and cardiac surgery patients actually demonstrated *higher* mortality rate in patients randomized to receive fresher units, although the two patient groups may have not been comparable.[42] Untoward effects of increased oxygen affinity may not be evident in relatively small-volume transfusions but might be expected to be more readily demonstrable in cases of massive transfusion, particularly if flow restrictions (eg, caused by atherosclerotic stenoses) were present or in cases of anemia that is initially more severe.[43,44] Opportunities to improve red cell storage to reduce the extent of the "storage lesion" and improve the preservation of 2,3-DPG continue to be pursued.[45]

ABO Matching

Although matching the patient and donor ABO groups will ensure compatibility in that blood group system, inventory considerations may suggest that an ABO-compatible rather than an ABO-identical unit should be transfused (Table 20-2). Although a compatible but non-identical unit will introduce some isoagglutinins directed against the recipient's A and/or B antigens, the small amount of plasma in an additive system or RBC unit (or even multiple units) is insufficient to cause hemolysis. Components containing larger amounts of plasma, such as platelets (see below) or Whole Blood units, raise the potential for these isoagglutinins to cause hemolysis. Consequently, Whole Blood, when used, would be transfused to an

TABLE 20-2. Selection of ABO-Compatible Red Blood Cell Units

Recipient Group	Compatible Red Blood Cells (additive solution units)
A	A, O
B	B, O
AB	AB, A, B, O
O	O

ABO-identical recipient. In the setting of ABO-incompatible heart transplantation to an infant, the transfusion service may be asked to plasma-reduce or wash an RBC unit. This is largely because the original protocol called for this modification, rather than solid evidence to indicate that incompatible passive ABO isoagglutinins can impair a new graft.[46]

Leukocyte Reduction

Whether all cellular components should have their white cells reduced in number remains controversial.[47-50] Although initially introduced in several European countries in the hope that it would decrease the transmission of prions, universal leukocyte reduction is most often spoken of as a way to reduce the risk of postoperative infection and improve posttransfusion survival through reduction in transfusion-related immunomodulation (TRIM). The benefit of removing leukocytes in patients who will be multitransfused and/or transplanted is clearly evident in terms of reduced rates of alloimmunization, decreased episodes of refractoriness to platelet transfusion, and fewer febrile reactions.[51-54] (Universal implementation of leukocyte reduction may not cause a measureable drop in febrile reaction rates, given the proportion of patients who are susceptible to such reactions.[55]) However, a positive clinical impact of universal leukocyte reduction has been difficult to identify and was not seen in the only large-scale, prospective randomized trial of its implementation.[56] Even in more defined situations, such as cardiac surgery, prospective trials have reached contradictory conclusions, even when performed by the same group.[57-60] The many retrospective analyses ascribing benefits to leukocyte reduction are often confounded,[61,62] although some do tantalize with strong arguments that removing leukocytes does lead to reduced length of stay, reduced infection, and improved outcome.[63,64] Other potential detriments associated with the presence of leukocytes in the component, such as increased red cell adhesive properties,[65] pose new questions about their impact. Several excellent meta-analyses and treatises offer a thorough examination of this complex subject.[66-69]

Many studies have investigated the possibility that leukocyte reduction can reduce the incidence of clinical outcomes caused by TRIM, but the results are contradictory.[61] One such proposal was that savings related to reduced immunomodulation could offset the costs of leukocyte reduction, but this was not demonstrable in a large prospective randomized trial.[63] Nonetheless, several countries have converted to a leukocyte-reduced blood supply, and this subject remains controversial.[64] Leukocyte reduction as a means of preventing cytomegalovirus (CMV) transmission has been well documented.[70]

The leukocyte content of units varies by their type[71-74] (Table 20-3). Current federal guidelines[73,74] and AABB *Standards for Blood Banks and Transfusion Services (Standards)*[75(pp26,28,29)] define a leukocyte-reduced component as one with $<5 \times 10^6$ residual donor leukocytes per final product (this includes RBCs, Apheresis Platelets, and Pooled Platelets). AABB *Standards*[75(p28)] requires $<8.3 \times 10^5$ leukocytes in Platelets Leukocytes Reduced, which are prepared from a single unit of Whole Blood, to achieve the requirement for a pool of 6 platelet units. Draft guidance from the Food and Drug Administration (FDA) recommends quality control to indicate with 95% confidence that at least 95% of units meet these criteria. By comparison, European guidelines define leukocyte-reduced components as those with $<1 \times 10^6$ residual leukocytes per unit and require that there should be no more than a 10% failure rate in the process.[76]

TABLE 20-3. Approximate Leukocyte Content of Blood Components (per unit)

Component	Leukocyte Content
Whole Blood	10^9
Red Blood Cells	10^8
Washed Red Blood Cells	10^7
Deglycerolized Red Blood Cells	10^6 to 10^7
Red Blood Cells Leukocytes Reduced (by filtration)*	$<5 \times 10^6$
Apheresis Platelets	10^6 to 10^8
Apheresis Platelets Leukocytes Reduced	$<5 \times 10^6$
Platelets†	10^7
Platelets Leukocyte Reduced	$<8.3 \times 10^5$
Pooled Platelets Leukocytes Reduced	$<5 \times 10^6$
Fresh Frozen Plasma (thawed)	$< 0.6 \times 10^6$ to 1.5×10^7

*Leukocyte reduction with third-generation leukocyte reduction filter.
†Derived from 1 unit of Whole Blood via platelet-rich plasma process.

Matching of Units to Patients' Hemoglobin Targets

For adult patients, the discussion of *when* or *whether* to transfuse red cells has usually not proceeded to a consideration of *how much* to transfuse. Although pediatricians commonly prescribe all medications, including blood components, based on the patient's size, the standard order for adult red cell transfusion has been 2 units regardless of patient size and usually without regard to a desired target hemoglobin. (The widely variable hemoglobin content of units is also usually not considered.[77]) Perhaps a more physiologic approach would be to identify the target hemoglobin desired *after* transfusion and then base the dose (ie, number of units or g of hemoglobin to be transfused) on the patient's current hemoglobin, any ongoing blood loss, and the calculated blood volume. The rationality of such an approach is acknowledged in the abandonment in recent years of automatic auditing for all transfusions of a single unit of RBCs, but the clinical import of such a change in transfusion philosophy remains to be investigated. In a pilot study based on this approach, however, it was shown that the number of units transfused to a group of patients could be reduced, thus reaping benefits in terms of inventory management as well as donor exposure rates.[78] It remains to be determined whether this approach can be implemented successfully across all patients in an institution, whether blood collection centers would be able to facilitate this effort by providing needed hemoglobin content information on all units, and whether the concept could be sustained in an era when more units are being produced by apheresis with a standardized hemoglobin content.

Emergency Transfusion

The unexpected need to transfuse (possibly a large amount of) red cells may require application of alternative procedures. Release of Group O red cells or antigen-negative uncrossmatched units may become necessary if waiting for completion of standard pretransfusion testing routines would risk anemic morbidity (see Chapter 15). An "emergency release" protocol might be used with one that allows rapid provision of a large number of units to accommodate the needs of patients who are bleeding rapidly. Elements of a "block release" system might include streamlined paperwork for multiple units, as well as "prepackaging" of these units to facilitate immediate delivery to the patient's side. The need for and components of such a system will vary according to the types of patients handled by the institution and the logistics of blood delivery. The expectations of clinicians (particularly surgeons, anesthesiologists, and emergency physicians) for rapid delivery of large volumes of red cells should be discussed so that appropriate requirements can be reliably met. In evaluating these clinical needs, attention should be given not only to the time required to issue blood from inventory to the door of the laboratory but also to the time required for it to finally reach the patient.

Transfusion When No Units Are "Compatible"

Occasionally, transfusion of red cells may be necessary when no serologically compatible RBC units are available for a patient. This most often occurs in patients with autoantibodies that typically react with all donors; however, so long as the presence of alloantibodies can be ruled out, the transfused cells would be expected to survive as long as autologous cells. The key point in ensuring a safe and successful transfusion in such a situation is the exclusion of the presence of alloantibodies. Because this may be difficult and the beneficial effects of the transfusion may be temporally limited, a conservative transfusion strategy is usually recommended in dealing with patients with autoimmune hemolytic anemia. Determination of the patient's phenotype before transfusion will simplify subsequent investigations for the presence of possible alloantibodies. (Chapters 15 through 17 contain a more complete discussion.)

Other situations in which all units appear incompatible include the presence of alloantibodies to high-frequency antigens and/or multiple antibody specificities.

If serologic testing fails to resolve the problem, or if the problem is identified but time is not sufficient for acquisition of compatible units, consultation between the transfusion service physician and the patient's clinician is advised to weigh the risks and benefits of transfusion and to consider what alternative therapies are suitable. If the need is sufficiently urgent, ABO-compatible but crossmatch-incompatible red cells may have to be given. Depending on the alloantibody's specificity (or the possible specificities that have not been ruled out), incompatible transfusion does not always result in immediate hemolysis, and the incompatible cells may remain in the circulation long enough to provide therapeutic benefit.[79]

If time permits and if equipment is available, the survival of a radiolabeled aliquot of the incompatible cells can be determined, but this is beyond the capability of most laboratories and is rarely needed. An "in-vivo crossmatch" can be performed by cautiously transfusing 25 to 50 mL of the incompatible cells, watching the patient's clinical response, and checking a 30-minute posttransfusion specimen for hemoglobin-tinged serum. Such assessment does not guarantee normal survival, but it can indicate whether an acute reaction will occur. If no adverse symptoms or hemolysis are observed, the remainder of the unit can be transfused slowly with careful clinical monitoring. If the transfusion need is life-threatening, RBC units may sometimes be given without special testing, but clinical staff should be prepared to treat any reaction that may result.

Red Cell "Substitutes"

A variety of means have been explored to provide hemoglobin's oxygen carrying capacity without using red cells. Development has proceeded furthest using hemoglobin solutions (derived from red cell lysates) in which the hemoglobin molecules have undergone one or more chemical modifications to optimize their oxygen dissociation and prevent renal damage. Two of the largest challenges with cell-free hemoglobin are its vasoconstrictive properties and its short half-life within the intravascular circulation. The goal of creating a hemoglobin substitute that the FDA considers to be as safe as donor red cells continues to be an elusive one.[80] (For a thorough review, see Winslow.[81])

PLATELET TRANSFUSION

Similar to the situation with red cells, there are many questions to be addressed when considering platelet transfusion.

Prophylactic vs Therapeutic Transfusion

Before the advent of platelet therapy, bleeding exceeded infection as the most common cause of death in patients with acute leukemia. The availability of platelet concentrates led to the natural consideration that prophylactic transfusion to prevent or limit the most severe depths of thrombocytopenia would prevent the onset of severe hemorrhage, and today, approximately 80% of all platelet transfusions are given to patients with hypoproliferative thrombocytopenia. However, the value of this approach has never been definitively documented. Early studies reached equivocal results or used statistical approaches that were less rigorous than would be expected today.[82,83] In fact, a randomized trial in leukemic children before the era of leukocyte reduction indicated that the use of prophylactic transfusion from the outset of chemotherapy increased the likelihood of bleeding (because of the development of refractoriness).[84] The alternative strategy of specifically directing platelet resources toward patients who are bleeding may be a wiser and more effective use of a limited resource.[85] In fact, a recent pilot study of prophylactic vs therapeutic platelet transfusions has suggested that the latter approach may not increase morbidity or mortality.[86] (This is being followed up with a more powerful study in an attempt to reach a definitive conclusion; an interim analysis is encouraging, indicating that a therapeutic transfusion strategy halves the number of platelet transfusions yet provides equivalent clinical outcomes.[87])

Overall, the role of prophylactic platelet transfusions for the prevention and control of thrombocytopenic bleeding is not yet clear. When identifying bleeding risk in thrombocytopenic patients, several factors in addition to platelet count should be considered. These include altered platelet function from intrinsic or acquired defects, and hemostatic defects involving the coagulation system. The disease process itself must also be considered. As an example, in acute leukemia, intracranial hemorrhage is more often associated with high circulating blast counts rather than low platelet counts.[88] The leukemic blasts may cause sludging of cells in capillaries and possible hemorrhagic infarction (particularly in the presence of a concomitant coagulopathy).

Transfusion Thresholds

If prophylactic transfusions are to be given to patients with hypoproliferative thrombocytopenia, what is the most appropriate threshold for transfusion? The first study to address this question sought to define a clinically useful threshold by observing and categorizing bleeding and to associate the risks of hemorrhage with patients' platelet counts.[88] These researchers were unable to define a clear platelet count threshold below which the risk of hemorrhage increased rapidly, but the paper was often cited as the source of the dictum that patients' platelet counts should be kept above 20,000/μL. (This study was conducted several years before the first observation of the effect of aspirin on platelet function.[89,90] Those neutropenic patients who were febrile undoubtedly received aspirin for their fevers, making the observations of the study not readily applicable to today's hematologic practice.[91]) Over the last decade several prospective studies using either historical or randomized control groups have documented successful application of 10,000/μL as a prophylactic transfusion threshold in inpatients.[84,92-96] These results parallel the finding that stool blood loss does not accelerate until a platelet count of approximately 5000/μL is reached.[97] Many institutions have now adopted 10,000/μL as their standard prophylactic transfusion threshold, but others have opted to combine laboratory data with the patient's clinical status to determine the most appropriate transfusion point[98] (Table 20-4). Furthermore, because platelets adsorb circulating thrombopoietin (TPO) and because higher platelet counts are associated with lower levels of free TPO,[99] maintaining patients at a lower platelet count has been suggested to lead to shorter intervals of thrombocytopenia, a potential additional benefit.

For patients who are already bleeding or who are about to undergo a hemostatic challenge (such as a surgical procedure), attempts are made to keep the platelet count higher, usually in the vicinity of 50,000/µL.[100] Although there are no trials to document this as the most appropriate level, it has become generally accepted as adequate.[101] An even higher target, up to 100,000/µL, is often used for intracerebral, pulmonary, and ophthalmic hemorrhage, not because 50,000/µL is inadequate to stop hemorrhage but because such a target gives a greater "cushion" to ensure adequate hemostasis in these vital and susceptible organs even if the platelet count should drop. Higher thresholds might also be used in massive transfusion or disseminated intravascular coagulation (DIC), where the platelet count may be dropping rapidly.

The role of anemia should also be considered in prevention (or treatment) of hemorrhage. Given their larger size and higher density, red cells tend to occupy the central (axial) portion of the blood flow, pushing platelets to the periphery in proximity with the vessel wall. This makes teleologic sense because it is only along the vessel wall that a rent in the endothelium can occur and where the platelets would then perform their hemostatic functions. In normal volunteers, reducing the hematocrit from 41% to 35% resulted in almost a doubling of their bleeding time, whereas decreasing their platelet count by a third had no effect.[102] Red cell transfusion or the administration of erythropoietin to increase the hematocrit in uremic patients similarly improved hemostasis.[103] Thus, although the patient's cardiovascular system might be tolerating the anemia associated with chemotherapy (or hemorrhage), the hemostatic system may be at a disadvantage.[104]

Transfusion to Correct Thrombocytopathy

Patients whose platelets are not able to complete all the complex metabolic steps necessary for activation, granular release, and aggregation may suffer from an increased likelihood of bleeding and/or an inability to respond to hemorrhage appropriately. These abnormalities may be congenital (eg, Glanzmann thrombasthenia) or may be acquired as the result of disease (eg, myelodysplasia) or drugs (eg, aspirin, GPIIb/IIIa antagonists). In addition, patients disconnecting from extracorporeal circulation (eg, cardiac bypass) may have platelet counts that appear to be adequate for hemostasis, but in fact their platelets may be dysfunctional because of prolonged exposure to

TABLE 20-4. Current Prophylactic Platelet Transfusion Thresholds

Patient Category	Platelet Count
All patients	10,000/µL
- or -	
Stable patient	5,000/µL
Patient with fever or recent hemorrhage (now stopped)	10,000/µL
Patient with coagulopathy, on heparin, or with anatomic lesion likely to bleed[98]	20,000/µL

Note: These levels are most commonly applied to inpatients. Adjustment of the transfusion threshold may be necessitated by unusual clinical situations.

roller pumps and foreign surfaces, leading to partial activation and degranulation.[105] In all of these circumstances, the decision to transfuse platelets will probably have to be based on the patient's clinical status rather than on the platelet count. Patients undergoing surgery while still under the effect of previously ingested aspirin do not necessarily bleed more than other patients, although physician knowledge that the patient has been taking aspirin has been associated with increased blood component usage.[106-111] The prophylactic use of platelets (and plasma) after cardiac surgery has been shown to be neither necessary nor beneficial, but a patient experiencing excessive blood loss postoperatively whose heparin has been completely reversed may benefit from a dose of platelets even before the postoperative platelet count is known. Patients who are given irreversible platelet antagonists (eg, clopidogrel) during cardiac catheterization and proceed directly to cardiac surgery may need one or more doses of platelets (as well as increased red cell transfusions) because their own platelets are no longer functional.[112,113] Such antiplatelet therapies continue to be used in catheterization because they appear to improve outcome even if the patient requires immediate surgery.[114] The effect of these drugs can be antagonized through pharmacologic intervention, including the use of desmopressin (DDAVP).[115]

Given the high proportion of patients receiving aspirin for a variety of reasons, bleeding patients on aspirin may be encountered frequently. Although the daily consumption of 81 mg aspirin for cardiac prophylaxis is unlikely to contribute to hemostatic difficulties, some patients are "hyperresponders" to aspirin and may have their bleeding times dramatically extended. Platelet transfusions are occasionally requested to correct the effect of aspirin. In these cases, only a small proportion (approximately 20%) of circulating platelets need to be functional in order to correct the deficiency,[116] so neither achievement of donor platelet levels of 50,000/μL nor a full therapeutic dose of platelets would be required in most patients to correct the situation.

Patients with significant renal disease (ie, a creatinine exceeding 3 mg/dL) may also have dysfunctional platelets. Transfusion of platelets into these patients is of little value, however, as the transfused platelets also rapidly succumb to the same metabolic derangement. DDAVP is usually recommended to augment the responsiveness of these platelets.[117] Alternatively, cryoprecipitate may provide the increased amount of von Willebrand factor that is believed helpful in activating these platelets[118] if tachyphylaxis to multiple doses of DDAVP precludes further treatment.[119] Dialysis to decrease the uremic environment is often indicated in clinical scenarios where optimal platelet function is desired.

Dosage

The amount of platelets to be considered a "therapeutic dose" remains undecided, but recent work is elucidating this topic.[120] Much early work was performed using platelet units with significantly lower platelet counts than units currently being produced. Initial platelet separation efficiencies were significantly lower than what has been achieved through evolutionary improvement in both component production processes and larger whole blood collections. Accordingly, many blood centers now report mean contents that are 20% to 40% above the required minimum of 5.5×10^{10} platelets per unit derived from whole blood. Thus, fewer units need to be pooled to obtain the same dose. At the same time, acceptance of lower platelet counts in patients has also facilitated the progressive reduction in the standard dose from 10 to 8 to 6 or even 4 units per pool (or transfusion).

The same question applies to platelets collected by apheresis. The standard of 3.0×10^{11} apheresis platelets per unit represents the amount that could be practically collected with early instruments, and it may also have represented the maximum time that donors would tolerate. These apheresis units gave an increment similar to the transfusion of a pool of 6 to 8 whole-blood-derived platelet components. However, since then, the increased efficiency of apheresis instruments allows the collection of two or even three times this quantity. Although blood centers derive a significant economic boost from "splitting" units, whether patients are better served by receiving larger units remains to be determined.

The question of optimal platelet dose has been approached in several ways. A mathematical model was used to calculate the fewest number of platelets that would need to be transfused if patients received just enough platelets to achieve the desired target level when they reached the transfusion threshold. This analysis argued for use of "small" therapeutic doses administered relatively more frequently.[121] The use of larger units in an actual clinical study resulted in longer intertransfusion intervals, although the relative size of this temporal increase was smaller than the increase in the number of platelets transfused.[122] In a paired study of marrow transplant patients, larger units were found to provide the expected lengthening of intertransfusion intervals and, unexpectedly, resulted in both count increments (CI) *and* corrected count increments (CCIs) that were higher than when using smaller units.[123]

The Strategies for Transfusion of Platelets (SToP) study[124] was a multicenter, prospective, randomized, controlled clinical trial that attempted to show that a lower dose for prophylactic platelet transfusions was not inferior to the standard dose usually given, with the outcome being incidence of bleeding categorized as World Health Organization (WHO) Grade 2 (or higher). Eligible hematopoietic stem cell transplant patients and nontransplant patients with chemotherapy-induced thrombocytopenia were enrolled. Subjects in the experimental arm received low-dose prophylactic platelet transfusions (1.5 to 2.9×10^{11} platelets per transfusion, defined as half the standard dose), and subjects in the control arm received a standard dose of platelets (3.0 to 6.0×10^{11} platelets per transfusion). Although sample size calculations indicated that approximately 270 patients would be necessary in each treatment arm, the study was stopped after enrollment of 130 patients. The study was stopped prematurely based on a preestablished safety threshold when the cumulative incidence of Grade 4 bleeding exceeded 5% between the two study arms. The main trends of this study suggested that the hypotheses that patients in the low-dose arm would require fewer units and have a shorter duration of thrombocytopenia were incorrect.

Another recent multicenter, prospective, randomized, controlled clinical trial called the Prophylactic Platelet Dose on Transfusion Outcomes (PLADO) study[125] did proceed to completion. Patients with hypoproliferative thrombocytopenia secondary to chemotherapy for hematologic malignancies or undergoing either autologous or allogeneic stem cell transplants were randomly assigned to receive one of three prophylactic platelet transfusion doses of 1.1 (low dose), 2.2 (medium dose), or 4.4×10^{11} (high dose) platelets/m^2. The patients were transfused with their assigned dose prophylactically for morning platelet counts of ≤10,000/µL. Additional platelet transfusions could be given for active bleeding or a planned invasive procedure. The primary endpoint of the study was the incidence of WHO Grade 2 or higher bleeding in patients stratified to receive one of three platelet doses. Of the 1272 patients who received at least one platelet transfusion, the percentage of patients in each group with at least one episode of such bleeding was 71%, 69%, and 70% in the low-, medium-, and high-dose groups, respectively. These results were not statistically different. Those in the low-dose arm did receive an average of one more platelet transfusion in their course, however.

As suggested by the above and previous studies, the life span of transfused platelets appears to be abnormally short in thrombocytopenic patients. Although platelets stored for 5 or 7 days and then reinfused autologously into normal subjects usually have survivals of more than 5 days, the life span of platelets in severely thrombocytopenic patients may only be about 2 days. This shortening may be attributable to the fixed loss of platelets from circulation of approximately 7100/µL/day for maintenance of normal hemostasis.[126] When the patient's platelet count is low (and of course still subject to daily reductions from senescence), this obligatory loss amounts to a large proportion of circulating platelets and leads to the need to transfuse every 2 to 3 days even in patients achieving good increments from transfusions.[127] More randomized, controlled clinical trials similar to the PLADO study are needed to clarify which dosage provides optimal hemostasis.

As with adult red cell transfusions, the size of the patients (and their spleens) are usually not considered in selecting the units to be transfused. One of the dose studies mentioned above attempted to set the dose based on patient weight, and the outcomes of the two studies may be helpful in determining the clinical importance of such a maneuver. The patient's size and the content of the unit are a routine part of the assessment of transfusion response through the CCI (Table 20-5). This measure, or a similar approach of calculating the "recovery" of transfused platelets based on content and blood volume,[128] can provide a yardstick to determine whether special efforts such as selection of antigen-negative units to combat alloimmunization may be helpful to the patient.

Unit Type and Age

The choice of which type of platelet unit to use for routine transfusion varies by institution. Currently, about 85% of platelet transfusions in the United States are derived from apheresis collections, and the usage rate of these platelets has increased in a steady, linear manner for two decades.[129] Local pricing policies and the preference of transfusion services to avoid the extra processing steps associated with whole-blood-derived units are probably significant factors in the choice (see Table 20-6). Some in-vitro measures identify a larger "platelet storage lesion" in platelets produced via the platelet-rich plasma (PRP) method than by apheresis,[130] and one paired reinfusion study has suggested superiority of apheresis platelets.[131] However, the radiolabeled autologous recovery and survival of the two types of platelets do not appear dissimilar even after 7

TABLE 20-5. Determination of Platelet Response

Corrected count increment (CCI)		
CCI = (CI × BSA)/unit content (× 10^{-11})		
Platelet recovery		
Platelet recovery (%) =	$\dfrac{\text{CI} \times (1000\ \mu\text{L/mL}) \times \text{blood volume in mL} \times 100}{\text{unit content}}$	
Sample calculations		
Patient mass = 80 kg: blood volume = 80 kg × 75 mL/kg = 6000 mL Patient body surface area: 2.0 m^2 (determined from a table or nomogram)		
Pretransfusion platelet count: Posttransfusion platelet count:	5000/µL 25,000/µL	➔ CI = 20,000/µL
Platelet count in unit: Volume of unit:	1.5 × 10^6/µL 267 mL	➔ Unit content = 4.0 × 10^{11} platelets
CCI = (20,000/µL × 2.0 m^2)/4.0 = 10,000		
Successful transfusion:	≥7500	
Refractory patient:	Two or more transfusions with CCI <5000	
Recovery = (20,000/µL × 1000 µL/mL × 6000 mL × 100%)/(4.0 × 10^{11}) = 30% Maximum achievable if patient has spleen: 65% to 70%		

TABLE 20-6. Comparison of Platelet Units Available in the United States

	Whole-Blood-Derived Platelets		
Characteristic	**Individual Unit**	**Prestorage Pooled***	**Apheresis Platelets**
Cost of preparation	Lower	Lower	Higher
Ease of bacteria testing	Lower	Higher	Higher
Ease of leukocyte reduction	Lower	Higher	Higher
Hospital preparation required	More	Less	Less
Donor exposures	Greater	Greater	Fewer
HLA selection possible	No	No	Yes
Platelet content known	No	No	Yes

*Storage of pools of platelets beyond 4 hours requires bacteria detection by an FDA-approved culture technique.

days of storage.[132,133] Platelets derived from whole blood buffy coats may have some advantages, such as less activation during centrifugal preparation steps, but these platelets are currently not available in the United States (although they are probably the most widely used platelet component around the world). From a clinical efficacy standpoint, all three platelet preparations give good clinical results.

All platelet unit types accumulate a "storage lesion" that leaves them less responsive to physiologic agonists. Typically, these platelets also bear markers of platelet activation, although none of these has proven a useful predictor of recovery or survival after transfusion.[134-137] Thus, studies using reinfusion of radiolabeled platelets at the limit of the storage period are commonly required for FDA licensure of new means of collecting or storing platelets. Both recovery and survival appear to shorten with increased storage time in such radiolabeling studies. However, not all series of clinical observations have been able to document a decrement in CCI with increased storage time, perhaps because of limited study sizes and the inherent variability between patients and between the outcomes of transfusions occurring at different points in the course of illness.[138,139] The useful observation that the response to platelet transfusions declines with increasing numbers of transfusions received (even in patients who are not alloimmunized) further complicates assessment of recipient response.[140,141] Therefore, transfusion of platelets in most institutions focuses on the most efficient use of the short-lived and scarce resource by transfusing the most appropriate unit that is closest to its outdate. Some patients may appear more sensitive to accumulation of the storage lesion than others and may benefit from receipt of platelets that have been stored for shorter periods; this can be determined only empirically.

"Out-of-Group" Transfusions

The importance of providing platelet transfusions using units of the same ABO group as the recipient is also an unresolved issue. There are several points to consider: 1) the presence of ABH antigens on platelets that could be targeted by the recipient's isoagglutinins; 2) the presence of plasma in the unit, which could lead to hemolysis of the recipient's red cells; and 3) the potential for immunologic effects of the incompatibility that could affect patient outcome. Typically, the presence of ABO-incompatible donor red cells in the platelet component is not a significant concern because they are present at very low levels.

Platelets bear ABO antigens both as intrinsic structures and as extrinsic ones, adsorbed from plasma.[142] They are thus subject to attack by recipient isoagglutinins. For the majority of patients, the posttransfusion recovery of ABO-compatible and -incompatible platelets are indistinguishable, but for a significant minority (20%-40%), possibly those with higher isoagglutinin titers encountering a unit with higher antigen expression,[143-145] a significantly lower recovery occurs when they receive platelets bearing incompatible ABO antigens, particularly from an A_1 donor.[146,147] Any diminution in response appears to be more pronounced with repeated out-of-group transfusions, possibly due to stimulation of higher isoagglutinin titers in the recipients.[148] If ABO-identical platelet units are transfused, this potential problem is avoided. Failure to achieve expected platelet increments with an out-of-group transfusion should prompt a trial of ABO-identical transfusions, particularly if the patient is not alloimmunized to platelet-specific or HLA antigens (see Fig 20-1).[149]

Until recently, all platelets transfused in the United States were suspended solely in plasma. An out-of-group platelet transfusion, such as a group O unit to a group A recipient, will result in the transfusion of about 300 mL of plasma containing isoagglutinins that are directed against antigens present on the recipient's red cells. Although it would not be considered standard practice to transfuse a group O plasma unit to a group A recipient, this practice *is* commonly performed under the rubric of platelet transfusion. Many patients show no signs or symptoms of the mismatch, although the majority may have a transiently positive direct antiglobulin test (DAT) that at least causes some immunohematologic confusion as to its source.[150] However, a donor with a high titer of isoagglutinins can cause hemolysis of recipient red cells that may be clinically significant and even fatal. This outcome may be more likely in situations where the recipient is smaller (and thus the volume transfused represents a greater proportion of the recipient's plasma volume), with apheresis units (where all the plasma is coming from the same donor and is not "diluted" by plasma of lower isoagglutinin titer from other units in the pool), and in situations of multiple transfusions.[151] The risk of hemolysis with apheresis platelet units is in the range of 1:3000 to 1:10,000.[152,153] The question of whether ABO-compatible but nonidentical plasma poses a

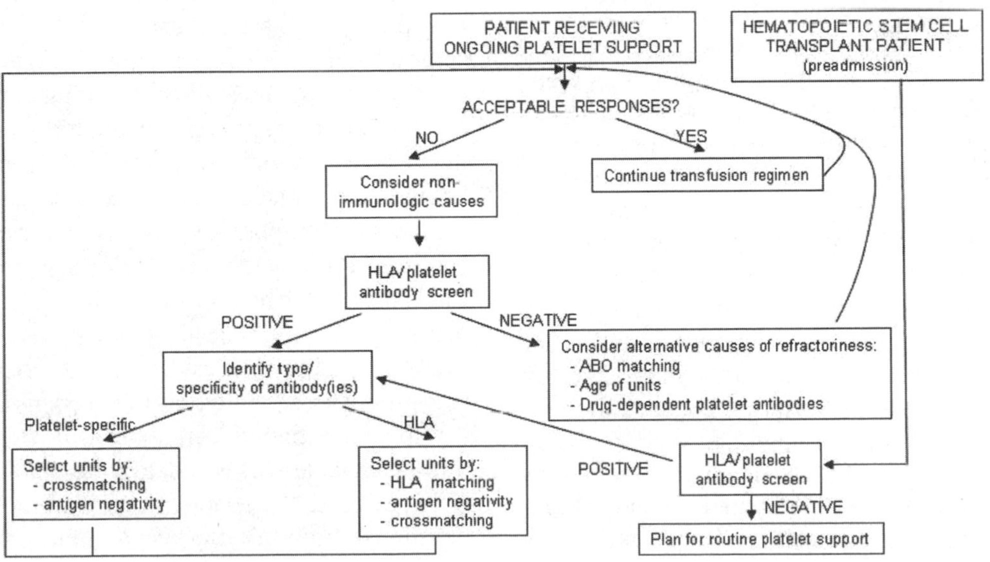

FIGURE 20-1. One approach to management of thrombocytopenic patients.

risk through circulating immune complexes has recently been raised.[154] The recent FDA approval of a platelet additive solution may eliminate some of these problems.

Different approaches may be used to prevent acute hemolysis when incompatible plasma must be transfused as part of a platelet transfusion. One approach is to limit the amount of plasma being transfused by centrifuging the unit and expressing off the majority of the plasma shortly before transfusion (see Method 6-14). This ameliorates the potential severity of any hemolysis but may not prevent it and, in any case, does result in the loss of some proportion of the platelet content of the unit. Another approach is to avoid out-of-group transfusion of units having a "dangerously high" titer of isoagglutinins. This approach usually involves identifying units with anti-A above a particular threshold, often a titer of 200. However, this approach lacks a solid evidence base, will vary by method,[155] and will not pick up all potentially "dangerous" donors.[156] Avoidance of out-of-group plasma or amelioration of the situation through volume reduction is an especially important issue for pediatric recipients, in whom the volume transfused is relatively greater, and in neonates, where hyperbilirubinemia may have particularly adverse consequences.

The possibility exists that the transfusion of incompatible plasma may also have other, less-immediate but still untoward effects on recipients' immune systems. For example, minimization of exposure to incompatible plasma was associated with improved survival probability in marrow transplant patients in one retrospective analysis, and another retrospective study suggested that such a strategy reduced in-hospital mortality after cardiac surgery by two-thirds.[157] This finding was not replicated in a subsequent, larger study, however.[158] There is also some suggestion that transfusion with ABO-incompatible platelets may hasten the development of alloimmunization and refractoriness[159] and may reduce survival after marrow transplantation.[160] Any delayed immunologic impact of the transfusion of mismatched plasma with platelets remains to be fully elucidated, although avoidance of out-of-group transfusion when possible would obviate concern. When transfusion is necessary, however, it should not be delayed to jeopardize the patient just for the sake of this issue.

Rh Matching

A small but immunogenic dose of red cells can be contained in a platelet transfusion. This is more likely in whole-blood-derived than apheresis platelet units (given their minuscule red cell content) but is at least theoretically possible with any platelet unit. Therefore, attempts are usually made to provide Rh-negative recipients with Rh-negative platelet units even though platelets themselves do not express or carry Rh antigens. When an Rh-negative patient must receive an Rh-positive unit of platelets, a dose of Rh Immune Globulin (RhIG) may be administered to prevent D alloimmunization.

The clinical magnitude of this issue is far less than one might expect. Most patients receiving platelets are severely immunosuppressed, and a primary response to the D or other red cell antigens is very uncommon.[161,162] Additionally, for most patients, the formation of anti-D would have minimal impact on their subsequent hemotherapy support. However, if the patient is a female of childbearing potential, the formation of anti-D could have a significant impact on her future pregnancies. Rather than provide RhIG to all Rh-negative recipients of Rh-positive platelets, many centers supply it only to premenopausal females. Given the 3-week half-life of IgG and the minimal red cell content in most platelet units, a single dose of RhIG would be expected to provide prophylaxis for multiple transfusions over a 2- to 4-week period (certainly for the period during which anti-D was detectable serologically). Because the recipient was (and probably still is) thrombocytopenic, an intravenous form of RhIG may be administered to avoid a hematoma (particularly if the platelet count remains below 50,000/µL).[163]

Alloimmunization: Prevention and Response

Although patients who are receiving multiple platelet transfusions are usually immunosuppressed by virtue of their underlying disease and/or the therapy they are receiving for it, they are still able to mount an immune response against antigens on platelets. This is usually seen as antibodies to HLA Class I antigens, but some patients may make antibodies to platelet-specific antigens. The former require presentation of the antigens via donor lymphocytes, and thus leukocyte reduction (of both platelet and red cells units transfused to these patients) has proven highly effective in reducing the risk of primary HLA alloimmunization.[51] However, if the patient has previously been sensitized, such as through pregnancy or a prior, non-leukocyte-reduced transfusion, the Class I antigens on the platelets themselves may be sufficient to provoke an anamnestic response and prompt the appearance of refractoriness.

For some patients who can be predicted to require multiple platelet transfusions, such as those slated for a hematopoietic stem cell transplant, advance knowledge of their (current) alloimmunization status may be helpful and allow one to prepare for provision of specially selected units. Usually, however, the hunt for alloantibodies begins when alloimmunization is suspected from poor responses to platelet transfusions not explicable on the basis of other, nonimmunologic factors, such as splenomegaly or sepsis. The availability of kits to screen for HLA and other platelet-directed antibodies by enzyme immunoassay or other, simple approaches has expanded the number of laboratories able to perform this testing and provide clinically useful information with a short turnaround time. Identification of the specificities of multiple HLA antibodies, however, may still require performance of lymphocytotoxicity testing in some circumstances.

Before such testing had become readily available, the detection or supposition of immunologic refractoriness led to a call for "HLA-matched" platelets.[164,165] Because even a donor registry of substantial size may not be able to provide a completely matched unit, many "HLA-matched" units actually bear antigens against which the patient may have an alloantibody. (The presence of serologic cross-reactive groups prevents recognition of some antigens as foreign but at the same time reduces the range of donors who are truly compatible.) Platelet crossmatching is another approach that can be used, the lack of in-vitro reactivity being taken as a predictor of good in-vivo compatibility. This technique is still used often when alloimmunization is directed at a platelet antigen because few blood collection agencies have phenotyped their donors for these antigens. However, neither approach has been able to guarantee a good result more than 50% to 80% of the time [a "good" HLA match (A or BU grade) provides the best prediction of transfusion success].[166] An alternative, simpler approach that parallels practice with patients who are alloimmunized against red cell antigens is the selection of platelet units that lack the antigen(s) against which the recipient is immunized (and those from cross-reacting groups).[167] (See Fig 20-1.)

Antibodies provoked by or directed at a wide variety of drugs can lead to thrombocytopenia.[168] These drug-dependent platelet antibodies (DDPAs) can lead to mild or profound thrombocytopenia and also to refractoriness to transfused platelets.[169] Although often thought of as a rare event, this phenomenon can be caused by many drugs and found in many patients. For example, in one study, approximately 10% of patients receiving gentamicin were noted to have a decrease in their platelet counts, and almost half of these (5.9% overall) had an antibody that interacted with platelets in the presence of gentamicin.[170] When refractoriness to platelet transfusion cannot be explained by the patient's condition or alloimmunization to HLA or platelet antigens, consideration should be given to the presence of DDPAs.

Managing the Refractory Patient

Responses to platelet transfusion are most often quantitated using the CCI at 1 hour after transfusion.[171] A sample taken 10 minutes after transfusion yields similar information and may be easier to obtain routinely.[172] The calculation is based on the count increment (CI = posttransfusion count – pretransfusion count), the platelet content of the unit (expressed as $\times 10^{-11}$), and the size of the patient (expressed as body surface area, or BSA, in m^2) (see Table 20-5 for calculation details).

A CCI above 7500 is considered evidence of a "successful" transfusion; two transfusions with CCIs below 5000 within 1 hour after transfusion are regarded as evidence of refractoriness. A similar, alternative approach calculates the recovery of platelets compared to the expected value.[128]

Occasionally, despite diligent efforts, no compatible platelets can be found to transfuse to a refractory patient. Alternative measures can be tried to stem or forestall hemorrhage, but these are of unpredictable benefit. Administration of antifibrinolytic agents—such as ε-aminocaproic acid [Amicar (Xanodyne Pharmaceuticals, Newport, KY)], either intravenously or, in the case of gingival bleeding, as a mouthwash—may allow the clot that is formed to be sustained.[128] Curiously, administration of intravenous immune globulin (IVIG), an effective therapy for *auto*immune thrombocytopenia appears to be of little benefit in *allo*immune refractoriness. IVIG can provide increased increments shortly after transfusion, but the durability of the response is limited, and by 24 hours after transfusion the patient has usually returned to baseline.[128] The claim that platelets accumulate at sites of bleeding even though they are not seen in circulation via a platelet count increment has not been substantiated and is unlikely.[128,173-175] Others have advocated administration of platelets by "slow drip," which may involve making aliquots of a therapeutic dose and administering it over 4 to 12 hours; however, the predicted benefit to the patient is based primarily on anecdotal experience.

Contraindications to Platelet Transfusion

Immune (autoimmune) thrombocytopenia (ITP, previously known as immune thrombocytopenic purpura) can cause profoundly low platelet counts, but patients with ITP (particularly children) rarely suffer hemorrhagic consequences.[176,177] Transfusion of platelets in the stable, nonbleeding ITP patient accomplishes no benefit (as the platelets are rapidly cleared by the circulating antibodies). In situations where the patient is bleeding, clinicians may feel compelled to take some actions, including use of antifibrinolytic agents and platelet transfusion. Success in stemming hemorrhage is not universal, but bleeding may slow or cease after transfusion in perhaps half or two-thirds of attempts,[178] making transfusion certainly worth trying, particularly when the bleeding is serious.

Thrombotic thrombocytopenic purpura (TTP) has traditionally been regarded as a contraindication to platelet transfusion.[179,180] Thrombocytopenia occurs in this disease as abnormally large multimers of von Willebrand factor incite (inappropriate) platelet activation without other cofactors and consume the platelets in thromboses.[181] The resulting thrombocytopenia may be protective, then, in slowing the formation of additional pathologic thromboses. Case reports describing development of coma in close temporal relationship to platelet transfusion led to the idea that platelets may "add fuel to the fire" and prompt further thromboses in critical sites. A recent review of the literature, accompanied by a prospective observational study of 54 patients with TTP, found no increased frequency of neurologic events or death in patients who received platelet transfusions.[180] Nonetheless, well-designed trials are needed to refute or deny the thinking that platelet transfusion is contraindicated in TTP. Platelet transfusion is also usually avoided in patients with heparin-induced thrombocytopenia, especially the immunologic (Type II) form, in order to forestall the development of limb- and life-threatening thromboses.[182]

Other Uses of Platelets

Autologous or allogeneic platelets may also be applied topically to an area of surgical reconstruction. The presence of platelet-derived growth factor through applications of PRP or platelet gels is thought to stimulate angiogenesis and promote more rapid tissue repair.[183,184]

PLASMA TRANSFUSION

Indications for Plasma

The current data supporting evidence-based guidelines for plasma transfusion are surprisingly weak. A systematic review of the available data, with subsequent development of guidelines by an expert panel, found the data to be sparse and of low quality.[185] The panel developed a "voluntary" guidance document after taking into account the potential benefit and harm demonstrated in the available data.[186] The primary supportable indications were in the settings of massive transfusion and reversal of warfarin anticoagulation in patients with intracranial hemorrhage. The panel regarded the data as insufficient for issuing a recommendation for an optimal ratio of red cells to plasma in massive transfusion. Likewise, in other clinical scenarios such as surgery without massive transfusion or warfarin reversal in the absence of intracranial hemorrhage, a guideline was not developed because of insufficient data. The panel recommended against plasma infusion in situations that have typically resulted in prophylactic plasma infusion, such as acute pancreatitis or in critically ill nonsurgical noncardiac patients. In these types of patients where coagulopathy or bleeding was absent, the risk of lung injury and possible increased mortality outweighed any perceived benefit.[185]

What Do Test Results Tell Us?

Although the diagnosis of a congenital hemostatic factor deficiency is straightforward using laboratory tests, the detection of the more common acquired deficits that may lead to hemostatic difficulties is much more problematic. The bleeding time test, for example, has been recognized as unable to predict surgical hemostasis and is no longer used for this purpose.[187] The venerated prothrombin time (PT) and partial thromboplastin time (PTT) assays have long ago been shown to have limited capabilities to predict who will bleed at surgery,[188] yet their results remain at the core of most clinicians' decision to administer plasma prophylactically.

The PT test is the most frequently abnormal test result in patients with a (potential) coagulopathy and is the test most frequently consulted when deciding whether to transfuse plasma. The introduction of standardization via the International Sensitivity Index (ISI) to express results as an international normalized ratio [INR; INR = $(\text{patient PT}/\text{mean normal PT})^{\text{ISI}}$] helped to standardize oral anticoagulant therapy and allowed laboratories to render comparable results. Before the creation of this approach to PT standardization, studies would often report the PT value used in the study as a multiple of either the midpoint or the upper end of the reference range as a means of standardization. In one of the early studies that helped define the difference between an abnormal (ie, out-of-reference-range) PT from one that was associated with a coagulopathy, trauma patients who were massively transfused were followed.[189] In this series, patients whose PTs (or PTTs) exceeded 1.3 times the upper limit of normal (ULN) were much more likely to suffer the oozing type of bleeding associated with a deficiency of procoagulants. In another study of patients undergoing percutaneous liver biopsy, those with normal PT and PTT and those whose values were abnormal but not exceeding 1.3 times the upper limit of the reference range experienced the same frequency of bleeding.[190] Many other similar studies have shown that abnormal coagulation studies do not predict an increased risk of hemorrhage.[191] These findings parallel older observations that therapeutic oral anticoagulation did not increase the risk of bleeding in major surgery,[192,193] and they are supported by a study in which the time required for the liver to stop bleeding after a needle biopsy under laparoscopy demonstrated no correlation to the patient's PT.[194]

Why are the standard coagulation screening tests such poor predictors of hemorrhage? Part of the answer may stem from the fact that they (particularly the PT) are inordinately sensitive to mild deficiencies of multiple procoagulants.[195] As a result, they become "abnormal" at factor levels that are not clinically associated with bleeding. Additional confusion arises with the recognition that the critical thresholds in these studies, 1.3 times the ULN or 1.5 times the midpoint of the reference range (usually almost exactly the same number), usually fall at an INR of about 1.5 to 2.0. Because the usual target for oral anticoagulation therapy is an INR of 2.0 to 3.0, some clinicians assume that patients with an INR close to 2.0 require correction of their "coagulopathy" before surgery. (Many clinicians and some textbooks recommend INRs of anywhere between 1.3 and 1.5 without citing any factual basis.) Patients with an INR of 2.0 may have reduced activity of their coagulation systems so that their congenital risk factor for hypercoagulability (eg, Factor V Leiden) or acquired abnormality (eg, prosthetic cardiac valve) is less likely to threshold unwanted clotting. However, that reduction does not imply that normal, physiologic thresholds of the clotting system will be unable to cause an appropriate thrombotic sequence. This distinction is important to make when deciding whether a patient requires correction of a slightly abnormal coagulation test result.

The guidelines for plasma administration of several professional associations, including the American Society of Anesthesiologists and the College of American Pathologists, recommend that correction of the coagulation test results by plasma transfusion before surgery or to facilitate thrombosis need occur only at the point that corresponds to an INR of approximately 1.5 to 2.0.[196,197] An association of British hematologists similarly noted the limited utility in attempting to correct mildly abnormal coagulation tests.[198] Their guidelines for correction of excessive anticoagulation as well as those published by the American College of Chest Physicians[199] (Table 20-7) notably avoid the use of plasma in lieu of administration of vitamin K until very abnormal INRs and bleeding are encountered. Administration of small doses of vitamin K can achieve correction of the warfarin excess promptly (6 to 24 hours) without complicating reestablishment of proper levels of anticoagulation.[200-202] Prothrombin complex concentrates (PCCs) can also be used to correct the effects of warfarin rapidly, but currently available PCCs in the United States have little Factor VII.[203] To compensate for this, the transfusion of 2 units of plasma has been combined with PCCs and reported with success for rapid reversal of overanticoagulation.[204] (This is discussed more fully below in the section on Factor IX complex concentrate.)

Patients with cirrhosis commonly have abnormalities of clotting tests because of their synthetic difficulties. They also often suffer gastrointestinal bleeding caused by increased portal vein pressure. However, one might expect much more frequent hemorrhage (and an inability to clot) in these patients based on observation of their PTs only. Why do cirrhotic patients not bleed? The answer to this question—which can also explain the intricate pro- and antithrombotic balances inherent in the clotting system—was recently elucidated by an observation that the amounts of thrombin generated in vitro in plasma from normal and cirrhotic patients were the same, but only with the addition of thrombomodulin to the test system (which activates protein C).[205] As the liver's synthetic production declines, the amount of procoagulants circulating in plasma decreases, but so does the level of certain *anti*coagulants, such as protein C. Less activity may be expected of a cirrhotic patient's procoagulant system, but at the same time there will be less of an opposing force from the coagulation's control system.

What happens if the decision is made to correct the patient's PT before a procedure? Often, surprisingly little. One study noted that the mean reduction in INR was only 0.03/unit of plasma transfused.[206] Another noted that the PT decreased to the normal range in less than 1% of plasma recipients who had mildly abnormal PTs before transfusion, and the difference to the ULN was reduced by half in only 14.5%.[207] The mean decrease was only 0.2 second, and there was no correlation between PT abnormality and subsequent red cell transfusion. This study also revealed that only 1 in 10 patients receiving plasma had their PT re-

TABLE 20-7. Guidelines for Correction of Excessive Oral Anticoagulation*

Clinical Situation	Guideline
INR >therapeutic but <5, no significant bleeding	Lower anticoagulant dosage.
	Temporarily discontinue drug if necessary.
INR >5 but <9, no significant bleeding	Omit 1-2 doses; monitor INR; resume when in therapeutic range.
	Alternative if patient at increased risk of hemorrhage: ◆ Omit a dose and give 1 to 2.5 mg vitamin K_1 orally. ◆ For rapid reversal before urgent surgery: give 2 to 4 mg vitamin K_1 orally; repeat dose with 1 to 2 mg at 24 hours if INR remains elevated.
INR >9, no significant bleeding	Omit warfarin; give 2.5-5.0 mg vitamin K_1 orally.
	Closely monitor INR; give additional vitamin K_1 if necessary.
	Resume warfarin at lower dose when INR is within therapeutic range.
Serious bleeding at any elevation of INR	Omit warfarin.
	Give 10 mg vitamin K_1 by slow intravenous infusion.
	Supplement with plasma or prothrombin complex concentrate depending on urgency of correction. Vitamin K_1 infusions can be repeated every 12 hours.
Life-threatening hemorrhage	Omit warfarin.
	Give prothrombin complex concentrate with 10 mg vitamin K_1 by slow intravenous infusion.
	Repeat as necessary, depending on INR.

*Adapted from Ansell et al[199]; guidelines developed and vetted by the American College of Chest Physicians.
INR = international normalized ratio.

checked within 8 hours—despite the fact that the ordering clinician felt that the correction was clinically important and the fact that the expected shortening occurred infrequently.

In cases of rapid bleeding, a more proactive approach may be beneficial. Reducing the magnitude of a potential problem (ie, a slightly abnormal coagulation parameter) before the abnormality worsens to the point that it is contributing to the patient's bleeding difficulties is recommended as an approach in massive transfusion. Correction of a true coagulopathy after it has become clinically manifest can be much more difficult and may lead to the need for increased transfusion of other components. Formulae giving proportions of blood components to be transfused or to predict when platelets or plasma will need to be transfused fail to recognize the individual patient's situation, and direct involvement of a transfusion medicine specialist can best guide hemotherapy in these complex, rapidly evolving situations. Such consultation can also take into account other important factors, such as reduced patient temperature and the presence of acidosis, both of which decrease the in-vivo activity of the coagulation system significantly.[208-211]

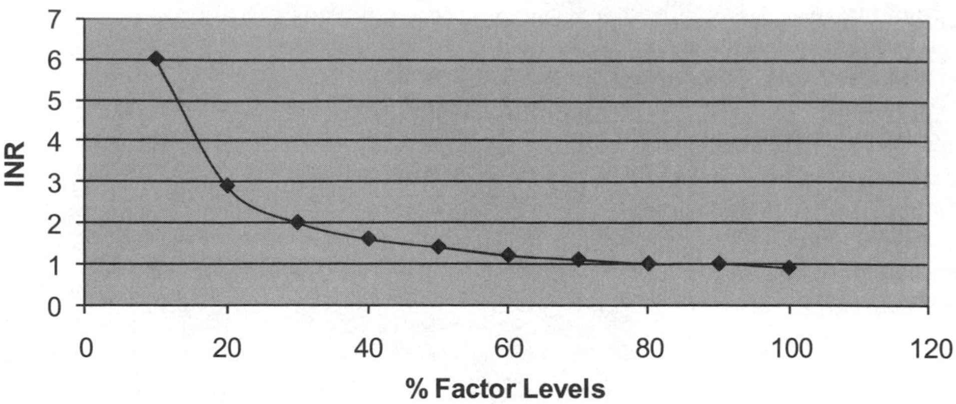

FIGURE 20-2. Exponential relationship of INR to percentages of factor levels. (Used with permission from Wayne Chandler, MD, University of Washington Department of Laboratory Medicine.)

Other in-vitro testing techniques can also be useful in identifying the need for plasma (or platelet) transfusion. For example, some centers have reported utility from use of the thromboelastograph (TEG) analysis of the blood's capability to clot.[212-215] When performed in a controlled manner and interpreted by one skilled in the meaning of the test's output, the TEG can assist in recognition of a problem and suggest the most appropriate approach for correction. The TEG may be particularly useful for recognizing states of fibrinolysis.

Dose and Timing of Plasma

Although the normal physiologic state varies widely between 50% and 150% activity of circulating clotting factors, numerous publications provide evidence that one has the ability to clot with significantly lower levels of factors.[216] For deficiencies of single factors such as VIII and IX, often a level of 30% activity is needed for hemostasis. For a state with multiple factor deficiencies such as trauma, factor levels closer to 40% may be needed for hemostasis (see Table 20-8 and Fig 20-2). Additionally, the further the patient's procoagulant activ-

TABLE 20-8. Coagulation Factor Half-Lives

Factor	In-Vivo Half-Life	Percent Needed for Hemostasis
I	3-6 days	12-50
II	2-5 days	10-25
V	5-36 hours	10-30
VII	2-5 hours	>10
VIII	8-12 hours	30-40
IX	18-24 hours	15-40
X	20-42 hours	10-40
XI	40-80 hours	20-30
XIII	12 days	<5

ity is from normal, the easier it is to effect a change in the PT because the relationship between factor activity and PT is more exponential than linear.[206,217] A usual dose of plasma is 10 to 20 mL/kg. This dose would be expected to increase the level of coagulation factors by 20% immediately after infusion. Precise prediction of the amount of plasma needed to be transfused to correct a particular coagulopathy exceeds current capabilities. Thus, posttransfusion repetition of the coagulation test that prompted transfusion is warranted.[206,207]

When attempting to correct a coagulopathy with plasma transfusion, the biologic half-life of procoagulants must also be considered. Factor VII has the shortest half-life in vivo (~5 hours), so if a transfusion had raised the patient's activity of this factor from 30% to 45%, for example, 5 hours later the activity would have dropped halfway back to the steady state that the patient was able to maintain (ie, to 37%). Additional attempts at correction then have to change the factor concentration in an enlarged plasma volume, and multiple repetitions of plasma transfusion risk development of pulmonary edema through fluid overload. In addition, if correction is truly required before a hemostatic challenge, such as major surgery, the plasma should be given shortly before the procedure in order for the benefit to be present at the time of the hemostatic challenge.

Types of Plasma

There are several types of plasma that may be available for transfusion, and for most situations, they can be used interchangeably. To use the name "Fresh Frozen Plasma," the unit must be frozen within 8 hours of collection and transfused within 24 hours of thawing, thus optimizing the levels of the most labile procoagulants, Factors V and VIII. However, congenital Factor V deficiency is a rarity, and most patients requiring plasma transfusion already have an elevated Factor VIII level because it is an acute phase reactant. Thus, Plasma Frozen Within 24 Hours After Phlebotomy has procoagulant contents that are equally capable of correcting most clinical coagulopathies.[218,219] Thawed Plasma made from Plasma Frozen Within 24 Hours After Phlebotomy and kept refrigerated after thawing can effectively be used throughout its 5-day shelf life because most coagulation factors remain at hemostatic levels.[220,221] Thawed plasma can be part of an effective strategy for reducing wastage of plasma, in combination with the institution of appropriate ordering practices.

Transfusion of Plasma for Other Indications

There are several other clinical situations where the transfusion of plasma is indicated under slightly different rationales.

Therapeutic plasma exchange (TPE) may call for partial or complete replacement of the removed volume of patient plasma. This may occasionally be necessitated by frequent (ie, daily) procedures that can deplete procoagulant levels faster than they can be replenished. However, most patients do not require such an aggressive TPE schedule, and the need to use plasma as factor replenishment is very unusual. TTP presents a different situation, however, because the plasma component's content of ADAMTS13 is therapeutic, replenishing the patient's supply that has been reduced by autoantibody or congenital deficiency, for example.[181]

Congenital deficiencies of procoagulants may require prophylactic or therapeutic replenishment via plasma transfusion, but these are rarities. Patients congenitally deficient in C1-esterase inhibitor are subject to angioedema, a potentially life-threatening activation of complement and inflammatory pathways that can occur from a variety of insults, including general anesthesia.[222] These patients are best identified preoperatively through careful family histories. Management may include administration of Cinryze (ViroPharma Inc, Exton, PA), a C1 inhibitor derived from human plasma. In emergent situations where this product is not available, plasma transfusion can be used as a source of C1 inhibitor.[223]

CRYOPRECIPITATED AHF

The discovery that certain proteins critical to the coagulation system could be concentrated by thawing frozen plasma at 4 C and centrifugally separating them from the supernatant provided the first truly effective treatment for patients with hemophilia A (congenital deficiency of Factor VIII). Ironically, Cryoprecipitated Antihemophilic Factor (Cryoprecipitated AHF, commonly called cryoprecipitate or CRYO) is rarely if ever used today for this original purpose, having been supplanted by other simpler and safer means of providing the deficient factor. Nevertheless, cryoprecipitate is an essential component in modern hemotherapy.

Although the regulatory requirements for the content of cryoprecipitate are written in terms of Factor VIII content (minimum: 80 U/unit), it is for its fibrinogen content that cryoprecipitate is most commonly used. When fibrinogen consumption (eg, DIC) and/or loss (eg, massive hemorrhage) are occurring, exogenous replacement may be necessary to maintain plasma's coagulation potential. The fibrinogen concentration necessary to maintain hemostasis is in the range of 50 to 100 mg/dL. However, coagulation test results that are depended on to follow patients through such situations usually become abnormal because of hypofibrinogenemia when the concentration decreases below 100 mg/dL; thus, maintaining fibrinogen above this level aids both the patient and those attempting to interpret the situation through laboratory testing. When fibrinogen levels are decreasing because of DIC or ongoing, high-volume hemorrhage, it may be wise to initiate transfusion (or at least prepare the component) as the critical point of 100 mg/dL is being approached (eg, at ~120 mg/dL).

Although the dosage of cryoprecipitate is traditionally stated in tens of units (eg, 10, 20, 30), the dosage required to achieve the desired effect is readily calculated from the difference between the current and desired (usually 200 mg/dL) concentration of fibrinogen, a projection of the patient's plasma volume [as (1 – hematocrit) × 0.7 dL/kg × body mass, or 30 dL if the patient's weight is unknown], and the usual fibrinogen content of cryoprecipitate (250 mg/unit):

Dose (units) = [Desired fibrinogen increment (mg/dL) × Plasma volume (dL)]/250 mg/unit

Although the small volume (5-15 mL) of each unit facilitates rapid thawing, the pooling of units (usually with rinsing of the bags to maximize recovery) can be time consuming. Planning ahead for rapid use later in a case of massive transfusion, for example, can certainly facilitate patient care. Some facilities have chosen to produce pools of cryoprecipitate using sterile technique before freezing the component. This component has a higher fibrinogen content and a shorter time to issue when needed.

Dysfibrinogenemias are rare congenital abnormalities that result in dysfunctional fibrinogen molecules that can lead to increased tendencies for thrombosis, bleeding, or both or can have no clinical manifestations.[224] Patients may require administration of cryoprecipitate to correct the deficiency. Some degree of dysfunctional fibrinogen is also produced in damaged or regenerating livers and in neonates, but this rarely results in the need to transfuse normal fibrinogen.[225] States of localized fibrinolysis can be induced during surgeries that disrupt the prostatic bed, urothelium, or salivary gland tissue because plasminogen activators are produced by these tissues. In these cases, cryoprecipitate may be warranted to stop bleeding, with or without the use of antifibrinolytic therapy. (It should be noted that bleeding from the urinary tract is a relative contraindication to antifibrinolytic therapy.) States of systemic fibrinolysis can occur with medical conditions such as widespread amyloidosis, or as a result of chemotherapy using L-asparaginase, typically for acute lymphoblastic leukemia.

Although no longer considered to be routine use because of the availability of concentrated plasma derivatives of copurified Factor VIII and von Willebrand factor (vWF), cryoprecipitate can be used as a source of vWF for patients with von Willebrand disease (vWD). The most common form of vWD is type 1, which results in a relative deficiency of a normal protein. Type 1 vWD most often can be managed using administration of DDAVP. Patients with Types 2 and 3 vWD should have bleeding managed with an exogenous source of vWF. Table 20-9 lists general factor replacement guidelines for the treatment of vWD.

Cryoprecipitate can also be applied topically on surfaces where suturing is ineffective to achieve hemostasis and surfaces that are slow to generate clot, such as the raw surface of traumatically injured liver.[228] When applied simultaneously with calcium and bovine thrombin (usually using two syringes), a thick, gelatinous mass quickly forms over the area and quells the bleeding. This approach can also be used to "glue" together structures, such as in surgery in the inner ear. However, use of bovine thrombin can stimulate the formation of antibodies against thrombin and other procoagulant proteins in xenogeneic products, including Factor V, that can cross-react with their human counterparts and lead to the development of "acquired inhibitors," clinically significant functional deficiencies, and bleeding.[229] These uses of cryoprecipitate have declined markedly with the introduction of virus-inactivated fibrinogen concentrates that are more readily stored (lyophilized) and packaged for ease of use.[230]

GRANULOCYTES

The development of apheresis technology several decades ago allowed the collection of granulocytes (neutrophils) to transfuse to neutropenic patients with serious infections. Most of these patients were not able to mount an appropriate response because of marrow hypoplasia (eg, resulting from chemotherapy). In addition, the therapy was applied to patients with congenital neutrophil dysfunction (eg, chronic granulomatous disease, or CGD). However, the benefit of this approach to these dire situations was not uniformly identified, with only modest improvements in outcome noted in a majority—but not all—of the trials.[231-235] (Strauss[236] and Price[237] provide a complete review of this and other topics related to granulocyte transfusion therapy.) With the development of more potent antimicrobial drugs and the availability of cytokines that promote more rapid marrow recovery of granulocyte production, differentiation, and function [products such as granulocyte colony-stimulating factor (G-CSF) and granulocyte/macrophage colony-stimulating factor (GM-CSF[238,239])], the frequency at which granulocyte transfusion therapy was used fell to very low levels. This low utilization was also prompted by the recognition that the amount of granulocytes that could be collected from a donor—even one "mobilized" with prior administration of a corticosteroid, on the order of 1×10^{10}—was only 1% to 10% of what a normal marrow would produce each day in response to a serious infection. The trials that had reported success in using granulocyte transfusion therapy were generally the ones in which higher doses of granulocytes had been transfused, but these higher yields were very difficult to obtain.

More recently, the concept of using components with a greater, "more-therapeutic" content has achieved renewed attention for granulocyte transfusion therapy. Despite newer antimicrobial agents, infection remains a common problem in patients undergoing rigorous chemotherapy regimens, especially those culminating in hematopoietic stem cell transplantation; more rigorous T-cell depletion schemes in allogeneic hematopoietic transplantation lead to an increased frequency of serious and fatal infections, particularly from yeasts and fungi.[240,241] Case reports of success in treating CGD patients who develop fungal infections during transplantation have also rekindled interest in this approach.[242,243] With the administration of 8 mg dexamethasone (orally) and 5 µg/kg G-CSF (subcutaneously) 8 to 16 hours before apheresis, yields of up to 10^{11} granulocytes (or more) have been reported.[244] (This use of G-CSF is not approved by the FDA, and specific donor informed consent should be obtained. In addition, the suggestion that corticosteroid administration may lead to posterior subcapsular cataracts has prompted some to consider foregoing the dexamethasone administration to donors even though this decreases yield by one-quarter.[245]) A clinical trial to document the effec-

TABLE 20-9. General Factor Replacement Guidelines for Treatment of Hemophilia A and von Willebrand Disease

Indication	Minimum Desired Factor Level (%)	Factor VIII Dose (IU/kg)	Factor IX Dose (IU/kg)	Duration (days)
Hemophilia*				
Severe epistaxis, oral mucosal bleeding[†]	20-30	10-15	20-30	1-2
Hemarthrosis, hematoma, persistent hematuria,[‡] gastrotintestinal bleeding, retroperitoneal bleeding	30-50	15-25	30-50	1-3
Trauma without signs of bleeding, tongue/retro-pharyngeal bleeding[†]	40-50	20-25	40-50	2-4
Trauma with bleeding, surgery,[§] intracranial bleeding[§]	100	50	100	10-14
von Willebrand Disease[‖]				
Major surgery	50	40-60, daily		
Minor surgery	30	30-50, daily or every other day		
Dental extractions	30	20-30, single		0.5
Spontaneous bleeding	30	20-30, single		

*Data from USP.[226] Dosing intervals based on a half-life for Factor VIII of 8 to 12 hours (2-3 doses/day) and a half-life for Factor IX of 18-24 hours (1-2 doses/day). Maintenance doses of one-half the initial dose (as shown) may be given at these intervals. The frequency depends on the severity of bleeding, with more frequent dosing for serious bleeding.

[†]In addition to antifibrinolytics.

[‡]Painless spontaneous hematuria usually requires no treatment. Increased oral or intravenous fluids are necessary to maintain renal output.

[§]Continuous factor infusion may be administered. Following the initial loading dose, a continuous infusion at a dose of 3 IU/kg/hour is given. Subsequent doses are adjusted according to measured plasma factor levels.

[‖]For concentrates labeled in terms of ristocetin cofactor, the recommended doses for adults, the number of infusions, and the target plasma levels are the same as those for Factor VIII:C.[227]

tiveness of these more potent components is under way through the Transfusion Medicine Hemostasis Clinical Trials Network of the National Heart, Lung, and Blood Institute. The potential utility of prophylactic granulocyte transfusions remains unclear at present, again owing to dosage considerations.[246]

Neonates born prematurely or after prolonged premature rupture of membranes are also at increased risk of bacterial sepsis. Their neutropenia is related to a temporary limitation on the production of neutrophils from a marrow "primed" to produce red cells. These patients have also been treated with granulocyte transfusions, either those derived from an apheresis procedure or from whole-blood-derived buffy coats. The latter can provide only a limited number of cells and has not been found to be clinically efficacious.[247] This intervention is used rarely at present, usually eschewed in favor of potent antibiotics. IVIG may also be given, because premature infants may be hypogammaglobulinemic,[248] although this administration may increase susceptibility to other potentially fatal infections.[249]

Severely neutropenic patients (absolute neutrophil count <500/µL) are considered for granulocyte therapy if the infection is not controllable with appropriate, bactericidal antimicrobials and if the period of neutropenia is temporary, such that recovery of endogenous production in a few days can be predicted. (Patients with CGD are usually considered for granulocyte transfusions if they have deep-seated abscesses and/or fungal infections that are not responding to antimicrobial therapy.) Components must be ABO compatible if the granulocyte collection contains 2 mL or more of red cells, as is often the case. If the patient requires CMV-reduced-risk transfusions, the donor should be CMV seronegative because, of course, leukocyte reduction cannot be used on these components. If the recipient is alloimmunized to HLA antigens, HLA-compatible donors will need to be found, or the cells risk rapid clearance without achieving their intended purpose (not to mention untoward reactions that may occur). If patients are at risk for transfusion-associated graft-vs-host disease (as is usually the case with neutropenic patients), units may be gamma irradiated. Donors often undergo infectious disease testing when they present for predonation stimulation, in order to facilitate rapid release of the collected component following documentation of ABO/Rh typing. Granulocyte units should be stored for the least time possible at room temperature without agitation and administered through regular blood component filters (eg, 170 microns). Drugs known to interact with granulocytes, such as amphotericin, are best given at times remote from the granulocyte transfusions (ie, 12 hours). Transfusions are usually given daily (sometimes more frequently if yields are low) until the patient recovers from the infection and/or neutrophil production returns.

PLASMA DERIVATIVES

From its origin as a means of expanding the blood volume of injured soldiers in World War II, the preservation of plasma proteins has evolved over the past half century into a multifaceted operation of separating, purifying, and virus inactivating a wide variety of specific proteins to accomplish specific tasks. Just as component therapy changed the face of transfusion medicine, the ability to target a specific condition with a (usually concentrated) form of a specific protein radically changed the course of treatment of several devastating diseases.

Plasma proteins are derived from both Source Plasma (ie, plasma collected specifically for the purpose of manufacturing plasma derivatives, about 6 million liters per year in the United States) and recovered plasma (ie, plasma separated from whole blood donations, about 2.5 million units per year). The plasma, delivered to the manufacturing facility frozen, is usually first converted to cryoprecipitate, which is directed to the production of Factor VIII concentrate, and a cryosupernatant from which a variety of other proteins are separated by manipulation of pH, alcohol content, and temperature as well as by passing through columns that separate proteins by physical and antigenic characteristics. The final products are subjected to one or more virus inactivation techniques (including heat, solvent/detergent treatment, and nanofiltration), and additional testing (eg, for hepatitis A virus or parvovirus) may be performed by nucleic acid amplification techniques to add an additional margin of safety. The prions associated with variant Creutzfeldt-Jakob disease (vCJD) appear to be successively removed through multiple steps in the separation process to beyond the limit of detection, and neither classical CJD nor vCJD cases have been reported as attributed to plasma derivatives.[250] Although these pathogen-inactivation techniques have an excellent record with respect to transmission of infectious diseases, the unfortunate infection of the majority of severe hemophiliacs with human immunodeficiency virus from Factor VIII preparations two decades ago has led to caution among recipients. Most US hemophilia patients now prefer Factor VIII or IX concentrates produced via recombinant DNA technology and, whenever possible, produced without any human proteins in the manufacturing process.

Immunoglobulin products have often been regarded as free of infectious risks because of the production method and/or the presence of neutralizing antibodies. Multiple examples of hepatitis C virus transmission[251-254] have raised doubts regarding this contention, but these products were usually prepared through nonstandard donor selection or production methods.

Albumin

Albumin was the first of the modern plasma proteins to be developed. It serves as a colloid, expanding plasma volume in approximately the volume administered (at the 5% concentration) with a half-life of approximately 16 hours.[255] Unless the container has been damaged, the pasteurization (60 C for 10 hours) of albumin prevents transmission of viruses or bacteria.

There are several obvious and accepted applications of albumin,[256] including 1) volume replacement unresponsive to crystalloids, 2) postparacentesis volume management unresponsive to colloids, 3) volume replacement in patients with severe necrotizing pancreatitis, 4) diarrhea (>2 L/day) in hypoalbuminemic (<2.0 g/dL) patients on enteral feedings unresponsive to short-chain peptide supplementation, and 5) TPE. Use of albumin infusions merely to raise the albumin concentration in cachectic or other chronically hypoalbuminemic patients is recognized as ineffective and inappropriate but may be helpful in treating its complications in acute illness if a concentration of at least 3.0 g/dL can be achieved.[257]

In most situations of hypovolemia, crystalloids are usually used as the primary means of volume replacement because of their effectiveness, availability, and cost. Questions about the safety of albumin as a volume replacement fluid were raised following a meta-analysis that identified a greater morbidity risk with the administration of albumin than crystalloid in critically ill patients.[258] However, a subsequent prospective randomized controlled trial intended to verify this projection failed to find outcome differences in patients receiving albumin.[259] At the same time, it should be noted that neither did this trial identify a benefit associated with the use of albumin in critically ill patients; thus the debate of crystalloid vs colloid support of hypovolemia continues. When colloid support *is* required, other, nonhuman sources, such as hydroxyethyl starch and dextran, may also be useful in both clinical and apheresis situations,[260] although the volume that can be administered in a day without affecting coagulation function may be restricted. These synthetic substitutes may (rarely) prompt an anaphylactic reaction and have been associated with a syndrome of pruritus beginning several weeks after administration in some patients.[261]

Clotting Factor Concentrates

A complete discussion of the treatment of hemophilia A and B (Factor VIII and IX deficiency, respectively) is beyond the scope of this text. Although the first effective treatment for hemophilia A was cryoprecipitate, patients with moderate (1%-5% Factor VIII activity) and severe (<1% activity) disease are now treated exclusively with a lyophilized concentrate. The same treatment has evolved for patients deficient in Factor IX, also an X-linked recessive condition. For both conditions, the necessary dose of the factor to be administered can be easily calculated based on the patient's plasma volume [body mass × 70 mL/kg × (1 – hematocrit)] multiplied by the desired increase in activity level. Thus a 70-kg male (hematocrit = 40%) with 1% activity needing to have his activity level raised by 99% (0.99 IU/mL) to 100% (1 IU/mL) would require approximately 2900 IU of Factor VIII to be administered. As the half-life of Factor VIII is 8 to 12 hours, repeat doses will be required to ensure hemostasis (ie, >30% activity) through surgery or a bleeding episode (often a period of at least 10 days). (See Table 20-9.) Because recovery of activity may vary by product and patient, close follow-up of patients with repetitive assays of factor activity is advised. Patients may also be maintained on regular prophylactic doses of Factor VIII to reduce the risk of spontaneous hemorrhage and preserve joint function,[262] although the value of this has been difficult to prove definitively because of the small size of most trials.[263] Nevertheless, prophylaxis is a widely recommended course of action.

About a third of patients with severe hemophilia A will develop antibodies against Factor VIII because they either do not produce it or produce a defective form that is immunologically dissimilar from that being infused. These patients can be very difficult to support, as it is impractical to attempt to overwhelm the inhibitor (antibody) with higher and higher doses of Factor VIII to stem hemorrhage. A variety of treatments have been tried, including a high-dose desensitization program; immunosuppression; and, when rapid reduction in inhibitor titers is needed, TPE. The advent of recombinant Factor VIIa (rFVIIa) to bypass the inhibition of Factor VIII activity has dramatically altered (and improved) the therapy of bleeding in this dreaded complication of hemophilia therapy. (See section on Factor VIIa below.)

Factor IX Complex Concentrate

Procoagulants that require vitamin K for appropriate carboxylation and normal activity—Factors II (prothrombin), VII, IX, and X—are called the vitamin-K-dependent factors. They have long been known to be separable from plasma by simple chemical means and have been available as a "Factor IX Complex Concentrate" or "Prothrombin Complex Concentrate." (This product should not be confused with a Factor IX concentrate used to treat hemophilia B. The latter, now also available as a recombinant product, contains only Factor IX.) The first means of producing this derivative resulted in activation of a substantial proportion of some of the procoagulants and could lead to unwanted thromboses. This complication precluded its routine use, but the product was found to be beneficial in bypassing the effect of Factor VIII inhibitors that occurred in some hemophilia A patients. This "activated" form of Factor IX Complex Concentrate was known for its Factor VIII inhibitor bypassing activity (FEIBA). Subsequent development of Factor IX Complex Concentrate with minimal amounts of activated factors has allowed its reconsideration for broader use, particularly as an antidote to warfarin overdosage.[203] When evaluating the literature, one needs to be aware that the factor concentrates available in the United States lack Factor VII. These are sometimes termed "three-factor PCCs." Studies performed outside the United States that demonstrate rapid correction of coagulation status with PCCs likely have been performed with a "four-factor PCC," not currently available in the United States. Because the concentrates available in the United States lack Factor VII, plasma should remain part of any protocol developed for the reversal of warfarin overdosage, and a combined approach of a small dose of plasma plus PCC has been shown to yield rapid correction of coagulation status.[204,264] The reduced capacity of a cirrhotic liver to clear the circulating byproducts of the coagulation cascade, such as D-dimers, may lead to DIC or other derangements of the coagulation system, and thus the use of PCC in liver disease remains risky.[198]

Factor VIIa

The production of the activated form of coagulation Factor VII via recombinant technology has led to exploration of this drug as a means of addressing a wide variety of hemorrhagic situations. The drug was developed and is approved for use as a means of bypassing antibodies against Factor VIII in hemophilia A patients and achieving hemostasis without having to achieve hemostatic levels of Factor VIII in the face of potent antibodies. It can also be used to address congenital deficiency of Factor VII.[265] Beyond these applications, it has been considered for use in a wide variety of situations where bleeding is difficult to control or is life threatening but that have nothing to do with hemophilia or Factor VII deficiency. For example, it has been used to counteract the effect of warfarin, replacing the inactive factor (produced in the presence of the vitamin K antagonist) with active rFVIIa that can immediately stimulate the "downstream" procoagulants and produce fibrin.[266] Its use has also received much attention in trauma, liver transplantation, and massive transfusion, where correction of procoagulant deficiency and achievement of hemostasis can be challenging.[267,268] The success in one study, where hemostasis was achieved in 80% of 40 massively bleeding patients, was tempered with a concern that has arisen in other studies—that of unwanted thromboses and thromboembolic disease.[269] For example, three patients in this group suffered thromboembolic events after rFVIIa administration. Use in liver biopsy patients similarly seemed to reduce bleeding but was associated with incitement of DIC in one case and portal vein thrombosis in another.[270] A registry that collected reports of adverse events after use of rFVIIa had its use listed as a contributing cause of death as a result of a large proportion of patient deaths.[271] However, in a review of 13 published trials, no increase in adverse outcomes was attributed to rFVIIa.[272] A recent evaluation of 17 randomized controlled trials involving the use of rFVIIa for nonhemophilia indications concluded that there is little evidence to support routine use of rFVIIa for patients with massive bleeding.[273] Given the open question of adverse events related to unwanted clotting and the exclusion of patients with a propensity to clot (including those with atherosclerotic disease) from many of the trials, it may be prudent to refrain from using this drug when the patient may be at increased risk of unwanted thrombosis.

The application of rFVIIa does not always result in the expected improvement in coagulation status and hemostasis. Trials in patients with upper gastrointestinal hemorrhage and in patients undergoing resection of hepatomas did not show benefit from rFVIIa.[274,275] A preliminary study suggesting that rFVIIa use in the setting of intracranial hemorrhage resulted in improved outcome and decreased mortality could not be confirmed in a follow-up study.[276] Several studies as well as practitioners have adopted the approach of ensuring adequate component replacement before adding rFVIIa, to ensure that it is really necessary and that sufficient procoagulants are available to complete the cascade. Additionally, the use of rFVIIa will be less effective in states of significant acidosis or hypothermia.

A substantial stumbling block in the consideration of rFVIIa has been its cost. If it is effective in substantially reducing hemorrhage or morbidity, then rFVIIa may pay for itself. Another approach is to adopt a practice of standardized rather than weight-based dosing; this reduces consumption while appearing to provide similar clinical results.[277] Clinical consultation from a transfusion medicine specialist may be very helpful in guiding the use of this product.[278]

Intravenous Immune Globulin

Concentrates of plasma immunoglobulins were developed to treat congenital immunodeficiencies and to treat (or provide prophylaxis against) certain viral exposures. Because immunoglobulins tend to polymerize during Cohn fractionation and purification, initial preparations had to be given intramuscularly to avoid severe hypotensive and/or anaphylactoid reactions. Subsequent development of a variety of chemical modifications has allowed the development of IVIG preparations that have low proportions of aggregates. These allow the administration of larger quantities over shorter intervals to achieve more pronounced clinical effects.

Although its initial intended use was to reduce infections in immunodeficient patients, the optimal dose for this purpose remains under discussion, and the clinical application of IVIG has extended far beyond this indication.[279] (See Table 20-10; see Durabi et al[280] for a thorough review.) When used for the treatment of hypogammaglobulinemia, a dose of 600 mg/kg (children: 800 mg/kg) every 4 weeks rather than the usual 300 mg/kg (children: 400) slightly reduces the frequency and duration of infections in patients with primary immune deficiencies.[281] However, the cost-effectiveness of increased dosages may be poor, and they would accelerate usage rates. The ever-increasing off-label use of IVIG poses an additional challenge to the adequacy of supply for treating the 50,000 congenital hypogammaglobulinemia patients in the United States. The FDA-approved indications for IVIG account for only 30% of its usage. The other situations in which IVIG is administered may have greater or lesser scientific underpinnings, but the usage rate in developed countries appears to be increasing at approximately 10% per year. The wide variability of usage rates, however—from <0.03 g per person in Australia to over 0.06 g per person in the United States and Canada, without concomitant variations in outcomes—raises questions about the true utility of some of these applications.

Administration of IVIG can be associated with a wide variety of adverse events (Table 20-11). Some of these appear to occur as idiosyncratic combinations of a particular product in a particular patient, and thus good advantage can be taken of the wide variety of available IVIG products to find a particular form of the medication that is well tolerated.[282] Slow rates of infusion and pretreatment with antihistamines and/or steroids usually obviate reactions. Clinically dramatic reactions are usually seen only in patients with agammaglobulinemia who have not previously been treated and who have an infection. IgA may be present in sufficient concentration in some preparations

TABLE 20-10. Applications of Intravenous Immune Globulin

Primary immune deficiencies
Hypo/agammaglobulinemia*
Selective antibody deficiency*
Class/subclass deficiency with recurrent infection*
Secondary (acquired) immune deficiencies
Chronic lymphocytic leukemia*
Multiple myeloma
Prevention of (CMV) pneumonitis after hematopoietic stem cell transplantation*
Reduction of bacterial infection in pediatric AIDS*
Immune cytopenias
(Auto)immune thrombocytopenia (ITP)*†
Pure red cell aplasia‡
Other cytopenias: NAIT, PTP, WAIHA
HIV-related ITP
(Presumed) autoimmune disorders
Kawasaki disease*
Guillain-Barré syndrome‡
Multiple sclerosis
Myasthenia gravis‡
Dermatomyositis‡
Systemic vasculitides
Factor VIII inhibitors (congenital/acquired hemophilia)
Prevention/treatment of infections
After hematopoietic stem cell transplantation
After solid organ transplantation and immunosuppression
Parvovirus infection
Neonatal sepsis
Other (presumed) immunologic conditions
Recurrent spontaneous abortion

(Continued)

TABLE 20-10. Applications of Intravenous Immune Globulin (Continued)

Graft-vs-host disease
Asthma
Myocarditis
Inflammatory bowel disease
Stevens-Johnson syndrome
Other conditions
Alzheimer disease
Atherosclerosis (predisposition)
Autism
Chronic fatigue syndrome
Multifocal motor neuropathy
Rh prophylaxis if patient cannot receive intramuscular product

*Approved indications.
†Usually used only in chronic ITP because most acute ITP cases are self-limited. (Many other agents potentially effective in ITP are being developed.[279])
‡Commonly accepted indications.
CMV = cytomegalovirus; NAIT = neonatal alloimmune thrombocytopenia; PTP = posttransfusion purpura; WAIHA = warm autoimmune hemolytic anemia; HIV = human immunodeficiency virus.

to prompt an anti-IgA reaction in sensitized patients. Although the antibody specificities contained in IVIG products represent the range (and relative concentrations) of the donors' immunoglobulin responses and thus may convey varying degrees of protection against particular pathogens, the large pool sizes used in manufacture reduce this variability. Hyperimmunoglobulins are manufactured from donors chosen for higher titers of activity against selected agents, such as hepatitis A or B virus, tetanus, rabies, varicella zoster, or cytomegalovirus, but they are usually available only in the intramuscular form.

The products may, on occasion, convey sufficient isoagglutinins or red cell alloantibodies of a particular specificity (usually anti-D) to cause a positive DAT in the recipient, but clinically detectable or significant hemolysis is rare.[283] Administration of a hyperimmune anti-D [WinRho (Cangene, Winnipeg, Canada)] to an Rh-positive patient for treatment of ITP may induce a life-threatening or fatal acute hemolysis, and the product carries a "black box" warning to remind physicians of this potential outcome.

Antithrombin

Antithrombin circulates in plasma as a serine protease inhibitor that inactivates the serine proteases of the coagulation system, including thrombin and Factors IXa, Xa, XIa, and XIIa, by covalently binding at their serine active site.[284] The ability of antithrombin to accomplish this inhibition is greatly accelerated by heparin, which induces a change in the polypeptide's

TABLE 20-11. Adverse Events Associated with Intravenous Immune Globulin Use

Infusion-associated	
Fever	Chest tightness
Chills	Dyspnea
Facial flushing	Wheezing
Tachycardia	Hypotension
Palpitations	Anxiety
Abdominal pain	Nausea
Headache	Vomiting
Lumbar pain	Urticarial rash
Other associations	
Volume overload	
Arterial thrombosis (myocardial infarction, stroke)	
Venous thromboembolism	
Disseminated intravascular coagulation	
Hemolysis (caused by alloantibodies/isoagglutinins)	
Nephrotoxicity	
Neutropenia	

conformation; hence its name as "heparin cofactor."

Patients who are congenitally deficient in antithrombin have an increased risk of developing thrombosis.[285] Acquired deficiency of antithrombin can also occur from reduced synthesis (as in hepatic disease), increased loss (as in a nephrotic syndrome), increased breakdown (as caused by L-asparaginase treatment), or increased consumption (in DIC, trauma, or surgery). In addition, the administration of heparin accelerates the metabolism of antithrombin and can lead to a relative resistance to heparin.[285]

Although antithrombin is stable in frozen or thawed plasma, deficiencies are usually addressed at present through the infusion of antithrombin concentrate. Congenital deficiency is rare, but antithrombin has also been used in the treatment of sepsis and DIC to stem thrombotic complications and in the treatment of patients with heparin for extracorporeal circulation when they fail to demonstrate the expected effect of heparin.

Activated Protein C

Protein C is a serine protease that acts with protein S to hydrolyze and thus inactivate Factors Va and VIIIa. It thus serves an antithrombotic regulatory function. It is normally activated along with the prothrombotic cascade, leading to an innate regulation of the clotting system. When given as an infusion over 96 hours to patients with sepsis, recombinant activated protein C concentrate reduced mortality by 19%, although the risk of serious bleeding almost doubled.[286]

α_1-Antitrypsin

α_1-Antitrypsin (also known as α_1-proteinase inhibitor, or A1PI) is a natural inhibitor of the elastase elaborated by activated polymorphonuclear leukocytes. If the activity of elastase is left unchecked, as in congenital deficiencies of α_1-antitrypsin, excessive damage to pulmonary parenchyma occurs after even minor infections, leading to development of fatal emphysema at an early age in the 100,000 US patients with this deficiency. Hepatic cirrhosis can also occur. Until the development of several plasma-derived replacements,[287] congenitally deficient patients could stem the advance of tissue destruction only by attempting to avoid and then rapidly treat respiratory infections. Periodic (usually weekly) infusions of α_1-antitrypsin can be administered prophylactically to prevent additional lung damage in these patients.

KEY POINTS

1. Each blood component has specific indications. Transfusion for other reasons generates risk for the recipient without conferring demonstrable benefit. Moreover, hypovolemia should be not be confused with anemia, nor symptomatic anemia with low hemoglobin.
2. Red cell transfusion thresholds should be set for each patient's unique situation. However, most current guidelines do not recommend considering transfusion of red cells unless the patient's hemoglobin is approaching 7 to 8 g/dL. Maintaining a patient's hemoglobin at levels above 8 to 9 g/dL may be detrimental.
3. Studies are inconclusive regarding the clinical effect of the red cell storage lesion.
4. Transfusion in the presence of an autoantibody that precludes a negative crossmatch is safe—and could be life-saving—providing that alloantibodies can be excluded.
5. Although prophylactic platelet transfusions during periods of aplasia are common practice, it is uncertain whether a prophylactic vs a therapeutic transfusion approach is optimal.
6. The most common prophylactic transfusion threshold is 10,000 platelets/μL. The current standard prophylactic dose of platelets (3 to 4 × 10^{11} for an adult) may be halved without generating increased risk of bleeding.

7. When platelets are transfused bearing ABO antigens that are foreign to the recipient, the response of the platelet count may be blunted or obliterated. When plasma in platelet units contains antibodies against A and/or B antigens expressed on the recipient's red cells, hemolysis may occur; steps are often taken to identify and avoid high-titer units and/or reduce the volume of plasma transfused, especially for pediatric recipients, when time permits.
8. Alloimmunized refractory recipients may be supported through platelet donors lacking the targeted epitope(s), either by phenotyping the donor (unit) or through provision of "HLA-matched" units (in the case of HLA alloimmunization).
9. There are very limited data to suggest there is benefit in transfusing plasma outside of intracranial hemorrhage after overanticoagulation or massive transfusion.
10. Patients with prothrombin times less than 1.5 times the midpoint of the reference range are not at increased risk of hemorrhage. (Note: This is *not* necessarily the same as an international normalized ratio of 1.5.)
11. Overanticoagulation with warfarin may be successfully treated, when indicated, with a combination of prothrombin complex concentrate and plasma.
12. The transfusion of plasma may have remarkably little effect on coagulation test abnormalities. If plasma transfusion is felt to be indicated, the effect of its transfusion should be documented.

REFERENCES

1. Weisel RD, Charlesworth DC, Mickleborough LL, et al. Limitations on blood conservation. J Thorac Cardiovasc Surg 1984; 88:26-38.
2. Skillman JJ, Olson JE, Lyons JH, Moore FD. The hemodynamic effect of acute blood loss in normal man, with observations on the effect of the Valsalva maneuver and breath holding. Ann Surg 1967;166:713-38.
3. Adamson J, Hillman RS. Blood volume and plasma protein replacement following acute blood loss in normal man. JAMA 1968;205:609-12.
4. Evans EI, James GW, Hoover MJ. Studies in traumatic shock. II. The restoration of blood volume in traumatic shock. Surgery 1944;15: 420-32.
5. Elizade JI, Clemente J, Marin JL, et al. Early changes in hemoglobin and hematocrit levels after packed red cell transfusion in patients with acute anemia. Transfusion 1997;37:573-6.
6. Weiskopf RB, Viele MK, Feiner J, et al. Human cardiovascular and metabolic response to acute, severe isovolemic anemia. JAMA 1998; 279:217-21.
7. Fontana JL, Welborn L, Mongan PD, et al. Oxygen consumption and cardiovascular function in children during profound intraoperative normvolemic hemodilution. Anesth Analg 1995;80:219-25.
8. Wilkerson DK, Rosen AL, Sehgal LR, et al. Limits of cardiac compensation in anemic baboons. Surgery 1988;103:665-70.
9. Adams RP, Dieleman A, Sain SM. A critical value for O_2 transport in the rat. J Appl Physiol 1982;53:660-4.
10. Rasanen J. Supply-dependent oxygen consumption and mixed venous oxyhemoglobin saturation during isovolemic hemodilution in pigs. Chest 1992;101:1121-4.
11. Weiskopf RB, Kramer JH, Viele M, et al. Acute severe isovolemic anemia impairs cognitive function and memory in humans. Anesthesiology 2000;92:1646-52.
12. vanWoerkens ECSM, Trouborst A, van Lanschot JJB. Profound hemodilution: What is the critical level of hemodilution at which oxygen-dependent oxygen consumption starts in an anesthetized human? Anesth Analg 1992;75: 818-21.
13. Carson JL, Duff A, Poses RM, et al. Effect of anaemia and cardiovascular disease on surgical mortality and morbidity. Lancet 1996;348: 1055-60.
14. Johnson RG, Thurer RL, Kruskall MS, et al. Comparison of two transfusion strategies after elective operations for myocardial revascular-

ization. J Thorac Cardiovasc Surg 1992;104: 307-14.

15. Spiess BD, Ley C, Body SC, et al. Hematocrit value on intensive care unit entry influences the frequency of Q-wave myocardial infarction after coronary artery bypass grafting. J Thorac Cardiovasc Surg 1998;116:460-7.
16. Messmer K, Lewis DH, Sunder-Plassman L. Acute normovolemic hemodilution. Eur Surg Res 1972;4:55-70.
17. Besarab A, Bolton WK, Browne JK, et al. The effects of normal as compared with low hematocrit values in patients with cardiac disease who are receiving hemodialysis and epoetin. N Engl J Med 1998;339:584-90.
18. Nelson AH, Fleisher LA, Rosenbaum SH. Relationship between postoperative anemia and cardiac morbidity in high-risk vascular patients in the intensive care unit. Crit Care Med 1993;21:860-6.
19. Carson JL, Terrin ML, Barton FB, et al. A pilot randomized trial comparing symptomatic vs hemoglobin-level-driven red blood cell transfusions following hip fracture. Transfusion 1998;38:522-9.
20. Grover M, Talwalkar S, Casbard A, et al. Silent myocardial ischemia and haemoglobin concentration: A randomized controlled trial on transfusion strategy in lower limb arthroplasty. Vox Sang 2006;90:106-12.
21. Fortune JB, Feustel PJ, Saifi J, et al. Influence of hematocrit on cardiopulmonary function after acute hemorrhage. J Trauma 1987;27:243-9.
22. Hébert PC, Yetisir E, Martin C, et al. Is a low transfusion threshold safe in critically ill patients with cardiovascular disease? Crit Care Med 2001;29:227-34.
23. Vincent JL, Baron JF, Reinhart K, et al. Anemia and blood transfusion in critically ill patients. JAMA 2002;288:1499-507.
24. Hébert PC, Blajchman MA, Cook DJ, et al. Do blood transfusions improve outcomes related to mechanical ventilation? Chest 2001;119: 1850-7.
25. Carson JL, Noveck H, Berlin J, Gould SA. Mortality and morbidity in patients with very low postoperative hemoglobin levels who decline blood transfusion. Transfusion 2002;42:812-18.
26. Bell EF, Strauss RG, Widness JA, et al. Randomized trial of liberal versus restrictive guidelines for red blood cell transfusion in preterm infants. Pediatrics 2005;115:1685-91.
27. Wu WC, Rathore SS, Wang Y, et al. Blood transfusion in elderly patients with myocardial infarction. N Engl J Med 2001;345:1230-6.
28. Rao SV, Jollis JG, Harrington RA, et al. Relationship of blood transfusion and clinical outcomes in patients with acute coronary syndromes. JAMA 2004;292:1555-62.
29. Rao SV, Harrington RA, Calif RM, Stamler JS. Blood transfusion in patients with acute coronary syndrome. JAMA 2005;293:673-4.
30. Perioperative red cell transfusion. Natl Inst Health Consens Dev Conf Consens Statement 1988;7:1-6.
31. Blood use benchmarking project executive summary 2002. Oak Brook, IL: University Health System Consortium, 2002.
32. Laine E, Steadman R, Calhoun L, et al. Comparison of RBCs and FFP with whole blood during liver transplant surgery. Transfusion 2003;43:322-7.
33. Heaton A, Keegan T, Holme S. In vivo regeneration of red cell 2,3-diphosphoglycerate following transfusion of DPG-depleted AS-1, AS-3 and CPDA-1 red cells. Br J Haematol 1989; 71:121-6.
34. Marik PE, Sibbald WJ. Effect of stored-blood transfusion on oxygen delivery in patients with sepsis. JAMA 1993;269:3024-9.
35. Reynolds JD, Ahearn GS, Angelo M, et al. S-nitrosohemoglobin deficiency: A mechanism for loss of physiological activity in banked blood. Proc Natl Acad Sci U S A 2007;104: 17058-62.
36. d'Almeida MS, Gray D, Martin C, et al. Effect of prophylactic transfusion of stored RBCs on oxygen reserve in reponse to acute isovolemic hemorrhage in a rodent model. Transfusion 2001;41:950-6.
37. Offner PJ, Moore EE, Biffi WL, et al. Increased rate of infection associated with transfusion of blood after severe injury. Arch Surg 2002;137: 711-17.
38. Vamvakas EC, Carven JH. Length of storage of transfused red cells and postoperative morbidity in patients undergoing coronary artery

bypass graft surgery. Transfusion 2000;40:101-9.

39. Vamvakas EC, Carven JH. Transfusion and postoperative pneumonia in coronary artery bypass graft surgery: Effect of the length of storage of transfused red cells. Transfusion 1999;39:701-10.
40. Koch CG, Li L, Sessler DI, et al. Duration of red-cell storage and complications after cardiac surgery. N Engl J Med 2008;358:1229-39.
41. Walsh TS, McArdle F, McLellan SA, et al. Does the storage time of transfused red blood cells influence regional or global indexes of tissue oxygenation in anemic critically ill patients? Crit Care Med 2004;32:364-71.
42. Hébert PC, Chin-Yee I, Fergusson D, et al. A pilot trial evaluating the clinical effects of prolonged storage of red cells. Anesth Analg 2005; 100:1433-8.
43. Woodson RD, Fitzpatrick JHJ, Costello DJ, Gilboe DD. Increased blood oxygen affinity decreases canine brain oxygen consumption. J Lab Clin Med 1982;100:411-24.
44. Raat NJ, Verhoeven AJ, Mik EG, et al. The effect of storage time of human red cells on intestinal microcirulatory oxygenation in a rat isovolemic exchange model. Crit Care Med 2005; 33:39-45.
45. Högman CF, Löf H, Meryman HT. Storage of red blood cells with improved maintenance of 2,3-bisphosphoglycerate. Transfusion 2006;46: 1543-52.
46. West LJ, Pollock-Barziv SM, Dipchand AI, et al. ABO incompatible heart transplantation in infants. N Engl J Med 2001;344:793-800.
47. Blumberg N. Deleterious clinical effects of transfusion immunomodulation: Proven beyond a reasonable doubt. Transfusion 2005; 45(Suppl 2):33S-40S.
48. Vamvakas EC. White-blood-cell-containing allogeneic blood transfusion, postoperative infection and mortality: A meta-analysis of observational "before-and-after" studies. Vox Sang 2004;86:111-19.
49. Vamvakas EC, Blajchman MA. Universal WBC reduction: The case for and against. Transfusion 2001;41:691-712.
50. Vamvakas EC. Deleterious clinical effects of transfusion immunomodulation: Proven beyond a reasonable doubt (letter). Transfusion 2006;46:492-4.
51. Leukocyte-reduction and ultraviolet B irradiation of platelets to prevent alloimmunization and refractoriness to platelet transfusions. The Trial to Reduce Alloimmunization to Platelets Trial Study Group. N Engl J Med 1997;337: 1861-9.
52. Blackall DP. Leukocyte reduction reduces the rate of febrile nonhemolytic transfusion reactions to platelets and red blood cells. Curr Hematol Rep 2004;3:435-6.
53. King KE, Shirey RS, Thoman SK, et al. Universal leukoreduction decreases the incidence of febrile nonhemolytic transfusion reactions to RBCs. Transfusion 2004;44:25-9.
54. Paglino JC, Pomper GJ, Fisch GS, et al. Reduction of febrile but not allergic reactions to RBCs and platelets after conversion to universal prestorage leuko-reduction. Transfusion 2004;44:16-24.
55. Uhlmann EJ, Isriggs E, Wallhermfechtel M, Goodnough LT. Prestorage universal WBC reduction of RBC units does not affect the incidence of transfusion reactions. Transfusion 2001;41:997-1000.
56. Dzik WH, Anderson JK, O'Neill EM, et al. A prospective, randomized clinical trial of universal WBC reduction. Transfusion 2002;42: 1114-22.
57. Wallis JP, Chapman CE, Orr KE, et al. Effect of WBC reduction of transfused RBCs on postoperative infection rates in cardiac surgery. Transfusion 2002;42:1127-34.
58. Van de Watering LM, Hermans J, Houbiers JG, et al. Beneficial effects of leukocyte depletion of transfused blood on postoperative complications in patients undergoing cardiac surgery—a randomized clinical trial. Circulation 1998;97:562-8.
59. Bilgin YM, van de Watering LM, Eijsman L, et al. Double-blind, randomized controlled trial on the effect of leukocyte-depleted erythrocyte transfusions in cardiac valve surgery. Circulation 2004;109:2755-60.
60. Bracey A, Radovancevic R, Nussmeier N, et al. Leukocyte-reduced blood in open heart surgery patients: Effects on outcome (abstract). Transfusion 2002;42(9S):5S.

61. Hébert PC, Fergusson D, Blajchman MA, et al. Clinical outcomes following institution of the Canadian universal leukoreduction program for red cell transfusions. JAMA 2003;289:1941-9.
62. Corwin HL, AuBuchon JP. Is leukoreduction of blood components for everyone? JAMA 2003; 289:1993-5.
63. Llewelyn CA, Taylor RS, Todd AA, et al. The effect of universal leukoreduction on postoperative infections and length of stay in elective orthopedic and cardiac surgery. Transfusion 2004;44:489-500.
64. Fung MK, Rao N, Rice J, et al. Leukoreduction in the setting of open heart surgery: A prospective cohort-controlled study. Transfusion 2004;44:30-5.
65. Anniss AM, Sparrow RL. Storage duration and white blood cell content of red blood cell (RBC) products increases adhesion of stored RBCs to endothelium under flow conditions. Transfusion 2006;46:1561-7.
66. Ratko TA, Cummings JP, Oberman HA, et al. Evidence-based recommendations for the use of WBC-reduced cellular blood components. Transfusion 2001;41:1310-19.
67. Vamvakas EC. WBC-containing allogeneic blood transfusion and mortality: A meta-analysis of randomized controlled trials. Transfusion 2003;43:963-73.
68. Vamvakas EC, Blajchman MA. Deleterious clinical effects of transfusion-associated immunomodulation: Fact or fiction? Blood 2001;97:1180-95.
69. Dzik S, AuBuchon J, Jeffries L, et al. Leukocyte reduction of blood components: Public policy and new technology. Transfus Med Rev 2000; 14:34-52.
70. Preiksaitis J. The cytomegalovirus-"safe" blood product: Is leukoreduction equivalent to antibody screening? Transfus Med Rev 2000;14: 112-36.
71. Stringham JC, Bull DA, Fuller TC, et al. Avoidance of cellular blood product transfusions in LVAD recipients does not prevent HLA allosensitization. J Heart Lung Transplant 1999;18: 160-5.
72. Gresens CJ, Paglieroni TG, Moss CB, et al. WBC populations in thawed fresh frozen plasma (abstract). Transfusion 1999;39(Suppl):99S.
73. Food and Drug Administration. Memorandum: Recommendations and license requirements for leukocyte-reduced blood products. (May 29, 1996) Rockville, MD: CBER Office of Communication, Outreach, and Development, 1996.
74. Food and Drug Administration. Draft guidance for industry: Prestorage leukocyte reduction with whole blood and blood components intended for transfusion. (January 23, 2001) Rockville, MD: CBER Office of Communication, Outreach, and Development, 2001.
75. Carson TH, ed. Standards for blood banks and transfusion services. 27th ed. Bethesda, MD: AABB, 2011.
76. European Commission Directive 2004/33/EC. Official Journal of the European Union, March 30, 2004. [Available at http://eur-lex.europa.eu/LexUriServ/LexUriServ.do?uri=OJ:L:2004:091:0025:0039:EN:PDF (accessed January 14, 2011).]
77. Högman CF, Meryman HT. Red blood cells intended for transfusion: Quality criteria revisited. Transfusion 2006;46:137-42.
78. Arslan O, Toprak S, Arat M, Kayalak Y. Hb content-based transfusion policy successfully reduces the number of RBC units transfused. Transfusion 2004;44:485-8.
79. Klein HG, Anstee DJ. Mollison's blood transfusion in clinical medicine. 11th ed. Malden, MA: Blackwell Science, 2005:406-54.
80. Natanson C, Kern SJ, Lurie P, et al. Cell free hemoglobin based blood substitutes and risk of myocardial infarction and death: A meta-analysis. JAMA 2008;299:2304-12.
81. Winslow RM. Current status of oxygen carriers ("blood substitutes"): 2006. Vox Sang 2006;91: 102-10.
82. Higby DJ, Cohen E, Holland JF, Sinks L. The prophylactic treatment of thrombocytopenic leukemic patients with platelets: A double blind study. Transfusion 1974;14:440-6.
83. Patten E. Controversies in transfusion medicine. Prophylactic platelet transfusion therapy: Con. Transfusion 1992;32:381-5.
84. Murphy S, Litwin S, Herring LM, et al. Indications for platelet transfusion in children with acute leukemia. Am J Hematol 1982;13:347-50.
85. Callum JL, Dzik WH. The use of blood components prior to invasive bedside procedures: A

critical appraisal. In: Mintz PD, ed. Transfusion therapy: Clinical principles and practice. 3rd ed. Bethesda, MD: AABB Press, 2011:1-35.
86. Wandt H, Frank M, Schaefer-Eckart K, Wilhelm M. Routine prophylactic platelet transfusions are not necessary in patients with acute myeloid leukemia—a therapeutic transfusion strategy is safe and cost effective (abstract). Blood 2005;106:129a.
87. Schaefer-Eckart K, Wendelin K, Wilhelm M, et al. Interim analysis of a prospective randomized study comparing a therapeutic platelet transfusion strategy with the prophylactic platelet transfusion standard in patients after autologous peripheral stem cell transplantation (ASCT) (abstract). Blood 2006;108:174a.
88. Gaydos LA, Freireich EJ, Mantel N. The quantitative relation between platelet count and hemorrhage in patients with acute leukemia. N Engl J Med 1962;266:905-9.
89. O'Brien JR. Effects of salicylates on human platelets. Lancet 1968;i:779-83.
90. Quick AJ. Salicylates and bleeding: The aspirin tolerance test. Am J Med Sci 1966;252:265-9.
91. Beutler E. Platelet transfusions: The 20,000/µL trigger. Blood 1993;81:1411-13.
92. Lawrence JB, Yomtovian R, Hammons T, et al. Lowering the prophylactic platelet transfusion threshold: A prospective analysis. Leuk Lymphoma 2001;41:67-76.
93. Heckman KD, Weiner GJ, Davis CS, et al. Randomized study of prophylactic platelet transfusion threshold during induction therapy for adult acute leukemia: 10,000/µL versus 20,000/µL. J Clin Oncol 1997;15:1143-9.
94. Rebulla P, Finazzi G, Marangoni F, et al. The threshold of prophylactic platelet transfusions in adults with acute myeloid leukemia. N Engl J Med 1997;337:1870-5.
95. Roy AJ, Jaffe N, Djerassi I. Prophylactic platelet transfusions in children with acute leukemia. A dose response study. Transfusion 1973;13:283-91.
96. Wandt H, Frank M, Ehninger G, et al. Safety and cost effectiveness of a 10×10^9/L trigger for prophylactic platelet transfusions compared with the traditional 20×10^9/L trigger; a prospective comparative trial in 105 patients with acute myeloid leukemia. Blood 1998;91:3601-6.
97. Slichter SJ, Harker LA. Thrombocytopenia: Mechanisms and management of defects in platelet production. Clin Haematol 1978;7:523-39.
98. Gmur J, Burger J, Schanz U, et al. Safety of a stringent prophylactic platelet transfusion policy for patients with acute leukemia. Lancet 1991;338:1223-6.
99. Deutsch VR, Tomer A. Megakaryocyte development and platelet production. Br J Haematol 2006;134:453-66.
100. Nuttall GA, Oliver WC, Ereth MH, Santrach PJ. Coagulation tests predict bleeding after cardiopulmonary bypass. J Cardiothorac Vasc Anesth 1997;11:815-23.
101. National Institutes of Health Consensus Development Conference. Platelet transfusion therapy. Transfus Med Rev 1987;1:195-200.
102. Valeri CR, Cassidy G, Pivacek LE, et al. Anemia-induced increase in the bleeding time: Implications for treatment of nonsurgical blood loss. Transfusion 200;41:977-83.
103. Moia M, Mannucci PM, Vizzotto L, et al. Improvement in the hemostatic defect of uraemia after treatment with recombinant human erythropoietin. Lancet 1987;ii:1227-9.
104. Escolar G, Garrido M, Mazzara R, et al. Experimental basis for the use of red cell transfusion in the management of anemic-thrombocytopenic patients. Transfusion 1988;28:406-11.
105. Hartmann M, Sucker C, Boehm O, et al. Effects of cardiac surgery on hemostasis. Transfus Med Rev 2006;20:230-41.
106. Tuman KJ, McCarthy RJ, O'Connor CJ, et al. Aspirin does not increase allogeneic blood transfusion in reoperative coronary artery surgery. Anesth Analg 1996;83:1178-84.
107. Korinth MC, Gilsbach JM, Weinzierl MR. Low-dose aspirin before spinal surgery: Results on a survey among neurosurgeons in Germany. Eur Spine J 2007;16:365-72.
108. Foss NB, Kehlet H. Hidden blood loss after surgery for hip fracture. J Bone Joint Surg Br 2006;88:1053-9.
109. Kennedy MT, Roche S, Fleming SM, et al. The association between aspirin and blood loss in hip fracture patients. Acta Orthoped Belg 1006;72:29-33.
110. Liu G, McNicol PL, Macall P, et al. The effect of preoperative aspirin and/or heparin therapy on coagulation and postoperative blood loss after coronary artery bypass surgery. Crit Care Resusc 1999;1: 139.

111. Slichter SJ. Platelet refractoriness and alloimmunization. Leukemia 1998;12(Suppl 1):S51-3.
112. Englberger L, Faeh B, Berdat PA, et al. Impact of clopidogrel in coronary artery bypass grafting. Eur J Cardiothorac Surg 2004;26:96-101.
113. Mehta RH, Roe MT, Mulgund J, et al. Acute clopidogrel use and outcomes in patients with non-ST-segment elevation acute coronary syndromes undergoing coronary artery bypass surgery. J Am Coll Cardiol 2006;48:281-6.
114. Nguyen CM, Harrington RA. Glycoprotein IIb/IIIa receptor antagonists: A comparative review of their use in percutaneous coronary intervention. Am J Cardiovasc Drugs 2003;3:423-36.
115. Reiter R, Jilma-Stohlawetz P, Horvath M, Jilma B. Additive effects between platelet concentrates and desmopressin in antagonizing the platelet glycoprotein IIb/IIIa inhibitor eptifibatide. Transfusion 2005;45:420-6.
116. Stuart MJ, Murphy S, Oski FA, et al. Platelet function in recipients of platelets from donors ingesting aspirin. N Engl J Med 1972;287:1105-9.
117. Watson AJS, Keogj JAB. Effect of 1-deamino-8-D-arginine vasopressin on the prolonged bleeding time in chronic renal failure. Nephron 1982;32:49-52.
118. Janson PA, Jubelirer SJ, Weinstein MJ, Deykin D. Treatment of the bleeding tendency in uremia with cryoprecipitate. N Engl J Med 1980; 303:1318-22.
119. Shattil S, Bennett JS. Acquired qualitative platelet disorders. In: Williams WJ, Beutler E, Erslev AJ, Lichtman M, eds. Hematology. New York: McGraw-Hill, 1990:1420-2.
120. Slichter SJ. Background, rationale, and design of a clinical trial to assess the effects of platelet dose on bleeding risk in thrombocytopenic patients. J Clin Apher 2006;21:78-84.
121. Hersh JK, Hom EG, Brecher ME. Mathematical modeling of platelet survival with implications for optimal transfusion practice in the chronically platelet transfusion-dependent patient. Transfusion 1998;38:637-44.
122. Norol F, Bierling P, Roudot-Thoraval F, et al. Platelet transfusion: A dose-response study. Blood 1998;92:1448-53.
123. Klumpp TR, Herman JH, Gaughan JP, et al. Clinical consequences of alterations in platelet transfusion dose: A prospective, randomized, double-blind trial. Transfusion 1999;39:674-81.
124. Heddle NM, Cook RJ, Tinmouth A, et al. A randomized controlled trial comparing standard and low dose strategies for transfusion of platelets (SToP) to patients with thrombocytopenia. Blood 2009;113:1564-73.
125. Slichter SJ, Kaufman RM, Assman SF, et al. Dose of prophylactic platelet transfusion and prevention of hemorrhage. N Engl J Med 2010; 362:600-13.
126. Hanson SR, Slichter SJ. Platelet kinetics in patients with bone marrow hypoplasia: Evidence for a fixed platelet requirement. Blood 1985;66: 1105-9.
127. Murphy S. Radiolabeling of PLTs to assess viability: A proposal for a standard. Transfusion 2004;44:131-3.
128. Slichter SJ. Mechanisms and management of platelet refractoriness. In Nance SJ, ed. Transfusion medicine in the 1990s. Arlington, VA: AABB, 1990:95-179.
129. Silva MA, Gregory KR, Carr-Greer MA, et al. Summary of the AABB Interorganizational Task Force on Bacterial Contamination of Platelets: Fall 2004 impact survey. Transfusion 2006;46:636-41.
130. Murphy S, Heaton WAL, Rebulla P, and the BEST Working Party of the International Society of Blood Transfusion. Platelet production in the Old World—and the New. Transfusion 1996;36:751-4.
131. Arnold DM, Heddle NM, Kulczycky M, et al. In vivo recovery and survival of apheresis and whole blood-derived platelets: A paired comparison in healthy volunteers. Transfusion 2006;46:257-64.
132. Dumont LJ, AuBuchon JP, Whitley P, et al. Seven-day storage of single-donor platelets: Recovery and survival in an autologous transfusion study. Transfusion 2002;42:847-53.
133. AuBuchon JP, Taylor H, Holme S, Nelson E. In vitro and in vivo evaluation of leukoreduced platelets stored for 7 days in CLX containers. Transfusion 2005;45:1356-61.
134. Holme S, Moroff G, Murphy S, for the BEST Working Party of the International Society of Blood Transfusion. A multi-laboratory evaluation of in vitro platelet assays: The tests for extent of shape change and response to hypotonic shock. Transfusion 1998;38:31-40.
135. Murphy S, Rebulla P, Bertolini F, et al. In vitro assessment of the quality of stored platelet concentrates. The BEST (Biomedical Excellence for Safer Transfusion) Task Force of the

International Society of Blood Transfusion. Transfus Med Rev 1994;8:29-36.

136. Rinder HM, Smith BR. In vitro evaluation of stored platelets. Is there hope for predicting posttransfusion platelet survival and function? Transfusion 2003;43:2-6.
137. Murphy S, Rinder HM, Smith BR. Utility of in vitro tests in predicting the in vivo viability of stored PLTs. Transfusion 2004;44: 618-19.
138. Peter-Salonen K, Bucher U, Nydegger UE. Comparison of post-transfusion recoveries achieved with either fresh or stored platelet concentrates. Blut 1987;54:207-12.
139. Leach MF, AuBuchon JP. The effect of platelet storage time on clinical response in marrow transplant recipients. Transfusion 1993;33: 661-4.
140. Slichter SJ, Davis K, Enright H, et al. Factors affecting posttransfusion platelet increments, platelet refractoriness, and platelet transfusion intervals in thrombocytopenic patients. Blood 2005;105:4106-14.
141. Davis KB, Slichter SJ, Corash L. Corrected count increments and platelet recoveries as measures of post-transfusion platelet response: Problems and a solution. Transfusion 1999;39:586-92.
142. Dunstan RA, Simpson MB, Knowles RW, Rosse WF. The origin of ABH antigens on human platelets. Blood 1985;65:615-19.
143. Julmy F, Achermann F, Schulzki T, et al. PLTs of blood group A1 donors express increased surface A antigen owing to apheresis and prolonged storage. Transfusion 2003;43:1378-85.
144. Hou M, Stockelberg D, Rydberg L, et al. Blood group A antigen expression in platelets is predominantly associated with glycoprotein Ib and Ib. Evidence for an A1/A2 difference. Transfus Med 1996;6:51-9.
145. Curtis BR, Edwards JT, Hessner MJ, et al. Blood group A and B antigens are strongly expressed on platelets of some individuals. Blood 2000; 96:1574-81.
146. Duquesnoy RJ, Anderson AJ, Tomasulo PA, Aster RH. ABO compatibility and platelet transfusions to refractory patients. Blood 1987;70: 23-30.
147. Heal JM, Rowe JM, McMican A, et al. The role of ABO matching in platelet transfusion. Eur J Haematol 1993;50:100-7.
148. Lee EJ, Schiffer CA. ABO compatibility can influence the results of platelet transfusion. Results of a randomized trial. Transfusion 1989; 29:384-9.
149. Heal JM, Blumberg N, Masel D. An evaluation of crossmatching, HLA, and ABO matching for platelet transfusions to refractory patients. Blood 1987;70:23-30.
150. Shanwell A, Ringden O, Wiechel B, et al. A study of the effect of ABO incompatible plasma in platelet concentrates transfused to bone marrow transplant recipients. Vox Sang 1991; 60:23-7.
151. Sadnai DT, Urbaniak SJ, Bruce M, Tighe JE. Repeat ABO-incompatible platelet transfusions leading to haemolytic transfusion reaction. Transfus Med 2006;16:375-9.
152. Larson LG, Welsh VJ, Ladd DJ. Acute intravascular hemolysis secondary to out-of-group platelet transfusion. Transfusion 2000;40:902-6.
153. Mair B, Benson K. Evaluation of changes in hemoglobin levels associated with ABO-incompatible plasma in apheresis platelets. Transfusion 1998;38:51-5.
154. Shanwell A, Andersson TM, Rostgaard K, et al. Post-transfusion mortality among recipients of ABO-compatible but non-identical plasma. Vox Sang 2009;96:316-23.
155. AuBuchon JP, de Wildt-Eggen J, Dumont L. Reducing the variation in performance of antibody titrations. Vox Sang 2008;95:57-65.
156. Fauzie D, Shirey RS, Thoman S, et al. The risk of hemolytic transfusion reactions due to passively acquired ABO antibodies: A retrospective study of non-group O adult recipients of Group O plateletpheresis transfusions (abstract). Transfusion 2004; 44(Suppl):36A.
157. Blumberg N, Heal JM, Kicks GL Jr, Risher WH. Association of ABO-mismatched platelet transfusions with morbidity and mortality in cardiac surgery. Transfusion 2001;41:790-3.
158. Lin Y, Callum JL, Coovadia AS, Murphy PM. Transfusion of ABO-nonidentical platelets is not associated with adverse clinical outcomes in cardiovascular surgery patients. Transfusion 2002;42:166-72.
159. Carr R, Hutton JL, Jenkins JA, et al. Transfusion of ABO-mismatched platelets leads to early platelet refractoriness. Br J Haematol 1990;75: 408-13.
160. Benjamin RB, Antin JH. ABO-incompatible bone marrow transplantation: The transfusion of incompatible plasma may exacerbate regimen-related toxicity. Transfusion 1999;39: 1273-4.
161. Molnar R, Johnson R, Sweat LT, Geiger TL. Absence of D alloimmunization in D– pediatric

oncology patients receiving D-incompatible single-donor platelets. Transfusion 2002;42: 177-82.

162. Huang ST, Huang Z, Boctor FN, Marques MB. Probability of anti-D development among Rh negative hospitalized patients receiving Rh positive apheresis platelets (abstract). Transfusion 2006;46(Suppl):158a.
163. Ewing CA, Rumsey DH, Langberg AF, Sandler SG. Immunoprophylaxis using intravenous Rh immune globulin should be standard practice when selected D-negative patients are transfused with D-positive random donor platelets. Immuno-hematol 1998;14:133-7.
164. Herzig RH, Herzig GP, Bull MI, et al. Correction of poor platelet transfusion responses with leukocyte-poor HL-A-matched platelet concentrates. Blood 1975;46:743-50.
165. Yankee RA, Grumet FC, Rogentine GN. Platelet transfusion therapy. The selection of compatible platelet donors for refractory patients by lymphocyte HL-A matching. N Engl J Med 1969;281:1208.
166. Moroff G, Garratty G, Heal JM, et al. Selection of platelets for refractory patients by LA matching and prospective crossmatching. Transfusion 1992;32:633-40.
167. Petz LD, Garratty G, Calhoun L, et al. Selecting donors of platelets for refractory patients on the basis of HLA antibody specificity. Transfusion 2000;40:1446-56.
168. AuBuchon JP, Leach MF. Investigating the possibility of drug-dependent platelet antibodies. Immunohematology 2009;25:136-40.
169. Leach MF, Cooper LK, AuBuchon JP. Detection of drug-dependent, platelet-reactive antibodies by solid-phase red cell adherence assays. Br J Haematol 1997;97:755-61.
170. Leach MF, AuBuchon JP. Coincidence of gentamycin induced drug-dependent platelet antibodies (abstract). Transfusion 1998;38(Suppl):29S.
171. Daly PA, Schiffer CA, Aisner J, Wiernik PH. Platelet transfusion therapy. One-hour posttransfusion increments are valuable in predicting the need for HLA-matched preparations. JAMA 1980;243:435-8.
172. O'Connell B, Lee EJ, Schiffer CA. The value of 10-minute posttransfusion platelet counts. Transfusion 1988;28:66-7.
173. Hirsch EO, Gardner FH. The transfusion of human blood platelets. J Lab Clin Med 1952;39: 556-69.
174. McFarland JG, Anderson AJ, Slichter SJ. Factors influencing the transfusion response to HLA-selected apheresis donor platelets in patients refractory to random platelet concentrates. Br J Haematol 1989;73:380-6.
175. Parker RD, Yamamoto LA, Miller WR. Interaction effects analysis of platelet transfusion data. Transfusion 1974;14:567-73.
176. Nakhoul IN, Kozuch P, Varma M. Management of adult idiopathic thrombocytopenic purpura. Clin Adv Hematol Oncol 2006;4:136-44.
177. Tarantino M. Recent advances in the treatment of childhood immune thrombocytopenic purpura. Semin Hematol 2006;43(3 Suppl 5):S11-7.
178. Carr JM, Kruskall MS, Kaye JA, Robinson SH. Efficacy of platelet transfusions in immune thrombocytopenia. Am J Med 1986;80:1051-4.
179. Fontana S, Kremer Hovinga JA, Lammle B, Mansouri Taleghani B. Treatment of thrombotic thrombocytopenic purpura. Vox Sang 2006;90:245-54.
180. Swisher KK, Terrell DR, Vesely SK, et al. Clinical outcomes after platelet transfusions in patients with thrombotic thrombocytopenic purpura. Transfusion 2009;49:873-87.
181. George JN. Clinical practice. Thrombotic thrombocytopenic purpura. N Engl J Med 2006; 354:1927-35.
182. Warkentin TE. Heparin-induced thrombocytopenia: Diagnosis and management. Circulation 2004;110:e454-8.
183. Leitner GC, Gruber R, Neumiller J, et al. Platelet content and growth factor release in platelet-rich plasma: A comparison of four different systems. Vox Sang 2006;91:135-8.
184. Everts PA, Knape JT, Weibrich G, et al. Platelet-rich plasma and platelet gel: A review. J Extra Corpor Technol 2006;38:174-87.
185. Murad MH, Stubbs JR, Gandhi MJ, et al. The effect of plasma transfusion on morbidity and mortality: A systematic review and meta-analysis. Transfusion 2010;50:1370-83.
186. Roback JD, Caldwell S, Carson J, et al. Evidence-based practice guidelines for plasma transfusion. Transfusion 2010;50:1227-39.
187. Peterson P, Hayes TE, Arkin CF, et al. The preoperative bleeding time test lacks clinical benefit: College of American Pathologists' and American Society of Clinical Pathologists' position article. Arch Surg 1998;133:134-9.
188. Suchman AL, Mushlin AI. How well does the activated partial thromboplastin time predict

postoperative hemorrhage? JAMA 1986;256: 750-3.

189. Counts RB, Haisch C, Simon TL, et al. Hemostasis in massively transfused trauma patients. Ann Surg 1979;190;91-9.
190. McVay PA, Toy PT. Lack of increased bleeding after liver biopsy in patients with mild hemostatic abnormalities. Am J Clin Pathol 1990;94: 747-53.
191. Segal JB, Dzik WH, Transfusion Medicine/Hemostasis Clinical Trials Network. Paucity of studies to support that abnormal coagulation test results predict bleeding in the setting of invasive procedures: An evidence-based review. Transfusion 2005;45:1413-25.
192. Rustad H, Myhre E. Surgery during anticoagulant treatment. The risk of increased bleeding in patients on oral anticoagulant treatment. Acta Med Scand 1963;173:115-19.
193. Storm O, Hansen AT. Mitral commissurotomy performed during anticoagulant prophylaxis with dicumarol. Circulation 1955;12:981-5.
194. Ewe K. Bleeding after liver biopsy does not correlate with indices of peripheral coagulation. Dig Dis Sci 1981;26:388-93.
195. Burns ER, Goldberg SN, Wenz B. Paradoxic effect of multiple mild coagulation factor deficiencies on the prothrombin time and activated partial thromboplastin time. Am J Clin Pathol 1993;100:94-8.
196. American Society of Anesthesiologists Task Force on Perioperative Blood Transfusion and Adjuvant Therapies. Practice guidelines for perioperative blood transfusion and adjuvant therapies: An updated report by the American Society of Anesthesiologists Task Force on Perioperative Blood Transfusion and Adjuvant Therapies. Anesthesiology 2006;105:198-208.
197. Fresh-Frozen Plasma, Cryoprecipitate, and Platelets Administration Practice Guidelines Development Task Force of the College of American Pathologists. Practice parameter for the use of fresh-frozen plasma, cryoprecipitate, and platelets. JAMA 1994;271:777-81.
198. O'Shaughnessy DF, Atterbury C, Bolton Maggs P, et al for the British Committee for Standards in Haematology, Blood Transfusion Task Force. Guidelines for the use of fresh-frozen plasma, cryoprecipitate and cryosupernatant. Br J Haematol 2004;126:11-28.
199. Ansell J, Hirsh J, Poller L, et al. The pharmacology and management of the vitamin K antagonists: The Seventh ACCP Conference on Antithrombotic and Thrombolytic Therapy. Chest 2004;126(3 Suppl):204S-33S.
200. Murphy PT, Casey MC, Abrams K. Audit of patients on oral anticoagulants with international normalized ratios of eight or above. Clin Lab Haematol 1998;20:253-7.
201. Makris M, Greaves M, Phillips WS, et al. Emergency oral anticoagulant reversal: The relative efficacy of infusions of fresh frozen plasma and clotting factor concentrate on correction of the coagulopathy. Thromb Haemost 1997; 77:477-80.
202. Yiu KH, Siu CW, Jim MH, et al. Comparison of the efficacy and safety profiles of intravenous vitamin K and fresh frozen plasma as treatment of warfarin-related over-anticoagulation in patients with mechanical heart valves. Am J Cardiol 2006;97:409-11.
203. Lankiewicz MW, Hays J, Friedman KD, et al. Urgent reversal of warfarin with prothrombin complex concentrate. J Thromb Haemost 2006;4:967-70.
204. Holland L, Warkentin TE, Refaai M, et al. Suboptimal effect of a three-factor prothrombin complex concentrate (Profilnine-SD) in correcting supratherapeutic international normalized ratio due to warfarin overdose. Transusion 2009;49:1171-7.
205. Tripodi A, Salerno F, Chantarangkul V, et al. Evidence of normal thrombin generation in cirrhosis despite abnormal conventional coagulation tests. Hepatology 2005;41:553-8.
206. Holland LL, Foster TM, Marlar RA, Brooks JP. Fresh frozen plasma is ineffective for correcting minimally elevated international normalized ratios. Transfusion 2005;45:1234-5.
207. Abdel-Wahab OI, Healy B, Dzik WH. Effect of fresh-frozen plasma transfusion on prothrombin time and bleeding in patients with mild coagulation abnormalities. Transfusion 2006; 46:1279-85.
208. Rohrer MJ, Natale AM. Effect of hypothermia on the coagulation cascade. Crit Care Med 1992;20:1402-5.
209. Meng ZH, Wolberg AS, Monroe DM 3rd, Hoffman M. The effect of temperature and pH on the activity of factor VIIa: Implications for the efficacy of high-dose factor VIIa in hypothermic and acidotic patients. J Trauma 2003;55: 886-91.
210. Ereth MH, Nuttall GA, Oliver WC Jr, et al. Temperature and duration of cardiopulmonary bypass influence transfusion requirements. J Clin Anesth 1998;10:588-92.

211. Engstrom M, Schott U, Romner B, Reinstrup P. Acidosis impairs the coagulation: A thromboelastographic study. J Trauma 2006;61:624-8.
212. Avidan, MS, Alcock EL, Da Fonseca J, et al. Comparison of structured use of routine laboratory tests or near-patient assessment with clinical judgement in the management of bleeding after cardiac surgery. Br J Anaesth 2004;92:178-86.
213. Anderson L, Quasim I, Soutar R, et al. An audit of red cell and blood product use after the institution of thromboelastometry in a cardiac intensive care unit. Transfus Med 2006;16:31-9.
214. De Gasperi A, Amici O, Mazza E, et al. Monitoring intraoperative coagulation. Transplant Proc 2006;38:815-17.
215. Samama CM, Djoudi R, Lecompte T, et al. Perioperative platelet transfusion. Recommendations of the French Health Products Safety Agency (AFSSAPS) 2003. Minerva Anestesiol 2006;72:447-52.
216. Suchman AL, Griner PF. Diagnostic uses of the activated partial thromboplastin time and prothrombin time. Ann Intern Med 1986;104: 810.
217. Orlin JB, Berkman EM. Partial plasma exchange using albumin replacement: Removal and recovery of normal plasma constituents. Blood 1980;56:1055-9.
218. Smith JF, Ness PM, Moroff G, Luban NL. Retention of coagulation factors in plasma frozen after extended holding at 1-6 degrees C. Vox Sang 2000;78:28-30.
219. O'Neill EM, Rowley J, Hannson-Wicher M, et al. Effect of 24-hour whole-blood storage on clotting factors. Transfusion 1999;39:488-91.
220. Scott E, Puca K, Hearly J, et al. Evaluation and comparison of coagulation factor activity in fresh-frozen plasma and 24-hour plasma at thaw and after 120 hours of 1 to 6 degrees C storage. Transfusion 2009;49:1584-91.
221. Sidhu RS, Le T, Brimhall B, Thompson H. Study of coagulation factor activities in apheresed thawed fresh frozen plasma at 1-6 degrees C for five days. J Clin Apher 2006;21:224-6.
222. Brach FA. Hereditary angioedema. Curr Opin Hematol 2005;12:493-8.
223. Cocchio C, Marzella N. Cinryze, a human plasma-derived C1 esterase inhibitor for prophylaxis of hereditary angioedema. PT 2009;34: 293-328.
224. Cunningham MT, Brandt JT, Laposata M, Olson JD. Laboratory diagnosis of dysfibrinogenemia. Arch Pathol Lab Med 2002;126:499-505.
225. Martinez J. Disorders of fibrinogen. In: Hoffman R, Benz EJ, Shattil SJ, et al, eds. Hematology: Basic principles and practice. 3rd ed. New York: Churchill Livingstone, 2000:1924-36.
226. The United States Pharmacopoeial Convention. Hemophilia management. Transfus Med Rev 1998;12:128-40.
227. Mannucci PM. How I treat patients with von Willebrand disease. Blood 2001;97:1915-19.
228. Lupinetti FM, Stoney WS, Alford WC Jr, et al. Cryoprecipitate-topical thrombin glue. Initial experience in patients undergoing cardiac operations. J Thorac Cardiovasc Surg 1985;90: 502-5.
229. Streiff MB, Ness PM. Acquired FV inhibitors: A needless iatrogenic complication of bovine thrombin exposure. Transfusion 2002;42:18-26.
230. Albala DM, Lawson JH. Recent clinical and investigational applications of fibrin sealant in selected surgical specialties. J Am Coll Surg 2006;202:685-97.
231. Graw RG Jr, Herzig G, Perry S, Henderson IS. Normal granulocyte transfusion therapy. N Engl J Med 1972;287:367-76.
232. Fortuny IE, Bloomfield CD, Hadlock DC, et al. Granulocyte transfusion: A controlled study in patients with acute non-lymphocytic leukemia. Transfusion 1975;15:548-58.
233. Higby DJ, Yates JW, Henderson ES, Holland JF. Filtration leukoapheresis for granulocyte transfusion therapy. N Engl J Med 1975;292: 761-7.
234. Vogler WR, Winton EF. A controlled study of the efficacy of granulocyte transfusions in patients with neutropenia. Am J Med 1977;63: 548-55.
235. Herzig RH, Herzig GP, Graw RG Jr, et al. Successful granulocyte therapy for gram-negative septicemia. N Engl J Med 1977;296:701-5.
236. Strauss RG. Granulocyte (neutrophil) transfusion therapy. In: Mintz PD, ed. Transfusion therapy: Clinical principles and practice. 3rd ed. Bethesda, MD: AABB Press, 2011:433-8.
237. Price TH. Granulocyte transfusion therapy. Transfusion 2006;46:1-5.
238. Gabrilove J. The development of granulocyte colony-stimulating factor and its various clinical applications. Blood 1992;80:1382-7.
239. Anderlini P, Przepiorka D, Champlin R, Körbling M. Biologic and clinical effects of granu-

locyte colony-stimulating factor in normal individuals. Blood 1996;88:2819-25.
240. Pirsch JD, Maki DG. Infectious complications in adults with bone marrow transplantation and T-cell depletion of donor marrow. Ann Intern Med 1986;104:619-32.
241. Morrison VA, Hakke RJ, Weisdorf DJ. Non-Candida fungal infections after bone marrow transplantation: Risk factors and outcomes. Am J Med 1994;96:497-503.
242. Ozsahin H, von Planta M, Muller I, et al. Successful treatment of invasive aspergillosis in chronic granulomatous disease by bone marrow transplantation, granulocyte colony-stimulating factor-mobilized granulocytes, and liposomal amphotericin-B. Blood 1998;92:2719-24.
243. Bielorai B, Toren A, Wolach B, et al. Successful treatment of invasive aspergillosis in chronic granulomatous disease by granulocyte transfusions followed by peripheral blood stem cell transplantation. Bone Marrow Transplant 2000;26:1025-8.
244. Liles WC, Rodger E, Dale DC. Combined administration of G-CSF and dexamethasone for the mobilization of granulocytes in normal donors: Optimization of dosing. Transfusion 2000;40:642-4.
245. Ghodsi Z, Strauss RG. Cataracts in neutrophil donors stimulated with adrenal corticosteroids. Transfusion 2001;41:1464-8.
246. Vamvakas EC, Pineda AA. Determinants of the efficacy of prophylactic granulocyte transfusions: A meta-analysis. J Clin Apher 1997;12:74-81.
247. Vamvakas EC, Pineda AA. Meta-analysis of clinical studies of the efficacy of granulocyte transfusions in the treatment of bacterial sepsis. J Clin Apher 1996;11:1-9.
248. Jenson HB, Pollock BH. The role of intravenous immunoglobulin for the prevention and treatment of neonatal sepsis. Semin Perinatol 1998;22:50-63.
249. Weisman LE, Weisman E, Lorenzetti PM. High intravenous doses of human immune globulin suppress neonatal Group B streptococcal immunity in rats. J Pediatr 1989;115:445-9.
250. Foster PR. Prions and blood products. Ann Med 2000;32:501-13.
251. Berger A, Doerr HW, Scharrer I, Weber B. Follow-up of four HIV-infected individuals after administration of hepatitis C virus and GBV-C/hepatitis G virus-contaminated intravenous immunoglobulin: Evidence for HCV but not GBV-C/HGV transmission. J Med Virol 1997;53:25-30.
252. Report of the tribunal of inquiry into the Blood Transfusion Service Board. Ireland: Government Publications, 1996.
253. Power JP, Davidson F, O'Riordan J, et al. Hepatitis C infection from anti-D immunoglobulin. Lancet 1995;346:372-3.
254. Yap PL. Intravenous immunoglobulin and hepatitis C virus: An overview of transmission episodes with emphasis on manufacturing data. Clin Ther 1996;18(Suppl B):43-58.
255. Doweiko JP, Nompleggi DJ. The role of albumin in human physiology and pathophysiology. Part III: Albumin and disease states. J Parenter Enteral Nutr 1991;15:476-83.
256. Vermeulen LC Jr, Ratko TA, Erstad BL, et al. A paradigm for consensus. The University Hospital consortium guidelines for the use of albumin, nonprotein colloid and crystalloid solutions. Arch Intern Med 1995;155:373-9.
257. Vincent JL, Dubois MJ, Navickis RJ, Wilkes MM. Hypoalbuminemia in acute illness: Is there a rationale for intervention? A metanalysis of cohort controlled trials. Ann Surg 2003;237:319-34.
258. Cochrane Injuries Group Albumin Reviewers. Human albumin administration in critically ill patients: Systematic review of randomized controlled trials. Br Med J 1998;317:235-46.
259. The SAFE study investigators. A comparison of albumin and saline for fluid resuscitation in the intensive care unit. N Engl J Med 2004;350:2247-56.
260. Brecher ME, Owen HG, Bandarenko N. Alternatives to albumin: Starch replacements for plasma exhange. J Clin Apher 1997;12:146-53.
261. Bork K. Pruritis precipitated by hydroxyethyl starch: A review. Br J Dermatol 2005;152:3-12.
262. Brown D, et al. Initial results of a randomized, prospective trial of prophylaxis to prevent joint disease in young children with factor VIII (FVIII) deficiency (abstract). Blood 2005;106:6a.
263. Stobart K, Iorio A, Wu JK. Clotting factor concentrates given to prevent bleeding and bleeding-related complications in people with hemophilia A or B. Cochrane Database Syst Rev 2006;19:CD003429.
264. Leissinger CA, Blatt PM, Hoots WK, Ewenstein B. Role of prothrombin complex concentrates in reversing warfarin anticoagulation: A review of the literature. Am J Hematol 2008;83:137-43.

265. Mariana G, Testa MG, Di Paolantonio T, et al, for the ad hoc study group. Use of recombinant, activated factor VII in the treatment of congenital factor VII deficiencies. Vox Sang 1999;77:131-6.
266. Deveras RA, Kessler CM. Reversal of warfarin-induced excessive anticoagulation with recombinant human factor VIIa concentrate. Ann Intern Med 2002;137:884-8.
267. Levy M, Peters M, Buller HR. Efficacy and safety of recombinant factor VIIa for treatment of severe bleeding. Crit Care Med 2005;33:883-90.
268. Niemann CU, Behrends M, Quan D, et al. Recombinant factor VIIa reduces the transfusion requirements in liver transplant patients with high MELD scores. Transfus Med 2006;16:93-100.
269. O'Connell NM, Perry DJ, Hodgson AJ, et al. Recombinant FVIIa in the management of uncontrolled hemorrhage. Transfusion 2003;43:1711-16.
270. Jeffers L, Chalasani N, Balart L, et al. Safety and efficacy of recombinant factor VIIa in patients with liver disease undergoing laparoscopic liver biopsy. Gastroenterology 2002;123:118-26.
271. O'Connell KA, Wood SS, Wise RP, et al. Thromboembolic adverse events after use of recombinant human factor VIIa. JAMA 2006;295:293-8.
272. Levy J, Fingerhut A, Brott T, et al. Recombinant factor VIIa in patients with coagulopathy secondary to anticoagulant therapy, cirrhosis, or severe traumatic injury: Review of safety profile. Transfusion 2006;46:919-23.
273. Johansson PI. Off-label use of recombinant factor VIIa for treatment of haemorrhage: Results from randomized controlled clinical trials. Vox Sang 2008;95:1-7.
274. Bosch J, Thabut D, Bendtsen F, et al for the European Study Group on rFVIIa in UGI Hemorrhage. Recombinant Factor VIIa for upper gastrointestinal bleeding in patients with cirrhosis: A randomized double-blind trial. Gastroenterology 2004;127:1123-30.
275. Lodge JP, Jonas S, Oussoultzoglou E. Recombinant coagulation factor VIIa in major liver resection: A randomized, placebo-controlled, double-blind clinical trial. Anesthesiology 2005;102:269-75.
276. Mayer SA, Brun NC, Begtrup K, et al. Efficacy and safety of recombinant activated factor VII for acute intracerebral hemorrhage. N Engl J Med 2008;358:2127-37.
277. Goodnough LT, Lublin DM, Zhang L, et al. Transfusion medicine service policies for recombinant factor VIIa administration. Transfusion 2004;44:1325-31.
278. Mathew P, Simon TL, Hunt KE, Crookston KP. How we manage requests for recombinant factor VIIa (NovoSeven). Transfusion 2007;47:8-14.
279. Bromberg ME. Immune thrombocytopenic purpura—the changing therapeutic landscape. N Engl J Med 2006;355:164-5.
280. Durabi K, Abdel-Wahab O, Dzik WH. Current usage of intravenous immune globulin and the rationale behind it: Massachusetts General Hospital data and a review of the literature. Transfusion 2006;46:741-53.
281. Eijkhout HW, van Der Meer JW, Kallenberg CG, et al for the Inter-University Working Party for the Study of Immune Deficiencies. The effect of two different dosages of intravenous immunoglobulin on the incidence of recurrent infections in patients with primary hypogammaglobulinemia. A randomized, double-blind, multicenter crossover trial. Ann Intern Med 2001;135:165-74.
282. Nydegger UE. Immunoglobulins. In: Simon TL, Snyder EL, Solheim BG, et al, eds. Rossi's principles of transfusion medicine. 4th ed. Bethesda, MD: AABB Press, 2009:260-72.
283. Schwartz J Spitalnik S, Grima KM. Severe hemolysis following administration of Rh_0(D) immune globulin in an ITP patient associated with anti-C. Blood 2006;107:2585.
284. Griffin JH. Control of coagulation reactions. In: Beutler E, Lichtman MA, Coller BS, et al, eds. Williams hematology. 6th ed. New York: McGraw-Hill, 2001:1435-49.
285. 285. Bucur SJ, Levy JH, Despotis GJ, et al. Uses of antithrombin III concentrate in congenital and acquired deficiency states. Transfusion 1998;38:481-98.
286. White B, Perry D. Acquired antithrombin deficiency in sepsis. Br J Haematol 2001; 112:26-31.
287. Kolarich D, Turecek PL, Weber A, et al. Biochemical, molecular characterization, and glycoproteomic analyses of α_1 proteinase inhibitor products used for replacement therapy. Transfusion 2006;46:1959-77.

Chapter 21

Administration of Blood Components

Bonnie L. S. Sink, BSN, RN, HP(ASCP)

THE ADMINISTRATION OF blood and blood components incorporates multiple personnel and hospital services. There should be collaboration between all parties in developing policies and procedures for the blood administration process. It involves not only the transfusion service but also surgeons, anesthesiologists, primary-care physicians, transporting personnel, and the nurse or transfusionist. The act of initiating a transfusion is critical in that procedures at this stage provide the last line of defense in the detection of errors before the infusion of the component to the patient. All personnel who contribute to this event should be provided training in their duties regarding what actions they can take to provide the safest transfusion for the patient.

EVENTS AND CONSIDERATIONS BEFORE DISPENSING THE COMPONENT

Once a patient has been identified by a licensed provider/prescriber as needing a transfusion, many steps and considerations are involved in the time before the component is dispensed.

Recipient Consent

AABB *Standards for Blood Banks and Transfusion Services (Standards)*[1(p41)] states that "the blood bank or transfusion service medical director shall participate in the development of policies, processes, and procedures regarding recipient consent for transfusion." The recipient consent document should contain indications, risks, possible side effects, and alternatives to transfusion of allogeneic blood components. (Note that some state laws contain specific required elements of consent.) The patient has the right to accept or reject a transfusion. The patient needs to have an opportunity to ask questions. Documentation of consent can be obtained with the use of a signed consent form or through the recording of verbal consent. Documentation of such consent must be maintained in the patient's medical record in the manner defined by the institution. If a patient refuses transfusion, this refusal must also be documented in the medi-

Bonnie L. S. Sink, BSN, RN, HP(ASCP), Clinical Nurse Specialist, National Institutes of Health, Department of Transfusion Medicine, Bethesda, Maryland
The author has disclosed no conflicts of interest.

cal record. Each institution needs to have a process for recording a patient's refusal to receive blood or blood components.

Recipient consent for the transfusion must be obtained from patients who are competent to make such decisions. If the patient is unable to give consent, a legally authorized representative or surrogate may provide consent (depending on local and state laws). If no one is available to give consent and the need for transfusion is considered to be a medical emergency, the component may be administered without consent. If consent is not obtained, the need to transfuse without obtaining consent needs to be documented in the medical record. Medical institutions should define which individuals within the institution are allowed to obtain the consent and the duration the consent remains in effect.

Patient Education and History

The patient needs to have the opportunity to ask questions. The physician or nurse starting the transfusion should discuss with the patient the symptoms to report that are suggestive of a reaction, indicate how long the patient should expect the transfusion event to last, and answer any other questions the patient may have.

It is important to take a history from the patient before the component is ordered so that it can be determined if the patient is at increased risk for a transfusion reaction. It is useful to ask whether the patient has had any previous transfusions and, if so, whether there were any adverse reactions.

If the patient has had previous reactions, the medical team should determine whether the patient needs to receive medication before the transfusion or whether special processing of the component is indicated to mitigate the risk of an adverse reaction.

Medical Order

Blood Component

A licensed care provider issues two orders for components to be administered. The first order, for the clinical laboratory, should request that units be prepared [eg, crossmatching of Red Blood Cell (RBC) units] for the patient. The second order, for the transfusionist, should indicate how the component should be administered. These orders should specify the following:

- The patient's name and other identifiers (eg, date of birth, medical record number).
- The component (eg, RBCs, Apheresis Platelets) to prepare or administer.
- Any special processing required of the component (eg, leukocyte reduction, irradiation, washing).
- The number of units or volume to be administered.
- The date and time for the infusion.
- The flow rate or period for administering the component (must be <4 hours).

Laboratory Testing

After receiving an order from a licensed provider, the transfusion service initiates a series of steps to ensure the provision of a compatible component. In order to issue blood components for a specifically identified patient (except in the case of an emergency transfusion), the laboratory must have a blood sample from the patient. Generally, the sample must be drawn within 3 days of the individual being transfused; the draw date is considered day 0.[1(p34)] Institutional policy may differ on how long the sample is acceptable for testing and crossmatching. For example, if the patient has not had a transfusion or been pregnant in the prior 3 months, the sample may be acceptable for longer than 3 days for testing purposes. The sample must be labeled at the patient's bedside using at least two unique identifiers, such as patient name and date of birth. The label should contain sufficient information for unique identification of the patient (eg, name, date of birth, patient identification number), the identification of the person collecting the sample, and the date the sample was collected.[1(pp32-33)]

The steps required to type and screen the recipient's blood for unexpected allo- and autoantibodies are described in detail in Chapters 15 and 16. The time interval from sample receipt to availability of the requested component can vary greatly, depending on a number of factors. For example, availability is highly dependent on the inventory of components maintained by the transfusing facility. Some components may need to be ordered from an outside provider. If the patient has developed an antibody to a red cell antigen, the laboratory may require additional time to identify the specificity of the antibody and find compatible units. Some components require thawing, pooling, relabeling, or other preparation before release. Communication between laboratory and transfusing personnel is needed to predict availability of components for administration. Components that require thawing have a shortened shelf life once thawed (4-24 hours), and transfusionists need to be aware of the shortened period during which the unit must be infused.

Venous Access

The transfusionist must determine whether the patient has a central line, peripheral intravenous line, implantable port, or peripherally inserted central catheter (PICC) in place that is acceptable for infusion of blood components. The acceptability of the catheter size is dependent on how quickly the blood needs to be administered. Acceptable intravenous catheter sizes for use in transfusing cellular blood components range from 22 to 14 gauge.[2] A 20- to 18-gauge intravenous catheter is a good compromise for the general adult population and provides adequate flow rates without excessive discomfort to the patient. In patients with small veins or in need of rapid flow rates, the catheter size should be adjusted accordingly. When transfusing an infant or a toddler, a 24- to 22-gauge intravenous catheter may be suitable but requires infusion through a syringe[3] (see Chapter 23). With the use of smaller catheters, blood dilution and a pump are helpful to administer the unit to prevent slow flow rates that lead to clogging of the intravenous catheter. Units suspended in a preservative solution such as Adsol usually do not require additional dilution. It is important that the infusion line be open and functioning well before the component is received at the patient's bedside.

Prophylactic Medications Given Before Transfusion

If a medication has been ordered before the infusion, it should be administered in advance of the component's arrival to the transfusion unit. Although antipyretics (acetaminophen) are commonly ordered to reduce the occurrence of febrile nonhemolytic transfusion reactions,[4] indications for their use are controversial. Some providers routinely use antipyretics in a prophylactic manner, whereas others wait until the patient has experienced at least one febrile transfusion reaction.[4-7] Others believe prophylactic use may mask the elevated temperature that results from a transfusion reaction, thus hiding a clinically relevant event, although evidence for this is limited. Antihistamines (diphenhydramine and/or an H2 blocker) may be ordered as a premedication for individuals who have had mild allergic or urticarial reactions to transfusions in the past. Meperidine (Demerol, Bayer Corp., Myerstown, PA) or corticosteroids are occasionally ordered for patients who have experienced severe rigors during a prior transfusion.[8] If the premedication is given orally, the transfusionist should wait 30 to 60 minutes before initiating the transfusion. If the premedication is given intravenously, a 10-minute period before transfusion is adequate.

Equipment

Blood Warmers

Blood warmers are rarely needed during routine transfusion situations. However, they can be useful when rapid transfusion of components is required, especially in trauma or surgery settings, because the infusion of cold components can cause hypothermia and cardiac complications, increasing morbidity and mortality for the patient.[9] The likelihood of clinically important hypothermia is increased when blood is transfused through a central venous device directly into the right atrium.

Other settings where blood warmers are advantageous include transfusions to neonates, where hypothermia can cause serious adverse effects in the infant. Opinions vary on the use of blood warmers in patients with cold agglutinins.[10,11]

AABB *Standards*[1(p6)] states that "warming devices shall be equipped with a temperature-sensing device and a warning system to detect malfunctions and prevent hemolysis or other damage to blood or blood components." Warming blood to temperatures >42 C may cause hemolysis.[12] The transfusion service should work with departments that use blood warmers to make sure the devices are approved by the Food and Drug Administration (FDA) for infusion of components. Warming devices should be validated, and maintenance and testing of alarms should be performed according to the manufacturer's suggestion. Blood should not be warmed by placing it in a microwave, on a heat source, or in hot water or by using other devices not specifically approved by the FDA for blood warming.

Infusion Systems

Infusion pumps or infusion systems are used to administer fluids, medications, blood, and components through clinically accepted routes of administration. An infusion pump or infusion system allows for a controlled infusion rate and, thus, controlled administration of volume over a desired period; it also provides an alarm system to notify care providers of problems with the infusion. Consequently, many providers prefer this method to simple gravity administration. However, there is potential for hemolysis of the cellular components infused through these pumps. The manufacturer of the pump should be consulted to determine if the pump is approved for infusion of blood components. If it is not approved, the institution should establish a validation plan to confirm that the pump does not injure components before its use if component therapy is allowed. Many of the electromechanical pump devices that are approved for blood administration have available specific administration sets with standard in-line filters.

With the use of infusion pumps and PICC lines for blood transfusion, the risk of exceeding the pounds per square inch allowed for the catheter should be taken into consideration. Each institution should ensure the infusion pump used does not generate pressure that exceeds the limits of the catheter.[13]

Syringe Infusion Pumps

A syringe infusion pump may be used for neonatal or pediatric patients. It requires the withdrawal of blood into the syringe and allows for the infusion of small volumes. For more details, see Chapter 23.

Pressure Devices

The use of an externally applied pneumatic pressure device may achieve flow rates of 70 to 300 mL per minute depending on the pressure applied.[2] The device should have a gauge to monitor the pressure. Pressure in excess of 300 mm Hg may cause the seams of the blood bag to leak or rupture. Pressure should be applied evenly over the entire bag. When using a pressure device, a large-gauge cannula should be used to prevent hemolysis. The application of an external pressure device to the blood bag to expedite the transfusion of RBCs causes minimal damage to the red cells and is a safe practice in the majority of patients.[14] However, the use of pressure devices has been reported to provide only a small increase in component flow rates. When rapid infusion is desired, an increase in cannula size typically provides better results.[15]

Availability of Emergency Equipment

The transfusionist should know how to obtain and administer emergency interventions. Items to be prepared or available for emergency use to respond to a transfusion reaction include the following:

- 0.9% sodium chloride intravenous (IV) solution and administration set to keep an IV line open.

- Medications to treat a reaction. There should be a mechanism to obtain emergency medications as prescribed in the event of an allergic reaction, shock, renal failure, hypotension, rigors, or circulatory overload.
- A mechanism to activate emergency resuscitation measures in the event of a severe reaction. Ventilatory assistance and an oxygen source should be available in case of transfusion-related acute lung injury or severe allergic reaction.

Baseline Assessment of Recipient

A baseline physical assessment should include vital signs and assessment for signs and symptoms existing before the transfusion that may mimic a transfusion reaction, such as shortness of breath, rash, pruritus, wheezing, and chills. A patient with renal or cardiopulmonary disease may indicate the need for a slower flow rate to prevent fluid overload.

The patient's vital signs should be taken before the initiation of the transfusion as a baseline for subsequent comparison. This helps to identify possible untoward reactions that may result from the transfusion. If the patient has an elevated temperature before transfusion, it may be difficult to ascertain later if a transfusion reaction presenting with an elevation of temperature has occurred during blood administration. In addition, a patient with an elevated temperature may destroy cellular components at an increased rate.[15] In patients with an elevated temperature, an antipyretic should be administered and given time to have an effect, as long as the transfusion can be postponed.

DISPENSING AND TRANSPORTATION

Delivery of Components to the Patient Area

Each institution must have an identified method for issuing components and ensuring that they are delivered and accepted in a timely manner by the receiving transfusionist. Before dispensing, transfusion service personnel should check the appearance of the unit. The blood should not be issued if it appears discolored or abnormally cloudy or foamy, or if clots, clumps or loss of bag integrity are detected. Components should not leave the controlled environment until the transfusion site for the patient has been identified, the patient has been properly prepared, and the transfusionist is ready to begin the infusion. There must be a mechanism to correctly identify the intended recipient and component at the time of the request to issue the component. Institutions should train staff to order components so that they arrive in an expedited manner and are not left outside a controlled environment. Institutions may use dedicated personnel or automated delivery systems to facilitate the delivery of components to their final destination. Whatever the system, the transfusion service should validate the procedure by which components are picked up and/or transported, to ensure that delivery occurs in a timely manner and with no damage to the units. With the exception of emergency or large-volume transfusion circumstances, transfusion services generally allow the issue of only 1 unit at a time.

At the time a unit is issued, AABB *Standards* requires a final clerical check of transfusion service records with each unit or component. Verification must include[1(p39)]:

1. The intended recipient's two independent identifiers (name, date of birth, or patient identification number and/or unique identifier given at the time the crossmatch sample is drawn), ABO group, and Rh type.
2. The donor unit or pool identification number, the donor ABO group, and, if required, the Rh type.
3. The interpretation of crossmatch tests, if performed.
4. Special transfusion requirements.
5. The expiration date and, if applicable, time.
6. The date and time of issue.

Standards requires that there be a process to confirm agreement of the above information and that discrepancies be resolved before issue.[1(p40)]

Delay in Starting Transfusion

If an unexpected occurrence does not allow for the prompt start of the component infusion, the unit should be returned to the transfusion service for proper storage. Transfusion services may set limits, based on validation, to the time that a unit can be out of the controlled storage environment before it is considered unsuitable for reissue (usually 30 minutes). Transfusion services may also have methods to determine if the component is suitable for reissue. Components should never be stored or held in a patient care unit unless there is a controlled, monitored environment for components. Trauma areas and surgical units may have arrangements with the transfusion service for controlled storage of units. If the temperature of a refrigerated component rises above 10 C, reissue is not permissible.

If a unit has been entered (spiked for transfusion), it may not be returned to the transfusion service for reissue. It must either be infused within 4 hours of the time it was spiked, or it must be discarded.

EVENTS AND CONSIDERATIONS BEFORE COMPONENT ADMINISTRATION

Identification of the Recipient and Correct Component

Once the unit is received, a qualified transfusionist should take it to the patient's bedside and perform several checks with another health-care provider qualified in performing identification verification. If two individuals are not available, automated identification technology (eg, a bar-code reader) may be used in place of one of the individuals.[16] The following items should be checked:

- **Appearance of the unit.** Units should be returned if there is discoloration, foaming, or bubbles in the component; abnormal cloudiness; presence of clots or clumps; or loss of integrity of the bag.
- **Identification of patient and unit.** The patient's name and identification number must match the label on the unit bag or tag and the medical order. The requirements of the institution for patient identification must be satisfied. Institutions often require an additional identification check to verify the identity of the unit with the same patient whose sample was collected for crossmatch.
- **Medical order.** The transfusionist should verify that the component is the one requested on the medical order and that any special processing was performed. In particular, the transfusionist should ensure that leukocyte reduction or irradiation was performed if ordered.
- **Blood type.** The patient's blood type should be compatible with the unit.
- **Expiration date (and time, if applicable).** The unit should not be transfused if the expiration date or time has passed.

The transfusion should be withheld if any discrepancy or abnormality is found. Requirements of The Joint Commission (2009NPSG.01.03.01)[16] state that hospitals should "eliminate transfusion errors related to patient misidentification."

Proper bedside identification of the recipient is the final step to prevent the administration of an incorrect blood component to a patient. Although individuals often worry about the possibility of exposure to infectious agents from transfusion, equal concern should be raised about the inadvertent transfusion of incompatible blood. Approximately 1 in every 19,000 units of RBCs are transfused to the wrong patient each year; 1 in 76,000 units results in an acute hemolytic transfusion reaction, and 1 in 1.8 million units of transfused RBCs results in death from an acute hemolytic transfusion reaction. A reduction in these avoidable deaths has been noted with the initiation of machine-readable information on blood container labels and systems for checking the identity of patients.[17]

To prevent the fatal consequences of misidentification, specific systems have been developed and marketed, including identification bracelets with bar codes and/or radiofrequency identification devices, biometric scanning, mechanical or electronic locks preventing access to bags assigned to other patients, and hand-held computers suitable for transferring blood request and administration data from the patient's bedside to the transfusion service information system in real time. Each system provides a method to bring staff toward self-correction during the procedure.[18,19] Studies show that rates of positive recipient identification can be increased by such systems. None of these systems negates the need for good quality management such as adequate standard operating procedures, regular training, periodic competency assessment, and system monitoring.

Infusion Sets

Components must be administered through special IV tubing with a filter designed to remove blood clots and particles potentially harmful to the patient. Standard blood administration tubing generally has a 170- to 260-micron filter, but this specific micron size is not mandated or required. The tubing can be rinsed or primed with either 0.9% sodium chloride or the component itself. The manufacturer's instructions should be reviewed for proper use. The IV setup should have a mechanism that allows bypass of the blood IV administration tubing to start 0.9% sodium chloride in the event of a reaction. A suggested mechanism is to have a "Y" port or three-way stopcock close to the infusion site that would allow the administration of 0.9% sodium chloride.

Microaggregate Filters

Microaggregate filters are not used for routine blood administration. These second-generation filters were originally developed to remove leukocytes and to complement or replace the clot screen in the 1970s.[20] They have since been replaced by more efficient third-generation leukocyte reduction filters.[21] Microaggregate filters have a screen filter of 20 to 40 microns and retain fibrin strands and clumps of dead cells. Red cells, which are 8 microns in diameter, can flow through the filters. Microaggregate filters are typically used for the reinfusion of shed autologous blood collected during or after surgery.

Leukocyte Reduction Filters

Leukocyte reduction filters are expected to reduce the number of leukocytes in red cell and platelet units to less than 5×10^6 cells per unit (greater than 99.9% of the leukocytes are removed from the unit). Leukocyte reduction decreases the incidence of febrile transfusion reactions, the risk of HLA alloimmunization, and the transmission of cytomegalovirus by cellular blood components[20,21] (see Chapter 6). These filters are provided by various manufacturers for prestorage use shortly after collection of the units in the transfusion service or for poststorage use at the bedside. Prestorage leukocyte reduction is generally preferred for a number of reasons, one of which is that leukocyte reduction efficacy can be monitored. It is important to verify that the filter being used is intended for use with the component being transfused (red cells or platelets) and to note the maximum number of units that can be administered through one filter. Filters designed for red cells or platelets may not be used interchangeably. The manufacturer's instructions should be followed for priming and administering blood components through the filter. Otherwise, leukocyte removal may be ineffective or an air lock may develop, preventing passage of the component through the filter. Leukocyte filters should never be used to administer granulocyte or mononuclear cell concentrates (eg, hematopoietic progenitor cells).

The use of bedside leukocyte reduction filters has been associated with dramatic hypotension in some individuals, often in the absence of other symptoms. This happens more frequently with patients taking angiotensin-converting enzyme (ACE) inhibitors. If a precipitous drop in blood pressure is noted, the transfusion should be stopped immediately.

The use of components that were filtered in the blood center or transfusion service before storage decreases the incidence of such reactions.[22]

Compatible IV Solutions

No medications or solutions other than 0.9% sodium chloride injection (USP) should be administered with blood components through the same tubing. Solutions containing dextrose alone may cause red cells to swell and lyse. Lactated Ringer's solution or other solutions containing high levels of calcium may overcome the buffering capacity of the citrate anticoagulant in the blood preservative solution and cause clotting of the component.[23]

AABB *Standards* allows exceptions to the above restrictions when 1) the drug or solution has been approved by the FDA for use with blood administration or 2) there is documentation available to show that the addition is safe and does not adversely affect the blood or component.[1(p42)] Acceptable solutions according to these criteria include ABO-compatible plasma, 5% albumin, or plasma protein fraction. Certain solutions are compatible with blood or blood components as noted in the package inserts reviewed by the FDA, including Normosol-R pH 7.4 (Hospira, Lake Forest, IL), Plasma-Lyte-A injection pH 7.4 (Baxter Healthcare, Deerfield, IL), and Plasma-Lyte 148 injection (Multiple Electrolytes Injection, Type 1, USP; Baxter Healthcare).[21] There are several formulations of Plasma-Lyte that are not isotonic or that contain calcium; package inserts must be checked to confirm compatibility with components.

The literature reports the safe use of morphine, hydromorphone (Dilaudid, Abbott Laboratories, Abbott Park, IL), and meperidine (Demerol) administered as a bolus in the same tubing as red cells during monitored periods of patient-controlled analgesia. However, high doses of meperidine added to the RBC bag have caused hemolysis.[24,25] The literature is not extensive, so this practice should be used with caution and only when there is no other venous access available to allow separate administration.

ADMINISTRATION

Starting the Transfusion

Once the identification of the unit and the recipient are verified, the unit is spiked using aseptic technique. At hospitals that use Joint Commission accreditation for deemed status purposes, Joint Commission requirements for the transfusionist apply (HR.01.02.01)[16]: "If blood transfusions and intravenous medications are administered by staff other than doctors of medicine or osteopathy, the staff members have special training for this duty."

The blood administration tubing should be filled with either 0.9% sodium chloride or with the contents of the blood component. If any solution or medication other than 0.9% sodium chloride is infused before component administration, the tubing should be flushed with 0.9% sodium chloride before the blood infusion. Furthermore, isotonic saline should be the last solution to flow through the tubing before blood infusion. The infusion should start slowly at approximately 2 mL per minute for the first 15 minutes while the transfusionist remains near the patient. Severe reactions may occur with as little as 10 mL transfused. Potentially life-threatening reactions most commonly occur within 10 to 15 minutes of the start of a transfusion.[26] If there is no sign of a reaction after the first 15 minutes, the flow rate can be increased to the designated infusion rate. The flow rate should be adjusted according to the volume that the patient's circulatory system can tolerate. Consideration should be give to the patient's size, blood volume, cardiac status, and hemodynamic condition. (See Table 21-1.)

Monitoring the Transfusion

The transfusionist should continue to monitor the patient throughout the infusion and check the IV site and flow rate. If the IV rate has slowed down, the transfusionist should take one or more of the following actions: 1) check to make sure that the IV site is patent and there is no swelling at the IV site; 2) attempt to administer the component through an infusion pump; 3) raise or elevate the unit; 4) examine the filter for air, excessive debris, or clots; or 5)

TABLE 21-1. Blood Component Transfusions in Nonemergency Settings

	Suggested Adult Flow Rate				
Component	**First 15 minutes**	**After 15 minutes**	**Special Considerations**	**ABO Compatibility**	**Filter**
Red Blood Cells (RBCs)	1-2 mL/min (60-120 mL/hour)	As rapidly as tolerated; approximately 4 mL/min or 240 mL/hour	Infusion should not exceed 4 hours For patients at risk of fluid overload, adjust flow rate to 1 mL/kg/hour	Whole blood: ABO identical RBCs: ABO compatible with recipient's plasma Crossmatch required	In-line (170-260 micron) Leukocyte reduction if indicated
Platelets	2-5 mL/min (120-300 mL/hour) during the first 5 minutes	300 mL/hour or as tolerated (after the first 5 minutes)	Generally given over 1 hour	Crossmatch not required ABO/Rh compatibility preferable but not required May be HLA matched	In-line (170-260 micron) Leukocyte reduction if indicated
Plasma	2-5 mL/min (120-300 mL/hour) during the first 5 minutes	As rapidly as tolerated (after the first 5 minutes); approximately 300 mL/hour	Thaw time may be needed before issue	Crossmatch not required ABO compatibility with recipient red cells	In-line (170-260 micron)
Granulocytes	1-2 mL/min (60-120 mL/hour)	120-150 mL/hour or as tolerated	Over approximately 2 hours Infuse as soon as possible after collection/release of product; irradiate	Crossmatch required ABO/Rh compatibility required May be HLA matched	In-line (170-260 micron) No leukocyte reduction filter or depth-type microaggregate filters
Cryoprecipitated AHF	As rapidly as tolerated		Infuse as soon as possible after thawing; pooling is preferred	Crossmatch and ABO compatibility not required	In-line (170-260 micron)

consider the addition of 0.9% sodium chloride as a diluent if the unit is too viscous. Frequent monitoring of vital signs during the infusion helps alert the transfusionist to a possible transfusion reaction. It is suggested that vital signs be taken within 5 to 15 minutes after beginning the transfusion, then according to institutional policy thereafter. There is little evidence to indicate a required routine frequency for vital-sign monitoring other than at baseline, early on after the start of the transfusion, and after transfusion.[27] Vital signs should be taken at once if there is a suspected transfusion reaction. The bag tag or other unit identifiers should never be removed during the transfusion.

The transfusionist should be knowledgeable about signs of an adverse reaction and able to act early when such signs arise (see Chapter 27). Visual observation of the patient is important, along with listening to the patient. The patient may experience symptoms before any changes in the vital signs.

If a transfusion reaction is suspected, the transfusion should be stopped and 0.9% sodium chloride administered. The 0.9% sodium chloride should be infused near the IV insertion site to avoid flushing the tubing with the residual component. The unit identification should be rechecked. The transfusionist should notify the patient's care provider of any suspected transfusion reaction and obtain emergency medication orders as needed for the suspected reaction. It is helpful for institutions to summarize and have readily available descriptions of common reactions and immediate steps to be taken in the event of certain symptoms. Once the patient is stable, the transfusion service should be notified of a suspected transfusion reaction, and institutional policy should be followed for return of the component bag and/or laboratory studies needed to evaluate the reaction.

Completing the Transfusion

At the completion of the transfusion event, the patient's vital signs are obtained. The bag and tubing are discarded in a biohazard container if the transfusion is uneventful.

Because patients can experience transfusion reactions several hours to days after the transfusion is complete, medical staff should continue to monitor the patient periodically for 4 to 6 hours after the end of the transfusion to detect febrile or pulmonary reactions that may be associated with blood administration. If the patient is not under direct medical supervision after the transfusion event, medical staff should provide written instructions to the patient and caregiver about signs and symptoms to be aware of and report, and they should ensure that the patient has a phone number to call or a person to contact should a reaction occur later.

Documentation of the transfusion event should be made in the patient's medical record. At a minimum, AABB *Standards* requires the following documentation[1(p42)]:

1. Medical order for transfusion.
2. Documentation of recipient consent.
3. Name or type of component.
4. Donor unit or pool identification number.
5. Date and time of transfusion.
6. Pre- and posttransfusion vital signs.
7. Volume transfused.
8. Identification of the transfusionist.
9. Any adverse events possibly related to the transfusion.

If another unit needs to be transfused, the institution's guidelines and/or manufacturer's recommendations should be consulted to determine if the same blood administration tubing may be used for subsequent units. If there are no contraindications from the manufacturer, institutions frequently allow the tubing to be used for a 4-hour period. Therefore, if more than 1 unit can be infused in 4 hours, blood administration tubing sets may be used for more than one component.

UNIQUE TRANSFUSION SETTINGS

See Chapter 23 for information about pediatric and neonatal patients and transfusion.

Operating Room and Trauma: Rapid Infusions

If components need to be administered rapidly, the use of pressure infusion, large-bore administration tubing, and 8-Fr intravenous catheters can decrease the infusion time without the occurrence of hemolysis.[28,29] Specific tubing sets are designed for rapid blood administration with appropriate filters. Flow rates as fast as 10 to 25 mL/second (600-1500 mL/minute) have been reported with such tubing. As multiple units are infused through the same tubing, the flow rate may decrease appreciably. At such rapid infusion rates, steps should be taken to avoid hypothermia.

Hypocalcemia has been noted with rapid transfusions. This is usually transient and dependent on the amount and rate of citrate infused. Calcium replacement may be based on the patient's ionized serum calcium level and the rate of citrate administration.[30]

Transfusion-associated hyperkalemic cardiac arrest has been reported with rapid administration of RBCs. It may develop with rapid RBC administration even with modest transfusion volume between 1 (in a neonate) and 54 units. Contributing factors are acidosis, hypoglycemia, hypocalcemia, and hypothermia at time of arrest.[31]

If components are urgently needed and a delay in transfusion could be detrimental to the patient, the transfusion service should have a process to provide components before all pretransfusion compatibility testing is completed. Uncrossmatched units are released with a signed statement from the requesting physician indicating that the clinical situation requires urgent release before the completion of testing. If components in the transfusion service inventory are not immediately accessible to trauma units or the operating room, a supply of group O red cells may be maintained at these sites. The transfusion service must ensure proper storage of components at satellite storage sites.

Out-of-Hospital Transfusion

Transfusing blood in a nonhospital setting requires a well-planned program that incorporates all the aspects of the hospital setting and emphasizes safety considerations. An outpatient surgery center, oncology clinic, or dialysis center is likely to be able to provide medical assistance in a timely manner in the event of an adverse reaction. Medical staff availability as well as medications and equipment to handle adverse reactions must be considered and arranged in advance. Staff should be comfortable with blood administration procedures and patient monitoring. Blood administration outside the hospital should be performed by personnel with substantial experience in this setting.

Transfusion in the home generally allows close monitoring of the transfusion event because the personnel-to-patient ratio is one to one. The disadvantage is that there is no trained assistant available in the event of a severe adverse reaction. Issues to consider when preparing for a transfusion in the home include the following:

- Availability of a competent adult in the home to assist in patient identification and summoning medical assistance if needed.
- A mechanism to obtain immediate physician consultation.
- A telephone to contact emergency personnel, and easy access for emergency vehicles.
- Documentation of prior transfusions unaccompanied by adverse reactions.
- The ability to properly dispose of medical waste.[32,33]

CONCLUSION

Blood administration policies should be written and performed with patient safety at the forefront. Following procedures and policies strictly can do much to prevent a transfusion reaction. Although in some cases reactions or adverse events cannot be prevented, close monitoring and early intervention can make a critical difference in the patient's recovery. The transfusion service should periodically audit the blood administration process to identify nonconformances, to analyze their causes, and to address actions to prevent them in the future.

KEY POINTS

1. Blood administration involves preparation of the recipient, administration of the appropriate product to the correct recipient, and careful observation of the recipient during and after the transfusion for any adverse reaction. All steps must be appropriately documented in the patient's medical record.
2. A licensed care provider should initiate requests for blood administration with an order for the appropriate blood component along with an order for the administration of the component(s). The recipient should be informed and educated about the upcoming administration of the blood component so that he or she can give consent. Just before the planned administration, the transfusionist must verify appropriate venous access, administration of any prophylactic medications required, and availability of the required equipment (eg, blood warmer, infusion pump, and pressure devices) and emergency equipment. A baseline assessment of the recipient should be performed for purposes of subsequent comparison.
3. Institutions should identify appropriate issuing and delivery mechanisms to ensure that the transfusionist receives the components in a timely manner. Transfusion services should ensure that other departments are aware of the requirement for timely return of components if delays in a transfusion are necessary.
4. Before starting a transfusion, double verification of recipient and component identification should be performed. The following items should be verified: appearance of the unit, identification of the recipient and unit, the medical order, the blood type, and the expiration date/time of the component. Components must be administered through the appropriate infusion sets and filter, if indicated. No solution other than 0.9% sodium chloride injection (USP) should be administered through the same tubing.
5. The infusion should start slowly at approximately 2 mL per minute for the first 15 minutes. During this time the transfusionist should remain near the patient. If no sign of reaction appears, the infusion rate can be increased. Infusions must be completed within 4 hours. The transfusionist monitors the patient throughout the infusion and stops the infusion in the event of an adverse reaction. After completion, the transfusionist takes the patient's vital signs. If the patient is not going to have direct medical supervision, the patient and caregiver should receive instruction about signs and symptoms to be aware of and to report.
6. The transfusion event must be documented in the patient's medical record with the following information, at a minimum: the medical order, consent, type of component, unit identification number, date and time of infusion, pre- and posttransfusion vital signs, volume transfused, identification of the transfusionist, and any adverse reaction if noted.

REFERENCES

1. Carson TH, ed. Standards for blood banks and transfusion services. 27th ed. Bethesda, MD: AABB, 2011.
2. De la Roche MR, Gauthier L. Rapid transfusion of packed red blood cells: Effects of dilution, pressure, and catheter size. Ann Emerg Med 1993;22:1551-5.
3. Barcelona SL, Vilich F, Cote CJ. A comparison of flow rates and warming capabilities of the Level 1 and Rapid Infusion System with various-size intravenous catheters. Anesth Analg 2003;97:358-63, table.
4. Kennedy LD, Case LD, Hurd DD, et al. A prospective, randomized, double-blind controlled trial of acetaminophen and diphenhydramine pretransfusion medication versus placebo for the prevention of transfusion reactions. Transfusion 2008;48:2285-91.
5. Ezidiegwu CN, Lauenstein KJ, Rosales LG, et al. Febrile nonhemolytic transfusion reactions. Management by premedication and cost im-

plications in adult patients. Arch Pathol Lab Med 2004;128:991-5.
6. Geiger TL, Howard SC. Acetaminophen and diphenhydramine premedication for allergic and febrile nonhemolytic transfusion reactions: Good prophylaxis or bad practice? Transfus Med Rev 2007;21:1-12.
7. Wang SE, Lara PN Jr, Lee-Ow A, et al. Acetaminophen and diphenhydramine as premedication for platelet transfusions: A prospective randomized double-blind placebo-controlled trial. Am J Hematol 2002;70:191-4.
8. Patterson BJ, Freedman J, Blanchette V, et al. Effect of premedication guidelines and leukoreduction on the rate of febrile nonhaemolytic platelet transfusion reactions. Transfus Med 2000;10:199-206.
9. Boyan CP, Howland WS. Cardiac arrest and temperature of bank blood. JAMA 1963;183: 58-60.
10. Donham JA, Denning V. Cold agglutinin syndrome: Nursing management. Heart Lung 1985; 14:59-67.
11. Iserson KV, Huestis DW. Blood warming: Current applications and techniques. Transfusion 1991;31:558-71.
12. Hirsch J, Menzebach A, Welters ID, et al. Indicators of erythrocyte damage after microwave warming of packed red blood cells. Clin Chem 2003;49:792-9.
13. Houck D, Whiteford J. Improving patient outcomes: Transfusion with infusion pump for peripherally inserted central catheters and other vascular access devices. J Infus Nurs 2007; 30:341-4.
14. Frelich R, Ellis MH. The effect of external pressure, catheter gauge, and storage time on hemolysis in RBC transfusion. Transfusion 2001; 41:799-802.
15. Klein H, Anstee D. Mollison's blood transfusion in clinical medicine. 11th ed. Oxford: Blackwell, 2005.
16. Comprehensive accreditation manual for hospitals. Oakbrook Terrace, IL: The Joint Commission, 2009.
17. Vamvakas EC, Blajchman MA. Transfusion-related mortality: The ongoing risks of allogeneic blood transfusion and the available strategies for their prevention. Blood 2009;113: 3406-17.
18. Pagliaro P, Rebulla P. Transfusion recipient identification. Vox Sang 2006;91:97-101.
19. Koshy R. Navigating the information technology highway: Computer solutions to reduce errors and enhance patient safety. Transfusion 2005;45(4 Suppl):189S-205S.
20. Wortham ST, Ortolano GA, Wenz B. A brief history of blood filtration: Clot screens, microaggregate removal, and leukocyte reduction. Transfus Med Rev 2003;17:216-22.
21. Lane TA. Leukocyte reduction of cellular blood components. Effectiveness, benefits, quality control, and costs. Arch Pathol Lab Med 1994; 118:392-404.
22. Zoon KC, Jacobson ED, Woodcock J. Hypotension and bedside leukocyte reduction filters. Int J Trauma Nurs 1999;5:121-2.
23. Dickson DN, Gregory MA. Compatibility of blood with solutions containing calcium. S Afr Med J 1980;57:785-7.
24. Birch C, Hogan C, Mahoney G. Co-administration of drugs and blood products. Anaesth Intensive Care 2001;29:137-40.
25. Yousef HM, Padmore RF, Neurath DD, Rock GA. The effect of patient-controlled analgesia on coadministered red blood cells. Transfusion 2006;46:372-6.
26. Bradbury M, Cruickshank JP. Blood transfusion: Crucial steps in maintaining safe practice. Br J Nurs 2000;9:134-8.
27. Oldham J, Sinclair L, Hendry C. Right patient, right blood, right care: Safe transfusion practice. Br J Nurs 2009;18:312, 314, 316-20.
28. Iserson KV, Knauf MA. Confirmation of high blood flow rates through 150 mu filter/high-flow tubing. J Emerg Med 1990;8:689-91.
29. Floccare DJ, Kelen GD, Altman RS, et al. Rapid infusion of additive red blood cells: Alternative techniques for massive hemorrhage. Ann Emerg Med 1990;19:129-33.
30. Denlinger JK, Nahrwold ML, Gibbs PS, Lecky JH. Hypocalcaemia during rapid blood transfusion in anaesthetized man. Br J Anaesth 1976; 48:995-1000.
31. Smith HM, Farrow SJ, Ackerman JD, et al. Cardiac arrests associated with hyperkalemia during red blood cell transfusion: A case series. Anesth Analg 2008;106:1062-9.
32. Fridey JL. Practical aspects of out-of-hospital transfusion. Am J Clin Pathol 1997;107(Suppl 1): S64-S71.
33. Evans CS. Out-of-hospital transfusion. Transfusion 1997;37:756-67.

Chapter 22

Perinatal Issues in Transfusion Practice

Melanie S. Kennedy, MD

HEMOLYTIC DISEASE of the fetus and newborn (HDFN), fetal/neonatal alloimmune thrombocytopenia (FNAIT), and immune thrombocytopenia (ITP, previously known as immune thrombocytopenic purpura) affect pregnant women, their fetuses, and newborns. The blood bank and transfusion service play critical roles in supporting the diagnosis and treatment of these conditions, including the appropriate provision of Rh Immune Globulin (RhIG).

HEMOLYTIC DISEASE OF THE FETUS AND NEWBORN

Pathophysiology

HDFN is the destruction of fetal and newborn red cells by maternal alloantibodies specific for inherited paternal red cell alloantigen(s). The maternal IgG antibody is transported across the placenta into the fetal circulation where it binds to the corresponding red cell antigen, targeting the antibody-coated red cells for destruction by macrophages in the fetal spleen. The fetal marrow initially responds by increasing erythropoiesis and releases many of the newly produced red cells into the circulation prematurely as nucleated precursors, leading to the term "erythroblastosis fetalis." With worsening anemia, erythropoiesis expands to the liver and spleen, causing organ enlargement and portal hypertension. A resulting decrease in liver production of albumin leads to reduced plasma colloid osmotic pressure, generalized edema, ascites, and effusions known as "hydrops fetalis." Untreated, hydrops fetalis, with its associated high-output cardiovascular failure, can lead to fetal death in the majority of cases. Severe disease can occur as early as 18 to 20 weeks' gestation, and severity usually increases in subsequent pregnancies.

Alloimmunization

Females can be alloimmunized to red cell antigens by previous transfusions and previous or current pregnancy. Hemorrhage of fetal red cells into the maternal circulation may occur spontaneously during pregnancy or with trauma, amniocentesis, cordocentesis, abortion, and other manipulations. Because exposure to fetal red cells and resulting maternal alloim-

Melanie S. Kennedy, MD, Associate Professor Emeritus and Transfusion Medicine Attending, Ohio State University Medical Center, Columbus, Ohio
The author has disclosed no conflicts of interest.

munization typically occur late during pregnancy and at delivery, the fetus and newborn of the first pregnancy are rarely affected.

Complex factors influence the ability of individuals to respond to red cell antigens. Rh(D) is the most potent immunogen, in that a 200-mL transfusion of red cells stimulates anti-D in about 85% of D-negative individuals, except in immunosuppressed recipients. About half of the remaining 15% will never become immunized, even after repeated challenges with D-positive red cells. Although as little as 0.1 to 1 mL of D-positive red cells can stimulate antibody production, the volumes of fetomaternal hemorrhage (FMH) are generally small, which contributes to relatively low alloimmunization rates in pregnancy.[1] For example, without prophylaxis, D alloimmunization occurs in only about 16% of D-negative mothers with D-positive infants. Approximately 1.5% to 2% become sensitized at the time of their first delivery, an additional 7% become sensitized within 6 months, and the final 7% become sensitized during the second affected pregnancy.[2] Immunization is reduced to about 1.5% to 2%[1] when the mother is ABO incompatible with the fetus, probably because of the shortened life span of the incompatible fetal red cells.[3(p188)] Almost all cases of D alloimmunization can be prevented by appropriate prophylaxis with RhIG.

Antibodies targeted against numerous antigens in addition to D can also cause HDFN. The most common are K, and c. Unlike HDFN caused by anti-D, HDFN caused by anti-K uniquely produces suppression of fetal erythropoiesis in addition to hemolysis.[4(p527)] Other antibodies that have been less commonly reported to cause moderate or severe disease include k, Kp^a, Kp^b, Ku, Js^a, Js^b, Jk^a, Fy^a, Fy^b, S, s, and U.[5]

Hemolysis

Hemolysis occurs when the maternal antibody binds to a fetal red cell antigen, causing attachment to the Fc receptor of macrophages in the spleen of the fetus. The rate of hemolysis and severity of disease are determined by the IgG subclass, amount of antibody, and the number of antigenic sites on the red cells.[6] The subclasses IgG1 and IgG3 are more efficient at causing hemolysis than IgG2 or IgG4. Transportation of IgG1 and IgG3 across the placenta is mediated by the Fc receptor beginning in the second trimester and continuing until birth.[7] Because IgG1 is transported across the placenta earlier and in larger amounts than IgG3, IgG1 is associated with more severe disease. After delivery, continuing destruction of red cells can cause progressive anemia and hyperbilirubinemia. However, the amount of maternal antibody present continues to decrease over the next 12 weeks, with a half-life of about 25 days.

During gestation, fetal red cell destruction releases hemoglobin. The hemoglobin is broken down into bilirubin, which passes into the maternal circulation and is conjugated by the maternal liver. Birth severs the connection with the mother, causing the bilirubin (resulting from red cell destruction) to remain in the neonatal circulation. However, the infant's immature liver cannot conjugate the bilirubin efficiently; thus, excess unconjugated bilirubin passes through the immature blood-brain barrier of the newborn and, in large amounts, can cause permanent damage to the brain. This is known as kernicterus.[8]

Diagnosis and Management

The diagnosis and management of HDFN involve the close cooperation of the patient, the obstetrician, and the laboratory personnel. During the first trimester, the obstetric and transfusion history should be obtained. A previously affected pregnancy alerts the obstetrician to possible problems in the current pregnancy.[9] Laboratory testing also plays an important role, as described below.

Serologic and Molecular Testing

During the first prenatal visit, ABO and Rh typing and antibody detection (screening) should be performed on a maternal sample. If a D-negative woman has an initial negative antibody screen, she is a candidate for RhIG.

The antibody screen should use techniques that detect IgG antibodies reactive at

37 C and use separate screening cells representing all clinically important specificities. To avoid detecting IgM antibodies, which do not cross the placenta, immediate-spin and/or room-temperature incubation and complement-containing antihuman globulin (AHG) should be omitted.[10] A positive antibody screen requires antibody identification. Antibodies such as anti-I, -P1, -Le^a, and -Le^b, whether IgM or IgG, may be ignored because these antigens are poorly developed at birth. Treatment of the mother's plasma with dithiothreitol (DTT) can help distinguish IgG from IgM antibodies. The most common significant antibodies are anti-D, -K, -c, -C, and -Fy^a.[11] However, numerous other IgG antibody specificities have been reported to cause HDFN and, rarely, warm-reactive autoantibodies have also been implicated.

After identifying a clinically significant antibody, the next step is establishing whether the father has the corresponding antigen and whether he is heterozygous or homozygous. If the father is homozygous for the corresponding antigen and paternity is ensured, the fetus is clearly at risk for HDFN. If the father is heterozygous for the antigen, then the genotype of the fetus may be determined by polymerase chain reaction (PCR) testing of samples obtained by amniocentesis, chorionic villus sampling, or cordocentesis.[12] The reported sensitivity and specificity of DNA testing by PCR are 98.7% and 100%, respectively, with a low false-negative rate (1%-3%).[13] Molecular typing of fetal DNA can also be performed on maternal plasma during the second trimester.[14,15] DNA probes are currently available for D, c, e, C, E, K, k, Fy^a, Fy^b, Jk^a, Jk^b, M, S, s, and other antigens.

The titer has been the mainstay of decision making for the alloimmunized pregnancy. Different methods have been used to determine the mother's antibody titer. The AABB-recommended method is saline AHG with a 60-minute incubation at 37 C (Method 5-3).[10] Others prefer using standard saline testing (to detect newly stimulated IgM antibody, which generally indicates an increase in IgG titer and worsening disease), followed by 37 C incubation and anti-IgG AHG. Many reports of HDFN in the literature are based on this approach. Recent data show that other methods, such as gel, result in titers several dilutions higher than the recommended method, which may lead to inappropriate tests (some invasive) for the mother and fetus. Each method should be validated to clinical data from the institution to ensure appropriate interpretation of the data by the obstetricians.

The selection of red cells for titration studies is also controversial.[10] Many believe red cells selected for testing should be obtained from heterozygous donors to mimic the red cells of the fetus. Others prefer to use red cells from homozygous donors for increased sensitivity. Whichever method is chosen by an institution should be carefully validated and used consistently. The antibody titer should be established in the first trimester to serve as a baseline, and the specimen should be frozen for future comparisons (see Method 5-3).[1]

Testing previously frozen serum samples in parallel with a current specimen minimizes the possibility that changes in the titer result from differences in technique and reagent red cell selection. The critical titer for anti-D (the level below which HDFN and hydrops fetalis are considered so unlikely that no further invasive procedures will be undertaken) should be selected at each facility and is usually 16 or 32 in the AHG phase.[16] As long as the titer is 8 or lower, except in the case of anti-K, the pregnancy can be followed by titers every 4 to 6 weeks until delivery.[16] A difference of two dilutions or a score of 10 (Method 3-7; Table 3-7-1) is considered a significant change. Once the titer reaches the facility's critical titer and the gestation is at least 18 weeks, an intervention such as ultrasound, color Doppler ultrasonography, amniocentesis, or cordocentesis is performed to establish the severity of disease (see below). These titer criteria apply to anti-D, to other Rh antibodies, and generally to other clinically significant antibodies, with Kell system antibodies being an exception. Kell system antigens are present on early red cell precursors, so even a maternal anti-K of relatively low titer can cause erythropoietic failure and severe anemia. A critical titer of 8 is generally accepted for anti-K.[5]

After birth, neonatal red cells can be typed using cord blood samples. The cord blood should be collected using a needle and syringe, which avoids contamination with Wharton's jelly and the need for additional washing of the cells. ABO typing includes the forward grouping only, as the ABO antibodies are all maternal. The D type on cord blood may be falsely negative if the cells are heavily coated with anti-D ("blocked D"). In this case, an eluate prepared from the fetal cells will contain anti-D. The neonatal D type may also be falsely negative because of repeated intrauterine transfusions of D-negative red cells. A positive direct antiglobulin test (DAT), using anti-IgG only, indicates IgG antibody is coating the infant's red cells but does not indicate the cause. The strength of the reaction does not correlate well with the severity of the disease. Infants may have a positive test without evidence of HDFN—for example, associated with RhIG given during the third trimester. A positive DAT with a negative maternal antibody screen may be caused by ABO antibodies or alloimmunization to a low-prevalence antigen. Generally, an elution of DAT-positive neonatal cells is not indicated unless the cause is unknown and clinically important.

Diagnosis of Anemia, Hydrops Fetalis, and Hemolysis

Ultrasound testing can detect early hydrops fetalis, which is associated with a high risk of fetal demise. A preferred, noninvasive method is color Doppler ultrasonography, which measures blood flow velocity. Fetal anemia results in increased cardiac output and decreased viscosity, which increases blood flow. For convenience, the fetal middle cerebral artery is chosen for study. The measurement, middle cerebral artery peak systolic velocity (MCA-PSV), has been shown to correlate with the severity of the anemia and predict the need for more invasive procedures, such as cordocentesis and red cell transfusion.[17] Studies have found good correlation between MCA-PSV, fetal hematocrit, and amniocentesis (ie, using the change in fluid optical density at 450 nm, or ΔOD_{450}) measurements.[18] In skilled hands, MCA-PSV is diagnostically equivalent or perhaps superior to amniocentesis, without the 1% risk of fetal morbidity and mortality.[9,19]

Before the development of color Doppler ultrasonography, the severity of HDFN was usually monitored by amniocentesis, typically performed with ultrasound guidance, to follow the level of bilirubin pigment in amniotic fluid. Amniocentesis is indicated when the placenta is anterior and access to the umbilical cord is difficult. The aspirated amniotic fluid is protected from light and tested by a scanning spectrophotometer for the ΔOD_{450}, which is proportional to bilirubin concentration. The result is then plotted on a graph according to gestational age.[20]

Liley[21] divided his graph into three zones: the top zone (zone 3), with the highest ΔOD_{450} (highest bilirubin concentration), indicates severe disease; the bottom zone (zone 1) indicates mild or no disease; and the middle zone (zone 2) indicates a moderately affected fetus. Liley's graph applies from 27 through 40 weeks' gestation. Queenan et al[20] described a graph including 14 to 25 weeks of gestation as well (Fig 22-1). They identified four zones, with early invasive intervention recommended in the highest zone. The severity of HDFN is more accurately predicted by trends established from serial ΔOD_{450} measurements. Normally, the ΔOD_{450} decreases during the third trimester; a steady or increasing level indicates increasing hemolysis. Ultrasound is important to establish the correct gestational age so that the test can be interpreted and the course of therapy for a particular ΔOD_{450} will be appropriate.[9] Because amniocentesis or cordocentesis may cause FMH, RhIG immunoprophylaxis should be administered after the procedure to D-negative women who do not have anti-D. Amniotic fluid analysis does not correlate well with the degree of fetal anemia in mothers with Kell system antibodies. For these patients, MCA-PSV and/or cordocentesis is indicated.

Intervention and Management

In cases of severe fetal anemia from hemolytic disease, fetal transfusion provides antigen-

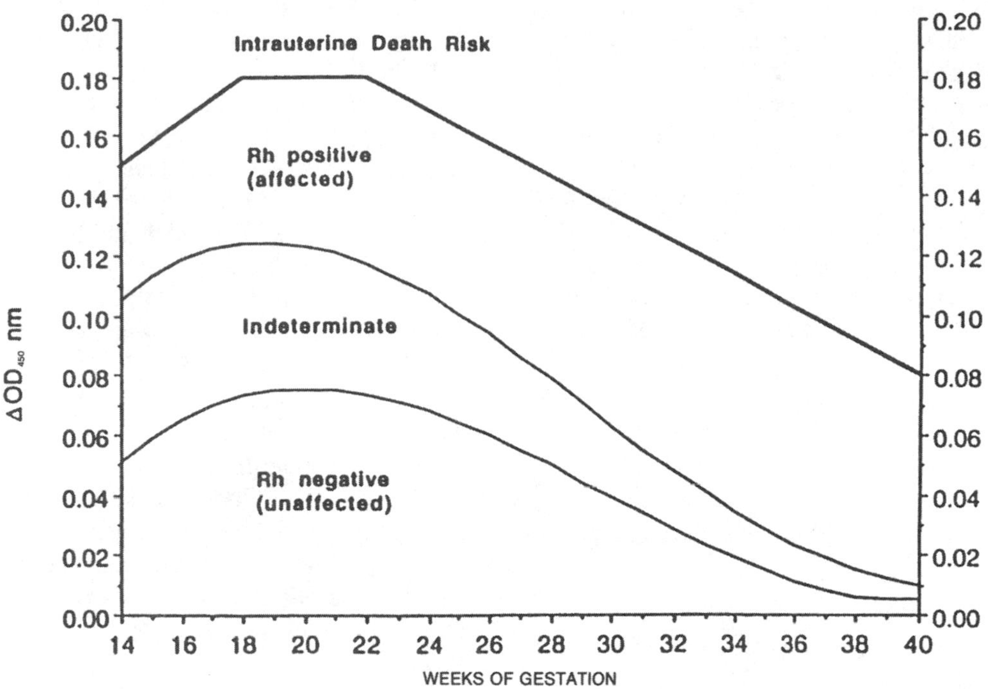

FIGURE 22-1. Amniotic fluid ΔOD_{450} management zones. (Adapted from Queenan et al.[20])

negative red cells to treat anemia. Intrauterine transfusions were originally performed by injecting blood into the fetal peritoneal space for uptake by the lymphatics into the circulation. This was an inefficient method, espccially when ascites and hydrops were present.[11] A superior approach for directly accessing the fetal circulation is cordocentesis, which is performed by inserting a needle into the umbilical vein using color Doppler enhancement of high-resolution sonography to guide the procedure. Transfusion by cordocentesis is more efficient in that the red cells immediately circulate and function, and larger transfusions are possible because the placenta is part of the total blood volume. Additionally, a sample of fetal blood is obtained at the same time to determine blood type, DAT, antigen type, hemoglobin, hematocrit, platelet count, and bilirubin. Cordocentesis is associated with a 1% to 2% risk of fetal morbidity and mortality and can be complicated by infection, bleeding, fetal bradycardia, and premature rupture of the membranes.

Selection of Blood

For intrauterine transfusion, the blood should be 1) irradiated to prevent transfusion-associated graft-vs-host disease in the immunologically immature fetus, 2) cytomegalovirus (CMV) reduced-risk (leukocyte reduced and/or CMV seronegative), and 3) known to lack hemoglobin S to prevent sickling under low oxygen tension. Donor group O red cells that are antigen negative for the mother's corresponding antibodies and crossmatch-compatible with maternal plasma are selected. Generally, Red Blood Cell (RBC) units that were collected within 7 days of use are preferred.

Rarely, the mother's antibody reacts with a high-prevalence antigen and no compatible blood is available. An alternative source is the mother's red cells, which should be washed to remove the mother's antibodies or may be frozen in small aliquots and deglycerolized before transfusion.[22] The mother's siblings or a rare donor registry may be additional sources for compatible units. If the clinical situation is sufficiently urgent and the above options are unavailable, incompatible donor blood can be used for the transfusion.

The volume of blood to be transfused can be calculated, as shown in the following example, by 1) determining the fetal and placental total blood volume by multiplying the ultrasound-estimated fetal weight in grams (eg, 1000 g) by 0.14 mL/g; 2) multiplying this answer (eg, 140 mL) by the difference in posttransfusion (desired) and pretransfusion hematocrit (eg, 40% –15% = 25%); and 3) dividing the result by the hematocrit of the RBC unit (in this case, 85%). The result is 41.2 mL.

Example:

$$\frac{(1000\text{ g}) \times (0.14\text{ mL/g}) \times (40\% - 15\%)}{85\%} = 41.2\text{ mL}$$

The blood volume transfused by cordocentesis should be adjusted to accommodate the clinical status of the fetus.[23] Transfusion is repeated according to the severity of the disease or based on an estimated decline in hematocrit of 1% per day, in an effort to maintain the fetal hematocrit at about 30%.[11] Intravascular transfusion allows gestation to continue to term and fetal lungs and liver to mature, reducing the need for exchange transfusion after birth.[11] In addition, the transfusions suppress erythropoiesis, reducing the amount of hemolysis.[11] Overall, survival is 74% of hydropic fetuses and 94% of nonhydropic fetuses.[24] In severe cases, intrauterine exchange transfusion has been performed, which has the additional advantage of removing antibody-coated fetal red cells and maternal antibody.[25]

Maternal plasma exchange and the administration of intravenous immune globulin (IVIG) have been attempted as alternatives to intrauterine transfusion.[2,9] Plasma exchange can temporarily reduce antibody levels by as much as 75%. Because its efficacy and safety have not been proven, the AABB and the American Society for Apheresis consider plasma exchange as treatment Category II for this indication in patients with a history of a severely affected pregnancy and if the fetus is less than 20 weeks' gestational age.[26] IVIG infusion has been shown to stabilize anti-D titers, with best results obtained when started before 28 weeks' gestation and when the fetus is not hydropic.[27]

During the first days after birth, close monitoring of the bilirubin level is necessary because of the threat of kernicterus, especially in premature neonates.[28] The infant may require ultraviolet (UV) wavelength phototherapy, which changes the elevated unconjugated bilirubin to nontoxic biliverdin. Additionally, IVIG may be given to the infant to help control hemolysis and, thus, elevated bilirubin. In neonates with elevated bilirubin levels unresponsive to UV light and IVIG, a double-volume exchange transfusion removes approximately 90% of the circulating fetal red cells and 50% of the bilirubin. Exchange transfusion is generally unnecessary if the infant received intrauterine transfusions. (See Chapter 23 for discussion of exchange transfusion in the newborn.)

Rh IMMUNE GLOBULIN

High-titered IgG D antibodies of human origin (RhIG) are commercially available for use in preventing alloimmunization to the D antigen. Both high-dose (300 μg) and mini-dose (50 μg) formulations are available, although many hospitals stock only the high-dose vials so that the mini-dose of RhIG is not inappropriately administered. The risk of a D-negative mother becoming immunized by a D-positive fetus can be reduced from about 16% to less than 0.1% by the appropriate administration of RhIG.[1,2]

Screening and Dosing for RhIG

Antepartum Administration

In a pregnancy where the mother is D-negative and the father is D-positive, the fetus may be D-positive and the mother may be at risk for D alloimmunization. Such females are candidates for RhIG prophylaxis to prevent alloimmunization. The following females are *not* candidates for RhIG: the D-negative female whose infant is known to be D negative, a D-negative female previously immunized to D, and any D-positive female. The decision to perform weak D testing is made by the medical director. Women with red cells that are clearly positive on the weak D test should be considered D positive and not receive RhIG, although rarely a positive weak D test can be caused by a partial D antigen. Very rare cases of HDFN have been reported in infants born to women with partial D antigen and alloanti-D.

In women at risk for D alloimmunization, the American College of Obstetricians and Gynecologists (ACOG) recommends initial RhIG administration at 28 weeks' gestation based on the observation that 92% of women who develop anti-D during pregnancy do so at or after 28 weeks.[1,29] Antenatal RhIG administration reduces the alloimmunization rate during gestation from about 1.5% to 0.1%. Indications for administration of additional doses of RhIG during pregnancy include invasive procedures such as amniocentesis and cordocentesis; manipulations such as version; abortion; and abdominal trauma.

Postpartum Administration

The D-negative mother who is not immunized to D should also receive an appropriate dose of RhIG after delivery of a D-positive infant. As soon as possible after delivery, cord blood from infants born to D-negative mothers should be tested for the D antigen. If the neonate is D negative, no further RhIG is necessary. However, if the infant tests D positive, the mother should have a postpartum blood sample screened for FMH in order to determine the appropriate RhIG dose.

The rosette test is a sensitive method to detect FMH of approximately 10 mL or more. The maternal sample is incubated with anti-D, and then indicator D-positive red cells are added. The indicator red cells will form agglutinates (rosettes) with the fetal D-positive red cells. The fetal cells must be D positive and the mother D negative for the test to be valid. The rosette test may be falsely positive if the mother is positive for the weak D phenotype, and falsely negative if the neonate is positive for weak D. If the rosette testing is negative, a dose of 300 µg RhIG (100 µg in the United Kingdom) is given, which is sufficient to prevent immunization after delivery in 99% of cases.[4(p531)] This dose suppresses immunization by 15 mL of red cells (5 mL in the United Kingdom) or 30 mL of whole blood. It is important to note that the presence of residual anti-D from antepartum RhIG does not indicate ongoing protection.

A positive rosette test indicates the occurrence of a large FMH. Although estimates suggest that only 0.3% of pregnancies are complicated by FMH greater than 30 mL, a large FMH is an important and preventable cause of failed immunoprophylaxis.[1] The AABB *Standards for Blood Banks and Transfusion Services* requires the transfusion service to have a policy for RhIG prophylaxis of Rh-negative patients identified to be at risk for immunization.[30(p43)] Thus, in patients with a positive rosette test, a quantitative test such as the Kleihauer-Betke (acid/elution) test or flow cytometry (which is the second most commonly used method for this purpose)[31] is performed to calculate the dose of RhIG. Flow cytometry can precisely measure fetal hemoglobin and/or D-positive red cells. The use of both markers avoids false-positive results from maternal red cells containing fetal hemoglobin.[32]

The principle of the Kleihauer-Betke test is the resistance of fetal hemoglobin to acid treatment (Method 5-2). A thin smear of maternal blood is made on a slide, treated with acid, rinsed, counterstained, and read microscopically. The maternal cells will appear as ghosts, and the fetal cells will be pink. The fetal cells and maternal cells are counted separately for a total of 2000 cells. The following formula can be used to calculate the fetal bleeding:

$$\frac{\text{Fetal cells} \times \text{maternal blood volume (mL)}}{\text{Total cells counted}} = \text{Fetal hemorrhage (mL)}$$

Example:

6 cells/2000 cells × 5000 mL = 15 mL fetal whole blood

Because a single 300-µg vial of RhIG will suppress alloimmunization by 30 mL of fetal whole blood, and in the present example the calculated fetal bleeding was 15 mL, the number of RhIG vials can be calculated as 15 mL/30 mL/vial = 0.5 vial. Because of the inherent wide estimate of the test, if the calculated dose to the right of the decimal point is ≥0.5 vial, it should be rounded up to the next whole number plus one vial; if <0.5, rounded down plus one vial (Table 22-1). In the above example, the dose to be given is two vials. Additional examples are shown as follows:

Examples:

1.6 vials calculated = 2 (round up) + 1 (add 1) = 3

1.4 vials calculated = 1 (round down) + 1 (add 1) = 2

Postpartum RhIG should be given within 72 hours of delivery. If prophylaxis is delayed, the likelihood of preventing alloimmunization is decreased. Nonetheless, the ACOG recommends that treatment still be administered, even if delayed past 72 hours, because some studies have found partial protection has occurred as late as 13 days after exposure and possibly as late as 28 days.[29] Furthermore, if the D type of the newborn is unknown or undetermined (eg, stillborn), RhIG should also be administered.

Depending on the preparation, RhIG can be given by intramuscular (IgM) or intravenous (IV) injection. Care must be taken that the IM-only preparation is not given by IV injection, as complement activation could occur. Multiple IM doses should be given at different sites or at different times within 72 hours. Alternatively, multiple doses of the IV preparation may be administered according to instructions in the package insert.

Serology and Mechanism

Administration of RhIG during pregnancy may produce a positive antibody screen in the mother, but the titer is rarely greater than 4 and thus poses no risk to the fetus. Occasionally, the DAT may be positive in the newborn without evidence of hemolysis. About 10% (20-30 μg) of the 28-week gestation dose will be present in the mother at delivery (half-life of IgG is 25 days) and can be detected and identified as anti-D. This anti-D should not be interpreted as active immunization, and the postpartum RhIG dose should be given if the newborn is D positive. Antibody titers in the mother do not correlate with the effectiveness of the RhIG or the amount of FMH. Anti-D can be detected in the maternal circulation for as long as 6 months. If it becomes necessary to distinguish passively administered RhIG from the anti-D formed by alloimmunization, laboratorians can take advantage of the fact that RhIG is entirely IgG, whereas active immunization produces an antibody response with an IgM component. Thus, anti-D produced by the mother can often be detected in saline phase and completely or partially inactivated

TABLE 22-1. RhIG Dosage for Fetomaternal Hemorrhage

		Dose	
% Fetal Cells	**Vials to Inject**	**μg (mcg)**	**IU**
0.3-0.8	2	600	3000
0.9-1.4	3	900	4500
1.5-2.0	4	1200	6000
2.1-2.6	5	1500	7500

Notes:

1. Based on a maternal blood volume of 5000 mL.
2. 1 vial of 300 μg (1500 IU) is needed for each 15 mL of fetal red cells or 30 mL of fetal whole blood.

by 2-mercaptoethanol or DTT treatment, whereas RhIG cannot. Additionally, passively acquired anti-D rarely achieves a titer above 4.

The mechanism of action of RhIG has not been completely elucidated. Current evidence shows that D-positive red cells are opsonized by RhIG and removed by macrophages, which release cytokines that result in immunomodulation.[33] The number of IgG molecules known to prevent immunization is much fewer than the D antigen sites on red cells.

ABO HEMOLYTIC DISEASE

With the widespread use of RhIG, ABO incompatibility has become the most common cause of HDFN. ABO HDFN may occur in the first or in any subsequent pregnancy. In the usual scenario, naturally occurring A,B IgG antibodies in a group O mother are transported across the placenta and bind to fetal red cells expressing A or B antigens. Despite the prevalence of ABO HDFN, destruction of fetal red cells only rarely leads to severe anemia, probably because fetal ABO antigens are poorly developed and antibody is neutralized by tissue and soluble antigens. After birth, hyperbilirubinemia generally can be successfully treated with phototherapy; rarely, exchange transfusion may be required.

IgG ABO antibodies of high titer are most frequent in group O mothers. Therefore, group A and B infants of group O mothers are more severely affected. In populations of European and Asian ethnicity, group A infants are most commonly affected; in those of African ethnicity, group B infants are likely to be affected. The overall incidence of ABO HDFN is higher in populations of African ancestry than in those of European ancestry.[4(p529)] The disease is not necessarily associated with a positive DAT or anti-A, anti-B, or anti-A,B in the eluate, although in severe disease the DAT is nearly always positive.[34]

If ABO HDFN is ruled out, antibodies against low-prevalence red cell antigens should be suspected. Testing an eluate from cord blood or maternal serum (if ABO compatible) against the father's red cells with an antiglobulin technique is often diagnostic. If either or both of these tests are positive, it indicates that the infant has an antigen of paternal origin that the mother lacks, causing her to make an IgG antibody directed against this antigen. If the DAT is positive but all attempts to characterize the antibody are consistently negative, causes of a false-positive DAT should be considered (see Chapter 17).

IMMUNE THROMBOCYTOPENIA

Maternal IgG antibodies to platelets can cross the placenta and cause severe thrombocytopenia. Two categories of immune thrombocytopenia are recognized: FNAIT and ITP. The diagnostic distinction between them is important therapeutically.

Fetal and Neonatal Alloimmune Thrombocytopenia

Pathophysiology

FNAIT is caused by antibodies specific for platelet antigens inherited from the father but absent in the mother. Platelet antigens represent specific polymorphisms in platelet membrane glycoproteins. In the United States, the platelet antigen most commonly implicated in FNAIT is human platelet antigen (HPA)-1a, formerly known as Pl^{A1}, accounting for approximately 80% of cases. Infrequently, other platelet antigens are involved.[35] About 10% of cases are caused by anti-HPA-5b, 4% by anti-HPA-1b, 2% by anti-HPA-3a, and 6% by other antibodies. HPA-1a is present in about 98% of the US population, which suggests that the approximately 2% of women who are HPA-1a negative should be at risk for FNAIT during pregnancy. However, the actual incidence of affected pregnancies is significantly lower, at approximately 1 per 1500 to 2000 pregnancies.[36] Studies have shown an association between the maternal HLA type DRw52a (*DRB3*0101*) and the development of anti-HPA-1a.[37]

Although FNAIT has similarities to HDFN, there are some distinct differences. In about 25% of FNAIT cases, the platelet antibody may develop sufficiently early during the first pregnancy for that fetus to be affected. The maternal antibody has been detected as early as 17 weeks' gestation, paralleling the development of fetal platelet antigens. In the affected pregnancies, the fetus may develop thrombocytopenia as early as 20 weeks' gestation. During the first pregnancy, the disease is often not discovered until birth, when the newborn presents with petechiae, ecchymoses, or intracranial hemorrhage. FNAIT is the cause of the majority of cases of intracranial hemorrhage caused by thrombocytopenia, greater than all the other etiologies of thrombocytopenia combined.[37] The incidence of intracranial hemorrhage is between 10% and 30%, with approximately half occurring in utero.[36] The risk of hemorrhage is inversely proportional to the platelet count, the greatest risk arising when the platelet count is less than 100,000/µL. In subsequent pregnancies, the fetus is also at risk for equivalent or more severe disease if the platelets carry the targeted antigen. The response of the fetal hematopoietic system to FNAIT is variable and may include compensatory extramedullary hematopoiesis. Rarely, fetal hydrops develops. Fetal anemia without red cell incompatibility can also occur.

Diagnosis and Management

In first pregnancies, the diagnosis is most likely at birth, when ecchymoses, petechiae, and (less often) intracranial hemorrhage are present. The infant's platelet count is decreased and may decrease more in the first few hours to days after birth. Platelet transfusion is generally needed, depending on the clinical condition and the platelet count. In the absence of bleeding, some obstetricians transfuse for platelet count <10,000/µL.[38] The maternal platelet count remains normal. In 2 to 3 weeks, once the antibody has been cleared, the infant's platelet count returns to normal. In subsequent pregnancies, the history of a newborn with thrombocytopenia can alert the obstetrician to a probable affected pregnancy. The presence or absence of severe thrombocytopenia and intracranial hemorrhage in the firstborn correlates with the outcome of subsequent pregnancies.[37] Routine screening of pregnant women for platelet alloantibodies is not generally practiced.

After a first affected pregnancy and with plans for a subsequent pregnancy, the mother and father should be typed for platelet antigens, and the mother screened for alloantibody. These tests are available through referral laboratories. DNA testing of the father can determine zygosity of the antigen involved, which thus determines the risk to future pregnancies.[39] During a subsequent pregnancy, the DNA genotype of the fetus can be determined using amniotic fluid or maternal plasma as early as 18 weeks' gestation. This gives a clear indication of the risk of FNAIT and the need for intensive monitoring. If indicated, assessment of the fetus should begin at or before 20 weeks' gestation, because severe thrombocytopenia and hemorrhage can occur by that time.

Cordocentesis can be used to determine the platelet count. Irradiated, CMV-reduced-risk, antigen-negative platelets should be available before the procedure is started. The platelet transfusion should be given prophylactically to treat thrombocytopenia and avoid hemorrhage and should be repeated weekly, as the platelet life span is 8 to 10 days. Many blood suppliers have identified HPA-1a-negative donors and can prepare platelets for intrauterine transfusion. An alternative donor is the mother, who is negative for the implicated platelet alloantigen. However, she must be able to donate, and her platelets must be washed to remove the offending alloantibodies. If platelet transfusions are needed urgently, incompatible platelets may be used.[40]

Generally, the mother is given IVIG after the fetus is determined to be affected. The dose is usually 1 g/kg each week. In a retrospective review of patients managed over time, noninvasive management appears to be as safe and effective as invasive management.41 However, even with IVIG treatment, the fetal platelet count may need to be monitored by cordocentesis because treatment failures may occur and platelet transfusions may be required.[42] The goal of both transfusion and IVIG is to avoid hemorrhage. Ultrasound monitoring to detect hemorrhage followed by therapeutic transfusions is not recommended because detection of intracranial hemorrhage generally indicates permanent brain damage.

Controversy exists about the use or avoidance of cordocentesis. Recently, IVIG without cordocentesis was given to pregnant mothers with a history of a child with intracranial hemorrhage. In three of seven pregnancies, cordocentesis was performed and platelet transfusions were given before delivery. None of the neonates had intracranial hemorrhage, although platelet counts were ≤50,000/μL.[43] However, (as discussed above) the risk of intracranial hemorrhage (10%-30%) must be weighed against the risk of cordocentesis (1%-2% morbidity and mortality).

Before delivery, the fetal platelet count should be determined. The platelet count should be >50,000/μL for vaginal delivery and should be kept above 20,000/μL after birth.

Immune Thrombocytopenia

Autoantibodies against platelets, which react with the patient's own platelets as well as donor or fetal platelets, is another significant cause of fetal and neonatal ITP. Thrombocytopenia in a pregnant mother is not uncommon and frequently is not associated with ITP. However, when present, ITP may cause thrombocytopenia in both the mother and fetus. Fortunately, only about 10% of these newborns will have platelet counts <50,000/μL, and only 1% to 2% have a risk of hemorrhage compared to infants with FNAIT.[44]

The mother with thrombocytopenia or a preexisting diagnosis of ITP should be tested for serum platelet autoantibody. The absence of circulating autoantibody in a pregnant woman generally indicates thrombocytopenia caused by other conditions and suggests that the fetus or neonate is not at risk. In contrast, the mother with significant thrombocytopenia and petechiae or other evidence of hemorrhage caused by autoantibody should be started on therapy similar to the nonpregnant woman with ITP.[44] Prednisone at a dose of 1 to 2 mg/kg is usually effective. However, with persistent maternal thrombocytopenia, IVIG 1 g/kg/day for 2 to 5 days is indicated. Although the maternal platelet count is often monitored in these cases, it does not correlate with the newborn's platelet count.[44] Generally, fetal blood sampling to determine platelet count is not recommended because the risk of morbidity and mortality from cordocentesis is higher or equal to the risk of severe bleeding in utero or at delivery. Platelet transfusions may be needed in about 15% of newborns.[44]

KEY POINTS

1. Hemolytic disease of the fetus and newborn (HDFN) is caused by maternal antibody specific for paternal red cell antigen. The maternal IgG antibody is transported across the placenta, destroying the fetal red cells.
2. Antibodies such as anti-I, -P1, -Le^a, and -Le^b can be ignored. The most common significant antibodies are anti-D, -K, -c, -C, and -Fy^a.
3. Molecular typing of fetal DNA can be performed on maternal plasma during the second trimester. DNA probes are currently available for D, c, e, C, E, K, k, Fy^a, Fy^b, Jk^a, Jk^b, M, S, s, and other antigens.
4. The recommended titer method is saline antihuman globulin with 60-minute incubation at 37 C. Methods such as those using gel result in higher titers, which may lead to misinterpretation by the obstetrician.
5. ABO typing of cord blood includes the forward grouping only. The D type on cord blood may be falsely negative because of intrauterine transfusion of D negative red cells. A positive direct antiglobulin test with negative maternal antibody screen may be caused by ABO antibodies.

6. Middle cerebral artery peak systolic velocity (MCA-PSV) predicts the need for cordocentesis and red cell transfusion. In skilled hands, MCA-PSV is diagnostically equivalent to amniocentesis, without the 1% risk of fetal morbidity and mortality.
7. For intrauterine transfusion, the blood should be irradiated, cytomegalovirus (CMV) reduced-risk, hemoglobin S negative, and generally group O, and less than 7 days old.
8. The rosette test is a sensitive method to detect fetomaternal hemorrhage of approximately 10 mL or more. Flow cytometry can precisely measure hemoglobin F and/or D-positive red cells.
9. Round up the calculated Rh Immune Globulin (RhIG) doses (if the number to the right of the decimal point is ≥0.5) or down (if <0.5) and add 1 vial. RhIG may opsonize D-positive red cells, which are removed by macrophages, releasing cytokines that result in immunomodulation.
10. Despite the prevalence of ABO HDFN, severe anemia rarely occurs. After birth, hyperbilirubinemia generally can be treated with phototherapy alone.
11. In fetal/neonatal alloimmune thrombocytopenia, the platelet antibody may develop around 17 weeks of gestation in the first pregnancy, and fetal thrombocytopenia as early as 20 weeks. Irradiated, CMV-reduced-risk, antigen-negative platelets should be given to treat thrombocytopenia and avoid hemorrhage.

REFERENCES

1. Bowman JM. The prevention of Rh immunization. Transfus Med Rev 1988;2:129-50.
2. Bowman JM. Controversies in Rh prophylaxis. Who needs Rh immune globulin and when should it be given? Am J Obstet Gynecol 1985; 151:289-94.
3. Klein HG, Anstee DJ. The Rh blood group system. In: Mollison's blood transfusion in clinical medicine. 11th ed. Oxford: Blackwell, 2005: 163-208.
4. Klein HG, Anstee DJ. Haemolytic disease of the fetus and newborn. In: Mollison's blood transfusion in clinical medicine. 11th ed. Oxford: Blackwell, 2005:496-545.
5. Vaughan JI, Manning M, Warwick RM, et al. Inhibition of erythroid progenitor cells by anti-Kell antibodies in fetal alloimmune anemia. N Engl J Med 1998;338:798-803.
6. Pollock JM, Bowman JM. Anti-Rh(D) subclasses and severity of Rh hemolytic disease of the newborn. Vox Sang 1990;59:176-9.
7. Firan M, Rawdon R, Radu C, et al. The MHC class I-related receptor, FcRn, plays an essential role in the maternal transfer of gammaglobulin in humans. Int Immunol 2001;13:993-1002.
8. Dennery PA, Seidman DS, Stevenson DK. Neonatal hyperbilirubinemia. N Engl J Med 2001; 344:581-90.
9. Moise KJ. Management of Rhesus alloimmunization in pregnancy. Obstet Gynecol 2002;100: 600-11.
10. Judd WJ. Practice guidelines for prenatal and perinatal immunohematology, revisited. Transfusion 2001;41:1445-52.
11. Bowman JM. RhD hemolytic disease of the newborn. N Engl J Med 1998;339:1775-7.
12. Bennett PR, Le Van Kim C, Colin Y, et al. Prenatal determination of fetal RhD type by DNA amplification. N Engl J Med 1993;329:607-10.
13. Van den Veyver IB, Beaudet AL. Comparative genomic hybridization and prenatal diagnosis. Curr Opin Obstet Gynecol 2006;18:185-91.
14. Lo YMD, Hjelm NM, Fidler C, et al. Prenatal diagnosis of fetal RhD status by molecular analysis of maternal plasma. N Engl J Med 1998;339: 1734-8.
15. Finning K, Martin P, Summers J, Daniels GL. Fetal genotyping for the K (Kell) and Rh C, c, and E blood groups on cell-free fetal DNA in maternal plasma. Transfusion 2007;47:2126-33.
16. Management of isoimmunization in pregnancy. ACOG educational bulletin #227. Washington, DC: American College of Obstetricians and Gynecologists, 1996.
17. Mari G, Deter RL, Carpenter RL, et al. Noninvasive diagnosis by Doppler ultrasonography

of fetal anemia due to maternal red cell alloimmunization. N Engl J Med 2000;342:9-14.

18. Nishie EN, Brizot ML, Liao AW, et al. A comparison between middle cerebral artery peak systolic velocity and amniotic fluid optical density at 450 nm in the prediction of fetal anemia. Am J Obstet Gynecol 2003;188:214-19.
19. Oepkes D, Seaward PG, Vanderbussche FPHA, et al. Doppler ultrasonography versus amniocentesis to predict fetal anemia. N Engl J Med 2006;355:156-64.
20. Queenan JT, Tomai TP, Ural SH, King JC. Deviation in amniotic fluid optical density at a wavelength of 450 nm in Rh-immunized pregnancies from 14 to 40 weeks' gestation: A proposal for clinical management. Am J Obstet Gynecol 1993;168:1370-6.
21. Liley AW. Liquor amnii analysis in the management of the pregnancy complicated by rhesus sensitization. Am J Obstet Gynecol 1961;82: 1359-70.
22. Gonsoulin WJ, Moise KJ, Milam JD, et al. Serial maternal blood donations for intrauterine transfusion. Obstet Gynecol 1990;75:158-62.
23. Rodunovic N, Lockwood CJ, Alvarez M, et al. The severely anemic and hydropic isoimmune fetus: Changes in hematocrit associated with intrauterine death. Obstet Gynecol 1992;79: 390-3.
24. Schumacher B, Moise KJ Jr. Fetal transfusion for red blood alloimmunization in pregnancy. Obstet Gynecol 1996;88:137-50.
25. Poissonnier MH, Brossard Y, Demedeiros N, et al. Two hundred intrauterine transfusions in severe blood incompatibilities. Am J Obstet Gynecol 1989;161:709-13.
26. Szczepiorkowski ZM, Winters JL, Bandarenko N, et al. Guidelines on the use of therapeutic apheresis in clinical practice—Evidence-based approach from the Apheresis Applications Committee of the American Society for Apheresis. J Clin Apher 2010;25:83-177.
27. Margulies M, Voto LS, Mathet E. High dose intravenous IgG for the treatment of severe Rhesus alloimmunization. Vox Sang 1991;61: 181-9.
28. American Academy of Pediatrics Subcommittee on Hyperbilirubinemia. Management of hyperbilirubinemia in the newborn 35 or more weeks gestation. Clinical practice guideline. Pediatrics 2004;114:297-316.
29. Prevention of Rh D alloimmunization. ACOG practice bulletin #4. Washington, DC: American College of Obstetricians and Gynecologists, 1999.
30. Carson TH, ed. Standards for blood banks and transfusion services. 27th ed. Bethesda, MD: AABB, 2011.
31. Duguid JKM, Bromilow IM. Laboratory measurement of fetomaternal hemorrhage and its clinical relevance. Transfus Med Rev 1999;13: 43-8.
32. Radel DJ, Penz CS, Dietz AB, Gastineau DA. A combined flow cytometry-based method for fetomaternal hemorrhage and maternal D. Transfusion 2008;48:1886-91.
33. Branch DR, Shabani F, Lund N, Denomme GA. Antenatal administration of Rh-immune globulin causes significant increases in the immunomodulary cytokines transforming growth factor- and prostaglandin E2. Transfusion 2006;48:1316-22.
34. Herschel M, Karrison T, Wen M, et al. Isoimmunization is unlikely to be the cause of hemolysis in ABO-incompatible but direct antiglobulin test-negative neonates. Pediatrics 2002;110:127-30.
35. Davoren A, Curtis BR, Aster RH, McFarland JG. Human platelet antigen-specific alloantibodies implicated in 1162 cases of neonatal alloimmune thrombocytopenia. Transfusion 2004; 44:1220-5.
36. Williamson LM, Hackett G, Rennie J, et al. The natural history of fetomaternal alloimmunization in the platelet-specific antigen HPA-1a (Pl^{A1}, Zw^{a}) as determined by antenatal screening. Blood 1998;92:2280-7.
37. Birchall JE, Murphy MF, Kroll H. European collaborative study of the antenatal management of feto-maternal alloimmune thrombocytopenia. Br J Haematol 2003;122:275-88.
38. Bassler D, Greinacher A, Okascharoen C, et al. A systematic review and survey of the management of unexpected neonatal alloimmune thrombocytopenia. Transfusion 2008;48:92-8.
39. Radder CM, Brand A, Kanhai HH. A less invasive treatment strategy to prevent intracranial hemorrhage in fetal and neonatal alloimmune thrombocytopenia. Am J Obstet Gynecol 2001; 185:683-8.
40. Kiefel V, Bassler D, Kroll H, et al. Antigen-positive platelet transfusion in neonatal alloimmune thrombocytopenia (NAIT). Blood 2006; 107:3761-3.
41. Van den Akker ESA, Oepkes D, Lopriore E, et al. Noninvasive antenatal management of fetal and neonatal alloimmune thrombocytopenia:

Safe and effective. Br J Obstet Gynaecol 2007; 114:469-73.
42. Silver RM, Porter TF, Branch DW, et al. Neonatal alloimmune thrombocytopenia: Antenatal management. Am J Obstet Gynecol 2000;182: 1233-8.
43. Kanhai HH, van den Akker ESA, Waither FJ, Brand A. Intravenous immunoglobulins without initial and follow-up cordocentesis in alloimmune fetal and neonatal thrombocytopenia at high risk of intracranial hemorrhage. Fetal Diag Ther 2006;21:55-60.
44. Webert KE, Mittal R, Sigouin C, et al. A retrospective 11-year analysis of patients with idiopathic thrombocytopenic purpura. Blood 2003;102:4306-11.

Chapter 23

Neonatal and Pediatric Transfusion Practice

Cassandra D. Josephson, MD

TRANSFUSION PRACTICE IN neonatal and pediatric patients differs from the practice in adults.[1] The differences are directly related to physiologic changes that occur during the transition from fetus to adolescent. Blood volume, hematologic values, immune system maturity, and physiologic responses to hypovolemia and hypoxia are widely variable in this heterogeneous population, contributing to the complexity and intricacies of pediatric transfusion practice. In addition, Red Blood Cells (RBCs) have recently been shown to be the most frequently transfused blood component in children.[2,3] These factors are the foundation for current transfusion practices detailed in this chapter.

This chapter discusses neonatal and pediatric transfusion practice in the context of two distinct periods: 1) infants up to 4 months of age and 2) older infants (greater than 4 months of age) and children. Although fetal (in-utero) transfusion practices overlap somewhat with those in the perinatal period, the former are discussed in detail in Chapter 22. The specific pediatric practices addressed in this chapter include 1) small-volume component preparation techniques; 2) transfusion indications for RBCs, platelets, plasma, and granulocytes; 3) transfusion administration and exchange transfusion protocols and procedures; 4) unique neonatal and pediatric situations; 5) transfusion support in specific diseases; and 6) the use of special processing methods to prevent adverse transfusion effects.

TRANSFUSION IN INFANTS LESS THAN 4 MONTHS OF AGE

Considerations in Component Preparation and Therapy

Blood centers, hospital blood banks, and transfusion services must be aware that patients less than 4 months of age have small blood volumes and immature organ function (eg, the immune system), which necessitate special approaches to component therapy. This is especially important for very low birth-

Cassandra D. Josephson, MD, Director of Blood and Tissue Services, Children's Healthcare of Atlanta, and Associate Professor, Pathology and Pediatrics, Emory University School of Medicine, Atlanta, Georgia

The author has disclosed no conflicts of interest.

weight (VLBW) infants (<1500 g) and extremely low birthweight (ELBW) infants (<1000 g).

Fetal and Neonatal Physiology Affecting Transfusion Practice

Healthy term neonates have a mean cord blood hemoglobin of 16.9 ± 1.6 g/dL, while that of preterm neonates is 15.9 ± 2.4 g/dL. The hemoglobin concentrations normally decline during the first few weeks of life. As a result, "physiologic anemia of infancy" occurs in newborns and "physiologic anemia of prematurity" occurs in preterm infants.[4] Both anemias are considered self-limited and are usually tolerated without any harmful effects. The rate of decline in hemoglobin is a function of gestational age at birth. At 4 to 8 weeks after birth, hemoglobin decreases to levels as low as 8.0 g/dL in preterm infants weighing 1000 to 1500 g, and 7.0 g/dL in neonates weighing less than 1000 g at birth.[5] The physiologic decrease in peripheral blood hemoglobin concentration is the result of several factors, including 1) a decrease in erythropoietin (EPO), resulting in diminished red cell production; 2) a decrease in survival of fetal red cells; and 3) an increasing blood volume due to rapid growth. Reduced EPO production results from increased oxygen delivery to tissues because of increased pulmonary blood flow, elevated arterial pO_2, and increased red cell 2,3-diphosphoglycerate (2,3-DPG) and hemoglobin A. This naturally occurring anemia requires treatment only if it causes symptoms in the patient.

Clinical Considerations Related to Infant Size and Blood Volume

Blood volumes of pediatric patients vary with body weight. A full-term newborn has a blood volume of approximately 85 mL/kg, and a preterm newborn, 100 mL/kg. Because of the small total blood volumes of the preterm infants (100 mL or less), blood banks and transfusion services need to be capable of providing smaller, appropriately sized blood components to meet their needs. Many factors, including iatrogenic blood loss from repeated phlebotomy, lead to frequent transfusions in this population. Hypovolemia is not tolerated as well in newborns as it is in adults because a newborn's left ventricular stroke volume decreases without an increase in heart rate when >10% of the blood volume is lost. Thus, newborns must physiologically increase their peripheral vascular resistance with decreasing cardiac output to maintain systemic blood pressure. Ultimately, poor tissue perfusion and oxygenation occur as well as metabolic acidosis.[6] However, although transfusion may be required in these patients, it is neither necessary nor acceptable to replace blood loss mL for mL; rather, transfusions can be administered to maintain a target hemoglobin level in certain clinical situations.[7] Once ill preterm and term neonates receive multiple transfusions, they will have proportionately lower levels of circulating fetal hemoglobin and an increase in adult hemoglobin.

Erythropoietic Response

The EPO response in newborns differs from that in adults and older children. In the latter groups, oxygen sensors in the kidney recognize decreases in oxygen delivery, which results in the release of EPO into the circulation. In contrast, in the fetus this sensor is located in the liver and is less sensitive, resulting in reduced EPO production in the face of hypoxia (hyporesponsiveness). This is likely a self-protective mechanism that prevents polycythemia of the fetus in the hypoxic intrauterine environment. Although EPO production eventually shifts from the liver to the kidney, the most premature infants produce the least amount of EPO for any degree of anemia.[8] As an alternative to transfusion, the use of recombinant human erythropoietin (rHuEPO) has been shown to reduce donor exposures in premature infants and minimize the severity of their anemia.[9] However, with greater compliance to strict criteria, clinicians have decreased phlebotomy rates in VLBW infants, thereby reducing anemia and transfusions and leaving in question the use of rHuEPO for the management of "anemia of prematurity." Thus, in most cases that approach achieves the same goal as EPO therapy (ie, to decrease transfusions and donor exposures) without expensive pharmacotherapy and the increased risk of potential adverse drug effects.

Cold Stress

Hypothermia in the neonate can trigger or exaggerate a number of responses, including 1) an increase in metabolic rate, 2) hypoglycemia, 3) metabolic acidosis, and 4) potential apneic events that may lead to hypoxia, hypotension, and cardiac arrest. Because blood at room temperature can decrease an infant's core temperature by 0.7 to 2.5 C, in-line blood warmers are required for all RBC exchange transfusions. A radiant heater should never be used to warm the blood because of the risk of hemolysis. Furthermore, to prevent hemolysis in neonates undergoing phototherapy, the blood administration tubing should be positioned to minimize exposure to phototherapy light.[10]

Immunologic Status

The infant's immature immune system predisposes it to infectious and noninfectious serious hazards of transfusion. In fact, much of the special processing and manipulation of products for preterm infants and neonates are directly related to their underdeveloped immune function. Most of their humoral immunity (antibody protection) is provided by the mother starting early in pregnancy (approximately 12 weeks) through placental transfer of immunoglobulins. Between 20 and 33 weeks of gestation, fetal IgG levels rise significantly because of selective transport system maturation in the placenta. IgG1 is the predominant maternal subclass crossing the placenta and is transported in the largest quantities.[11] In contrast, maternal IgM and IgA do not cross the placenta to the fetus in significant amounts. The breakdown of IgG occurs at a slower rate in the fetus than in the mother, enabling conservation of the transplacental maternal antibody during the neonatal period. Unexpected red cell alloantibodies of either IgM or IgG class are rarely formed during the neonatal period. The lack of red cell alloantibody production during this period is not well understood but has been postulated to be attributed to deficient T-helper function, enhanced T-suppressor activity, and poor antigen-presenting cell function.[12]

Cellular immune responses are also incompletely developed during this period and may make the infant susceptible to transfusion-associated graft-vs-host disease (TA-GVHD). TA-GVHD has been reported most frequently in the newborn with confirmed or suspected congenital immunodeficiency. The majority of TA-GVHD cases reported in nonimmunocompromised infants have occurred after intrauterine transfusion and subsequent postnatal exchange transfusion.[13,14] There have also been rare cases of TA-GVHD associated with extreme prematurity, neonatal alloimmune thrombocytopenia, and extracorporeal membrane oxygenation (ECMO).[13,15] Neonates with TA-GVHD clinically present following a prolonged latent period, with fever first occurring at an average of 28 days after exposure, as compared to 10 days for affected adults. Once TA-GVHD has occurred, there is more than a 90% chance of associated mortality. Fortunately, TA-GVHD can be completely prevented by pretransfusion irradiation of blood components for individuals with suspected and/or documented T-cell immunodeficiency as well as for all patients receiving directed-donor units from biologic relatives.[15,16] This is discussed in more detail later in this chapter.

Metabolic Problems

In the infant less than 4 months of age, large-volume transfusions of whole blood or plasma may result in acidosis or hypocalcemia because of the inability of the infant's immature liver to effectively metabolize citrate. The immature kidneys also contribute to these complications secondary to a reduced glomerular filtration rate and concentrating ability that lead to difficulties in excreting excess potassium, acid, and/or calcium.

POTASSIUM. Small-volume, simple transfusions administered slowly have been shown to have little effect on serum potassium concentrations in infants less than 4 months of age despite elevated potassium levels in the plasma of stored RBCs. In calculating levels of infused potassium, Strauss[16,17] determined that an RBC unit (80% hematocrit) in an extended storage medium for 42 days would deliver 2 mL of plasma containing only 0.1 mMol/L of potassium when transfused at 10 mL/kg. This amount is much less than the daily requirement of potassium of 2 to 3 mMol/L for a patient weighing 1 kg. It must be stressed that this calculation does not hold true for the transfusion of large volumes of RBCs because serum potassium may rise rapidly in these small patients particularly during surgery, exchange transfusion, or ECMO and is dependent on the plasma potassium levels in the blood and manipulation of the blood components.[18,19]

The type of anticoagulant-preservative solution used to store RBCs at collection will determine the amount of potassium leak. For instance, a unit of RBCs preserved in additive solution (AS) such as AS-1, AS-3, or AS-5 will deliver less extracellular potassium than RBCs stored in citrate-phosphate-dextrose-adenine-1 (CPDA-1).[16,20] In addition, special processing of the component, such as irradiation, can potentiate the potassium leak. If such components are stored for more than 24 hours, washing may be required to remove the excess potassium before transfusion.[15] This washing practice is supported by several reports of infants who received either older RBC units or units that had been irradiated (more than 1 day before transfusion) and showed severe adverse effects, including cardiac arrest and death, after receiving such components via a central line or an intracardiac line.[21,22]

2,3-DIPHOSPHOGLYCERATE. Levels of 2,3-DPG in RBCs are known to rapidly decline after the first week of RBC storage. This deficit does not negatively affect older children and adult recipients because of their ability to replace the missing 2,3-DPG and to compensate for hypoxia by increasing their heart rate. Infants younger than 4 months are not able to do this as effectively secondary to decreased levels of intracellular 2,3-DPG that reach even lower levels with respiratory distress syndrome or septic shock. Thus, if a large proportion of the neonate's blood volume is composed of transfused 2,3-DPG-depleted blood, the resulting shift in the hemoglobin oxygen dissociation curve will further increase oxygen affinity for hemoglobin and reduce oxygen availability to the tissues. Therefore, the recommended therapy for newborns is an exchange transfusion with the freshest blood conveniently available (up to 14 days). However, the medical need for fresh RBC units for small-volume transfusions has not been established and has even been suggested as unnecessary.[7,16,19] A prospective randomized controlled trial on RBC storage duration is necessary in this population.[23]

RBC Transfusion Support

Ill neonates are more likely to receive RBC transfusions than any other patient age group, and RBCs are the component most often transfused during the neonatal period.[7] RBC replacement is considered for sick neonates when approximately 10% of the patient's blood volume has been lost or they have symptomatic anemia.

Indications

Several guidelines have been published over the past 15 years regarding the indications for RBC transfusion in the neonate.[24-28] Most of the recommendations are based on the experience acquired in clinical practice rather than on evidence-based medicine. To this end, a critical need exists for future clinical studies in this area.[29] Table 23-1 lists the most recently published guidelines in this area.[25,28]

Compatibility Testing

AABB *Standards for Blood Banks and Transfusion Services*[30(pp36-37)] allows limited pretransfusion serologic testing for infants less than 4 months of age. Initial patient testing must include ABO and D typing of their red cells and a screen for unexpected red cell antibodies, using either plasma or serum from the infant or mother. During any one hospitalization, crossmatch compatibility testing and repeat ABO

TABLE 23-1. Transfusion Guidelines for RBCs in Infants Less than 4 Months of Age[25,28]

1.	Hematocrit <20% with low reticulocyte count and symptomatic anemia (tachycardia, tachypnea, poor feeding).	
2.	Hematocrit <30% and any of the following:	
	a.	On <35% oxygen hood.
	b.	On oxygen by nasal cannula.
	c.	On continuous positive airway pressure and/or intermittent mandatory ventilation on mechanical ventilation with mean airway pressure <6 cm of water.
	d.	With significant tachycardia or tachypnea (heart rate >180 beats/minute for 24 hours, respiratory rate >80 beats/minute for 24 hours).
	e.	With significant apnea or bradycardia (>6 episodes in 12 hours or 2 episodes in 24 hours requiring bag and mask ventilation while receiving therapeutic doses of methylxanthines).
	f.	With low weight gain (<10 g/day observed over 4 days while receiving ≥100 kcal/kg/day).
3.	Hematocrit <35% and either of the following:	
	a.	On >35% oxygen hood.
	b.	On continuous positive airway pressure/intermittent mandatory ventilation with mean airway pressure ≥6-8 cm of water.
4.	Hematocrit <45% and either of the following:	
	a.	On extracorporeal membrane oxygenation.
	b.	With congenital cyanotic heart disease.

and D typing may be omitted as long as all of the following criteria are met: the antibody screen is negative; transfused red cells are group O, ABO identical, or ABO compatible; and transfused cells are either D negative or the same D type as the patient. Testing the infant's reverse type for anti-A and/or anti-B is not necessary. However, before non-group-O RBCs can be issued, testing of the infant's plasma or serum is required to detect passively acquired maternal anti-A or anti-B and should include the antiglobulin phase. If the antibody is present, ABO-compatible RBCs must be used until the acquired antibody is no longer detected.

If an unexpected non-ABO alloantibody is detected in the infant's or mother's specimen, it is required that the infant receive RBC units lacking the corresponding antigen(s), or units compatible by antiglobulin crossmatch. This regimen should continue until the maternal antibody is no longer detected in the infant's plasma or serum. The policy of the hospital transfusion service will determine the frequency for reevaluating the patient for antibodies. Once a negative antibody screen is obtained, crossmatches and use of antigen-negative blood are no longer required up to 4 months of age because of the immature immunologic status of these infants. Multiple observational studies have shown that alloimmunization to red cell antigens is rare during the neonatal period.[12,31,32] Thus, repeated type-and-screen testing, as required for adults and children older than 4 months, is unnecessary in this population and merely contributes to iatrogenic and significant blood loss. Of importance, the transfusion service should avoid the transfusion of any components that may passively transfer unexpected alloantibodies or ABO-incompatible antibodies to the recipient.[33]

Components for Neonatal Transfusion

Advances in neonatology permitting the survival of extremely premature infants with the use of surfactant therapy, nitric oxide therapy, high-frequency ventilators, and compliance with transfusion practice guidelines have substantially decreased the number of RBC transfusions administered. Most neonatal transfusions are now given to ELBW infants weighing less than 1000 g.[7]

Aliquoting for Small-Volume Transfusion

The purpose of creating small-volume aliquots is to limit donor exposures and potentially decrease donor-related risks.[34-38] Several technical approaches are acceptable to accomplish these two goals and to minimize blood wastage.[39]

Small-volume RBC transfusion aliquots are commonly made with a multiple-pack system.[39,40] Quad packs, employed mostly by blood centers, are produced from a single unit of whole blood that is diverted into a primary bag with three integrally attached smaller bags. Each of the smaller units has the same expiration date as the original unit because the system's original seal remained intact, maintaining a "closed system" throughout the manufacturing process. The plasma is then separated and diverted into one bag during component preparation, resulting in small-volume aliquots for storage. A hospital transfusion service can then remove (either by heat sealer or metal clips) each aliquot as needed. For hospital transfusion services without a sterile connecting device (Fig 23-1), this method provides three aliquots from a single unit.[39] However, wastage of the product may still occur as a result of large-sized aliquots or an

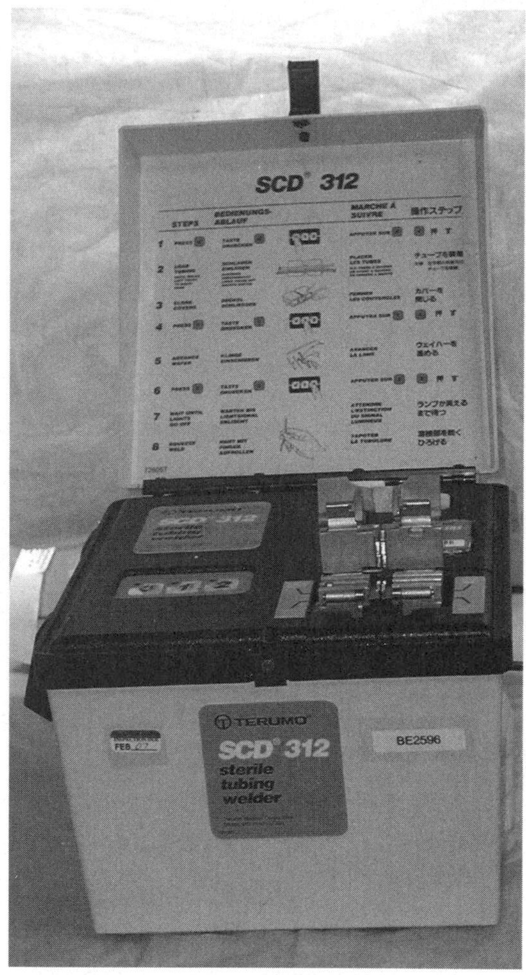

FIGURE 23-1. A sterile tubing welder (reproduced with permission from Terumo Medical Corp., Somerset, NJ).

aliquot that exceeds the actual dose written for each patient based on body weight.

Hospital transfusion services that have a sterile connecting device have multiple additional options to produce aliquots, such as transfer packs (eg, PEDI-PAK system from Genesis BPS, Hackensack, NJ; Fig 23-2), small-volume bags, or tubing with integrally attached syringes.[39] Syringe sets (Fig 23-3) offer the greatest accuracy for obtaining the desired volume to be transfused based on volume-per-weight calculations.[39] Some syringe sets have filters attached (150-micron in-line filters) such that, when issued by the blood bank, the

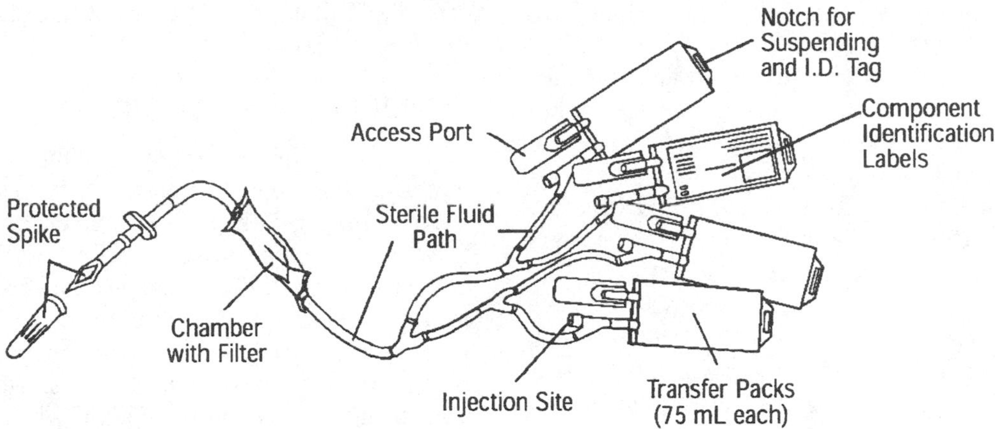

FIGURE 23-2. Diagram of PEDI-PAK (reproduced with permission of Genesis BPS, Hackensack, NJ).

cells have been filtered during the aliquoting process and are ready to be placed on a syringe pump without further manipulation of the component at the bedside. The advantage of this process is that it eliminates the need for the nurse to transfer blood from the pack to a syringe at the bedside in order to be delivered by a syringe pump. Removing this additional step reduces the risk of contamination, mislabeling, or damage to the unit that could result in loss or spillage of blood.[39]

Once an aliquot is produced at either the blood center or the hospital blood bank, it requires labeling with the expiration date and recording of the origin and disposition of each smaller unit. Reducing donor exposures is more readily accomplished by this technique, whereby a recipient can receive multiple small-volume transfusions from a single unit until it reaches its expiration date.[39,40] In order to maximize the above-mentioned benefits, many hospital transfusion services assign a single unit of RBCs to one or more infants based on their weight.[35-41]

RBC Additive Solution

Historically, transfused RBCs for pediatric patients contained CPDA-1 anticoagulant-pre-

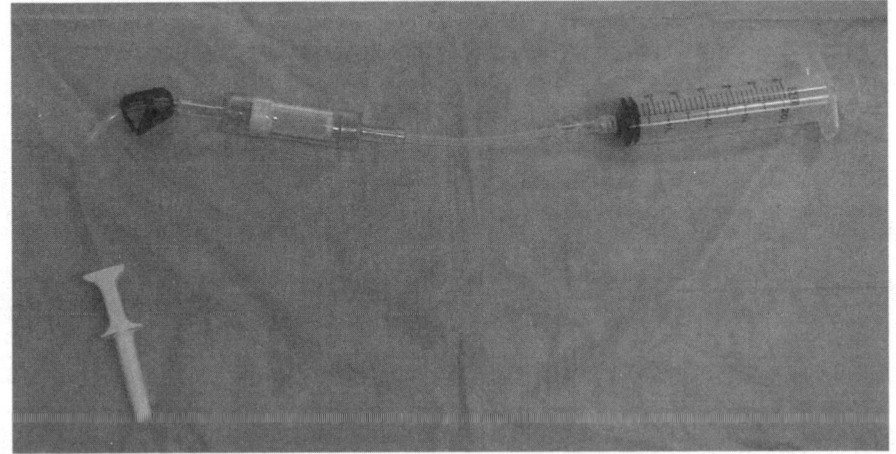

FIGURE 23-3. Syringe with filter (reproduced with permission from Charter Medical, Ltd, Winston-Salem, NC).

servative solution.[41] However, as AS (see Chapter 6) has evolved to extend the shelf life of RBCs, many have begun to question its safety in neonates. One concern is the large amount of adenine and mannitol in AS and its relation to renal toxicity. Moreover, mannitol is a potent diuretic with effects on fluid dynamics that can result in fluctuations in the cerebral blood flow of preterm infants.

Most evidence suggests that small-volume transfusions (5 to 15 mL/kg) containing AS are safe for this patient population. Specifically, when AS-1 and AS-3 were compared, no harmful effects were observed in neonates receiving small-volume, simple transfusions. These transfusions were shown to be as effective as CPDA-1 RBCs in increasing hemoglobin levels in recipients.[41-43] Luban et al further described theoretical calculations in a variety of clinical settings to demonstrate that RBCs preserved in extended-storage media present no substantive risk when used for small-volume transfusions.[44] However, for infants with renal or hepatic insufficiency, they recommended that AS solution be removed, particularly if multiple transfusions from the same unit are expected. The safety of AS-preserved RBCs in trauma-related massive transfusions, cardiac surgery, or exchange transfusions in this population has not been investigated. Thus, AS-preserved RBC units should be used with caution in these settings.[23,43-46]

Specific Indications for RBCs

In neonates, symptomatic anemia is the major indication for simple transfusion. Specifically, a venous hemoglobin of <13 g/dL in the first 24 hours of life necessitates clinical consideration of a red cell transfusion.[47] Red cell transfusion in this population should also be considered when approximately 10% of a sick neonate's blood volume has been removed or lost. When transfusing 10 mL/kg of red cells with a hematocrit of >80%, the expected increase in hemoglobin concentration in the neonate should be approximately 3 g/dL. A similar volume of red cells with AS usually has a hematocrit of 65% and will result in a projected posttransfusion hemoglobin increase of <3 g/dL (see Table 23-2 for dosing of blood components and expected results).[48]

Over the past 5 years, two randomized controlled trials have been completed: 1) the Premature Infants in Need of Transfusion (PINT) study and its follow-up, PINT-OS, and 2) the Iowa Study. These focused on restrictive (hemoglobin 7 g/dL) vs liberal (hemoglobin 10 g/dL) RBC transfusion thresholds in VLBW infants.[49-51] The Iowa trial revealed a decrease in transfusion events (3.3 vs 5.2; p = 0.025) overall

TABLE 23-2. Blood Components and Dosing of Small Volumes in Neonatal and Pediatric Patients[48]

Component	Dose	Expected Increment
Red Blood Cells	10-15 mL/kg	Hemoglobin increase 2-3 g/dL*
Fresh Frozen Plasma	10-15 mL/kg	15%-20% rise in factor levels (assuming 100% recovery)
Platelets [whole-blood-derived (WBD) or apheresis]	5-10 mL/kg or 1 WBD unit/10 kg (patients ≥10 kg)	50,000/µL rise in platelet count (assuming 100% recovery)†
Cryoprecipitated AHF	1-2 units/10 kg	60-100 mg/dL rise in fibrinogen (assuming 100% recovery)

*Dependent on anticoagulant-preservative solution: with 3 g/dL increment for CPD and CPDA-1 and 2 g/dL for AS-1, AS-3, and AS-5.

†Assumes ≥5.5 × 10^{10} platelets in 50 mL of plasma (whole-blood-derived) and ≥3.0 × 10^{11} platelets in 250-300 mL plasma (apheresis).

CPD = citrate-phosphate-dextrose; CPDA-1 = citrate-phosphate-dextrose-adenine-1; AS = additive solution.

with the restrictive strategy. However, there was a reported increase in periventricular leukomalacia and deaths (secondary outcomes) in the restrictive arm. In the PINT study, a composite endpoint was examined, revealing no significant difference between the two arms (restrictive vs liberal) in the composite outcome of death or any of the following: bronchopulmonary dysplasia; retinopathy of prematurity, stage >3; or brain injury (periventricular leukomalasia, intraventricular hemorrhage grade 4, or ventriculomegaly).[49,51] Of note, the PINT-OS follow-up study revealed, for those same infants enrolled in the PINT study, that at 18 to 24 months after birth there was an increase in neurodevelopmental impairments in the more restrictive RBC transfusion arm.[49,50] In summary, all three studies suggest a common theme: maintenance of higher hemoglobin levels in low-birthweight infants may be protective neurologically in the long term. Whether a restrictive or liberal strategy for transfusion of red cells in this population should be broadly implemented is not clear and requires further prospective randomized controlled trial data.

Exchange Transfusion for Hyperbilirubinemia

Exchange transfusion in neonates involves replacement of one to two whole blood volumes. The primary use of this therapy is to treat excessively high levels of unconjugated bilirubin, or hyperbilirubinemia. In high concentrations, bilirubin may cross the blood-brain barrier, concentrate in the basal ganglia and cerebellum of preterm and term infants, and cause irreversible damage to the central nervous system known as kernicterus. Preterm and term infants are susceptible to this complication because of their immature livers, which poorly conjugate bilirubin, as well as their incompletely developed blood-brain barriers, which allow bilirubin transit. Phototherapy, which uses fluorescent ultraviolet light, is the current treatment of choice, and exchange transfusion is reserved for patients who fail phototherapy.

Excessively high unconjugated bilirubin concentrations may occur in several conditions, including immune-mediated hemolysis, nonimmune hemolysis, bile excretion defects, and impaired albumin binding. Two critical objectives accomplished with exchange transfusions are the removal of unconjugated bilirubin and maximization of albumin binding to residual bilirubin. In addition, in antibody-mediated hemolytic processes, exchange therapy removes both free antibody and antibody-coated red cells, replacing them with antigen-negative red cells. Exchange transfusion needs to be performed before the development of kernicterus. For example, in term infants, kernicterus rarely develops at bilirubin levels less than 25 mg/dL. However, in sick VLBW infants, kernicterus has occurred at bilirubin levels as low as 8 to 12 mg/dL.[52] Rather than using a single bilirubin level as a decision point, most practitioners base their decisions to perform exchange transfusion on the rate at which the bilirubin is increasing. A double-volume exchange transfusion (two 85-mL/kg transfusions for term infants and two 100-mL/kg transfusions for VLBW infants) removes approximately 70% to 90% of the circulating red cells and approximately 50% of the total bilirubin.[53] However, after the first exchange transfusion, bilirubin levels may rise again because of a reequilibration of the extravascular tissue and plasma bilirubin, which may necessitate another exchange transfusion.[54]

Exchange Transfusion for Other Causes

Occasionally exchange transfusion is used to eliminate toxins, drugs, or chemicals when they have been administered to the mother near the time of delivery, when toxic doses have been administered to the infant, or if they accumulate at high levels in the infant as a result of prematurity and/or an inborn error of metabolism.[55,56] Beyond the scope of this chapter are other uses of this therapy in the neonatal period, which require evaluation of each individual case guided by established standards for practice.

Technique of Exchange Transfusion

COMPONENT CHOICE AND PHYSIOLOGIC EFFECTS. Typically, red cells are resuspended in ABO-compatible thawed Fresh Frozen Plasma (FFP) for an exchange transfusion. No single method of combining components has been shown to be superior to another. Most often, red cells less than 5 to 7 days old and stored in CPDA-1 are used to avoid high levels of potassium and to maximize red cell survival.[57] When using AS-RBC units, some blood banks elect to remove the additive-containing plasma in order to reduce the volume transfused. Most transfusion services provide red cells that are 1) hemoglobin S-negative to avoid potential intravascular sickling, 2) cytomegalovirus (CMV) seronegative to prevent virus transmission, and 3) irradiated to prevent TA-GVHD. Irradiation should be performed just before exchange if possible to prevent potentiation of the potassium storage lesion. Some experts recommend washing or removing the supernatant of red cells that were irradiated (from many hours to several days before their administration) in order to avoid complications of hyperkalemic cardiac arrhythmias.[58]

The glucose load administered during exchange transfusion has been noted to be extremely high in some cases. This stimulates the infant's pancreas to release insulin, which may result in rebound hypoglycemia. Thus, plasma glucose levels should be monitored during the first few hours following exchange transfusion.

Because unconjugated bilirubin binds to albumin, infusion of albumin is frequently used to increase intravascular binding. Theoretically, with additional albumin in the circulation, bilirubin from the extravascular space diffuses to the intravascular space. This, in turn, should increase the total quantity of bilirubin removed during the exchange. There have been conflicting results, however, regarding the efficacy of administering albumin either before or during exchange to enhance bilirubin removal. A study that compared 15 hyperbilirubinemic neonates given albumin with 27 who received none found similar efficiency of bilirubin removal in both groups.[59] Infusing albumin raises the colloid osmotic pressure and increases intravascular volume. Therefore, it should be given cautiously, if at all, to neonates or infants who are severely anemic, have increased central venous pressure, or are in renal or congestive heart failure.

VOLUME AND HEMATOCRIT CONSIDERATIONS. A double-volume exchange in neonates rarely necessitates the infusion of more than one unit of RBCs. Clinicians should aim for a final hematocrit of approximately 45% to 60% for the component, with sufficient plasma to provide clotting factors (the plasma volume is based on estimated blood volume).[58] If the neonate's situation necessitates a higher postexchange transfusion hematocrit, a small-volume red cell transfusion may be given, or a unit with a higher hematocrit can be used for the initial exchange transfusion. The reconstituted blood should be well mixed in order to sustain the intended hematocrit throughout the exchange. The infant's hematocrit and bilirubin can be measured by removing the last aliquot of the exchange.

VASCULAR ACCESS. Just after birth, umbilical venous catheters are typically used to achieve exchange transfusions in preterm and term infants. Catheterization is easiest soon after birth, yet access to this site is possible for several days. Radio-opaque catheters are used to facilitate x-ray monitoring of proper line placement before procedures. In the event that umbilical venous catheters are not available, small saphenous catheters may be used.

TECHNIQUES. Two exchange transfusion techniques are commonly employed: isovolumetric and manual push-pull. The former involves vascular access through two catheters of identical size that allow simultaneous withdrawal and infusion of blood and are regulated by a single peristaltic pump. The umbilical vein is typically used for infusion, and the umbilical artery for withdrawal. The latter technique uses a single vascular access portal with a three-way stopcock joining the unit of blood, the patient, and a graduated discard container. A standard filter and in-line blood warmer are recommended. The absolute maximum volume of each withdrawal and infusion is dependent on the infant's body weight and hemodynamic status. Usually no more than 5 mL/kg body weight or 5% of the infant's blood volume is removed and replaced during a 3- to 5-minute cycle.[57] The exchange transfusion should not be performed rapidly because sudden hemodynamic changes may affect cerebral blood flow and shift intracranial pressure, contributing to intraventricular hemorrhage.[60] A total double-volume exchange transfusion generally takes 90 to 120 minutes.[57]

Platelet Transfusion Support

Mild to moderate thrombocytopenia (platelet count <150,000/µL) is the most common hemostatic abnormality in sick preterm and full-term infants, and it affects approximately 20% of the infants in the neonatal intensive care unit.[61] Thrombocytopenia may have several causes, including impaired production, increased destruction, abnormal distribution, or dilution (of platelets) secondary to massive transfusion. The most common cause is increased destruction of platelets generally associated with a variety of self-limited conditions.

Indications

Most platelet transfusions in preterm and term infants are performed therapeutically, for platelet counts less than 50,000/µL in the presence of active bleeding.[62]

Prophylactic platelet transfusions in this population are controversial (see Table 23-3 for specific transfusion indications and thresholds).[29,63] Unlike adult patients who rarely have severe bleeding complications until platelet counts decline to less than 10,000/µL, preterm infants with other complicating illnesses may bleed at higher platelet counts. This increased risk may be attributable to 1) lower concentrations of plasma coagulation factors, 2) circulation of an anticoagulant that potentiates thrombin inhibition, 3) intrinsic or extrinsic platelet dysfunction (eg, hyporeactiv-

TABLE 23-3. Transfusion Guidelines for Platelets in Neonates and Older Children[25,28]

With Thrombocytopenia
1. Platelet count 5,000 to 10,000/µL with failure of platelet production.
2. Platelet count <30,000/µL in neonate with failure of platelet production.
3. Platelet count <50,000/µL in stable premature infant:
a. With active bleeding, or
b. Before an invasive procedure, with failure of platelet production.
4. Platelet count <100,000/µL in sick premature infant:
a. With active bleeding, or
b. Before an invasive procedure in patient with DIC.
Without Thrombocytopenia
1. Active bleeding in association with qualitative platelet defect.
2. Unexplained excessive bleeding in a patient undergoing cardiopulmonary bypass.
3. Patient undergoing ECMO with:
a. A platelet count of <100,000/µL, or
b. Higher platelet counts and bleeding.

DIC = disseminated intravascular coagulation; ECMO = extracorporeal membrane oxygenation.

ity), or 4) increased vascular fragility.[62] A complication of great concern is intraventricular hemorrhage, which occurs in approximately 40% of preterm neonates in the first 72 hours of life. Although prophylactic platelet transfusions may increase platelet counts and shorten bleeding times, this approach has not been shown to reduce the incidence of intraventricular hemorrhage.[61] Hence, the use of platelets in this situation as well as appropriate dosing remain controversial.[64] Posttransfusion platelet counts taken 15 to 60 minutes after transfusion will help clinicians evaluate survival of platelets; however, these counts are not good predictors of hemostatic efficacy.

Components and Dose

The use of whole-blood-derived platelets, specifically platelet doses of 5 to 10 mL/kg body weight, have been demonstrated to raise the platelet count of an average full-term newborn by 50,000 to 100,000/µL, depending on the concentration of the platelet component used.[17,61] A similar dosing regimen is typically used with apheresis platelets. When possible, the platelet component should be ABO group specific/compatible and should not contain clinically significant unexpected red cell antibodies. Transfusion of ABO-incompatible plasma should be avoided in pediatric patients and especially in infants because of their small blood and plasma volumes.[33] If it becomes necessary to administer ABO-incompatible platelets to an infant, plasma may be removed either by volume reduction or washing (see Method 6-14). The platelets may then be resuspended in saline or compatible plasma. However, routine centrifugation to remove plasma from platelets should be avoided because it is unnecessary and harmful to the platelets.[61,62] In addition, when platelets are stored in a syringe, the pH has been shown to rapidly decrease, a potential problem for an already ill and acidotic recipient.[65,66] Thus, when volume reduction in an open system is used and the product is placed in a syringe, the processing should be completed as close to the time of issuance as possible and the product infused within 4 hours.

Plasma Transfusion Support to Enhance Hemostasis

Infants must synthesize their own coagulation factors because significant amounts are not transferred in the prenatal period from the mother. However, infants are typically unable to produce the required amounts of these proteins in the early postnatal period. Physiologically low levels of vitamin K-dependent factors (II, VII, IX, and X) and the contact factors (XI, XII, prekallikrein, and high-molecular-weight kininogen) contribute to the long prothrombin and partial thromboplastin times seen in infants.[67] In addition, the naturally occurring vitamin-K-dependent anticoagulants (proteins C and S) and the non-vitamin-K-dependent antithrombin protein are also at low levels at birth. Despite these issues, the procoagulant and anticoagulant systems are usually in a fine balance in healthy newborns, which is why spontaneous bleeding and thrombosis are rarely observed. However, the reserve capacity for both systems to respond to pathologic insult is quite limited. Thus, serious bleeding may occur in sick premature infants during the first week of life. Cryoprecipitated AHF and FFP can be used to treat bleeding or clotting complications, such as disseminated intravascular coagulation (DIC), that result from an imbalance in the two systems.[68]

Fresh Frozen Plasma

FFP is frequently used to replace coagulation factors in preterm and term infants (Table 23-4), particularly if multiple factors are deficient—for example, in "hemorrhagic disease of the newborn" or vitamin K deficiency. The common dose for FFP is 10 to 15 mL/kg, which is expected to increase all factor activity levels by 15% to 20%, unless there is a marked consumptive coagulopathy.[63,65] To limit donor exposure for each recipient while minimizing wastage of plasma, blood can be collected into a system with multiple, integrally attached bags, creating aliquots ready to freeze.[28] Once thawed, the aliquots can be subdivided further for several patients if they can be used within a 24-hour period. In addition, it is important that FFP for infants be ABO compatible, unlike

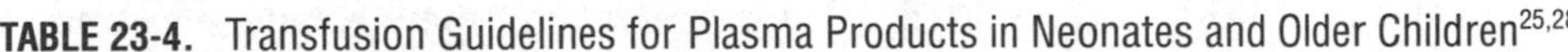

TABLE 23-4. Transfusion Guidelines for Plasma Products in Neonates and Older Children[25,28]

Fresh Frozen Plasma (FFP)
1. Support during treatment of disseminated intravascular dissemination.
2. Replacement therapy:
a. When specific factor concentrates are not available, including, but not limited to, antithrombin; protein C or S deficiency; and Factor II, Factor V, Factor X, and Factor XI deficiencies.
b. During therapeutic plasma exchange when FFP is indicated (cryopoor plasma, plasma from which the cryoprecipitate has been removed).
3. Reversal of warfarin in an emergency situation, such as before an invasive procedure with active bleeding.
Note: FFP is not indicated for volume expansion or enhancement of wound healing.
Cryoprecipitated AHF
1. Hypofibrinogenemia or dysfibrinogenemia with active bleeding.
2. Hypofibrinogenemia or dysfibrinogenemia while undergoing an invasive procedure.
3. Factor XIII deficiency with active bleeding or while undergoing an invasive procedure in the absence of Factor XIII concentrate.
4. Limited directed-donor cryoprecipitate for bleeding episodes in small children with hemophilia A (when recombinant and plasma-derived Factor VIII products are not available).
5. In the preparation of fibrin sealant.
6. von Willebrand disease with active bleeding, but only when both of the following are true:
a. Deamino-D-arginine vasopressin (DDAVP) is contraindicated, not available, or does not elicit response.
b. Virus-inactivated plasma-derived Factor VIII concentrate (which contains von Willebrand factor) is not available.

in adults, and free of clinically significant unexpected antibodies because transfused antibodies can reach high concentrations in infants and children with very small plasma volumes. A common practice at some institutions is to use group AB FFP because a single unit can provide multiple small-volume doses for several neonates.

Cryoprecipitated AHF

Cryoprecipitate is used primarily to treat conditions resulting from decreased or dysfunctional fibrinogen or Factor XIII deficiency. Cryoprecipitate is usually given in conjunction with platelets and FFP to treat DIC in newborns. Typically, 1 unit is sufficient to achieve hemostatic levels in an infant. Although cryoprecipitate transfusions in adults are not required to be ABO compatible with the recipient, these components should be ABO compatible with neonatal recipients because of their smaller blood volumes. Cryoprecipitate is not recommended for patients with Factor VIII deficiency because the standard therapy is to treat with recombinant Factor VIII products or virus-inactivated, monoclonal-antibody-purified, plasma-derived products.[68,69] Furthermore, cryoprecipitate should be used to treat von Willebrand disease (vWD) only if desmopressin is not an option and if plasma-derived, virus-inactivated concentrates containing von Willebrand factor are not available. (See Table 23-4 for other guidelines regarding cryoprecipitate use.[63])

Granulocyte Transfusion Support

Indications

The role of granulocyte transfusion for sepsis in neonates is unclear; however, there are certain clinical situations where it may be considered as adjunct therapy to antibiotics. Because neonatal neutrophil function is often abnormal, the current thinking is that providing well-functioning granulocytes may be beneficial.[17,70-74] It is important to establish the following factors before the transfusion of granulocytes: 1) strong evidence of bacterial or fungal septicemia, 2) absolute neutrophil count less than 3000/µL, and 3) diminished narrowing of the storage pool (such that 7% of nucleated cells in the marrow are granulocytes that are metamyelocytes or more mature).[18,75] (See Table 23-5 for guidelines on granulocyte transfusion support.)

Components and Dose

Granulocyte concentrates are produced by standard apheresis techniques or by pooling buffy coats from whole blood. A typical dose for infants is 10 to 15 mL/kg body weight, which is approximately 1×10^9 to 2×10^9 polymorphonuclear cells/kg.[18,71] Treatment should be administered daily until an adequate neutrophil count is achieved and/or the patient shows clinical improvement. According to AABB *Standards*, these components must be irradiated when the patient is at risk for TA-GVHD,[30(p38)] and the components should be obtained from CMV-seronegative donors to prevent virus transmission. Granulocytes must be ABO compatible with the recipient infant because of the significant amount of red cell content in these components (containing >2 mL red cells).[30(p35)] Many institutions also provide D-compatible components to decrease Rh alloimmunization.

Intravenous immune globulin in the treatment of early neonatal sepsis has also been studied, but there is a lack of agreement on its regular application to this patient population.[71,76-80]

TABLE 23-5. Transfusion Guidelines for Granulocytes in Neonates and Older Children[25,28]

1.	Neonates or children with neutropenia or granulocyte dysfunction with bacterial sepsis and lack of responsiveness to standard therapy.
2.	Neutropenic neonates or children with fungal disease not responsive to standard therapy.

Transfusion Administration

Vascular Access

Vascular access is the most difficult aspect of transfusion administration in patients less than 4 months of age, particularly in preterm infants who require long-term or continuous intravenous infusions. The umbilical vein is most frequently cannulated after birth to administer fluids and transfusions and to monitor central venous pressure.[81] Vascular catheters (24-gauge) and small needles (25-gauge) have been safely used for RBC transfusion, without causing hemolysis, if constant flow rates are applied. Smaller gauge needles and catheters have not been evaluated.

Pumps and Warming

When administered slowly, small-volume transfusions typically do not require a blood warmer; however, control of the rate and volume transfused is important. Electromechanical syringe delivery pumps administer the blood at a constant rate and are able to provide adequate control. These pumps cause minimal hemolysis.[82,83] Although several devices can be used to transfuse blood components, it is important to test and validate the mechanical system chosen for component administration.

Transfusion Sets and Filters

All blood component transfusions should go through a standard filter between 170 and 260 microns, even if the components have undergone leukocyte reduction before storage or at the bedside. The plastic tubing in the administration sets can add significant dead volume to the transfusion. Pediatric infusion sets created for platelets and other small-volume components have less dead space than standard sets because of their small tubing and 170-micron filter. Microaggregate filters (20 to 40 microns) are sometimes used for simple transfusion because of their small priming volume. However, providers should be aware that hemolysis may occur when stored RBCs are administered through these filters using negative pressure filtration.[84]

Administration Rates

A lack of clinical studies and evidence-based practices has led to variability both in rates of transfusion and selection of devices among institutions. The rate of RBC and other component administration is dictated by the clinical needs of the pediatric patient. Despite concerns from neonatologists that rapid blood infusion rates may adversely affect intravascular volume and electrolyte levels, an increased risk for intraventricular hemorrhage in these small and fragile patients has not been clearly demonstrated. Thus, a simple transfusion administered over 2 to 4 hours is adequate in nonemergent situations. However, in states of shock or severe bleeding, a rapid infusion is often required.

Unique Therapies and Situations in Neonates

Polycythemia

Neonatal polycythemia is defined as a venous hematocrit greater than 65% or a hemoglobin level greater than 22 g/dL any time during the first week of life. Approximately 5% of all newborns will develop polycythemia, a risk that may be higher in small-for-gestational-age neonates and infants of diabetic mothers. Once the hematocrit rises above 65%, viscosity increases and oxygen transport decreases. However, in neonates the exponential rise in viscosity can occur at hematocrits as low as 40%.[85] Congestive heart failure can result because infants have limited capability for increasing their cardiac output to compensate for hyperviscosity. Central nervous system abnormalities, pulmonary and renal failure, and necrotizing enterocolitis (NEC) can occur from the resultant decreased blood flow. A partial exchange is used to normalize the hematocrit to 55% to 60% and improve tissue perfusion while maintaining blood volume. This exchange is accomplished by removing whole blood and replacing it with normal saline or other crystalloid solutions. Plasma is not used to replace whole blood because NEC has been reported as a complication of the use of plasma.[86] The formula below can be used to approximate the volume of whole blood that must be withdrawn, and the volume of crystalloid infused:

$$\text{Volume} = \frac{\text{Blood volume (observed HCT} - \text{desired HCT)}}{\text{observed HCT}}$$

Extracorporeal Membrane Oxygenation

ECMO is a prolonged treatment in which blood is removed from the patient's venous circulation, circulated through a machine to remove CO_2 (waste), and replenished with O_2 before it is returned to the patient. ECMO has been successfully used since the early 1980s to provide gas exchange independent of a patient's lungs. ECMO allows patients to recover without exposure to aggressive ventilator support that can cause barotrauma and permanent lung damage[87] and to maintain circulation of oxygenated blood during cardiac surgery or disease when other forms of treatment fail.[88] In neonates and children, ECMO has become a lifesaving advance in the treatment of meconium aspiration syndrome, persistent pulmonary hypertension of the newborn, congenital diaphragmatic hernia, and respiratory failure caused by sepsis. It is also used for postoperative support following cardiac surgery.

Because standardized guidelines for transfusion practice in ECMO have not been established, individual centers typically establish their own criteria. Table 23-6 provides some guidelines on this subject.[89] Bleeding complications are frequent during ECMO treatment and may be caused by any of the following factors: 1) systemic heparinization, 2) platelet dysfunction, 3) thrombocytopenia, 4) other coagulation defects, and 5) the nonendothelial surface of the ECMO circuitry. Hospital blood banks and transfusion services must be in close communication with the ECMO staff and be in agreement with local protocols to ensure safe, efficient, and consistent care.

ECMO typically requires 1 to 2 units of ABO and Rh group-specific and crossmatch-compatible RBCs for blood priming. In addition, 1 unit of group-specific FFP should be allocated for the ECMO patient. RBC units are usually negative for hemoglobin S, relatively fresh (less than 5 to 7 days old),[44] irradiated, and CMV seronegative and/or leukocyte reduced.

TRANSFUSION IN OLDER INFANTS (MORE THAN 4 MONTHS OF AGE) AND CHILDREN

RBC Transfusion Support

RBC transfusions in infants older than 4 months and children are similar to transfusions in adults. The most significant differences between this young group and adults are 1) blood volume, 2) the ability to tolerate blood loss, and 3) age-appropriate hemoglobin and hematocrit levels. In these infants and children, the most common indication for RBC transfusion is for the treatment or prevention of tissue hypoxia caused by decreased red cell mass, typically seen in surgery, anemia of chronic diseases, or hematologic malignancies. Additionally, their hemoglobin and hematocrit levels are inherently lower than in adults; thus, they may remain asymptomatic despite extremely low hemoglobin concentrations, especially if the anemia develops slowly. Chronic RBC transfusions are the treatment of choice for children with sickle cell disease (SCD) and thalassemia. These transfusions are administered to combat tissue hypoxia as well

TABLE 23-6. Blood Component Protocols for ECMO[89]

Clinical Scenario	Urgency	Components	Blood Groups	Storage
Cardiac arrest	5-10 min	2 units RBCs	O-neg RBCs	<14 days, AS
ECMO circuit disruption	5-10 min	2 units RBCs	O-neg RBCs	<14 days, AS
Progressive septic shock (nonneonate)	30 min	2 units RBCs	O-neg RBCs or type specific	<10 days, any preservative
Neonate transferred for ECMO	1-2 hours	2 units RBCs 1 unit FFP 1 unit platelets	O-neg RBCs AB plasma	<10 days, CPD or CPDA
Cardiac ICU	30-60 min	2 units RBCs	Type specific	<7 days, AS
Gradual respiratory or cardiac failure on conventional support	Hours to days	2 units RBCs	Type specific	<10 days, CPD

ECMO = extracorporeal membrane oxygenation; RBCs = Red Blood Cells; AS = additive solution; FFP = Fresh Frozen Plasma; CPD = citrate-phosphate-dextrose; CPDA = citrate-phosphate-dextrose-adenine; ICU = intensive care unit.

as to suppress endogenous hemoglobin production. Table 23-7 can help guide transfusion decisions in patients older than 4 months of age.

Before receiving any RBC transfusion, all pediatric patients older than 4 months require ABO and Rh testing and screening for the presence of clinically significant antibodies. Compatibility testing should be performed according to AABB *Standards*.[30(pp36-37)]

Sickle Cell Disease

In patients with SCD, chronic transfusion therapy reduces the risk of stroke by decreasing the percent of red cells containing hemoglobin S in order to reduce sickling and prevent an increase in blood viscosity.[90-93] Chronic transfusions can reduce the risk of recurrent stroke to less than 10% if hemoglobin levels are maintained between 8 and 9 g/dL with a hemoglobin S level less than 30%. The method can be a simple, additive, or partial exchange transfusion, once every 3 to 4 weeks. Erythrocytapheresis has also been used to prevent iron overload in SCD patients. Chronic transfusion therapy is indefinite because cessation can lead to a stroke.[90,91] Table 23-7 lists other complications of SCD necessitating either simple or chronic RBC transfusions. Of note, RBCs for patients with SCD should ideally be screened for hemoglobin S and leukocyte reduced to prevent HLA alloimmunization and decrease platelet refractoriness in preparation for possible stem cell transplantation.

TABLE 23-7. Transfusion Guidelines for RBCs in Patients >4 Months of Age[25,28]

1. Emergency surgical procedure in patient with significant postoperative anemia.
2. Preoperative anemia when other corrective therapy is not available.
3. Intraoperative blood loss >15% total blood volume.
4. Hematocrit <24% and:
a. In perioperative period, with signs and symptoms of anemia.
b. While on chemotherapy/radiotherapy.
c. Chronic congenital or acquired symptomatic anemia.
5. Acute blood loss with hypovolemia not responsive to other therapy.
6. Hematocrit <40% and:
a. With severe pulmonary disease.
b. On extracorporeal membrane oxygenation.
7. Sickle cell disease and:
a. Cerebrovascular accident.
b. Acute chest syndrome.
c. Splenic sequestration.
d. Aplastic crisis.
e. Recurrent priapism.
f. Preoperatively when general anesthesia is planned (target hemoglobin 10 mg/dL).
8. Chronic transfusion programs for disorders of red cell production (eg, β-thalassemia major and Diamond-Blackfan syndrome unresponsive to therapy).

RED CELL ALLOIMMUNIZATION IN SCD. The frequency of humoral immunization to foreign red cell antigens in patients who are chronically transfused varies with each child's disease process, age of first transfusion, and number of transfusions received, as well as the ethnic background of both donors and the recipient.

Patients with SCD have the highest rates of alloimmunization of any patient group.[94-96] These antibodies are produced against common Rh, Kell, Duffy, and Kidd system antigens. Many sickle cell treatment centers perform thorough phenotype analysis of a patient's red cells before beginning transfusion therapy. This testing helps to reduce the rate of alloimmunization by allowing preferential selection of phenotypically similar units.[91,97,98] However, particularly for patients who are not yet alloimmunized, this process remains controversial because phenotypically compatible units may be difficult to obtain.[81,90]

In academic institutions in the United States and Canada, the most common protocol followed for nonalloimmunized patients is pretransfusion phenotypic matching for C, E, and K antigens to prevent alloimmunization.[99] Once patients have developed a red cell antibody, extension of matching to additional red cell antigens (Fy, Jk, S) is often used to prevent further alloimmunization.[100] In a recently published retrospective study, children with SCD demonstrated a decrease in RBC transfusion requirements during matched-sibling-donor marrow transplantation when they received units matched phenotypically for minor red cell antigen compatibility.[101] Method 2-23 can be used to perform red cell phenotyping on autologous red cells of recently transfused patients with SCD.

Another strategy aimed at preventing alloimmunization in patients with SCD is to develop donor recruitment programs specifically for donors of African ethnicity in order to decrease the number of antigenically different RBC units transfused to SCD patients. This approach decreases the exposure to the major antigenic differences of red cells from donors of European ethnicity and is thought to reduce the alloimmunization of SCD recipients. Leukocyte reduction is also beneficial to these patients because it reduces HLA alloimmunization and prevents a potential platelet refractory state.[102] For patients receiving phenotypically matched RBC units, leukocyte reduction is also used to avoid wasting a matched unit whose leukocytes might cause a febrile nonhemolytic transfusion reaction.[103] Leukocyte reduction as a means of preventing alloimmunization to red cell antigens remains controversial.[104,105] However, recently HLA alloimmmuization has been demonstrated to occur more frequently in SCD patients who already have red cell alloimmunization.[106]

OTHER COMPLICATIONS OF RED CELL TRANSFUSIONS IN SCD. The benefits of transfusion therapy in patients with SCD must be weighed against the complications of transfusion, such as iron overload and minor red cell antigen alloimmunization, as well as the risks of increased donor exposure during erythrocytapheresis. Some practitioners have proposed that a clinically successful course of transfusions that maintains the hemoglobin S level below 30% could, after several years, be transitioned to a strategy of more limited transfusions with a hemoglobin S target of 40% to 50% to reduce the risks of iron overload.[92] Patients with SCD may also be at risk for life-threatening delayed hemolytic transfusion reactions. Furthermore, if a patient's hemoglobin level is observed to decrease after transfusion, one may suspect a "hyperhemolytic" syndrome. This phenomenon is characterized by destruction of the patient's own red cells along with transfused cells. The mechanism is not well understood. If hyperhemolytic syndrome is suspected, one should consider stopping transfusion and administering corticosteroids in combination with intravenous immune globulin as noted in reported case studies.[107,108] These patients should also be monitored closely for the formation of autoantibodies, which is known to occur in this population.[109]

Thalassemia

Thalassemia with severe anemia is treated with transfusion to improve tissue oxygenation and suppress extramedullary erythropoiesis in the liver, spleen, and marrow.

Through this approach, many of the complications of thalassemia are mitigated. By maintaining target hemoglobin levels of 8 to 9 g/dL, normal growth and development can occur in these patients. Supertransfusion protocols aim for higher target hemoglobin levels (11 to 12 g/dL). Iron overload is a potential complication of this RBC transfusion protocol that cannot be prevented and should be treated with chelation therapy beginning early in childhood.[110,111]

Platelet and Plasma Support

The indications for platelet and plasma transfusion support are similar for older infants, children, and adults. Tables 23-3 and 23-4 identify indications for the use of platelets, FFP, and cryoprecipitate. In older infants and children, platelets are most often prophylactically administered during chemotherapy. The transfusion threshold for these patients is 10,000 to 20,000/µL, although the platelet count should not be the sole determinant for transfusion. The use of ABO-compatible platelets has been shown to be associated with better clinical outcomes than non-ABO-matched platelets.[33,112-114]

Granulocyte Support

For children older than 4 months, the indications for granulocyte transfusions are similar to those previously mentioned for the younger (<4 months) age group—that is, persistent neutropenia or granulocyte dysfunction in conjunction with bacterial and/or fungal infections. The minimum granulocyte dose for larger children and adults is 1×10^{10} cells/kg.[26,71] Granulocyte components should be irradiated, ABO compatible, CMV seronegative, and crossmatch compatible with the recipient. Granulocytes are also most effective if used within 24 hours of collection. To obtain higher doses of granulocytes for larger patients, donors can be mobilized with a combination of steroids and growth factors, such as granulocyte colony-stimulating factor, which leads to three to four times more granulocytes in the collection than components from donors receiving steroid stimulation alone.

PREVENTION OF ADVERSE EFFECTS OF TRANSFUSION IN NEONATES AND OLDER CHILDREN

Cytomegalovirus Prevention

CMV may be acquired in a number of ways—for example, in utero, during the birth process, by breast feeding, by close contact with mothers or nursery staff, or by transfusion. With current technologies, the risk of acquiring CMV from transfusion is between 1% and 3%.[115] Manifestation of CMV infection in neonates is quite variable, ranging from asymptomatic seroconversion to death. Studies have revealed that the rate of symptomatic transfusion-transmitted CMV infection in infants is low compared to the high incidence of seropositivity in adults. Moreover, symptomatic CMV infection is uncommon in neonates born to seropositive mothers.[116] The risk of transfusion-transmitted CMV infection is higher in multitransfused low-birthweight infants (<1200 g) born to seronegative mothers.[16,115,117] For this reason, it is recommended that low-birthweight infants born to CMV-seronegative mothers receive CMV-reduced-risk blood for transfusion. One approach is to use blood from CMV-seronegative donors. Alternatively, because CMV is associated with leukocytes, leukocyte-reduced components can also be used effectively to reduce the risk of transfusion-transmitted CMV.[17,118,119] Although deglycerolized and washed RBCs have been shown to reduce the risk of transfusion-transmitted CMV infection as well, this approach is logistically more difficult than filtration for removing leukocytes.

Leukocyte Reduction

Leukocyte-reduced components provide potential benefits for neonates, as described above, but their routine use still remains controversial for these patients. For example, transfusion reactions are infrequent in neonates younger than 4 months old, and infants rarely become alloimmunized to red cells or HLA antigens because of their immature immune system. Nonetheless, one benefit to providing leukocyte-reduced components is, as mentioned above, to reduce the risk of transfusion-transmitted CMV.[16,118,120] A recent study from Canada evaluating the clinical outcomes of premature infants (weighing <1250 g) before and after nationwide implementation of universal leukocyte reduction revealed no change in mortality or rate of bacteremia. However, the investigators observed a decrease in retinopathy of prematurity and bronchopulmonary dysplasia as well as a shorter length of hospitalization as a result of implementation.[121]

Irradiation

Cellular blood components are irradiated to prevent TA-GVHD in immunocompromised recipients. Mortality rates associated with TA-GVHD can reach 90% or more, and no effective treatments are available. Consequently, identifying vulnerable groups and individuals before transfusion is critical in preventing this noninfectious hazard of transfusion. Table 23-8 provides guidance for identifying groups who should receive irradiated cellular blood components. It should be noted that there are differing expert opinions and practices in this area, and local protocols should be based on patient populations served, equipment availability, and best practices at each institution. The processes of irradiation and irradiator quality control are beyond the scope of this chapter but are addressed in Chapters 9 and 27.

Volume Reduction

Reduction in the volume of the transfused component is generally used with premature infants who have renal ischemia or compromised cardiac function. In 1993, the AABB Committee on Pediatric Hemotherapy stated that volume reduction of platelet concentrates should be reserved for special infants who have total body fluid restrictions.[62] Methods for platelet volume reduction have been published[122] (see Method 6-14).

Washing

Saline-washed RBCs and platelets are administered in an effort to reduce the risk of adverse reactions to certain components from plasma, anticoagulant-preservative solutions, and high levels of potassium. Transfusion of unwashed RBCs or platelet components procured from the mother is strongly discouraged.[28] The importance of washing out maternal plasma lies in the prevention of hemolytic disease of the fetus and newborn and neonatal alloimmune thrombocytopenia as well as potential reduction of the lifelong risk of transfusion-related acute lung injury.

TABLE 23-8. Irradiation Guidelines for Neonates and Older Children Requiring Cellular Blood Components[25,28]

1. Premature infants weighing <1200 g at birth.
2. Any patient with:
a. Known or suspected cellular immune deficiency.
b. Significant immunosuppression related to chemotherapy or radiation treatment.
3. Any patient receiving:
a. Components from blood relatives.
b. HLA-matched or crossmatched platelet components.

KEY POINTS

1. Red Blood Cells (RBCs) are the most frequently transfused blood component in children, often because of frequent blood loss, including iatrogenic losses from repeated phlebotomy.
2. Symptomatic anemia or a target hemoglobin level (or both) is a preferred strategy for neonatal RBC transfusion, rather than an mL-for-mL replacement of blood lost.
3. A full-term newborn has a blood volume of approximately 85 mL/kg, whereas a preterm newborn has a total blood volume of 100 mL/kg.
4. In infants <4 months of age, initial patient testing must include ABO and D typing of their red cells and a screen for unexpected red cell antibodies, using either plasma or serum from the infant or mother. During any one hospitalization, crossmatch compatibility testing and repeat ABO and D typing may be omitted as long as certain conditions are met.
5. Small-volume simple RBC transfusions (regardless of storage solution), when administered slowly, have been shown to have little effect on serum potassium concentrations in infants <4 months of age despite elevated potassium levels in the plasma of stored RBCs.
6. When making aliquots during component preparation, if the smaller product is made with a sterile connecting device, it is considered a "closed system," and the original unit's expiration date can be used for the new aliquot product.
7. Dosing of RBC units with additive solution (AS) such as AS-1, AS-3, and AS-5 should not exceed 10 to 15 mL/kg for neonates.
8. Transfusion of ABO-incompatible plasma should be avoided in pediatric patients and especially in infants because of their small blood and plasma volumes. If ABO out-of-group platelet transfusion becomes necessary in pediatrics, plasma may be removed either by volume reduction or washing.
9. Chronic RBC transfusion therapy reduces the risk of stroke in patients with sickle cell disease (SCD) by decreasing the percentage of red cells containing hemoglobin S in order to reduce sickling and prevent an increase in blood viscosity. Hemoglobin levels should be maintained at approximately 8 to 9 g/dL, with a hemoglobin S level of <30%.
10. Patients with SCD have the highest rates of alloimmunization to red cell minor antigens of any other patient group. The most commonly formed antibodies are those to Rh, Kell, Duffy, and Kidd system antigens. Many sickle cell treatment centers try to prevent red cell alloimmunization by prophylactically matching for phenotypically similar antigen profiles, but this strategy is controversial.
11. Currently it is recommended that low-birthweight infants born to cytomegalovirus (CMV)-seronegative mothers receive CMV-reduced-risk components for transfusion. These units could be from CMV-seronegative donors or CMV-positive donors whose donations have been leukocyte reduced.

REFERENCES

1. Hillyer CD, Mondoro T, Josephson CD, et al. Pediatric transfusion medicine (PTM): Development of a critical mass (editorial). Transfusion 2009;49:596-601.
2. Slonim AD, Joseph JG, Turenne WM, et al. Blood transfusions in children: Multi-institutional analysis of practices and complications. Transfusion 2008;48:73-80.
3. Gauvin F, Champagne MA, Robillard P, et al. Long-term survival rate of pediatric patients after blood transfusion. Transfusion 2008;48: 801-8.
4. Blanchette V, Doyle J, Schmidt B, Zipursky A. Hematology. In: Avery GB, Fletcher MA, MacDonald MG, eds. Neonatology: Pathophysiology and management of the newborn. 4th ed. Philadelphia: JB Lippincott, 1994:952-99.

5. Brugnara C, Platt OS. The neonatal erythrocyte and its disorders. In: Nathan DG, Orkin SH, ed. Nathan and Oski's hematology of infancy and childhood. 5th ed. Philadelphia: WB Saunders, 1998:19-52.
6. Wallgren G, Hanson JS, Lind J. Quantitative studies of the human neonatal circulation. Acta Paediatr Scand 1967;179(Suppl):43-54.
7. Hume H, Bard H. Small volume red blood cell transfusions for neonatal patients. Transfus Med Rev 1995;9:187-99.
8. Ohls RK. Evaluation and treatment of anemia in the neonate. In: Christensen RD, ed. Hematologic problems of the neonate. Philadelphia: WB Saunders, 2000:137-69.
9. Ohls RK. Erythropoietin to prevent and treat the anemia of prematurity. Curr Opin Pediatr 1999;11:108-14.
10. Luban NLC, Mikesell G, Sacher RA. Techniques for warming red blood cells packaged in different containers for neonatal use. Clin Pediatr 1985;24:642-5.
11. Simister NE. Placental transport of immunoglobulin G. Vaccine 2003;21:3365-9.
12. DePalma L. Red cell antibody formation in the neonate and infant: Considerations for current immunohematologic practice. Immunohematology 1992;8:33-7.
13. Sanders MR, Graeber JE. Posttransfusion graft-versus-host disease in infancy. J Pediatr 1990; 117:159-63.
14. Heiko R, Bein G, Sachs U. Transfusion-associated graft-versus-host disease. Transfusion 2009;23:62-71.
15. Ohto H, Anderson KC. Posttransfusion graft-versus-host disease in Japanese newborns. Transfusion 1996;36:117-23.
16. Strauss RG. Data-driven blood banking practices for neonatal RBC transfusions. Transfusion 2000;40:1528-40.
17. Strauss RG. Transfusion therapy in neonates. Am J Dis Child 1991;145:904-11.
18. Strauss RG. Neonatal transfusion. In: Anderson KC, Ness PN, eds. Scientific basis of transfusion medicine: Implications for clinical practice. 2nd ed. Philadelphia: WB Saunders, 2000:321-6.
19. Strauss RG. Routinely washing irradiated red cells before transfusion seems unwarranted. Transfusion 1990;30:675-7.
20. McDonald TB, Berkowitz RA. Massive transfusion in children. In: Jefferies LC, Brecher ME, eds. Massive transfusion. Bethesda, MD: AABB, 1994:97-119.
21. Harris B, Lumadue J, Luban NLC, Pollack M. Transfusion-related hyperkalemic arrest from irradiated packed red blood cells (abstract). Transfusion 1998;38(Suppl):69S.
22. Hall TL, Barnes A, Miller JR, et al. Neonatal mortality following transfusion of red cells with high plasma potassium levels. Transfusion 1993;33:606-9.
23. Strauss RG. 2008 Emily Cooley Memorial Lecture: Lessons learned from pediatric transfusion medicine clinical trials ... a little child shall lead them. Transfusion 2009;49:1996-2004.
24. Batton DG, Goodrow D, Walker RH. Reducing neonatal transfusion. J Perinatol 1992;12:152-5.
25. Roseff SD, Luban NLC, Manno CS. Guidelines for assessing appropriateness of pediatric transfusion. Transfusion 2002;42:1398-413.
26. Warwick R, Modi N. Guidelines for the administration of blood products. Arch Dis Child 1995;72:379-81.
27. Voak D, Cann R, Finney RD, et al. Guidelines for administration of blood products: Transfusion of infants and neonates. British Committee for Standards in Haematology Blood Transfusion Task Force. Transfus Med 1994;4:63-9.
28. Wong ECC, Paul W. Intrauterine, neonatal, and pediatric transfusion therapy. In: Mintz PD, ed. Transfusion therapy: Clinical principles and practice. 3rd ed. Bethesda, MD: AABB Press, 2011:209-63.
29. New HV, Standworth SJ, Engelfriet CP, et al. Neonatal transfusions. International Forum. Vox Sang 2009;96:62-85.
30. Carson TH, ed. Standards for blood banks and transfusion services. 27th ed. Bethesda, MD: AABB, 2011.
31. Strauss RG. Selection of white cell-reduced blood components for transfusions during infancy. Transfusion 1993;33:352-7.
32. Ludvigsen C, Swanson JL. Thompson TR, McCullough J. The failure of neonates to form red cell alloantibodies in response to multiple transfusions. Am J Clin Pathol 1987;87:250-1.
33. Josephson CD, Castillejo MI, Grima K, Hillyer CD. ABO-mismatched platelet transfusions: Strategies to mitigate patient exposure to naturally occurring hemolytic antibodies. Transfus Apher Sci 2010;42:83-8.
34. Strauss RG, Burmeister LF, Johnson K, et al. AS-1 red cells for neonatal transfusions: A randomized trial assessing donor exposure and safety. Transfusion 1996;36:873-8.

35. Wang-Rodriguez J, Mannino FL, Liu E, et al. A novel strategy to limit blood donor exposure and blood waste in multiply transfused premature infants. Transfusion 1996;36:64-70.
36. Liu EA, Mannino FL, Lane TA. Prospective randomized trial of the safety and efficacy of a limited donor exposure transfusion program for premature neonates. J Pediatr 1994;125:92-6.
37. Bednarek FJ, Weisberger S, Richardson DK, et al. Variations in blood transfusions among newborn intensive care units. J Pediatr 1998; 133:601-7.
38. Maier RF, Sonntag J, Walka MW, et al. Changing practices of red blood cell transfusions in infants with birth weights less than 1000 g. J Pediatr 2000;136:220-4.
39. Roseff SD. Pediatric blood collection and transfusion technology. In: Herman JK, Manno CS, eds. Pediatric transfusion therapy. Bethesda, MD: AABB Press, 2002:217-47.
40. Levy GJ, Strauss RG, Hume H, et al. National survey of neonatal transfusion practices, I: Red blood cell therapy. Pediatrics 1993;91:523-9.
41. Strauss RG, Burmeister LF, Johnson K, et al. Feasibility and safety of AS-3 red blood cells for neonatal transfusions. J Pediatr 2000;136: 215-19.
42. Goodstein MH, Herman JH, Smith JF, et al. Metabolic consequences in very low birth weight infants transfused with older AS-1 preserved erythrocytes. Pediatr Pathol Lab Med 1999;18:173-85.
43. Rock G, Poon A, Haddad R, et al. Nutricel as an additive solution for neonatal transfusion. Transfus Sci 1999;31:229-35.
44. Luban NLC, Strauss RG, Hume HA. Commentary on the safety of red cells preserved in extended-storage media for neonatal transfusions. Transfusion 1991;31:229-35.
45. Tuchschid P, Mieth D, Burger R, et al. Potential hazard of hypoalbuminemia in newborn babies after exchange transfusion with Adsol red blood cell concentrates (letter). Pediatrics 1990;85:234-5.
46. Brecher ME, ed. Collected questions and answers. 6th ed. Bethesda, MD: AABB, 2000:73-5.
47. Pridjian G. Fetomaternal interactions: Placental physiology, the in-utero environment, and fetal determinants of adult disease. In: MacDonald MG, Seshia MM, Mullett MD, eds. Avery's neonatology. Pathophysiology and management of the newborn. 6th ed. Philadelphia: Lippincott Williams & Wilkins, 2005:149-65.
48. Wong E, Roseff SD, eds. Pediatric transfusion data card. Bethesda, MD: AABB, 2009.
49. Kirpalani H, Whyte RK, Andersen C, et al. The Premature Infants in Need of Transfusion (PINT) study: A randomized, controlled trial of a restrictive (low) versus liberal (high) transfusion threshold for extremely low birth weight infants. J Pediatr 2006;149:301-7.
50. Whyte RK, Kirpalani H, Asztalos EV, et al. Neurodevelopmental outcome of extremely low birth weight infants randomly assigned to restrictive or liberal hemoglobin thresholds for blood transfusion. Pediatrics 2009;123:207-13.
51. Bell EF, Strauss RG, Widness JA, et al. Randomized trial of liberal versus restrictive guidelines for red blood cell transfusion in preterm infants. Pediatrics 2005;115:1685-91.
52. Behrman RE, Kleigman RM, Jenson HB, eds. Nelson's textbook of pediatrics. 16th ed. Philadelphia: WB Saunders, 2000.
53. Vales T. Bilirubin distribution and dynamics of bilirubin removal by exchange transfusion. Acta Paediatr Scand 1963;52S:149.
54. Koenig JM. Evaluation and treatment of erythroblastosis fetalis in the neonate. In: Christensen RD, ed. Hematologic problems of the neonate. Philadelphia: WB Saunders, 2000: 185-207.
55. Ballard RA, Vincour B, Reynolds JW, et al. Transient hyperammonemia of the preterm infant. N Engl J Med 1978;299:920-5.
56. Leonard JV. The early detection and management of inborn errors presenting acutely in the neonatal period. Eur J Pediatr 1985;143: 253-7.
57. Wong EC, Pisciotto PT. Technical considerations/mechanical devices. In: Hillyer CD, Strauss RG, Luban NLC, eds. Handbook of pediatric transfusion medicine. London, UK: Elsevier Academic Press, 2004:121-8.
58. Luban NLC. Massive transfusion in the neonate. Transfus Med Rev 1995;9:200-14.
59. Chan G, Schoff D. Variance in albumin loading in exchange transfusions. J Pediatr 1976;88: 609-13.
60. Bada HS, Chua C, Salmon JH, Hajjar W. Changes in intracranial pressure during exchange transfusion. J Pediatr 1979;94:129-32.
61. Blanchette VS, Kuhne T, Hume H, Hellman J. Platelet transfusion therapy in newborn infants. Transfus Med Rev 1995;9:215-30.

62. Andrew M, Vegh P, Caco C, et al. A randomized, controlled trial of platelet transfusions in thrombocytopenic premature infants. J Pediatr 1993;123:285-91.
63. Poterjoy BS, Josephson CD. Platelets, frozen plasma, cryoprecipitate: What is the clinical evidence for their use in the neonatal intensive care unit? Semin Perinatol 2009;33:66-74.
64. Josephson C, Su L, Christensen R, et al. Platelet transfusion practices among neonatologists in the United States and Canada: Results of a survey. Pediatrics 2009;123:278-85.
65. Strauss RG, Levy GJ, Sotelo-Avila C, et al. National survey of neonatal transfusion practices: II. Blood component therapy. Pediatrics 1993;91:530-6.
66. Pisciotto P, Snyder EL, Snyder JA, et al. In vitro characteristics of leukocyte-reduced single unit platelet concentrates stored in syringes. Transfusion 1994;34:407-11.
67. Andrew M, Paes B, Johnston M. Development of the hemostatic system in the neonate and young infant. Am J Pediatr Hematol Oncol 1990;12:95-104.
68. Andrew M. Transfusion in the newborn: Plasma products. In: Kennedy M, Wilson S, Kelton J, eds. Perinatal transfusion medicine. Arlington, VA: AABB, 1990:145-77.
69. Pressey JG, Manno CS. Therapy for hemophilia and von Willebrand disease. In: Herman JK, Manno CS, eds. Pediatric transfusion therapy. Bethesda, MD: AABB Press, 2002:355-82.
70. Vamvakas EC, Pineda AA. Meta-analysis of clinical studies of the efficacy of granulocyte transfusions in the treatment of bacterial sepsis. J Clin Apher 1996;11:1-9.
71. Price TH. The current prospects for neutrophil transfusion for the treatment of granulocytopenic infected patients. Transfus Med Rev 2000;14:2-11.
72. Cairo MS, Rucker R, Bennetts GA, et al. Improved survival of newborns receiving leukocyte transfusions for sepsis. Pediatrics 1984;74:887-92.
73. Cairo MS, Worcester CC, Rucker RW, et al. Randomized trial of granulocyte transfusions versus intravenous immune globulin therapy for neutropenia and sepsis. J Pediatr 1992;120:281-5.
74. Hubel K, Dale DC, Liles WC. Granulocyte transfusion therapy: Update on potential clinical applications. Curr Opin Hematol 2001;8:161-4.
75. Christensen RD, Bradley PP, Rothstein G. The leukocyte left shift in clinical and experimental neonatal sepsis. J Pediatr 1981;98:101-5.
76. Sweetman RW, Cairo MS. Blood component and immunotherapy in neonatal sepsis. Transfus Med Rev 1995;9:251-8.
77. Rosenthal J, Cairo MS. Neonatal myelopoiesis and immunomodulation of host defenses. In: Petz LD, Swisher SN, Kleinman S, et al, eds. Clinical practice of transfusion medicine. 3rd ed. New York: Churchill Livingstone, 1996:685-703.
78. Jenson HB, Pollack BH. The role of intravenous immunoglobulins for the prevention and treatment of neonatal sepsis. Semin Perinatol 1998;22:50-63.
79. Sandberg K, Fasth A, Berger A, et al. Preterm infants with low immunoglobulin G levels have increased risk of neonatal sepsis but do not benefit from prophylactic immunoglobulin G. J Pediatr 2000;137:623-8.
80. Hill HR. Additional confirmation of the lack of effect of intravenous immunoglobulin in prevention of neonatal infection (editorial). J Pediatr 2000;137:595-7.
81. Ehrenkranz RA. The newborn intensive care unit. In: Oski FA, ed. Principles and practice of pediatrics. 2nd ed. Philadelphia: JB Lippincott, 1994;19:322.
82. Burch KJ, Phelps SJ, Constance TD. Effect of an infusion device on the integrity of whole blood and packed red blood cells. Am J Hosp Pharm 1991;48:92-7.
83. Criss VR, DePalma L, Luban NLC. Analysis of a linear peristaltic infusion device for the transfusion of red cells to pediatric patients. Transfusion 1993;33:842-4.
84. Longhurst DM, Gooch W, Castillo RA. In vitro evaluation of a pediatric microaggregate blood filter. Transfusion 1983;23:170-2.
85. Lindemann R, Haga P. Evaluation and treatment of polycythemia in the neonate. In: Christiansen RD, ed. Hematologic problems of the neonate. Philadelphia: WB Saunders, 2000:171-83.
86. Black VD, Rumack CM, Lubchenko LD, Koops BL. Gastrointestinal injury in polycythemic infants. Pediatrics 1985;76:225-31.
87. Kevy SV. Extracorporeal therapy for infants and children. In: Petz LD, Swisher SN, Kleinman S, et al, eds. Clinical practice of transfusion medicine. 3rd ed. New York: Churchill Livingstone, 1996:733-55.

88. Bartlett RH, Andrews AF, Toomasian JM, et al. Extracorporeal membrane oxygenation for newborn respiratory failure: Forty-five cases. Surgery 1982;92:425-33.
89. Friedman DF, Montenegro LM. Extracorporeal membrane oxygenation and cardiopulmonary bypass. In: Hillyer CD, Strauss RG, Luban NLC. Handbook of pediatric transfusion medicine. London, UK: Elsevier Academic Press, 2004;17: 181-9.
90. Sharon BI. Management of congenital hemolytic anemias. In: Simon TL, Snyder ES, Solheim BG, et al, eds. Rossi's principles of transfusion medicine. 4th ed. Bethesda, MD: AABB Press, 2009:448-69.
91. Cohen AR, Norris CF, Smith-Whitley K. Transfusion therapy for sickle cell disease. In: Capon SM, Chambers LA, eds. New directions in pediatric hematology. Bethesda, MD: AABB, 1996:39-88.
92. Adams DM, Schultz WH, Ware RE, Kinney TR. Erythrocytapheresis can reduce iron overload and prevent the need for chelation therapy in chronically transfused pediatric patients. J Pediatr Hematol Oncol 1996;18:3-7.
93. Adams RJ, McKie VC, Hsu L, et al. Prevention of a first stroke by transfusions in children with sickle cell anemia and abnormal results on transcranial Doppler ultrasonography. N Engl J Med 1998;339:5-11.
94. Rosse WF, Gallagher D, Kinney TR, et al. Transfusion and alloimmunization in sickle cell disease. Blood 1990;76:1431-7.
95. Spanos T, Karageorge M, Ladis V, et al. Red cell alloantibodies in patients with thalassemia. Vox Sang 1990;58:50-5.
96. Rosse WF, Telen M, Ware RE. Transfusion support for patients with sickle cell disease. Bethesda, MD: AABB Press, 1998.
97. Smith-Whitley K. Alloimmunization in patients with sickle cell disease. In: Herman JK, Manno CS, eds. Pediatric transfusion therapy. Bethesda, MD: AABB Press, 2002:240-82.
98. Hillyer KL, Hare VW, Josephson CD, et al. Partners for Life: The transfusion program for patients with sickle cell disease. Immunohematol 2006;22:108-11.
99. Afenyi-Annan A, Brecher ME. Pre-transfusion phenotype matching for sickle cell disease patients (letter). Transfusion 2004;44:619-20.
100. Tahan HR, Holbrook CT, Braddy LR, et al. Antigen-matched donor blood in the transfusion management of patients with sickle cell disease. Transfusion 1994;34:562-9.
101. McPherson M, Anderson AR, Haight AE, et al. Transfusion management of HLA-matched sibling bone marrow transplant (BMT) recipients with sickle cell disease (SCD). Transfusion 2009;49:1977-86.
102. Friedman DF, Lukas MB, Jawad A, et al. Alloimmunization to platelets in heavily transfused patients with sickle cell disease. Blood 1996; 88:3216-22.
103. Lane TA, Anderson KC, Goodnough LT, et al. Leukocyte reduction in blood component therapy. Ann Intern Med 1992;117:151-62.
104. Blumberg N, Heal JM, Gettings KF. Leukoreduction of red cell transfusions is associated with a decreased incidence of red cell alloimmunization. Transfusion 2003;43:945-52.
105. Van de Watering L, Jermans J, Witvliet M, et al. HLA and RBC immunization after filtered and buffy coat-dependent blood transfusion in cardiac surgery: A randomized controlled trial. Transfusion 2003;43:765-71.
106. McPherson M, Anderson A, Castillejo MI, et al. HLA alloimmunization is associated with RBC antibodies in multiply transfused patients with sickle cell disease. Pediatr Blood Cancer 2010;54:552-8.
107. Petz LD, Calhoun L, Shulman IA, et al. The sickle cell hemolytic transfusion reaction syndrome. Transfusion 1997;37:382-8.
108. Win N, Doughty H, Telfer P, et al. Hyperhemolytic transfusion reaction in sickle cell disease. Transfusion 2001;41:323-8.
109. Garratty G. Autoantibodies induced by blood transfusion (editorial). Transfusion 2004;44:5-9.
110. Hoffbrand AV, Al-Refaie F, Davis B, et al. Long-term trial of deferiprone in 51 transfusion-dependent iron overload patients. Blood 1998; 91:295-300.
111. Oliveri NF, Brittenham GM. Iron-chelating therapy and the treatment of thalassemia. Blood 1997;89:739-61.
112. Larsson LG, Welsh VJ, Ladd DJ. Acute intravascular hemolysis secondary to out-of-group platelet transfusion. Transfusion 2000;40:902-6.
113. Heal JM, Blumberg N. The second century of ABO: And now for something completely different. Transfusion 1999;39:1155-9.

114. Blumberg N, Heal JM, Hicks GL, Risher WH. Association of ABO-mismatch platelet transfusions with morbidity and mortality in cardiac surgery. Transfusion 2001;41:790-3.
115. Bowden RA, Slichter SJ, Sayers M, et al. A comparison of filtered leukocyte-reduced and cytomegalovirus (CMV) seronegative blood products for the prevention of transfusion-associated CMV infection after marrow transplant. Blood 1995;86:3598-603.
116. Mussi-Pinhata MM, Yamamoto AY, Rego MAC, et al. Perinatal or early-postnatal cytomegalovirus infection in preterm infants under 34 weeks gestation born to CMV-seropositive mothers within a high-seroprevalence population. J Pediatr 2004;145:685-8.
117. Bradley MT, Milam JD, Anderson DC. Use of deglycerolized red blood cells to prevent post-transfusion infection with cytomegalovirus in neonates. J Infect Dis 1984;150:334-9.
118. Gilbert GL, Hayes K, Hudson H, et al. Prevention of transfusion-associated cytomegalovirus infection in infants by blood filtration to remove leukocytes. Lancet 1989;i:1228-31.
119. Adler SP, Chandrika T, Lawrence L, Baggett J. Cytomegalovirus infections in neonates acquired by blood transfusions. Pediatr Infect Dis 1983;2:114-18.
120. Strauss RG. Selection of white cell-reduced blood components for transfusions during early infancy. Transfusion 1993;33:352-7.
121. Fergusson D, Hebert PC, Lee SK, et al. Clinical outcomes following institution of universal leukoreduction of blood transfu-sions in premature infants. JAMA 2003;289:1950-6.
122. Moroff G, Friedman A, Robkin-Kline L, et al. Reduction of the volume of stored platelet concentrates for use in neonatal patients. Transfusion 1984;24:144-6.

Chapter 24

Patient Blood Management

Jonathan H. Waters, MD

FOR MANY HOSPITAL laboratories, the largest budgetary cost is that of providing blood components. As these costs escalate, many hospitals are looking for ways of better handling their blood supply. Methods developed with such an outlook have been termed "blood management," now referred to as "patient blood management" (PBM), which can take many forms, from monitoring of crossmatch-to-transfusion ratios to the development of preoperative anemia management centers. It is important to differentiate PBM from "bloodless medicine." Bloodless medicine specifically addresses patients for whom blood transfusion is not an option. For the majority of these patients, transfusion is not an option because of religious objections adopted by the Jehovah's Witnesses, who refuse all major blood components. Those who practice bloodless medicine have been able to gain significant experience in managing patients without blood and have been able to transfer much of this knowledge to the general population. For patients who will accept blood, transfusion is an option, but one that is widely used inappropriately and can easily be contained either with improved outcome or without any detrimental effects to the patient. Another potential benefit in addition to better patient outcomes is reduction in hospital expenditures.

BEHAVIORAL CHANGES

Several behavioral changes in hospital care can result in significant reductions of blood usage, including adoption of a systematic transfusion algorithm or guide, administration of single-unit transfusions, and reduction of blood draws by eliminating those that are merely routine.

Transfusion Thresholds

The term "transfusion trigger" is a misnomer. The decision to transfuse has long been one of the most complex medical decisions, and reliance on a single number (usually generated by a laboratory) strips this decision of its stature. Many guidelines for red cell transfusion have been recommended by a number of organizations, including the National Institutes of Health,[1] American College of Physicians,[2] American College of Critical Care Medicine,[3]

Jonathan H. Waters, MD, Chief of Anesthesia Services, Magee-Womens Hospital, University of Pittsburgh Medical Center, and Medical Director, Perioperative Blood Management Program, University of Pittsburgh Health Systems, Pittsburgh, Pennsylvania

The author has disclosed no conflicts of interest.

and the American Society of Anesthesiologists.[4] In general, these guidelines are consistent across organizations and typically state that a red cell transfusion might be indicated when a patient's hemoglobin drops below 6.0 g/dL if the patient has no cardiopulmonary disease and has mechanisms of increasing heart rate and oxygen extraction to compensate for anemia. In patients who have cardiopulmonary disease, a higher threshold of 10 g/dL has been suggested. Since development of these guidelines, results of the Transfusion Requirements in Critical Care trials have been published and suggest that even some critically ill patients have better outcomes when a restrictive transfusion approach is applied.[5]

Auditing

It has been recommended that selective auditing of compliance with hospital-developed transfusion guidelines be performed; however, the success of behavioral change through such auditing is questionable.[6] Auditing can be performed in a retrospective or prospective fashion. In a prospective audit, barriers (by computer at the time of the transfusion order, or manual barriers before issue) can be placed to limit the administration of components outside the recommended guidelines. Retrospective audits review charts after the administration has taken place, evaluating compliance to the recommended guidelines. With the retrospective audit, transfusions are frequently vigorously defended by the treating clinician because of circumstances not reflected by a chart audit. Chapter 28 discusses blood utilization auditing in detail.

Single-Unit Transfusions

For decades, students and resident physicians have been taught to transfuse units of Red Blood Cells (RBCs) in groups of two, although the rationale behind this practice is unclear. A unit of blood has varying effects on measured parameters, depending on the size of the patient's blood volume as well as dynamic changes of the blood volume related to anesthesia and shifts in fluid between fluid compartments. For these reasons, transfusion practice may overshoot recommended guides. Many have advocated a paradigm shift away from duplicate transfusion to teach single-unit transfusion with assessment of patient hemoglobin and cardiorespiratory status between each unit.

Benchmarking

A powerful tool for behavioral modification is the creation of benchmarks for transfusion based on the type of surgical procedure. In many surgical procedures, significant variation exists in transfusion behavior across hospitals as well as among surgeons. By determining an average blood use statistic and publicizing the average for a specific diagnosis-related group (DRG), the competitive nature of surgeons can be harnessed to reduce blood usage. All surgeons who perform a specific procedure should be compared and averaged, and the results should be distributed to each of them. Frequent objections to this benchmarking will occur because of a perception that different surgeons perform surgery at different levels of difficulty and patient morbidity. Adjustments can be made for this consideration by using all-patient-refined DRGs or by applying similar risk adjustment tools. To date, published data from multiple US hospitals attest that transfusion in cardiac surgery can be reduced with little effect on outcome, emphasizing that many transfusions are inappropriate.[7]

Quality Assurance Measurement

Occasionally in the course of managing a surgical patient in the postoperative period, there is unexpected profound blood loss. Laboratory tests that point to a surgical cause of bleeding are frequently ignored. Generally, these patients are treated with multiple rounds of blood products with the hope that the bleeding will stop. Ultimately, it may be recognized that the bleeding does not stop on its own and that the patient needs to be taken back to the operating room for management of an unrecognized arterial or venous hemorrhage. This behavior of denying the need for returning the patient to the operating room is fostered through a surgical quality assurance measure for "operating room take-backs," which discourages the surgeon from returning a patient to the operating room. Better quality assurance measures such as a low threshold for take-backs should also include monitoring of blood utilization by DRG.

Blood Draws as Needed

All blood draws should have a specific reason, which implies that care would change based on results, rather than the draw being treated as a routine screen. Therefore, a change that should be adopted is the cessation of routine daily blood draws. It has been well documented that intensive care patients lose approximately 1 to 2 units of red cells per week from routine draws.[8] Blood should be drawn as needed, when justified, and the least amount of blood possible should be removed.[9] Transition to this practice can be aided through the use of many point-of-care laboratory testing devices, which provide laboratory data with blood samples as small as 10 µL. With samples this small, useful patient management information can be obtained without creating iatrogenic anemia.

In addition to the blood sample size and the frequency of the draws, the process of drawing the blood can often be a cause of lost blood. When using an arterial line or central line as the source of a blood sample, approximately 10 mL of blood is drawn from the line before the actual sample is taken. This practice is performed to prevent the laboratory sample from being diluted by flush solution in the arterial or central line system. The 10 mL of blood is subsequently discarded. During some intensive care unit (ICU) stays, blood draws can take place every hour. With 10 mL being lost with each blood draw, sizeable volume losses occur in a short period. To remedy this loss, devices are available (eg, VAMP System, Edwards Lifesciences, Irvine, CA) that allow for this 10 mL to be drawn into a closed, sterile system so that it can be reinjected once the undiluted blood sample is obtained.

PREOPERATIVE ANEMIA MANAGEMENT

The prevalence of preoperative anemia is surprisingly high. Depending on the comorbidity, it is found in 5% to 75% of elective surgical patients.[10,11] Preoperative anemia is the most important predictor of perioperative transfusion.[12,13] Historically, this anemia has often been ignored, and surgery has proceeded with allogeneic transfusion as needed. This may be perceived as the least labor-intensive option for managing these patients, but it is not the option that most patients would choose for themselves. Patients presenting for elective surgical procedures that are expected to result in significant blood loss should have their hemoglobin checked; if anemia is detected, an internist should follow up.[14] In many menstruating women, the source of the anemia is related to chronic iron deficiency. In others, an occult gastrointestinal malignancy might be present. A patient scheduled for an elective hip replacement, for example, is better served to have an occult malignancy detected and treated. Thus, the mechanism of the anemia is best elucidated and treated appropriately before any elective surgery.

The use of recombinant erythropoietin has been advocated for correcting a patient's low hemoglobin (anemia) before a surgical procedure where major blood loss is anticipated, but it should be administered with caution. Increasing rates of thromboembolic events have been seen in patients who received recombinant erythropoietin. Such thromboembolic events have been detected in studies of patients using this agent for chronic renal insufficiency or patients receiving chemotherapy for malignancy.[15] The Food and Drug Administration (FDA) has recently warned that agents such as recombinant erythropoietin should be used at the lowest possible dosage and the shortest duration, especially in cancer populations.

Because the majority of preoperative anemia is related to iron deficiency, simple iron replacement is indicated. The rate at which iron supplementation replenishes the red cell mass can be enhanced through intravenous administration. Iron delivered with iron dextran has been associated with high rates of anaphylaxis, so other forms of intravenous iron are typically advocated (see Table 24-1).[16]

PERIOPERATIVE AUTOTRANSFUSION PROGRAM

The intraoperative environment offers the greatest opportunities for blood use reduction. In general, use of a single technique is not as effective as multiple strategies used together.[17] Numerous techniques and devices are available for reducing the loss of blood during surgical procedures (see Table 24-2). In addition to devices available to the surgeon, a vast array of topical hemostatic agents is available to reduce localized blood loss (see Table 24-3). Through attention to these options, blood transfusion can often become unnecessary.

In some procedures, major blood loss is inevitable. (A list of procedures where major blood loss can be anticipated is provided in Table 24-4.) Nonetheless, several strategies can present alternatives to red cell, platelet, and plasma transfusion. Quality control approaches to perioperative transfusion are not yet as well developed as for other aspects of transfusion medicine. Current AABB requirements are described in the *Standards for Perioperative Autologous Blood Collection and Administration*[31]; also, the AABB *Guidelines for Blood Management and Utilization* and *Guidelines for Blood Recovery and Reinfusion in Surgery and Trauma* reflect recent developments.[32,33] Quality requirements will almost certainly be expanded in the future.

Alternatives to Red Cell Transfusion

Preoperative Autologous Donation

Historically, the primary technique used to reduce red cell transfusion was preoperative autologous donation (PAD). In this technique, the patient donates blood several weeks before the operative procedure. Conceptually, the technique may seem sound, but patients who donate preoperatively without receiving recombinant erythropoietin are often unable to rebuild their red cell mass before surgery and are more likely to receive a transfusion during the perioperative course.[34]

Intraoperative blood loss is unpredictable, and half of the PAD units are typically discarded. Such donation without subsequent use presents a sizeable waste of resources for many hospitals. As a result, many hospitals discourage this technique.[35]

Blood Recovery

As an alternative to PAD, blood recovery can be offered. Simply put, blood recovery is the collection and reinfusion of shed blood. Shed blood can be readministered after concentrat-

TABLE 24-1. Available Intravenous Iron Formulations

Iron Formulation	Brand Name	Elemental Iron per Ampule	Test Dose?	FDA Warnings	Anaphylactic Reactions?
Sodium ferric gluconate	Ferrlecit*	62.5 mg	No	General†	No
Iron sucrose	Venofer‡	100 mg	No	Bolded§	No
Iron dextran	INFeD* Dexferrum‡	50 mg	Yes	Black box‖	Yes

*Sanofi Aventis, Bridgewater, NJ

†Routine warnings (see full prescribing information for warning, precautions and adverse reactions).

‡American Regent, Shirley, NY.

§A particular side effect has been bolded in the *Circular of Information* to indicate a severe reaction.

‖The most significant of the FDA warnings is surrounded by a black box.

TABLE 24-2. Surgical Techniques for Minimizing Blood Loss

Method/Device	Product Name and/or Manufacturer	Method of Action	Function
Ultrasonic surgical aspirator	CUSA EXcel system (Integra LifeSciences, Plainsboro, NJ)	Two rupturing effects at the tissue interface: 1) Tip forces impacted tissue to vibrate, accelerate, and decelerate 2) Tip produces localized pressure waves that cause vapor pockets around cells	Tissue fragmentation, leaving intact vessels and portal ducts
Water jet	Multiple manufacturers	High-pressure pump transfers energy to a liquid jet	Jet-cutting of parenchymal tissue
Staplers	Multiple manufacturers	Metal staple across tissue surface	Division of major veins
Electrosurgical devices	Multiple manufacturers	Converts standard electrical current frequency of 60 cycles per second to 300,000 cycles per second with a variety of waveforms and tissue effects	To cut, coagulate, or vaporize tissue
Bovie electrocautery	Multiple manufacturers	High-power electrocautery	To score tissue and seal off small blood vessels (1-2 mm)
Radio frequency electrosurgery	Tissue Link (Tissue Link Medical, Denver, CO)	Radio frequency electrical energy with a low irrigation of saline to conduct energy	To seal structures up to 6 mm
Bipolar vessel sealing device	LigaSure (Tyco), Valleylab (Boulder, CO)	High-current, low-voltage output	To seal vessels up to 7 mm
Argon beam coagulator	ConMed Corp. (Utica, NY)	Conduction of high-frequency current to target tissue via a plasma arc	To limit or stop bleeding from large open surfaces
Ultrasonic shear devices	Ethicon Endo-Surgery [(division of Johnson & Johnson) New Brunswick, NJ]	Coaptive coagulation at low temperatures ranging from 50 to 100 C	To seal vessels up to 6 mm

TABLE 24-3. Absorbable Hemostatic Agents

Topical Agent	Manufacturer	Composition
Avitene	Davol (Cranston, RI)	Microfibrillar bovine collagen
FloSeal	Baxter (Deerfield, IL)	Flowable bovine gelatin matrix and thrombin
Gelfoam	Pfizer (New York, NY)	Porcine gelatin sponge
Helistat	Integra LifeSciences (Plainsboro, NJ)	Bovine collagen sponge
Helitene	Integra NeuroSciences (Andover, United Kingdom)	Bovine deep tendon collagen
Instat	Ethicon Biosurgery, a division of Johnson & Johnson (Somerville, NJ)	Bovine dermal collagen
Surgicel	Ethicon Biosurgery, a division of Johnson & Johnson (Somerville, NJ)	Oxidized regenerated cellulose
Surgifoam	Ethicon Biosurgery, a division of Johnson & Johnson (Somerville, NJ)	Porcine gelatin sponge
Vitagel	Orthovita (Malvern, PA)	Flowable bovine collagen and thrombin

ing and washing (washed recovered blood) with a blood recovery device, or it can be filtered and readministered (unwashed recovered blood). Unwashed recovered blood is usually reserved for the postoperative environment, where small quantities of blood are collected and reinfused.

With washed recovered blood, the economic impact can be controlled, making it a desirable alternative to PAD and erythropoietin. Collection of shed blood can take place in anticipation of major blood loss. Collection of the shed blood requires an anticoagulant, a sterile suction line, and a collection reservoir—together termed a "standby" setup. These three parts typically cost around US$50. If the blood loss is large, a centrifugation system can be implemented for processing and washing. The processing system adds approximately US$100 of additional cost as well as technician time for processing. Another economic advantage to blood recovery is that once the cost of disposables has been expended, units of blood can be repetitively produced with little additional cost.[36] This emphasizes the need to adequately strategize the use of blood recovery in procedures where the chance of needing transfusion is realistic. The need is variable from hospital to hospital and depends on the surgeon and, to some extent, the anesthetic technique.[37]

To maximize red cell capture and return, several management steps need to be taken. For instance, blood from the surgical field should be suctioned with the lowest negative pressure tolerated by the surgeon.[38] High pressures subject the red cells to significant mechanical forces, thus destroying them. In addition, suctioning of blood from pools is preferred to skimming of blood. Skimming or

TABLE 24-4. Surgical Procedures Where Large Blood Loss Can Be Anticipated

Type of Surgery	Procedures
Cardiac[18-21]	Valve replacement Coronary artery bypass grafting
Orthopedic[22,23]	Bilateral knee replacements Hip replacement revision Hemipelvectomy Major spine surgery (including anterior/posterior fusion, scoliosis/congenital surgery, tumor decompression, and infection debridement/fusion)
Urology	Radical retropubic prostatectomy (blood loss varies, depending on surgical skill) Cystectomy (limited to patients with prior radiation therapy to the pelvis) Nephrectomy with inferior vena cava thrombus
Cranial neurosurgery	Giant (>3 cm) and basilar aneurysm resection Arteriovenous malformations (must be complex type, ie, deep and extensive)
Vascular[24-27]	Thoraco-abdominal aneurysm repair Ruptured aortic aneurysm repair
Transplant[28,29]	Liver transplantation
Pregnancy-related	Ectopic pregnancy Cesarean section with placenta accreta/percreta/increta
Pediatric	Craniosynostosis repair[30]

suctioning small quantities of blood from a surface creates a blood:air interface, which further damages the red cells.

Another practice that can optimize red cell return is rinsing the sponges used to wipe blood from the surgical field.[39] On average, a fully soaked laparotomy sponge contains 100 mL of red cells. By taking these sponges and rinsing them in a basin of saline solution, approximately 75% of these cells can be harvested. Care must be taken to avoid mechanical hemolysis of the red cells. When the saline solution is grossly bloody, the surgical technician can suction the solution into the blood recovery system for processing.

Blood recovery should be implemented in adherence to the AABB perioperative blood management and transfusion standards.[31] Failure to do so could place the patient in significant jeopardy. Blood recovery has been associated with fatal air embolism[40] and the cell salvage syndrome.[41] An air embolus can occur when the blood recovery system's primary reinfusion bag is connected directly to the patient's intravenous line. Frequently, the reinfusion bag is pressurized to speed blood administration. Over time, the reinfusion bag will fill with air, which is undetectable with a pressure bag covering. To avoid this problem, blood should be dropped into a secondary administration bag, with the air expelled back into the primary system. The secondary administration bag can then be given to the anesthesia provider in the same way that a unit of allogeneic blood would be provided.

The cell salvage syndrome generally results from multiple factors. Probably the most common problem is suctioning the blood with high negative pressures, causing high levels of hemolysis, which can confuse the electronic eye in the blood recovery system. The electronic eye senses when the processing bowl is full. If it prematurely senses a "full" bowl, a partial bowl is washed, resulting in inadequate washout of particulate contaminates.[42] Readministration of large quantities of partial bowls can lead to coagulopathy.

Placing the circulating nurse in charge of the blood recovery equipment can also lead to the cell salvage syndrome. The nurse is busiest when the blood loss is greatest; thus, processing takes place when it is convenient (ie, when the nurse is passing by the machine while performing another task). As a result, processing occurs unobserved. If high suction pressures have been used, significant hemolysis can occur and free hemoglobin and red cell stroma remains in the finished product. For this reason, washing should always be closely observed for adequate washout of these products. This is easily accomplished by observing the color of the effluent waste line. When the effluent is as clear as the wash solution, the technician can assume that adequate washing has occurred. Reliance on a specific wash volume is frequently inadequate for sufficient removal of contaminants.

Many contraindications to the use of blood recovery systems have been described (see Table 24-5). Unfortunately, many of these contraindications are not based on the true risks presented by the procedure. The primary areas where blood recovery can result in significant reduction in blood use are in obstetrics and in surgery for malignancy. Several investigators have described the safe application of blood recovery in these areas.[43] Some have advocated the use of a leukocyte-reduction filter in conjunction with washing to remove cellular contaminants that might be present in these two environments.[44,45]

TABLE 24-5. Commonly Listed Contraindications for Blood Recovery

Pharmacologic agents
Clotting agents (Avitene,* Surgicel,† Gelfoam,‡ etc)
Irrigating solutions (Betadine,§ antibiotics meant for topical use)
Oxymetazoline (Afrin‖)
Epinephrine
Methylmethacrylate
Contaminants
Urine
Bone chips
Fat
Bowel contents
Infection
Amniotic fluid
Malignancy
Hematologic disorders
Sickle cell disease
Thalassemia
Miscellaneous
Carbon monoxide (electrocautery smoke)
Catecholamines (pheochromocytoma)

*C.R. Bard, Murray Hill, NJ.
†Ethicon Biosurgery, Somerville, NJ.
‡Pfizer, New York, NY.
§Purdue Pharma, Cranbury, NJ.
‖Schering-Plough HealthCare Products, Kenilworth, NJ.

Normovolemic Hemodilution

Acute normovolemic hemodilution (ANH) involves removal of whole blood just before the start of surgery so that blood shed during surgery has a lower concentration of red cells. The harvested whole blood is then returned upon completion of surgery. The technique has been compared with PAD but involves use of fresh autologous whole blood vs banked autologous blood. Patients undergoing ANH are monitored minute to minute, in contrast to PAD patients. ANH is associated with significantly reduced cost.[46-48] In addition, mathematical models have shown that hemodilution can help limit red cell use.[49,50]

Technically, hemodilution requires the removal of whole blood followed by infusion of colloid, crystalloid, or both to maintain blood volume and adequate perfusion. Oxygen delivery is maintained through increases in tissue oxygen extraction, increases in cardiac output, and decreased blood viscosity. As with single-unit donation, adequate access is necessary to harvest the blood. Ideally, a large central line such as a 9 Fr introducer should be used. Multilumen central-line catheters are generally inadequate because of the gauge of the lumen and the length of the catheter. It is better to use large-bore catheters where blood flow is rapid. Alternative sites for blood harvest are an arterial line or a large-gauge peripheral intravenous catheter. With an arterial line, the blood removal should take place at the hub of the catheter rather than downstream at the arterial line stopcock. Like the multilumen central line, long tubing slows the blood flow. A peripheral catheter can also be used. Ideally, this would take placc through a 14-gauge catheter.

The recommended degree of hemodilution is controversial. Some physicians remove blood to a hemoglobin level of 6 g/dL, whereas others are concerned with putting patients at risk for ischemic events and limit their dilution to much higher hemoglobin concentrations. To achieve a drop in hemoglobin level from 15 g/dL to 6 g/dL in a normal 70-kg individual requires a significant blood harvest.

Alternatives to Platelet and Plasma Transfusion

Normovolemic Hemodilution

An added benefit of ANH is that the whole blood that is removed contains plasma and functional platelets. Approximately 1 liter of whole blood contains enough plasma and platelets to correct even a severe coagulation defect. It is important to readminister this blood at the end of the surgical procedure rather than at the point of coagulation abnormality if the goal is to avoid allogeneic transfusion. If hemodilution is combined with blood recovery, hemoglobin concentrations can be maintained with blood recovery. Microvascular oozing can be tolerated until wound closure, at which time the presurgically removed blood is returned.

Plasma and Platelet Sequestration

ANH can be modified so that the whole blood that is removed is fractionated into its components. In essence, the patient can be used as his or her own blood bank. This fractionation can be performed with standard blood recovery equipment. The fractionation can take place through either a direct draw or an indirect draw technique.

In the direct draw, the blood is removed from a large central line and is transferred directly into the centrifugation bowl. During this technique, the blood flow is typically at the rate of 100 mL/minute. The autotransfusionist needs to keep in close contact with the anesthesia provider when performing this technique. At this flow rate, significant hypovolemia can occur rapidly. Some operating rooms are equipped with satellite monitors that can allow the autotransfusionist to directly monitor the effect of the blood removal. In addition to maintaining hemodynamic stability, it is critical to maintain adequate anticoagulation of the blood as it is being removed.

In an indirect draw technique, blood is drawn from the patient in single units and placed into a standard citrated donor bag. After the blood has been collected, it is disconnected from the patient and moved to the blood recovery machine for fractionation.

When performing intraoperative component sequestration, it is important to collect sufficient platelets and plasma to adequately correct platelet or factor deficiencies. Studies of this technique have shown no reduction of allogeneic blood transfusion when less than 4 units of platelets have been collected (see Table 24-6). Stated in other terms, approximately 1 unit should be collected for every 20 kg of body weight.

Adjunctive Techniques

Deliberate Hypotension

The reduction of blood pressure through pharmacologic means can reduce blood loss by reducing the driving pressure in the patient's system. In general, a mean arterial pressure of 50 mm Hg is desired. This pressure is thought to be on the low end of brain autoregulation. Deliberate hypotension can be achieved through a number of different agents, ranging

TABLE 24-6. Studies Comparing Yields from Plateletpheresis

Author	Outcome	Platelet Yield	
		Units	Kg/Unit
Noon et al[51]	+	9.8	7
Davies et al[52]	+	7.0	11
Christenson et al[53]	+	7.0	#
Wajon et al[54]	–	6.4	12
Al-Rashidi et al[55]	+	6.0	15
Stover et al[56]	+	5.6	14
Hiramatsu et al[57]	+	5.2	#
Harke et al[58]	+	5.0	13
Jones et al[59]	+	5.0	14
Boldt et al[60]	+	4.8	16
Ford et al[61]	–	4.5	#
Boldt et al[62]	+	3.9	20
Tobe et al[63]	–	3.6	29
Armellin et al[64]	+	3.4	20
Giordano et al[65,66]	+	3.0	23
Ferrari et al[67]	+ / –	2.9	28
Triulzi et al[68]	–	2.8	30
Ereth et al[69]	–	2.7	29
Wong et al[70]	–	2.5	33
Shore-Lesserson et al[71]	–	2.4	29
Boey et al[72]	–	0.6	110

+ = significant reduction of allogeneic transfusion occurred; – = no significant allogeneic reduction occurred; # = no weight was reported.

from nitroprusside to inhalational anesthetic agents.

Positioning

In spinal surgery, placing pressure on the abdominal contents will obstruct inferior vena cava blood flow. As a result, venous return to the heart takes an alternative route through the epidural venous plexus, making these veins engorged and prone to bleed.[73] Thus, the abdomen should be padded in such a fashion that it is not under pressure. Certain spinal tables will allow for the abdomen to hang freely.

Temperature Regulation

As body temperature falls, various aspects of coagulation function decline. As temperature drops below 34 C, the partial thromboplastin time (PTT) increases linearly with further decreases in temperature.[74] Likewise, platelet function declines below 33 C.[75] Therefore, efforts to maintain body temperature are imper-

TABLE 24-7. Pharmacologic Therapies to Assist Coagulation Function

Drug	Brand Name	Mechanism of Action	Suggested Dose
Aminocaproic acid	Amicar (Xanodyne, Newport, KY)	Inhibits the proteolytic activity of plasmin	5 g bolus followed by 1 g/hour infusion
Desmopressin	DDAVP (Sanofi-Aventis, Bridge-water, NJ)	Increases Factor VIII release	0.3 µg/kg
Recombinant Factor VIIa*	Novoseven (Novo Nordisk, Princeton, NJ)	Activates coagulation cascade	Approximately 50-100 µg/kg†
Tranexamic acid	Cyklokapron (Pfizer, New York, NY)	Inhibits the proteolytic activity of plasmin	10 mL/kg every 6-8 hours

*The use of recombinant Factor VIIa is considered by some to be controversial for this indication.
†Inadequate outcome data to determine effective dose in surgical patients.

ative. This is achieved through forced-air warmers, warming of intravenous fluids before infusion, and maintaining warmth of the patient's extremities before entering the operating room.

Acidosis

Like temperature, deviation from homeostasis leads to coagulation dysfunction. As pH falls, Factor Xa/Va complex decreases the speed of Factor IIa conversion.[76] Acidosis can arise from multiple sources. For example, it can occur from hypovolemia and hypotension with a resulting lactic acidosis. A less commonly recognized mechanism is excessive normal saline administration. Normal saline creates a hyperchloremic metabolic acidosis because of high chloride load.[77]

Point-of-Care Monitoring

Point-of-care testing involves coagulation monitoring at the patient's bedside. When blood is sent to a central laboratory, any delay in getting results impairs rational blood component usage. By placing coagulation monitoring devices at the bedside, quantitative information can be used to make transfusion decisions.[78] Platelet function monitoring today is often assessed through viscoelastometry [thromboelastography, with Sonoclot (Sienco, Arvada, CO)].[79] Prothrombin time and PTT monitoring can be performed with an I-stat monitor (Abbott Laboratories, Abbott Park, IL). Both of these devices allow for monitoring with microliter samples, thus obviating blood loss through blood testing.

Drug Therapies

Several drugs have been advocated to assist in coagulation during surgery (see Table 24-7).[80] These drugs include tranexamic acid, aminocaproic acid, recombinant Factor VIIa, and desmopressin. Outcome reports on the use of these drugs present controversy about the efficacy of the drugs in slowing hemorrhage and about resultant complications (eg, thromboembolic events or renal failure). Many studies comparing use of these drugs have outcomes that may have been influenced by drug company sponsorship and/or investigator bias.

ACKNOWLEDGMENT

The author would like to acknowledge the contribution of Aryeh Shander, MD, for proof reading and assistance with wording in several sections of this chapter.

KEY POINTS

1. Behavioral change in the health-care team can result in significant reduction of blood usage. Such change should incorporate adoption of evidence-based transfusion thresholds, single-unit transfusions, and a reduction in daily blood draws.
2. Comparing blood use by provider across high-volume surgical procedures can be a powerful tool in behavioral modification.
3. Preoperative anemia is the greatest predictor for whether a patient will be transfused during a surgical procedure. Identifying patients who are anemic before surgery and optimizing their hemoglobin can be a useful approach for reducing allogeneic use.
4. Intraoperative blood recovery can be effective during high blood loss procedures; however, it can lead to patient injury if misapplied. For this reason, the adoption of a quality program should be undertaken that prescribes safe practices.
5. Intraoperative blood recovery is a more cost-effective alternative to providing autologous blood for a patient when compared to preoperative autologous donation.
6. Normovolemic hemodilution is similar to preoperative autologous donation, but it is performed at the time of surgery. The effectiveness of this technique is equivalent for sparing blood use, and it is less expensive than preoperative autologous donation.
7. Point-of-care hemoglobin testing and coagulation function monitoring allow the clinician to make timely decisions based on quantitative data rather than make guesses about surgical blood loss.

REFERENCES

1. Consensus conference: Perioperative red blood cell transfusion. JAMA 1988;260:2700-3.
2. American College of Physicians. Practice strategies for elective red blood cell transfusion. Ann Intern Med 1992;116:403-6.
3. Napolitano LM, Kurek S, Luchette FA, et al. Clinical practice guideline: Red blood cell transfusion in adult trauma and critical care. Crit Care Med 2009;37:3124-57.
4. Practice guidelines for blood component therapy: A report by the American Society of Anesthesiologists Task Force on Blood Component Therapy. Anesthesiology 1996;84:732-47.
5. Hebert PC, Wells G, Marshall J, et al. Transfusion requirements in critical care. A pilot study. Canadian Critical Care Trials Group. JAMA 1995;273:1439-44.
6. Tinmouth A, Macdougall L, Fergusson D, et al. Reducing the amount of blood transfused: A systematic review of behavioral interventions to change physicians' transfusion practices. Arch Intern Med 2005;165:845-52.
7. Bennett-Guerrero E, Zhao Y, O'Brien SM, et al. Variation in use of blood transfusion in coronary artery bypass graft surgery. JAMA 2010; 304:1568-75.
8. Corwin HL, Parsonnet KC, Gettinger A. RBC transfusion in the ICU. Is there a reason? Chest 1995;108:767-71.
9. Smoller BR, Kruskall MS. Phlebotomy for diagnostic laboratory tests in adults. Pattern of use and effect on transfusion requirements. N Engl J Med 1986;314:1233-5.
10. Shander A, Knight K, Thurer R, et al. Prevalence and outcomes of anemia in surgery: A systematic review of the literature. Am J Med 2004;116(Suppl 7A):58S-69S.
11. Bierbaum BE, Callaghan JJ, Galante JO, et al. An analysis of blood management in patients having a total hip or knee arthroplasty. J Bone Joint Surg Am 1999;81:2-10.
12. Millett PJ, Porramatikul M, Chen N, et al. Analysis of transfusion predictors in shoulder arthroplasty. J Bone Joint Surg Am 2006;88-B: 1223-30.
13. Faris PM, Spence RK, Larholt KM, et al. The predictive power of baseline hemoglobin for transfusion risk in surgery patients. Orthopedics 1999;22:s135-40.
14. Goodnough LT, Shander A, Spivak JL, et al. Detection, evaluation, and management of anemia in the elective surgical patient. Anesth Analg 2005;101:1858-61.

15. Bohlius J, Wilson J, Seidenfeld J, et al. Recombinant human erythropoietins and cancer patients: Updated meta-analysis of 57 studies including 9353 patients. J Natl Cancer Inst 2006; 98:708-14.
16. Michael B, Fishbane S, Coyne DW, et al. Drug insight: Safety of intravenous iron supplementation with sodium ferric gluconate complex. Nat Clin Pract Nephrol 2006;2:92-100.
17. Society of Thoracic Surgeons Blood Conservation Guideline Task Force, Society of Cardiovascular Anesthesiologists Special Task Force on Blood Transfusion, et al. Perioperative blood transfusion and blood conservation in cardiac surgery: The Society of Thoracic Surgeons and The Society of Cardiovascular Anesthesiologists clinical practice guideline. Ann Thorac Surg 2007;83(5 Suppl):S27-86.
18. Ottesen S, Froysaker T. Use of Haemonetics cell saver for autotransfusion in cardiovascular surgery. Scand J Thorac Cardiovasc Surg 1982; 16:263-8.
19. Young JN, Edker RR, Moretti RL, et al. Autologous blood retrieval in thoracic, cardiovascular, and orthopedic surgery. Am J Surg 1982; 144:48-52.
20. Breyer RH, Engelman RM, Rousou JA, Lemeshow S. Blood conservation for myocardial revascularization: Is it cost effective? J Thorac Cardiovasc Surg 1987;93:512-22.
21. McCarthy PM, Popovsky MA, Schaff HV, et al. Effect of blood conservation efforts in cardiac operations at the Mayo Clinic. Mayo Clinic Proc 1988;63:225-9.
22. Paul JE, Ling E, Lalonde C, Thabane L. Deliberate hypotension in orthopedic surgery reduces blood loss and transfusion requirements: A meta-analysis of randomized controlled trials. Can J Anaesth 2007;54:799-810.
23. Santoro JE, Eastlack RK, Miroca JM, Bugbee WD. Impact of erythropoietin on allogeneic blood exposure in orthopedic surgery. Am J Orthop 2007;36:600-4.
24. Cali RF, O'Hara PJ, Hertzer NR, et al. The influence of autotransfusion on homologous blood requirements during aortic reconstruction. Clev Clin Q 1983;51:143-8.
25. Tawes RL, Scribner RG, Duval TB, et al. The cell saver and autologous transfusion: An underutilized resource in vascular surgery. Am J Surg 1986;152:105-9.
26. Hallett JW Jr, Popovsky M, Ilstrup D. Minimizing blood transfusions during abdominal aortic surgery: Recent advances in rapid autotransfusion. J Vasc Surg 1987;5:601-6.
27. Stanton PE, Shannon J, Rosenthal D, et al. Intraoperative autologous transfusion during major aortic reconstructive procedures. South Med J 1987;80:315-19.
28. Hendriks HG, van der Meer J, Klompmaker IJ, et al. Blood loss in orthotopic liver transplantation: A retrospective analysis of transfusion requirements and the effects of autotransfusion of cell saver blood in 164 consecutive patients. Blood Coagul Fibrinolysis 2000;11(Suppl): S87-93.
29. Phillips SD, Maguire D, Deshpande R, et al. A positive study investigating the cost effectiveness of intraoperative blood salvage during liver transplantation. Transplantation 2006;81: 536-40.
30. Di Rocco C, Tamburrini G, Pietrini D. Blood sparing in craniosynostosis surgery. Semin Pediatr Neurol 2004;11:278-87.
31. Ilstrup SJ, ed. Standards for perioperative autologous blood collection and administration. 4th ed. Bethesda, MD: AABB, 2009.
32. Waters JH, Dyga RM, Yazer MH, for the Scientific Section Coordinating Committee. Guidelines for blood recovery and reinfusion in surgery and trauma. Bethesda, MD: AABB, 2010.
33. Becker J, Shaz B for the Clinical Transfusion Medicine Committee and the Transfusion Medicine Section Coordinating Committee. Guidelines for blood management and utilization. Bethesda, MD: AABB, 2011 (in press).
34. Henry DA, Carless PA, Moxey AJ, et al. Pre-operative autologous donation for minimizing perioperative allogeneic blood transfusion. Cochrane Database Syst Rev 2002;(2): CD003602.
35. Brecher ME, Goodnough LT. The rise and fall of preoperative autologous blood donation (editorial). Transfusion 2001;41:1459-62.
36. Waters JR, Meier HH, Waters JH. An economic analysis of costs associated with development of a cell salvage program. Anesth Analg 2007; 104:869-75.
37. Szpisjak DF, Potter PS, Capehart BP. Economic analysis of an intraoperative cell salvage service. Anesth Analg 2004;98:201-5.
38. Waters JH, Williams B, Yazer MH, Kameneva MV. Modification of suction-induced hemolysis during cell salvage. Anesth Analg 2007;104: 684-7.
39. Haynes SL, Bennett JR, Torella F, McCollum CN. Does washing swabs increase the efficien-

cy of red cell recovery by cell salvage in aortic surgery? Vox Sang 2005;88:244-8.
40. Linden JV, Kaplan HS, Murphy MT. Fatal air embolism due to perioperative blood recovery. Anesth Analg 1997;84:422-6.
41. Bull MH, Bull BS, Van Arsdell GS, Smith LL. Clinical implications of procoagulant and leukoattractant formation during intraoperative blood salvage. Arch Surg 1988;123:1073-8.
42. Szpisjak DF. Debris elimination from partially-filled cell salvage bowls. Anesth Analg 2001;92:1137-8.
43. Waters JH. Indications and contraindications of cell salvage. Transfusion 2004;44(12 Suppl):40S-44S.
44. Waters JH, Biscotti C, Potter PS, Phillipson E. Amniotic fluid removal during cell salvage in the cesarean section patient. Anesthesiology 2000;92:1531-6.
45. Perseghin P, Vigano M, Rocco G, et al. Effectiveness of leukocyte filters in reducing tumor cell contamination after intraoperative blood salvage in lung cancer patients. Vox Sang 1997;72:221-4.
46. Goodnough LT, Despotis GJ, Merkel K, Monk TG. A randomized trial comparing acute normovolemic hemodilution and preoperative autologous blood donation in total hip arthroplasty. Transfusion 2000;40:1054-7.
47. Goodnough LT, Monk TG, Despotis GJ, Merkel K. A randomized trial of acute normovolemic hemodilution compared to preoperative autologous blood donation in total knee arthroplasty. Vox Sang 1999;77:11-16.
48. Monk TG, Goodnough LT, Brecher ME, et al. A prospective randomized comparison of three blood conservation strategies for radical prostatectomy. Anesthesiology 1999;91:24-33.
49. Feldman JM, Roth JV, Bjoraker DG. Maximum blood savings by acute normovolemic hemodilution. Anesth Analg 1995;80:108-13.
50. Weiskopf RB. Mathematical analysis of isovolemic hemodilution indicates that it can decrease the need of allogeneic blood transfusion. Transfusion 1995;35:37-41.
51. Noon GP, Jones J, Fehir K, Yawn DH. Use of preoperatively obtained platelets and plasma in patients undergoing cardiopulmonary bypass. J Clin Apher 1990;5:91-6.
52. Davies GG, Wells DG, Mabee TM, et al. Plateletleukocyte plasmapheresis attenuates the deleterious effects of cardiopulmonary bypass. Ann Thorac Surg 1992;53:274-7.
53. Christenson JT, Reuse J, Badel P, et al. Autologous platelet sequestration in patients undergoing coronary artery bypass grafting. Eur J Cardiothorac Surg 1996;10:1083-9.
54. Wajon P, Gibson J, Calcroft R, et al. Intraoperative plateletpheresis and autologous platelet gel do not reduce chest tube drainage or allogeneic blood transfusion after reoperative coronary artery bypass. Anesth Analg 2001;93:536-42.
55. Al-Rashidi F, Bhat M, Pierre L, Koul B. Acute plateletpheresis and aprotinin reduces the need for blood transfusion following Ross operation. Interact Cardiovasc Thorac Surg 2007;6:618-22.
56. Stover EP, Siegel LC, Hood PA, et al. Platelet-rich plasma sequestration, with therapeutic platelet yields, reduces allogeneic transfusion in complex cardiac surgery. Anesth Analg 2000;90:509-16.
57. Hiramatsu T, Okamura T, Imai Y, et al. Effects of autologous platelet concentrate reinfusion after open heart surgery in patients with congenital heart disease. Ann Thorac Surg 2002;73:1282-5.
58. Harke H, Tanger D, Furst-Denzer S, et al. [Effect of a preoperative separation of platelets on the postoperative blood loss subsequent to extracorporeal circulation in open heart surgery (author's translation).] Anaesthesist 1977;26:64-71.
59. Jones JW, McCoy TA, Rawitscher RE, Lindsley DA. Effects of intraoperative plasmapheresis on blood loss in cardiac surgery. Ann Thorac Surg 1990;49:585-9.
60. Boldt J, von Bormann B, Kling D, et al. Preoperative plasmapheresis in patients undergoing cardiac surgery procedures. Anesthesiology 1990;72:282-8.
61. Ford SMS, Unsworth-White MJ, Aziz T, et al. Platelet pheresis is not a useful adjunct to blood-sparing strategies in cardiac surgery. J Cardiothorac Vasc Anesth 2002;16:321-9.
62. Boldt J, Zickmann B, Ballesteros M, et al. Influence of acute preoperative plasmapheresis on platelet function in cardiac surgery. J Cardiothorac Vasc Anesth 1993;7:4-9.
63. Tobe CE, Vocelka C, Sepulvada R, et al. Infusion of autologous platelet rich plasma does not reduce blood loss and product use after coronary artery bypass. A prospective, randomized, blinded study. J Thorac Cardiovasc Surg 1993;105:1007-13.

64. Armellin G, Sorbara C, Bonato R, et al. Intraoperative plasmapheresis in cardiac surgery. J Cardiothorac Vasc Anesth 1997;11:13-17.
65. Giordano GF Sr, Giordano GF Jr, Rivers SL, et al. Determinants of homologous blood usage utilizing autologous platelet-rich plasma in cardiac operations. Ann Thorac Surg 1989;47: 897-902.
66. Giordano GF, Rivers SL, Chung GK, et al. Autologous platelet-rich plasma in cardiac surgery: Effect on intraoperative and postoperative transfusion requirements. Ann Thorac Surg 1988;46:416-19.
67. Ferrari M, Zia S, Valbonesi M, et al. A new technique for hemodilution, preparation of autologous platelet-rich plasma and intraoperative blood salvage in cardiac surgery. Int J Artif Organs 1987;10:47-50.
68. Triulzi DJ, Gilmor GD, Ness PM, et al. Efficacy of autologous fresh whole blood or platelet-rich plasma in adult cardiac surgery. Transfusion 1995;35:627-34.
69. Ereth MH, Oliver WC Jr, Beynen FM, et al. Autologous platelet-rich plasma does not reduce transfusion of homologous blood products in patients undergoing repeat valvular surgery. Anesthesiology 1993;79:540-7.
70. Wong CA, Franklin ML, Wade LD. Coagulation tests, blood loss, and transfusion requirements in platelet-rich plasmapheresed versus nonpheresed cardiac surgery patients. Anesth Analg 1994;78:29-36.
71. Shore-Lesserson L, Reich DL, DePerio M, Silvay G. Autologous platelet-rich plasmapheresis: Risk versus benefit in repeat cardiac operations. Anesth Analg 1995;81:229-35.
72. Boey SK, Ong BC, Dhara SS. Preoperative plateletpheresis does not reduce blood loss during cardiac surgery. Can J Anaesth 1993;40: 844-50.
73. Park CK. The effect of patient positioning on intra-abdominal pressure and blood loss in spinal surgery. Anesth Analg 2000;91:552-7.
74. Rohrer MJ, Natale AM. Effect of hypothermia on the coagulation cascade. Crit Care Med 1992;20:1402-5.
75. Wolberg AS, Meng ZH, Monroe DM 3rd, Hoffman M. A systematic evaluation of the effect of temperature on coagulation enzyme activity and platelet function. J Trauma 2004;56:1221-8.
76. Meng ZH, Wolberg AS, Monroe DM 3rd, Hoffman M. The effect of temperature and pH on the activity of Factor VIIa: Implications for the efficacy of high-dose Factor VIIa in hypothermic and acidotic patients. J Trauma 2003;55: 886-91.
77. Waters JH, Gottlieb A, Schoenwald P, et al. Normal saline versus lactated Ringer's solution for intraoperative fluid management in patients undergoing abdominal aortic aneurysm repair: An outcome study (see comment). Anesth Analg 2001;93:817-22.
78. Nuttall GA, Oliver WC, Santrach PJ, et al. Efficacy of a simple intraoperative transfusion algorithm for nonerythrocyte component utilization after cardiopulmonary bypass. Anesthesiology 2001;94:773-8.
79. Shore-Lesserson L, Manspeizer HE, DePerio M, et al. Thromboelastography-guided transfusion algorithm reduces transfusions in complex cardiac surgery. Anesth Analg 1999;88: 312-19.
80. Ozier Y, Schlumberger S. Pharmacological approaches to reducing blood loss and transfusions in the surgical patient. Can J Anaesth 2006;53(Suppl):S21-9.

Chapter 25

Transfusion Support for Hematopoietic Stem Cell Transplant Recipients

◆

Christopher A. Tormey, MD

◆25

THE PURPOSE OF this chapter is to familiarize the reader with aspects of transfusion support for recipients of hematopoietic stem cell transplantation (HSCT). HSCT recipients are unique patients who present a distinct set of challenges for blood banks and transfusion services. When considering transfusion for the recipient of an HSCT, one has to consider not only the complexities associated with the patient's underlying condition, immunosuppression, and preexisting immunohematologic features but also, depending on the type of transplant, the potential for changes in the expressed blood group systems, alloantibodies, and passenger lymphocytes. Over the past two decades, the field of transplantation medicine has seen not only a significant growth in the number of transplantations performed but also continued evolution in the preparative regimens for transplantation and in the cellular sources used for transplantation. Many patients are now seen in their community hospitals for extensive post-transplant care. Thus, issues regarding the complexity of transfusion support for HSCT recipients are no longer relegated to large, academic medical centers.

HSCTs can be categorized as either autologous or allogeneic based on the relationship between the recipient and the donor. In autologous transplants, hematopoietic progenitor cells (HPCs) are derived directly from the patient, while in allogeneic transplants HPCs are obtained from a donor. Whether collected from autologous or allogeneic sources, donor HPCs can be obtained: 1) through their mobilization into the peripheral circulation using selected agents to promote mobilization [eg, granulocyte colony-stimulating factor (G-CSF)], with subsequent collection by apheresis; 2) by harvesting directly from the marrow; or 3) through collection of cord blood. According to recent data,[1] the majority of allogeneic transplantations use HPCs derived from apheresis [HPC, Apheresis—abbreviated herein as HPC(A)], followed by HPCs from marrow [HPC, Marrow—abbreviated herein as HPC(M)] and HPCs from cord blood [HPC,

Christopher A. Tormey, MD, Assistant Professor of Laboratory Medicine, Yale University School of Medicine, New Haven, Connecticut

The author has disclosed no conflicts of interest.

Cord—abbreviated herein as HPC(C)]. [Please note that the terms HPC(A), HPC(M), and HPC(C) are used here only as abbreviations and are not intended to be used in the labeling process or on product labels.] Likewise, the cellular products used in autologous transplantation are most commonly HPC(A), followed by HPC(M) and, on very rare occasions, HPC(C). Of note, HPC(C) are an increasingly common source of cells for allogeneic HSCTs. Transplantation in the allogeneic setting can be further categorized by the myeloablative effect, which is related to the intensity of the preparative regimen—fully myeloablative or reduced-intensity transplantation (also called mini-transplant). A reduction in the intensity of the preparative regimen allows HSCT to be performed in older patients with decreased transplant-related mortality.

Given the growing number of patients undergoing HSCT and the wide variety of clinical conditions that are currently treated with this approach, it is imperative that transfusion medicine specialists be prepared to address the challenges associated with transfusion support for these patient populations. Primary challenges that may affect some, if not all, transfusion services include the following: 1) incompatibilities in ABO and other red cell antigens, 2) support of patients with HLA and/or platelet antibodies, 3) support of neutropenic patients, 4) support of highly immunocompromised patient populations, 5) transplant-associated microangiopathy, and 6) communication between transplant centers and other health-care providers in the posttransplant period. This chapter seeks to address many of these issues and to provide an up-to-date summary for blood bank physicians and medical practitioners.

ABO AND NON-ABO RED CELL ANTIGEN INCOMPATIBLE TRANSPLANTATION

The ABO blood group antigen system, an essential consideration in the everyday practice of transfusion medicine, is not necessarily a barrier to successful HSCT. The red cell antigens, including ABO, are not part of the HLA system nor are they major histocompatibility antigens. Unlike in solid organ transplantation, ABO compatibility is generally not considered critical in the selection of potential HPC donors because pluripotent and early-committed HPCs lack ABO antigens. Thus, engraftment of HPCs is uninhibited even in the presence of circulating ABO antibodies. Nonetheless, discrepancies in ABO and non-ABO antigens between donor and recipient do play an important role in transplantation and can become a major complicating factor in the transfusion support of HSCT recipients.

The relationship between the ABO types of the donor and recipient can fall into one of four categories: compatible, incompatible in the major crossmatch, incompatible in the minor crossmatch, and incompatible bidirectionally.[2-4] Table 25-1 lists all potential ABO combinations between donors and recipients, with an indication of the associated compatibility. A major incompatibility occurs when the recipient has antibodies against blood group antigen(s) present on the surface of the donor's red cells (eg, donor is group A, and recipient is group O with naturally occurring anti-A). Minor incompatibilities are defined as the presence of donor antibodies against blood group antigen(s) present on the recipient's red cells (eg, donor is group O with naturally occurring anti-A, and recipient is group A). A bidirectional incompatibility is the existence of both major and minor incompatibilities (eg, donor is group A and recipient is group B; each possesses a naturally occurring antibody directed against the corresponding antigen). Although the terms *major, minor,* and *bidirectional incompatibility* are most frequently used in the context of the ABO system, they are also applicable to describe the presence of other red cell alloantibodies, such as anti-K or anti-D, in the plasma of the donor and/or recipient. Although ABO incompatibilities are not a critical consideration in graft selection, they are present in 20% to 40% of donor/recipient pairs and thus can influence which blood components are selected for transfusion.[2,5,6]

TABLE 25-1. Compatibility for Hematopoietic Stem Cell Transplantation According to ABO Blood Group of Donor and Recipient

Recipient ABO Status	Donor ABO Status			
	O	**A**	**B**	**AB**
O	C	M	M	M
A	m	C	Bi	M
B	m	Bi	C	M
AB	m	m	m	C

C = compatibility; M = major incompatibility due to a naturally occurring antibody (or antibodies) in the recipient; m = minor incompatibility due to a naturally occurring antibody (or antibodies) in the donor graft product; Bi = bidirectional incompatibility due to naturally occurring antibodies in both the donor and recipient.

Major ABO Incompatibility

Major ABO incompatibility creates two challenges: 1) the potential for acute intravascular hemolysis when ABO-incompatible donor red cells are infused with the graft to the recipient and 2) the continued production of circulating ABO antibodies directed against donor red cells and erythroid progenitors produced by the engrafted HPCs. The first challenge is typically addressed during the processing of collected HPCs. Techniques such as red cell depletion allow for the removal of incompatible red cells from the graft product to minimize the risk of hemolysis during infusion. There is no general consensus about the threshold level of incompatible red cells that may be safely infused. However, the currently acceptable volumes range from 10 to 20 mL. In addition, many HPC products are cryopreserved (frozen) before administration, which also helps to curb hemolysis because incompatible donor red cells are typically lysed as a result of the freezing process. As suggested by some, the titer of the recipient antibody may also be used in guiding facility policy.[2] In the absence of red cell depletion or cryopreservation, plasmapheresis of the recipient immediately before graft infusion may be warranted to reduce the circulating titer of ABO antibodies.

More complex for clinicians is the second challenge accompanying major ABO incompatibility, that is, the continuous production of antibodies against A and/or B antigens of engrafted donor HPCs. This process may occur for periods as long as 3 to 4 months after HPC infusion. As a result, delays in erythropoiesis are often encountered, with red cell engraftment potentially delayed up to 40 days after transplantation. The typical findings include the presence of antibody directed against donor red cells, with accompanying anemia. In severe cases, pure red cell aplasia (PRCA) can develop. PRCA is determined to be present when a marrow biopsy demonstrates adequate myeloid, lymphoid, and megakaryocyte populations in the setting of absent or nearly absent erythroid precursors and profound peripheral reticulocytopenia.[6] The risk of PRCA varies but may be as high as 50%. Thus, HSCT involving major ABO incompatibility may render some recipients transfusion-dependent for many months following transplantation. Fortunately, major incompatibility tends not to severely affect production of other cells in the myeloid lineage (eg, platelets and granulocytes).

Minor ABO Incompatibility

In contrast to major ABO incompatibility, the manipulation of the graft in the setting of minor incompatibility is relatively straightforward. Analogous to red cell depletion for major incompatibility, donor red cell antibodies can be readily removed by depletion of plasma from the graft product. Even if isoagglutinins are not completely removed, the ensuing hemolysis is typically mild and self-limited. A more significant problem results from the ongoing production of anti-A and/or -B by donor lymphocytes against the circulating residual recipient red cells. Approximately 5 to 12 days after infusion of HPC(A) [and 9 to 16 days after infusion of HPC(M)], the patient may experience acute hemolysis that can result in severe morbidity and even mortality. However, in most cases the hemolysis is not particularly severe and eventually subsides, typically lasting no longer than 2 weeks, correlating with the loss of recipient red cells. From a laboratory standpoint, patients with minor ABO incompatibility typically demonstrate a positive direct antiglobulin test and an eluate with panreactivity against red cells possessing the patient's ABO antigen(s). This observation is consistent with the production of antibodies against the patient's cells by the passenger B lymphocytes present in the graft. If hemolysis is severe and potentially life threatening, rapid institution of erythrocytapheresis to exchange incompatible recipient red cells with donor-compatible red cells can be therapeutic and lifesaving. In some transplant centers, prophylactic erythrocytapheresis is also performed, although this is not a routine approach to minor incompatibility.

Bidirectional ABO Incompatibility

In bidirectional ABO incompatibility, the complications arising from both major and minor ABO-incompatible HSCT can be seen in the recipient. As such, the processing of the HPC graft should include depletion of both red cell and plasma content. Also, the posttransplant period can be complicated by the acute onset of hemolysis within days or weeks (as seen in minor incompatibility caused by passenger lymphocytes and antibodies against the recipient) and/or the delayed engraftment of red cells and, in some cases, PRCA (as seen in major incompatibility caused by recipient antibodies targeting engrafting HPCs).

Clinical Outcomes and Complications of ABO-Incompatible Transplants

Although ABO incompatibilities are not as significant as mismatches in the HLA system, some have questioned whether ABO incompatibilities between donor and recipient may have had previously unrecognized influences on transplant outcome. Many authors have reported that ABO incompatibility does not adversely affect patient survival, although it may be associated with prolonged erythroid aplasia and immediate and/or delayed hemolysis. For example, Kim et al noted that the time of neutrophil, platelet, and red cell engraftment; transfusion requirements; incidence of acute or chronic graft-vs-host disease (GVHD); relapse; and survival were not influenced by ABO incompatibility after allogeneic HSCT from HLA-matched sibling donors.[7] Similarly, data from pediatric populations indicate that major or minor ABO mismatches had no significant effect on outcome when compared with ABO-identical transplants.[8]

In contrast, Stussi et al performed a retrospective analysis of the consequences of ABO incompatibility in allogeneic HSCT at two centers.[9] In a total of 562 consecutive patients (including 361 undergoing ABO-identical HSCTs, and 98 minor, 86 major, and 17 bidirectional ABO-incompatible HSCTs), survival was significantly associated with ABO compatibility. Compared to ABO-identical HSCT, bidirectional ABO incompatibility increased the risk significantly, whereas the survival of patients with major or minor ABO-incompatible HSCT was not significantly different. Delayed red cell engraftment was associated with major ABO incompatibility, while a higher incidence of mild acute GVHD was seen in minor ABO incompatibility. In this analysis, survival and the rate of mild GVHD were negatively affected by ABO incompatibility. A more recent study by Kimura et al suggests that rates of survival for ABO-identical transplantations were higher than those for major and minor ABO mismatches.[10] In that study of approximately 5600 HSCT recipients, 1-year survival was 63.0% for patients receiving ABO-identical transplants vs 56.9% for those with a major ABO mismatch. Additionally, Kimura et al noted delayed engraftment of myeloid-lineage cells and an increased risk for GVHD in major-ABO-mismatch recipients. Data from Resnick et al also suggest an increase in nonrelapse mortality for major-ABO-mismatched transplants.[11] Thus, it is likely that as additional data are collected, the adverse effects and outcomes associated with major ABO mismatch may need to be reconsidered. As such, traditional thinking regarding the risks and disadvantages associated with ABO-mismatched transplants may change.[12]

An interesting angle on outcomes related to major-ABO-incompatible transplants is the underlying disease of the transplant recipient. Benjamin et al retrospectively analyzed a cohort of 292 allogeneic transplant recipients and reported an increased risk of death, by as much as 85% within 100 days of transplantation, in the subgroup of patients with myelodysplastic syndrome who received ABO-incompatible HPC(M).[13] Both ABO-major- and ABO-minor-mismatched recipients were at risk. This observation was not seen in the larger group of 112 patients who received transplants for chronic myelogenous leukemia (CML) performed in the same center. The authors concluded that in their experience, ABO-incompatible transplants may be associated with increased complications, but only in a selected group of patients.[13] Canals et al looked at the impact of ABO incompatibility on allogeneic HSCT in the subgroup of patients undergoing reduced-intensity conditioning.[14] They evaluated 77 consecutive HSCTs, including 22% major- and 10% minor-ABO-mismatched transplantations, and found that approximately 40% of patients in both groups experienced transient mild hemolysis. PRCA was observed in only one patient who received a major-ABO- and Jk^a-incompatible transplant. The authors concluded that reduced-intensity conditioning in ABO-incompatible HSCT is not associated with an increased risk of hemolysis and adverse clinical outcomes.[14]

Management of ABO incompatibility is not standardized. In a survey conducted in Italy, Raimondi et al reported a high degree of heterogeneity concerning the pretransplant tests, methods to overcome infusion of ABO-incompatible marrow, and posttransplant transfusion policy and monitoring.[15] The authors cited lack of evidence-based guidelines as one of the reasons behind the observed results. Despite clear evidence-based guidelines, new approaches in the prevention and treatment of the side effects of major and minor ABO incompatibility continue to be reported. For instance, Stussi et al recently demonstrated that PRCA associated with bidirectional ABO incompatibility could be ameliorated with pretransplantation plasmapheresis to reduce anti-A and/or anti-B titers.[16] In addition, Helbig et al have reported on their successful attempts to overcome PRCA with the use of monoclonal anti-CD20 therapy.[17] Further studies such as these will be necessary in order to develop more broad and evidence-based approaches to management of ABO incompatibility.

Incompatibility Related to Non-ABO Antigens

RBC antigens of other blood group systems can present challenges similar to the ones described for ABO-incompatible transplants. Overall, they are generally less frequently encountered, but the presence of red cell antibodies in the patient (more common) and/or in the donor (less common) requires attention and approaches similar to those outlined above for major and minor ABO incompatibility.

Voluntary Standards

Accreditation organizations such as the AABB and the Foundation for the Accreditation of Cellular Therapy (FACT) have long been interested in ensuring safety and minimizing adverse effects related to HSCTs involving incompatible ABO or other red cell antigens. Both organizations cite specific requirements for donor and patient testing and labeling of the final products.[18,19] In principle, the standards are identical and require that the donor and recipient be ABO typed. ABO typing of the product is also required. Any identified red cell incompatibilities in ABO or other red cell antigens should be discussed with the patient's physician and appropriate steps taken to minimize the risk of complications. Transplant centers that are members of National Marrow Donor Program (NMDP) are required to have policies and procedures addressing incompatibilities of ABO and other red cell antigens.

BLOOD COMPONENT CONSIDERATIONS

Red Cell Support

The majority of HSCT patients require transfusion support regardless of incompatibilities or blood group antigen mismatches. Transfusion support is most often required after transplantation and before red cell engraftment, which may take up to 6 weeks and sometimes even longer, as described above. However, many HSCT patients also receive multiple red cell units before transplantation in order to support courses of chemotherapy. The decision to initiate red cell transfusion is typically based on symptomatic anemia because there have been no trials performed specifically in HSCT transplant recipient populations to define a hemoglobin or hematocrit threshold below which red cell transfusion is appropriate or necessary. In the absence of symptomatic anemia, "threshold" hemoglobin or hematocrit levels defined in other patient populations have been applied to HSCT transplant recipients. As such, hemoglobin levels below 7 to 9 g/dL typically qualify a patient for red cell transfusion, particularly if the patient has a history of coexisting cardiac or peripheral vascular disease.[20,21]

Although red cell transfusion strategies for HSCT transplant patients do not currently differ markedly from other patient groups, the mechanisms underlying some of the anemia associated with HSCT are sufficiently unique to warrant further discussion. The intrinsic production of erythrocytes is under the control of erythropoietin (EPO).[22] It is well established that serum EPO levels rise in response to anemia. Similarly, after intensive chemotherapy, serum EPO levels increase rapidly and peak in the first week after treatment. Although recipients of autologous HSCT maintain adequate EPO levels throughout the posttransplant course and require less intensive red cell support during the posttransplant period, the situation is quite different in the recipients of allogeneic HSCT. In this setting there is a prolonged period of inappropriately low endogenous EPO levels.[23] Because a low level of EPO after allogeneic transplantation is quite common, red cell transfusions may be required for up to a year following engraftment. Thus, it would also seem that exogenous replacement of EPO would be of benefit in overcoming prolonged anemia associated with HSCT.

Despite physiologic mechanisms suggesting a potential benefit, placebo-controlled trials have not definitively shown early reduction of transfusion requirements or immediate reversal of anemia. For instance, Baron et al enrolled 34 allogeneic HSCT recipients in three small trials that varied by the timing of administration, dose of EPO, and hemoglobin goal.[24] The hemoglobin target was set at 13 to 14 g/dL. The authors of this report noted that early administration of EPO (ie, immediately after transplantation) is not beneficial, while delayed administration (ie, at least 35 days after transplantation) resulted in decreased red cell usage in this selected population of anemic HSCT recipients. More recently, Fox et al demonstrated that low-dose EPO therapy *was* ultimately an effective means to overcome anemia and reduce transfusion requirements for recipients of allogeneic HSCT.[22] However, in this study, like that reported by Baron et al, the benefits of EPO administration were obtained only after a delay in commencement of therapy (the median time to commencement of therapy was 61 days after transplantation). Thus, it remains unclear if EPO has a role to play in addressing the anemia initially encountered in the first days and weeks following HSCT. Alternatively, some investigators have incorporated EPO treatment into regimens used to overcome PRCA. One strategy, reported by Helbig et al in a small population of HSCT recipients, resulted in resolution of PRCA in five out of six cases.[25] Larger studies are necessary to determine if EPO is capable of consistently preventing complications of HSCT such as PRCA.

The Food and Drug Administration (FDA) has recently strengthened the warnings associated with EPO use after studies showed adverse effects of EPO treatment in patients with chronic renal failure (increased risk of death, blood clots, strokes, and heart attacks) as well as in cancer patients (decreased survival and/or tumor progression).[26] Although no studies have specifically linked EPO to poor outcomes in HSCT patient populations, clinicians should be mindful of this potential risk of EPO usage.

Platelet Support

Platelet recovery after allogeneic HSCT has been studied extensively. Several factors are strongly associated with the rate at which patients become platelet transfusion independent. Some of these factors include relationship between donor and recipient (related vs unrelated), the presence of GVHD, cytomegalovirus (CMV) infection, and the HPC CD34+ cellular dose.[27-29] In one study, recipients of unrelated grafts had a significantly lower platelet count on day 50 after transplantation than recipients of related or syngeneic grafts.[30] The platelet count also varied with acute GVHD grade. With Grade 0, patients had a platelet count of 153,000/µL, while patients with Grade III and IV GVHD had platelet counts of 32,000/µL and 22,000/µL, respectively. In the same study, active CMV infection with high antigenemia was associated with significantly lower platelet counts. The authors concluded that low platelet counts were a predictor of transplant-related mortality.[30] Pulanic et al recently provided an excellent review outlining the effects of *chronic* GVHD on platelet count and poor survival in HSCT recipients.[31] Clearly, more research is needed to better understand the relationship between GVHD, thrombocytopenia, and survival.

In an earlier study of thrombocytopenia after HSCT, Nash et al retrospectively reviewed data on 1468 recipients of autologous and allogeneic transplants.[32] Delayed platelet engraftment in autologous HSCT recipients was associated with the use of HPC(M) rather than HPC(A) as a source of stem cells, diagnosis of acute myelogenous leukemia (AML) rather than other diseases, positive CMV serology, and the presence of infection before engraftment. Risk factors associated with delayed platelet engraftment after allogeneic marrow transplantation included unrelated as opposed to related donor transplants, transplantation for diseases other than CML, increased age, onset of acute GVHD, male gender, the administration of methotrexate for GVHD prophylaxis, and the presence of infection before engraftment. Also noteworthy was the observation that delayed platelet recovery was associated with decreased overall survival after both autologous and allogeneic transplants. There is increasing evidence to suggest that the source [eg, HPC(A) vs HPC(C)] of an allogeneic transplant is also predictive of time to platelet engraftment. Several studies have shown that the median time to platelet engraftment for HPC(C) transplants is, on average, several times longer than for recipients of HPC(A) or HPC(M).[33-36] Thus, longer-term dependence on platelet transfusion is more likely to be necessary for recipients of cord transplants.

Plasma, including the significant volume of plasma in platelets, contains variable amounts of isoagglutinins such as anti-A and anti-B. Although transfusion of ABO-incompatible plasma and platelets is a common practice for routine transfusion, it cannot be readily applied to the recipients of allogeneic HSCT without careful consideration of the potential risks. As discussed above, infusion of isoagglutinins (eg, anti-A) may precipitate or exacerbate hemolysis.[37] Some researchers have reported that ABO-incompatible platelet transfusions combined with the use of melphalan correlated with development of hepatic veno-occlusive disease.[38] The authors concluded that transfusion of platelet concentrates containing ABO-incompatible plasma increases the risk of hepatic veno-occlusive disease in young children treated with a busulfan-containing regimen, possibly caused by binding of A and/or B antigens expressed on the surface of hepatic endothelial cells. They also recommended that transfusion of platelet concentrates containing ABO-incompatible plasma should be avoided in these children.[38]

In some centers it has become an institutional policy to transfuse only ABO-identical red cells and platelet concentrates to the recipients of HSCT. Heal et al noted that this policy may be associated with improved patient survival.[39] The authors consequently speculated that provision of ABO-identical blood components, including removal of incompatible plasma from other components when necessary, may result in reduced morbidity and mortality in HSCT recipients. There is an obvious need for additional prospective studies to address this provocative issue.[39] In ABO-incompatible HSCT, the plasma-containing components should also be compatible with both the donor and the recipient, whenever possible. Recommendations for component selection are more fully detailed below and in Table 25-2.

In the context of platelet transfusion in HSCT recipients, several additional issues require more extensive discussion: 1) the role of prophylactic vs therapeutic platelet transfusion, 2) the platelet transfusion "threshold," and 3) the appropriate transfusion dose.

Prophylactic vs Therapeutic Platelet Transfusion

Platelet concentrates are most frequently transfused as prophylaxis to prevent an acute hemorrhage rather than for actual bleeding in the setting of chemotherapy or HSCT. However, Wandt et al examined the assumption that prophylactic platelet transfusion could be replaced with therapeutic transfusion. In this study of 140 autologous HSCT recipients, therapeutic transfusions were provided when patients were in stable clinical condition but with active bleeding.[40] Minor or moderate bleeding was observed in 26 patients (19%) with no life-threatening hemorrhage. The median platelet dose was 1 unit (range = 0-18), and total platelet usage was half that seen in a historical control group. The authors advocated more widespread study and adoption of therapeutic platelet transfusion protocols.[40] Studies such as this one and others may help to reveal the true benefit of prophylactic platelet transfusions.

Platelet Transfusion Threshold

The dosing and the acceptable threshold for prophylactic transfusion of platelets have been studied for over 20 years. In the past, studies supported a prophylactic transfusion threshold of 20,000/µL for patients undergoing chemotherapy and HSCT. More recent investigations have studied the impact of lowering the threshold for prophylactic platelet transfusions on bleeding and platelet use in allogeneic HSCT recipients. One study has demonstrated that the platelet threshold could be safely set at 5000/µL in the absence of fever or bleeding and at 10,000/µL if such complications exist.[41] Two randomized controlled trials directly compared transfusion triggers of 10,000/µL and 20,000/µL in patients with acute leukemia. There was no increased risk of bleeding at 10,000/µL. On the basis of these data, a threshold of 10,000/µL in uncomplicated thrombocytopenia (ie, in patients without coexisting conditions such as fever, bleeding, or bacteremia/sepsis) is widely accepted.[42,43]

A systematic analysis of available literature on prophylactic platelet transfusion after chemotherapy and stem cell transplantation has recently been published.[44] The review includes eight completed published trials with a total of 390 participants in the intervention groups and 362 participants in the control groups. Three studies addressing the transfusion threshold (10,000/µL vs 20,000/µL) were included in a subanalysis that revealed no statistically significant differences between the groups with regard to mortality, remission rates, number of participants with severe bleeding events, or red cell transfusion requirements. The authors questioned whether the studies had sufficient power, even in combination, to demonstrate noninferiority of the lower threshold (10,000/µL) in terms of safety. Also, the authors concluded that the randomized trials undertaken to date are insufficient to make clinically relevant conclusions about the effect of different platelet doses. At the same time, however, the authors did not advo-

TABLE 25-2. Transfusion Support for Patients Undergoing HSCT According to the Type of ABO Incompatibility and the Transplant Stage

		ABO Blood Group Selection		
Type of Incompatibility	**Transplant Stage**	**Red Cells Compatible with**	**Platelets Compatible with**	**Plasma/Cryoprecipitate Compatible with**
Major incompatibility	Preparative regimen	Recipient	Donor	Donor
	Transplantation	Recipient	Donor	Donor
	Recipient antibodies detected	Recipient	Donor	Donor
	Recipient antibodies no longer detected	Donor	Donor	Donor
Minor incompatibility	Preparative regimen	Donor	Recipient	Recipient
	Transplantation	Donor	Recipient	Recipient
	Recipient cells circulating	Donor	Recipient	Recipient
	Recipient cells no longer circulating	Donor	Donor	Donor
Bidirectional incompatibility	Preparative regimen	Group O	Group AB	Group AB
	Transplantation	Group O	Group AB	Group AB
	Recipient antibodies detected; recipient cells circulating	Group O	Group AB	Group AB
	Recipient antibodies no longer detected; recipient cells no longer circulating	Donor	Donor	Donor

cate any changes to current practice as described above.[44]

In a prospective randomized trial, Zumberg et al evaluated bleeding incidence among 159 HSCT recipients when transfusion thresholds of 10,000/µL (10K arm) or 20,000/µL (20K arm) were used for prophylactic transfusions.[45] The authors analyzed the number of prophylactic and therapeutic transfusions, and the incidence of minor and major bleeding. There were no significant differences in bleeding incidence or its severity. Fourteen percent of patients in the 10K arm compared to 17% in the 20K arm experienced major bleeding. Three such episodes involved the central nervous system—two in the 10K arm and one in the 20K arm. There was no difference in the number of transfused platelet concentrates (10.4 vs 10.2 units)—most likely the result of additional safety measures incorporated into this study.[45] In a more recent study by Diedrich et al, 166 HSCT recipients were randomly assigned to prophylactic platelet transfusions at a low threshold (ie, platelet count below 10,000/µL; 79 patients) or a high threshold (ie, platelet count below 30,000/µL; 87 patients).[46] The number of red cell and platelet transfusions as well as the number of bleeding complications were monitored. No significant differences were found between the groups in clinical outcome variables (ie, bacteremia, engraftment, GVHD, hospital stay, death, and survival). The median number of transfused red cell units was also not different. The bleeding rate was 18% and 15% in low- and high-threshold groups, respectively.[46] The type of bleeding was similar as well. The only identified difference was the total number of platelet units transfused, with a median of 4 (range = 0-32) and 10 (range = 0-48) in the low- and high-threshold groups, respectively. The authors concluded that the lower threshold is safe for transfusion support of HSCT recipients.[46]

A provocative study of HSCT recipients by Nevo et al raises questions about the safety of a 10,000/µL threshold. In that study, patients infused at the "conservative" level of 10,000/µL demonstrated significantly increased mortality and reduced survival when compared to those infused at counts less than 20,000/µL.[47] Nevo et al did not include deaths associated with hemorrhage; thus the increased mortality for the 10K arm could be unrelated to hemorrhagic sequelae. As such, these findings suggest that provision of platelets to meet higher baseline counts may be associated with a survival benefit unrelated to hemostasis.[47] Despite the findings of this intriguing study, the majority of published literature to date suggest that the continued use of a platelet count of 10,000/µL for prophylactic transfusion in uncomplicated HSCT is prudent. However, it is imperative that data continue to be collected in order to determine if 10,000/µL is appropriate for mortality related to all causes.

Platelet Dose

Another question frequently associated with platelet transfusion is the optimal platelet dose per transfusion episode. One of the first studies to address this issue was reported by Tinmouth et al.[48] This study, a randomized controlled trial, examined the effectiveness of low-dose platelets in thrombocytopenic patients with acute leukemia or undergoing autologous HSCT. One hundred eleven patients were enrolled and randomly assigned to receive low-dose (3 platelet units) or standard-dose (5 platelet units) transfusions. The patients were then monitored daily for bleeding and received platelet transfusions prophylactically. Major bleeding was observed in 10.7% and 7.3% of patients receiving low-dose and standard-dose platelets, respectively. Two additional bleeding events occurred in the low-dose platelet group, despite their platelet counts being above 100,000/µL. The authors concluded that low-dose platelet transfusion appears to be safe, but equivalency of the doses could not be established in this study.[48] More recently, the results of a trial conducted by the Biomedical Excellence for Safer Transfusion (BEST) Collaborative were reported.[49] In this study, the Strategies for Transfusion of Platelets (SToP), investigators performed a multicenter, randomized controlled trial in thrombocytopenic patients with hypoproliferative marrow; the study group included both

HSCT recipients and patients with thrombocytopenia not undergoing HSCT. Platelet transfusion recipients were randomly assigned to either "low-dose" units (containing 1.5 - 3.0 × 10^{11} platelets/product) or "standard-dose" units (containing 3.0 - 6.0 × 10^{11} platelets/product) and then followed for development of bleeding after prophylactic transfusions. The results of the study showed that low-dose platelets were associated with a higher risk for the development of World Health Organization (WHO) Grade 4 bleeding; differences in risk for lower grade bleeding were not clearly evident. Furthermore, the authors did not find that a "low-dose" strategy reduced the number of transfusion exposures in HSCT recipients.[49] Based on this study alone, it would not seem prudent to recommend a change from current dosing strategies, particularly as lower doses were apparently associated with a higher risk for development of WHO Grade 4 bleeding. However, a recently published, large randomized trial sponsored by the National Heart, Lung, and Blood Institute (NHLBI) compared low (1.1 × 10^{11} platelets per square meter of body surface area), medium (2.2 × 10^{11} platelets), and high (4.4 × 10^{11} platelets) doses in patients with platelet counts less than 10,000/µL and produced a conflicting outcome regarding lower doses of platelets.[50] In this study, *no* differences in bleeding across the platelet dosages provided for WHO Grade 2 hemorrhages or higher were observed. Significantly, and unlike the SToP trial, patients were dosed for transfusion according to body surface area, which may help to explain the lack of increased bleeding for even lower platelet dosages. With appropriate dosing strategies based on body surface area, it may be possible to provide lower doses of platelets without leading to an increased risk for hemorrhage. Drawbacks to a lower dosing regimen would include a lower platelet increment after infusion and a potential for a greater number of platelet transfusions over time.[50] Clearly as more trials are performed and more data collected, clinicians may still better refine the approach to platelet transfusion in HSCT recipients.

Plasma, Cryoprecipiated AHF, and Factor Concentrate Support

The use of plasma, cryoprecipitate, and factor concentrates is not particularly unique to the recipients of HSCT. In fact, there are no specific recommendations regarding the usage of any of these products for HSCT patients. As discussed above and outlined in Table 25-2, the most rigorous guidelines necessary for transfusion of plasma products relate to respecting the ABO group of the recipient and of engrafting cells. However, for HSCTs complicated by GVHD, there has been interest in determining whether plasma-derived products and/or recombinant factor concentrates could particularly be of use for bleeding complications; dysregulation of hemostasis is a well-known complication of GVHD. Some investigators have examined recombinant concentrates such as activated Factor VII [NovoSeven (Novo Nordisk, Zurich, Switzerland)] as a potential therapy for bleeding related to HSCT. The largest study, a multicenter, randomized controlled trial by Pihusch et al, examined the use of this product at three doses (40, 80, and 160 µg/kg) in comparison to control groups for bleeding associated primarily with GVHD in the setting of HSCT.[51] The trial found that there was no difference in bleeding score for any of the dosing regimens vs control groups and that the transfusion requirements were the same across all patient cohorts. As such, the results of this trial indicate that recombinant Factor VIIa is likely to be ineffective as a first-line therapy to address bleeding complications associated with HSCT.[51] However, recombinant Factor VIIa may still be useful as a "last resort" approach in patients with intractable bleeding, and its use for this type of hemorrhage is encountered in many medical institutions. Clearly, further studies are necessary to better define the role of Factor VIIa for bleeding HSCT recipients. Another possibility for hemostasis therapy arises from the fact that GVHD results in the depletion of Factor XIII, increasing the risk for and severity of gastrointestinal hemorrhage.[52] As such, the high concentration of Factor XIII in cryoprecipitate and the small volume of this blood component make it a potentially useful therapy in GVHD-related hemorrhage. Formal studies are required to determine the efficacy of such an approach.

Selection of Blood Components

Selection of appropriate components is particularly problematic for recipients of allogeneic HSCT; autologous recipients can receive components that are ABO identical (or ABO compatible) without significant concern for adverse effects. When determining transfusion requirements for an allogeneic HSCT recipient, it is vital that the blood bank or transfusion service keep exquisite records documenting pretransplant ABO group and the ABO group of the donor. It is also imperative to determine the stage of the transplant (ie, preparative period, immediate posttransplant period, and postengraftment period with absence of recipient red cells and/or antibodies).[53] Recommendations for optimal component selection at each point in the transplant process are shown in Table 25-2. With regard to Rh(D), obviously there is no concern if HSCT donor and recipient are a match; the recipient can continue to receive the same type of components transfused before transplantation. However, if the recipient is Rh negative and the donor Rh positive, or vice versa, only Rh-negative components should be used (including platelets). For the above scenarios, provision of Rh-negative components will prevent alloimmunization to the potently immunogenic D-antigen.

HSCT RECIPIENTS WITH HLA AND/OR PLATELET ANTIBODIES

Some patients scheduled to undergo HSCT have antibodies against HLA antigens and/or human platelet antigens (HPAs), both of which may affect the efficacy of platelet transfusion. Although the vast majority of HSCT donors and recipients are HLA matched, this is not true for platelet donors. Thus, it is possible that the transfusion of platelets positive for antigens against which the patient has antibodies could result in a lower corrected count increment (CCI). For example, Balduini and colleagues found that alloimmunization was one of the primary factors affecting posttransfusion platelet increments in pediatric patients undergoing allogeneic HSCT.[54]

The issue of HPA and HLA matching of donor-patient pairs has been raised by several groups. It has been postulated that mismatches between donor and recipient for HPA (which may serve as minor histocompatibility antigen) increase the risk of GVHD. It is also speculated that these same mismatches potentially inhibit thrombopoiesis via platelet antibodies and destruction of megakaryocyte precursors. Leitner et al analyzed 53 donor-recipient pairs for platelet antigen (HPA-1, HPA-2, HPA-3, and HPA-5) allotypes and screened for platelet antibodies before HSCT and weekly thereafter until day 100.[55] The patients were also monitored for GVHD. In this limited study the authors did not find any effect of platelet mismatch on the frequency of GVHD or the onset of thrombopoiesis. The CCI and frequency of platelet transfusions were not affected by platelet antigen mismatch. The authors concluded that the HPA match is not likely to affect the outcome of HSCT. Similar results were reported by Garcia-Malo et al, who studied 77 identical allogeneic HSCTs. The authors concluded that incidence of GVHD, platelet utilization, or platelet engraftment are not affected by platelet antigen mismatch.[56]

Lapierre et al observed increased early expression of anti-HLA in the HSCT recipients who received HPC(A) rather than HPC(M). A similar observation was reported for the increased titer of ABO antibodies.[57] The use of HPC(A) was associated with anti-HLA appearing earlier and in more patients after transplantation [11 of 24 HPC(A) recipients vs 4 of 27 HPC(M) recipients]. The difference was less pronounced when complement-dependent cytotoxicity rather than flow cytometry was used as a detection method. The use of HPC(A) was associated with decreased platelet use despite an increase in circulating anti-HLA. The risk of bleeding in patients undergoing HSCT was studied by Toor et al in 39 consecutive AML patients, of whom 12 received allogeneic related grafts, and 27 received autologous grafts.[58] All patients received high-dose chemotherapy. In this series, HLA alloimmunization in autologous HSCT recipients was associated with very significantly increased platelet utilization, delayed bleeding, and poor outcome following transplantation.

NEUTROPENIC PATIENTS WITH INFECTION UNRESPONSIVE TO ANTIMICROBIAL THERAPY

Traditionally, infusions of fresh granulocytes have been used to treat severe, antibiotic-refractory bacterial or fungal infections in patients with absolute neutrophil counts less than 500/µL. Immunosuppression of this type is particularly relevant to the recipients of HSCTs. Only patients with a reasonable chance at sustainable marrow recovery after resolution of the underlying infection are candidates for granulocyte components.[53] In the past, the most significant barrier to the use of granulocytes was obtaining an adequate dose from a healthy donor. Because of the development of G-CSF and improvements in apheresis technology, white cell collection efficiency yields have increased, allowing granulocyte transfusion to be a more practical and efficacious therapy. Over the last 10 to 15 years, a number of trials have been performed to evaluate the safety and efficacy of granulocyte transfusion using G-CSF stimulation in healthy donors. Studies performed in both adult and pediatric populations have found that granulocyte transfusion leads to significant improvement in patients with fungal infections refractory to antimicrobial drugs.[59-61] Granulocyte doses in these studies were typically 5 to 10 × 10^{10} and resulted in increases in peripheral white cell counts of approximately 2000 to 5000/µL. To determine the true efficacy of granulocyte transfusion in the setting of HSCT, an ongoing multicenter randomized controlled trial sponsored by NHLBI will study neutropenic patients who have ongoing infection unresponsive to antimicrobial therapy. The results of this study will be helpful in understanding the benefit of granulocyte infusion such that it may be applied in a more rigorous and evidence-based way to HSCT patients. In addition to studies documenting the use of granulocyte infusions for the treatment of active infections, a number of investigators have reported on the successful use of this therapy to prevent onset or recurrence of severe infection.[62,63] Published experiences in this approach have been primarily limited to case reports and series. As such, the role of granulocytes as prophylaxis for primary infection remains unclear, and further studies are necessary.

SPECIAL PROCESSING OF BLOOD COMPONENTS FOR THE RECIPIENTS OF HSCT

The irradiation of cellular blood products and components (eg, red cells and platelets) is intended to inhibit the proliferation of donor lymphocytes, thereby preventing transfusion-associated GVHD.[53] Although it is generally accepted that immunosuppressed HSCT recipients require irradiation of components for at least 1 year after transplantation, it is unclear whether these patients require irradiation beyond this point. Despite absence of definitive evidence indicating that it is absolutely essential after this time has elapsed, many institutions (including this author's) indefinitely provide irradiated products to HSCT recipients. This is likely a prudent policy given the potential for lifelong immunosuppression associated with HSCT and the possibility for relapse of malignancies for which the patient was initially transplanted.

The situation is much more complex with regard to CMV. CMV is particularly relevant because infections can lead to high morbidity and mortality in HSCT recipients. It has been generally accepted that prestorage leukocyte reduction of components is equally as efficacious in the prevention of CMV spread when compared with use of components collected from donors lacking antibodies to CMV ("CMV seronegative" donors). However, in a recent review of the literature accompanied by a meta-analysis, Vamvakas analyzed a total of 829 recipients of CMV-seronegative components in 11 studies and a total of 878 recipients of leukocyte-reduced components in 12 studies.[64] Among HSCT recipients, the risk of CMV infection was, respectively, 1.63% (11/674) and 3.01% (21/697). He noted that in the subset of studies integrated in the meta-analysis, CMV-seronegative and leukocyte-reduced components were virtually equivalent to each other when they were compared with CMV-unscreened/non-leukocyte-reduced components. The risk reduction of CMV infection was 93.1% and 92.3%, respectively. In three studies that directly compared both approaches, CMV-seronegative components were associated with 58% reduction in risk as compared to leukocyte-reduced components.

These results suggest that CMV-seronegative components may be more efficacious than leukocyte-reduced components in preventing transfusion-acquired CMV infection. However, in the absence of a large supply of CMV-seronegative components, it is likely warranted to consider leukocyte-reduced units to be "CMV reduced risk." The CMV status of the recipient and the donor should also be considered before a decision is made regarding transfusion of leukocyte-reduced vs CMV-seronegative units. Some hospitals provide CMV-seronegative units exclusively to HSCT recipients who are CMV seronegative and who received a transplant from a CMV-seronegative donor. In other possible combinations, such as a CMV-seropositive donor and a CMV-seronegative recipient, leukocyte-reduced components are typically provided.

Patients demonstrating repeated reactions to transfusion may also benefit from modification of components. HSCT recipients chronically dependent on red cell or platelet transfusions may frequently exhibit allergic symptoms such as pruritis, urticaria, or wheezing. It is also not uncommon for such reactions to increase in severity over time. One approach to these repeated reactions is to "wash" components to remove supernatant plasma. This can be accomplished by automated methods with red cells or by centrifugation and saline resuspension for platelets. These modifications, in conjunction with timely premedication regimens, often help to ameliorate or even completely eliminate recurrent transfusion reactions.

OTHER PRACTICAL CONSIDERATIONS

As mentioned above, transfusion reactions are not uncommon in patients undergoing HSCT. Of particular concern is the occurrence of transfusion-associated GVHD. Because of their immunosuppression, HSCT transplant recipients are particularly vulnerable to this type of reaction. Transfusion-associated GVHD is especially ominous because if it occurs, it is almost uniformly fatal. Thus, blood banks and transfusion services should be rigorous in their maintenance of irradiation for cellular components provided to HSCT recipients. Part of this vigilance is the development of systems or policies to ensure that patients requiring irradiated products are recognized upon admission to a hospital. One approach to help reduce the likelihood of inadvertently releasing a nonirradiated unit is to employ universal irradiation of blood components. For instance, at this author's institution all platelet products are irradiated upon receipt from its regional blood center. In this way, elimination of GVHD associated with platelet transfusion is essentially guaranteed. This is also a prudent policy for platelets because so many of the recipients of this component are hematology/oncology patients. Although this strategy may not be practical for other components such as red cells because of the decreased shelf life of a unit after irradiation, other approaches may be developed. For example, some institutions irradiate all components issued to their inpatient hematology/oncology wards and outpatient clinics. This more selective strategy is also helpful in reducing the opportunity for transfusion-associated GVHD.

Other than GVHD, HSCT recipients are not necessarily at increased risk for other forms of reactions. However, the evaluation of suspected transfusion reactions in this patient population can be complex, given the substantial immunosuppression associated with transplantation and the evolution of blood group antigens and antibodies during the engraftment process. There are some subtle clinical hints that may help clinicians distinguish between a true transfusion reaction and an underlying disease process. For instance, in the setting of a fever temporally associated with transfusion, temperature increases occurring within 2 hours of the initiation or cessation of transfusion are more likely to be related to the transfusion; temperature increases occurring more than 2 hours after stopping a transfusion are much more likely to be from another cause.[53] In addition, patients demonstrating any fever during the 24 hours preceding transfusion should be evaluated for another cause for their temperature increase, as this pattern may suggest an underlying infection or inflammatory process.[53] Blood banks can also take some broad measures to help prevent adverse events associated with transfusion. It has been repeatedly demonstrated that leukocyte reduction reduces febrile reactions associated with red cell and platelet transfusion.[65,66] Thus, in addition to preventing HLA alloimmunization and CMV spread, implementation of universal leukocyte reduction can also help patients to better tolerate transfusion therapy.

Yet another consideration is the fact that many patients will undergo HSCT far from their "home" medical institution. Eventually, these patients will return for follow-up care with their own hematology/oncology and primary care physicians. Supporting such patients constitutes a significant challenge for the transfusion service. The flow of information from the transplant center to local providers is rarely perfect; with increased complexity of care, some critical data such as donor ABO group can be overlooked. Some institutions have created a process to deal with such situations. These processes are also helpful in standardization of care within each transplant center. The transfusion service needs to play an active role in obtaining necessary information and should develop a mechanism for gathering pertinent data for patients who underwent transplantation at other facilities. When the HSCT recipient is scheduled to be seen for the first time after transplantation, the process of contacting the transplant center and obtaining all required information should be initiated. The final completed worksheet should be made available to all parties involved in provision of health care to the patient.

KEY POINTS

1. Hematopoietic stem cell transplantation (HSCT) recipients are unique patients with distinct transfusion challenges because of their immunosuppression, preexisting disease, type of transplant, and potential for changes in expressed blood group systems.
2. ABO compatibility is not critical in the selection of potential HSCT donors because pluripotent and early-committed hematopoietic progenitor cells (HPCs) lack ABO antigens. Thus, engraftment of HPCs is uninhibited even in the presence of circulating ABO antibodies. ABO incompatibility does, however, influence transfusion decisions.
3. ABO incompatibilities are present in 20% to 40% of donor/recipient pairs and can fall into one of three categories: incompatible in the major crossmatch, incompatible in the minor crossmatch, and incompatible bidirectionally.
4. ABO incompatibilities have the potential to produce acute and ongoing intravascular hemolysis. They can be partially mitigated by red cell and/or plasma depletion of the graft before infusion.
5. Some evidence suggests that ABO-incompatible transplants may be associated with increased complications, but only in a select group of patients.
6. Accreditation organizations such as the AABB are focused on ensuring safety and minimizing adverse effects related to HSCTs involving incompatible ABO or other red cell antigens.

7. Factors associated with return to adequate platelet production in HSCT recipients include the relationship between donor and recipient (related vs unrelated), the presence of graft-vs-host disease (GVHD), cytomegalovirus (CMV) infection, and the HPC CD34+ cellular dose.
8. Platelet concentrates are most frequently transfused to HSCT recipients as prophylaxis to prevent an acute hemorrhage rather than for actual bleeding. A threshold of 10,000/µL in uncomplicated thrombocytopenia is widely accepted as safe practice.
9. Cellular blood components are irradiated to inhibit the proliferation of donor lymphocytes, thereby preventing transfusion-associated GVHD. Many services indefinitely provide irradiated components to HSCT recipients.
10. Prestorage leukocyte-reduced red cell and platelet components have been generally considered equivalent to CMV-seronegative units in terms of CMV transmission risks. Some studies, however, suggest that seronegative units may be marginally safer.

REFERENCES

1. Karanes C, Nelson GO, Chitphakdithai P, et al. Twenty years of unrelated donor hematopoietic cell transplantation for adult recipients facilitated by the National Marrow Donor Program. Biol Blood Marrow Transplant 2008;14(9 Suppl):8-15.
2. Rowley SD. Hematopoietic stem cell transplantation between red cell incompatible donor-recipient pairs. Bone Marrow Transplant 2001;28:315-21.
3. Stussi G, Halter J, Schanz U, Seebach JD. ABO-histo blood group incompatibility in hematopoietic stem cell and solid organ transplantation. Transfus Apher Sci 2006;35:59-69.
4. Kaufman RM, Sloan SR. Transfusion to bone marrow or solid organ transplant recipients. In: Hillyer C, Silberstein LE, Ness PM, et al, eds. Blood banking and transfusion medicine: Basic principles and practice. 2nd ed. Philadelphia: Churchill Livingstone/Elsevier, 2007: 539-50.
5. Sniecinski IJ, O'Donnell MR. Hemolytic complications of hematopoietic cell transplantation. In: Thomas ED, Blume KG, Forman SJ, eds. Hematopoietic cell transplantation. 2nd ed. Malden, MA: Blackwell Science, 1999:674-84.
6. Bolan CD, Leitman SF, Griffith LM, et al. Delayed donor red cell chimerism and pure red cell aplasia following major ABO-incompatible nonmyeloablative hematopoietic stem cell transplantation. Blood 2001;98:1687-94.
7. Kim JG, Sohn SK, Kim DH, et al. Impact of ABO incompatibility on outcome after allogeneic peripheral blood stem cell transplantation. Bone Marrow Transplant 2005;35:489-95.
8. Helming AM, Brand A, Wolterbeek R, et al. ABO incompatible stem cell transplantation in children does not influence outcome. Pediatr Blood Cancer 2007;49:313-17.
9. Stussi G, Muntwyler J, Passweg JR, et al. Consequences of ABO incompatibility in allogeneic hematopoietic stem cell transplantation. Bone Marrow Transplant 2002;30:87-93.
10. Kimura F, Sato K, Kobayashi S, et al. Japan Marrow Donor Program. Impact of ABO-blood group incompatibility on the outcome of recipients of bone marrow transplants from unrelated donors in the Japan Marrow Donor Program. Haematologica 2008;93:1686-93.
11. Resnick IB, Tsirigotis PD, Shapira MY, et al. ABO incompatibility is associated with increased non-relapse and GVHD related mortality in patients with malignancies treated with a reduced intensity regimen: A single center experience of 221 patients. Biol Blood Marrow Transplant 2008;14:409-17.
12. Rozman P, Kosir A, Bohinjec M. Is the ABO incompatibility a risk factor in bone marrow transplantation? Transpl Immunol 2005;14: 159-69.
13. Benjamin RJ, McGurk S, Ralston MS, et al. ABO incompatibility as an adverse risk factor for survival after allogeneic bone marrow transplantation. Transfusion 1999;39:179-87.
14. Canals C, Muniz-Diaz E, Martinez C, et al. Impact of ABO incompatibility on allogeneic peripheral blood progenitor cell transplantation after reduced intensity conditioning. Transfusion 2004;44:1603-11.
15. Raimondi R, Soli M, Lamparelli T, et al. ABO-incompatible bone marrow transplantation: A

GITMO survey of current practice in Italy and comparison with the literature. Bone Marrow Transplant 2004;34:321-9.

16. Stussi G, Halter J, Bucheli E, et al. Prevention of pure red cell aplasia after major or bidirectional ABO blood group incompatible hematopoietic stem cell transplantation by pretransplant reduction of host anti-donor isoagglutinins. Haematologica 2009;94:239-48.
17. Helbig G, Stella-Holowiecka B, Krawczyk-Kulis M, et al. Successful treatment of pure red cell aplasia with repeated, low doses of rituximab in two patients after ABO-incompatible allogeneic haematopoietic stem cell transplantation for acute myeloid leukaemia. Haematologica 2005;90(Suppl):ECR33.
18. Fontaine M, ed. Standards for cellular therapy product services. 5th ed. Bethesda, MD: AABB, 2011.
19. Warkentin P, ed. Standards for hematopoietic progenitor cell collection, processing and transplantation. 2nd ed. Omaha, NE: Foundation for the Accreditation of Cellular Therapy, 2002.
20. Corwin H. Anemia and red blood cell transfusion in the critically ill. Semin Dial 2006;19: 513-16.
21. Carson J, Ferreira G. Transfusion triggers: How low can we go? Vox Sang 2004;87:218-21.
22. Fox CP, Pacey S, Das-Gupta EP, et al. Low dose erythropoietin is effective in reducing transfusion requirements following allogeneic HSCT. Transfus Med 2005;15:475-80.
23. Gaya A, Urbano-Ispizua A, Fernández-Avilés F, et al. Anemia associated with impaired erythropoietin secretion after allogeneic stem cell transplantation: Incidence, risk factors, and response to treatment. Biol Blood Marrow Transplant 2008;14:880-7.
24. Baron F, Sautois B, Baudoux E, et al. Optimization of recombinant human erythropoietin therapy after allogeneic hematopoietic stem cell transplantation. Exp Hematol 2002;30: 546-54.
25. Helbig G, Stella-Holowiecka B, Wojnar J, et al. Pure red-cell aplasia following major and bidirectional ABO-incompatible allogeneic stem-cell transplantation: Recovery of donor-derived erythropoiesis after long-term treatment using different therapeutic strategies. Ann Hematol 2007;86:677-83.
26. Blau C. Erythropoietin in cancer: Presumption of innocence. Stem Cells 2007;25:2094-7.
27. Chang YJ, Xu LP, Liu DH, et al. The impact of CD34+ cell dose on platelet engraftment in pediatric patients following unmanipulated haploidentical blood and marrow transplantation. Pediatr Blood Cancer 2009;53:1100-6.
28. Pulsipher MA, Chitphakdithai P, Logan BR, et al. Donor, recipient, and transplant characteristics as risk factors after unrelated donor PBSC transplantation: Beneficial effects of higher CD34+ cell dose. Blood 2009;114:2606-16.
29. Jansen J, Hanks SG, Akard LP, et al. Slow platelet recovery after PBPC transplantation from unrelated donors. Bone Marrow Transplant 2009;43:499-505.
30. Dominietto A, Raiola AM, van Lint MT, et al. Factors influencing haematological recovery after allogeneic haemopoietic stem cell transplants: Graft-versus-host disease, donor type, cytomegalovirus infections and cell dose. Br J Haematol 2001;112:219-27.
31. Pulanic D, Lozier JN, Pavletic SZ. Thrombocytopenia and hemostatic disorders in chronic graft versus host disease. Bone Marrow Transplant 2009;44:393-403.
32. Nash RA, Gooley T, Davis C, Appelbaum FR. The problem of thrombocytopenia after hematopoietic stem cell transplantation. Stem Cells 1996;14(Suppl 1):261-73.
33. Diaz MA, Gonzalez-Vicent M, Ramirez M, et al. Allogeneic cord blood transplantation in children with hematological malignancies: A long-term follow-up single-center study. Pediatr Hematol Oncol 2009;26:165-74.
34. Petterson TE, Gabriel M, Tiedemann K, et al. Outcome following unrelated cord blood transplant in 136 patients with malignant and non-malignant diseases: A report from the Australian and New Zealand children's haematology and oncology group. Bone Marrow Transplant 2009;43:207-15.
35. Kurtzberg J, Prasad VK, Carter SL, et al. Results of the Cord Blood Transplantation Study (COBLT): Clinical outcomes of unrelated donor umbilical cord blood transplantation in pediatric patients with hematologic malignancies. Blood 2008;112:4318-27.
36. Cornetta K, Laughlin M, Carter S, et al. Umbilical cord blood transplantation in adults: Results of the prospective Cord Blood Transplantation (COBLT). Biol Blood Marrow Transplant 2005;11:149-60.
37. Sadani DT, Urbaniak SJ, Bruce M, Tighe JE. Repeat ABO-incompatible platelet transfusions

leading to haemolytic transfusion reaction. Transfus Med 2006;16:375-9.
38. Lapierre V, Mahe C, Auperin A, et al. Platelet transfusion containing ABO-incompatible plasma and hepatic veno-occlusive disease after hematopoietic transplantation in young children. Transplantation 2005;80:314-19.
39. Heal JM, Liesveld JL, Phillips GL, Blumberg N. What would Karl Landsteiner do? The ABO blood group and stem cell transplantation. Bone Marrow Transplant 2005;36:747-55.
40. Wandt H, Schaefer-Eckart K, Frank M, et al. A therapeutic platelet transfusion strategy is safe and feasible in patients after autologous peripheral blood stem cell transplantation. Bone Marrow Transplant 2006;37:387-92.
41. Gmur J, Burger J, Schanz U, et al. Safety of stringent prophylactic platelet transfusion policy for patients with acute leukaemia. Lancet 1991;338:1223-6.
42. Heckman KD, Weiner GJ, Davis CS, et al. Randomized study of prophylactic platelet transfusion threshold during induction therapy for adult acute leukemia: 10,000/µL versus 20,000/µL. J Clin Oncol 1997;15:1143-9.
43. Wandt H, Frank M, Ehninger G, et al. Safety and cost effectiveness of a 10×10^9/L trigger for prophylactic platelet transfusions compared with the traditional 20×10^9/L trigger: A prospective comparative trial in 105 patients with acute myeloid leukemia. Blood 1998;91:3601-6.
44. Stanworth SJ, Hyde C, Heddle N, et al. Prophylactic platelet transfusion for haemorrhage after chemotherapy and stem cell transplantation. Cochrane Database Syst Rev 2004;(4): CD004269.
45. Zumberg MS, del Rosario ML, Nejame CF, et al. A prospective randomized trial of prophylactic platelet transfusion and bleeding incidence in hematopoietic stem cell transplant recipients: 10,000/µL versus 20,000/µL trigger. Biol Blood Marrow Transplant 2002;8:569-76.
46. Diedrich B, Remberger M, Shanwell A, et al. A prospective randomized trial of a prophylactic platelet transfusion trigger of 10×10^9 per L versus 30×10^9 per L in allogeneic hematopoietic progenitor cell transplant recipients. Transfusion 2005;45:1064-72.
47. Nevo S, Fuller AK, Zahurak ML, et al. Profound thrombocytopenia and survival of hematopoietic stem cell transplant patients without clinically significant bleeding, using prophylactic platelet transfusion triggers of 10×10^9 or 20×10^9 per L. Transfusion 2007;47:1700-9.
48. Tinmouth A, Tannock IF, Crump M, et al. Low-dose prophylactic platelet transfusions in recipients of an autologous peripheral blood progenitor cell transplant and patients with acute leukemia: A randomized controlled trial with a sequential Bayesian design. Transfusion 2004;44:1711-19.
49. Heddle NM, Cook RJ, Tinmouth A, et al. A randomized controlled trial comparing standard- and low-dose strategies for transfusion of platelets (SToP) to patients with thrombocytopenia. Blood 2009;113:1564-73.
50. Slichter SJ, Kaufman RM, Assmann SF, et al. Dose of prophylactic platelet transfusions and prevention of hemorrhage. N Engl J Med 2010; 362:600-13.
51. Pihusch M, Bacigalupo A, Szer J, et al. Recombinant activated factor VII in treatment of bleeding complications following hematopoietic stem cell transplantation. J Thromb Haemost 2005;3:1935-44.
52. Pihusch M. Bleeding complications after hematopoietic stem cell transplantation. Semin Hematol 2004;41(Suppl 1):93-100.
53. Tormey CA, Snyder EL. Transfusion support for the oncology patient. In: Simon TL, Snyder EL, Solheim BG, et al, eds. Rossi's principles of transfusion medicine. 4th ed. Bethesda, MD: AABB, 2009:482-97.
54. Balduini CL, Salvaneschi L, Klersy C, et al. Factors influencing post-transfusional platelet increment in pediatric patients given hematopoietic stem cell transplantation. Leukemia 2001;15:1885-91.
55. Leitner GC, Tanzmann A, Stiegler G, et al. Influence of human platelet antigen match on the success of stem cell transplantation after myeloablative conditioning. Bone Marrow Transplant 2003;32:821-4.
56. Garcia-Malo MD, Corral J, Gonzalez M, et al. Human platelet antigen systems in allogeneic peripheral blood progenitor cell transplantation: Effect of human platelet antigen mismatch on platelet engraftment and graft-versus-host disease. Transfusion 2004;44:771-6.
57. Lapierre V, Auperin A, Tayebi H, et al. Increased presence of anti-HLA antibodies early after allogeneic granulocyte colony-stimulating factor-mobilized peripheral blood hematopoietic stem cell transplantation compared with bone marrow transplantation. Blood 2002;100:1484-9.

58. Toor AA, Choo SY, Little JA. Bleeding risk and platelet transfusion refractoriness in patients with acute myelogenous leukemia who undergo autologous stem cell transplantation. Bone Marrow Transplant 2000;26:315-20.
59. Price TH, Bowden RA, Boeckh M, et al. Phase I/II trial of neutrophil transfusions from donors stimulated with G-CSF and dexamethasone for treatment of patients with infections in hematopoietic stem cell transplantation. Blood 2000;95:3302-9.
60. Hubel K, Carter RA, Liles WC, et al. Granulocyte transfusion therapy for infections in candidates and recipients of HPC transplantation: A comparative analysis of feasibility and outcome for community donors versus related donors. Transfusion 2002;42:1414-21.
61. Grigull L, Pulver N, Goudeva L, et al. G-CSF mobilised granulocyte transfusions in 32 paediatric patients with neutropenic sepsis. Support Care Cancer 2006;14:910-16.
62. Mousset S, Hermann S, Klein SA, et al. Prophylactic and interventional granulocyte transfusions in patients with haematological malignancies and life-threatening infections during neutropenia. Ann Hematol 2005;84:734-41.
63. Kerr JP, Liakopolou E, Brown J, et al. The use of stimulated granulocyte transfusions to prevent recurrence of past severe infections after allogeneic stem cell transplantation. Br J Haematol 2003;123:114-18.
64. Vamvakas EC. Is white blood cell reduction equivalent to antibody screening in preventing transmission of cytomegalovirus by transfusion? A review of the literature and meta-analysis. Transfus Med Rev 2005; 19:181-99.
65. Paglino JC, Pomper GJ, Fisch GS, et al. Reduction of febrile but not allergic reactions to RBCs and platelets after conversion to universal prestorage leukoreduction. Transfusion 2004;44:16-24.
66. Tormey CA, Sweeney JD, Champion MH, et al. Analysis of transfusion reactions associated with prestorage-pooled platelet components. Transfusion 2009;49:1242-7.

Chapter 26

Therapeutic Apheresis

Robertson D. Davenport, MD

THERAPEUTIC APHERESIS IS a branch of transfusion medicine encompassing the treatment of diseases through removal of blood components or specific blood substances. It is distinct from blood component collection by apheresis, which is covered in Chapter 7. The AABB provides standards for voluntary compliance for apheresis activities.[1] The American Society for Apheresis (ASFA) has published additional guidelines and recommendations for the use of therapeutic apheresis in clinical practice.[2] All personnel involved with apheresis activities should be familiar with these sources and should have documentation that they are qualified by training and experience to perform apheresis. Guidelines for therapeutic apheresis clinical privileges and for documentation of therapeutic apheresis procedures in the medical record by apheresis physicians have been published by ASFA.[3,4]

PRINCIPLES

Apheresis is the process in which whole blood is withdrawn from a person's circulation, a component such as plasma is separated out and retained, and the remainder is returned to the patient usually with some replacement fluid. In therapeutic apheresis the goal is to remove a pathologic element from the blood. This element may be a plasma protein such as an autoantibody as in myasthenia gravis, red cells as in sickle cell anemia, leukocytes as in hyperleukocytosis accompanying acute leukemia, or platelets as in marked thrombocytosis. Therapeutic plasma exchange (TPE) is the separation and removal of plasma from whole blood with replacement by a colloid solution (typically albumin or plasma) or a combination of crystalloid/colloid solution. Cytapheresis is the removal of cellular blood elements. If red cells are removed and replaced with donor Red Blood Cells (RBCs), it is called red cell exchange.

The effectiveness of apheresis in removing a pathologic substance depends on the concentration in blood, the volume of blood processed, and the equilibrium between blood and the extravascular volume of distribution. Apheresis is most efficient at the beginning of the procedure and least efficient at the end. In principle, exchange of a single blood volume will eliminate approximately two-thirds of a substance if it does not move from extravascular sites to the intravascular space (Fig 26-1). However, continued production of the sub-

Robertson D. Davenport, MD, Medical Director, Blood Bank and Transfusion Service, and Associate Professor, University of Michigan Health System, Ann Arbor, Michigan

The author has disclosed no conflicts of interest.

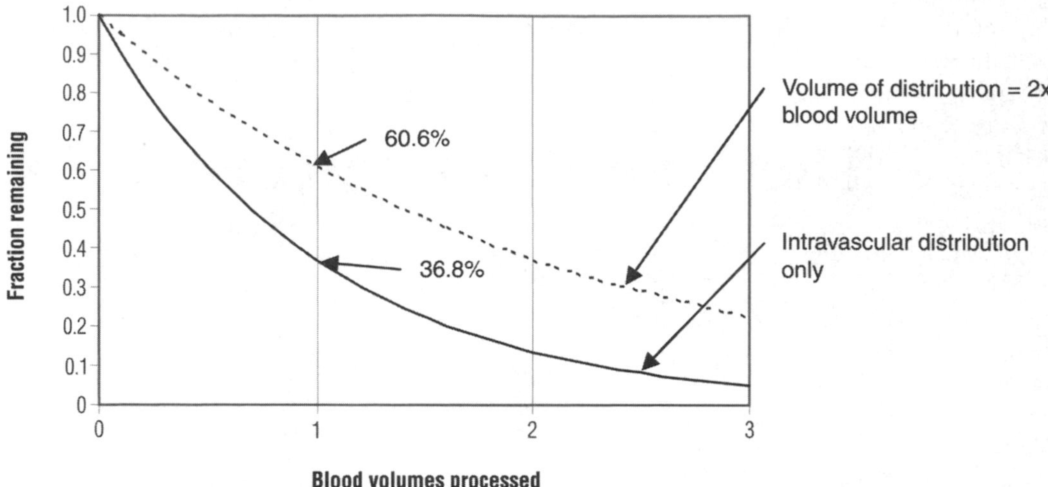

FIGURE 26-1. Theoretical removal of a substance by apheresis. For a substance that is strictly intravascular, 36.8% of the initial concentration will remain after a single blood volume exchange by apheresis. However, if the substance is also present in the extravascular space with a total volume of distribution equal to twice the blood volume, for example, 60.6% will remain after processing a single blood volume.

stance or mobilization from tissues into the intravascular space will result in less apparent reduction despite an equal or even greater total amount removed. For example, if the volume of distribution is twice the blood volume and there is equilibrium between the intravascular and extravascular compartments, a one-blood-volume apheresis procedure will remove only 40% of the substance.

TPE is usually limited to 1 or 1.5 plasma volumes, or approximately 40 to 60 mL plasma exchanged per kg of body weight in patients with normal hematocrit and average body size. Although larger volume exchange causes greater initial diminution of the pathologic substance, overall it is less efficient and requires considerably more time. Larger volume exchanges can increase the risk of coagulopathy, citrate toxicity, or electrolyte imbalance, depending on the replacement fluid.

MODALITIES

Manual plasma exchange is performed by first removing whole blood, typically the equivalent of a single unit donation. The blood is centrifuged, and the plasma is expressed into an attached bag and discarded. The cells are then reinfused to the patient along with an appropriate volume of replacement fluid, and the process is repeated. While effective, manual plasma exchange has been largely superseded by automated techniques that are faster and more efficient. Manual red cell exchange can be accomplished similarly by discarding whole blood, or the cellular component, and replacing with donor red cells.

In automated apheresis, a specialized device is used that controls the rate of blood withdrawal, anticoagulation, separation, replacement fluids, and blood return. Blood component separation is accomplished by centrifugation or filtration.

Continuous-flow centrifuge devices have a rotating channel designed so that whole blood is introduced at one site, and the blood elements subsequently separate by density as blood flows through the channel. The resulting layers of plasma, platelets, leukocytes, or red cells can be removed selectively. The component to be removed is diverted into a collection bag, while the remaining blood components are mixed with the replacement fluid and returned to the patient. The device controls the flow rates of blood withdrawal, anticoagulant solution, and replacement fluid as well as centrifuge speed to achieve optimal separation. This is the most commonly used method for therapeutic apheresis.

Intermittent centrifugation devices use an alternative method where a specified volume of whole blood is first withdrawn into a centrifuge bowl. Blood withdrawal is then stopped, and the extracorporeal blood product is processed. The procedure is then similar to the continuous-flow process in that the blood is centrifuged, the selected component is diverted into a waste bag, and the remainder is returned to the patient with appropriate replacement fluid. The process can be repeated for a certain number of cycles. Intermittent centrifugation is most commonly used for photopheresis.

Filtration devices also operate by continuous flow. The anticoagulated whole blood is passed through a microporous filter that allows plasma to pass and retains blood cells. The separated plasma can then be diverted into a waste bag, or as in the case of selective adsorption, further processed and returned to the patient. This type of device is not suitable for cytapheresis. A variant of this technique is rheopheresis, or double filtration TPE, in which high-molecular-weight molecules—primarily fibrinogen, low-density lipoprotein (LDL), fibronectin, and von Willebrand factor (vWF)—are removed. This results in reduced blood and plasma viscosity, reduced platelet and red cell aggregation, and enhanced red cell membrane flexibility, which in turn may increase perfusion and oxygen delivery to critical tissues such as the retinal pigment epithelium. Although there is limited experience with rheopheresis to date, encouraging results have been seen in clinical trials in age-related macular degeneration and sudden sensorineural hearing loss.[5,6]

In selective adsorption, blood or plasma is passed through a medium that has a high affinity for a specific component, such as IgG or LDL, and the effluent is returned to the patient. This has the advantage of highly specific removal of the element of interest. However, it is restricted to only a few conditions for which affinity adsorbers have been developed.

INDICATIONS

Although there are many case reports of successful treatment of a large variety of diseases and conditions by apheresis, there have been few high-quality trials. ASFA has published a categorization of indications for apheresis based on the best available evidence.[2]

- Category I: Apheresis is standard and acceptable as a primary therapy or in conjunction with other therapies. This designation does not imply that apheresis is mandatory in all cases.
- Category II: Apheresis is accepted as supportive therapy, either as a standalone treatment or in conjunction with other modes of treatment.
- Category III: The optimal role of apheresis therapy is not established. Decision making should be individualized.
- Category IV: Published evidence demonstrates or suggests that apheresis is ineffective or harmful in these disorders. If apheresis treatment is undertaken in these circumstances, institutional review board approval is desirable.

Therapeutic Plasma Exchange

The goal of TPE is to remove a pathogenic molecule, protein, antibody, or high-molecular-weight complex from plasma. Additionally, TPE may be used to provide a deficient normal substance, such as an enzyme or coagulation factor. Indications for TPE are listed in Table 26-1. Diseases in which a pathogenic autoantibody is targeted include acute and chronic inflammatory demyelinating polyradiculoneuropathy (AIDP and CIDP), antiglomerular basement membrane antibody disease (Goodpasture syndrome), and myasthenia gravis. Conditions in which the goal is to remove an alloantibody include renal transplantation with presensitization, and antibody-mediated organ transplant rejection.

TABLE 26-1. Indications for Therapeutic Plasma Exchange[2]

Indication	Category
ABO-incompatible hematopoietic stem cell transplantation	
Marrow	II
Peripheral hematopoietic progenitor cells	II
ABO-incompatible solid organ transplantation	
Kidney	II
Heart (<40 months of age)	II
Liver, perioperative	III
Acute disseminated encephalomyelitis	II
Acute inflammatory demyelinating polyneuropathy (Guillain-Barré syndrome)	I
Acute liver failure	III
Amyloidosis, systemic	IV
Amyotrophic lateral sclerosis	IV
Antiglomerular basement membrane disease	
Dialysis-independent	I
Diffuse alveolar hemorrhage (DAH)	I
Dialysis-dependent and no DAH	IV
Antineutrophil cytoplasmic antibody (ANCA)-associated rapidly progressive glomerulonephritis	
Dialysis-dependent	I
DAH	I
Dialysis-independent	III
Aplastic anemia	III
Autoimmune hemolytic anemia	
Warm autoimmune hemolytic anemia	III
Cold agglutinin disease (life-threatening)	II
Burn shock resuscitation	IV
Cardiac allograft antibody-mediated rejection	III
Catastrophic antiphospholipid syndrome	II
Chronic focal encephalitis (Rasmussen encephalitis)	II
Chronic inflammatory demyelinating polyradiculoneuropathy (CIDP)	I
Coagulation factor inhibitors	IV
Cryoglobulinemia, severe/symptomatic	I
Dermatomyositis or polymyositis	IV
Dilated cardiomyopathy, New York Heart Association Class II-IV	III
Familial hypercholesterolemia	
Homozygotes with small blood volume	II

TABLE 26-1. Indications for Therapeutic Plasma Exchange[2] (Continued)

Indication	Category
Focal segmental glomerulosclerosis, recurrent	I
Hemolytic uremic syndrome (HUS)	
Atypical HUS due to complement factor gene mutations	II
Atypical HUS due to autoantibody to factor H	I
Diarrhea-associated HUS or typical HUS	IV
Hypertriglyceridemic pancreatitis	III
Hyperviscosity in monoclonal gammopathies	
Treatment of symptoms	I
Prophylaxis for rituximab	I
Immune thrombocytopenia (ITP)	IV
Immune complex rapidly progressive glomerulonephritis	III
Inclusion body myositis	IV
Lambert-Eaton myasthenic syndrome	II
Multiple sclerosis	
Acute central nervous system inflammatory demyelinating disease unresponsive to steroids	II
Chronic progressive	III
Myasthenia gravis	
Moderate to severe	I
Prethymectomy	I
Myeloma cast nephropathy	II
Nephrogenic systemic fibrosis	III
Neuromyelitis optica (Devic syndrome)	II
Overdose, venoms, and poisoning	
Mushroom poisoning	II
Invenomation	III
Monoclonal antibody with progressive multifocal leukoencephalopathy	III
Other compounds	III
Paraneoplastic neurologic syndromes	III
Paraproteinemic polyneuropathies	
IgG/IgA	I
IgM	I
Multiple myeloma	III
Pediatric autoimmune neuropsychiatric disorders associated with streptococcal infections (PANDAS)	I
Pure red cell aplasia	II
Pemphigus vulgaris	IV

(Continued)

TABLE 26-1. Indications for Therapeutic Plasma Exchange[2] (Continued)

Indication	Category
Phytanic acid storage disease (Refsum disease)	II
POEMS (polyneuropathy, organomegaly, endocrinopathy, M protein, and skin changes)	IV
Posttransfusion purpura	III
Psoriasis	IV
Red cell alloimmunization in pregnancy	
Before intrauterine transfusion availability	II
Renal transplantation	
Antibody-mediated rejection (AMR)	I
Desensitization, living-donor, positive crossmatch due to donor-specific HLA antibody	II
High panel-reactive antibody; cadaveric donor	III
Rheumatoid arthritis, refractory	IV
Schizophrenia	IV
Scleroderma (progressive systemic sclerosis)	III
Sepsis with multiorgan failure	III
Stiff-person syndrome	IV
Sydenham chorea	I
Systemic lupus erythematosus	
Severe (eg, cerebritis, diffuse alveolar hemorrhage)	II
Nephritis	IV
Thrombotic microangiopathy, drug-associated	
Ticlopidine/clopidogrel	I
Cyclosporine/tacrolimus	III
Gemcitabine	IV
Quinine	IV
Thrombotic microangiopathy, hematopoietic stem cell transplant-associated	III
Thrombotic thrombocytopenic purpura (TTP)	I
Thyroid storm	III
Wilson disease, fulminant hepatic failure with hemolysis	I

In myeloma with hyperviscosity, the goal is to remove an excessive paraprotein (M protein). Measurement of plasma viscosity is useful in guiding therapy. For some pathologic proteins, plasma viscosity is highly temperature dependent, so viscosity should be measured at 37 C. Normal plasma viscosity ranges from 1.4 to 1.8 cP. Because most patients are not symptomatic until the plasma viscosity is more than 4.0 or 5.0 cP, patients with mild elevations may not require treatment. In general, hyperviscosity becomes a concern when M protein concentrations reach 3 g/dL for IgM, 4 g/dL for IgG, and 6 g/dL for IgA.[7] Patients receiving rituximab (anti-CD20) therapy for IgM myeloma may experience a transient increase in M protein levels. Patients with pretreatment IgM greater than 5 g/dL are at particular risk of developing symptomatic hyperviscosity.[8]

Data have been conflicting regarding the efficacy of TPE for treatment of acute renal failure in myeloma. A randomized controlled trial of TPE vs conventional care showed no difference in mortality or renal function at 6 months.[9] However, among dialysis-dependent patients, 43% in the TPE group and none in the control group recovered renal function. Another randomized clinical trial showed no benefit to TPE in a composite outcome measure of death, dialysis dependence, and glomerular filtration rate.[10] However, biopsy confirmation of the renal diagnosis was not required in this trial. Similarly, a recent retrospective cohort study showed no benefit of TPE in either reducing mortality or preserving renal function.[11] If TPE is to be undertaken, biopsy confirmation of cast nephropathy may be advisable.

Diseases in which immune complexes may be pathogenic and can be removed by apheresis include rapidly progressive glomerulonephritis, cryoglobulinemia, and vasculitis. Other indications include removal of protein-bound drugs or toxins or high-concentration lipoproteins.

In thrombotic thrombocytopenic purpura (TTP), a deficiency of the vWF-cleaving metalloprotease ADAMTS13 results in accumulation of high-molecular-weight vWF multimers with subsequent intravascular platelet activation.[12] In many cases, an inhibitor of ADAMTS13 can be demonstrated. Plasma exchange is first-line treatment for TTP, with the goal of removing both the inhibitor and large vWF multimers while simultaneously replacing the deficient enzyme. Secondary forms of microangiopathic hemolytic anemia associated with systemic lupus erythematosus (SLE), hematopoietic progenitor cell transplantation, chemotherapy, or immunosuppressive medications may be clinically indistinguishable from idiopathic TTP. However, in many cases ADAMTS13 activity has been shown to be normal or moderately reduced, and the response to plasma exchange is typically poor. Transplant-associated microangiopathic hemolysis rarely responds to apheresis and probably represents a different disease process.[13]

TPE in TTP is typically performed daily until the platelet count and lactate dehydrogenase (LDH) are in the normal range, but the intensity and duration of treatment should be guided by the individual patient's course. After response has been achieved, intermittent apheresis or plasma infusion taper may be instituted, but the efficacy of this approach in preventing relapse has not been established.[14] TPE therapy has greatly improved the survival rate in TTP; however, treatment failures do occur and cause major morbidity or death.[15]

Hemolytic uremic syndrome (HUS) is a similar condition that occurs more commonly in children than adults. HUS may follow diarrheal infections with verotoxin-secreting strains of *Escherichia coli* (strain 0157:H7) or *Shigella*. Compared to patients who have classic TTP, those with HUS have more renal dysfunction and less prominent neurologic and hematologic findings. Most patients with HUS do not have antibody to ADAMTS13 and have normal activity of this protease. Although diarrhea-associated HUS rarely responds to TPE, atypical HUS caused by complement factor deficiencies or autoantibodies to factor H may respond.

The role of TPE in treatment of central nervous system (CNS) demyelinating disorders is controversial. Experience in treating chronic progressive multiple sclerosis with TPE has been discouraging. However, a randomized clinical trial in acute CNS inflammatory demyelinating diseases unresponsive to steroids showed benefit of TPE.[16] Early initiation of TPE is predictive of response, and some clinical responses may not manifest until later in follow-up.[17] TPE may be effective in neuromyelitis optica, even in the absence of NMO antibodies.[18]

In focal segmental glomerulosclerosis (FSGS), a circulating factor that increases glomerular permeability with resultant proteinuria has been demonstrated.[19] The molecular characteristics of this factor have not been elucidated. FSGS frequently recurs after renal transplantation and can result in allograft failure. TPE has been shown to effectively remove the permeability factor and induce remission in posttransplant recurrent FSGS. Response to TPE in the primary form of the disease has not been well studied.

TPE may be an adjunct to immunosuppression in the treatment or prevention of antibody-mediated rejection (AMR) of solid organ transplants. Shorter time from transplantation to the occurrence of AMR is predictive of response to TPE.[20] TPE before renal transplantation of an ABO-incompatible kidney can prevent hyperacute AMR, although delayed AMR and delayed graft function may occur.[21,22]

TPE in conjunction with immunomodulatory therapies, such as intravenous immune globulin (IVIG), before transplantation can reduce the risk of rejection in HLA-alloimmunized patients.

Cytapheresis

The goal of cytapheresis is to remove excessive or pathogenic leukocytes, platelets, or red cells. In addition, in red cell exchange, donor red cells are used for replacement of oxygen-carrying capacity and, in sickle cell disease, hemoglobin A. Indications for cytapheresis are listed in Table 26-2.

In settings of acute leukemia, high blast counts (typically >100,000/µL) can result in microvascular stasis with headache, mental status changes, visual disturbances, or dyspnea. The leukocyte count at which a patient may become symptomatic is variable. Typically, patients with acute or chronic lymphocytic leukemia tolerate higher cell counts than patients with myelogenous leukemia, and cytapheresis is not required. Cytapheresis commonly re-

TABLE 26-2. Indications for Cytapheresis[2]

Indication	Procedure	Category
Babesiosis		
Severe	Red cell exchange	I
High-risk population	Red cell exchange	II
Dermatomyositis or polymyositis	Leukocytapheresis	IV
Hereditary hemochromatosis	Erythrocytapheresis	III
Hyperleukocytosis		
Leukostasis	Leukocytapheresis	I
Prophylaxis	Leukocytapheresis	III
Inclusion body myositis	Leukocytapheresis	IV
Inflammatory bowel disease	Adsorptive cytapheresis	II
Malaria, severe	Red cell exchange	II
Polycythemia vera	Erythrocytapheresis	III
Secondary erythrocytosis	Erythrocytapheresis	III
Sickle cell disease		
Acute stroke	Red cell exchange	I
Acute chest syndrome	Red cell exchange	II
Stroke prophylaxis; prevention of iron overload	Red cell exchange	II
Multiorgan failure	Red cell exchange	III
Thrombocytosis		
Symptomatic	Thrombocytapheresis	II
Prophylactic or secondary	Thrombocytapheresis	III

sults in a less-than-predicted reduction in leukocyte count, despite excellent collection, because of mobilization and reequilibration of cells from extravascular sites. Myelogenous leukemia cells commonly have a higher density than lymphocytic cells and can be difficult to separate from red cells. Use of hydroxyethyl starch enhances red cell sedimentation by rouleaux formation and can improve the efficiency of cytapheresis in acute myelogenous leukemia. Massive thrombocytosis, typically >1,000,000/μL, can occur in essential thrombocythemia, in polycythemia vera, or occasionally as a reactive phenomenon. Such patients may be at risk of thrombosis. Reduction in platelet count is commonly less than predicted because of mobilization of platelets to the peripheral blood, primarily from the spleen.

Red cell exchange is most commonly performed in the setting of sickle cell anemia. Here the goal is both to reduce the burden of hemoglobin S and to provide donor red cells containing hemoglobin A. Acute chest syndrome is a serious complication of sickle cell disease, presenting as dyspnea, chest pain, and cough, often accompanied by fever, leukocytosis, decreasing hematocrit, and pulmonary infiltrates. Respiratory failure can develop, and death occurs in about 3% of cases.[23] Exchange transfusion is indicated for progressive infiltrates and hypoxemia refractory to conventional therapy and simple transfusion.[24,25] The goal is to reduce hemoglobin S to less than 30% with a final hematocrit not higher than 30%. Red cell exchange may also be indicated for prevention of stroke in sickle cell anemia. For patients with elevated cerebral blood flow velocity, transfusion reduces the risk of stroke.[26,27] Chronic red cell exchange, typically every 4 to 6 weeks, can be effective in controlling cerebral blood flow while reducing the problems of iron overload. The role of red cell exchange in other sickle cell syndromes, including priapism and pain crisis, has not been established. Red cell exchange for priapism has been associated with adverse neurologic events (ASPEN syndrome).[28] In the setting of malaria or babesiosis with a heavy parasite burden, red cell exchange may also be used to prevent complications.

Photopheresis

Photopheresis is a specialized procedure in which the buffy-coat layer is collected from peripheral blood, treated with 8-methoxypsoralen (8-MOP) and ultraviolet light, and reinfused into the patient. The treatment causes crosslinking of leukocyte DNA, which prevents replication and induces apoptosis. The procedure was developed for the treatment of cutaneous T-cell lymphoma, although it is increasingly used for other indications (Table 26-3). Photopheresis has complex immunomodulatory effects, including induction of monocyte differentiation to dendritic cells, alteration of T-cell subsets, and changes in cytokine production profiles.[29] Depending on the setting, these effects may be proinflammatory or tolerogenic. There is encouraging evidence for the efficacy of photopheresis in chronic graft-vs-host disease (GVHD) and organ transplant rejection, but the precise role for this therapy remains to be established.[30,31] In general, skin GVHD tends to respond better than involvement of other sites such as the gastrointestinal

TABLE 26-3. Indications for Photopheresis[2]

Indication	Category
Cardiac allograft rejection	
Prophylaxis	I
Treatment of rejection	II
Cutaneous T-cell lymphoma; mycosis fungoides; Sézary syndrome	
Erythrodermic	I
Nonerythrodermic	III
Graft-vs-host disease	
Skin (chronic)	II
Skin (acute)	II
Nonskin (acute/chronic)	III
Lung allograft rejection	II
Nephrogenic systemic fibrosis	III
Pemphigus vulgaris	III
Scleroderma (progressive systemic sclerosis)	IV

tract. Extracorporeal photochemotherapy (ECP) for organ transplant rejection has been best studied in cardiac transplantation. In randomized clinical trials, prophylactic ECP in conjunction with standard immunosuppression (cyclosporine, azathioprine, and prednisone) resulted in fewer rejection episodes, decreased HLA antibodies, and reduced coronary artery intimal thickness, but no difference in time to first episode, incidence of hemodynamic compromise, or survival at 6 or 12 months.[32,33] In recurrent cardiac rejection, ECP may decrease severity of rejection and allow for reduced dosage of immunosuppressives.[34] However, the role of ECP with current immunosuppression has not been studied. There is limited evidence regarding ECP in other solid organ transplants.[35]

TABLE 26-4. Indications for Selective Adsorption[2]

Indication	Category
Chronic focal encephalitis (Rasmussen encephalitis)	II
Coagulation factor inhibitors	III
Cryoglobulinemia	
Secondary to hepatitis C virus	II
Dilated cardiomyopathy	
New York Heart Association Class II-IV	III
Familial hypercholesterolemia	
Homozygous	I
Heterozygous	II
Paraneoplastic neurologic syndromes	III
Paraproteinemic polyneuropathies	
IgG/IgA or IgM	III
Rheumatoid arthritis, refractory	II

Selective Adsorption

There are presently few established indications for selective adsorption of plasma proteins (Table 26-4) and few devices that have received approval from the Food and Drug Administration (FDA).

Selective removal of LDL can be accomplished by passing heparinized plasma over a dextran sulfate column (Liposorber, Kaneka Pharma America, New York, NY); by precipitation of heparin-LDL complexes in acidified plasma, known as heparin extracorporeal LDL precipitation (HELP System, B. Braun Medical Inc, Bethlehem, PA); or by passing whole blood over beads coated with anionic polyacrylate ligands (DALI, Fresenius Medical Care AG, Bad Homburg, Germany). The first two systems are FDA approved for the treatment of familial hypercholesterolemia refractory to maximal medical management. LDL apheresis markedly reduces LDL levels with minimal impact on high-density lipoprotein. Because LDL production continues, apheresis treatments must be repeated, typically at 2-week intervals, indefinitely. There is good evidence that LDL apheresis reduces the incidence of major coronary events and stroke.[36] In addition, atherosclerotic plaque regression can occur in some patients.[37] Secondary effects of LDL apheresis that may be beneficial include reduction in C-reactive protein, fibrinogen, tissue factor, and soluble adhesion molecules.[38,39]

IgG can be selectively removed by passing plasma over a column of staphylococcal protein A bound to silica. One such device (Prosorba, Fresenius HemoCare, Redmond, WA) is FDA-approved for treatment of refractory immune thrombocytopenic purpura and treatment of rheumatoid arthritis in patients who have failed methotrexate or other second-line drugs.[40-42] The column binds approximately 1 g of IgG and immune complexes. The putative mechanism of action is the removal of pathogenic autoantibodies or immune complexes, although there is some controversy.[43] Staphylococcal protein A adsorption treatment can be performed manually or in conjunction with automated TPE. However, at present no manufacturer is marketing protein A columns in the United States.

Selective removal of leukocytes in the treatment of inflammatory bowel disease is controversial. Selective removal of granulocytes and monocytes can be accomplished with either a column containing cylindrical nonwoven polyester fibers (Cellsorba, Asahi Kasei Kuraray Medical, Tokyo, Japan) or cellulose acetate beads (Adacolumn, JIMRO, Takasaki, Japan). Several randomized clinical trials have shown efficacy in treatment of ulcerative colitis and Crohn disease.[44] However, in many of these trials, treatment allocation was not concealed from the subjects. Of note, two Phase III randomized, double-blind, sham-controlled trials in patients with moderate-to-severe ulcerative colitis or moderate-to-severe Crohn disease did not demonstrate efficacy for induction of clinical remission or response.[45,46] These devices are not currently FDA approved.

ANTICOAGULATION

Sodium citrate, the most commonly used anticoagulant for therapeutic apheresis, acts by chelating ionized calcium and preventing clot formation. Current automated apheresis devices control the administration rate of citrate to achieve anticoagulation while minimizing the risk for hypocalcemia. Heparin anticoagulation is necessary for LDL apheresis and may be desirable for selected patients undergoing TPE who are particularly susceptible to hypocalcemia, such as small children. With citrate anticoagulation, coagulation monitoring is not necessary, although monitoring of ionized calcium may be helpful for selected patients (see "Adverse Effects"). The infused citrate in the returned blood is rapidly metabolized and rarely causes systemic anticoagulation. For procedures in which heparin is used, monitoring the activated clotting time can be helpful in guiding dosage.

REPLACEMENT FLUIDS

Considerations in the selection of replacement fluid include the type of procedure, the indication, and the patient's coagulation status. Five-percent albumin is the most commonly used replacement fluid for TPE. Albumin has a long shelf life, carries minimal risk of infectious disease transmission, and provides normal oncotic pressure. Albumin lacks coagulation factors, ADAMTS13, immunoglobulins, and calcium. During intensive TPE with albumin replacement, depletion of other plasma proteins can occur (see "Adverse Effects"), which may require temporary use of plasma as a replacement fluid.

Plasma replacement is specifically indicated for the treatment of TTP or in the treatment of patients with coagulation factor deficiencies or bleeding risks. For patients without an underlying coagulopathy who are undergoing intensive TPE, albumin can be used for the first part of the procedure and the final liter replaced with plasma. The use of plasma should be limited because of the risks of allergic reactions and transfusion-related acute lung injury (TRALI) in addition to a small, finite risk of infectious disease transmission.

Cryoprecipitate-reduced plasma (CRP) is an alternative to plasma for the treatment of TTP. CRP is manufactured by refreezing the supernatant plasma after the removal of cryoprecipitate. It is relatively deficient in the high-molecular-weight forms of vWF and retains normal ADAMTS13 activity. CRP thus would appear to be preferable to plasma in plasma exchange for TTP. However, presently there is no definitive evidence for the superiority of CRP.[47] A comparison of replacement fluids for TPE is shown in Table 26-5.

RBCs are required for replacement in red cell exchange. In addition to compatibility with ABO and any known alloantibodies, in the treatment of patients with sickle cell anemia, the RBCs should be matched for C, E, and K.[48] It is desirable to use comparatively fresh units to maximize posttransfusion red cell survival. Units containing either citrate-phosphate-dextrose-adenine (CPDA)-1 or additive solutions (AS) may be used. AS units have a greater volume, but this is seldom clinically significant. It is desirable that all units used in a given procedure contain the same anticoagulant solution so that they have similar hematocrits. This simplifies calculation of the replacement volume required. RBCs may also be used to prime the apheresis circuit when treating small patients (ie, <10 kg) in whom the extracorporeal volume is a substantial fraction of the blood volume. Red cell exchange carries

TABLE 26-5. Comparison of Replacement Fluids

Replacement Solution	Advantages	Disadvantages
Crystalloids	Low cost Nonallergenic No viral risk	2-3 volumes required Hypo-oncotic Lacks coagulation factors and immunoglobulins
Albumin	Iso-oncotic Low risk of reactions	Higher cost Lacks coagulation factors and immunoglobulins
Plasma	Iso-oncotic Normal levels of coagulation factors, immunoglobulins and other plasma proteins	Viral transmission risk Citrate load ABO compatibility required Risk of allergic reactions
Cryoprecipitate-reduced plasma	Iso-oncotic Reduced HMW vWF Normal levels of most other plasma proteins	Same as plasma

HMW vWF = high-molecular-weight von Willebrand factor.

the same risks of transfusion reactions and infectious disease transmission as red cell transfusion.

ADVERSE EFFECTS

Although therapeutic apheresis is very safe, complications do occur. Some adverse event occurs in about 4% of procedures (Table 26-6), the great majority of which are mild.[49,50] The frequency of reactions is similar for TPE and cytapheresis. Complications are less common with photopheresis, most likely because citrate is not used and the flow rates are lower. Symptomatic hypocalcemia from infusion of citrate with the returned blood is the most common adverse effect of apheresis. Perioral and digital paresthesias are the most common symptoms. Nausea may also occur. Tetany is rare. Cardiac arrhythmia is very rare, but patients with preexisting hypocalcemia or significant prolongation of the QT interval should be monitored carefully. Calcium supplementation may alleviate the symptoms of citrate toxicity. A typical supplementary dose is 10 mL of 10% calcium gluconate per liter of albumin. Citrate also chelates ionized magnesium, so it is possible that hypomagnesemia contributes to the symptoms of citrate toxicity. However, one randomized clinical trial showed no benefit to adding magnesium during leukapheresis with continuous intravenous calcium supplementation.[51] The metabolism of citrate leads to a mild metabolic alkalosis, which can exacerbate hypocalcemia and may cause hypokalemia.[52]

Allergic reactions are most common with plasma replacement, although they may occur with albumin as well. Most reactions are mild, such as urticaria or cutaneous flushing. More severe reactions can involve the airways with dyspnea, wheezing, and (rarely) stridor. Most allergic reactions respond quickly to intravenous diphenhydramine. Anaphylaxis is very rare but can occur. Patients with TTP who receive large volumes of plasma are most at risk of allergic reactions. Premedication with an antihistamine, or possibly a steroid, is not necessary for routine apheresis but may be indicated for patients with repeated or previous severe reactions.

Respiratory difficulty during or immediately following apheresis can have many causes, such as pulmonary edema, pulmonary em-

TABLE 26-6. Reported Frequency of Adverse Reactions to Apheresis

Reaction	Frequency (%)
Paresthesia	1.30
Hypotension	0.91
Urticaria	0.63
Nausea	0.39
Shivering	0.29
Flushing	0.16
Dyspnea	0.15
Vertigo	0.17
Arrhythmia	0.11
Abdominal pain	0.12
Anaphylaxis	0.02
Total	4.26

Adapted from Norda et al.[49]

bolism, air embolism, obstruction of the pulmonary microvasculature, anaphylactic reactions, and TRALI.[53] Hemothorax or hemopericardium due to vascular erosion by a central venous catheter is rare, but when it occurs it is typically unsuspected and may be fatal.[54] Pulmonary edema that results from volume overload or cardiac failure is usually associated with dyspnea, an increase in the diastolic blood pressure, and characteristic chest radiograph findings. Acute pulmonary edema may also arise from damage to alveolar capillary membranes secondary to an immune reaction or to vasoactive substances in plasma or colloid solutions prepared from human plasma. Predominantly ocular (periorbital edema, conjunctival swelling, and tearing) reactions have occurred in donors sensitized to the ethylene oxide gas used to sterilize disposable plastic apheresis kits.[55,56]

Hypotension during apheresis can be a sign of citrate toxicity, hypovolemia, a vasovagal reaction, an allergic reaction, a drug reaction, or a transfusion reaction. Hypovolemia can occur early in a treatment of a small patient when the return fluid consists of the saline used to prime the apheresis circuit. Vasovagal reactions are characterized by bradycardia and hypotension. Such reactions usually respond well to a fluid bolus and placing the patient in the Trendelenburg position. When hypotension occurs during plasma or red cell exchange, a transfusion reaction such as TRALI, acute hemolysis, bacterial contamination, or anti-IgA-related anaphylaxis should be considered. Hypotension is more frequent in children, the elderly, neurology patients, anemic patients, and those treated with intermittent-flow devices that have large extracorporeal volumes. Continuous-flow devices typically do not require large extracorporeal volumes but can produce hypovolemia if return flow is inadvertently diverted to a waste collection bag, either through operator oversight or device malfunction. Hypovolemia may also be secondary to inadequate volume or protein replacement. During all procedures, it is essential to maintain careful and continuous records of the volumes removed and returned.

When plasma is exposed to foreign surfaces of plastic tubing or filtration devices, the kinin system can be activated, resulting in production of bradykinin. Infusion of plasma containing bradykinin can cause abrupt hypotension. Patients taking angiotensin-converting enzyme (ACE) inhibitors are more susceptible to the hypotensive reactions because the drugs block enzymatic degradation of bradykinin. Hypotensive reactions are more likely during selective adsorption procedures because the devices expose plasma to a very large surface area. Because some ACE inhibitors have a long duration of action, stopping the drug 1 day or less before the procedure may not be sufficient to prevent a reaction.

Intensive TPE without plasma replacement causes depletion of coagulation factors. A one-plasma-volume exchange will typically reduce coagulation factor levels by 25% to 50%, though Factor VIII levels are less affected.[57] Fibrinogen, a large molecule without extravascular distribution, will be reduced by about 66%. If the patient has normal hepatic synthetic function, coagulation factor levels return to near normal within 2 days, so many patients can tolerate TPE every other day for 1 or 2 weeks without developing coagulopathies that require replacement.

Bleeding as a consequence of coagulation factor depletion is very rare but has been reported. For patients at risk, plasma can be used for replacement at the end of the procedure. TPE can also cause thrombocytopenia. Typically an acute decrease in platelet count by 25% can be expected after a one-plasma-volume exchange. Clinically significant thrombocytopenia is very unusual unless the patient has suppressed marrow function. Intensive TPE can cause hypogammaglobulinemia. Serum levels of IgG and IgM recover to about 40% to 50% of the preapheresis level at 48 hours.[57] The absolute immunoglobulin level at which a patient becomes at risk for infections has not been established, but immunoglobulin replacement in the form of IVIG after apheresis may be advisable for some patients. Protein-bound drugs are effectively removed by TPE. This can result in a patient becoming subtherapeutic for their medications unless dosage adjustments are made. Particular care should be taken with anticonvulsants such as phenytoin, as abrupt reduction in plasma levels can precipitate a seizure. High-molecular-weight biologicals such as IVIG, antithymocyte globulin, and monoclonal antibodies such as rituximab have a long intravascular half-life and are readily removed by apheresis. TPE shortly after administration of such drugs should be avoided because it may significantly impair their effectiveness. Additionally, intensive apheresis reduces the concentration of potentially diagnostic plasma constituents, so blood for testing should be drawn before initiating a course of treatment.

Collapsed or kinked tubing, malfunctioning pinch valves, or improper threading of tubing may damage red cells in the extracorporeal circuit. Machine-related hemolysis has been reported in 0.06% of therapeutic apheresis procedures.[50] Hemolysis can also occur with incompatible replacement fluids such as D5W (eg, D5W used to dilute 25% albumin) or ABO-incompatible plasma. The operator should carefully observe plasma collection lines for pink discoloration suggestive of hemolysis. Other types of equipment failure such as problems with the rotating seal, leaks in the plastic, and roller pump failure are rare.

Fatalities during apheresis are rare. Death has been reported in 0.006% to 0.09% of therapeutic procedures.[50,58] Most fatalities are attributable to underlying medical conditions.

VASCULAR ACCESS

Therapeutic apheresis requires good vascular access to achieve adequate flow rates. Peripheral access generally requires at least a 17-gauge needle for blood withdrawal and at least an 18-gauge catheter for return. Patients without adequate peripheral veins or who require multiple frequent procedures may require central venous catheters. Central venous catheters for apheresis must be rigid walled to accommodate the negative pressure generated in the withdrawal line. Catheters designed for hemodialysis usually work well. Peripherally inserted central catheters (PICC lines) should be avoided. At least two lumens are required for continuous-flow procedures, although single-lumen catheters can be used for intermittent-flow procedures, such as photopheresis.

The choice of placement site for a central catheter is influenced by the expected length of treatment. Subclavian or internal jugular access is generally preferable for treatments lasting up to several weeks. Femoral access should only be used temporarily. Patients requiring long-term treatment usually have a tunneled catheter. With proper care, tunneled catheters can be used for a year or more.

Good catheter care is very important to maintain patency and prevent complications. Catheters need to be flushed regularly. Heparin is usually placed in each lumen after each use to prevent occlusion by clots. Alternative methods are available for patients in whom heparin is contraindicated. If a port becomes clotted, instillation of a fibrinolytic agent such as urokinase may restore patency. Routine dressing care is essential to prevent insertion site infections. An arteriovenous (AV) fistula can also be used for apheresis, but apheresis personnel should be suitably trained before attempting to access an AV fistula.

Apheresis Service Evaluation Form

Name: ______________________ **Location** ____________

Reg. No.: ______________________ **Age:** ________ **M/F:** ________

Attending Physician: ______________________

Procedure Requested: ______________________

Indication: ______________________

Recent Medical History: ______________________

____

____

PE: ________ BP: ________ Pulse: ________ Height: ________ Weight: ________

Allergies: ______________________ Transfusion Rxn: ____________

Neuro: ______________________

Cardiac: ______________________

Pulmonary: ______________________

Renal: ______________________

Hematology: ______________________

Venous Access: Peripheral Dialysis Catheter A-V fistula (CRF)

Pertinent Laboratories: ABO/RH ____________

CBC: Electrolytes: PT/PTT ____________

Total Protein ____________

Albumin ____________

Ionized CA++ ____________

Other: ______________________

____

Medications*: ______________________

____

FIGURE 26-2. Sample apheresis evaluation form. (Courtesy Robertson D. Davenport, MD)
*ACE-Inhibitors (Lotensin/Benazepril, Capoten/Captopril, Vasotec/Enalopril, Monopril/Fosinopril, Zestril/Prinivil/Linsinopril, Accupril/Quinapril, Univasc/Moesipril, Altace/Ramipril, Movik/Trandolopril). Diabetic (eat before procedure): Insulin, oral hypoglycemics. Protein-bound Drugs: Dilantin, Valproic Acid, Digitoxin, Warfarin, Propranolol, Mycophenolate (check others). Biologicals: Thymoglobulin, ATGAM, IVIG, rituximab.

Venous access devices may cause further vascular damage, sometimes resulting in thrombosis. Infrequently, they may result in severe complications such as pneumothorax or perforation of the heart or great vessels. Other complications include arterial puncture, deep hematomas, and AV fistula formation. Bacterial colonization often complicates long-term placement and may lead to catheter-associated sepsis, especially in patients who are receiving steroids or other immunosuppressants. Inadvertent disconnection of catheters may produce hemorrhage or air embolism.

PATIENT EVALUATION

All patients should be evaluated by a physician familiar with apheresis before starting treatment. The indication, type of procedure, frequency and number of treatments, and the goal or endpoint should be documented in the patient's medical record. The nature of the procedure, the expected benefits, the possible risks, and the available alternatives should be explained to the patient by a knowledgeable individual, and the patient's consent should be documented. The procedure should be performed only in a setting where there is ready access to care for untoward reactions; such a setting includes equipment, medications, and personnel trained in managing serious adverse events such as anaphylaxis.

The assessment should include evaluation of the indication, medical conditions that may affect the ability of the patient to tolerate apheresis, vascular access, and medications. An example of an evaluation form is shown in Fig 26-2. Some points to consider include the following:

- *Transfusion history:* history of transfusion reactions; special blood component requirements.
- *Neurologic status:* mental status; ability to consent and cooperate; history of seizures.
- *Cardiorespiratory status:* adequate ventilation and oxygenation; hyper- or hypovolemia; cardiac arrhythmia.
- *Renal and metabolic status:* fluid balance; electrolyte abnormalities, including hypocalcemia, hypokalemia, and hypomagnesemia.
- *Hematologic status:* significant anemia or thrombocytopenia; coagulopathy; bleeding or thrombosis.
- *Medications:* protein-bound drugs; immunoglobulin and biologicals.

Appropriate laboratory monitoring is dictated by the indication, type and frequency of procedures, and concomitant medical conditions. In general, it is wise to obtain a complete blood cell count (CBC), type and screen, and electrolytes assessment before starting treatment. If at all possible, diagnostic studies such as for infectious disease, pregnancy, ADAMTS13 activity, glomerular basement membrane antibody, or acetylcholine receptor antibody should be obtained before the first treatment, particularly if plasma is used for replacement. Coagulation monitoring may be appropriate when albumin is used for replacement during frequently repeated procedures. Therapeutic drug monitoring is helpful in guiding dosage of protein-bound drugs, especially anti-seizure medications. Periodically checking immunoglobulin levels is appropriate for patients receiving long-term treatment.

KEY POINTS

1. Therapeutic apheresis treats disease by removal of pathologic plasma substances, white cells, platelets, or red cells, and may be accomplished by continuous centrifugation, filtration, selective adsorption, or photopheresis.
2. The American Society for Apheresis (ASFA) has published guidelines and recommendations for the use of therapeutic apheresis in clinical practice.
3. Anticoagulation is usually accomplished with citrate, although heparin may be used, particularly for selective adsorption and photopheresis.

4. Albumin is the most commonly used replacement fluid for therapeutic plasma exchange, but plasma may be indicated for patients with thrombotic thrombocytopenic purpura or coagulopathies.
5. Adverse effects of apheresis are usually mild but may include symptomatic hypocalcemia, hypotension, urticaria, nausea, and pain. Complications of apheresis can include coagulopathy, hypogammaglobulinemia, thrombocytopenia, and removal of protein-bound drugs and biologicals.
6. Vascular access for apheresis may be accomplished through peripheral veins, but a central venous catheter or an arteriovenous fistula are required for some patients.
7. Medical evaluation of the apheresis patient should focus on the indication, type of procedure, frequency and number of treatments, therapeutic goal, ability of the patient to tolerate apheresis, vascular access, and medications. Appropriate laboratory monitoring is dictated by the indication, type and frequency of procedures, and concomitant medical conditions.

REFERENCES

1. Carson TH, ed. Standards for blood banks and transfusion services. 27th ed. Bethesda, MD: AABB, 2011.
2. Szczepiorkowski ZM, Winters JL, Bandarenko N, et al. Guidelines on the use of therapeutic apheresis in clinical practice—evidence-based approach from the Apheresis Applications Committee of the American Society for Apheresis. J Clin Apher 2010;25:83-177.
3. Guidelines for therapeutic apheresis clinical privileges. J Clin Apher 2007;22:181-2.
4. Guidelines for documentation of therapeutic apheresis procedures in the medical record by apheresis physicians. J Clin Apher 2007;22:183.
5. Koss MJ, Kurz P, Tsobanelis T, et al. Prospective, randomized, controlled clinical study evaluating the efficacy of rheopheresis for dry age-related macular degeneration. Dry AMD treatment with Rheopheresis Trial-ART. Graefes Arch Clin Exp Ophthalmol 2009;247: 1297-306.
6. Mosges R, Koberlein J, Heibges A, et al. Rheopheresis for idiopathic sudden hearing loss: Results from a large prospective, multicenter, randomized, controlled clinical trial. Eur Arch Otorhinolaryngol 2009;266:943-53.
7. Somer T. Rheology of paraproteinaemias and the plasma hyperviscosity syndrome. Baillieres Clin Haematol 1987;1:695-723.
8. Treon SP, Branagan AR, Hunter Z, et al. Paradoxical increases in serum IgM and viscosity levels following rituximab in Waldenstrom's macroglobulinemia. Ann Oncol 2004;15:1481-3.
9. Johnson WJ, Kyle RA, Pineda AA, et al. Treatment of renal failure associated with multiple myeloma. Plasmapheresis, hemodialysis, and chemotherapy. Arch Intern Med 1990;150:863-9.
10. Clark WF, Stewart AK, Rock GA, et al. Plasma exchange when myeloma presents as acute renal failure: A randomized, controlled trial. Ann Intern Med 2005;143:777-84.
11. Movilli E, Guido J, Silvia T, et al. Plasma exchange in the treatment of acute renal failure of myeloma. Nephrol Dial Transplant 2007;22: 1270-1.
12. Terrell DR, Williams LA, Vesely SK, et al. The incidence of thrombotic thrombocytopenic purpura-hemolytic uremic syndrome: All patients, idiopathic patients, and patients with severe ADAMTS-13 deficiency. J Thromb Haemost 2005;3:1432-6.
13. George JN, Li X, McMinn JR, et al. Thrombotic thrombocytopenic purpura-hemolytic uremic syndrome following allogeneic HPC transplantation: A diagnostic dilemma. Transfusion 2004;44:294-304.
14. Bandarenko N, Brecher ME, for the United States Thrombotic Thrombocytopenic Purpura Apheresis Study Group (US TTP ASG): Multicenter survey and retrospective analysis of current efficacy of therapeutic plasma exchange. J Clin Apher 1998;13:133-41.
15. Howard MA, Williams LA, Terrell DR, et al. Complications of plasma exchange in patients treated for clinically suspected thrombotic thrombocytopenic purpura-hemolytic uremic syndrome. Transfusion 2006;46:154-6.
16. Weinshenker BG, O'Brien PC, Petterson TM, et al. A randomized trial of plasma exchange in acute central nervous system inflammatory

demyelinating disease. Ann Neurol 1999;46: 878-86.
17. Llufriu S, Castillo J, Blanco Y, et al. Plasma exchange for acute attacks of CNS demyelination: Predictors of improvement. Neurology 2009;73:949-53.
18. Bonnan M, Valentino R, Olindo S, et al. Plasma exchange in severe spinal attacks associated with neuromyelitis optica spectrum disorder. Mult Scler 2009;15:487-92.
19. Savin VJ, Sharma R, Sharma M, et al. Circulating factor associated with increased glomerular permeability to albumin in recurrent focal segmental glomerulosclerosis. N Engl J Med 1996;334:878-83.
20. Al-Badr W, Kallogjeri D, Madaraty K, et al. A retrospective review of the outcome of plasma exchange and aggressive medical therapy in antibody mediated rejection of renal allografts: A single center experience. J Clin Apher 2008;23:178-82.
21. Sivakumaran P, Vo AA, Villicana R, et al. Therapeutic plasma exchange for desensitization before transplantation in ABO-incompatible renal allografts. J Clin Apher 2009;24:155-60.
22. Tobian AAR, Shirey RS, Montgomery RA, et al. Therapeutic plasma exchange reduces ABO titers to permit ABO incompatible renal transplantation. Transfusion 2009;49:1248-54.
23. Vichinsky EP, Neumayr LD, Earles AN, et al. Causes and outcomes of the acute chest syndrome in sickle cell disease. National Acute Chest Syndrome Study Group. N Engl J Med 2000;342:1855-65.
24. Lawson SE, Oakley S, Smith NA, Bareford D. Red cell exchange in sickle cell disease. Clin Lab Haematol 1999;21:99-102.
25. Stuart MJ, Setty BN. Sickle cell acute chest syndrome: Pathogenesis and rationale for treatment. Blood 1999;94:1555-60.
26. Adams RJ, McKie VC, Hsu L, et al. Prevention of a first stroke by transfusions in children with sickle cell anemia and abnormal results on transcranial Doppler ultrasonography. N Engl J Med 1998;339:5-11.
27. Lee MT, Piomelli S, Granger S, et al. Stroke Prevention Trial in Sickle Cell Anemia (STOP): Extended follow-up and final results. Blood 2006;108:847-52.
28. Siegel JF, Rich MA, Brock WA. Association of sickle cell disease, priapism, exchange transfusion and neurological events: ASPEN syndrome. J Urol 1993;150:1480-2.
29. Bladon J, Taylor PC. Extracorporeal photopheresis: A focus on apoptosis and cytokines. J Dermatol Sci 2006;43:85-94.
30. Chan KW. Extracorporeal photopheresis in children with graft-versus-host disease. J Clin Apher 2006;21:60-4.
31. Messina C, Locatelli F, Lanino E, et al. Extracorporeal photochemotherapy for paediatric patients with graft-versus-host disease after haematopoietic stem cell transplantation. Br J Haematol 2003;122: 118-27.
32. Barr ML, Baker CJ, Schenkel FA, et al. Prophylactic photopheresis and chronic rejection: Effects on graft intimal hyperplasia in cardiac transplantation. Clin Transplant 2000;14:162-6.
33. Barr Ml, Meiser BM, Eisen HJ, et al. Photopheresis for the prevention of rejection in cardiac transplantation. Photopheresis Transplantation Study Group. N Engl J Med 1998; 339:1744-51.
34. Dall'Amico R, Montini G, Murer L, et al. Extracorporeal photochemotherapy after cardiac transplantation: A new therapeutic approach to allograft rejection. Int J Artif Organs 2000;23: 49-51.
35. Marques MB, Tuncer HH. Photopheresis in solid organ transplant rejection. J Clin Apher 2006;21:72-7.
36. Masaki N, Tatami R, Kumamoto T, et al. Ten-year follow-up of familial hypercholesterolemia patients after intensive cholesterol-lowering therapy. Int Heart J 2005;46:833-43.
37. Matsuzaki M, Hiramori K, Imaizumi T, et al. Intravascular ultrasound evaluation of coronary plaque regression by low density lipoprotein-apheresis in familial hypercholesterolemia: The Low Density Lipoprotein-Apheresis Coronary Morphology and Reserve Trial (LACMART). J Am Coll Cardiol 2002;40:220-7.
38. Wang Y, Blessing F, Walli AK, et al. Effects of heparin-mediated extracorporeal low-density lipoprotein precipitation beyond lowering proatherogenic lipoproteins—reduction of circulating proinflammatory and procoagulatory markers. Atherosclerosis 2004;175:145-50.
39. Kobayashi S, Oka M, Moriya H, et al. LDL-apheresis reduces P-Selectin, CRP and fibrinogen—possible important implications for improving atherosclerosis. Ther Apher Dial 2006; 10:219-23.
40. Felson DT, LaValley MP, Baldassare AR, et al. The Prosorba column for treatment of refractory rheumatoid arthritis: A randomized, dou-

ble-blind, sham-controlled trial. Arthritis Rheum 1999;42:2153-9.

41. Snyder HW Jr, Bertram JH, Henry DH, et al. Use of protein A immunoadsorption as a treatment for thrombocytopenia in HIV-infected homosexual men: A retrospective evaluation of 37 cases. AIDS 1991;5:1257-60.
42. Snyder HW Jr, Cochran SK, Balint JP Jr, et al. Experience with protein A-immunoadsorption in treatment-resistant adult immune thrombocytopenic purpura. Blood 1992;79:2237-45.
43. Silverman GJ, Goodyear CS, Siegel DL. On the mechanism of staphylococcal protein A immunomodulation. Transfusion 2005;45:274-80.
44. Habermalz B, Sauerland S. Clinical effectiveness of selective granulocyte, monocyte adsorptive apheresis with the Adacolumn device in ulcerative colitis. Dig Dis Sci 2010;55:1421-8.
45. Sands BE, Sandborn WJ, Feagan B, et al. A randomized, double blind, sham controlled study of granulocyte/monocyte apheresis for active ulcerative colitis. Gastroenterology 2008;135: 400-9.
46. Otsuka America Pharmaceutical, Inc. Study for the treatment of Crohn's disease with adacolumn (monograph). [Available at http://clinicaltrials.gov/ct2/show/NCT00162942 (accessed November 9, 2010).]
47. Rock G, Shumak KH, Sutton DM, et al. Cryosupernatant as replacement fluid for plasma exchange in thrombotic thrombocytopenic purpura. Members of the Canadian Apheresis Group. Br J Haematol 1996;94:383-6.
48. Vichinsky EP, Luban NLC, Wright E, et al. Prospective RBC phenotype matching in a stroke-prevention trial in sickle cell anemia: A multicenter transfusion trial. Transfusion 2001;41: 1086-92.
49. Norda R, Berseus O, Stegmayr B. Adverse events and problems in therapeutic hemapheresis. A report from the Swedish registry. Transfus Apher Sci 2001;25:33-41.
50. McLeod BC, Sniecinski I, Ciavarella D, et al. Frequency of immediate adverse effects associated with therapeutic apheresis. Transfusion 1999;39:282-8.
51. Haddad S, Leitman SF, Wesley RA, et al. Placebo-controlled study of intravenous magnesium supplementation during large-volume leukapheresis in healthy allogeneic donors. Transfusion 2005;45: 934-44.
52. Marques MB, Huang ST. Patients with thrombotic thrombocytopenic purpura commonly develop metabolic alkalosis during therapeutic plasma exchange. J Clin Apher 2001;16:120-4.
53. Askari S, Nollet K, Debol SM, et al. Transfusion-related acute lung injury during plasma exchange: Suspecting the unsuspected. J Clin Apher 2002;17:93-6.
54. Duntley P, Siever J, Korwes ML, et al. Vascular erosion by central venous catheters. Clinical features and outcome. Chest 1992;101:1633-8.
55. Leitman SF, Boltansky H, Alter HJ, et al. Allergic reactions in healthy plateletpheresis donors caused by sensitization to ethylene oxide gas. N Engl J Med 1986;315:1192-6.
56. Purello D'Ambrosio F, Savica V, Gangemi S, et al. Ethylene oxide allergy in dialysis patients. Nephrol Dial Transplant 1997;12:1461-3.
57. Orlin JB, Berkman EM. Partial plasma exchange using albumin replacement: Removal and recovery of normal plasma constituents. Blood 1980;56:1055-9.
58. Kiprov DD, Golden P, Rohe R, et al. Adverse reactions associated with mobile therapeutic apheresis: Analysis of 17,940 procedures. J Clin Apher 2001;16:130-3.

Chapter 27

Noninfectious Complications of Blood Transfusion

◆

Catherine A. Mazzei, MD; Mark A. Popovsky, MD; and Patricia M. Kopko, MD

ALTHOUGH THE BLOOD supply today is thought to be the safest it has ever been, patients still worry when a doctor tells them they need a transfusion. Concerned about viral diseases such as hepatitis and AIDS, some patients request blood from directed donors (family members or friends asked to donate specifically for the patient), and others, if able, donate autologous blood. Nevertheless, statistically the greatest risk to the patient lies in the other, noninfectious, complications of blood transfusion. In fact, transfusion-related acute lung injury (TRALI) and hemolytic transfusion reactions (HTRs) are two of the three most-reported causes of transfusion-related mortality.[1] It is these noninfectious complications of transfusion that are addressed in this chapter.

HEMOVIGILANCE

Hemovigilance may be defined as the collection of information on the complications of transfusion, analysis of the data, and subsequent data-driven improvement in transfusion practices. One of the main purposes of developing a hemovigilance program is to improve reporting of transfusion-related adverse events. It is widely believed that the major noninfectious complications of transfusion are both underrecognized and underreported. The increasing incidence of reported cases of TRALI, including unreported cases discovered through look-back studies, further emphasizes the need for hemovigilance.

Many countries have implemented successful hemovigilance programs that allow them to compare data and choose the safest blood components and procedures available. The United States is aware of the need for such a program. An interorganizational task force on biovigilance was formed that includes the AABB. Biovigilance also includes organ and tissue transplant safety, but transfusion safety was addressed first. The National Healthcare

Catherine A. Mazzei, MD, Associate Medical Director, BloodSource, Sacramento, California; Mark A. Popovsky, MD, Associate Clinical Professor, Harvard Medical School, Boston, Massachusetts, and Vice President and Chief Medical Officer, Haemonetics Corporation, Braintree, Massachusetts; and Patricia M. Kopko, MD, Chief Medical Officer, BloodSource, Sacramento, California

C. Mazzei and P. Kopko have disclosed no conflicts of interest. M. Popovsky has disclosed a financial relationship with Haemonetics Corporation.

Safety Network (NHSN) hemovigilance module is available online from the Centers for Disease Control and Prevention (CDC).[2]

Definitions and classification schemes are outlined in detail in the appendices of the NHSN Biovigilance Component Protocol, with the goal of improving the quality of national surveillance data.[2(p5)] The pilot study was completed in early 2010, and all interested hospitals may now participate. Results will be published by the CDC in an annual public health surveillance report after 12 to 24 months. This time frame allows sufficient participation for benchmarks to be established.[3,4]

In addition, as increasing amounts of data have become available from various hemovigilance programs outside the United States, efforts to decrease the risk of noninfectious complications of blood transfusion have expanded beyond component safety. Blood management issues, including liberal vs restrictive transfusion strategies as well as the impact of the age of components, have recently been studied in an effort to provide the highest level of patient safety.[5]

RECOGNITION AND EVALUATION OF A SUSPECTED TRANSFUSION REACTION

Identification of a Transfusion Reaction

Although clinicians and laboratorians try to ensure that transfusion of blood and blood components is as safe as possible and use blood only when necessary, some adverse effects cannot be accurately predicted or completely avoided. It is therefore important that physicians be aware of such risks when discussing the need for transfusion with a patient. Informed consent for transfusion may include a discussion of infectious disease risk and the risk of serious noninfectious complications such as TRALI and HTRs.[6] Furthermore, nurses and transfusionists administering components should be well aware of the signs and symptoms of a possible reaction and be prepared to take steps to mitigate the current episode as well as prevent future similar reactions when possible. Many common clinical signs and symptoms are associated with more than one type of adverse reaction (see Table 27-1). Early recognition, prompt cessation of the transfusion, and further evaluation are keys to a successful outcome.

Signs and symptoms that may be indicators of a transfusion reaction include the following:

- Fever, generally defined as 1 C rise in temperature above 37 C[7(p907)] (the most common sign of an acute HTR, or AHTR).
- Chills with or without rigors.
- Respiratory distress, including wheezing, coughing, dyspnea, and cyanosis.
- Hyper- or hypotension.
- Abdominal, chest, flank, or back pain.
- Pain at the infusion site.
- Skin manifestations, including urticaria, rash, flushing, pruritus, and localized edema.
- Jaundice or hemoglobinuria.
- Nausea/vomiting.
- Abnormal bleeding.
- Oliguria/anuria.

The differential diagnosis of a transfusion reaction can be divided into acute or immediate reactions vs delayed reactions. These two types may be further classified as immune-mediated or nonimmune-mediated reactions, as detailed later in this chapter.

Clinical Evaluation and Management of a Transfusion Reaction

The evaluation of a suspected transfusion reaction involves a two-pronged investigation combining clinical evaluation of the patient with laboratory verification and testing. The role of the nurse or tranfusionist is threefold in that he or she 1) recognizes the possibility of a transfusion reaction, 2) treats the patient and administers supportive care at the direction of the physician, and 3) discontinues transfusion of the implicated component and contacts the blood bank for direction in the investigation. When the nurse or transfusionist suspects an AHTR, several steps must be taken immediately.

TABLE 27-1. Categories and Management of Adverse Transfusion Reactions*

Type	Incidence	Etiology	Presentation	Diagnostic Testing	Therapeutic/Prophylactic Approach
Acute (<24 hours) Transfusion Reactions—Immunologic					
Hemolytic	◆ ABO/Rh mismatch—1:40,000 ◆ AHTR—1:76,000 ◆ Fatal HTR—1:1.8 million	Red cell incompatibility	Chills, fever, hemoglobinuria, hypotension, renal failure with oliguria, DIC (oozing from IV sites), back pain, pain along infusion vein, anxiety	◆ Clerical check ◆ DAT ◆ Visual inspection (free Hb) ◆ Repeat patient ABO, pre- and posttransfusion sample ◆ Further tests as indicated to define possible incompatibility ◆ Further tests as indicated to detect hemolysis (LDH, bilirubin, etc)	◆ Keep urine output >1 mL/kg/hour with fluids and IV diuretic (furosemide) ◆ Analgesics (may need morphine) ◆ Pressors for hypotension (low-dose dopamine) ◆ Hemostatic components (platelets, CRYO, FFP) for bleeding
Febrile, nonhemolytic	0.1%-1% with universal leukocyte reduction	◆ Accumulated cytokines in platelet unit ◆ Antibody to donor WBCs	Fever, chills/rigors, headache, vomiting	◆ Rule out hemolysis (DAT, inspect for hemoglobinemia, repeat patient ABO) ◆ Rule out bacterial contamination ◆ WBC antibody screen	◆ Leukocyte-reduced components ◆ Antipyretic premedication (acetaminophen, no aspirin)
Urticarial	1:100-1:33 (1%-3%)	Antibody to donor plasma proteins	Urticaria, pruritis, flushing	◆ Rule out hemolysis (DAT, inspect for hemoglobinemia, repeat patient ABO)	◆ Antihistamine, treatment or premedication (PO or IV) ◆ May restart unit slowly after antihistamine if symptoms resolve

(Continued)

TABLE 27-1. Categories and Management of Adverse Transfusion Reactions* (Continued)

Type	Incidence	Etiology	Presentation	Diagnostic Testing	Therapeutic/Prophylactic Approach
Anaphylactic	1:20,000-1:50,000	◆ Antibody to donor plasma proteins (includes IgA, haptoglobin, C4) ◆ Cytokines	Hypotension, urticaria, bronchospasm (respiratory distress, wheezing), local edema, anxiety	◆ Rule out hemolysis (DAT, inspect for hemoglobinemia, repeat patient ABO) ◆ Anti-IgA ◆ IgA, quantitative	◆ Trendelenberg (feet up) position ◆ Fluids ◆ Epinephrine (adult dose: 0.2-0.5 mL of 1:1000 solution SC or IM; in severe cases, 1:10,000 IV, initial rate 1 μg/min) ◆ Antihistamines, corticosteroids, beta-2 agonists ◆ IgA-deficient blood components
Transfusion-related acute lung injury	1:1200-1:190,000	WBC antibodies in donor (occasionally in recipient) or other WBC-activating agents in components	Hypoxemia, respiratory failure, hypotension, fever, bilateral pulmonary edema	◆ Rule out hemolysis (DAT, inspect for hemoglobinemia, repeat patient ABO) ◆ Rule out cardiogenic pulmonary edema ◆ WBC antibody screen in donor and recipient. If positive, antigen typing may be indicated ◆ WBC crossmatch ◆ Chest x-ray	◆ Supportive care until recovery ◆ Defer implicated donors

Acute (<24 hours) Transfusion Reactions—Nonimmunologic

Transfusion-associated sepsis	Varies by component (see Chapter 8)	Bacterial contamination	Fever, chills, hypotension	◆ Gram's stain ◆ Culture of component ◆ Patient culture ◆ Rule out hemolysis (DAT, inspect for hemoglobinemia, repeat patient ABO)	◆ Broad spectrum antibiotics (until sensitivity testing is completed) ◆ Treat complications (eg, shock)
Hypotension associated with ACE inhibition	Dependent on clinical setting	Inhibited metabolism of bradykinin with infusion of bradykinin (negatively charged filters) or activators of prekallikrein	Flushing, hypotension	◆ Rule out hemolysis (DAT, inspect for hemoglobinemia, repeat patient ABO)	◆ Withdraw ACE inhibition ◆ Avoid albumin volume replacement for plasmapheresis ◆ Avoid bedside leukocyte filtration
Transfusion-associated circulatory overload	<1%	Volume overload	Dyspnea, orthopnea, cough, cyanosis, tachycardia, hypertension, headache	◆ Chest x-ray ◆ Rule out TRALI	◆ Upright posture ◆ Oxygen ◆ IV diuretic (furosemide) ◆ Phlebotomy (250-mL increments)
Nonimmune hemolysis	Rare	Physical or chemical destruction of blood (heating, freezing, hemolytic drug or solution added to blood)	Hemoglobinuria, hemoglobinemia	◆ Rule out patient hemolysis (DAT, inspect for hemoglobinemia, repeat patient ABO) ◆ Test unit for hemolysis	◆ Identify and eliminate cause
Air embolus	Rare	Air infusion via line	Sudden shortness of breath, acute cyanosis, pain, cough, hypotension, cardiac arrhythmia	◆ X-ray for intravascular air	◆ Place patient on left side with legs elevated above chest and head

(Continued)

TABLE 27-1. Categories and Management of Adverse Transfusion Reactions* (Continued)

Type	Incidence	Etiology	Presentation	Diagnostic Testing	Therapeutic/Prophylactic Approach
Hypocalcemia (ionized calcium/citrate toxicity)	Dependent on clinical setting	Rapid citrate infusion (massive transfusion of citrated blood, delayed metabolism of citrate, apheresis procedures)	Paresthesia, tetany, arrhythmia	◆ Ionized calcium ◆ Prolonged QT interval on electrocardiogram	◆ PO calcium supplement for mild symptoms during therapeutic apheresis procedures ◆ Slow calcium infusion while monitoring ionized calcium levels in severe cases
Hypothermia	Dependent on clinical setting	Rapid infusion of cold blood	Cardiac arrhythmia	Central body temperature	◆ Employ blood warmer
Delayed (>24 hours) Transfusion Reactions—Immunologic					
Alloimmunization, RBC antigens	1:100 (1%)	Immune response to foreign antigens on red cells	Positive blood group antibody screening test	◆ Antibody screen ◆ DAT	◆ Avoid unnecessary transfusions ◆ Give leukocyte-reduced components
Alloimmunization, HLA antigens	1:10 (10%)	WBCs and platelets (HLA)	Platelet refractoriness, delayed hemolytic reaction, HDFN	◆ Platelet antibody screen ◆ Lymphocytotoxicity test	◆ Avoid unnecessary transfusions ◆ Give leukocyte-reduced components
Hemolytic	1:2500-11,000	Anamnestic immune response to red cell antigens	Fever, decreasing hemoglobin, new positive antibody screening test, mild jaundice	◆ Antibody screen ◆ DAT ◆ Tests for hemolysis (visual inspection for hemoglobinemia, LDH, bilirubin, urinary hemosiderin as clinically indicated)	◆ Identify antibody ◆ Transfuse compatible red cells as needed

Graft-vs-host disease	Rare	Donor lymphocytes engraft in recipient and mount attack on host tissues	Erythroderma, maculopapular rash, anorexia, nausea, vomiting, diarrhea, hepatitis, pancytopenia, fever	◆ Skin biopsy ◆ HLA typing ◆ Molecular analysis for chimerism	◆ Corticosteroids, cytotoxic agents ◆ Irradiation of blood components for patients at risk (including related-donor and HLA-selected components)
Posttransfusion purpura	Rare	◆ Recipient platelet antibodies (apparent alloantibody, usually anti-HPA-1) destroy autologous platelets	Thrombocytopenic purpura, bleeding, 8-10 days after transfusion	◆ Platelet antibody screen and identification	◆ IVIG ◆ HPA-1-negative platelets ◆ Therapeutic plasma exchange
Delayed (>24 hours) Transfusion Reactions—Nonimmunologic					
Iron overload	Typically after >100 RBC units	Multiple transfusions with obligate iron load in transfusion-dependent patient	Diabetes, cirrhosis, cardiomyopathy	◆ Serum ferritin ◆ Liver enzymes ◆ Endocrine function tests	◆ Iron chelators

*For platelet refractoriness, see Chapter 18 on platelet and granulocyte antigens and antibodies; for septic transfusion reactions, see Chapter 8 on transfusion-transmitted diseases; for a recent summary of transfusion reactions, see Hendrickson.[5]

ACE = angiotensin-converting enzyme; AHTR = acute HTR; antibody screen = blood group antibody screening test; CRYO = cryoprecipitate; DAT = direct antiglobulin test; DIC = disseminated intravascular coagulation; FFP = Fresh Frozen Plasma; Hb = hemoglobin; HPA = human platelet antigen; HTR = hemolytic transfusion reaction; IV = intravenous; IVIG = intravenous immune globulin IM = intramuscular; LDH = lactate dehydrogenase; PO = by mouth; RBC = Red Blood Cell; SC = subcutaneous; TRALI = transfusion-related acute lung injury; WBC = white (blood) cell.

Patient-focused steps are as follows:

1. Stop the transfusion immediately but keep the line open with saline.
2. Document the clerical recheck between the patient and the component. The labels on the component, patient records, and patient identification should be examined to detect any identification errors. Transfusing facilities may require repeat ABO determination or grouping of the patient on a new sample.[8(p82)] (See "Standard Laboratory Investigations of Transfusion Reactions" section below.)
3. Contact the treating physician immediately for instructions for patient care.

Component-focused steps are as follows:

1. Contact the transfusion service for directions for investigation. Most transfusion services use a standardized form to document all of the information available for both the patient and the component.
2. Obtain instructions concerning the return of any remaining component, associated intravenous (IV) fluid bags, and tubing.
3. Determine appropriate samples (blood and urine) to be sent to the laboratory.
4. The transfusion service determines whether the blood provider should be notified.

Most serious transfusion reactions, such as AHTRs caused by ABO incompatibility and anaphylaxis, occur within the first 15 minutes of transfusion. Therefore, a slow initial infusion rate with continuous monitoring of the patient during the early stages of a transfusion allows the reaction to be discovered in a timely manner. Some other serious reactions, such as TRALI and transfusion-associated circulatory overload (TACO), may occur during or within 1 to 2 hours after transfusion. For serious reactions, IV access should be maintained with normal saline, and other agents should be administered as directed by the patient's physician. The physician will evaluate the patient to determine what type of reaction has occurred, consult with blood bank and laboratory personnel as needed, and direct further treatment, if any, of the patient. The patient may still require transfusion, and the patient's physician may consult with the transfusion service medical director to determine the safest approach.

Identification errors may be discovered at the bedside or in the laboratory. When such an error is identified, the transfusion service must be notified immediately so that any "companion errors" may be avoided. Companion errors occur when patient identification, sample identification labels, or component labels are switched. The occurrence of a transfusion reaction may be the first indication that a switch has occurred, and, by identifying the other party involved, a second reaction may be prevented.

The laboratory will provide instructions regarding laboratory issues, often included as part of a standard transfusion reaction form, on how to proceed. Once the patient is stabilized, the laboratory will likely need a blood sample as well as the returned component. In cases of suspected ABO incompatibility, or as required by the transfusion service, a urine specimen may be requested. In these cases it is often a good idea to monitor the patient's urine output and color over the next several hours. Additional patient treatment options are included in the treatment sections of the various types of transfusion reactions discussed in this chapter.

Hospital policies may vary, and in the case of urticaria and sometimes volume overload, postreaction blood samples may not be required for laboratory evaluation. The requirements for these exceptions should be clearly covered in the procedures and/or forms used in the investigation of a transfusion reaction. If it is not clear at the time of the reaction, the transfusion service or laboratory staff should be consulted.

Standard Laboratory Investigation of a Transfusion Reaction

When the laboratory receives notice of a possible transfusion reaction, several steps are performed by technologists:

1. Clerical check of the component bag, label, paperwork, and patient sample.
2. Repeat ABO testing on the posttransfusion sample.
3. Visual check of pre- and posttransfusion samples to look for evidence of hemolysis (hemolysis may not be visible if <50 mg/dL of hemoglobin is present).
4. Direct antiglobulin test (DAT) on a posttransfusion sample.
5. Findings reported to the blood bank supervisor or medical director, who may request additional studies or tests.

The clerical check for identification errors must be performed as soon as a transfusion reaction is suspected in order to identify the potential for an ABO incompatibility as well as to prevent any associated companion errors from resulting in further complications.

The posttransfusion blood sample should be examined for visual evidence of hemolysis. Comparison of the supernatant in the patient's pre- and posttransfusion specimens may aid in assessing any hemolysis that may have occurred. Destruction of red cells and release of free hemoglobin result in a pink to red appearance of the supernatant. Detectable hemoglobinemia may result from hemolysis of only 2.5 to 5 mL of red cells; therefore, care must be taken to obtain a postreaction venous sample that was collected properly. Hemolysis may also be caused by other medical interventions. If proper collection of the posttransfusion sample is in question, a second posttransfusion sample should be drawn and examined. Myoglobinemia, seen in trauma patients, may be confused with hemoglobinemia. Examination of a postreaction urine specimen may aid in the diagnosis of acute hemolysis. Free hemoglobin in the urine is indicative of intravascular hemolysis. Hematuria, or intact red cells in the urine, and myoglobinuria both have other causes.

If the DAT is positive on the patient's posttransfusion specimen, a DAT should also be performed on a pretransfusion specimen (unless already completed as a part of the pretransfusion testing). In most cases where the pretransfusion DAT is negative, a positive DAT after transfusion indicates the presence of remaining incompatible red cells. If the posttransfusion DAT, or both DATs, are positive, further workup is necessary, as indicated below. Sometimes hemolysis is brisk, destroying all of the transfused red cells, and the posttransfusion DAT is negative. A negative DAT may also occur with nonimmune causes of hemolysis.

Additional laboratory evaluation may be required when an HTR is suspected:

1. Human error should be ruled out, primarily in the area of patient and sample identification. Repeat ABO and Rh testing should be performed on the unit of blood or available segment, pretransfusion specimen, and posttransfusion sample to exclude any clerical errors or sample mixups.
2. Antibody detection studies should be performed on the pre- and posttransfusion samples to look for any previously undetected alloantibodies. Enhancement techniques may be required to demonstrate the antibody, particularly in the pretransfusion specimen. If a DAT is positive after transfusion, an elution may need to be performed to detect newly formed antibody. If an alloantibody is identified, samples from any recently transfused red cells should be tested for the corresponding antigen. In a delayed HTR (DHTR), the antibody may be just beginning to increase as a result of the anamnestic immune response. Rarely, hemolysis may occur from passive transfer of antibody in the unit of blood, usually when group O platelets are given to a non-group-O patient. The crossmatch should be repeated with both pre- and posttransfusion specimens using an indirect antiglobulin test (IAT) method, which has increased sensitivity over the immediate-spin crossmatch.[9(pp241-77)] This may indicate the presence of an antibody to a low-prevalence antigen.
3. When laboratory evidence of hemolysis is not evident, demonstration of decreased red cell survival may aid in the diagnosis.

Serial hemoglobin levels may be adequate, or red cell survival studies may be required in more complex cases. Phenotypic differences between the donor and the patient can be identified and followed using flow cytometry.[10] The patient may be evaluated by serial measurement of certain laboratory values, such as haptoglobin, lactate dehydrogenase (LDH), and unconjugated bilirubin levels. An increase in bilirubin may begin as early as 1 hour after the reaction, peak at 5 to 7 hours, and disappear within 24 hours if liver function is normal.

4. Finally, examination of the returned components may yield important information concerning possible traumatic or mechanical causes of hemolysis. Both the blood bag and the administration tubing should be included in the examination. Hemolysis in both the component container and administration set could result from a process that affected the unit of blood, such as inappropriate warming of the unit. If the hemolysis was present only in the administration set, a faulty infusion pump, if used, could be the cause.

The transfusion service must retain any patient records that are related to transfusion reactions, clinically significant antibodies, and special transfusion requirements.[8(pp69-71)] Additional information regarding special products, such as irradiated or washed components required for a particular patient, may be retained by the transfusion service as well. In an increasingly mobile society, it is typically not a failure to keep adequate records that contributes significantly to the difficulties of transfusion but rather the patient's need for treatment in a location other than where his or her records reside. When the patient is able to give a thorough history, transfusion services are able to share medical information in a timely manner. If the patient is unable to give a medical history, medical warning bracelets or wallet identification cards may be of some benefit, particularly for patients with multiple alloantibodies whose strength may decrease over time.

Specialized Laboratory Investigations for Selected Reactions

Additional laboratory evaluation may be required in the investigation of some nonhemolytic transfusion reactions, as described in the following sections.

Anaphylaxis

In cases of suspected anaphylaxis, the patient should be tested for antibodies to immunoglobulin A (anti-IgA), and quantitative IgA levels should be assessed. IgA-deficient patients should be transfused with components from IgA-deficient donors (see "Allergic Reactions"). Washed cellular blood components are also appropriate in these patients as well as in patients with a history of severe allergic reactions caused by other allergens.

Sepsis

Visual examination of the returned component should be conducted in suspected cases of posttransfusion sepsis. Particular attention should be paid to any color changes, especially brown or purple discoloration in a red cell component, and bubbles/frothiness in a platelet component. A Gram's stain should be performed on the returned component, and cultures should be performed on both the component and the patient's posttransfusion blood sample.

Transfusion-Related Acute Lung Injury

In cases of suspected TRALI, the collecting facility should be consulted to coordinate the approach to posttransfusion testing. Patient samples should be obtained at the time of the reaction because they may not be available at a later date. A serum sample should be drawn for antibody studies, and an acid-citrate-dextrose tube should be drawn for HLA typing. The collecting facility may obtain a sample of the donor's serum to test for HLA and neutrophil antibodies.

ACUTE OR IMMEDIATE TRANSFUSION REACTIONS

Acute or immediate transfusion reactions occur within 24 hours of the administration of a component, and often during the transfusion itself. Acute transfusion reactions include hemolysis, both immune- and nonimmune-mediated; transfusion-related sepsis; TRALI; severe allergic reactions, including anaphylaxis; TACO; complications of massive transfusion; and air embolism. Other acute transfusion reactions, usually of little clinical significance, include febrile nonhemolytic transfusion reactions (FNHTRs) and mild allergic reactions such as urticaria or rash. The clinical significance of an acute transfusion reaction often cannot be determined by clinical history or signs and symptoms alone but requires laboratory evaluation.

Acute Hemolytic Transfusion Reactions

Presentation

Rapid hemolysis of as little as 10 mL of incompatible blood can produce symptoms of an AHTR. The most common presenting symptom is fever with or without accompanying chills or rigors. In a mild reaction, the patient may have abdominal, chest, flank, or back pain. In a severe AHTR, hypotension, dyspnea, and flank pain may be present and in some cases progress to shock, with or without accompanying disseminated intravascular coagulation (DIC). Red or dark urine may be the first sign of intravascular hemolysis, particularly in the anesthetized or unconscious patient, who may also present with oliguria or, rarely, DIC. The severity of symptoms of this reaction is related to the amount of incompatible blood transfused. Prompt recognition of the reaction and immediate cessation of the transfusion can prevent grave consequences.

Differential Diagnosis

Many of the signs and symptoms of an immune-mediated AHTR are common to other acute transfusion reactions. Fever, with or without chills, accompanied by hypotension may also be seen in transfusion-related sepsis and TRALI. Hemolysis, although not seen in sepsis or TRALI, may not be detected immediately. Respiratory difficulty is not typically a symptom of an AHTR. Immediate treatment of acute hemolysis is identical to that of sepsis—stopping the transfusion and maintaining hemodynamic stability—and can be instituted while the diagnosis is being determined.

The patient's underlying disease process can make the diagnosis of any AHTR extremely difficult. Patients with glucose-6-phosphate dehydrogenase (G6PD) deficiency may experience hemolysis after transfusion. Transfusion of patients with autoimmune hemolytic anemia or sickle cell disease presents a particularly complicated situation when symptoms such as fever and hypotension occur. In these patients, autoantibodies and multiple alloantibodies will delay the serologic diagnosis of an AHTR and make identification of the responsible antibody a challenge. Acute hemolysis may also result from nonimmune mechanisms, as described later.

Pathophysiology

The interaction of preformed antibodies with red cell antigens is the immunologic basis for AHTRs. The most severe reactions are associated with transfusion of red cells that are ABO incompatible with the recipient's isohemagglutinins, resulting in acute intravascular destruction of the transfused cells. Alternatively, transfusion of ABO-incompatible plasma, as found in apheresis platelets, has been shown to cause hemolysis of the patient's red cells. Although this form of acute hemolysis is not usually clinically significant or characterized by typical hemolytic symptoms, it can be severe if donors have high titers of ABO antibodies. Although rare, the most common circumstance is when group O platelets from donors with high titers of anti-A are transfused to group A patients.[11,12]

When preformed IgM or IgG antibodies recognize corresponding red cell antigens, complement activation may occur, resulting in intravascular hemolysis, hemoglobinemia, and eventually hemoglobinuria. IgM antibodies are strong activators of complement, and IgG antibodies, when present at sufficient concentrations, may activate complement as well. Complement activation involves C3 cleavage, with the ensuing production of C3a, an anaphylatoxin, which is released into the plasma, and C3b, which coats the red cells. If complement activation proceeds to completion, which is characteristic of ABO antibodies, a membrane attack complex is assembled on the red cell surface, and intravascular lysis occurs. C5a, an anaphylatoxin 100 times more potent than C3a, is produced as a part of this hemolysis. C3a and C5a promote the release of histamine and serotonin from mast cells, leading to vasodilation and smooth muscle contraction, particularly bronchial and intestinal. These anaphylatoxins are recognized by many other cell types as well, including monocytes, macrophages, endothelial cells, platelets, and smooth muscle, and are involved in the production and release of cytokines, leukotrienes, free radicals, and nitric oxide. The end result may include wheezing, flushing, chest pain or tightness, and gastrointestinal symptoms. These symptoms may also be caused by release of bradykinin and norepinephrine caused by antigen-antibody complex stimulation. Phagocytosis of IgG-coated red cells leads to cytokine release, which plays a role in producing the effects of acute hemolysis.[13] Interleukin-8 (IL-8, CXCL8), which activates neutrophils, and tumor necrosis factor alpha (TNFα), which activates the coagulation cascade, have also been demonstrated after in-vitro incubation of incompatible group O whole blood and group A or B red cells.[14] Other cytokines involved in the pathogenesis of AHTRs include IL-1β, IL-6, and monocyte chemoattractant protein-1 (MCP-1, CCL2). In a mouse model of HTR, transfusion of incompatible red cells resulted in very high plasma levels of MCP-1 and IL-6 with lower levels of TNFα.[15]

If complement activation does not proceed to completion, which typically happens with non-ABO antibodies, the red cells can undergo extravascular hemolysis where cells coated with C3b and/or IgG are rapidly removed from the circulation by phagocytes. In extravascular hemolysis, the consequences of complement activation, including release of anaphylatoxins and opsonization of red cells, may still have adverse effects.

Coagulation abnormalities associated with AHTRs may be caused by various mechanisms. The "intrinsic" pathway of the clotting cascade may be activated by antigen-antibody interaction, resulting in activation of Factor XII, or Hageman factor. Activation of the Hageman factor can result in hypotension through its effect on the kinin system, which produces bradykinin, which in turn increases vascular permeability and causes vasodilation. Activated complement, as well as TNFα and IL-1, may increase the expression of tissue factor. Tissue factor, expressed by leukocytes and endothelial cells, can activate the "extrinsic" pathway and is associated with the development of DIC. DIC is an often life-threatening consumptive coagulopathy. Its characteristics include microvascular thrombi formation with ischemic organ and tissue damage; consumption of platelets, fibrinogen, and coagulation factors; and activation of fibrinolysis with resultant production of fibrin-degradation products. The end result of these activations can vary from generalized oozing to uncontrolled bleeding.

Shock may be a component of DIC. Hypotension, caused by the release of vasoactive amines, kinins, and other mediators, produces a compensatory vasoconstrictive response, further aggravating organ and tissue damage. Renal failure may occur as well. Historically, it was thought that free hemoglobin led to renal failure; thus, importance was placed on good hydration in treating an AHTR. Although free hemoglobin does impair renal function, compromised renal cortical supply is thought to be the major contributing factor in developing renal failure. Additionally, antigen-antibody complex deposition as well as vasoconstriction and thrombus formation contribute to the development of renal vascular compromise.

Frequency

The frequency of AHTRs is not easy to determine. In large retrospective studies, the incidence of red cell components transfused to the wrong patient ranges from 1:12,000 to 1:19,000.[10] Taking into account the possibility of chance ABO-compatible transfusion despite administration to the wrong patient, authors of one study estimated the residual rate of mistransfusion to be 1:14,000.[11] Other studies have estimated that the rate of ABO/Rh mismatches is 1:6000 to 1:20,000 transfusions.[16,17] Of the fatalities reported to the Food and Drug Administration (FDA) from 2005 to 2009, 27% (68 patients) were caused by HTRs.[1] More recent data gathered from hemovigilance studies in several countries have indicated the following risk rates: AHTRs in 1:76,000; fatal HTRs in 1:1.8 × 10^6; clinical and or laboratory evidence of hemolysis in 1:80,000; and ABO-incompatible transfusion in 1:40,000.[18,19]

Treatment

Prompt recognition of an AHTR with immediate cessation of the transfusion is critical to a successful outcome. The unit of blood should be returned to the blood bank for the transfusion reaction investigation, and infusion of saline should be continued. The infusion of saline serves to treat hypotension as well as help ensure adequate renal blood flow, with a goal of urine flow rate >1 mL/kg/hour. Saline infusion also maintains venous access, which is likely to be important if additional therapy is needed. Saline infusion alone may not be adequate therapy, and the urine output must be carefully monitored so as not to cause volume overload in the patient. It has long been accepted that low-dose dopamine hydrochloric acid (1-5 µg/kg/minute) combines an inotropic cardiac effect with renal vasodilation to selectively improve renal blood flow. However, the use of dopamine in acute renal failure has become controversial, in part because of the lack of published controlled trials. Recent review articles conclude that low-dose dopamine may improve renal function initially, but no solid evidence exists that it can prevent renal failure. However, these studies, which did not include patients with AHTRs, did show a 25% increase in urine output in the acute setting.[20] Thus, low-dose dopamine may still have a role in treating the complications of an AHTR, but no recommendations regarding its use may be made.

The addition of the diuretic furosemide (40-80 mg intravenously in adults, 1-2 mg/kg in children) promotes increased urine output and further enhances renal cortical blood flow.[21] If urine output remains diminished after a liter of saline has been infused, acute tubular necrosis may have occurred, and the patient may be at risk for developing pulmonary edema. At this point, a nephrologist should be consulted for further management of the patient. Oliguric renal failure may be complicated by hyperkalemia and subsequent cardiac arrest; therefore, these patients should be placed on telemetry. Metabolic acidosis and uremia often necessitate the institution of dialysis.

DIC is an equally serious component of an AHTR. DIC is extremely difficult to treat and may be the first indication that hemolysis has occurred in an anuric or anesthetized patient. Traditional therapy for DIC includes treating or removing the underlying cause and providing supportive care via the administration of platelets, frozen plasma, and cryoprecipitated antihemophilic factor (AHF). The administration of heparin in the treatment of DIC associated with HTRs is controversial. First, the underlying condition for which the patient required transfusion may be a contraindication for heparin administration. For example, with recent surgery or active bleeding, heparin can exacerbate bleeding. Second, there is some thought that because the precipitating event is limited to hemolysis of the volume of blood transfused, the risks of administering heparin are not justified. Those in favor of heparin point out, however, that the most unstable patients (with the most severe reactions) are those who received larger volumes of incompatible blood and are thus the most likely to develop DIC.[22] In the worst cases, DIC can become a self-sustaining vicious cycle of inflammation and consumptive coagulopathy. Recent studies of optimal treatment for

DIC have looked at targeting various components of the inflammatory and coagulation cascades. Activated protein C has shown some benefit in septic patients with DIC; however, no new therapeutic agents have been added to the arsenal to treat DIC associated with AHTRs at this time.[23,24]

Unconscious or anesthetized patients may receive multiple units of incompatible blood before acute hemolysis is recognized. Because the severity of an AHTR is related to the amount of incompatible red cells transfused, red cell exchange transfusion may be considered. Some severe reactions to a single unit of strongly incompatible blood may require exchange transfusion as well. Antigen-negative blood must be used for the red cell exchange. In the case of acute hemolysis caused by a non-ABO antibody, the blood bank must be given adequate time in order to identify the appropriate units for further transfusion. This holds true for simple red cell transfusion as well as for planned red cell exchange. Plasma and platelets likewise should be chosen so that they will not contribute to hemolysis.

Prompt initiation of therapy to aggressively manage hypotension, renal blood flow, and DIC provides the greatest chance for a successful outcome. Furthermore, consultation with appropriate medical specialists early in the course of treatment will ensure that the patient receives hemodialysis, cardiac monitoring, and mechanical ventilation when needed.

Prevention

The most common events leading to the transfusion of a component in error are the very things that the laboratory evaluates when an AHTR is suspected. Clerical and human errors involving proper patient, sample, and blood unit identification are the most common causes of mistransfusion and, therefore, AHTRs. Institutional policies and procedures should be in place to minimize such errors, and corrective and preventive action programs should target continual reduction of such errors. AABB *Standards for Blood Banks and Transfusion Services* requires facilities to have a peer-review program to monitor patient identification, sample collection, labeling, and near-miss events.[8(p85)] Resulting data reveal a mislabeling rate of 1:71 to 1:165, with a wrong-blood-in-tube rate of 1:2000 to 1:2800.[25] In 1 in 15,000 transfusions, the wrong blood is given, and the risk of a near miss is 1 in 1000.[18] In a more recent study of ABO-incompatible Red Blood Cell (RBC) transfusions, all were due to error, with 62% of the errors occurring at the bedside.[26] Although new patients with no blood type on record may not be adequately captured, these monitoring programs are an important step among others in the right direction toward improved transfusion safety. Even though these policies can help reduce the number of such errors, no one method is foolproof. Fortunately, new products are becoming available to increase patient safety. Among the most promising technology-based solutions are radiofrequency identification chips, handheld bar-code scanners, and "smart" refrigerators similar to systems used for pharmacologic agents. The prevention of hemolysis from the administration of minor ABO-incompatible platelets remains a challenge, particularly as the number of patients with HLA antibodies increases. A number of options, including anti-A or anti-B titering of product, limitations of the total amount of incompatible plasma transfused from platelets, and volume reduction may offer some benefit. Platelet additive solutions, while not approved for use in the United States, are also promising approaches because they allow for greater removal of ABO-incompatible plasma.[27]

Nonimmune-Mediated Hemolysis

Transfusion-associated hemolysis can also occur from several nonimmune-mediated causes. Before units are issued, improper shipping or storage temperatures as well as incomplete deglycerolization of frozen red cells can lead to hemolysis. At the time of transfusion, using a needle with an inappropriately small bore size or employing a rapid pressure infuser can cause mechanical hemolysis, which may be seen with the use of roller pumps as well.

Improper use of blood warmers or the use of microwave ovens and hot waterbaths can cause temperature-related hemolysis. It is important to stress that only a few fluids are approved for transfusion with RBCs.[8(p42)] Infusion of RBCs simultaneously through the same tubing with hypotonic solutions or some pharmacologic agents may cause osmotic hemolysis; for safe administration, these should be given via alternate venous access locations. Rarely, hemolysis may be caused by bacterial contamination of the RBC unit. Not infrequently, patients may also experience hemolysis as part of their underlying disease process.

When both immune and nonimmune causes of hemolysis have been excluded, the possibility of an intrinsic red cell membrane defect in the recipient or even in the transfused cells should be considered. Cells with these defects, such as G6PD deficiency, have increased fragility when challenged with particular stressors and may undergo coincidental hemolysis.

Treatment

Hemolysis from nonimmune etiologies may cause symptoms with severity depending on the degree of hemolysis and amount of component transfused. In all cases, the transfusion should be discontinued and appropriate care administered. (See the previous section on the treatment of AHTRs for details on managing hypotension and declining renal function.)

Prevention

As is true for the mitigation of any type of transfusion reaction, written procedures for all aspects of the manufacture and transfusion of blood and components should be followed. Prompt recognition of nonimmune hemolysis and robust root-cause analysis may prevent additional occurrences.[28]

Transfusion-Related Sepsis

Presentation

Fever (particularly 38.5 C or 101 F) and shaking chills and hypotension during or shortly after transfusion are the most frequent presenting symptoms in transfusion-related sepsis. In severe cases, the patient may develop shock with accompanying renal failure and DIC.

Differential Diagnosis

The abruptness of onset and severity of the signs and symptoms associated with transfusion-related sepsis may be very similar to those seen in AHTRs. Mild cases may be confused with FNHTRs. The key to diagnosing transfusion-related sepsis is culturing the same organism from both the patient and the remainder of the component. Any concomitantly administered IV solutions should be cultured at this time as well.

Treatment

If transfusion-related sepsis is suspected, the transfusion should be immediately stopped and supportive care of the patient should be initiated. Broad-spectrum antibiotics may be started, and preliminary Gram's stain results may be of some use. (See Chapter 8 for more detailed discussion about bacterial contamination of transfused blood, including frequency data and prevention strategies.)

Febrile Nonhemolytic Transfusion Reactions

Presentation

An FNHTR is defined as the occurrence of >1 C rise in temperature above 37 C, associated with transfusion, for which no other cause is identifiable. Note that in some patients, a reaction preexisting fever may mask a febrile transfusion reaction, although in others the fever may still increase by >1 C. Accompanying symptoms may include shaking, chills, an increased respiratory rate, a change in blood pressure, and anxiety. Symptoms usually occur during transfusion but may occur 1 to 2 hours later. Most FNHTRs are benign, although they may cause significant discomfort and even hemodynamic or respiratory effects.

Differential Diagnosis

The symptoms associated with an FNHTR may be seen in several other types of transfusion reactions, the most serious of which are HTRs, sepsis, and TRALI. Each of these other reactions has signs, symptoms, and associated laboratory results that help distinguish them from an FNHTR once an investigation is begun; FNHTR is a diagnosis of exclusion. Fever may commonly occur as a component of a patient's underlying illness. In a patient who has been experiencing spiking fevers during the course of admission, it may be difficult to rule out an FNHTR. Hemolysis, along with any other signs or symptoms of a serious reaction, must be ruled out in a patient who experiences fever associated with transfusion.

Pathophysiology

As early as the 1950s, it was recognized that leukocyte antibodies could cause febrile transfusion reactions not accompanied by hemolysis.[9(pp487-508)] Studies found that as few as 0.25×10^9 leukocytes could produce a temperature elevation in the recipient. FNHTRs may also be the result of accumulated cytokines in a cellular blood component.[29] This mechanism may be particularly relevant in reactions seen after the transfusion of platelets. Some FNHTRs are attributable to recipient antibodies, particularly HLA antibodies, that react with antigens on transfused lymphocytes, granulocytes, or platelets. Cytokine release in the recipient in response to these antigen-antibody reactions may contribute to the severity of the reaction. Whatever the initiating cause, cytokine release is the common event leading to symptoms of FNHTRs.

Treatment

When an FNHTR is suspected, the transfusion should be discontinued and a transfusion reaction workup initiated. Antipyretics (acetaminophen) should be administered, and the patient may be safely transfused once symptoms subside. In general, the remainder of the implicated component should not be transfused. Many times, an FNHTR does not develop until after the transfusion has been completed. If a portion of the component remains, the laboratory workup to exclude hemolysis must be completed before resuming transfusion. This may be difficult to accomplish within an acceptable amount of time. Among the few valid situations in which transfusion of the remainder should be considered is the case of a medically indicated rare unit if a significant volume remains untransfused. In that circumstance, the blood bank's medical director should be consulted before proceeding with caution because bacterial contamination of the component may have been the underlying cause of the reaction.[30,31]

Prevention

Prestorage leukocyte reduction decreases the number of residual leukocytes to less than 5×10^6 in Apheresis Platelets and RBCs[8(p24)] and significantly decreases the frequency of FNHTRs.[32] Premedication with acetaminophen may be beneficial in further reducing the residual rate of FNHTRs and has not been shown to impair the ability to detect serious complications of transfusion.[31]

Allergic Reactions

Presentation

Most allergic transfusion reactions are mild, but the spectrum can range from a simple allergic reaction (urticaria) to life-threatening anaphylaxis. Symptoms generally occur within seconds or minutes of the start of the transfusion. Rarely, the symptoms may take several hours to develop. An allergic transfusion reaction is diagnosed much like any other allergic reaction.

The mildest form of an allergic transfusion reaction is urticaria. Urticaria, also known as hives, is an outbreak of swollen, raised, red areas (wheals) on the skin that appears suddenly as a result of the body's adverse reaction to an allergen—in this case, something in the blood. Hives usually cause itching (pruritus) but may also burn or sting. Hives can appear anywhere on the body and vary in size from less than a centimeter to very large areas that may coalesce. They can last for hours or up to several days before fading but often respond quickly to treatment with antihistamines. More extensive cases may be accompanied by angioedema.

Angioedema is similar to urticaria, but the swelling is caused by fluid accumulation beneath the skin instead of on the surface. It is characterized by deep swelling, often around the eyes and lips, and generally lasts longer than urticaria. Angioedema can, rarely, involve the throat, tongue, or lungs, causing respiratory distress.

More serious are anaphylactic or anaphylactoid transfusion reactions, which share the same clinical presentation. Anaphylaxis includes the symptoms of urticaria and angioedema in the majority of cases.[33] Severe hypotension, shock, and loss of consciousness may also occur. In addition, the respiratory system is often involved, with patients experiencing dyspnea, wheezing, and stridor. Other common symptoms affecting approximately 30% of these patients include gastrointestinal disturbances such as nausea, vomiting, diarrhea, and cramping. Cardiovascular manifestations, in addition to hypotension, may include tachycardia, arrhythmia, or cardiac arrest.

Differential Diagnosis

As mentioned above, anaphylaxis and anaphylactoid reactions have similar presentations. Both respond to the same treatment as well, so it is not necessary to distinguish between them clinically. It is, however, important to distinguish anaphylaxis from other reactions characterized by hypotension, dyspnea, and/or loss of consciousness. The most common reaction that may be mistaken for anaphylaxis is a vasovagal reaction, characterized by hypotension, diaphoresis, nausea/vomiting, weakness, bradycardia, and sometimes loss of consciousness. Urticaria, angioedema, pruritus, and respiratory symptoms such as wheezing or stridor are symptoms of anaphylaxis but do not occur in vasovagal reactions. The respiratory symptoms of anaphylaxis may be suggestive of an acute asthma attack or TRALI, but again the classic symptoms of allergy, including urticaria, angioedema, and pruritus, do not occur in either of these instances. Fever, a prominent symptom of HTRs and bacterial contamination, is not a feature of anaphylaxis.

Patients who take angiotensin-converting enzyme (ACE) inhibitors and who undergo plasma exchange have developed hypotensive reactions mimicking anaphylaxis when albumin is used as a replacement fluid.

Pathophysiology

Allergic reactions are hypersensitivity reactions to allergens in the component and are less commonly caused by antibodies from an allergic donor. Preformed IgE antibody in the patient or recipient interacts with the allergen, usually a plasma protein in the component. Mast cells are activated by the binding of allergen to the IgE bound to the mast cells (type I hypersensitivity).[34] Activation results in degranulation, with the release of preformed histamine, chemotactic factors, proteases, and proteoglycans. Secondary mediators—including cytokines and lipid mediators such as arachidonic acid metabolites, leukotrienes, and prostaglandin D2, as well as platelet-activating factor—are generated and released in response to mast cell activation.[35]

When the allergen is introduced systemically, as in the case of transfusion, anaphylaxis or a systemic type I hypersensitivity response may occur. When similar reactions result from non-IgE-mediated release of mast cell mediators, they are called "anaphylactoid" but, as mentioned earlier, have essentially the same presentation and treatment.

Transfusion-related allergic reactions that progress beyond urticaria may be seen in IgA-deficient patients. These anaphylactoid reactions are caused by anti-IgA in the recipient. Although IgA deficiency is found in approximately 1:700 people of European ancestry, only a small percentage of these people ever make antibodies against IgA. Those who do have been divided into two groups based on IgA levels as well as the type of antibody formed. Those with absolute IgA deficiency (<0.05 mg/dL) may form class-specific antibodies (eg, IgE anti-IgA), which are often associated with anaphylactoid reactions. Those with decreased but detectable amounts of IgA, or relative IgA deficiency, can form subclass-specific antibodies (eg, anti-IgA1, anti-IgA2) or allotype-specific antibodies [anti-IgA2m(1), anti-IgA2m(2)] depending on which IgA determinants are lacking.[36]

Although precautions should be taken when transfusing an IgA-deficient patient, it must be kept in mind that the majority of anaphylactic or anaphylactoid reactions are caused by allergens other than IgA.[37] Other known triggers of anaphylactic or anaphylactoid reactions have included patient antibodies against haptoglobin,[38] penicillin, the C4 determinant of complement,[39] and ethylene oxide, which was used in the gas sterilization of medical supplies such as IV tubing and apheresis kits.[40]

Patients taking ACE inhibitors can experience transfusion reactions that are thought to be the result of dual actions on bradykinin: inhibition of its catabolism by the ACE inhibitor and activation of bradykinin by low levels of prekallikrein activity in plasma protein fraction. A similar mechanism is thought to be responsible for hypotensive reactions reported in recipients on ACE inhibitors who were transfused using bedside leukocyte reduction filters, as well as in association with plasma that has been in contact with charged dialysis membranes and low-density lipoprotein or staphylococcal protein A adsorption columns.

Frequency

Allergic reactions to transfusion are quite common, with an overall frequency of approximately 1% to 3% of transfusions. Allergic reactions also represent a significant proportion of transfusion reactions, from 13% to 33% of all reactions.[41,42] Urticaria is relatively common, whereas anaphylaxis and anaphylactoid reactions occur much less often. As with any allergic reaction, anaphylaxis occurs most commonly during the transfusion of plasma or platelets; it has an incidence of 1:20,000 to 1:50,000 transfusions.[41,43] Of the transfusion-associated fatalities reported to the FDA from 2005 to 2009, 3% (six patients) were caused by anaphylaxis.[1]

Treatment

Urticaria is the only transfusion reaction in which the administration of the component may be routinely resumed after prompt treatment. When a patient develops symptoms, the transfusion should be paused so that antihistamines, typically 25 mg to 50 mg diphenhydramine, may be administered. Once the symptoms have dissipated, the transfusion may be resumed, and laboratory workup need not be initiated.[42]

If the symptoms do not subside—or, in the case of severe urticaria or urticaria accompanied by hypotension, if dyspnea, significant edema, or gastrointestinal symptoms do not subside—the transfusion must be stopped and the reaction promptly treated. Severe urticarial reactions may require treatment with methylprednisolone (125 mg intravenously) or prednisone (50 mg orally). Once a severe reaction or developing anaphylaxis is identified, action should be promptly initiated to maintain oxygenation and stabilize hypotension. Epinephrine (1:1000) may be administered intramuscularly or subcutaneously, using an adult dose ranging from 0.2 mL to 0.5 mL or a pediatric dose of 0.01 mL/kg. If symptoms persist, the dose may be repeated every 5 to 15 minutes, up to three times, unless palpitations, extreme anxiousness, or tremors occur. If the patient is unconscious or in shock, epinephrine may be given intravenously at a dilution of 1:10,000 (100 µg/mL) at an initial rate of 1 µg/minute. Such patients ideally receive cardiac monitoring because of the arrhythmic potential of the epinephrine.

Supplemental oxygen should be administered, and the airway maintained. Hypotensive patients should be placed in the Trendelenburg position and supported with crystalloids. If bronchospasm is present, respiratory symptoms may not respond to the epinephrine, and addition of a beta II agonist or aminophylline may be required. Refractory patients, who may not respond because of the presence of a beta adrenergic blocker or an ACE inhibitor, may respond to the addition of glucagon as a 1-mg bolus given intravenously or by continuous infusion.[33,44]

Prevention

Premedication with antihistamines (25 mg to 50 mg diphenhydramine) 30 minutes before transfusion may be helpful in patients with a history of multiple or severe urticarial transfusion reactions. Routine prophylaxis may also be beneficial for patients undergoing multiple transfusions, as in plasma exchange; however, routine antihistamine premedication of all patients receiving transfusion has not been shown to decrease the risk of allergic reaction.[45] If antihistamines are not sufficient, prednisone (20-50 mg orally) or parenteral steroids may be of benefit. For patients whose reactions are severe, unrelenting, and unresponsive to premedication, washing red cells or platelets may be considered. Alternatively, the administration of deglycerolized RBCs has met with some success when reactions have occurred despite washing red cells with 2 L of saline.

Plasma transfusions for patients with diagnosed IgA deficiency who produce anti-IgA should be from IgA-deficient donors (<0.05 mg/dL). If the local blood center cannot provide these components, they may be available through the American Rare Donor Program (see Method 3-13). Other cellular components (RBCs and Platelets) can be depleted of plasma proteins through a washing procedure. IgA deficiency without the presence of anti-IgA or without a history of an anaphylactoid/anaphylactic reaction would not merit the use of IgA-deficient or plasma-depleted components. Intravenous immune globulin (IVIG) products from various manufacturers have differing IgA content. The manufacturer should be contacted for detailed information concerning a particular product and lot number.[46] Autologous donation programs may also be considered for these patients once they have recovered.

Transfusion-Related Acute Lung Injury

Presentation

Clinical signs and symptoms of TRALI typically include fever, chills, dyspnea, cyanosis, hypotension, and new onset of bilateral pulmonary edema.[47] An increase in blood pressure followed by hypotension is not uncommon. TRALI can be life-threatening or fatal. Symptoms arise within 6 hours of transfusion, with most cases becoming evident within 1 to 2 hours after the end of transfusion. In addition to the signs and symptoms traditionally associated with TRALI, there is a growing appreciation that the disorder can be associated with a dramatic transient neutropenia or leukopenia.[48]

All plasma-containing components, including Whole Blood, RBCs, Platelets, Cryoprecipitated AHF, and Fresh Frozen Plasma (FFP), have been implicated in TRALI. Transfusion volumes as small as 15 mL have led to cases of TRALI.

TRALI is a form of acute lung injury (ALI). The American-European Consensus Conference on ARDS defined ALI as acute hypoxemia with a PaO_2/FiO_2 ratio of 300 mm Hg and bilateral pulmonary edema on frontal chest radiograph.[49] The Canadian Consensus Conference relied on this definition of ALI when forming its diagnostic criteria for TRALI[50]: 1) ALI with hypoxemia and PaO_2/FiO_2 300 or SpO_2 <90% on room air, 2) no preexisting ALI before transfusion, 3) onset of symptoms within 6 hours of transfusion, and 4) no temporal relationship to an alternative risk factor for ALI. The panel also defined possible TRALI using the same criteria as for TRALI, with the exception that possible TRALI occurs in the setting of an alternative risk factor for ALI.

Although the lung injury in ALI is commonly irreversible, the lung injury in TRALI is most often transient. Approximately 80% of affected patients will improve within 48 to 96 hours. Even so, in one of the largest studies of TRALI patients, 100% of the patients required oxygen support, with 72% requiring mechanical ventilation.[51] The remaining 20% of patients who do not improve rapidly will either have a protracted clinical course or a fatal outcome.

Differential Diagnosis

The three main conditions that need to be distinguished from TRALI are 1) anaphylactic transfusion reactions, 2) TACO, and 3) transfusion-related sepsis. In anaphylactic transfusion reactions, bronchospasm, laryngeal edema, severe hypotension, erythema (often confluent), and urticaria are prominent symptoms. Fever and pulmonary edema are not associated with anaphylactic reactions. The clinical presentation of TACO is very similar to TRALI, with respiratory distress, tachypnea, and cyanosis as the most prominent features. The key distinction between the two entities is that the pulmonary edema in TACO is cardiogenic, whereas it is noncardiogenic in TRALI. High fever with hypotension and vascular collapse are prominent features in transfusion-related sepsis. Respiratory distress is infrequently associated with these reactions. With rapid onset of respiratory distress, in addition to TACO and TRALI, coincident myocardial infarction and pulmonary embolus as well as other possible causes of ALI should also be considered.

Pathophysiology

The precise mechanism of lung injury in TRALI has not been determined. TRALI has been associated with the infusion of antibodies to leukocyte antigens and the infusion of biologic response modifiers (BRMs).[51,52] Infusion of either is thought to initiate a sequence of events that results in cellular activation and damage of the basement membrane. Pulmonary edema occurs secondary to leakage of protein-rich fluid into the alveolar space.

Antibodies to HLA Class I antigens, HLA Class II antigens, and human neutrophil antigens (HNA) have been associated with TRALI. These antibodies can be formed after exposure to foreign antigens via pregnancy, transfusion, or transplantation. In the majority of cases with antibodies, the source of the antibody is the donor, not the patient. It has been hypothesized that TRALI has been associated more frequently with antibodies in the donor than antibodies in the patient because infused antibodies are able to react with the entire intravascular pool of recipient leukocytes.[53] If the recipient possesses the antibody, the antibody can interact only with the leukocytes in the transfused component.

BRMs accumulate in some cellular components during storage. BRMs enhance the polymorphonuclear cell oxidative burst. They are soluble in chloroform and consist of a mixture of lysophosphatidylcholines.[54]

A two-event model of the mechanism of TRALI has been hypothesized.[54] In the first event, generation of biologically active compounds activates pulmonary vascular endothelial cells and primes neutrophils. This results in sequestration of neutrophils in the pulmonary microvasculature. This first event can result from a variety of physiologic stressors, including sepsis, surgery, and massive transfusion, and predisposes the patient to develop TRALI if a second event is experienced. The infusion of BRMs or antibodies is the second of the two events in this model of TRALI. These stimuli, which ordinarily would not activate neutrophils, activate the primed neutrophils in the pulmonary microvasculature. Neutrophil activation results in pulmonary endothelial damage, capillary leakage, and pulmonary edema.

Frequency

The true incidence of TRALI is unknown. Estimates of frequency range from 1:1300 to 1:5000 transfusions. TRALI is the leading cause of transfusion-related mortality reported to the FDA, with more than 20 cases reported per year from 2003 to 2005.[55] Recent efforts to decrease the amount of transfusable plasma collected from female donors appears to be decreasing the number of TRALI fatalities in the United States.[1]

In 2006, the year before many blood centers implemented measures to reduce the risk of TRALI from plasma, 35 fatal cases of TRALI, 22 of which were associated with transfusion of FFP, were reported to the FDA. In 2008, the year after many blood centers implemented such measures, only 16 fatal cases of TRALI, four of which were associated with transfusion of FFP, were reported.

Treatment

Treatment of TRALI consists of respiratory and circulatory support. Treatment should be as intensive as dictated by the clinical picture. Oxygen supplementation, with or without mechanical ventilation, is required in almost all cases. Pressor agents may be needed to support blood pressure. Diuretics are not indicated because TRALI is not related to volume overload. Administration of corticosteroids has not been shown to improve clinical outcome in TRALI or acute respiratory distress syndrome.[56]

Prevention

Strategies to reduce the risk of TRALI are complicated by a number of factors. Although approximately 10% of blood donations contain HLA and/or HNA antibodies, TRALI occurs in fewer than 1:1000 transfusions.[51,54] There is no mechanism to identify which patients are at risk of developing TRALI. In 2006, the AABB issued a nonbinding *Association Bulletin* recommending that blood collection facilities complete measures to reduce the risk of TRALI from plasma components by November 2007.[57] The bulletin left the decisions regarding how this should be accomplished up to the individual blood center. A variety of means to reduce the amount of transfusable plasma from female donors have been implemented, including 1) using male-donor plasma exclusively for transfusion and diverting female-donor plasma for fractionation, 2) using female-donor plasma for transfusion only if there is no male-donor plasma available (predominantly male plasma), 3) using male-donor and nulliparous female donor plasma for transfusion, and 4) testing female plasma donors for HLA antibodies. These efforts appear to have resulted in a decrease in the number of TRALI fatalities reported to the FDA in 2008.[1]

In 2007, AABB subsequently issued an *Association Bulletin* recommending that blood collection facilities initiate measures to reduce the risk of TRALI from apheresis platelets by November 2008.[58] Reducing the risk of TRALI from apheresis platelets will be more difficult to accomplish than reducing the risk from plasma because of the significantly shorter shelf life of platelets (5 days vs 1 year for plasma) and lack of excess platelets in the blood supply. Several blood centers have begun screening female platelet donors for HLA antibodies if they are multiparous or have ever been pregnant. Data from the Retrovirus Epidemiology Donor Study II, Leukocyte Antibody Prevalence Study[59] found a similar prevalence of HLA antibodies in never-pregnant females and transfused and untransfused males, suggesting screening these donors for HLA antibodies may not be beneficial in reducing the risk of TRALI. This study demonstrated an increased prevalence of HLA antibodies in female blood donors with each additional pregnancy up to four pregnancies, which was the limit of the study.

Although these measures will reduce the risk of TRALI, it is important to recognize they will not eliminate TRALI. These measures do not decrease the risk of TRALI from RBCs, platelet concentrates, or cryoprecipitate. HLA antibody screening addresses only the risk of TRALI from HLA antibodies. A practical test to screen the blood supply for HNA antibodies is not available. In addition, none of these risk-reduction measures addresses the risk of TRALI from BRMs.

Transfusion-Associated Circulatory Overload (TACO)

Presentation

It is well known that transfusion can precipitate acute pulmonary edema caused by volume overload, but only recently has this problem been recognized as an important complication. Patients over 70 years old and infants are at greatest risk, although all transfusion recipients are susceptible to some degree.[60] Although large volumes of components and nonblood fluids are most frequently implicated, modest volumes can also precipitate TACO. High flow rates are frequently cofactors. There are no diagnostic signs or symptoms. Within 1 to 2 hours of transfusion, patients may develop any or all of the following: gallop, jugular venous distension, elevated central venous pressure, dyspnea, orthopnea, new ST segment and T wave changes on electrocardiogram, and elevated serum troponin.[61] Increased blood pressure characterized by a widening of the pulse pressure is characteristic. Radiographs show a widened cardiothoracic ratio.

Differential Diagnosis

TACO is frequently confused with TRALI because a key feature of both is pulmonary edema. It is possible for these complications to occur concurrently in the same patient. The timelines and the clinical presentation are similar, but hypertension is a constant feature in TACO whereas it is only an infrequent and transient manifestation in TRALI. Furthermore, rapid improvement with diuresis or inotropic agents is consistent with TACO. Recently, a cardiac marker, brain natriuretic peptide (BNP) has been introduced as a diagnostic tool. In congestive heart failure, BNP levels are elevated. Several studies have shown that a posttransfusion-to-pretransfusion BNP ratio of 1.5 with a posttransfusion level at least 100 pg/mL as a cutoff yielded a sensitivity and specificity above 80% in TACO.[62] On the other hand, a recent study in the intensive care setting found that BNP was only of moderate value in differentiating TACO and TRALI.[63] With rapid onset of respiratory distress, possible causes of ALI such as coincident myocardial infarction, pulmonary embolus, and others should be considered in addition to TACO and TRALI.

Frequency

The incidence is unknown, but several studies suggest that TACO is much more frequent than previously appreciated. In the general population, one group found TACO in 1:707 recipients of RBCs, with 20% of the affected patients receiving a single unit of RBCs. In studies of older orthopedic patients undergoing hip or knee replacement, TACO was found in 1% and 8%, respectively.[64,65] In one report from the Quebec hemovigilance network, an incidence of 1:5000 components was reported, with 1.3% of the cases resulting in death.[66] In the critical care setting, 1:356 units transfused resulted in TACO.[67] From 2005 to 2008, 8% of the transfusion-associated fatalities reported to the FDA (17 patients) were a consequence of TACO.[1]

Treatment

As soon as symptoms suggest TACO, the transfusion should be stopped. The symptoms are treated by placing the patient in a seated position, providing supplementary oxygen, and reducing the intravascular volume with diuretics. If symptoms persist in confirmed TACO, administration of additional diuretics or therapeutic phlebotomy in 250-mL increments is appropriate.

Prevention

In the absence of ongoing and rapid blood loss, components should be administered slowly, particularly in patients at risk for TACO (pediatric patients, patients with severe anemia, and patients with congestive heart failure). A rate of 2 to 4 mL/minute and 1 mL/kg of body weight per hour are the most cited figures, despite a paucity of data on appropriate infusion rates. Total fluid input and output should be monitored.

Complications of Massive Transfusion

The potential complications of massive transfusion, generally defined as receiving more than 10 units of RBCs within 24 hours, include metabolic and hemostatic abnormalities, immune hemolysis, and air embolism. Metabolic abnormalities can depress ventricular function. Hypothermia from refrigerated blood, citrate toxicity, and lactic acidosis from underperfusion and tissue ischemia, which are often complicated by hyperkalemia, can contribute to this effect. Although metabolic alkalosis caused by citrate metabolism may occur, it is not likely to be clinically significant. Patients who are losing blood rapidly may have preexisting or coexisting hemostatic abnormalities or develop them during resuscitation. Hemostatic abnormalities may include dilutional coagulopathy, DIC, and liver and platelet dysfunction.

Citrate Toxicity

PATHOPHYSIOLOGY AND MANIFESTATIONS. Plasma, whole blood, and platelets contain citrate as an anticoagulant. When large volumes of these components are transfused rapidly, particularly in the presence of liver disease, plasma citrate levels may rise, binding calcium and ionized calcium and resulting in hypocalcemia. In patients with a normally functioning liver, citrate is rapidly metabolized; thus, these symptoms are transient.[68] Hypocalcemia is more likely to cause manifestations in patients who are hypothermic or in shock.

A decrease in ionized calcium increases neuronal excitability, which in the conscious patient leads to symptoms of perioral and peripheral tingling, shivering, and lightheadedness, followed by a diffuse sense of vibration, muscle cramps, fasciculations, spasm, and nausea. In the central nervous system, hypocalcemia is thought to increase the respiratory center's sensitivity to carbon dioxide, causing hyperventilation. Because myocardial contraction is dependent on the intracellular movement of ionized calcium, hypocalcemia depresses cardiac function.[69]

TREATMENT AND PREVENTION. Massively transfused patients, particularly those with severe liver disease, may benefit from calcium replacement. It should be noted that empiric replacement therapy in the era before prompt and accurate monitoring of ionized calcium was available was associated with iatrogenic mortality.[70] Unless the patient has a predisposing condition that hinders citrate metabolism, hypocalcemia caused by citrate overload can usually be treated by slowing the infusion. Calcium replacement should be considered when the calcium concentration falls below 50% of its normal value and the symptoms of hypocalcemia are evident.[71]

Hyperkalemia and Hypokalemia

PATHOPHYSIOLOGY. When RBCs are stored at 1 to 6 C, the intracellular potassium gradually leaks into the supernatant plasma or additive solution. Although the concentration in the plasma/anticoagulant portion of an RBC unit may be high (see Chapter 6) because of the small volume of supernatant fluid, the total extracellular potassium load is less than 0.5 mEq for fresh RBC units and only 5 to 7 mEq for units at expiration. This rarely causes problems in the recipient because rapid dilution, redistribution into cells, and excretion blunt the effect. However, hyperkalemia can be a problem in patients with renal failure, in premature infants, and in newborns receiving large transfusions, such as in cardiac surgery or exchange transfusion; otherwise, it is typically a transient effect during very rapid transfusions.

Hypokalemia is observed more frequently than hyperkalemia after transfusion because potassium-depleted donor red cells reaccumulate this ion intracellularly, and citrate metabolism causes further movement of potassium into the cells in response to the consumption of protons. Catecholamine release and aldosterone urinary loss can also trigger hypokalemia in the setting of massive transfusion.[72]

TREATMENT AND PREVENTION. No treatment or preventive strategy is usually necessary, provided the patient is adequately resuscitated from whatever underlying condition required massive transfusions.[73] For infants receiving small-volume transfusions infused slowly, units may be used safely until the expiration date.[74] Although washing of RBC units results in very low levels of potassium, there is no evidence that routine red cell transfusions require manipulation to lower potassium levels, even in patients with impaired renal function.[75]

Hemostatic Abnormalities in Massive Transfusion

PATHOPHYSIOLOGY. Coagulopathy can be observed in massive transfusion, particularly when the lost blood is initially replaced with red cells and asanguinous fluids. Massive transfusion may be defined as 10 or more units of RBCs transfused within 24 hours. Coagulopathy in this situation is frequently ascribed to dilution of platelets and clotting factors, which occurs as patients lose hemostatically active blood and enzymatic activity is reduced, along with cooling of the core body temperature if a blood warmer is not used. Mortality rates range from 20% to 50%.[76] The high rate of mortality results from hypothermia, metabolic acidosis, and coagulopathy.[77] Studies of military and civilian trauma patients demonstrated a progressive increase in the incidence of microvascular bleeding (MVB) characteristic of a coagulopathy with increasing transfusion, typically occurring after replacement of two to three blood volumes (20 to 30 units).[78,79] Although platelet counts, coagulation parameters, and levels of selected clotting parameters correlate with the volume transfused, contrary to expectations from a simple dilutional model, the relationship is marked by tremendous variability. Moreover, there is frequently discordance between the laboratory assessment and the clinical evidence of bleeding. It has been suggested that the platelet deficits were more important in causing the bleeding than were the coagulation deficiencies. MVB typically occurred when the platelet count fell below 50,000 to 60,000/µL.[80] On the other hand, no simple relationship could be determined between a patient's coagulation test results and the onset of bleeding. The etiology of bleeding (elective surgery vs massive trauma) may play a role as well.[80]

Subsequent studies have refined these observations. Significant platelet dysfunction has been demonstrated in massively transfused patients.[81,82] In the studies of Counts and coworkers,[79] low fibrinogen and platelet counts were better predictors of hemostatic failure than were elevations of prothrombin time (PT) and partial thromboplastin time (PTT), suggesting that consumption coagulopathy was an important factor in addition to dilution. A similar conclusion was reached by Harke and Rahman, who showed that the degree of platelet and clotting abnormalities correlated with the length of time the patient was hypotensive, suggesting that shock was the most important cause of DIC.[83] In aggregate, Collins concluded that "coagulopathy in heavily transfused patients was due to hypoperfusion, not transfusion."[84] More recently, more powerful hemostatic assays have been introduced that may be more predictive of blood component requirements.[85]

These data may not be generalizable to patients undergoing massive transfusion in the "clean" setting of the operating room, where hypotension caused by volume loss is prevented. In this context, coagulation factor levels may have priority over platelet problems. Murray et al documented that excessive bleeding in elective surgical patients transfused with greater than one blood volume (RBCs and crystalloid) corresponded to a prolongation in PT and PTT compared to patients with normal hemostasis.[80]

TREATMENT AND PREVENTION. The dilutional model of coagulopathy in massive transfusion would suggest that prophylactic replacement of hemostatic components based on the volume of red cells or whole blood transfused would prevent development of a bleeding diathesis. No specific regimen has yet been shown to be superior in prospective studies.[86] This is a controversial subject. Recent studies using 1:1 ratios of red cells to plasma in severe trauma point to improved survival.[87] Other studies suggest otherwise. Rice et al found that platelet counts and coagulation parameters were similar between patients receiving RBCs and those receiving whole blood, illustrating that routine administration of a set number of FFP units per number of RBC units transfused is not warranted.[88] Recent AABB guidelines stated that there are insufficient data to recommend for or against a 1:1 red cell to plasma transfusion ratio in massive transfusion.[89] Until recently, the predominant thinking was that the replacement of platelets and coagulation factors in the massively transfused surgical and trauma patient should be based on identification of a specific abnormality by use of platelet counts, international normalized ratio, activated PTT (aPTT), and fibrinogen levels. Frequent monitoring of these laboratory values serves to avoid overuse of platelets and plasma products (FFP and Cryoprecipitated AHF) by anticipating the specific component needs, while avoiding dilutional coagulopathy. It is imperative that the laboratory provide results rapidly. Intraoperative and postoperative laboratory testing such as thromboelastography may be useful.

USE OF RECOMBINANT FACTOR VIIA IN MASSIVE TRANSFUSIONS. Recombinant Factor VIIa (rFVIIa), a 50-kDa analog of Factor VIIa, is licensed in the United States for the treatment of bleeding in hemophilia patients (hemophilia A and B) with inhibitors. However, the off-label use of rFVIIa is growing in several areas, including hemorrhagic bleeding in trauma and surgery.[90,91] The recombinant product works by targeting the site of tissue damage, where it binds to tissue factor. This complex activates Factor X to Factor Xa and ultimately Factor IXa. In hemophilia patients, rFVIIa bypasses the need for Factor VIII or Factor IX through the activation of the small amounts of Factor X on activated platelet surfaces at the site of injury. Studies of the efficacy of rFVIIa have produced mixed results.[92,93] In the absence of definitive data, transfusion services should establish guidelines on the reasonable use of rFVIIa.

Air Embolism

Air embolism can occur if blood in an open system is infused under pressure, or if air enters a central catheter while containers or blood administration sets are being changed. It has been reported in association with intraoperative and perioperative blood recovery systems that allow air into the blood infusion bag.[16] The minimum volume of air embolism that is potentially fatal for an adult is approximately 100 mL.[94] Symptoms include cough, dyspnea, chest pain, and shock.

If air embolism is suspected, the patient should be placed on the left side with the head down to displace the air bubble from the pulmonic valve. Aspiration of the air is sometimes attempted. However, proper use and inspection of infusion pumps, equipment for blood recovery or apheresis, and tubing couplers are still essential to prevent this complication.

Hypothermia

Blood warmers may be used to prevent hypothermia. Proper procedures for the use of blood warmers should be followed because overheating may damage or destroy red cells, causing hemolysis and serious transfusion reactions, including fatalities. Blood warmers must have a temperature monitor and warning system to decrease the risk of such a reaction.[8(p6)]

DELAYED TRANSFUSION REACTIONS

Delayed transfusion reactions occur days to months or even years after transfusion. As with acute transfusion reactions, the consequences may be severe but are often treatable.

Delayed Hemolytic Transfusion Reactions

Presentation

Fever and anemia occurring days to weeks after transfusion of a red cell component are characteristic of a DHTR. The hemolysis associated with a DHTR is usually not brisk, but some patients may develop jaundice and leukocytosis. In a DHTR, the hemolysis is primarily extravascular, so although hemoglobinuria may occur rarely, acute renal failure and DIC are not generally seen. In some cases, the hemolysis occurs without causing clinical symptoms. These patients present with unexplained anemia or do not experience an increase in hemoglobin following transfusion.

Differential Diagnosis

Fever with hemolysis occurring well after transfusion may also be seen when the component has been contaminated with an intracellular red cell parasite, as in the case of posttransfusion malaria or babesiosis. Intravascular hemolysis of both donor and recipient red cells occurs. Examination of thick film blood smears and antibody titers to specific parasites should be performed to confirm the diagnosis. Fever without hemolysis may be an indication of graft-vs-host disease (GVHD, described in a subsequent section) or transfusion-transmitted viral disease (see Chapter 8). Hemolysis resulting from antibody production by donor passenger lymphocytes may occur after transplantation of a minor ABO-incompatible organ (eg, a group A patient receives a group O liver).

Pathophysiology

After transfusion or transplantation or, as seen in hemolytic disease of the fetus and newborn, after pregnancy, a patient may make an antibody to a red cell antigen he or she lacks. Red cell antibodies may cause a delayed transfusion reaction if the patient subsequently receives a unit of blood that expresses the corresponding red cell antigen. Primary alloimmunization may occur anywhere from days to months after transfusion of antigen-positive red cells, depending on the immunogenicity and dose of the antigen. Approximately 1% to 1.6% of red cell transfusions are associated with antibody formation, excluding anti-D. D-negative blood is usually transfused to D-negative patients, so although anti-D is capable of causing DHTRs, the frequency attributable to anti-D is relatively low. Newly formed alloantibodies are routinely detected during pretransfusion screening (see Chapters 15 and 16). Recently transfused or pregnant patients must have samples drawn for compatibility testing within 3 days of the scheduled transfusion to ensure identification of any potential new alloantibodies.[8(p34)] A 5-year retrospective study of alloimmunization showed that 11 of 2932 patients (0.4%) had developed new antibodies within 3 days of their transfusion, including anti-E, anti-K, and anti-Jk^a.[95]

DHTRs and delayed serologic transfusion reactions (DSTRs, the rapid development of alloantibody in the absence of laboratory evidence of hemolysis) rarely, if ever, occur as a result of primary immunization and are generally associated with subsequent transfusions. Antibody titers may slowly decrease after the initial immune response, with as many as 30% to 40% of alloantibodies becoming undetectable over periods ranging from months to years. Antibodies against some blood group systems, such as the Kidd system, are notorious for exhibiting this behavior. Subsequent transfusion of an antigen-positive unit triggers an anamnestic response, with production of antibodies occurring over the next several days to weeks after transfusion. The rapidity of antibody production and hemolytic potential of the antibody combine to influence the clinical presentation. Blood group antibodies associated with DHTRs/DSTRs include those of the Kidd, Duffy, Kell, and MNS systems, in order of decreasing frequency.[9(pp358-89)] In a DHTR/DSTR, antibodies may be found in the serum, on the transfused red cells, or both. Routine antibody screening and antibody identification should be possible. If transfused red cells are still present, the DAT may be positive. When the DAT is positive, an eluate should be performed and the antibody identified. If a segment from the unit is available, antigen typing of the red cells may confirm the diagnosis.

Frequency

As in the case of AHTRs, the estimated rate of DHTRs varies widely from study to study. Some of this variation is the result of the practice of considering DSTRs and DHTRs as one category; also, improvements in laboratory techniques have contributed to the increased number of DSTRs detected. It is known that these reactions occur much more frequently than AHTRs, with estimates of approximately 1:2500 for either type of delayed reaction.[17,96] These reactions are likely very much underrecognized, as most patients do not undergo red cell antibody screening following transfusion.[97]

Treatment

The treatment of DHTRs consists of monitoring the patient and providing appropriate supportive care. The most frequent therapy is correction of the anemia by transfusing antigen-negative red cells as needed. When a DSTR is identified by the laboratory, the patient's physician and the transfusion service director should be notified so that any unrecognized hemolysis may be appropriately identified and treated.

Prevention

Prevention of DHTRs/DSTRs caused by known antibody specificities is accomplished by transfusion of antigen-negative red cells. It is essential to obtain prior transfusion records[3] because alloantibodies may have been identified that are no longer detectable but represent cause for supplying blood that is negative for all corresponding antigens. Many institutions have programs to provide at least partially phenotypically matched blood for sickle cell patients and other select patients who have developed multiple alloantibodies. This is clinically important in patients with sickle cell disease who may develop a complication known as sickle cell HTR ("bystander hemolysis"), where autologous cells are destroyed as well as allogeneic cells.

Refractoriness to Platelet Transfusions

See Chapter 18.

Transfusion-Associated Graft-vs-Host Disease

Presentation

The clinical manifestations of transfusion-associated GVHD (TA-GVHD) typically begin 8 to 10 days after transfusion. Symptoms can occur as early as 3 days and as late as 30 days after transfusion. Signs and symptoms include a maculopapular rash, fever, enterocolitis with watery diarrhea, elevated liver function tests, and pancytopenia. The rash begins on the trunk and progresses to involve the extremities. In severe cases, bullae may develop.[98]

Unlike GVHD after allogeneic marrow transplantation, TA-GVHD leads to profound marrow aplasia, with the mortality rate greater than 90%. The time course of the disease is very rapid; death typically occurs within 1 to 3 weeks of the first symptoms.

Differential Diagnosis

Because the clinical manifestations of TA-GVHD appear several days after transfusion, it may be difficult to associate the patient's symptoms with transfusion. The symptoms can easily be attributed to other conditions, including drug reactions and viral illness. In cases of TA-GVHD, skin biopsy reveals a superficial perivascular lymphocytic infiltrate, necrotic keratinocytes, compact orthokeratosis, and bullae formation. Molecular studies may aid in diagnosis. If the donor has any HLA antigens not present in the recipient, HLA typing by molecular methods will reveal the presence of both donor and recipient HLA antigens.[99] If the donor is homozygous for an HLA haplotype shared with the recipient, molecular HLA typing will not aid in the diagnosis. However, other molecular techniques, including analysis of short tandem repeats, can be used in making the diagnosis.[100]

Pathophysiology

Billingham has proposed three requirements for GVHD to develop in a patient.[101] First, there must be differences in the HLA antigens expressed between the donor and the recipient. Second, immunocompetent cells must be present in the graft. Finally, the host must be incapable of rejecting the immunocompetent cells.

In TA-GVHD, viable transfused lymphocytes mount an immunologic attack against the transfusion recipient. Consistent with Billingham's work, the three primary factors that determine the risk of developing TA-GVHD are the degree of recipient immunodeficiency, the number of viable T cells in the transfusion, and the degree of a population's genetic diversity. Immunodeficient states that are risk factors for developing TA-GVHD include leukemia, lymphoma, use of immunosuppressive drugs administered for transplant or myeloablative chemotherapy, congenital immunodeficiency disorders, and the neonatal state.[102,103] The number of viable lymphocytes in a transfusion can be affected by the age, leukocyte reduction status, and irradiation status of the component.[104] The fresher the component, the more viable T cells it will contain. Unfortunately, the minimum number of viable lymphocytes required to cause TA-GVHD is unknown. Although current leukocyte reduction technologies significantly reduce the number of lymphocytes present in a component, leukocyte reduction does not eliminate the risk of TA-GVHD. There are well-documented cases in which transfusion of leukocyte-reduced blood components has caused TA-GVHD.[105] Irradiation of components, with no area of the bag receiving less than 15 Gy, is the only reliable way to ensure reduction of the number of viable lymphocytes to a level guaranteed to prevent TA-GVHD.[106]

Although patients who are immunocompromised are at risk of developing TA-GVHD, the disorder has been reported also in transfusion recipients with an intact immune system.[100,107] This can occur after transfusion from a donor who is homozygous for an HLA haplotype to a heterozygous recipient (one-way haplotype match). In this circumstance, the recipient's immune system is unable to recognize the HLA homozygous transfused lymphocytes as foreign. In contrast, the transfused lymphocytes are able to recognize the host cells as foreign and are able to mount an immunologic attack on the host. One-way haplotype matches are not uncommon in families because of shared HLA antigens.

The degree of genetic diversity in a population also affects the risk of developing TA-GVHD. The estimated risk of developing TA-GVHD ranges from 1:874 in Japan to 1:16,835 in France.[106] The difference is a result of the decreased diversity in HLA antigen expression in the Japanese population.

Treatment

Treatment of TA-GVHD has been attempted with a variety of immunosuppressive agents. Unfortunately, the disorder is almost uniformly fatal; only rare cases of successful treatment have been reported. Therefore, emphasis is placed on prevention of the disorder.

Prevention

TA-GVHD may be prevented by irradiation of cellular blood components. AABB standards require a minimum dose of 25 Gy (2500 cGy) delivered to the central portion of the container and a minimum of 15 Gy (1500 cGy) dose elsewhere.[8(p24)] AABB standards require irradiation of cellular blood components when 1) the patient is identified as being at risk for TA-GVHD, 2) the donor is a blood relative of the recipient, or 3) the donor is selected for HLA compatibility by typing or crossmatching.[8(p38)] These standards represent minimum requirements for irradiation of cellular blood components. Institutions may choose to include additional categories of patients who should receive irradiated components (see Table 27-2).

Posttransfusion Purpura

Presentation

Posttransfusion purpura (PTP) is a relatively uncommon complication of transfusion. Nonetheless, more than 200 cases are reported in the literature, and data from the Serious Hazards of Transfusion (SHOT) program in the United Kingdom suggest the disorder may be more common than previously appreciated.[105] Participating hospitals reported a total of 44 cases of PTP in 8 years. An additional report of cases estimates the frequency to be 1:24,000 blood components transfused.[108]

Patients typically present with wet purpura and thrombocytopenia at a mean of 9 days after transfusion (range = 1-24).[109] The thrombocytopenia is often profound, with platelet counts <10,000/µL. Bleeding from mucous membranes and the gastrointestinal and urinary tracts is common. Mortality rates in large case series range from 0 to 12.8%,[83,84] with the primary cause being intracranial hemorrhage.

PTP has most commonly been associated with the transfusion of RBCs or whole blood; however, the disorder has also been associated with the transfusion of platelets or plasma.

Differential Diagnosis

The differential diagnosis of PTP includes other causes of thrombocytopenia, such as autoimmune thrombocytopenic purpura, thrombotic thrombocytopenic purpura, heparin-induced thrombocytopenia, DIC, and drug-induced thrombocytopenia. Although the diagnosis of PTP can be obvious in patients with previously normal platelet counts and no other significant medical abnormalities (eg, a sur-

TABLE 27-2. Clinical Indications for Irradiated Components

Well-documented indications
Intrauterine transfusions
Premature, low-birthweight infants
Newborns with erythroblastosis fetalis
Congenital immunodeficiencies
Hematologic malignancies or solid tumors (neuroblastoma, sarcoma, Hodgkin disease)
Peripheral blood stem cell or marrow transplantation
Components that are crossmatched, HLA matched, or directed donations (from family members or related donors)
Fludarabine therapy
Granulocyte components
Potential indications
Other malignancies, including those treated with cytotoxic agents
Donor-recipient pairs from genetically homogeneous populations
Usually not indicated
Patients with human immunodeficiency virus
Term infants
Nonimmunosuppressed patients

gical patient presenting with wet purpura a week after hospital discharge), it can be a challenge in patients with multiple medical problems. Platelet serology studies may aid in the diagnosis.

Pathophysiology

The pathogenesis of PTP is related to the presence of platelet-specific alloantibodies in a previously exposed patient. The female-to-male ratio in affected patients is 5 to 1. Almost all patients have been exposed to platelet antigens via pregnancy or transfusion. Antibodies against human platelet antigen 1a (HPA-1a), located on glycoprotein IIIa, are identified in about 70% of PTP cases. Antibodies to HPA-1b, other platelet antigens, and HLA antigens have also been implicated in PTP.[109]

The reason for the concomitant destruction of autologous platelets in this disorder is unclear; three theories have been advanced. In the first, immune complexes bind to platelets through the Fc receptor, causing destruction of platelets.[110] In the second theory, the patient's platelets absorb a soluble platelet antigen from donor plasma, making them susceptible to immune destruction. In the third, the platelet alloantibody has autoreactivity that develops when a patient is reexposed to a foreign platelet-specific antigen.[109] The third theory currently has the most support.

The use of leukocyte reduction filters may decrease the incidence of PTP. In the 3 years before implementation of universal leukocyte reduction in the United Kingdom, there were 10.3 cases of PTP per year and 2.3 cases per year afterward ($p < 0.001$).[105] In addition, a higher number of cases after universal leukocyte reduction were associated with recent platelet transfusion. The decrease in PTP may be secondary to removal of platelets during leukocyte reduction of RBCs.

Treatment

Because the duration of thrombocytopenia in untreated patients is about 2 weeks, it can be difficult to assess the effectiveness of therapies reported to treat PTP. It has been difficult to determine whether the change in platelet count is secondary to treatment or to the natural disease process running its course. Steroids, whole blood exchange, and plasma exchange have all been used as treatments for PTP. The current treatment of choice for PTP is IVIG.[111,112] The average patient responds within 4 days; some respond within hours.

Prevention

PTP typically does not recur with subsequent transfusions. However, there are four case reports of PTP recurrence. Therefore, for patients with previously documented PTP, efforts should be made to obtain components from antigen-matched donors. Autologous donations and directed donations from antigen-matched donors and family members may be the most appropriate sources of blood for these patients. Because PTP has also occurred after transfusion of Deglycerolized Rejuvenated or Washed RBCs, such manipulations are not indicated for the prevention of recurrence.[109]

Iron Overload

A unit of RBCs contains approximately 250 mg of iron. The average rate of excretion of iron is approximately 1 mg per day. As red cells are destroyed, the majority of the released iron cannot be excreted and is stored in the body as hemosiderin and ferritin. Transferrin becomes saturated after the administration of 10 to 15 units of RBCs to a nonbleeding patient.[113] As iron accumulates in the reticuloendothelial system, liver, heart, spleen, and endocrine organs, tissue damage leading to heart failure, liver failure, diabetes, and hypothyroidism may occur. Patients who are chronically transfused for diseases such as thalassemia, sickle cell disease, and other chronic anemias are at the greatest risk for iron overload. A cumulative dose of 50 to 100 units of RBCs can cause significantly greater morbidity and mortality than the underlying anemia.[114] Prevention of the accumulation of these toxic levels of iron by reducing the body's iron stores through the use of iron chelators is therefore extremely important.

In iron chelation, an agent binds to iron in the body and tissues and helps remove it through the urine and/or feces. The development of iron-chelating drugs, such as parenteral deferoxamine and the oral agent deferiprone, greatly reduced the complications of iron overload in chronically transfused patients, leading to an improved quality of life. Deferiprone is more effective than deferoxamine in reducing myocardial siderosis.[115] The newest agent, deferasirox, has a much longer half-life than deferoxamine and may be administered in one daily oral dose. The use of deferasirox is expected to greatly enhance the acceptance of iron chelation therapy, especially for children, as the tablets are dissolved in a

TABLE 27-3. How to Notify the Food and Drug Administration

Method	Contact Details
E-mail	fatalities2@fda.hhs.gov
Telephone/voice-mail	301-827-6220
Fax	301-827-6748
Express mail	Food and Drug Administration Center for Biologics Evaluation and Research Director, Office of Compliance and Biologics Quality Attn: Fatality Program Manger (HFM-650) 1401 Rockville Pike, Suite 200N Rockville, MD 20852-1448

glass of juice or water. Although in-vivo studies are in early stages, deferasirox shows similar rapid access to intracellular iron stores in cultured myocytes as deferiprone.[116] Unlike deferiprone, which has occasionally been associated with agranulocytosis, the most frequent side effects of deferasirox are transient gastrointestinal distress and mildly increased creatinine levels, rarely of clinical significance. Deferasirox has shown efficacy in children and adults with sickle cell disease, resulting in a significant dose-dependent decline in their serum ferritin levels. No new adverse events were reported in the study, which covered a median 2.7-year treatment period.[117]

FATALITY REPORTING REQUIREMENTS

When the death of a patient results from a transfusion reaction or complication of transfusion, current good manufacturing practice regulations require reporting of the fatality to the FDA by the facility that performed the compatibility testing.[118] The director of the Office of Compliance and Biologics Quality for the Center for Biologics Evaluation and Research (CBER) must be notified as soon as possible by telephone, express mail, or electronic means (facsimile or electronic mail), followed by a written report within 7 days. Table 27-3 lists the contact information for the FDA. The report should contain the patient's medical records, including laboratory reports, and the autopsy results when available. The patient's underlying illness may make determination of the cause of death difficult. If there is any clinical suspicion that the transfusion may have contributed to the patient's death, an investigation into that possibility should be performed. Most transfusion-associated fatalities are caused by acute hemolysis, TRALI, anaphylaxis, or sepsis. Investigation in these cases must attempt to rule out laboratory, transfusion service, or blood administration error.[119]

KEY POINTS

1. Blood today is safer than ever. Hemovigilance and blood management programs should decrease the risk of noninfectious complications of transfusion even further.
2. Many transfusion reactions have signs or symptoms that may be present in more than one type of reaction. Early recognition, prompt cessation of the transfusion, and further evaluation are the keys to a successful resolution.
3. Acute intravascular hemolytic reactions are often caused by sample or patient misidentification and are thus, for the most part, preventable. Symptoms commonly include fever and range from chills to disseminated intravascular coagulation.
4. Allergic reactions range from urticaria (hives) to anaphylaxis. Patients suffering severe reactions should be checked for IgA deficiency and transfused accordingly.
5. Transfusion-related acute lung injury (TRALI) is a diagnosis of exclusion. Most patients will recover with supportive care. It is thought that TRALI has historically been underrecognized and underreported.
6. Transfusion-associated circulatory overload (TACO) can be confused with TRALI, as both feature pulmonary edema. TACO should be suspected in nonbleeding patients and those subject to congestive heart failure.
7. The most common complications of massive transfusion are hemostatic abnormalities. Each institution should develop its own massive transfusion protocol, taking into account the availability of appropriate laboratory testing.
8. Transfusion-associated graft-vs-host disease (TA-GVHD) has a much more acute and severe course compared to GVHD after marrow or stem cell transplantation. It is >90% fatal and is prevented by irradiation of blood components.

9. Posttransfusion purpura (PTP) is a serious but rare complication; antibodies to human platelet antigens result in destruction of autologous and allogeneic platelets.
10. Iron overload is perhaps the longest-lasting long-term complication of transfusion. Oral iron chelators greatly increase compliance with therapy.
11. The most and least common causes of transfusion-related mortality reported to the US Food and Drug Administration (FDA) are TRALI and PTP, respectively.
12. When the death of a patient results from a transfusion reaction or complication of transfusion, the fatality must be reported to the FDA by the facility that performed the compatibility testing.

REFERENCES

1. Fatalities reported to FDA following blood collection and transfusion: Annual summary for fiscal year 2009. Rockville, MD: Office of Communication, Outreach, and Development, 2010. [Available at http://www.fda.gov/BiologicsBloodVaccines/SafetyAvailability/ReportaProblem/TransfusionDonationFatalities/ucm113649.htm (accessed January 5, 2011).]
2. Centers for Disease Control and Prevention. The National Healthcare Safety Network (NHSN) manual: Biovigilance component. (July 2010) Atlanta, GA: CDC Division of Healthcare Quality Promotion, 2010. [Available at http://www.cdc.gov/nhsn/PDFs/hemovigModuleProtocol_current.pdf (accessed January 16, 2011).]
3. Williams L. The U.S. Biovigilance Network: Improving patient safety and donor health. AABB News 2009;11(10):8-16.
4. Staropoli A. The importance of being vigilant. AABB News 2009;11(10):18-22.
5. Hendrickson JE, Hillyer CD. Noninfectious serious hazards of transfusion. Anesth Analg 2009;108:759-69.
6. Eder AF, Chambers LA. Noninfectious complications of blood transfusion. Arch Pathol Lab Med 2007;131:708-18.
7. Jenner PW, Holland PV. Diagnosis and management of transfusion reactions. In: Petz LD, ed. Clinical practice of transfusion medicine. 3rd ed. New York: Churchill Livingstone, 1996: 905-29.
8. Carson TH, ed. Standards for blood banks and transfusion services. 27th ed. Bethesda, MD: AABB, 2011.
9. Mollison PL, Engelfriet CP, Contreras M. Blood transfusion in clinical medicine. 10th ed. Oxford, UK: Blackwell Science, 1997.
10. Mock DM, Lankford GL, Widness JA, et al. Measurement of red cell survival using biotin-labeled red cells: Validation against ^{51}Cr-labeled red cells. Transfusion 1999;39:156-62.
11. Josephson CD, Mullis NC, Van Demark C, et al. Significant numbers of apheresis-derived group O platelet units have “high-titer” anti-A/A,B: Implications for transfusion policy. Transfusion 2004;44:805-8.
12. Sapatnekar S, Sharma G, Downes KA, et al. AHTR in a pediatric patient following transfusion of apheresis platelets. J Clin Apher 2005; 20:225-9.
13. Davenport RD. Hemolytic transfusion reactions. In: Popovsky MA, ed. Transfusion reactions. 3rd ed. Bethesda, MD: AABB Press, 2007: 1-55.
14. Davenport RD, Strieter RN, Standiford TJ, et al. Interleukin-8 production in red cell incompatibility. Blood 1990;76:2439-42.
15. Hod EA, Cadwell CM, Liepkalms JS, et al. Cytokine storm in a mouse model of IgG-mediated hemolytic transfusion reactions. Blood 2008; 112:891-4.
16. Linden JV, Wagner K, Voytovich AE, et al. Transfusion errors in New York state: An analysis of 10 years’ experience. Transfusion 2000; 40:1207-13.
17. Spiess BD. Risks of transfusion: Outcome focus. Transfusion 2004;44(12 Suppl):4S-14S.
18. Vamvakas EC, Blajchman MA. Transfusion-related mortality: The ongoing risks of allogeneic blood transfusion and the available strategies for their prevention. Blood 2009;113:3406-417.
19. Alter HJ, Klein HG. The hazards of blood transfusion in historical perspective. Blood 2008; 112:2617-25.
20. Friedrich JO, Adhikari N, Herridge MS, et al. Meta-analysis: Low-dose dopamine increases urine output but does not prevent renal dys-

function or death. Ann Intern Med 2005;142: 510-24.
21. Ludens JH, Hook JB, Brody MJ, et al. Enhancement of renal blood flow by furosemide. J Pharmacol Exp Ther 1968;163:456-60.
22. Goldfinger D. Acute hemolytic transfusion reactions—a fresh look at pathogenesis and considerations regarding therapy. Transfusion 1977;17:85-98.
23. Toh CH, Dennis M. Disseminated intravascular coagulation: Old disease, new hope. Br Med J 2003;327:974-7.
24. Norman KE. Alternative treatments for disseminated intravascular coagulation. Drug News Perspect 2004;17:243-50.
25. Monitoring and preventing the occurrence of deviations and near-miss events in pretransfusion testing: Mislabeling/wrong blood in tube. Association bulletin #06-05. Bethesda, MD: AABB, 2006. [Available at http://www.aabb.org>ResourceCenter>Publications>Association Bulletins (accessed November 12, 2010).]
26. Janatpour KA, Kalmin ND, Jensen HM, Holland PV. Clinical outcomes of ABO-incompatible RBC transfusions. Am J Clin Pathol 2008; 129:276-81.
27. Fung MK, Downes KA, Shulman IA. Transfusion of platelets containing ABO-incompatible plasma: A survey of 3156 North American laboratories. Arch Pathol Lab Med 2007;131:909-16.
28. Dubey A, Verma A, Sonker A, et al. Transfusion medicine illustrated. Sudden increased incidence of transfusion reactions reported from a ward: Root cause analysis. Transfusion 2009; 49:409-10.
29. Brand A. Passenger leukocytes, cytokines, and transfusion reactions (editorial). N Engl J Med 1994;331:670-1.
30. Oberman HA. Controversies in transfusion medicine: Should a febrile transfusion response occasion the return of the blood component to the blood bank? Con. Transfusion 1994;34:353-5.
31. Ezidiegwu CN, Lauenstein KJ, Rosales LG, et al. Febrile nonhemolytic transfusion reactions. Management by premedication and cost implications in adult patients. Arch Pathol Lab Med 2004;128:991-5.
32. Paglino JC, Pomper GJ, Fisch GS, et al. Reduction of febrile but not allergic reactions to RBCs and platelets after conversion to universal prestorage leukoreduction. Transfusion 2004;44:16-24.
33. Tang AW. A practical guide to anaphylaxis. Am Fam Physician 2003;68:1325-32.
34. Hennino A, Berard F, Guillot I, et al. Pathophysiology of urticaria. Clin Rev Allergy Immunol 2006;30:3-11.
35. Cotran RS, ed. Robbins pathologic basis of disease. 5th ed. Philadelphia: WB Saunders, 1994: 178.
36. MedlinePlus medical encyclopedia: Selective deficiency of IgA. Atlanta, GA: A.D.A.M., 2007. [Available at http://www.nlm.nih.gov/medlineplus/ency/article/001476.htm (accessed November 12, 2010).]
37. Sandler SG, Mallory D, Malamut D, et al. IgA anaphylactic transfusion reactions. Transfus Med Rev 1995;9:1-8.
38. Shimada E, Odagiri M, Chaiwong K, et al. Detection of Hp^{del} among Thais, a deleted allele of the haptoglobin gene that causes congenital haptoglobin deficiency. Transfusion 2007;47: 2315-21.
39. Lambin P, Le Pennec PY, Hauptmann G, et al. Adverse transfusion reactions associated with a precipitating anti-C4 antibody of anti-Rodgers specificity. Vox Sang 1984;47:242-9.
40. Leitman SF, Boltansky H, Alter HJ, et al. Allergic reactions in healthy plateletpheresis donors caused by sensitization to ethylene oxide gas. N Engl J Med 1986;315:1192-6.
41. Domen RE, Hoeltge GA. Allergic transfusion reactions: An evaluation of 273 consecutive reactions. Arch Pathol Lab Med 2003;127:316-20.
42. Vamvakas EC. Allergic and anaphylactic reactions. In: Popovsky MA, ed. Transfusion reactions. 3rd ed. Bethesda, MD: AABB Press, 2007: 105-56.
43. Stainsby D, Jones H, Asher D, et al. Serious hazards of transfusion: A decade of hemovigilance in the UK. Transfus Med Rev 2006;20: 273-82.
44. Brown SGA, Mullins RJ, Gold MS. 2. Anaphylaxis: Diagnosis and management. Med J Aust 2006;185:283-9.
45. Kennedy LD, Case LD, Hurd DD, et al. A prospective, randomized, double-blind controlled trial of acetaminophen and diphenhydramine pretransfusion medication versus placebo for the prevention of transfusion reactions. Transfusion 2008;48:2285-91.
46. Sandler SG. How do I manage patients suspected of having had an IgA anaphylactic transfusion reaction? Transfusion 2006;46: 10-13.

47. Popovsky MA, Haley NR. Further characterization of transfusion-related acute lung injury: Demographics, clinical and laboratory features and morbidity. Immunohematology 2000; 16:157-9.
48. Nakagawa M, Toy P. Acute and transient decrease in neutrophil count in transfusion-related acute lung injury: Cases at one hospital. Transfusion 2004;44:1689-94.
49. Bernard GR, Artigas A, Brigham KL, et al. The American-European Consensus Conference on ARDS. Definitions, mechanisms, relevant outcomes, and clinical trial coordination (review). Am J Respir Crit Care Med 1994;149:818-24.
50. Kleinman S, Caulfield T, Chan P, et al. Toward an understanding of transfusion-related acute lung injury: Statement of a consensus panel. Transfusion 2004;44:1774-89.
51. Popovsky MA, Moore SB. Diagnostic and pathogenetic considerations in transfusion-related acute lung injury. Transfusion 1985;25: 573-7.
52. Silliman CC, Ambruso DR, Boshkov LK. Transfusion-related acute lung injury. Blood 2005; 105:2266-73.
53. Popovsky MA, Chaplin HC Jr, Moore SB. Transfusion-related acute lung injury: A neglected, serious complication of hemotherapy. Transfusion 1992;32:589-92.
54. Silliman CC, Boshkov LK, Mehdizadehkashi Z, et al. Transfusion-related acute lung injury: Epidemiology and a prospective analysis of etiologic factors. Blood 2003;101:454-62.
55. Kopko PM, Popovsky MA. Transfusion-related acute lung injury. In: Popovsky MA, ed. Transfusion reactions. 3rd ed. Bethesda, MD: AABB Press, 2007:207-28.
56. Steinberg KP, Hudson LD, Goodman RB, et al. Efficacy and safety of corticosteroids for persistent acute respiratory distress syndrome. N Engl J Med 2006;354:1671-84.
57. Transfusion-related acute lung injury. Association bulletin #06-07. Bethesda, MD: AABB, 2006. [Available at http://www.aabb.org>ResourceCenter>Publications>AssociationBulletins (accessed November 12, 2010).]
58. Clarifications to recommendations to reduce the risk of TRALI. Association bulletin #07-03. Bethesda, MD: AABB, 2007. [Available at http://www.aabb.org>ResourceCenter>Publications>Association Bulletins (accessed November 12, 2010).]
59. Triulzi D, Kleinman S, Kakaiya R, et al. The effect of previous pregnancy and transfusion on HLA alloimmunization in blood donors: Implications for a transfusion-related acute lung injury risk reduction strategy. Transfusion 2009;49:1825-35.
60. Robillard P, Itaj NK, Chapdelaine A. Increasing incidence of transfusion-associated circulatory overload reported to the Quebec Hemovigilance System, 2000-2006 (abstract). Transfusion 2008;48(Suppl):204A.
61. Pomper GJ. Febrile, allergic, and non-immune transfusion reactions. In: Simon TL, Snyder EL, Solheim BG, et al, eds. Rossi's principles of transfusion medicine. 4th ed. Bethesda, MD: AABB Press, 2009:826-46.
62. Zhou L, Giacherion D, Cooling L, et al. Use of B-natriuretic peptide as a diagnostic marker in the differential diagnosis of transfusion-associated circulatory overload. Transfusion 2005; 45:1056-63.
63. Li G, Daniels CE, Kojicic M, et al. The accuracy of natriuretic peptides (brain natriuretic peptide and N-terminal pro-brain natriuretic) in the differentiation between transfusion-related acute lung injury and transfusion-related circulatory overload in the critically ill. Transfusion 2009;49:13-20.
64. Popovsky MA, Audet AM, Andrzejewski C. Transfusion-associated circulatory overload in orthopedic surgery patients: A multi-institutional study. Immunohematology 1996;12:87-9.
65. Bierbaum BE, Callaghan JJ, Galante JO. An analysis of blood management in patients having a total hip or knee arthroplasty. J Bone Joint Surg Am 1999;81:2-10.
66. Robillard P, Itaj KI, Chapdelaine AC. Incidence of TRALI and respiratory complications in the Quebec Hemovigilance System (abstract). Vox Sang 2006;91(Suppl 3):229.
67. Rana R, Fernandez-Perez E, Khan SA, et al. Transfusion-related acute lung injury and pulmonary edema in critically ill patients: A retrospective study. Transfusion 2006;46:1478-83.
68. Dzik WH, Kirkley SA. Citrate toxicity during massive blood transfusion. Transfus Med Rev 1988;2:76-94.
69. Olinger GN, Hottenrott C, Mulder DG, et al. Acute clinical hypocalcemic myocardial depression during rapid transfusion and postoperative hemodialysis: A preventable complication. J Thorac Cardiovasc Surg 1976;72:503-11.

70. Howland WS, Jacobs RG, Goulet AH. An evaluation of calcium administration during rapid blood replacement. Anesth Analg 1960;39:557-63.
71. Dzik WH. Massive transfusion in the adult patient: Lessons from liver transplantation. In: Jeffries LC, Brecher ME, eds. Massive transfusion. Bethesda, MD: AABB, 1994:65-93.
72. Wilson RF, Binkley LE, Sabo FM, et al. Electrolyte and acid-base changes with massive transfusion. Am Surg 1992;58:535-44.
73. Collins JA. Problems associated with the massive transfusion of stored blood. Surgery 1974; 174:274-95.
74. Liu EA, Manino FL, Lane TA. Prospective, randomized trial of the safety and efficacy of a limited donor exposure program for premature neonates. J Pediatr 1994;125:92-6.
75. Bansal I, Calhoun BW, Joseph C, et al. A comparative study of reducing the extracellular potassium concentration in red blood cells by washing and by reduction of additive solutions. Transfusion 2007;47:248-50.
76. Malone DL, Hess JR, Fingerhut A. Massive transfusion practices around the globe and a suggestion for a common massive transfusion protocol. J Trauma 2006:60(Suppl):S91-6.
77. Engstrom M, Schott U, Rommer B, Reinstrup P. Acidosis impairs the coagulation: A thromboelastographic study. J Trauma 2006;61:624-8.
78. Miller RD, Robbins TO, Tong MJ, et al. Coagulation defects associated with massive blood transfusion. Ann Surg 1971;174:794-801.
79. Counts RB, Haisch C, Simon TL, et al. Hemostasis in massively transfused trauma patients. Ann Surg 1979;190:91-9.
80. Murray DJ, Pennell BJ, Weinstein SL, et al. Packed red cells in acute blood loss: Dilutional coagulopathy as a cause of surgical bleeding. Anesth Analg 1995;80:336-42.
81. Lim RC, Olcott C, Robinson AJ, et al. Platelet response and coagulation changes following massive blood replacement. J Trauma 1973;13: 577-82.
82. Harrigan C, Lucas CE, Ledgerwood KAT, et al. Serial changes in primary hemostasis after massive transfusion. Surgery 1985;98:836-43.
83. Harke H, Rahman S. Haemostatic disorders in massive transfusion. Bibl Haematol 1980;46: 179-88.
84. Collins JA. Recent developments in the area of massive transfusion. World J Surg 1987;11:75-81.
85. Plotkin AJ, Wade CE, Jenkins DH, et al. A reduction in clot formation rate and strength assessed by thromboelastography is indicative of transfusion requirements in patients with penetrating injuries. J Trauma 2008;64:S64-8.
86. Reed RI, Ciaverella D, Heimbach DM, et al. Prophylactic platelet administration during massive transfusion: A prospective, randomized double-blinded clinical study. Ann Surg 1986;203:40-8.
87. Borgman MA, Spinella PC, Perkins JG, et al. The ratio of blood products transfused affects mortality in patients receiving massive transfusions at a combat support hospital. J Trauma 2007;63:805-13.
88. Rice CI, John DA, Smith DE. Coagulation changes with packed red cell versus whole blood transfusion (abstract). Crit Care Med 1978;6:118.
89. Roback JD, Caldwell S, Carson J, et al. Evidence-base practice guidelines for plasma transfusion. Transfusion 2010;50:1227-39.
90. Hedner U, Erhardson E. Potential role for rFVIIa in transfusion medicine. Transfusion 2002; 42:114-24.
91. Uhl L. Complications of massive transfusion. In: Popovsky MA, ed. Transfusion reactions. 3rd ed. Bethesda, MD: AABB Press, 2007:435-57.
92. Dutton RP, Hess JR, Scalea TM. Recombinant factor VIIa for control of hemorrhage: Early experience in critically ill trauma patients. J Clin Anesth 2003;15:184-8.
93. Clark AD, Gordon WC, Walker ID, et al. "Last-ditch" use of recombinant factor VIIa in patients with massive hemorrhage is ineffective. Vox Sang 2006;86:120-4.
94. O'Quin RJ, Lakshminarayan S. Venous air embolism. Arch Intern Med 1982;142:2173-7.
95. Schonewille H, van de Watering LMG, Loomans DSE, Brand A. Red blood cell alloantibodies after transfusion: Factors influencing incidence and specificity. Transfusion 2006;46: 250-6.
96. Vamvakas EC, Pineda AA, Reisner R, et al. The differentiation of delayed hemolytic and delayed serologic transfusion reactions: Incidence and predictors of hemolysis. Transfusion 1995;35:26-32.
97. Schonewille H, van de Watering LMG, Brand A. Additional red blood cell alloantibodies after blood transfusions in a nonhematologic alloimmunized patient cohort: Is it time to take

precautionary measures? Transfusion 2006;46: 630-4.

98. Rhl H, Bein G, Sachs UJH. Transfusion-associated graft-versus-host disease. Transfus Med Rev 2009;23:62-71.
99. Hutchinson K, Kopko PM, Muto KN, et al. Early diagnosis and successful treatment of a patient with transfusion-associated GVHD with autologous peripheral blood progenitor cell transplantation. Transfusion 2002;42:1567-72.
100. Triulzi D, Duquesnoy R, Nichols L, et al. Fatal transfusion-associated graft-versus-host disease in an immunocompetent recipient of a volunteer unit of red cells. Transfusion 2006; 46:885-8.
101. Billingham R. The biology of graft-versus-host reactions. In: The Harvey lecture series, 1966-1967. Orlando, FL: Academic Press, 1968; 62:21-78.
102. Anderson KC, Weinstein HJ. Transfusion-associated graft-versus-host disease. N Engl J Med 1990;323:315-21.
103. Leitman SF, Tisdale JF, Bolan CD, et al. Transfusion-associated GVHD after fludarabine therapy in a patient with systemic lupus erythematosus. Transfusion 2003;43:1667-71.
104. Klein HG. Transfusion-associated graft-versus-host disease: Less fresh blood and more gray (Gy) for an aging population. Transfusion 2006;46:878-80.
105. Williamson LM, Stainsby D, Jones H, et al. The impact of universal leukodepletion of the blood supply on hemovigilance reports of posttransfusion purpura and transfusion-associated graft-versus-host disease. Transfusion 2007;47:1455-67.
106. Alyea EP, Anderson KC. Transfusion-associated graft-versus-host disease. In: Popovsky MA, ed. Transfusion reactions. 3rd ed. Bethesda, MD: AABB Press, 2007:229-49.
107. Petz LD, Calhoun L, Yam P, et al. Transfusion-associated graft-vs-host disease in immunocompetent patients: Report of a fatal case associated with transfusion of blood from a second-degree relative, and a survey of predisposing factors. Transfusion 1993;33:742-50.
108. Shtalrid M, Shvidel L, Vorst E, et al. Post-transfusion purpura: A challenging diagnosis. Isr Med Assoc J 2006;8:672-4.
109. McFarland JG. Posttransfusion purpura. In: Popovsky MA, ed. Transfusion reactions. 3rd ed. Bethesda, MD: AABB Press, 2007:275-99.
110. Shulman NR, Aster RH, Leitner A, et al. Immunoreactions involving platelets. V. Post-transfusion purpura due to a complement-fixing antibody against a genetically controlled platelet antigen. A proposed mechanism for thrombocytopenia and its relevance in "autoimmunity." J Clin Invest 1961;40:1597-620.
111. Ziman A, Klapper E, Pepkowitz S, et al. A second case of post-transfusion purpura caused by HPA-5a antibodies: Successful treatment with intravenous immunoglobulin. Vox Sang 2002;83:165-6.
112. Woelke C, Eichler P, Washington G, et al. Post-transfusion purpura in a patient with HPA-1a and GPIa/IIa antibodies. Transfus Med 2006;16:69-72.
113. Ley TJ, Griffith P, Nienhuis AW. Transfusion haemosiderosis and chelation therapy. Clin Haematol 1982;11:437-64.
114. Sharon BI. Management of congenital hemolytic anemias. In: Simon TL, Snyder EL, Solheim BG, et al, eds. Rossi's principles of transfusion medicine. 4th ed. Bethesda, MD: AABB Press, 2009:448-69.
115. Cario H, Janka-Schaub G, Jarisch A, et al. Recent developments in iron chelation therapy. Klin Padiatr 2007;219:158-65.
116. Neufeld EJ. Oral chelators deferasirox and deferiprone for transfusional iron overload in thalassemia major: New data, new questions. Blood 2006:3436-41.
117. Hampton T. Strides made in red blood cell disorders, but substantial barriers to care remain. JAMA 2008;299:395-6.
118. Food and Drug Administration. Guidance for industry: Notifying FDA of fatalities related to blood collection or transfusion. (September 22, 2003) Rockville, MD: CBER Office of Communication, Outreach, and Development, 2003.
119. Code of federal regulations. Adverse reaction file. Title 21, CFR Part 606.170(a). Washington, DC: US Government Printing Office, 2010 (revised annually).

Chapter 28

Approaches to Blood Utilization Auditing

Alan Tinmouth, MD, FRCPC, MSc, and

Simon Stanworth, MD, DPhil

AUDITING THE USE of blood transfusions is a required and necessary function for all hospital transfusion services.[1] Both The Joint Commission and the AABB require health-care institutions to monitor the use of blood components at their facilities. The Joint Commission requires hospitals to collect data to monitor the performance of processes that involve risks or may result in sentinel events, which includes the use of blood and blood components (Standard PI.3.1.1).[2] The AABB requires all facilities to have a peer-review program to monitor transfusion practices for all categories of blood and components, including monitoring of usage and discard and appropriateness of use.[3(p85)] In addition, federal regulations pertaining to Medicare and Medicaid require that hospitals make recommendations to the medical staff regarding improvements in transfusion procedures.[1] Other countries have similar requirements for processes to audit and monitor transfusion practice. For example, in the United Kingdom, through the Department of Health, its Better Blood Transfusion initiatives, and the Care and Quality Commission, there is a requirement to participate in national audits, including the National Comparative Audit of Blood Transfusion program.

Several different methods can be employed to meet the requirements to monitor or audit blood transfusion use, but the general objective of all blood utilization programs is to ensure the appropriate use of blood components. Historically, audits of component use have concentrated on controlling or reducing the total number of components transfused and/or individual "overtransfusion." This focus is based on the assumption that inappropriate use is primarily overtransfusion. How-

Alan Tinmouth, MD, FRCPC, MSc, Head, General Medicine and Transfusion Medicine, The Ottawa Hospital, and Scientist, University of Ottawa Centre for Transfusion Research, Clinical Epidemiology Program, Ottawa Hospital Research Institute, Ottawa, Ontario, Canada, and Simon Stanworth, MD, DPhil, Consultant Hematologist, National Health Service Blood and Transplant, Oxford Radcliffe Hospitals, University of Oxford, Oxford, United Kingdom

(Alan Tinmouth is supported by a Research Award from the Department of Medicine, The Ottawa Hospital.)
The authors have disclosed no conflicts of interests.

ever, with increased attention on limiting patients' exposure to blood components, undertransfusion now may be an issue. In addition, examining the dose of the blood transfusion request, which may result in overuse or underuse, might need to be assessed in audits. Nevertheless, neither of these issues has historically been a major focus in the monitoring of blood transfusion utilization.[4]

The specific methods used to audit blood component use should depend partially on the desired objectives. Monitoring trends in the total number of components transfused, perhaps to control ordering or inventory management, requires a different process than that required when the primary aim is to limit individual inappropriate transfusion requests. In all instances, the transfusion service (technologists and/or physicians) and the institutional transfusion medicine or blood utilization committee should work together to perform the appropriate audit(s) and follow-up.

RATIONALE FOR MONITORING BLOOD UTILIZATION

The primary motivation for monitoring blood utilization is to identify instances when component use is less than optimal. Interventions can then be undertaken to change transfusion practice. This emphasizes the need to couple audits or monitoring with a recognized process to effectively provide feedback of the findings to the appropriate health-care professionals.

Improving or ensuring optimal use of blood transfusions is important for a number of reasons. Blood is a biologic agent associated with many possible adverse events, which include both infectious and noninfectious complications.[5,6] Many of these complications are well known; others are not generally recognized by physicians or the general population, and other potential complications are still not fully understood. Unnecessary complications from inappropriate blood transfusions need to be avoided. Moreover, blood components are a scarce and expensive resource. Transfusing a single unit of Red Blood Cells (RBCs) has been estimated to cost from US$400[7] to US$760[8] when all the associated costs are included, and many regions have experienced shortages of blood products.[6]

Through monitoring of component use, instances of inappropriate use can be identified, and corrective actions can be taken. If a "real-time," or prospective, audit system is being used, a member of the transfusion medicine service can intervene, which may result in a change to the transfusion request before the issue of a component. A retrospective review does not alter the current transfusion episode but identifies issues that can be addressed through interventions designed to change future transfusion practice.

A variety of different interventions have been used to change transfusion practice (Table 28-1). The most common interventions for change have included audit and feedback, which is defined by the Cochrane Effective Practice and Organisation of Care Group as "any summary of clinical performance of health care over a specified period of time." There is less understanding about the effective "ingredients" in audit and feedback or how the feedback should be best structured to deliver the change in behavior in different settings. Following the delivery of an intervention, ongoing monitoring then allows for an assessment of the intervention's sustained effectiveness and of the need for ongoing or additional intervention. In summary, audits serve the dual function of identifying areas of concern in the use of blood and then monitoring any interventions or changes in the identified areas.

TYPES OF TRANSFUSION AUDITS

Audits of transfusion practice can examine individual blood transfusion requests and/or aggregate transfusion data. The individual review can be performed either prospectively in real time or retrospectively. Review of individual transfusions may also be performed (retrospectively) very shortly after the event (usually within 24 hours); this has been termed a concurrent review, as it still affords the ability to provide timely feedback on individual transfusion episodes.[9] More remote retrospective au-

TABLE 28-1. Use of Interventions to Change Transfusion Practice with Different Types of Audits

Intervention	Prospective Audit	Concurrent Audit	Retrospective Audit
Individual education/feedback	++	++	+
Group education/feedback/teaching	–	–	++
Guideline dissemination	+	+	+
Incorporation of reminders/guidelines into transfusion request form or computerized order entry system	++	++	+

++ = very complementary to audit type; + = can be complementary to audit type; – = less complementary or not complementary to audit type.

dits allow for the review of aggregate transfusion data, which can then be analyzed in a number of ways. Reviews of individual and aggregate transfusion data are not mutually exclusive. As they may serve different functions or purposes, they can in fact be complementary.

Prospective ("Real-Time") Audit

In a prospective audit, the transfusion requests are reviewed in real time (ie, review of individual transfusion requests before issue of the component). An electronic review using a computer-based algorithm, a manual review by technologists, or both is undertaken whereby the request is compared to local transfusion audit criteria. Clinical data (eg, hematocrit and indication for red cell transfusion) is required to perform the review. Ideally, this information is obtained from the clinical staff as part of the transfusion request process. Alternatively, laboratory staff can obtain some of this data from the laboratory information system. Transfusions that do not meet the audit criteria are flagged, and the requesting physician is contacted by the transfusion medicine service before issuing the component, to discuss the need for the transfusion.

A prospective audit system should be organized such that undue delays in filling transfusion requests do not occur. Delays in laboratory results and the uncertainties of clinical cases also need to be understood and reflected in the audit process. Given these issues and constraints, the criteria used as part of the prospective audit may need to be less rigid than guidelines for the optimal utilization of components, as prospective audits might delay some urgent transfusions that fail to meet audit criteria for appropriateness but are nevertheless necessary. Therefore, a mechanism should be in place to ensure that emergency and urgent transfusions are not unduly delayed. Specific clinical areas such as emergency departments and operating suites, where delays in filling transfusion requests might result in adverse clinical events, are often excluded from prospective transfusion audits.

It is important to understand that prospective audits have the potential to raise animosity from the ordering physician when a transfusion request is questioned. Engaging the requesting physician groups and broadly consulting in the development of the audit guidelines and the audit process can help reduce friction and ensure long-term success of a prospective audit system. Another consideration is that because the interaction with the requesting physician often requires the involvement of a transfusion medicine physician or, at least, a senior technologist, the time requirements of technologists and physicians in a prospective audit system can be substantial. To reduce the potential for this to become onerous, selective audits of specific clinical areas (eg, obstetrics, orthopedics), specific periods, or both may be used.

The potential benefits of a prospective audit are obvious. A prospective audit provides the ability to intervene directly and change a specific transfusion request before the component is issued. This may stop an unnecessary transfusion or lead to a change in the request such that a more appropriate component or dose is ordered. Ideally, the immediate intervention in a prospective audit also results in long-term changes in the transfusion practice of the ordering physician. However, the benefits from this immediate intervention need to be weighed against the additional work required by the transfusion medicine service, including the transfusion medicine physician.

A number of reports from single institutions have demonstrated the effectiveness of prospective audits in reducing the total number units transfused,[10-13] the number of units transfused per patient,[12,14,15] the proportion of patients transfused,[16] and the number of inappropriate transfusions[12,17] (Table 28-2). Eight of these nine studies[10-14,16,17,20] used prospective audits in conjunction with other interventions to change transfusion practice. Although these reports attest to the potential utility of prospective audits to change transfusion practice, the sustainability of the changes in transfusion practice resulting from the introduction of a prospective audit is not known. In one study, the initial reduction in inappropriate transfusions following the implementation of a prospective audit system did not persist when reexamined 3 years later.[20]

Concurrent Audit

A concurrent audit is a review of individual transfusion requests that occurs in the 12 to 24 hours following the transfusion episode.[9] As such, it involves similar processes as the prospective audit, but as a posttransfusion review, the individual transfusion event cannot be altered. Therefore, the concurrent audit seeks only to alter future transfusion practice. Nevertheless, follow-up with the requesting physician occurs while the transfusion event remains fresh in his or her memory. It is hoped that this immediate contact improves the chance of changing the physician's future transfusion behavior.

As with the prospective audit, the concurrent review can be performed either by a computer algorithm or manually using transfusion audit criteria. The review may occur at the time of the transfusion or shortly after the request is filled. Requests that do not meet the audit criteria are flagged for subsequent review by a senior technologist or transfusion medicine physician. When performing the review, the transfusion medicine physician may have access to additional laboratory results that help to determine appropriateness. However, the review should also consider that these additional results were not available to the ordering physician at the time of the request. Because the concurrent audit does not delay the filling of the transfusion request, the audit can assess urgent transfusions and use stricter criteria for appropriateness as compared to a prospective audit.

Following the identification of an inappropriate transfusion request, the ordering physician may be contacted by phone or e-mail to discuss the case while the details are fresh in the mind of the ordering physician. The less immediate nature of the request and the ability to use written communication may reduce any potential animosity from the ordering physician. This may result in a more meaningful dialogue. One study by Shanberge et al reported a 77% reduction in the number of Fresh Frozen Plasma units transfused after the introduction of a concurrent audit system combined with a new guideline and an education program.[28]

Concurrent audits are still time consuming and they usually require a transfusion medicine physician to review inappropriate transfusion requests and follow up with the requesting physicians. For this reason, performing a concurrent audit on all transfusion requests may not be feasible. Using selective audits as discussed with prospective audits is an option to reduce workload. The use of concurrent audits may be particularly relevant in certain patient groups—such as trauma patients or other patients in the emergency department, where there is urgent need for

TABLE 28-2. Studies Evaluating the Effectiveness of Prospective and Retrospective Audits to Change Transfusion Practice

Study	Interventions	Blood Components	Reduction in Inappropriate Transfusions (%)	Reduction in Proportion of Patients Transfused (%)	Reduction in Number of Units per Patient (%)	Reduction in Total Number of Units Transfused (%)
Sarode (2010)[10]	Prospective audit; guideline; education	RBCs	—	—	—	13
		FFP	—	—	—	60
		Platelets	—	—	—	25
Yeh (2006)[11]	Prospective audit; retrospective audit	RBCs	—	—	—	15
		FFP	—	—	—	74
		Platelets	—	—	—	14
Rubin (2001)[18]	Audit/feedback; education	RBCs	2	—	—	—
Capraro (2001)[19]	Retrospective audit; education	RBCs	—	26	—	—
		FFP	—	7	—	—
		Platelets	—	6	—	—
Tobin (2001)[20]	Prospective audit; guidelines	RBCs	+4	—	—	—
		FFP	+13	—	—	—
		Platelets	+14	—	—	—
Hameedullah (2000)[21]	Retrospective audit; guideline; education	FFP	—	21	—	—
Rehm (1998)[14]	Prospective audit; form	RBCs	—	—	26	—
Joshi (1997)[22]	Retrospective audit; guideline	RBCs	21	50	—	—
Tuckfield (1997)[17]	Prospective audit; form	RBCs	13	—	—	—
		FFP	10	—	—	—
		Platelets	10	—	—	—

(Continued)

TABLE 28-2. Studies Evaluating the Effectiveness of Prospective and Retrospective Audits to Change Transfusion Practice (Continued)

Study	Interventions	Blood Components	Reduction in Inappropriate Transfusions (%)	Reduction in Proportion of Patients Transfused (%)	Reduction in Number of Units per Patient (%)	Reduction in Total Number of Units Transfused (%)
Cheng (1996)[12]	Prospective audit; form	FFP	7	—	35	31
		Platelets	10	—	22	17
Littenberg (1995)[16]	Prospective audit; guideline	RBCs	—	4	—	1
Brandis (1994)[23]	Retrospective audit; education	RBCs	—	—	29	19
Hawkins (1994)[15]	Prospective audit	FFP	—	—	55	—
Morrison (1993)[24]	Retrospective audit; education; guideline; form	RBCs	—	—	12	62
Rosen (1993)[25]	Retrospective audit; form; guideline	RBCs	—	—	27	21
		FFP	—	—	18	9
		Platelets	—	—	23	15
Ayoub (1989)[26]	Retrospective audit; education; guideline	FFP	—	—	—	46
Giovanetti (1988)[27]	Retrospective audit; guideline	RBCs	67	11	—	—
Solomon (1988)[13]	Prospective audit; retrospective audit; guideline; education; form	FFP	—	—	—	52
Shanberge (1987)[28]	Concurrent audit; education; guideline	FFP	—	—	—	77
Handler (1983)[29]	Retrospective audit; education	RBCs	—	79	—	—

RBCs = Red Blood Cells; FFP = Fresh Frozen Plasma; — = not studied; + = increased by.

blood—but the recording of accurate timelines, which might not be readily determined in retrospective audits, is needed to determine the appropriate activation of massive transfusion protocols or communication with the transfusion service.

Retrospective Audit

Retrospective audits of blood utilization are commonly performed by hospital teams or transfusion services. Results should be reviewed by the transfusion medicine committee. The frequency of such audits varies from one institution to another. Computerized information technology systems may facilitate an ongoing program of utilization review across many specialties. In contrast to prospective and concurrent reviews, a retrospective audit can look at aggregate transfusion data and trends in transfusion utilization, which may be informative for understanding wider differences in transfusion practice across different specialty groups. Individual transfusion requests can also be reviewed for appropriateness as part of a retrospective audit, but this may be cumbersome unless the data are collected prospectively or the laboratory information system can link transfusion events and laboratory results.

The retrospective review can analyze the data in a variety of manners. The simplest analysis would examine the total number of components transfused and the total number of patients transfused. However, these data might show considerable temporal variability that limits meaningful analysis. Further analysis is required to make observations regarding differences in blood utilization. The mean or median number of units transfused per hospitalized patient and/or procedure provides a more meaningful summary of component use. Merely dividing the total number of units by the total number of patients is not an appropriate statistical analysis; any observed changes in total blood use, particularly during a short period, could be skewed by a small number of individuals who required a large number of units. The proportion of patients transfused should also be determined. The proportion transfused could be further examined by procedure or clinical specialty. These would represent the minimum analyses required to monitor differences in component use. Additional analyses could include assessment of appropriate and inappropriate transfusion rates, although this would require collecting additional clinical data and individual review of transfusion requests, which may be a labor-intensive exercise.

Generally, a retrospective review is less labor intensive than a prospective or concurrent review, particularly as it involves less immediate attention from a technologist or a transfusion medicine physician. The amount of time required to perform the review will depend on the amount of detail desired. Utilization trends by individual component, individual physician, or clinical service can be analyzed. For health-care institutions with multiple sites, similar clinical services at different sites can also be compared. These additional layers of analysis may provide important information to identify variation in practice and detect inappropriate transfusion practices. Such areas could then be targeted for an intervention to improve transfusion practice.

The use of retrospective audits and dedicated feedback to clinicians has been effective in a number of studies in reducing the total number of units transfused,[11,13,23-26] the number of units transfused per patient,[23-25] the proportion of patients transfused,[19,21,22,27,29] and the number of inappropriate transfusions[18,22,27] (Table 28-2). The durability of these changes in transfusion practice following the introduction of a retrospective audit has not been evaluated.

INTERVENTIONS TO CHANGE TRANSFUSION PRACTICE

As previously described, the results of transfusion audits should ideally be used in conjunction with specific interventions to effect change and improve transfusion practice. Thus, audits should be considered as a critical component of a larger process to optimize the use of components. This process can be more widely conceived as "dissemination," "knowledge translation," or "implementation" work, where the goal is to increase the uptake of research or best knowledge into daily practice.[30] The process of closing the gap between knowledge and action involves first distilling knowledge, usually in the form of guidelines. National or international guidelines can be wholly adopted; however, local modification of guidelines with the involvement of local stakeholders may increase adherence to guidelines.[31] Audits then serve the purpose of identifying areas of gaps between the guidelines (best knowledge) and current practice (action). When important gaps are identified through audits, interventions can then be developed toward changing practice. To improve the chance of achieving meaningful and lasting change in practice, the intervention should be carefully chosen and designed. Unfortunately, the process of identifying the best interventions has not been well defined. Ideally, the facilitators and barriers to change are first identified so that any selected intervention would target these identified factors.[32,33] Although 1) prospective audits with approval for requests outside of guidelines and 2) concurrent or retrospective audits with feedback are both common interventions, other interventions—including dissemination of guidelines,[13,21,24-28] education,[13,24,26,29] and the introduction of new transfusion request forms or computer order entry[24,25]—have been used in conjunction with audits.[34,35] Again, either a prospective audit or a concurrent audit where feedback is provided to individual physicians is an intervention in itself. Both retrospective[36] and prospective[15] audits have been effective as solitary interventions in changing transfusion practice.

EFFECTIVENESS OF MONITORING AND INTERVENTIONS TO CHANGE TRANSFUSION PRACTICE

The published studies evaluating the effect of prospective and retrospective audits on transfusion practice have generally demonstrated a reduction in either the total amount of blood transfused or the proportion of inappropriate transfusions (Table 28-2). Such reduction was seen in one study that used a prospective audit alone[15] and one study that used only a retrospective audit and feedback.[36] The former study showed a reduction in RBC and frozen plasma utilization, but not platelets.[15] The latter study showed only a reduction in RBC utilization, not frozen plasma or platelet utilization.[36] The results from these two studies might suggest that prospective and retrospective audits, when used in conjunction with other interventions, are more effective in improving blood component utilization. However, the magnitude of the changes observed in the two studies, which used only audits, was not qualitatively different than that of studies that combined audits with other interventions. In fact, the poor design of the studies that have examined interventions to change transfusion practice (almost exclusively uncontrolled, single-center, before-and-after studies) and the possibility of publication bias (ie, studies with an intervention that did not result in an improvement in transfusion practice are not published) do not allow the true or relative effectiveness of individual interventions or combinations of interventions to be inferred.[34,35]

SELECTING AN AUDIT PROCESS TO MONITOR TRANSFUSIONS

Determining how transfusions should be monitored depends on a number of factors specific to each institution.[37] The first step is to decide which types of audits to use. The prospective and concurrent audits serve identical purposes and are mutually exclusive for an individual transfusion episode. Prospective audits require the greatest amount of time from laboratory staff and transfusion medicine physicians, including 24-hour coverage, and support from the laboratory information system. This may present difficulties for smaller hospitals and very busy transfusion medicine services, respectively. In general, concurrent reviews would be more practical in smaller hospitals or hospitals with limited resources

TABLE 28-3. Implementing a Prospective Audit System to Monitor Blood Component Utilization

1. Determine the extent and frequency of the audit process.
◆ The audit may be performed on all blood components or only on specific components.
◆ Areas with urgent need for transfusion (emergency rooms, operating theaters) may be excluded to avoid delays in transfusion for those cases.
◆ To limit resource demands, a selective audit may be used. For example, transfusion requests may be audited from only a single ward, selected on a rotating basis for high transfusion volume or because of a perceived problem in transfusion practice.
◆ Similarly, audits may be restricted to specific hours to limit off-hour work by laboratory staff and transfusion medicine physicians.
2. Implement a requirement for clinical information at the time of the transfusion request. This may be provided on a request form (Appendix 28-1) or by computer order entry.
3. Produce guidelines or criteria for appropriate or inappropriate indications for transfusions.
◆ Audit criteria should be less stringent than optimal transfusion guidelines, to reduce both audit workload and conflict with requesting physicians.
◆ Audit criteria should be produced in conjunction with the transfusion medicine committee and various medical specialties that use significant amounts of blood components, to increase acceptance of transfusion audits.
4. Screen transfusion requests with review by laboratory staff, transfusion nurses, or a computer algorithm to identify "inappropriate" transfusion requests.
5. Contact the requesting physician for all inappropriate transfusion requests.
◆ Contact is usually made by the transfusion medicine physician or senior technologist.
◆ Transfusion service protocols provide a predefined mechanism to override or bypass the review if blood is required urgently, which avoids unacceptable delays in filling transfusion requests.
6. Make a decision to change the transfusion request, when necessary, in conjunction with the ordering physician.

for laboratory staff or transfusion medicine physicians such that transfusions can be reviewed in the 12 to 24 hours following transfusion. If a universal prospective audit on all blood components is not feasible, then the prospective audit could also be limited to particular products (eg, specialty products such as intravenous immune globulin or recombinant Factor VIIa) or specific clinical areas. Retrospective reviews supplement the audit of indi-

TABLE 28-4. Implementing a Concurrent Audit System to Monitor Blood Component Utilization

1-4. These steps are the same as those for the prospective audit (Table 28-3).
5. Save all inappropriate transfusion requests for subsequent review by senior laboratory staff or a transfusion medicine physician who will contact the requesting physician to discuss the transfusion request.
◆ Contact with the requesting physician is made within 24 hours of the transfusion so that the physician remembers the clinical details. This represents an optimal time to provide feedback and potentially change future transfusion behavior.
◆ Contact can be made by phone or via electronic means.

vidual transfusions (either prospective or concurrent) by identifying trends in the use of transfusions.

An outline of the steps for implementing prospective (Table 28-3), concurrent (Table 28-4), and retrospective (Table 28-5) reviews are provided. A redesigned transfusion request form or order entry system incorporating guidelines or requesting clinical information (or both) can aid either prospective or concurrent audits in identifying inappropriate transfusion requests (Appendix 28-1).[38] Similarly the laboratory information system and computer algorithms can be used for all types of audits to screen transfusions for appropriateness. The frequency of the review may increase for larger transfusion services or decrease for smaller hospitals. The retrospective data can allow smaller hospitals to compare their transfusion practice with other similar institutions (eg, number of units transfused per patient by diagnosis-related group).

CONCLUSION

Auditing transfusion practice is a required function for all transfusion services. However, there is little guidance regarding how monitoring should be undertaken and how the results should be used. Audits combined with guidelines are clearly essential to evaluate transfusion practice at individual institutions. They permit the identification of suboptimal transfusion practice. Although feedback provided from audits can be used to change transfusion practice, other interventions can also be used to change transfusion practice. Ideally, the selection of audits and interventions should be based on assessment of local barriers and facilitators and on well-designed studies assess-

TABLE 28-5. Implementing a Retrospective Audit System to Monitor Blood Component Utilization

1. Determine the extent and frequency of the audit process.
◆ The frequency of the data review needs to be determined on the basis of the volume of transfusions and the resources available. Review periods should not extend beyond 6 months.
◆ The orders chosen for review will need to be determined; at a minimum, the review should include all conventional components and any other frequently transfused components.
2. Determine the outcomes to be monitored.
◆ Merely totaling the number of transfusions and the number of patients transfused represents the simplest approach but provides limited understanding and ability to monitor changes in blood utilization. Tracking utilization by patient (mean or median number of units per patient) and proportion of patients transfused provides greater understanding of utilization.
◆ The appropriateness of transfusions can also be noted if clinical and/or laboratory data are available. This can be aggregate data from prospective or concurrent reviews, or the laboratory information system can link laboratory data to transfusion events.
3. Review the audit data.
◆ Audit data should be reviewed by the transfusion medicine service and the transfusion medicine committee.
◆ Data may be analyzed by individual physician, department, or diagnosis.
◆ Data may be compared within one institution or with other similar institutions to compare overall utilization rates for blood components.
◆ Data should be shared with relevant departments and physicians.
4. Determine if any additional interventions to optimize transfusion practice are warranted.

ing the effectiveness of different interventions. Further audits would then allow for monitoring any changes in transfusion practice. Unfortunately, the current literature provides little rationale for selecting specific interventions, and there are few data to indicate which interventions are the most effective in changing transfusion practice. Future studies are required to determine what interventions are likely to be the most effective in certain circumstances. Nonetheless, audits remain a critical part of the process to evaluate the utilization of blood components and to improve transfusion practice.

KEY POINTS

1. Auditing the use of blood components is a necessary function for all transfusion medicine services and is required by AABB and The Joint Commission. The main purpose of auditing blood utilization is to assess the appropriate use of components and help optimize their use.
2. Different forms of audits (prospective, concurrent, or retrospective) may be used depending of the objectives of the audit and the resources available. In all cases, providing feedback to the users, using other interventions, or both are necessary to effect change in transfusion practice.
3. Prospective audits require the review of transfusion requests before issue of components, which permits the opportunity to intervene and stop or change an inappropriate transfusion request. Individual transfusion requests are reviewed using prespecified audit criteria (eg, guidelines).
4. Concurrent audits review individual transfusion requests in the 12 to 24 hours following a transfusion episode and involve similar processes as the prospective audit. The individual transfusion events cannot be altered, as they have already occurred, but feedback to the physician within a short period after the transfusion offers the opportunity to change future transfusion practice.
5. Retrospective audits of transfusion offer the opportunity to review aggregate transfusion data. Reviewing individual transfusions for appropriateness may be more difficult, given the remoteness of the transfusion event. Feedback to individual clinicians or clinical services should be part of a retrospective audit process to help ensure the optimal use of components.
6. All forms of audits can be used alone to effect changes in transfusion practice. Audits may also be combined with other interventions such as dissemination of guidelines, education, and the introduction of new transfusion request forms. Ideally the selection of interventions includes local stakeholders and an assessment of local factors that may affect the effectiveness of interventions.
7. Published studies evaluating the effect of prospective and retrospective audits on transfusion practice have generally demonstrated a reduction in either the total amount of blood transfused or the proportion of inappropriate transfusions. Because of the poor quality of published studies, the true or relative effectiveness of individual interventions or combinations of interventions cannot be inferred.

REFERENCES

1. Mintz PD. Quality assessment and improvement of blood transfusion practices. In: Mintz PD, ed. Transfusion therapy: Clinical principles and practice. 3rd ed. Bethesda, MD: AABB Press, 2011:813-36.

2. Comprehensive accreditation manual for hospitals (CAMH): The official handbook. Oak-Brook Terrace, IL: The Joint Commission, 2010.
3. Carson TH, ed. Standards for blood banks and transfusion services. 27th ed. Bethesda, MD: AABB, 2011.
4. Saxena S, Wehrli G, Makarewicz K, et al. Monitoring for underutilization of RBC components and platelets. Transfusion 2001;41:587-90.
5. Popovsky M, ed. Transfusion reactions. 3rd ed. Bethesda, MD: AABB Press, 2007.
6. Tinmouth AT, Fergusson DA, Chin-Yee IH, et al. Clinical consequences of red cell storage in the critically ill. Transfusion 2006;46:2014-27.
7. Amin M, Fergusson D, Wilson K, et al. The societal unit cost of allogenic red blood cells and red blood cell transfusion in Canada. Transfusion 2004;44:1479-86.
8. Shander A, Hofmann A, Ozawa S, et al. Activity-based costs of blood transfusions in surgical patients at four hospitals. Transfusion 2010;50: 753-65.
9. Becker J, Shaz B for the Clinical Transfusion Medicine Committee and the Transfusion Medicine Section Coordinating Committee. Guidelines for blood management and utilization. Bethesda, MD: AABB, 2011 (in press).
10. Sarode R, Refaai MA, Matevosyan K, et al. Prospective monitoring of plasma and platelet transfusions in a large teaching hospital results in significant cost reduction. Transfusion 2010;50:487-92.
11. Yeh CJ, Wu CF, Hsu WT, et al. Transfusion audit of fresh-frozen plasma in southern Taiwan. Vox Sang 2006;91:270-4.
12. Cheng G, Wong HF, Chan A, et al. The effects of a self-educating blood component request form and enforcements of transfusion guidelines on FFP and platelet usage. Queen Mary Hospital, Hong Kong. British Committee for Standards in Hematology (BCSH). Clin Lab Haematol 1996;18: 83-7.
13. Solomon RR, Clifford JS, Gutman SI. The use of laboratory intervention to stem the flow of fresh-frozen plasma. Am J Clin Pathol 1988; 89:518-21.
14. Rehm JP, Otto PS, West WW, et al. Hospital-wide educational program decreases red blood cell transfusions. J Surg Res 1998;75: 183-6.
15. Hawkins TE, Carter JM, Hunter PM. Can mandatory pretransfusion approval programmes be improved? Transfus Med 1994;4:45-50.
16. Littenberg B, Corwin H, Gettinger A, et al. A practice guideline and decision aid for blood transfusion. Immunohematology 1995;11:88-94.
17. Tuckfield A, Haeusler MN, Grigg AP, et al. Reduction of inappropriate use of blood products by prospective monitoring of transfusion request forms. Med J Aust 1997;167:473-6.
18. Rubin GL, Schofield WN, Dean MG, et al. Appropriateness of red blood cell transfusions in major urban hospitals and effectiveness of an intervention. Med J Aust 2001;175:354-8.
19. Capraro L, Syrjala M. Advances in cardiac surgical transfusion practices during the 1990s in a Finnish university hospital. Vox Sang 2001; 81:176-9.
20. Tobin SN, Campbell DA, Boyce NW. Durability of response to a targeted intervention to modify clinician transfusion practices in a major teaching hospital. Med J Aust 2001;174:445-8.
21. Hameedullah, Khan FA, Kamal RS. Improvement in intraoperative fresh frozen plasma transfusion practice—impact of medical audits and provider education. J Pak Med Assoc 2000;50:253-6.
22. Joshi G, McCarroll M, O'Rourke P, et al. Role of quality assessment in improving red blood cell transfusion practice. Ir J Med Sci 1997;166:16-19.
23. Brandis K, Richards B, Ghent A, et al. A strategy to reduce inappropriate red blood cell transfusion. Med J Aust 1994;160:721-2.
24. Morrison JC, Sumrall DD, Chevalier SP, et al. The effect of provider education on blood utilization practices. Am J Obstet Gynecol 1993; 169:1240-5.
25. Rosen NR, Bates LH, Herod G. Transfusion therapy: Improved patient care and resource utilization. Transfusion 1993;33:341-7.
26. Ayoub MM, Clark JA. Reduction of fresh frozen plasma use with a simple education program. Am Surg 1989;55:563-5.
27. Giovanetti AM, Parravicini A, Baroni L, et al. Quality assessment of transfusion practice in elective surgery. Transfusion 1988;28:166-9.
28. Shanberge JN. Reduction of fresh-frozen plasma use through a daily survey and education program. Transfusion 1987;27:226-7.
29. Handler S. Does continuing medical education affect medical care? A study of improved transfusion practices. Minn Med 1983;66:167-80.

30. Graham ID, Logan J, Harrison MB, et al. Lost in knowledge translation: Time for a map? J Contin Educ Health Prof 2006;26:13-24.
31. Harrison MB, Graham ID, Fervers B. Adapting knowledge to a local context. In: Straus S, Tetroe J, Graham ID, eds. Knowledge translation in health care. Oxford: Blackwell Publishing, 2009:73-82.
32. Cabana MD, Rand CS, Powe NR, et al. Why don't physicians follow clinical practice guidelines? A framework for improvement. JAMA 1999;282:1458-65.
33. Legare F, O'Connor AM, Graham ID, et al. Primary health care professionals' views on barriers and facilitators to the implementation of the Ottawa Decision Support Framework in practice. Patient Educ Couns 2006;63:380-90.
34. Wilson K, MacDougall L, Fergusson D, et al. The effectiveness of interventions to reduce physician's levels of inappropriate transfusion: What can be learned from a systematic review of the literature. Transfusion 2002;42:1224-9.
35. Tinmouth A, MacDougall L, Fergusson D, et al. Reducing the amount of blood transfused: A systematic review of behavioral interventions to change physicians' transfusion practices. Arch Intern Med 2005; 165:845-52.
36. Lam HT, Schweitzer SO, Petz L, et al. Are retrospective peer-review transfusion monitoring systems effective in reducing red blood cell utilization? Arch Pathol Lab Med 1996;120: 810-16.
37. Toy PT, Fiebig E. Blood utilization review. In: Saxena S, Shulman IA, eds. The transfusion committee: Putting patient safety first. Bethesda, MD: AABB Press, 2006:59-66.
38. Hannon T. Transfusion guidelines: Development and impact on blood management. In: Saxena S, Shulman IA, eds. The transfusion committee: Putting patient safety first. Bethesda, MD: AABB Press, 2006:115-30.

◆ APPENDIX 28-1
Example of a Transfusion Order Form*

- **Use this form for all blood component transfusion orders.**
- Check off at least one indication for each type of blood component order.
- The minimal effective dose of all blood components should be used; SINGLE UNIT Red Blood Cell (RBC) transfusions are often effective.
- Compliance with transfusion guidelines will be monitored by the transfusion committee.
- The blood bank phone # is XXX-XXX-XXXX.

☐ Blood Transfusion Consent signed

TRANSFUSION ORDER (indicate type and amount):______________________________

Request for special RBC components: _______ Irradiated _______ Washed _______ CMV negative

Patient location (ICU, OR, PACU, etc)

____

Utilization review ☐

INDICATION (check all that apply):

<u>Red Blood Cells</u> Most recent hemoglobin _____g/dL or hematocrit_____%

One RBC unit in an adult, 8 mL/kg pediatric dose, will increase hematocrit by approximately 3% and hemoglobin by 1 g/dL.

☐ Hematocrit ≤21% or hemoglobin ≤7 g/dL

☐ Hematocrit ≤24% or hemoglobin ≤8 g/dL in a patient with coronary artery disease and unstable angina/myocardial infarction/cardiogenic shock

☐ Rapid blood loss with >30% to 40% of estimated blood volume (>1500 to 2000 mL) not responding to appropriate volume resuscitation, or with ongoing blood loss

☐ The patient has been determined to be normovolemic and there is evidence to support the need for increased oxygen-carrying capacity as witnessed by (indicate):

NOTE: *These indications will be tracked and may be peer reviewed.*

☐ Tachycardia, hypotension not corrected by adequate volume replacement alone

☐ PVO_2 <25 torr, extraction ratio >50%, VO_2 <50% of baseline—
*specify*____________________________

☐ Other—
*specify*____

☐ Autologous preoperatively donated red cells: same criteria as above

<u>Platelets</u> Most recent platelet count ________/ µL

A single dose of platelets (adult: one apheresis or six concentrates; pediatric dose 1 unit/10 kg) will increase the platelet count by 25,000 to 35,000/µL

☐ Platelet count ≤10,000/µL prophylactically in a patient with failure of platelet production

☐ Platelet count ≤20,000/µL and signs of hemorrhagic diasthesis (petechiae, mucosal bleeding)

☐ Platelet count ≤50,000/µL in a patient with—
specify____

☐ Active hemorrhage

♦ APPENDIX 28-1 (CONTINUED)

Example of a Transfusion Order Form*

- ☐ Invasive procedure (recent, in-progress, planned)
- ☐ Platelet dysfunction as documented by—*specify*__________________________

Fresh Frozen Plasma **Most recent coag. studies: PT___ INR ___ PTT ___ Fibrinogen _____**

A dose of 10-15 mL/kg is usually adequate to correct a coagulopathy. **Patient weight ______ kg**

- ☐ Abnormal coagulation studies and significant hemorrhage
- ☐ Prophylactic use for PT/aPTT >1.5 times the mean of the reference range
- ☐ Emergent reversal of coumadin

Cryoprecipitate **Most recent coag. studies: PT___ INR ___ PTT ___ Fibrinogen _____**

One unit per 10 kg is usually adequate when cryoprecipitate is required. **Patient weight ______ kg**

- ☐ Fibrinogen ≤100 mg/dL
- ☐ Fibrinogen ≤150 mg/dL with active hemorrhage

___________________________/

___________________________ ________________

_________ ______________ ________________

Physician's signature / printed name

Pager # Date Time

*Modified from Hannon T. Transfusion guidelines: Development and impact on blood management. In: Saxena S, Shulman IA, eds. The transfusion committee: Putting patient safety first. Bethesda, MD: AABB Press, 2006:115-30.

CMV = cytomegalovirus; ICU = intensive care unit; OR = operating room; PACU = postanesthesia care unit; PVO_2 = peripheral venous oxygen; VO_2 = venous oxygen; PT = prothrombin time; INR = international normalized ratio; PTT = partial thromboplastin time; aPTT = activated PTT.

Chapter 29

Collecting and Processing Marrow Products for Transplantation

◆

Janice Davis-Sproul, MAS, MT(ASCP)SBB;
N. Rebecca Haley, MD; and John D. McMannis, PhD

HEMATOPOIETIC STEM CELLS are cells capable of self-renewal and differentiation into all blood cell lineages. In sufficient numbers, they give rise to complete sustained hematopoietic engraftment. In contrast, hematopoietic progenitor cells are committed to a blood cell lineage. They do not have the capacity for sustained self-renewal or the ability to differentiate into all hematopoietic lineages.[1] Both cell populations are referred to as hematopoietic progenitor cells (HPCs) in this chapter.

HPC transplantation can be classified as autologous, allogeneic, syngeneic, and xenogeneic. The classification depends on who the donor is.

Autologous HPC transplantation is technically not transplantation but, rather, the "rescue" of a patient's hematopoietic system with the patient's own HPCs, which are collected and stored (either refrigerated or cryopreserved) before treatment of the patient with myeloablative irradiation and/or chemotherapy. Autologous HPCs are reinfused after treatment to repopulate the patient's marrow.

Allogeneic HPC transplantation involves the infusion of HPCs from another individual into the patient. When the transplant uses an identical twin as the donor, it is referred to as a *syngeneic* transplant. Allogeneic cells may be derived from related or unrelated donors and may be HLA matched or mismatched.

Xenogeneic HPC transplantation, by definition, involves the transplantation into a human recipient of either 1) live HPCs from a nonhuman animal source or 2) human cells that have had ex-vivo contact with live nonhuman animal cells. There are immunologic barriers, disease concerns, and regulatory issues associated with xenotransplantation. The Food and Drug Administration (FDA) has a Xenotransplantation Action Plan to provide approaches to the regulation of this field.

Janice Davis-Sproul, MAS, MT(ASCP)SBB, Manager, Cell Therapy Laboratory, Johns Hopkins Medical Institute, Baltimore, Maryland; N. Rebecca Haley, MD, Associate Professor of Medicine, and Program Director, Cell Therapy Core, Duke Translational Medicine Institute, Duke University Medical Center, Durham, North Carolina; and John D. McMannis, PhD, Professor, University of Texas M.D. Anderson Cancer Center, Houston, Texas

The authors have disclosed no conflicts of interest.

Before the administration of the HPC product, the recipient is "conditioned." In patients with neoplastic diseases in both the allogeneic and autologous settings, the purpose of the conditioning regimen is to reduce the tumor burden. In the allogeneic setting, the conditioning regimen also creates "space" for the transplanted cells via myeloablation and suppresses the patient's immune system to allow for engraftment of the donor cells.[2]

Recently, conditioning regimens have been classified as 1) myeloablative, 2) reduced-intensity, or 3) nonmyeloablative. The categories are based on the duration of cytopenia and on the requirement for stem cell support.[3]

Sources of hematopoietic progenitor cells used clinically include marrow [HPC, Marrow; or HPC(M)], peripheral blood [HPC, Apheresis; or HPC(A)], and umbilical cord blood [HPC, Cord Blood; or HPC(C)].[4,5] [Please note that the terms HPC(M), HPC(A), and HPC(C) are used here only as abbreviations and are not intended to be used in the labeling process or on product labels.] The focus of this chapter will be the use of HPC(M) as a source of hematopoietic stem and progenitor cells. Peripheral blood and cord blood will be covered in subsequent chapters of this manual. In addition, the use of marrow is under investigation in support of nonhematopoietic transplant indications. An overview is presented by Janssens.[6]

Once collected, HPC(M) may be subjected to ex-vivo processing—for example, reduction of incompatible red cells, plasma, and T cells, and/or cell enrichment or tumor purging—before infusion. In some procedures, certain cell populations are "positively" selected (enriched). The classic example is the enrichment of CD34+ cells to theoretically eliminate or reduce contaminating CD34– malignant cells from an autologous product. In the allogeneic transplant setting, positive selection of CD34+ cells has been used to indirectly deplete the product of T cells. Alternatively, some cell populations may be "negatively selected" (removed, reduced, or destroyed). For example, antibody-mediated lysis has been used to destroy malignant cells in the autologous setting and to deplete T cells in the allogeneic setting.

DISEASES TREATED WITH HEMATOPOIETIC CELL TRANSPLANTATION

Many diseases have been treated with HPC transplantation (Table 29-1).[7-10] Malignant diseases are the most common indication. Although many nonmalignant diseases have also been treated with transplantation, as a group they represent less than 10% of all transplantations.[11]

Newer transplant trends include use in inborn disorders of metabolism, sickle cell disease, beta thalassemia major, and autoimmune disorders. The success rate of HPC transplantation depends on the disease of the patient being treated; the stage of the disease; the degree of prior treatment; the age and condition of the patient; and, in the case of allogeneic transplantation, the degree of HLA match between the donor and the patient.

AUTOLOGOUS HEMATOPOIETIC CELL TRANSPLANTATION

Whether a marrow transplant can be used for autologous rescue after high-dose chemo/radiotherapy depends on the overall "health" of the marrow. Heavy infiltration with malignant cells, lack of normal HPCs (ie, in patients with genetic diseases, fibrosis), or necrotic infiltrates limit the use of marrow as a transplant product. Prior pelvic irradiation, poor anesthesia risk, obesity, or patient refusal for marrow collection can also limit consideration of marrow as an option. In these cases, other sources of HPCs may be used.

ALLOGENEIC HEMATOPOIETIC CELL TRANSPLANTATION

Allogeneic transplants avoid many of the problems associated with the use of an autologous product for patients with malignant diseases, marrow failure, and genetic diseases such as immunodeficiency, inborn disorders of metabolism, or hemoglobinopathy. However, allogeneic transplantation is associated with a major risk of graft-vs-host disease

TABLE 29-1. Possible Indications for Hematopoietic Transplantation

Congenital immune deficiencies
Severe combined immunodeficiency disease
Wiskott-Aldrich syndrome
Marrow failure syndromes
Severe aplastic anemia
Fanconi anemia
Diamond-Blackfan anemia (congenital hypoplastic anemia)
Inborn disorders of metabolism
Mucopolysaccharidoses (eg, Hunter or Hurler syndrome)
Leukodystrophies (eg, adrenoleukodystrophy)
Glycoprotein disorders (eg, fucosidosis, mannosidosis)
Lysosomal disorders (eg, Gaucher, Pompe, Neimann-Pick disease)
Osteopetrosis
Osteogenesis imperfecta
Hemoglobinopathies
Thalassemia
Sickle cell disease
Malignant or clonal diseases of marrow
Acute leukemia
Chronic myelogenous leukemia
Hodgkin and non-Hodgkin lymphoma
Myelodysplatic syndromes
Myeloproliferative disorders
Multiple myeloma
Chronic lymphocytic leukemia
Solid tumors
Breast cancer
Ovarian cancer
Renal cell carcinoma
Testicular cancer
Childhood solid tumors
Wilm tumor
Neuroblastoma

(Continued)

TABLE 29-1. Possible Indications for Hematopoietic Transplantation (Continued)

Rhabdomyosarcoma
Ewing sarcoma
High-grade gliomas (eg, medulloblastoma)
Other
Paroxysmal nocturnal hemoglobinuria
Acquired aplastic anemia
Multiple sclerosis
Systemic lupus erythematosus
Autoimmune disorders

(GVHD), caused by immunocompetent donor T cells reacting against recipient tissue.[12] In addition to GVHD, mature donor T cells also have an immunologic anti-tumor effect, often referred to as graft-vs-tumor or -leukemia effect (GVT or GVL). The study of T cell subsets responsible for GVHD and GVT is an area of active investigation.

Even in HLA-identical donor/recipient pairs (10 of 10 alleles matched), a low percentage of grafts will fail, and GVHD will occur in 20% to 60% of cases—despite immunosuppressive therapy administered for several months after the procedure. This is most likely related to minor histocompatibility mismatches that are not linked to the major histocompatibility complex antigens.[13]

The best chance of finding a 10-of-10-allele HLA match is among the patient's full genetic siblings. There is a 25% chance of a sibling being a complete match (10 of 10), a 50% chance of a haplotype match (5 of 10), and a 25% chance of a complete mismatch. Parents and siblings will be at least a haplotype match. In the rare instance a recipient has an identical twin, a syngeneic transplant may be preferred because the donor and recipient cells are genotypically identical, and the risk of GVHD is reduced. However, syngeneic grafts may not provide the GVT effect found in allogeneic transplants.[14]

UNRELATED DONOR TRANSPLANTATION

Unrelated donor searches are often initiated for the 60% to 70% of candidates without an HLA-matched related donor. Several marrow donor databases are available worldwide. The largest is the National Marrow Donor Program (now named the Be The Match Registry), founded in 1986. Approximately 13 million adult donors and greater than 400,000 cord blood units are currently listed in the Be The Match Registry, which facilitates more than 4800 transplantations a year. A directory of transplant centers with outcome results and costs is available from the registry's website.[15]

HISTOCOMPATIBILITY

Currently, DNA-based typing methods define an individual's HLA genotype (DNA-defined alleles). Nucleic acid techniques provide greater resolution than historical serologic-based techniques (see Chapter 19). The direction of HLA mismatching between a donor and recipient has clinical implications for graft failure and acute GVHD. In addition, in the unrelated donor setting, the total number of HLA mismatches has additive effects, and different risks are associated with mismatching at different HLA loci.[16]

GRAFT-VS-HOST DISEASE

Traditionally, GVHD is characterized in two forms, acute and chronic. For myeloablated recipients, acute GVHD typically presents anywhere from a few days to 100 days after transplantation. The skin, the gastrointestinal tract, and the liver are most commonly involved, although usually not all three systems concurrently.[12,17] The site and severity determine the clinical grade of acute GVHD. The risk of GVHD is greater with unrelated and related mismatched transplants than with HLA-identical transplants.[13,18]

Chronic GVHD characteristically occurs months after transplantation and may either evolve from active or remitted acute GVHD (generally after posttransplant day 50) or arise de novo. In addition to the symptoms found in the acute form, chronic autoimmune-type disorders such as biliary cirrhosis, Sjogren syndrome, and systemic sclerosis may develop. Chronic GVHD occurs in 30% to 40% of allogeneic transplant patients who survive beyond day 100.[19,20]

Both forms of GVHD predispose the patient to infections, which may severely affect the patient's quality of life and cause transplant-related mortality. To prevent or control GVHD, patients are treated prophylactically with a variety of immunosuppressive drug therapies.

Chronic GVHD has been associated with decreased relapse of malignant disease and therefore improved overall survival in patients with aggressive leukemias and other diseases. Such an effect is believed to be secondary to the graft attacking residual malignant cells—the GVT or GVL effect.[21] A major clinical challenge is to maximize the GVL effect while minimizing the adverse sequelae of GVHD. The mechanism of GVL is not completely understood, but donor-derived cytotoxic T lymphocytes specific for the patient's minor histocompatibility antigens may contribute to the effect.

Donor lymphocyte infusion (DLI, ie, therapeutic T cells) in relapsed patients without concurrent, active GVHD after allogeneic transplantation has been used to induce a GVL effect.[22,23] Data conflict as to whether a GVL effect can occur independently of GVHD. The optimal number of donor lymphocytes capable of inducing a GVL effect without significant GVHD is not known. Immunosuppression, number of T cells transfused, T-cell phenotype, myelosuppression, and the timing of the DLI infusion all play a role in the balance between the GVL effect and GVHD.

DONOR ELIGIBILITY

Autologous Donors

Screening

In the autologous setting, the major concern regarding suitability for transplantation arises from the medical condition of the patient (ie, absence of high-risk comorbidities), the sensitivity of the malignancy to the myeloablative regimen, and the possibility of tumor cells in the harvested marrow. Another area of concern is whether a sufficient number of cells can be collected from the patient to reconstitute the marrow after myeloablation. Patients being considered for an autologous transplant should have their marrow assessed for residual malignancy and marrow cellularity and undergo an extensive history and physical examination to identify the risks and potential adverse events from the marrow harvest and myeloablative transplantation.

Testing

Autologous donors should be tested for infectious diseases as required by cellular therapy accrediting organizations.[24,25]

Allogeneic Donors

Donor Selection

In the allogeneic transplant setting, many issues are involved in selecting a donor. These factors are influenced by the specific type of transplantation being performed.[13,26] Initially, donor selection is based on HLA compatibility between the donor and the recipient. Ideally, a full 10-of-10-allele HLA match should be found; however, transplant procedures have been performed successfully using allele-mismatched and haploidentical donors.

It is important to ascertain the cytomegalovirus (CMV) status of the donor and the recipient before transplantation because CMV infection is one of the leading causes of posttransplant mortality in the allogeneic setting.[27] A recipient can develop primary CMV infection if he or she is CMV negative and receives a CMV-positive product. Recipients who are CMV positive may experience reinfection or reactivation. Patients who are CMV positive or who receive marrow from a seropositive donor are closely monitored for viral reactivation during the posttransplant period. Given the high morbidity and the need for prolonged antiviral treatment associated with CMV infection, the CMV status of the donor is noted in the donor selection process.

The use of multiparous females as donors is associated with an increased risk of GVHD, as is a history of transfusion in the donor.[28] Therefore, when more than one HLA-identical donor is available, the preferred donor would be CMV negative (in the case of a CMV-negative recipient); and if female, nonparous; and untransfused.[26,28]

Screening

Allogeneic donors should be screened as required in the current standards developed by the cellular therapy accrediting organizations in addition to the FDA guidance document on donor screening.[24,25,29] This screening includes evaluation of general physical and health history, risk factors for relevant communicable diseases, anesthesia risks, and pregnancy in female donors. A donor screening questionnaire is available from the AABB.[30]

Testing

Allogeneic donors should be tested for infectious diseases as required by the current accreditation standards in addition to applicable FDA regulations.[24,25,31] All allogeneic HPC donors must undergo blood testing for human immunodeficiency virus (HIV), types 1 and -2; human T-cell lymphotropic virus (HTLV), types I and II; hepatitis B and C viruses; *Treponema pallidum*; and CMV within 30 days before collection. Donors who are confirmed positive for HIV should not be used. Other positive disease markers do not necessarily prohibit use of collections from a particular donor (eg, positive for antibodies to hepatitis B core antigen). Components from such donors may be used with the informed consent of the donor (to release the results of the testing), the recipient, and the attending physician, as well as formal documentation of justification for "urgent medical need."

MARROW HARVEST

The technique for marrow harvest is the same for an allogeneic donor as for an autologous patient.[32] The procedure is performed under sterile conditions in the operating room. The posterior iliac crest provides the most practical and productive site for marrow collection. Prior radiation therapy to an aspiration site may result in hypocellular yields, and in general, previously irradiated sites should be avoided. Once aspirated, the marrow should be mixed with an anticoagulant (usually heparin and/or acid-citrate-dextrose). Some centers also add an electrolyte solution to the collection container. The marrow aspirates are transferred to a sterile vessel or a harvest collection bag equipped with filters of graduated pore size. The marrow is then transferred to a sterile blood bag and transported to the processing laboratory, and samples are removed for product evaluation (quality control testing). The product may proceed to further processing, cryopreservation, and/or infusion.

COLLECTION TARGETS

The recipient's body weight and the type of product manipulation, if any, will determine the target total nucleated cell dose and volume of marrow to be collected. Cell dose is recognized as a limiting factor for engraftment and survival.[33-35] A frequently used minimum target for autologous transplants is 2.0×10^8 nucleated cells per kilogram of recipient body weight. Marrow harvests in autologous patients who have received alkylating agents as therapy may yield fewer progenitor cells relative to the total nucleated cells collected. In these cases, extra marrow should be obtained if possible. If the harvested product is to be processed in an effort to remove tumor cells, the protocol may request that additional marrow be collected. For most allogeneic harvests, the target dose is 3×10^8 nucleated cells per kg of recipient weight. Allogeneic donors harvested for the Be The Match Registry will have specific marrow prescriptions (target nucleated dose) based on the recipient's body weight and type of processing required.[36] The Be The Match Registry limits the volume harvested from its donors to a maximum of 20 mL/kg donor weight. Many centers use the cell number (cells/kg) requested for transplantation and the cell count (cells/mL) on the product obtained approximately midway through the collection to determine the final collection volume.

CLINICAL CONSIDERATIONS

The age of the donor and, in the autologous setting, the underlying disease and previous treatment regimen influence the total nucleated cell and progenitor cell yield. Because of the volume of marrow removed, Red Blood Cell (RBC) transfusions may be required for both autologous and allogeneic donors. Frequently, allogeneic marrow donors will have an autologous RBC unit collected 2 to 3 weeks before the harvest. Most RBC transfusions occur after the harvest to avoid marrow dilution. Allogeneic blood components should be irradiated if given before or during the procedure, to prevent any lymphocytes from the component from causing GVHD in the event that those lymphocytes are aspirated into the harvested marrow. In transplantations that require marrow manipulation, the recovered red cells may be returned to the donor. Common complications of marrow harvests include bruising and local discomfort lasting less than 3 weeks.[32]

CD34 ANTIGEN

CD34 is the cluster designation given to a transmembrane glycoprotein on immature hematopoietic cells, some mature endothelial cells, and stromal cells.[37] The antigen has an approximate molecular weight of 110 kD and carries a negative charge. Cells expressing the CD34 antigen encompass the lineage-committed cells as well as the pluripotent stem cells. Less than 1% to 3% of normal marrow cells express this antigen. CD34+ cells purified from marrow are capable of trilineage reconstitution in humans.

PROCESSING OF HPC(M) PRODUCTS

A marrow harvest may result in a product with a volume of up to 1500 mL or greater. HPC(M) products contain red cells, white cells, hematopoietic stem and progenitor cells, mesenchymal stem cells, platelets, plasma, bony spicules, and fat globules. In the case of an autologous transplant, the product is stored (either refrigerated[38] or frozen[39]) while the patient undergoes myeloablative therapy. A laboratory may process the HPC(M) to facilitate cryopreservation, preparing either a buffy-coat or density/mononuclear cell (MNC)-enriched product before cryopreservation. The reduced product volume requires less dimethylsulfoxide (DMSO) for cryopreservation, resulting in fewer DMSO-related toxicities at infusion. In addition, red cells and granulocytes may not be effectively preserved during cryopreservation; therefore, their removal before freezing is desirable. The infusion of lysed red cells may result in renal or other hemolysis-related toxicities.[40] The by-products of granulocyte breakdown as well as the presence of platelets can result in clumping of the thawed product and decreased progenitor cell recovery.[41] Concentrating a product can also reduce the amount of costly reagents required for a tumor cell purge. In the case of allogeneic HPC(M) products, it may be necessary to reduce the volume of incompatible red cells or plasma before infusion to prevent hemolytic reactions (see "Processing in the Presence of Red Cell Incompatibilities"). The endpoint of basic marrow processing is often the preparation of a buffy-coat-enriched product (white cell concentrate) with a modest reduction of red cells and volume. This product is generally prepared by centrifugation of the marrow using a variety of manual or automated techniques.

Manual Buffy-Coat Preparations

Manual buffy-coat enrichment procedures involve the centrifugation of marrow in conical tubes[42] or transfer bags.[43] Once the marrow is centrifuged, the supernatant is removed, followed by the collection of the buffy-coat (white) cells. Remaining red cells may be pooled and washed for reinfusion to the donor. Buffy-coat-enriched products collected in this fashion often recover >75% of the original nucleated cells. A disadvantage of using the conical tube method for buffy-coat preparation is the risk of bacterial contamination inherent in open-system processing. Hence, many laboratories use a transfer bag method in addition to the sterile connecting device to maintain a closed system.

Automated Buffy-Coat Preparations

Several cell washers and apheresis instruments have been adapted for the semiautomated and automated processing of marrow.[44] The recoveries using automated or semiautomated methods vary according to instrument and operator. The COBE 2991 Cell Processor (CaridianBCT, Lakewood, CO) has been used for the collection of buffy-coat-enriched products with a recovery of >80% of the nucleated cells and a reduction of the total volume of up to 80%. Although buffy-coat-enriched products contain the majority of the harvested nucleated cells and progenitor cell colonies (colony-forming units, or CFUs), the products also contain granulocytes and a variable amount of red cells.

Automated Mononuclear Cell Preparations

MNC enrichment can be performed using a clinical-grade good manufacturing practice density gradient reagent (eg, Ficoll-Hypaque), which will significantly reduce the red cell and granulocyte content. An alternative to the use of density gradient solutions (clinical or research grade) is the use of selected apheresis devices to prepare MNC-enriched products.[44] The Caridian (COBE) Spectra has been used to process HPC(M), with reported MNC recoveries of greater than 79% and greater than 96% reduction in red cells.[45,46] Employment of such apheresis devices for processing HPC(M) yields density/MNC-enriched products with CFU recoveries and red cell content comparable to products prepared using density gradient solutions.[47] Regardless of the processing method selected, process validation should be performed before use.

Cell Enrichment

Cell populations can be enriched based on phenotypic cell surface molecules. As a hematopoietic stem cell undergoes differentiation and maturation, CD34 antigen levels on the surface of the cell decrease.[37] This property, coupled with the use of monoclonal antibodies (MoAbs) specific for the different epitopes of the CD34 molecule, permits the isolation or enrichment of CD34+ cells using physical separation procedures, such as fluorescence-activated cell sorting (FACS)[48] and the use of immunomagnetic beads.[49] Another antigen used to enrich for stem/progenitor cells is CD133, which is expressed on primitive cell populations, such as CD34+ hematopoietic stem and progenitor cells.[50]

As previously stated, enrichment of CD34+ cells may reduce the number of CD34– tumor cells in the infused product in the autologous transplant setting or can be used to reduce the T-cell content of allogeneic products to reduce the risk of GVHD.

Another strategy for cell enrichment relies on a stem cell function rather than phenotype.[51] Storms et al [52] described a fluorescent substrate of aldehyde dehydrogenase (ALDH) that can be used to isolate cells with increased ALDH activity. Enrichment of these cells is an area of active clinical investigation. [53]

Immunomagnetic separation and FACS are methods used to enrich specific cell populations and are based on antibody binding to an antigen present on the cells of interest.

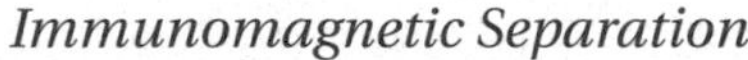

Immunomagnetic Separation

This method uses an antibody coupled to a magnetic bead. This bead complex is incubated with product, and the cells expressing the antigen bind to the antibody-coated beads. A magnet is applied to separate the bound cells from the unbound cells. The CliniMACS (Miltenyi Biotec, Bergisch Gladbach, Germany) is used for clinical isolation of CD34+ cells.[49] The magnetic particles used in the CliniMACs system are nanoparticles and therefore can be left on the cell surface after selection. Before clinical use of this system, the applicable federal regulatory requirements should be determined.

Fluorescence-Activated Cell Sorting

A fluorescence-activated cell sorter combines a flow cytometer with a physical separation methodology (such as droplet or fluid switch sorting) that segregates individual cells based on binding to fluorochrome-conjugated antibodies with the predefined properties.[48] Although this technique is sensitive, it is not commonly employed for large-scale purification of marrow products because of the length of time required to perform the isolation.

Autologous Tumor Cell Purging

Tumor purging refers to the removal or destruction of tumor cells that may contaminate an autologous product. In patients with hematopoietic disease or malignancies that frequently involve the marrow (eg, lymphomas, leukemias), residual disease in the product may contribute to relapse.[54] Whether tumor purging effectively decreases the likelihood of relapse is controversial. However, because most autologous transplants are performed using HPC(A) products, the controversy along with the practice of purging autologous marrow products has faded from the transplant arena.

T-Cell Reduction

As previously stated, in allogeneic HPC transplantation, GVHD is a significant transplant complication. Processing strategies have been developed that target and remove or reduce the T-cell content of the product in an effort to decrease the incidence, or at least lessen the severity, of GVHD. Many of the techniques outlined for CD34+ cell enrichment can also be applicable to T-cell depletion (Table 29-2).[55]

Two major areas of concern related to the use of T-cell-depleted/reduced products are graft failure and relapse. Most instances of graft failure (early or late) are caused by immunologic rejection; host T cells or natural killer cells react against donor cells. In addition to the increased risk of graft failure observed with the use of T-cell-reduced products, early transplant studies using T-cell-reduced marrow in patients with chronic myelogenous leukemia showed a 50% or greater relapse rate. This was in contrast to patients who developed GVHD and had lower relapse rates.[21,55] Clinical research and development efforts have focused on determining the optimal level of T-cell reduction to balance the challenges of ensuring engraftment and maintaining the GVL effect while minimizing the severity of GVHD.

RED CELL INCOMPATIBILITIES

Although HLA compatibility is crucial in the successful engraftment of myelosuppressed or myeloablated patients, ABO compatibility is

TABLE 29-2. Methods of T-Cell Depletion

Nonimmunologic
Counterflow centrifugal elutriation
Soybean agglutination and sheep red cell rosetting
Pharmacologic or cytotoxic drugs
Immunologic
Monoclonal antibodies with or without complement
Immunotoxins
Immunomagnetic beads

not, because ABO and HLA antigens are inherited independently. Pluripotent and very early committed HPCs do not possess ABH antigens, allowing engraftment to occur successfully regardless of the ABO compatibility between the recipient and donor. ABO incompatibility does not affect neutrophil or platelet engraftment, graft failure, or rejection.[56] However, delayed red cell engraftment may occur following major-ABO-incompatible myeloablative transplantation, and delayed hemolysis may occur following minor-ABO-incompatible myeloablative transplantation (Table 29-3).[57]

Major Red Cell Incompatibility

Red cell incompatibility, which includes ABO major incompatibility, occurs when the recipient has antibodies against donor red cell antigens. Donor red cells present in the aspirated marrow may be rapidly hemolyzed at the time of infusion. Fortunately, HPC(M) products can be processed to remove/reduce the red cell volume.[45,46] A group O recipient who receives a group A product may continue to produce anti-A and anti-B for 3 to 4 months, or longer in rare instances. The presence of anti-A may delay erythropoiesis by the group A donor marrow; group A red cells appear in the circulation when the recipient's anti-A disappears. Red cell engraftment may therefore be delayed to 40 days after the transplantation in this setting.[58] Granulocyte and platelet production are not affected.[59] Red cells used for transfusion of the recipient must be compatible with both the donor and the recipient. In some centers, group O red cells are given to all major-ABO-incompatible transplant recipients in order to avoid confusion. Recommendations for optimal blood component selection are given in Chapter 25.

Minor Red Cell Incompatibility

Minor ABO incompatibility occurs when the donor has antibodies against recipient red cell antigens (such as a group O donor to a non-group-O recipient). Before infusion of the marrow product from a minor-ABO-incompatible donor, the plasma volume may be reduced to avoid infusion of preformed antibodies. Plasma reduction can also be performed when the donor has an antibody to non-ABO red cell antigens that are found on the recipient's red cells.

Recipients of minor-ABO-incompatible transplants may experience delayed hemolysis mediated by donor lymphocytes 7 to 14 days after infusion. Donor lymphocytes, often referred to as "passenger lymphocytes," produce isoagglutinins capable of destroying the recipient's red cells and resulting in varying degrees of hemolysis. The incidence of hemolysis varies and may relate to the degree of patient conditioning (myeloablative vs nonmyeloablative), the type of posttransplant immunosuppression, the type of product [HPC(M) vs HPC(A)], and the type of processing (eg, T-cell reduction).[60-62] If the direct antiglobulin test (DAT) is positive, anti-A and/or anti-B can be recovered in the eluate, and hemoglobinemia and/or hemoglobinuria may occur. Some transplant recipients develop a positive DAT without experiencing gross hemolysis. In all cases, plasma used for transfusion should be compatible with both the donor and the recipient. It is recommended that RBC transfusions be of donor type from the start of the conditioning regimen.

Processing in the Presence of Red Cell Incompatibilities

Each facility should have a policy regarding HPC(M) processing in the presence of ABO and other red cell antigen incompatibilities. At a minimum, this policy should address the maximum red cell volume and/or dose as the level that requires physician notification, processing, or both.

Major Red Cell Incompatibility

Two approaches have been used in the medical management of major-ABO-incompatible donor/recipient pairs: 1) the rarely used approach—removal of or decrease in the isoagglutinin level in the recipient, or 2) the commonly used approach—reduction of the red cell content of the marrow product. Attempts

TABLE 29-3. Potential Problems with ABO- and Rh-Incompatible HPC Transplantation*

Incompatibility	Donor	Patient	Potential Problems
ABO (major)	Group A	Group O	Hemolysis of infused donor red cells, failure or delay of red cell engraftment, hemolysis at the time of donor group A red cell engraftment
ABO (minor)	Group O	Group A or Group B	Hemolysis of patient red cells from infused donor plasma or hemolysis of patient red cells 7-10 days after transplantation, resulting from passenger-lymphocyte-derived isohemagglutinins
Rh	Negative	Positive	Hemolysis of patient red cells by donor anti-D produced after engraftment
	Positive	Negative (with anti-D)	Hemolysis of infused donor red cells, hemolysis at the time of donor Rh-positive red cell engraftment

*These are illustrative examples. See Chapter 25 for more detailed discussion.

HPC = hematopoietic progenitor cell.

to remove or decrease the isoagglutinin titer in recipients involve the use of large-volume plasma exchange with or without the subsequent infusion of donor type red cells as a secondary effort to absorb any additional isoagglutinins.[63]

The second approach focuses on the product instead of the recipient. Several methods of red cell reduction have been used. One method is red cell sedimentation.[44,64] This procedure is relatively quick and inexpensive and can be performed in a closed system. The most common sedimenting agent is 6% hydroxyethyl starch (HES), although dextran can be used. HES is combined with marrow in a ratio of 1:5 to 1:8. Once combined, the marrow/HES mixture is allowed to sediment for 45 to 90 minutes. HES promotes rouleaux formation, causing the red cells to settle and leaving the nucleated cells in the plasma. After the red cells have settled, they are drained into a secondary bag. This process allows for the retention of 76% to 80% of the initial nucleated cells and 60% to 99% of the granulocyte-macrophage colonies (CFU-GM).[64,65] Some institutions accomplish red cell reduction using the Caridian (COBE) 2991 Cell Processor; others use continuous-flow apheresis machines such as the Caridian (COBE) Spectra or the Fenwal CS-3000 Plus (Fenwal, Lake Zurich, IL).[44] Whatever method is selected, a facility should validate the process before implementation. A maximum red cell volume for infusion should be determined by the appropriate medical staff.

Minor Red Cell Incompatibility

Circulating isoagglutinins in the donor marrow are not always predictive of posttransplant hemolysis. The amount of incompatible plasma can be reduced in the product by centrifugation. After process validation, each laboratory and transplant program should define acceptable cell recovery ranges. Plasma reduction may also be performed as a means of volume reduction for small recipients or for patients with fluid-sensitive conditions.

SHORT- AND LONG-TERM STORAGE

Conditions for HPC storage vary with the length of time between collection and infusion as well as the type of processing the product will undergo. Facilities should have validated processes for product storage.

Allogeneic Products

The collection of allogeneic marrow is generally timed to coincide with the completion of the recipient's preparative regimen. However, under unusual circumstances in which the donor is not available on the required collection date, allogeneic products may be cryopreserved.

The ability to store unmanipulated marrow for up to 3 days at either 2 to 8 C or 18 to 24 C[66] is vital where unrelated-donor marrow products are collected and then transported great distances before transplantation. In a series of 938 transplants using unrelated marrow, reported by Lazarus et al[67] in 2009, the median time from the end of collection to infusion was 14 hours. It was reported that mortality rates were higher in recipients of HLA-mismatched marrow when the interval from the end of collection to receipt at the transplant center was 20 hours. The article urged a general review of current transport practices and supported efforts to minimize the time from collection to infusion.

Autologous Products

Depending on the length of time required for treatment, autologous products may be refrigerated[38] or cryopreserved[39] until the time of infusion. HPC(M) may also be collected and cryopreserved while a patient is in remission and then stored for later use in the event of relapse. At present, no expiration date has been defined for HPC(M); marrow stored for 11 years has been used for transplantation, with sustained engraftment.[68]

Cryopreservation

The purpose of cryopreservation is to freeze HPC(M) products in such a way as to maintain stem and progenitor cell viability and potency.[69] The main obstacle to maintaining viability during cryopreservation is the formation of intracellular ice crystals and dehydration, both resulting in cell lysis. The time required for phase change (the shift from the liquid state to the solid state) and the postphase change freezing rate are important aspects of cryopreservation.[39,69]

The adverse effects caused by the formation of intracellular ice crystals or by cell dehydration can be minimized by a slow cooling rate and the addition of cryoprotective agents. DMSO is a small molecule that penetrates the cell membrane and moderates the osmotic balance within the cell, thereby decreasing the amount of water absorbed by the ice crystals. One cryoprotectant formulation used to preserve HPC(M) consists of 20% DMSO and 20% plasma or albumin prepared in a buffered electrolyte solution. The cryoprotectant is then combined with an equal volume of cells immediately before freezing to yield a final concentration of 10% DMSO. Another cryoprotectant uses DMSO and HES.[70] If nonclinical-grade HES is used, an investigational new drug (IND) application should be submitted to the FDA. Some protocols require that each component (freezing media and cell product) be chilled before mixing. Whatever cryoprotectant or mixing process is used, process validation must be performed before use.

The cell damaging effects of phase change and postphase change freezing rate can be minimized by a slow controlled freeze.[69] One method of freezing uses a computer-controlled programmable freezer. Another method uses a mechanical –80 C freezer, in which the combination of the metal canisters that the bags are placed in, the bag configuration, and the volume of product produce a freezing rate of approximately 3 C/minute, which is in line with the rates programmed into a controlled-rate freezer.[70] Investigators report that the mechanical freezer method is a viable and cost-effective alternative to the use of programmable freezing chambers.[70,71] Whatever method is chosen, a laboratory must validate the method before use.

Storage of Cryopreserved HPC(M)

In accordance with FDA regulations, storage areas should be controlled to prevent mix-ups, contamination, and cross-contamination of products and to prevent the improper release of a product for distribution.[31] One consideration for the use of liquid nitrogen storage is whether to store products in liquid or vapor phase. In liquid phase, storage temperatures are easily maintained at –180 C and colder. Products are completely immersed in liquid nitrogen; therefore, temperature fluctuations within the freezer and within the products themselves are minimal. Should an electrical or liquid nitrogen supply crisis occur, enough liquid nitrogen is present in the freezer to sustain adequate storage conditions for several days. In vapor phase, the storage temperature that can be achieved, although not as cold as liquid phase, averages –145 C to –185 C, a temperature that has been shown to allow for viable long-term marrow storage.[68] The major drawbacks to vapor-phase storage are the potential fluctuation in temperature when the freezer is opened and possible variations in storage temperature throughout the freezer itself. The allowable reaction time in cases of electrical or liquid nitrogen supply emergencies is significantly shorter with a vapor-phase storage system than with a liquid-phase storage system. However, the important advantage of vapor-phase storage is the decreased risk of cross-contamination between bags.[72-74] In some facilities, products are stored in a mechanical freezer. It has been reported that HPC(M) products stored at –80 C have successfully engrafted in patients after 2 years of storage.[70]

Storage of Untested or Infectious Products

Samples for infectious disease testing of HPC donors should be collected within 30 days of collection.[24,25] Facilities should have policies regarding the storage of untested or infectious products. One approach to reduce the risk of cross-contamination is to store all products in vapor phase; another is to use an overwrap bag, that is, placing the cryobag inside another plastic bag that is sealed before storage.

TRANSPORTATION AND SHIPPING

In some situations, a marrow product must be transported from one facility to another.[75] In all cases, precautions should be taken to protect the component from rough handling, extremes of temperature and pressure, x-ray examination, breakage, and spillage. In the case of cryopreserved components, the use of a liquid-nitrogen "dry shipper" is preferred. Such "dry shippers" have liquid-nitrogen absorbent material between the walls of the container. When kept in the upright position, the inside of the shipper can maintain temperatures around –180 C for up to 10 to 14 days. Current standards require that 1) shipping containers be validated and 2) for cryopreserved products, a temperature monitor be placed in the shipper to provide continuous monitoring during transit.[24,25]

THAWING AND INFUSION

For all components, laboratories should have procedures in place for the distribution of cellular therapy products.[76] Before a product is issued, the medical order for product issue must be reviewed. For many years, DMSO was thought to be toxic to HPCs at room temperature. It has been reported that DMSO, at the concentration used for HPC product cryopreservation, is nontoxic to cells after short-term room-temperature exposure (up to 1 hour).[77] However, this report should not encourage the routine storage of thawed, *unwashed* HPC(M) at room temperature. To control postthaw storage conditions, facilities may thaw one bag at a time near the bedside or patient's room. Some centers place product bags in secondary containment bags before thawing; others immerse the bag (all but the access ports) directly in sterile water or saline at 37 to 40 C. The bag is kneaded gently until all solid clumps have thawed. Final identification of the product is performed by the appropriate medical staff performing the infusion according to institutional policies. Cell flow through the central venous catheter is confirmed, and the cells are infused by gravity drip, calibrated pump, or manual push with or without an in-line filter (a standard 170-micron red cell infusion filter is acceptable). The cells are then infused (usually 10-15 mL per minute). Products may also be washed in the laboratory before infusion to reduce DMSO infusion-related toxicities.

Side effects associated with infusions include nausea, diarrhea, flushing, bradycardia, hypertension, and abdominal pain. In general, such side effects may justify slowing, but not halting, the infusion until the symptoms pass. Sudden and severe hypotension can occur in the absence of adequate antihistamine premedication.[41] The patient may be hydrated and the urine "alkalinized" before infusion. This facilitates the clearance of hemoglobin caused by red cell lysis, which occurs during freezing, and reduces the risk of renal complications.[40] If the total infusion volume contains greater than 1 g/kg of DMSO, it is recommended that the product be infused over 2 days. For reference, 100 mL of cryopreserved cells in a 10%-DMSO-based cryoprotectant contains 10 g of DMSO.

EVALUATION AND QUALITY CONTROL OF HEMATOPOIETIC PRODUCTS

Cell Counts

Each marrow product is analyzed to determine the total nucleated cell concentration, which is used to calculate the number of nucleated cells per kilogram (of recipient body weight). In addition, nucleated cell counts can be used to calculate the percentage of nucleated cell recovery after processing, thereby providing a quality control measure for processing procedures and equipment.[78]

In general, automated cell counts provide the most rapid and accurate value. However, platelet/cellular aggregates or fat globules in specimens can falsely decrease or increase cell counts.[79,80] In such cases, postprocessing recoveries may appear out-of-range as a result of inaccurate starting cell counts. Because cell dose is important to assess product quality, consideration for the accuracy of the cell count is essential.

Viability

Viability assays assess the percentage of live cells in a cellular therapy product and are based on the loss of membrane integrity during necrotic cell death. Multiple methods are in clinical use with a range of equipment requirements.[81] Reagents include trypan blue dye, fluorescent dyes such as acridine orange and propidium iodide, and 7-amino-actinomycin-D (7-AAD), which requires the use of a flow cytometer.

Microbial Cultures

HPC(M) products are tested for sterility.[82] Because marrow is collected using multiple aspirations through the skin, culture-positive results have been reported.[83-85] Bacterial or fungal growth can result from contamination during collection or processing or as a result of patient or donor sepsis. Skin commensals are the predominant isolates from these cultures. It is important to identify the sources, the degree of contamination, the causative organism, and its antibiotic sensitivity to assist the medical staff with infusion-related decisions. Each product should be tested at defined points for microbial contamination (bacterial and fungal cultures).[24,25] A positive culture result in a HPC(M) product does not necessitate immediate discard of the product, as these are frequently irreplaceable cells. However, caution should be used for certain contaminants, especially gram-negative bacteria.[84] Culture-positive results should be reviewed by the appropriate physician(s) according to the applicable facility policy.

CD34 Analysis/Enumeration

As hematopoietic stem cells differentiate, they gain and lose surface markers. In the case of the CD34 antigen, expression diminishes as the stem cell differentiates. Stages of differentiation may be studied by the expression or coexpression of other antigens—for example, CD38. The CD34 antigen has been used to evaluate the "quality" of HPC products.[86] Flow cytometry can be used to determine the percentage of CD34+ cells in the product. The percentage and nucleated cell dose is then used to calculate the CD34+ dose (the number of CD34+ cells per kilogram of recipient body weight that are in a product).

Measurement of Cytoplasmic Aldehyde Dehydrogenase

Intracellular ALDH is an enzyme that has been found to be in high levels in early hematopoietic, long-term repopulating cells.[87] This finding led to the development of a flow-cytometry-based test kit for the quantitation of cytoplasmic ALDH. It has been reported that the number of ALDH-bright cells in a stem cell graft correlates with the speed of neutrophil engraftment.[88]

Colony-Forming Cell Assays

Culture assays are available that can demonstrate in-vitro proliferative capacity in HPC(M) samples.[89] It is thought that committed progenitor cells are responsible for short-term engraftment (within 2-4 weeks after transplantation), and pluripotent stem cells are responsible for long-term, sustained engraftment. Hematopoietic cultures, examined after 12 to 14 days of incubation, may be used to assess the short-term engraftment potential of the product. However, culture techniques and colony identification may vary from laboratory to laboratory, and therefore comparison of colony results between facilities may be difficult. Reported CFU-GM doses below which engraftment may be delayed range from 1.5×10^5 to 5.0×10^5/kg.[90] Routine use of this assay to evaluate HPC(M) products is controversial.

Long-term cultures,[91] which measure primitive stem cells, are not routinely used to evaluate clinical products because of the 5- to

8-week assay incubation requirements. However, these assays may be useful when evaluating developmental procedures involving product manipulation.

Bioluminescence Assays

Cell proliferation can be correlated with intracellular adenosine triphosphate (i-ATP) concentration.[92] Assays have been developed that measure i-ATP concentration using bioluminescence.

Tumor Cell Detection

Tumor cell detection techniques have been developed to screen HPC products suspected of tumor cell contamination. The majority of these assays use monoclonal antibodies that specifically bind tumor antigens. Detection and quantitation can use flow cytometry, immunofluorescence, or immunohistochemical staining; sensitivity varies with technique.

Engraftment Data

Ultimately, engraftment of neutrophils, platelets, and red cells is the primary determinant of product "quality," yet engraftment is dependent on multiple clinical factors beyond the product such as the use of hematopoietic growth factors after transplantation.[93] Monitoring and documenting time to engraftment is required by the cellular therapy accrediting organizations.[24,25] Each institution should have a policy in which engraftment is defined and monitored.

REGULATIONS

In the United States, minimally manipulated marrow collected from unrelated donors is overseen by the Health Resources and Services Administration. However, if the marrow product is used for nonhomologous use (regardless of the extent of manipulation) or if the product is more than minimally manipulated, then an IND application must be submitted to the FDA. Applicable regulations would apply [good tissue practice (21CFR 1271)[31] and good manufacturing practice (21 CFR 211)[94]].

STANDARDS

The AABB and the Foundation for the Accreditation of Cellular Therapy (FACT) have published separate, but substantially similar, standards (for accreditation) for HPCs.[24,25] The AABB *Standards for Cellular Therapy Product Services* address the collection, processing, storage, and distribution of cellular therapy products. In addition to collection, processing, storage, and distribution, FACT standards address clinical transplant program requirements. Other organizations, such as the Be The Match Registry,[36] publish voluntary standards. International efforts to harmonize standards have begun with the formation of the Alliance for Harmonization of Cellular Therapy Accreditation. To address the terminology and labeling of cellular therapy products, a multi-organizational effort has resulted in the publication of terminology and labeling standards.[95] These international collaborative efforts are important and support the safe distribution of unrelated-donor products around the world.

KEY POINTS

1. Hematopoietic progenitor cell (HPC) transplantation can be classified as autologous, allogeneic, syngeneic, or xenogeneic, depending on who is the donor.
2. Conditioning regimens are classified as myeloablative, reduced-intensity, or nonmyeloablative, based on the duration of cytopenia and on the requirement for stem cell support.
3. Malignant diseases are the most common indication for transplantation. Newer transplant trends include the following as indications: inborn disorders of metabolism, sickle cell disease, beta thalassemia major, and autoimmune disorders.

4. ABO compatibility is not required for successful allogeneic engraftment.
   a. ABO incompatibility does not affect neutrophil or platelet engraftment, graft failure, or graft rejection.
   b. Delayed red cell engraftment may occur following major-ABO-incompatible myeloablative transplantation.
   c. Delayed hemolysis may occur following minor-ABO-incompatible myeloablative transplantation.
5. HPC, Marrow [HPC(M)] product processing can include the following:
   a. Red cell reduction (buffy-coat or mononuclear cell enrichment).
   b. Plasma reduction.
   c. Cell enrichment or depletion based on phenotypic cell markers.
   d. Cryopreservation.
6. Each facility should have a policy regarding HPC(M) processing in the presence of ABO and other red cell antigen incompatibilities.
7. The AABB, the National Marrow Donor Program (Be The Match Registry), and the Foundation for the Accreditation of Cellular Therapy publish standards for HPC(M) products. These standards include donor screening and testing and quality control requirements.
8. Food and Drug Administration regulations for HPC(M) apply only to products considered as biologics under investigational new drug regulations.
9. The Health Resources and Services Administration oversees unrelated-donor HPC(M) products.

REFERENCES

1. Williams DA. Stem cell model of hematopoiesis. In: Hoffman R, Benz ES, Shattil SJ, et al, eds. Hematology: Basic principles and practices. 3rd ed. London: Churchill Livingstone, 2000:126-38.
2. Bolanos-Meade J, Jones RJ. Conditioning regimens. In: Wingard JR, Gastineau D, Leather H, et al, eds. Hematopoietic stem cell transplantation: A handbook for clinicians. Bethesda, MD: AABB, 2009:51-60.
3. Bacigalupo A, Ballen K, Rizzo D, et al. Defining the intensity of conditioning regimens: Working definitions. Biol Blood Marrow Transplant 2009;15:1628-33.
4. Bacigalupo A, Frassoni F, Van Lint MT. Bone marrow or peripheral blood as a source of stem cells for allogeneic transplants. Curr Opin Hematol 2000;7:343-7.
5. Grewal SS, Barker JN, Davies SM, Wagner JE. Unrelated donor hematopoietic cell transplantation: Marrow or umbilical cord blood? Blood 2003;101:4233-44.
6. Janssens S. Stem cells in the treatment of heart disease. Annu Rev Med 2010;61:287-300.
7. To LB, Haylock DN, Simmons PJ, Jutner CA. The biology and clinical uses of blood stem cells. Blood 1997;89:2233-58.
8. McGlave P. Overview of stem cell transplantation. In: Hoffman R, Benz ES, Shattil SJ, et al, eds. Hematology: Basic principles and practices. 3rd ed. London: Churchill Livingstone, 2000:1550-2.
9. Horowitz MM. Uses and growth of hematopoietic cell transplantation. In: Blume KG, Forman SJ, Appelbaum FR, eds. Thomas' hematopoietic cell transplantation. 3rd ed. Malden, MA: Wiley-Blackwell; 2004:9-15.
10. Section I: Issues relevant to the pre-transplant period: Clinical indications (Chapter 1-19). In: Ball ED, Lister J, Law P, eds. Hematopoietic stem cell therapy. Philadelphia: Churchill Livingstone, 2000:2-224.
11. Diseases treatable by hematopoietic cell transplant. Minneapolis, MN: National Marrow Donor Program, 2010. [Available at http://www.marrow.org/PHYSICIAN/Tx_Indications_Timing_Referral/Diseases_Treatable_by_HCT/index.html (accessed November 26, 2010).]

12. Cutler C. Acute graft-vs-host disease. In: Wingard JR, Gastineau D, Leather H, et al, eds. Hematopoietic stem cell transplantation: A handbook for clinicians. Bethesda, MD: AABB, 2009:331-44.
13. Petersdorf EW. Risk assessment in haematopoietic stem cell transplantation: Histocompatibility. Best Pract Res Clin Haematol 2007; 20:155-70.
14. Gale RP, Horowitz MM, Ash RC, et al. Identical-twin bone marrow transplants for leukemia. Ann Intern Med 1994:120:646-52.
15. Be The Match. U.S. NMDP transplant centers. Minneapolis, MN: National Marrow Donor Program, 2010. [Available at http://www.marrow.org/PATIENT/Plan_for_Tx/Choosing_a_TC/US_NMDP_Transplant_Centers/tc_list_by_state.pl (accessed January 2, 2011).]
16. Petersdorf EW. HLA. In: Wingard JR, Gastineau D, Leather H, et al, eds. Hematopoietic stem cell transplantation: A handbook for clinicians. Bethesda, MD: AABB, 2009:61-76.
17. Goker H, Haznedaroglu IC, Chao NJ. Acute graft-vs-host disease: Pathobiology and management. Exp Hematol 2001;29:259-77.
18. Ottinger HD, Ferencik S, Beelen DW, et al. Hematopoietic stem cell transplantation: Contrasting the outcome of transplantations from HLA-identical siblings, partially HLA-mismatched related donors, and HLA-matched unrelated donors. Blood 2003;102:1131-7.
19. Pusic I, Vogelsang GB, Pavletic S. Chronic graft-vs-host disease. In: Wingard JR, Gastineau D, Leather H, et al, eds. Hematopoietic stem cell transplantation: A handbook for clinicians. Bethesda, MD: AABB, 2009:345-64.
20. Shulman HM, Kleiner D, Lee SJ, et al. Histopathologic diagnosis of chronic graft-versus-host disease: National Institutes of Health consensus development project on criteria for clinical trials in chronic graft-versus-host disease: II. Pathology Working Group report. Biol Blood Marrow Transplant 2006;12:31-47.
21. Van der Straaten HM, Fijnheer R, Dekker AW, et al. Relationship between graft-versus-host disease and graft-versus-leukaemia in partial T cell-depleted bone marrow transplantation. Br J Haematol 2001;114:31-5.
22. Kolb H, Buhmann R. Donor lymphocyte infusion and graft-vs-leukemia effects of allogeneic transplantation. In: Wingard JR, Gastineau D, Leather H, et al, eds. Hematopoietic stem cell transplantation: A handbook for clinicians. Bethesda, MD: AABB, 2009:555-72.
23. Levine JE, Braun T, Penza SL, et al. Prospective trial of chemotherapy and donor leukocyte infusions for relapse of advanced myeloid malignancies after allogeneic stem cell transplantation. J Clin Oncol 2002;20:405-12.
24. Fontaine M, ed. Standards for cellular therapy product services. 5th ed. Bethesda, MD: AABB, 2011.
25. FACT-JACIE international standards for cellular therapy product collection, processing, and administration. 4th ed. Omaha, NE: Foundation for the Accreditation of Cellular Therapy, 2008.
26. Be The Match. HLA matching: Finding the best donor or cord blood unit. Minneapolis, MN: National Marrow Donor Program, 2010. [Available at http://www.marrow.org/PATIENT/Donor_Select_Tx_Process/The_Search_Process/HLA_Matching_Finding_the_Best_/index.html (accessed January 2, 2011).]
27. Boeckh M, Leather H. Viral infections after engraftment. In: Wingard JR, Gastineau D, Leather H, et al, eds. Hematopoietic stem cell transplantation: A handbook for clinicians. Bethesda, MD: AABB, 2009:293-312.
28. Flowers MED, Pepe MS, Longton G, et al. Previous donor pregnancy as a risk factor for acute graft-versus-host disease in patients with aplastic anemia treated by allogeneic marrow transplantation. Br J Haematol 1990; 74:492-6.
29. Food and Drug Administration. Guidance for industry: Eligibility determination for donors of human cells, tissues, and cellular and tissue-based products. (August 2007) Rockville, MD: CBER Office of Communication, Outreach, and Development, 2007. [Available at http://www.fda.gov/cber/gdlns/tissdonor.htm (accessed November 26, 2010).]
30. Donor history questionnaire for allogeneic HPC, Apheresis and HPC, Marrow (HPC-DHQ). Version 1.2. Bethesda, MD: AABB, 2009. [Available at http://aabb.org>ResourceCenter>Blood Donation Information>Donor History Questionnaires> HPC Donor History Questionnaire (accessed November 26, 2010).]
31. Code of federal regulations. Title 21, CFR Part 1271. Human cells, tissues, and cellular and tissue-based products. Washington, DC: US Government Printing Office, 2010 (revised annually).
32. Spitzer T. Bone marrow collection. In: Areman EM, Loper K, eds. Cellular therapy: Principles,

methods, and regulations. Bethesda, MD: AABB, 2009:236-50.

33. Bacigalupo A, Piaggio G, Podesta M, et al. Influence of marrow CFU-GM content on engraftment and survival after allogeneic bone marrow transplantation. Bone Marrow Transplant 1995;15:221-6.
34. Mavroudis D, Read E, Cottler-Fox M, et al. CD34+ cell dose predicts survival, post transplant morbidity, and rate of hematologic recovery after allogeneic marrow transplants for hematologic malignancies. Blood 1996;88: 3223-9.
35. Bittencourt H, Rocha V, Chevret S, et al. Association of CD34 cell dose with hematopoietic recovery, infections, and other outcomes after HLA-identical sibling bone marrow transplantation. Blood 2002;99:2726-33.
36. National Marrow Donor Program standards. 20th ed. Minneapolis, MN: NMDP, 2009. [Available at http://www.marrow.org/ABOUT/Who_We_Are/NMDP_Network/Maintaining_NMDP_Standards/Standards_PDF/NMDP%2020th%20Ed.% 20Stds.pdf (accessed November 26, 2010).]
37. Krause DS, Fackler MJ, Civin CI, et al. CD34: Structure, biology, and clinical utility. Blood 1996:87:1-13.
38. Preti RA, Razis E, Ciavarella D, et al. Clinical and laboratory comparison study of refrigerated and cryopreserved bone marrow for transplantation. Bone Marrow Transplant 1994;13: 253-60.
39. Berz D, McCormack EM, Winer ES, et al. Cryopreservation of hematopoietic stem cells. Am J Hematol 2007;82:463-72.
40. Smith DM, Weisenburger DD, Bireman P, et al. Acute renal failure associated with autologous bone marrow transplantation. Bone Marrow Transplant 1987;2:196-201.
41. Rowley SD. Storage of hematopoietic cells. In: Sacher RA, AuBuchon JP, eds. Marrow transplantation: Practical and technical aspects of stem cell reconstitution. Bethesda, MD: AABB, 1992:105-27.
42. Dickson LG, Hill MG. Buffy coat concentration/buffy coat preparation. In: Areman EM, Deeg JH, Sacher RA, eds. Bone marrow and stem cell processing: A manual of current techniques. Philadelphia: FA Davis, 1992:101-3.
43. Areman EM. Manual buffy coat separation using transfer bags. In: Areman EM, Deeg JH, Sacher RA, eds. Bone marrow and stem cell processing: A manual of current techniques. Philadelphia: FA Davis, 1992:104-6.
44. Croskell M, Loper K, McKenna DH. Basic cellular therapy manufacturing procedures. In: Areman EM, Loper K, eds. Cellular therapy: Principles, methods, and regulations. Bethesda, MD: AABB, 2009:299-302.
45. Guttridge MG, Sidders C, Booth-Davey E, et al. Factors affecting volume reduction and red blood cell depletion of bone marrow on the COBE Spectra cell separator before haematopoietic stem cell transplantation. Bone Marrow Transplant 2006;38:175-81.
46. Larghero J, Rea D, Esperou H, et al. ABO-mismatched marrow processing for transplantation: Results of 114 procedures and analysis of immediate adverse events and hematopoietic recovery. Transfusion 2006;46:398-402.
47. Davis JM, Schepers KF, Eby LL, et al. Comparison of progenitor cell concentration techniques: Continuous flow separation versus density-gradient isolation. J Hematother 1993; 2:314-20.
48. Larsen JK. Principles, capacity, and limitations of immunofluorescent flow sorting of rare cell species. In: Wunder E, Sovalat H, Henon P, Serke S, eds. Hematopoietic stem cells: The Mullhouse manual. Dayton, OH: AlphaMed Press, 1995:133-40.
49. Karandish S. Graft modification: Cell enrichment or depletion. In: Areman EM, Loper K, eds. Cellular therapy: Principles, methods, and regulations. Bethesda, MD: AABB, 2009:398-409.
50. Miraglia S, Godfrey W, Yin AH, et al. A novel five-transmembrane hematopoietic stem cell antigen: Isolation, characterization, and molecular cloning. Blood 1997;90:5013-21.
51. Jones RD, Barber JP, Vala MS, et al. Assessment of aldehyde dehydrogenase in viable cells. Blood 1995;85:2742-6.
52. Storms RW, Trujiool AP, Springer JB, et al. Isolation of primitive human hematopoietic progenitors on the basis of aldehyde dehydrogenase activity. Proc Natl Acad Sci U S A 1999;96: 9118-23.
53. Hickerson D, Fiordalisi M, Reese M, et al. Modification of a commercial cell sorter to support efficient and reliable preparation of ALDH-bright cells for clinical use. Cytotherapy 2007; 9:562-8.
54. Brenner MK, Rill DR, Moen RC, et al. Genemarking to trace origin of relapse after autolo-

gous bone-marrow transplantation. Lancet 1993:341:85-6.
55. Champlin R, Kyoung L. T-cell depletion to prevent graft-versus-host disease following allogeneic bone marrow transplantation. In: Areman EM, Deeg HJ, Sacher RA, eds. Bone marrow and stem cell processing: A manual of current techniques. Philadelphia: FA Davis, 1992:163-70.
56. Mielcarek M, Leisenring W, Toror-Storb B, Storb R. Graft-versus-host disease and donor-directed hemagglutinin titers after ABO-mismatched related and unrelated marrow allografts: Evidence for a graft-versus-plasma effect. Blood 2000;96:1150-6.
57. Lopez-Plaza I, Triulzi DJ. Transfusion support in HSCT. In: Ball ED, Lister J, Law P, eds. Hematopoietic stem cell therapy. Philadelphia: Churchill Livingstone, 2000:589-97.
58. Worel N, Greinix HT, Schneider B, et al. Regeneration of erythropoiesis after related and unrelated donor BMT or peripheral blood HPC transplantation: A major ABO mismatch means of problems. Transfusion 2000;40:543-60.
59. Long GD, Blume KG. Allogeneic and autologous bone marrow transplantation. In: Beutler E, Lichtman MA, Coller BS, Kipps TL, eds. Williams hematology. 5th ed. New York: McGraw-Hill, 1995:172-94.
60. Rowley SD, Liang PS, Ulz L. Transplantation of ABO-incompatible bone marrow and peripheral blood stem cell components. Bone Marrow Transplant 2000;26:749-57.
61. Canals C, Muniz-Diaz E, Marinez C, et al. Impact of ABO incompatibility on allogeneic peripheral blood progenitor cell transplantation after reduced intensity conditioning. Transfusion 2004;44:1603-11.
62. Badros A, Tricot G, Toor A, et al. ABO mismatch may affect engraftment in multiple myeloma patients receiving nonmyeloablative conditioning. Transfusion 2002;42:205-9.
63. Buckner CD, Clift RA, Sanders JE, et al. ABO incompatible marrow transplants. Transplantation 1978;26:233-8.
64. Dinsmore RE, Reich LM, Kapoor N, et al. ABH incompatible bone marrow transplantation: Removal of erythrocytes by starch sedimentation. Br J Haematol 1983;54:441-9.
65. Warkentin PI, Hilden JM, Kersey JH, et al. Transplantation of major ABO-incompatible bone marrow depleted of red cells by hydroxyethyl starch. Vox Sang 1985;48:89-104.
66. Antonenas V, Garvin F, Webb M, et al. Fresh PBSC harvests, but not BM, show temperature related loss of CD34 viability during storage and transport. Cytotherapy 2006;8:158-65.
67. Lazarus HM, Kan F, Tarima S, et al. Rapid transport and infusion of hematopoietic cells is associated with improved outcome after myeloablative therapy and unrelated donor transplant. Biol Blood Marrow Transplant 2009;15:589-96.
68. Aird W, Laborpin M, Gorin NC, Anten JH. Long term cryopreservation of human stem cells. Bone Marrow Transplant 1992;9:487-90.
69. Hubel A. Cryopreservation of cellular therapy products. In: Areman EM, Loper K, eds. Cellular therapy: Principles, methods, and regulations. Bethesda, MD: AABB, 2009:342-57.
70. Stiff PJ, Koester AR, Weidner MK, et al. Autologous bone marrow transplantation using unfractionated cells cryopreserved in dimethylsulfoxide and hydroxyethyl starch without controlled-rate freezing. Blood 1987;70:974-8.
71. McCullough J, Haley R, Clay M, et al. Long-term storage of peripheral blood stem cells frozen and stored with a conventional liquid nitrogen technique compared with cells frozen and stored in a mechanical freezer. Transfusion 2010;50:808-19.
72. Tedder RS, Zuckerman MA, Goldstone AH, et al. Hepatitis B transmission from contaminated cryopreservation tank. Lancet 1995;346:137-40.
73. Fountain D, Ralston M, Higgins N, et al. Liquid nitrogen freezers: A potential source of microbial contamination of hematopoietic stem cell products. Transfusion 1997;37:585-91.
74. Husebekk AM, Skaug K, Kolstad A, et al. Hepatitis B virus-infected peripheral blood progenitor cell harvests in liquid nitrogen freezer containing non-infectious products. Transfusion 2005;44:942-3.
75. Regan D. Transportation and shipping of cellular therapy products. In: Areman EM, Loper K, eds Cellular therapy: Principles, methods, and regulations. Bethesda, MD: AABB, 2009:362-74.
76. Delany M, Haspel R. Thawing and infusing cellular therapy products. In: Areman EM, Loper K, eds. Cellular therapy: Principles, methods, and regulations. Bethesda, MD: AABB, 2009:375-96.
77. Rowley SD, Anderson GL. Effect of DMSO exposure without cryopreservation on hemato-

poietic progenitor cells. Bone Marrow Transplant 1993;11:389-93.

78. Keever-Taylor CA. Cell counts and differentials of cellular therapy products. In: Areman EM, Loper K, eds. Cellular therapy: Principles, methods, and regulations. Bethesda, MD: AABB, 2009:528-37.
79. Bentley SA, Taylor MA, Killian DE, et al. Correction of bone marrow nucleated cell counts for the presence of fat particles. Am J Clin Pathol 1995;140:60-4.
80. Read EJ, Carter CS, Cullis HM. Bone marrow cell counting: Methodological issues. In: Gee AP, ed. Bone marrow processing and purging: A practical guide. Boca Raton, FL: CRC Press, 1991:107-19.
81. Greco N, O'Donnell L. Assessment of viability and apoptosis in cellular therapy products. In: Areman EM, Loper K, eds. Cellular therapy: Principles, methods, and regulations. Bethesda, MD: AABB, 2009:563-72.
82. Khuu H. Assessing cellular therapy products for microbial contamination. In: Areman EM, Loper K, eds. Cellular therapy: Principles, methods, and regulations. Bethesda, MD: AABB, 2009:604-11.
83. Kelly M, Roy DC, Labbe AC, Laverdiere M. What is the clinical significance of infusing hematopoietic cell grafts contaminated with bacteria? Bone Marrow Transplant 2006;38: 183-8.
84. Klein MA, Kadidlo D, McCullough J, et al. Microbial contamination of hematopoietic stem cell products: Incidence and clinical sequelae. Biol Blood Marrow Transplant 2006;12:1142-9.
85. Padley D, Dietz AB, Gastineau DA. Sterility testing of hematopoietic progenitor cell products: A single-institution series of culture-positive rates and successful infusion of culture-positive products. Transfusion 2007;47:636-43.
86. Sutherland DR, Keeney M. Enumeration of CD34+ cells by flow cytometry. In: Areman EM, Loper K, eds. Cellular therapy: Principles, methods, and regulations. Bethesda, MD: AABB, 2009:538-54.
87. Haley NR. Assessing the function of cellular therapy products by measurement of cytoplasmic aldehyde dehydrogenase. In: Areman EM, Loper K, eds. Cellular therapy: Principles, methods, and regulations. Bethesda, MD: AABB, 2009:592-7.
88. Fallon P, Gentry T, Balber AE, et al. Mobilized peripheral blood SSCL0ALDHbr cells have the phenotypic and functional properties of primitive haematopoietic cells and their number correlates with engraftment following autologous transplantation. Br J Haematol 2003;122: 99-108.
89. Clarke E. Colony-forming cell assays for determining potency of cellular therapy products. In: Areman EM, Loper K, eds. Cellular therapy: Principles, methods, and regulations. Bethesda, MD: AABB, 2009:573-80.
90. Davis JM, Schepers KG. Quality control of hemapoietic progenitor cell products. In: Brecher ME, Lasky LC, Sacher RA, Issitt LA, eds. Hematopoietic progenitor cells: Processing, standards, and practice. Bethesda, MD: AABB, 1995:159-81.
91. Petzer AL, Hogge DE, Lansdorp PM, et al. Self-renewal of primitive human hematopoietic cells (long-term culture-initiating cells) in vitro and their expansion in defined medium. Proc Natl Acad Sci U S A 1996;93:1470-4.
92. Hall KM, Rich IN. Bioluminescence assays for assessing potency of cellular therapy products. In: Areman EM, Loper K, eds. Cellular therapy: Principles, methods, and regulations. Bethesda, MD: AABB, 2009:581-91.
93. O'Donnell PV. Engraftment. In: Wingard JR, Gastineau D, Leather H, et al, eds. Hematopoietic stem cell transplantation: A handbook for clinicians. Bethesda, MD: AABB, 2009:163-80.
94. Code of federal regulations. Title 21, CFR Part 211. cGMP in manufacturing, processing, packaging, or holding drugs and finished pharmaceuticals. Washington, DC: US Government Printing Office, 2010 (revised annually).
95. Ashford P, Distler P, Gee A, et al. Standards for the terminology and labeling of cellular therapy products. Transfusion 2007;42:1319-27.

Chapter 30

Hematopoietic Progenitor Cells Collected by Apheresis

Thomas A. Lane, MD, and John D. McMannis, PhD

HEMATOPOIETIC PROGENITOR cells (HPCs) collected by apheresis (HPC, Apheresis; also referred to as peripheral blood stem/progenitor cells) are currently the most common type of hematopoietic graft that is used for autologous hematopoietic transplantation because of ease of acquisition and rapid engraftment. HPC, Apheresis [HPC(A)] collections are also commonly used for syngeneic or allogeneic transplantation from related or unrelated donors.[1] [Please note that the terms HPC(A); HPC(M), for HPC, Marrow; and HPC(C), for HPC, Cord Blood are used here only as abbreviations and are not intended to be used in the labeling process or on product labels.] HPC(A) grafts are harvested by leukocyte apheresis following the "mobilization" of HPCs from marrow stem cell niches into the peripheral blood using a variety of pharmacologic methods, including myelosuppressive therapy, hematopoietic growth factors, and adhesion-receptor blockade. Nearly all normal healthy donors mobilize HPCs sufficiently well to enable the collection of an adequate HPC(A) graft, but marked differences exist in the mobilization potential among autologous marrow transplant patients. This difference is chiefly the result of prior myelosuppressive therapy for malignancy and possibly genetic factors, and despite the approval of new mobilizing agents, it continues to represent a challenge in collecting sufficient HPC(A) for some autologous transplant patients.

The cellular content of HPC(A) grafts includes a variable number of HPCs (measured by CD34+ cell content) and other leukocytes, and the content differs significantly from marrow-derived HPC grafts as described in a later section. HPC(A) grafts typically require minimal laboratory processing before infusion, but they are generally volume-reduced if the grafts are to be cryopreserved before transplantation. Additional manipulations such as T-cell reduction may be performed if necessary, according to study protocols. Procedures for the routine handling, processing, and storage of an HPC(A) graft are sufficiently well characterized to reliably result in excellent cell recovery

Thomas A. Lane, MD, Medical Director, Transfusion Services and Stem Cell Processing, University of California at San Diego, School of Medicine, La Jolla, California, and John D. McMannis, PhD, Professor and Director, Cell Therapy Laboratory, University of Texas MD Anderson Cancer Center, Houston, Texas

T. Lane has disclosed a financial relationship with Fenwal, and J. McMannis has disclosed financial relationships with BioSafe Medical Technologies, Pall Corporation, and BioE Corporation.

and viability when performed by well-trained staff in a well-designed facility, but careful quality control testing is nevertheless required to verify the safety, potency, and content of each HPC(A) product and to fulfill accreditation and regulatory requirements.

This chapter describes the methods of mobilizing HPC(A); the characteristics, clinical uses, selection, processing, and storage of HPC(A) products; the important differences in the harvest and content of HPC(A) compared with HPC(M); and how those differences translate into differences in patient outcome. General apheresis considerations and techniques are discussed in Chapter 7.

BIOLOGY OF HPC MOBILIZATION

The biology of HPC adherence to marrow sites has become of critical practical importance since the discovery of agents that can directly modulate HPC adherence. HPCs of varying stages of differentiation and lineage commitment are thought to normally reside in specialized hematopoietic "niche" spaces in the marrow.[2] The precise nature of the hematopoietic niche is the subject of intensive investigation and may in part be composed of osteoblasts, marrow stromal cells, vascular cells, and their associated matrixes. HPC adherence to the niche is mediated by a variety of adhesion molecule interactions, including the binding of a receptor, CXCR4 on HPCs, to stromal-cell-derived factor 1 (SDF1); the binding of beta-1 integrin adhesion molecules (eg, VLA4 on HPCs) to vascular cell adhesion molecule 1 (VCAM1) on stromal cells and to fibronectin; and the binding of HPC CD44 to hyaluronic acid, among others.[3] HPC mobilization involves a temporary increase in the dissociation rate of HPCs from the niche through the disruption of those adhesive interactions and the migration of HPCs into the marrow and then into the peripheral blood circulation.[2,3]

Physiologic processes that lead to dissociation of HPC adhesive interactions may be initiated by myelosuppressive chemotherapy or by administration of hematopoietic growth factors, both of which typically require several days to generate increases in circulating HPCs. Both types of regimen are associated with the release of metalloproteases (eg, MMP9, elastase, and cathepsin G) that are hypothesized to cleave one or more receptor-ligand pairs (eg, SDF1) and to release HPC tethers to their stroma.[1,3] In contrast, agents or antibodies that directly disrupt or block HPCs or stromal adhesive receptors such as VLA4 antibodies, or oligopeptides that block CXCR4, are associated with increases in circulating HPCs in a matter of minutes to hours.[1] Combined modality mobilization—for example, administration of chemotherapy and hematopoietic growth factors—typically results in an additive increase in circulating CD34+ cell responses. That finding has clinical implications for the design of mobilizing regimens, and it suggests that different classes of mobilizing agents act by nonoverlapping mechanisms. Wide variability exists in the HPC mobilization response among individuals, presumably reflecting marrow reserve of HPCs and possibly genetic variations. Factors reported to affect HPC mobilization include the patient's age and gender; the presence of marrow disease; the extent of prior myelotoxic therapy (eg, cancer chemo- or radiotherapy or treatment of hepatitis C virus with interferon-γ); the type of prior cancer chemotherapy (eg, marrow irradiation and busulfan are irreversibly toxic to hematopoietic stem cells); the dose, schedule, and type of mobilizing regimen used; the patient's underlying disease (eg, autoimmune vs cancer); and the patient's genetic polymorphisms.[1,4-6]

CLINICAL MOBILIZATION REGIMENS

Chemotherapy

Myelotoxic chemotherapy is used only for HPC mobilization of patients who are scheduled for autologous transplantation. The initial discovery that HPCs can be mobilized into the peripheral blood was made by recognizing that circulating myeloid colony-forming cells increased up to 20-fold at the same time that leukocytes rebounded after chemotherapy-induced leukopenia.[7] Since that time, a host of cancer chemotherapy regimens have been described that are effective in mobilizing HPCs, and all are characterized by inducing varying degrees of transient myelosuppression and peripheral blood neutropenia.[8] The regimens may be administered either on a single day or over several days, and there is a general relationship between the severity of neutropenia induced by the regimen and the extent of subsequent HPC mobilization. Thus, as the leukocyte count increases after the neutropenic phase (about 10 to 20 days), HPCs typically increase more than 50-fold and remain elevated for 3 to 5 days, during which time HPCs are collected by apheresis. Chemotherapy alone mobilizes HPCs sufficiently well in many patients to collect an adequate dose of HPCs in one or more apheresis procedures. A possible advantage of some disease-specific chemotherapy-based regimens is the potential for "in-vivo purging" of tumor cells that might otherwise contaminate the HPC(A) product and/or the ability to keep rapidly progressive disease in check during the time required to mobilize and collect HPC(A) and to prepare the patient for the high-dose antineoplastic therapy (see later this chapter).

The side effects and complications associated with chemotherapy regimens used for HPC mobilization are predictably the same as those of similar doses of the drugs when they are used in that population for cancer therapy. Consequently, nearly all such regimens are associated with treatment-intensity-dependent thrombocytopenia, with an increased risk of bleeding, and neutropenia, with an increased risk of infection. Febrile neutropenia and/or infection frequently requires hospitalization for effective treatment and remains an important cause of the morbidity and mortality that is associated with these procedures.[9] In addition, central venous line complications, including clotting or infections, are more common after chemotherapy mobilization regimens, with each occurring in 5% to 15% of patients. Infections usually require antibiotic therapy and line replacement and are a frequent cause of microbial contamination of HPC(A).[10]

Another practical challenge associated with mobilization regimens that use chemotherapy is the timing of the increase in blood leukocyte count and HPC count, which may vary considerably among different regimens and among different patients.[11] That variability translates into the need to monitor the patient's counts daily during the expected window of HPC mobilization, and the need for apheresis, cell processing, and flow cytometry services to be promptly available with a minimum of lead time. Those problems may be managed to some extent by performing leukocyte and CD34+ counts on a daily basis once the leukocyte count begins to increase and/or by initiating apheresis when the count reaches a defined threshold, which is typically above 1000 to 10,000 white cells or 5 to 20 CD34+/μL of peripheral blood. Knowledge of the peripheral blood CD34+ cell count before apheresis makes it possible to predict the number of CD34+ cells that will be collected with some accuracy.[1,12] Some automated cell counters report an "HPC" parameter that may also serve as a rough guide of HPC mobilization but that lacks sufficient accuracy to reliably predict apheresis yield.[13] Alternatively, investigators have defined certain specific mobilization regimens (eg, combined chemotherapy plus growth factor) that result in predictable and reliable leukocyte and CD34+ cell mobilization. Thus, apheresis collection may be initiated on a predetermined day—for example, 11 days following initiation of mobilizing chemotherapy.[14,15]

Assessment of when to discontinue HPC(A) collection by apheresis is ideally based on the viable CD34+ cells available in the combined total of all processed apheresis components, and such assessments require the rapid availability of flow cytometry results, sometimes late in the day. For programs that lack such readily available cytometry services, especially after normal hours, an alternative method to assess apheresis yields is to measure the CD34+ cell content of the cells collected by apheresis approximately midway through the apheresis procedure and to extrapolate the final yield. When carefully used, that method has been reported to permit accurate decisions regarding whether to continue apheresis for another day or to discontinue it, without waiting for the final HPC(A) CD34+ cell count to be available. That approach may avoid unnecessary growth factor injections and apheresis procedures.[16] Currently, most chemotherapy regimens that are used for HPC mobilization also use growth factors because these combinations are capable of generating additive increases in circulating CD34+ cells.[8]

Hematopoietic Growth Factors

Granulocyte colony-stimulating factor (G-CSF) and granulocyte-macrophage colony-stimulating factor (GM-CSF) are the principal hematopoietic growth factors used for HPC mobilization in allogeneic, syngeneic, and autologous donors. G-CSF is more potent as a mobilizing agent and is far more widely used than GM-CSF, which is typically used in combination regimens.[17-19] G-CSF administration to normal or autologous donors results in dose-dependent increases in leukocyte, lymphocyte, and HPC counts. G-CSF is typically administered once daily subcutaneously in doses ranging from 5 to 20 µg/kg/day, although higher doses may be used in poor mobilizers (see below).[20] Some reports suggest that divided doses of G-CSF permit higher doses, result in improved mobilization with fewer side effects, or both, but those findings are not universal.[21,22] G-CSF results in increases in circulating HPCs and leukocytes that are predictable and are sufficient to collect HPC(A) beginning about 3 to 4 days after the first dose. The increases typically persist for 3 to 5 days, depending on the dose and patient-specific factors, as described above. When used alone, G-CSF is ideally administered at least 4 hours before scheduled HPC collection because of a transient decrease in HPC levels that occurs shortly after G-CSF administration.[23] A single dose of long-acting, pegylated G-CSF has been reported to result in satisfactory allogeneic or autologous donor HPC mobilization, but this drug is not currently approved for HPC mobilization.[24]

Hematopoietic growth factor administration is nearly always accompanied by side effects, albeit effects that are usually tolerable. The most common symptoms associated with G-CSF administration are bone pain (long bones or chest) that is dependent on dose and treatment duration; headache and muscle aches, which may be treated by nonsteroidal anti-inflammatory drug (NSAID) therapy; fatigue or malaise; insomnia; nausea; flu-like symptoms; sweating; anorexia; and less commonly, abdominal pain and rash.[17,18,25,26] (See Table 30-1.) Symptoms may require dose reduction or omission, and they typically disappear within a day or two after discontinuing G-CSF. Female donors are reported to have more

TABLE 30-1. Adverse Events among 2408 Unrelated Donors of Peripheral Blood Stem Cells

Sign or Symptom	Percentage of Donors*
Bone pain	80
Myalgia	70
Headache	70
Fatigue	70
Insomnia	40
Flu-like symptoms	30
Nausea	30
Sweats	20
Anorexia	20
Fever	10
Chills	10
Local symptoms	5
Emesis	5
Skin	5
Allergy	1

Data from Pulsipher et al.[26]

*Approximate percentage of donors reporting adverse events at any time during mobilization and collection.

bone pain and other symptoms and greater transient increases in levels of alkaline phosphatase, alanine aminotransferase (ALT), and lactate dehydrogenase (LDH).[26] An asymptomatic increase in spleen size is commonly observed during G-CSF administration in normal donors.[27] Impaired pulmonary exchange has also been reported in normal donors receiving G-CSF.[28] Leukocyte counts in some donors may increase to >50,000/μL, and platelet counts may decrease by more than 50% during G-CSF mobilization, the latter at least in part as a result of the apheresis procedure. A consensus report found that when used in normal donors, G-CSF doses >10 μg/kg/day are of uncertain benefit and are associated with increased side effects. Most centers avoid leukocyte counts >70,000/μL by dose reduction if necessary, and platelet counts >80,000/μL are desirable before apheresis, especially for normal allogeneic donors.[29]

Intolerance is rare, and although severe symptoms caused by G-CSF are unusual, dose reduction, omission, or discontinuation may be necessary. Of 2408 normal unrelated donors mobilized with 10 μg/day G-CSF for 5 days, 15 (0.6%) had severe adverse events related to G-CSF and/or apheresis (most requiring hospitalization), including headache, nausea, chest or back pain, bleeding, citrate toxicity, or thrombocytopenia.[26] Rare adverse events reported in normal donors treated with G-CSF include allergic reactions, splenic rupture (incidence: 1/5000 to 1/10,000),[26] myocardial ischemia, stroke, iritis, immune thrombocytopenia (ITP), capillary leak syndrome, anaphylaxis, and other life-threatening events.[25,26,30-33] G-CSF should be used with extreme caution (if used at all) in patients with sickle cell disease or sickling disorders, but G-CSF administration has been reported to be safe in small studies of patients with sickle trait.[34,35] G-CSF is typically used in combination with myelosuppressive chemotherapy when mobilizing patients with autoimmune or inflammatory disease because of the concern regarding disease flare-up.[6,36] More frequent angina accompanies the use of G-CSF in patients with coronary artery disease, and G-CSF should be used with caution in that population.[37] Follow-up with 2408 normal donors for 1 to 4 years and a smaller group up to 6 years after mobilization using G-CSF showed normal blood counts[26] and no adverse events that were thought to be caused by G-CSF.[38] A significant increase in the rate of AML/MDS has been reported in women who received G-CSF support during intensive therapy for breast cancer.[25] The potential for G-CSF to cause myeloid leukemia or other malignancies is also a concern associated with its administration to normal donors, and rare case reports (three) exist of related donors developing leukemia several years after receiving G-CSF. However, after more than 10 years of use in normal related and unrelated donors and after tens of thousands of donor treatments, no increase in the risk of leukemia after mobilization with G-CSF has been identified.[25,26,39]

GM-CSF is a poor mobilizing agent when used alone, but it has been effectively used along with G-CSF or after chemotherapy to augment mobilization.[17] Several additional agents that support HPC mobilization have been described, such as dextran, human growth factor, interleukin-8, erythropoietin (EPO), thrombopoietin (TPO), and stem cell factor (SCF, or ckit ligand). However, those agents are not used in the clinic because of limited efficacy, lack of availability, or side effects. Additional agents that induce hematopoietic stem cell mobilization by interfering with their adhesive properties to the niche are currently under investigation.

Adhesion-Blocking Agents and Cytokines

Plerixafor, or AMD3100 [Mozobil (Genzyme, Cambridge, MA)], was recently approved for use in combination with G-CSF for the mobilization of CD34+ cells in autologous transplant patients with non-Hodgkin lymphoma or multiple myeloma. It is being studied to support mobilization in other conditions (eg, Hodgkin disease), but it is not approved for use in patients with leukemia or in normal donors.[40-42] Mozobil is a synthetic SDF1-like molecule that blocks the adhesive interaction between SDF1 on marrow stromal cells and CXCR4 on CD34+

cells. It is unique among clinical CD34+ cell mobilizing agents in that it stimulates the release of CD34+ cells within several hours after administration. In both normal experimental subjects and autologous hematopoietic transplantation donors, Mozobil is approximately as active as G-CSF in mobilizing CD34+ cells when used alone. Mozobil's additive effects increase circulating CD34+ cells and T cells when it is administered in combination with G-CSF or myelosuppressive agents. The FDA-approved protocol for HPC mobilization using Mozobil and G-CSF combined calls for 10 µg/kg G-CSF to be administered each morning and for 0.24 mg/kg Mozobil to be administered subcutaneously (in patients with normal renal function) on day 4 of G-CSF mobilization, approximately 11 hours before leukapheresis.[40] The combined use of G-CSF and Mozobil has been reported to increase the number of HPCs collected per apheresis procedure, to decrease the number of apheresis procedures required to collect a target dose of HPCs, and to improve the mobilization of HPCs in poor mobilizers (see below).[40,41,43] The most common adverse reactions reported during HPC mobilization and apheresis using Mozobil with G-CSF were diarrhea (37%), nausea (34%), fatigue (27%), injection site reaction (34%), headache (22%), arthralgia (13%), dizziness (11%), and vomiting (10%).[40] Long-term side effects of Mozobil in patients and normal donors have not been well studied. The economics of selected vs universal use of combined Mozobil and G-CSF is under investigation, as are alternative strategies to add Mozobil by algorithm during a CD34+ cell mobilization attempt in patients who are shown to be mobilizing insufficiently.[43] Additional novel adhesion-blocking agents and cytokines are currently undergoing investigation.

Combined Growth Factor and Chemotherapy

The combined use of myelosuppressive chemotherapy followed by growth factor administration for autologous HPC(A) mobilization results in improved HPC mobilization when compared with either treatment alone, with 10-fold to 100-fold increases in circulating CD34+ cells, and with a mean 3.5-fold increase in circulating colony-forming units, compared with growth factor alone.[8,44] Additional advantages of combined modality mobilization include the potential to reduce the probability of disease progression during the time required to perform HPC(A) mobilization, collection, and scheduling for transplant, and possibly to reduce the frequency or level of contamination of malignant cells in the autologous graft (in-vivo purging, as mentioned earlier). Consequently, disease-specific, combined modality HPC mobilization regimens are often used for those purposes, as described below.[45] As with chemotherapy-alone regimens, combined modality regimens have the potential to result in chemotherapy-induced cytopenias, the frequency of which varies depending on the intensity of the chemotherapy regimen and on the patient's marrow reserve. Also, the administration of growth factor in combination with chemotherapy may diminish the duration of neutropenia.[44] One widely used combined modality regimen (cyclophosphamide plus G-CSF) results in predictable mobilization with few side effects.[14] The combination of Mozobil after chemotherapy with or without G-CSF has also been reported to further enhance HPC(A) mobilization.

Poor Mobilizers

Poor HPC mobilization is defined in a wide variety of ways—for example, as the failure to achieve a minimum level of 5 to 20 CD34+ cells/µL in peripheral blood after completion of the mobilization regimen, or as the inability to collect at least 1 to 2 × 10^6 CD34+ cells/kg during a single apheresis procedure, or as the failure to collect a total of 5 × 10^6 CD34+ cells/kg in all collections.[4,46] Poor mobilization has thus been reported in 2% to 20% of mobilization attempts in normal donors (the latter is based on failure to achieve 20 CD34+ cells/µL) and in 10% to 50% of autologous transplantation donors (the latter is based on failure to achieve 5 × 10^6 CD34+ cells/kg).[4,47,48] The management of patients who fail to mobilize well remains a challenging problem and is a common reason that otherwise eligible patients (eg, acute leukemia patients) do not receive an autologous transplant.[49] This is because patients transplanted with low doses of HPCs have prolonged times to engraftment, higher rates of graft failure and posttransplant complications, and poorer outcomes.[50] Factors noted in Table 30-2 and other factors, such as the premobilization peripheral blood CD34+ cell count, flt3 ligand level, or platelet count, have been reported to correlate with and to predict postmobilization CD34+ cell counts, but they are not widely used.[51]

No current consensus exists on the optimal management of poor mobilizers, but recent trials indicate that either adding Mozobil on day 4 for myeloma or lymphoma patients who are poorly mobilizing with G-CSF[43] (see above) or remobilizing with growth factor and Mozobil are effective in most myeloma and non-Hodgkin lymphoma patients who mobilize poorly.[52,53] Historically, attempts to remobilize extensively treated, poorly mobilizing, multiple-myeloma patients using the same protocol were unsuccessful.[54] Remobilization with growth factor alone at the same or an increased dose,[55] different chemotherapy regimens (with or without growth factor)[56,57] at variable time delays after the first failed regimen, or both, were effective in 40% to 70% of poor mobilizers. Immediate administration of 32 µg/kg/day of G-CSF for 4 days led to acceptable mobilization in 80% of a heterogeneous group of poorly mobilizing autologous patients.[48] Large-volume leukapheresis, in which four to six patient blood volumes are processed, may also improve overall HPC(A) collection in those patients.[58]

Finally, combining additional HPCs collected by marrow harvest with a suboptimal dose of HPC(A) was reported as effective in some,[59] but not other, studies in poorly mobilizing patients.[57] Pretreatment of HPC(M) donors with G-CSF for 2 to 5 days before marrow harvest has been reported to increase the yield of HPC(M) and to improve engraftment speed after autologous transplantation.[60] Transplantation of autologous HPC(M) collected after marrow harvesting in poor HPC(A) mobilizers was also reported to enable marrow transplantation, albeit with variable rates of engraftment speed.[61]

In summary, there is no universally accepted method of managing poor mobilizers. The specific contribution of second attempts at mobilization using modified mobilization regimens (or of marrow collection) vs the simple benefit of spontaneous marrow recovery during the interim between the first and second HPC collections has not been studied but may also play an important role in the success of remobilization.[62] Historically, acceptable grafts were obtained from about half of the patients who mobilize poorly, but engraftment rates after autologous transplantation, especially for platelets, were prolonged in patients who received borderline doses of CD34+ cells. The novel mobilizing agent Mozobil is expected both to diminish the frequency of poor initial mobilization and to mobilize HPCs more reliably in myeloma and non-Hodgkin lymphoma patients during a second mobilization attempt.[52,53]

TABLE 30-2. Factors Reported to Affect the Mobilization of HPC, Apheresis

Factor
◆ Mobilization method
– Chemotherapy: degree of transient myelosuppression
– Growth factors: type, schedule, dose
– Combined chemotherapy and growth factors
◆ Extent and type of prior chemotherapy, radiotherapy, or certain drugs (interferon-γ, lenalidomide)
◆ Patient or donor age
◆ Patient or donor diagnosis
◆ Patient or donor gender
◆ Presence of marrow disease or metastases

PREPARATION AND ADMINISTRATION OF HPC(A)

Processing, Cryopreservation, and Storage of HPC(A)

HPC(A) products typically require minimal processing before infusion or cryopreservation.[63] Processing may include volume reduction to minimize the space needed to cryopreserve the product. In some allotransplants, reduction of the incompatible plasma or red cell content of HPC(A) may be required to minimize HPC(A) infusion-related hemolysis. A variety of other processing steps may be required in specific settings, such as CD34 selection, T-cell depletion, and (rarely) tumor purging. Overnight storage of HPC(A) at 4 C to 15 C before processing has been reported to be associated with normal graft quality and engraftment. Current National Marrow Donor Program guidelines permit HPC(A) products to be stored for up to 48 hours before infusion.[64] Cryopreservation of HPC(A) is typically accomplished by suspending the cells in autologous plasma or in another source of protein and by adding a final concentration of 10% dimethylsulfoxide (DMSO) before controlled-rate freezing, which is typically 1 to 2 C/minute to –30 C to –50 C, then 2 to 10 C/minute to –90 C. However, many acceptable variations have been reported to be equally effective in preserving HPC(A) viability, including the use of lower concentrations of DMSO, with or without hydroxyethyl starch, and so-called "dump" freezing in a –70 C to –130 C freezer.[65] Cryopreserved HPC(A) products may be stored in either mechanical freezers at <–70 C or in liquid-nitrogen freezers (–196 C in liquid or <–150 C in vapor phase) for several years and will still maintain sufficient viability to support rapid, stable, trilineage engraftment (leukocytes, platelets, and red cells) after administration. In contrast, marrow harvests nearly always require laboratory processing in order to generate an acceptable graft volume, red cell content, or both, as a result of the large collection volume and of the greater red cell and plasma content.

Thawing and Infusion of HPC(A)

Thawing and infusion of HPC(A) have been reviewed.[66] HPC(A) may be thawed (frequently inside a sterile overwrap in case of bag leakage) in a 37 C waterbath immediately before infusion at the bedside or may be thawed and sometimes also washed in the laboratory and transported to the bedside for infusion.[66] The advantage of laboratory thawing and washing is reduction of DMSO infusion toxicity, but laboratory thawing and washing require excellent communications with the bedside caregivers to ensure that the thawed cells are infused without undue delay and without loss of cell viability.[65,67] HPC(A) may be infused rapidly if the patient's condition permits—for example, at 5 to 20 mL/minute with or without an in-line, 170- to 210-micron screen filter. If filters are used, the staff should be carefully trained to ensure that the proper filter is selected and that leukocyte reduction filters are not used, because they may remove HPCs and could result in graft failure.

Infusion reactions are common during HPC(A) administration, more so with infusion of cryopreserved and unwashed products, presumably caused by DMSO (which frequently causes an unpleasant taste) and possibly also caused by cell lysis products, especially in grafts that contain large numbers of neutrophils.[66,68-70] The most frequently reported reactions include nausea, vomiting, hypertension, hypotension, flushing, fever, chest tightness, cramps, and bradycardia (see Table 30-3).[71,72] Doses of DMSO >0.8 to 1 g/kg may be associated with delayed (up to 8 hours) cardiac dysfunction and fatal dysrhythmias and may be avoided by separating multiple bag infusions over 2 days.[73] Concern has been expressed that children are more susceptible to adverse reactions caused by DMSO infusion; one report demonstrated a high rate of HPC infusion reactions in children, but direct comparisons between children and adults are lacking.[74,75] Removal of DMSO by washing the cell product may diminish certain infusion reactions (eg, nausea and vomiting), albeit with some loss of cell numbers.[66,67] Commonly employed prein-

TABLE 30-3. Signs and Symptoms Reported to Accompany HPC(A) Infusion in Adults[71,72]

Sign or Symptom	Percentage of Patients
Nausea	45
Vomiting	8 to 22
Hypertension	22 to 36
Flushing	22
Hypotension	21
Fever	12
Chest tightness	1 to 9
Abdominal cramps	9
Arrhythmia	3
Bradycardia	3 to 4.5

fusion medications include antihistamines to counteract DMSO-induced histamine release, and antiemetics, antipyretics, and/or corticosteroids to diminish emesis, cramps or fever, and allergic symptoms, although controlled studies to support their use are not available.[66] Simple administration of a flavored lozenge may diminish nausea and vomiting.

Bacterial contamination has recently been reported to occur in 0.2% to 4% of HPC(A) collections.[76] The vast majority of contaminants consist of skin bacteria, typically coagulase-negative *Staphylococcus*, but many other organisms have been encountered.[66,76,77] The investigation of contaminated HPCs should include consideration of subclinical donor bacteremia, which is typically the result of an infected central line and requires prompt management, or contamination of the HPCs during collection, during processing, or even during culture inoculation. If there are insufficient uncontaminated HPCs available, the decision to infuse a contaminated HPC component should take into consideration the risk of its infusion vs the risks of attempting to procure additional HPCs, including the risk of disease relapse while the patient is remobilized. Contaminated HPCs have been infused with or without antibiotic coverage of the relevant organism. Although septic events and fatalities have been rarely reported with the contaminating organism, the vast majority of such infusions have been well tolerated in patients who have been adequately covered by administration of effective antibiotics before HPC(A) infusion.[66,76,77] In addition, a positive culture renders an HPC(A) a nonconforming component, the infusion of which first requires careful assessment, by the laboratory/medical director and the patient's responsible physician, of the risk vs benefit to the patient of infusing such a product; then, informed consent of the patient and assessment of the applicability of regulatory requirements are also necessary.

In view of the frequent HPC infusion-related adverse events, the patient's vital signs are typically monitored frequently during and for a period after HPC infusion. It has been recommended that infusion of HPCs that may be associated with an increased risk of adverse events (eg, volumes of cryopreserved HPCs that contain DMSO approaching 1 g/kg/day) justifies more intensive and prolonged patient monitoring or dividing the infusion over 2 days.[66,72]

CLINICAL USE OF HPC(A)

Autologous Transplantation

The vast majority of candidates for autologous transplantation are patients with malignant conditions 1) who are in partial or complete clinical remission, 2) whose type of disease has been shown to benefit from high-dose anticancer therapy with hematopoietic rescue, and 3) whose marrow and blood ideally do not contain viable malignant cells. However, autologous transplantation is also under investigation for autoimmune diseases.[6] Autologous donors may be mobilized using hematopoietic growth factors, myelosuppressive chemotherapy, and Mozobil.

The apheresis collection goal of CD34+ cells to support a single autologous transplantation typically ranges from a minimum of 2 $\times 10^6$ CD34+ cells/kg to a more preferable 5 $\times 10^6$ CD34+ cells/kg.[78-83] The ability to achieve this goal is influenced by institution-specific protocols for patient therapy and mobilization, the extent of prior therapy in an individual patient, local variations in CD34+ cell measurement, HPC(A) storage and processing, and the perception of need for high-dose therapy. Higher administered doses of CD34+ cells increase the speed of engraftment for both neutrophils and platelets, especially in heavily pretreated patients.[78,79] The speed of engraftment is measured by the number of days after infusion of the graft until a defined threshold of circulating neutrophils (polymorphonuclear cells, or PMNs) or platelets is reached, typically the first of 3 days for PMNs >500/µL and platelets >20,000/µL, without transfusion. Administration of $>5 \times 10^6$ viable CD34+ cells/kg is generally not advantageous, and administration of $<2 \times 10^6$ CD34+ cells/kg may compromise both the probability and speed of engraftment.[50,80,81]

Engraftment speed is important because short engraftment times are associated with fewer infections, fewer transfusions, shorter hospital stays, and lower cost. The administration of G-CSF after transplantation has been reported to speed neutrophil engraftment regardless of CD34+ cell dose. TPO-mimetic drugs are available, but their effect on platelet engraftment after marrow transplantation has not been studied, and they are not approved for use after marrow transplantation. Apart from CD34+ dose, additional factors that have been reported to affect engraftment after autologous transplantation include the type and extent of previous myelotoxic therapy [ie, engraftment is slower after total body irradiation (TBI) or busulfan] and whether the patient was a poor HPC mobilizer (see Table 30-4).[80,82,83] The empirical limit of engraftment speed with optimal CD34+ cell dose and growth factor administration is approximately 9 days. Preliminary clinical studies suggest that the time of 9 days may be shortened in the future by coadministration with HPCs that have been expanded, activated ex vivo, or both.[84] However, a high CD34+ cell dose may not always translate into improved survival. It was reported that in autologous recipients with acute myelogenous leukemia (AML), patients who mobilized poorly and thus received small HPC(A) doses actually had improved relapse-free survival compared with those who mobilized very well and thus received the highest CD34+ doses, presumably because the grafts in the latter group also contained higher numbers of residual clonogenic AML cells.[85]

The possible contamination of mobilized HPC(A) with malignant cells is of special concern in autologous transplantation. Viable malignant cells may circulate in the blood to a variable extent in a variety of malignant diseases. Malignant cells may be present and even increase after mobilization and may thus contaminate HPC(A) grafts for autologous patients.[86,87] Gene-marked malignant cells that were present in HPC(A) have subsequently been identified after autologous transplantation in sites of metastatic tumor.[88,89] Although randomized studies in certain diseases (eg, myeloma, lymphoma, and selected AML patients) show a clear clinical benefit from autologous transplantation in terms of disease-free survival vs chemotherapy without autologous transplantation, disease relapse still remains the major impediment to long-term cure of those malignant conditions by hematopoietic transplantation.[90,91] A variety of "ex-vivo purging" techniques (chemical, physical, and immunologic) have been investigated in an effort to reduce or eliminate malignant cells from autologous HPC(A). Some retrospective studies of ex-vivo purging vs historical controls suggested that patients whose HPC(A) dona-

TABLE 30-4. Factors Reported to Affect the Rate of Neutrophil and/or Platelet Engraftment

◆ Infused dose of viable CD34+ cells/kg
◆ Use of posttransplant growth factor
◆ Type of pretransplant preparative regimen (aka "conditioning")
◆ Ease of mobilizing the donor
◆ Extent and type of prior chemotherapy or radiotherapy
◆ Patient or donor age

tions were rendered negative for the malignant cell marker by purging techniques before transplantation had improved disease-free survival after transplantation when compared with patients whose purged HPC(A) still tested positive for tumor cells.[92] However, given the retrospective nature of these studies, patients who had tumor-positive HPCs after ex-vivo purging may have also had a higher or more resistant tumor burden. Moreover, the few randomized clinical trials of ex-vivo purging failed to show a clinical benefit in disease-free or overall survival.[93] Consequently, ex-vivo purging of HPC(A) is infrequently performed and has largely given way to the concept of in-vivo purging, whereby patients who are candidates for autologous transplantation are treated with effective chemotherapy before mobilization of HPC(A) in an effort to minimize or to eliminate malignant cells in the marrow or are treated by the use of disease-specific chemotherapy regimens (typically with hematopoietic growth factor) that serve not only to mobilize HPCs but also to concomitantly minimize tumor contamination of HPC(A).[94,95] Toward that goal, a host of chemotherapy regimens that are tailored to the patient's malignant disease, most of which also use G-CSF or GM-CSF to augment HPC mobilization, have been reported to have such a compound effect.[96,97] The potential benefits of in-vivo purging by chemotherapy may in some cases be balanced by higher rates of poor mobilization.[46]

Allogeneic or Syngeneic Transplantation

Allogeneic donors, who may be either related or unrelated to the recipient and who may be fully or partially tissue matched with the recipient, and syngeneic donors are mobilized using growth factors alone because of concerns about the safety of using myelosuppressive and potentially mutagenic chemotherapy in normal persons. G-CSF alone is typically used because of its fewer side effects and its improved efficacy when compared with GM-CSF. Doses range from 5 to 16 μg/kg/day in single or split doses for 4 days followed by collection of HPC(A) starting on day 5. Collection of an acceptable CD34+ cell dose is nearly always accomplished by 1 or 2 days of apheresis. In retrospective surveys including >1000 normal HPC(A) donors, 5% to 20% of normal donors required central catheters for venous access (more commonly in females[26]), and complications were identified in 0% to 1%, one-third of which were catheter related.[17,18,26,39] Although G-CSF is generally well tolerated in normal donors, side effects are common; donors should be well informed about the side effects to prevent undue alarm (see earlier section on hematopoietic growth factors). The HPC(A) collection goal range for allogeneic transplantation is similar to that for autologous transplantation (2 to 5×10^6 CD34+ cells/kg). However, because of the generally longer time to neutrophil engraftment and especially to platelet engraftment associated with allogeneic transplantation and with unrelated donors in comparison with autologous patients, a higher HPC(A) dose (at least 4×10^6 CD34+ cells/kg) is preferred.[98,99] Administration of higher doses of CD34+ cells from related or unrelated, fully or partially matched donors that are given to adults or children is consistently associated with more rapid neutrophil and platelet engraftment. Higher doses are also associated with a higher frequency and severity of chronic, but usually not acute, graft-vs-host disease (GVHD) in some, but not all, related-donor myeloablative transplants.[99] In some studies of allogeneic transplantation, CD34+ cell dose was also associated with decreased transplant-related mortality and relapse, as well as with improved overall patient survival.[99,100] However, survival benefits are controversial because studies of adult or pediatric patients who received allogeneic HPC(A) transplants from sibling donors for ablative therapy show that very high CD34+ doses (>8 $\times 10^6$/kg) were associated with increased morbidity resulting from chronic GVHD, a common cause of severe morbidity and mortality after allogeneic transplantation—and with no improvement in survival.[98,101] Concerns have also been raised by observations of increased chronic GVHD in patients who received HPC(A) grafts compared with marrow grafts from unrelated donors.[102] However, graft selection and CD34+ cell dose should be individualized, because reports also indicate that increased CD34+ cell doses are associated with more rapid full-donor chimerism and may improve survival in high-risk leukemia patients who undergo nonmyeloablative regimens using HPC(A) from HLA-identical sibling donors or in standard- to high-risk patients after ablative or nonablative marrow transplantation using matched unrelated donors.[99,103]

Selection of an HPC(A) Graft vs an HPC(M) Graft

HPC(A) grafts are currently the principal source of HPCs for both autologous and allogeneic transplantation in adults. HPC(M) is also used for transplantation, mostly for allogeneic procedures. HPC(C) is used almost exclusively for allogeneic transplantation. Historically, marrow grafts were derived from multiple aspirations from the donors' iliac crests. However, not all patients (or normal donors) are candidates for marrow harvesting because of problems such as prior pelvic irradiation, metastatic tumor, obesity, or severe back pain. Patients who are at high risk for general anesthesia are also not good candidates for HPC(M). Early attempts to use hematopoietic grafts consisting of HPC(A) from "unmobilized" donors (ie, without prior treatment to increase the level of circulating HPCs) met with graft failures, slow engraftment, or both. HPC(A) became a practical alternative to marrow grafts only after the advent of pharmacologic methods to reliably mobilize HPCs from the donor's marrow into the peripheral blood.

Compared with HPC(M), HPC(A) grafts from mobilized donors typically contain nearly 10-fold more total nucleated cells and T cells, more than fivefold greater numbers of CD34+ cells and primitive colony-forming cells, and far fewer red cells [hematocrit typically <10% vs 20% to 30% for HPC(M)].[104-106] Those differences can be explained by observations that most HPC mobilization regimens elevate the peripheral blood levels not only of CD34+ cells but also of total leukocytes and lymphocytes. The apheresis harvesting procedure, although effective in excluding most red cells, is poorly selective in collecting mononuclear cells and CD34+ cells vs other leukocytes and platelets. In addition, it is practical to perform daily HPC collections until a target dose of CD34+ cells or HPC(A) has been attained, whereas it is impractical to perform repeated attempts at marrow harvesting.

Adequate access to venous blood is critical for HPC(A) collection. Patients who are scheduled for autologous transplantation typically have central intravenous lines placed for ease of drawing blood and administering chemotherapy, and many of those lines can also be used for apheresis. Most normal allogeneic donors have acceptable peripheral veins and do not require catheter insertion, but catheters are more frequently required in female donors.

Compared with HPC(A) harvesting, marrow collection may be perceived by some as less convenient for both donor and physician because HPC(M) harvesting typically requires the use of an operating or procedure room; the administration of general anesthesia, local anesthesia, or both, to the donor; the presence of one or more physicians and staff personnel to perform the collection, to prepare the syringes, and to filter the marrow; and typically an overnight hospital stay for the donor. Some hospitals collect autologous blood from the donor before HPC(M) harvesting because up to 2 L of marrow may be harvested, thereby resulting in a significant decrease in red cell counts. During marrow collection, total leukocyte counts are obtained on samples from the filtered marrow collection bag to guide the progress of an individual marrow harvest, but repeat marrow harvests on following days are rarely performed to obtain a target number of progenitor cells. In addition, donor morbidity, which consists mostly of prolonged back pain, and absence from work are greater after marrow harvest when compared with HPC(A) collection. Hence, given the choice, most well-informed donors prefer to donate by HPC mobilization and apheresis collection.[106,107]

CLINICAL TRANSPLANTATION OUTCOMES OF HPC(A) VS HPC(M) GRAFTS

Autologous Transplantation

As a result of the administration of higher progenitor cell doses, autologous transplantation using HPC(A) grafts is associated with shorter times to neutrophil and platelet engraftment than HPC(M) grafts—with fewer transfusions; fewer infections; shorter hospital stays; and, in some studies, lower overall costs.[103,108] Immunologic recovery is also more rapid using HPC(A) when compared with HPC(M).[109] In contrast to early hopes, HPC(A) collections mobilized from patients with malignancy have essentially the same level of cancerous cells as HPC(M) harvests. That problem has been somewhat mitigated by in-vivo purging before HPC mobilization.[110] Despite the advantage of rapid engraftment, most studies do not report either a disease-free or overall survival benefit after autologous transplantation using HPC(A) grafts when compared with HPC(M).[110,111] However, taken together, the differences between HPC(M) and HPC(A) mentioned earlier have made HPC(A) the graft of choice for nearly all autologous transplants. HPC(M) is typically used only if the patient mobilizes HPCs poorly and if an insufficient dose of HPC(A) is collected. However, the quality and efficacy of HPC(M) grafts in patients who have failed mobilization are controversial.[1,57] The administration of G-CSF to the donor 2 to 4 days before marrow harvesting has been reported to result in HPC(M) grafts with significantly higher numbers of cells and engraftment rates that are equal to or greater than those of HPC(A) grafts, and that technique has also been reported effective in patients who mobilized poorly.[60,61]

Allogeneic Transplantation

Studies in related-donor allogeneic transplantation in adults who received myeloablative conditioning also show that HPC(A) grafts are associated with shortened time to neutrophil and platelet engraftment with fewer transfusions, fewer infections, and shorter hospital stays when compared with HPC(M).[112,113] Immunologic recovery may be prolonged for up to a year, especially when the donor is unrelated, and prolonged immunologic recovery is associated with increased infections.[114,115] Recovery of immune cells and function are both more rapid after HPC(A) transplantation compared with HPC(M), both after related and matched unrelated allogeneic transplantation.[115] In most studies not using graft T-cell depletion, the frequency of acute GVHD was not significantly increased after using HPC(A) compared with HPC(M).[112,113] However, numerous studies report that chronic GVHD, both limited and extensive, is increased after allogeneic transplantation (including related nonmyeloablative, unrelated, and pediatric) using HPC(A) and may result in a longer duration of GVHD treatment.[113,116,117] In selected patient groups [eg, chronic myelogenous leukemia (CML), standard- or high-risk AML, and myelodysplastic syndrome (MDS)] HPC(A) grafts from related[112,116,117] or unrelated donors[118] have been reported to impart improved overall and disease-free survival compared with HPC(M) grafts, especially in patients with advanced disease.

Improved survival after allogeneic grafting with unrelated-donor HPC(A) is not a common finding, however,[113,119] and this may be due in part to the higher incidence of chronic GVHD after transplantation with HPC(A) when compared with HPC(M). GVHD may be perceived as beneficial, especially in high-risk patients who undergo transplantation for CML and advanced AML, because studies show a reduced relapse rate and improved survival in such leukemia patients who have mild GVHD after transplantation, presumably resulting from a concomitant graft-vs-leukemia effect.[117] However, the graft-vs-malignancy effect is attenuated or unapparent in other malignant conditions (eg, acute lymphocytic leukemia) and is both unnecessary and detrimental in hematopoietic transplantation for nonmalignant conditions, such as aplastic anemia. Consequently, the engraftment speed advantage of HPC(A) in patients who are unlikely to benefit from the graft-vs-malignancy effect must be balanced against the possible excess morbidity and mortality associated with chronic GVHD. It is noteworthy that recent large retrospective registry studies have reported that in related-donor myeloablative therapy for patients with severe aplastic anemia or acute leukemia who were less than 20 years of age, the use of HPC(M) grafts was associated with improved overall survival when compared with a similar group of patients who received HPC(A) grafts. The difference was presumably the result of a lower rate of chronic GVHD in the former group.[102,120] Consequently, the rationale for the widespread use of HPC(A) as a source of allogeneic grafts has been challenged.[117] A randomized clinical trial has recently been completed in adults to determine the advantages and disadvantages of both sources of HPC grafts for allogeneic transplantation in different diseases. Initial reports suggest that the advantages of rapid engraftment speed and disadvantages of chronic GVHD appear to apply as well to unrelated-donor or nonmyeloablative conditioning using HPC(A) vs HPC(M) grafts according to observational studies.[121] Following an evidence-based review, an expert panel recommended the preferential use of HPC(M) for matched related-donor transplantation in pediatric patients who have AML and are in first remission, but no recommendation was made for unrelated-donor marrow transplantation.[122]

In summary, the selection of an HPC(A) vs an HPC(M) graft for allogeneic transplantation should take into account not only the speed of engraftment, the donor and physician preferences for HPC harvesting, the risk factors for general anesthesia vs G-CSF administration, and the possible need for central line placement, but also the patient's disease risk status, age, type of disease, and, possibly, type of conditioning regimen. The graft source, the pharmacologic exposure, and possibly the graft content have an impact on transplantation outcome. In addition to the advances in conditioning regimens and supportive care, the findings also indicate there is much more to be learned regarding the optimal composition of HPC grafts.

SELECTION OF AN HPC(A) OR HPC(M) GRAFT VS AN HPC(C) GRAFT

Selection of HPC(A) vs HPC(C) is relevant to allogeneic unrelated-donor transplantation and to the far less common setting of prospective banking of HPC-C by a family member for a patient who has a disease that may be treated by hematopoietic transplantation. As of 2010, there were no randomized prospective comparisons of HPC(A) grafts vs HPC(C) grafts, and the results of a recently completed comparison of HPC(A) vs HPC(M) are not yet available. However, according to the results of large-scale retrospective comparisons of unrelated-donor marrow transplantation using HPC(A), HPC(M), or HPC(C), the potential advantages of HPC(A) or HPC(M) include more rapid engraftment, fewer graft failures, and an ability to obtain additional cells if they are needed because of poor recipient engraftment or disease relapse. The potential advantages of HPC(C) include a shorter time to obtain the graft, decreased GVHD, and the ability to identify an acceptably HLA-matched graft for a patient whose donor search identified no acceptable HPC(A) or HPC(M) donor. Retrospective studies of unrelated-donor transplantation in adults with leukemia reported faster engraftment and improved overall 5-year survival rates[123] or similar overall 2-year survival rates[124] using HPC(M) grafts as compared with HPC-C grafts. A recent retrospective registry study in adults with acute leukemia who received marrow transplantation using HPC(C) (165 patients), HPC(A) (888), or HPC(M) (472) also showed equivalent overall survival but increased transplant-related mortality in recipients of HPC(C).[125] Thus, in adults, a matched unrelated HPC(A) or HPC(M) graft is preferable to an HPC(C) graft. A retrospective study of unrelated-donor HPC(C) and HPC(M) in children with leukemia also reported that the 5-year leukemia-free survival of 503 recipients of HPC(C) was equal to that of 282 recipients of HPC(M).[126]

KEY POINTS

1. Hematopoietic progenitor cells collected by apheresis (HPC-A) are currently the most common type of hematopoietic graft used for autologous transplantation.
2. HPC-A grafts are harvested by leukocyte apheresis following the "mobilization" of HPCs from marrow stem cell niches into the peripheral blood. Mobilization can involve myelosuppressive therapy, hematopoietic growth factors [granulocyte colony-stimulating factor (G-CSF), granulocyte-macrophage colony-stimulating factor (GM-CSF)], and/or adhesion-receptor blockade (Mozobil); these agents act by nonoverlapping mechanisms.
3. Growth factor administration is nearly always accompanied by side effects, including bone pain, headache and muscle aches, fatigue, nausea, and flu-like symptoms. More severe findings have included an increase in spleen size, impaired pulmonary exchange, and leukocyte counts >50,000/µL.
4. Mozobil is a synthetic SDF1-like molecule that blocks the adhesive interaction between SDF1 on marrow stromal cells and CXCR4 on CD34+ cells. It is unique among mobilizing agents in that it stimulates the release of CD34+ cells within several hours after administration.
5. Mozobil is approximately as active as G-CSF in mobilizing CD34+ cells when used alone. Mozobil has additive effects on increasing circulating CD34+ cells and T cells when administered in combination with G-CSF or myelosuppressive agents.
6. Poor HPC mobilization has been reported in 2% to 20% of mobilization attempts in normal donors and in 10% to 50% of autologous transplantation donors. There is no universally accepted method of managing poor mobilizers.
7. HPC-A products commonly require minimal processing before infusion or cryopreservation. Cryopreservation typically uses 10% dimethylsulfoxide (DMSO) and controlled-rate freezing. Cryopreserved HPC-A may be stored for several years before use, without impaired engraftment.
8. Cryopreserved HPC-A may be thawed in a 37 C waterbath immediately before infusion and then infused rapidly at 5 to 20 mL/minute. Infusion reactions are commonly attributable to DMSO.
9. Shorter engraftment times are associated with fewer infections, fewer transfusions, shorter hospital stays, and lower cost. The empirical limit for engraftment is approximately 9 days.
10. The selection of an HPC-A vs HPC, Marrow (HPC-M) graft should take into account a number of factors, including the speed of engraftment, the donor and physician preferences for HPC harvesting, the risk factors for general anesthesia (HPC-M) vs G-CSF (HPC-A), and the patient's disease risk status.

REFERENCES

1. Cottler-Fox MH, Lapidot T, Petit I, et al. Stem cell mobilization. Hematology Am Soc Hematol Educ Program 2003;419-37.
2. Yin T, Li L. The stem cell niches in bone. J Clin Invest 2006;116:1195-201.
3. Papayannopoulou T. Current mechanistic scenarios in hematopoietic stem/progenitor cell mobilization. Blood 2004;103:1580-5.
4. Anderlini P, Przepiorka D, Seong C, et al. Factors affecting mobilization of CD34+ cells in normal donors treated with filgrastim. Transfusion 1997;37:507-12.
5. Benboubker L, Watier H, Carion A, et al. Association between the SDF1-3'A allele and high levels of CD34(+) progenitor cells mobilized into peripheral blood in humans. Br J Haematol 2001;113:247-50.
6. Statkute L, Verda L, Oyama Y, et al. Mobilization, harvesting, and selection of peripheral blood stem cells in patients with autoimmune

diseases undergoing autologous hematopoietic stem cell transplantation. Bone Marrow Transplant 2007;39:317-29.
7. Richman CM, Weiner RS, Yankee RA. Increase in circulating stem cells following chemotherapy in man. Blood 1976;47:1031-9.
8. Lane TA. Peripheral blood progenitor cell mobilization and collection. In: Ball E, Lister J, Law P, eds. Hematopoietic stem cell therapy. Philadelphia: Churchill Livingstone, 2000:269-86.
9. Goldschmidt H, Hegenbart U, Haas R, Hunstein W. Mobilization of peripheral blood progenitor cells with high-dose cyclophosphamide (4 or 7 g/m2) and granulocyte colony-stimulating factor in patients with multiple myeloma. Bone Marrow Transplant 1996;17:691-7.
10. Goldberg SL, Mangan KF, Klumpp TR, et al. Complications of peripheral blood stem cell harvesting: Review of 554 PBSC leukaphereses. J Hematother 1995;4:85-90.
11. Ho AD, Gluck S, Germond C, et al. Optimal timing for collections of blood progenitor cells following induction chemotherapy and granulocyte-macrophage colony-stimulating factor for autologous transplantation in advanced breast cancer. Leukemia 1993;7:1738-46.
12. Armitage S, Hargreaves R, Samson D, et al. CD34 counts to predict the adequate collection of peripheral blood progenitor cells. Bone Marrow Transplant 1997;20:587-91.
13. Lee JL, Kim SB, Lee GW, et al. Clinical usefulness of the hematopoietic progenitor cell counts in predicting the optimal timing of peripheral blood stem cell harvest. J Korean Med Sci 2003;18:27-35.
14. Meisenberg B, Brehm T, Schmeckel A, et al. A combination of low-dose cyclophosphamide and colony-stimulating factors is more cost-effective than granulocyte-colony-stimulating factors alone in mobilizing peripheral blood stem and progenitor cells. Transfusion 1998;38:209-15.
15. Bashey A, Donohue M, Liu L, et al. Peripheral blood progenitor cell mobilization with intermediate-dose cyclophosphamide, sequential granulocyte-macrophage colony-stimulating factor and granulocyte colony-stimulating factor and scheduled commencement leukapheresis in 225 patients undergoing autologous transplantation. Transfusion 2007;47: 2153-60.
16. Lane TA, Bashey A, Carrier E, et al. Improving the efficiency of PBPC collection by pre-apheresis peripheral blood and mid-apheresis product measurements of CD34 cells. Cytotherapy 2004;6:318-27.
17. Lane TA, Law P, Maruyama M, et al. Harvesting and enrichment of hematopoietic progenitor cells mobilized into the peripheral blood of normal donors by granulocyte-macrophage colony-stimulating factor (GM-CSF) or G-CSF: Potential role in allogeneic marrow transplantation. Blood 1995;85:275-82.
18. Lane TA, Ho AD, Bashey A, et al. Mobilization of blood-derived stem and progenitor cells in normal subjects by granulocyte-macrophage and granulocyte colony-stimulating factors. Transfusion 1999;39:39-47.
19. Koc ON, Gerson SL, Cooper BW, et al. Randomized cross-over trial of progenitor-cell mobilization: High-dose cyclophosphamide plus granulocyte colony-stimulating factor (G-CSF) versus granulocyte-macrophage colony-stimulating factor plus G-CSF. J Clin Oncol 2000;18:1824-30.
20. Weaver CH, Birch R, Greco FA, et al. Mobilization and harvesting of peripheral blood stem cells: Randomized evaluations of different doses of filgrastim. Br J Haematol 1998;100:338-47.
21. Anderlini P, Donato M, Lauppe MJ, et al. A comparative study of once-daily versus twice-daily filgrastim administration for the mobilization and collection of CD34+ peripheral blood progenitor cells in normal donors. Br J Haematol 2000;109:770-2.
22. Kroger N, Sonnenberg S, Cortes-Dericks L, et al. Kinetics of G-CSF and CD34+ cell mobilization after once or twice daily stimulation with rHu granulocyte-stimulating factor (lenograstim) in healthy volunteers: An intraindividual crossover study. Transfusion 2004;44:104-10.
23. Watts MJ, Addison I, Ings SJ, et al. Optimal timing for collection of PBPC after glycosylated G-CSF administration. Bone Marrow Transplant 1998;21:365-8.
24. Bruns I, Steidl U, Kronenwett R, et al. A single dose of 6 or 12 mg of pegfilgrastim for peripheral blood progenitor cell mobilization results in similar yields of CD34+ progenitors in patients with multiple myeloma. Transfusion 2006;46:180-5.
25. Tigue CC, McKoy JM, Evens AM, et al. Granulocyte-colony stimulating factor administration to healthy individuals and persons with

chronic neutropenia or cancer: An overview of safety considerations from the Research on Adverse Drug Events and Reports project. Bone Marrow Transplant 2007;40:185-92.

26. Pulsipher MA, Chitphakdithai P, Miller JP, et al. Adverse events among 2408 unrelated donors of peripheral blood stem cells: Results of a prospective trial from the National Marrow Donor Program. Blood 2009;113:3604-11.
27. Stiff P, Bensinger W, Abidi M, et al. Clinical and ultrasonic evaluation of spleen size during peripheral blood progenitor cell mobilization by filgrastim. Biol Blood Marrow Transplant 2009; 15:827-34.
28. Yoshida I, Matsuo K, Teshima T, et al. Transient respiratory disturbance by granulocyte colony-stimulating factor administration in healthy donors of allogeneic peripheral blood progenitor cell transplantation. Transfusion 2006;46:186-92.
29. Anderlini P, Korbling M, Dale D, et al. Allogeneic blood stem cell transplantation: Considerations for donors. Blood 1997;90:903-8.
30. Nuamah NM, Goker H, Kilic YA, et al. Spontaneous splenic rupture in a healthy allogeneic donor of peripheral-blood stem cell following the administration of granulocyte colony-stimulating factor (g-csf). A case report and review of the literature. Haematologica 2006;91: ECR08.
31. Arimura K, Inoue H, Kukita T, et al. Acute lung injury in a healthy donor during mobilization of peripheral blood stem cells using granulocyte colony-stimulating factor alone. Haematologica 2005;90:ECR10.
32. Keung YK, Suwanvecho S, Cobos E. Anaphylactoid reaction to granulocyte colony-stimulating factor used in mobilization of peripheral blood stem cell. Bone Marrow Transplant 1999;23:200-1.
33. Cassens U, Baumann C, Hillmann H, et al. Circulatory arrest during PBPC apheresis in an unrelated donor. Transfusion 2003;43:736-41.
34. Kang EM, Areman EM, David-Ocampo V, et al. Mobilization, collection, and processing of peripheral blood stem cells in individuals with sickle cell trait. Blood 2002;99:850-5.
35. Kamble RT, Tin U, Carrum G. Successful mobilization and transplantation of filgrastim mobilized hematopoietic stem cells in sickle cell-hemoglobin C disease. Bone Marrow Transplant 2006;37:1065-6.
36. Burt RK, Fassas A, Snowden J, et al. Collection of hematopoietic stem cells from patients with autoimmune diseases. Bone Marrow Transplant 2001;28:1-12.
37. Sinha S, Poh KK, Sodano D, et al. Safety and efficacy of peripheral blood progenitor cell mobilization and collection in patients with advanced coronary heart disease. J Clin Apher 2006;21:116-20.
38. Cavallaro AM, Lilleby K, Majolino I, et al. Three to six year follow-up of normal donors who received recombinant human granulocyte colony-stimulating factor. Bone Marrow Transplant 2000;25:85-9.
39. Anderlini P, Rizzo JD, Nugent ML, et al. Peripheral blood stem cell donation: An analysis from the International Bone Marrow Transplant Registry (IBMTR) and European Group for Blood and Marrow Transplant (EBMT) databases. Bone Marrow Transplant 2001;27:689-92.
40. DiPersio JF, Micallef IN, Stiff PJ, et al. Phase III prospective randomized double-blind placebo-controlled trial of plerixafor plus granulocyte colony-stimulating factor compared with placebo plus granulocyte colony-stimulating factor for autologous stem-cell mobilization and transplantation for patients with non-Hodgkin's lymphoma. Clin Oncol 2009;27: 4767-73.
41. DiPersio JF, Stadtmauer EA, Nademanee A, et al. Plerixafor and G-CSF versus placebo and G-CSF to mobilize hematopoietic stem cells for autologous stem cell transplantation in patients with multiple myeloma. Blood 2009; 113:5720-6.
42. Mozobil prescribing information (package insert). Cambridge, MA: Genzyme Corp., 2010. [Available at http://www.mozobil.com/document/Package_Insert.pdf (accessed February 17, 2011).]
43. Costa LJ, Alexander ET, Hogan KR, et al. Development and validation of a decision-making algorithm to guide the use of plerixafor for autologous hematopoietic stem cell mobilization. Bone Marrow Transplant 2011;46:64-9.
44. Haas R, Hohaus S, Egerer G, et al. Recombinant human granulocyte-macrophage colony-stimulating factor (rhGM-CSF) subsequent to chemotherapy improves collection of blood stem cells for autografting in patients not eligible for bone marrow harvest. Bone Marrow Transplant 1992;9:459-65.
45. Cremer FW, Kiel K, Wallmeier M, et al. Leukapheresis products in multiple myeloma: Lower tumor load after mobilization with cyclophos-

phamide plus granulocyte colony-stimulating factor (G-CSF) compared with G-CSF alone. Exp Hematol 1998;26:969-75.

46. Olavarria E, Kanfer EJ. Selection and use of chemotherapy with hematopoietic growth factors for mobilization of peripheral blood progenitor cells. Curr Opin Hematol 2000;7:191-6.
47. Ings SJ, Balsa C, Leverett D, et al. Peripheral blood stem cell yield in 400 normal donors mobilised with granulocyte colony-stimulating factor (G-CSF): Impact of age, sex, donor weight and type of G-CSF used. Br J Haematol 2006;134:517-25.
48. Gazitt Y, Freytes CO, Callander N, et al. Successful PBSC mobilization with high-dose G-CSF for patients failing a first round of mobilization. J Hematother 1999;8:173-83.
49. Ewing JC, Robertson JD, Kell WJ, et al. Autologous peripheral blood stem cell transplantation in first remission adult acute myeloid leukaemia—an intention to treat analysis and comparison of outcome using a predictive model based on the MRC AML10 cohort. Hematology 2003;8:83-90.
50. Pavone V, Gaudio F, Console G, et al. Poor mobilization is an independent prognostic factor in patients with malignant lymphomas treated by peripheral blood stem cell transplantation. Bone Marrow Transplant 2006;37:719-24.
51. Cottler-Fox M, Lapidot T. Mobilizing the older patient with myeloma. Blood Rev 2006;20:43-50.
52. Micallef IN, Stiff PJ, DiPersio JF, et al. Successful stem cell remobilization using plerixafor (Mozobil) plus granulocyte colony-stimulating factor in patients with non-hodgkin lymphoma: Results from the plerixafor NHL phase 3 study rescue protocol. Biol Blood Marrow Transplant 2009;15:1578-86.
53. Calandra G, McCarty J, McGuirk J, et al. AMD3100 plus G-CSF can successfully mobilize CD34+ cells from non-Hodgkin's lymphoma, Hodgkin's disease and multiple myeloma patients previously failing mobilization with chemotherapy and/or cytokine treatment: Compassionate use data. Bone Marrow Transplant 2008;41:331-8.
54. Prince HM, Imrie K, Sutherland DR, et al. Peripheral blood progenitor cell collections in multiple myeloma: Predictors and management of inadequate collections. Br J Haematol 1996;93:142-5.
55. Fraipont V, Sautois B, Baudoux E, et al. Successful mobilization of peripheral blood HPCs with G-CSF alone in patients failing to achieve sufficient numbers of CD34+ cells and/or CFU-GM with chemotherapy and G-CSF. Transfusion 2000;40:339-47.
56. Bashey A, Corringham S, Gilpin E, et al. Simultaneous administration of G-CSF and GM-CSF for remobilization in patients with inadequate initial progenitor cell collections for autologous transplantation. Cytotherapy 2000;2:195-200.
57. Goterris R, Hernandez-Boluda JC, Teruel A, et al. Impact of different strategies of second-line stem cell harvest on the outcome of autologous transplantation in poor peripheral blood stem cell mobilizers. Bone Marrow Transplant 2005;36:847-53.
58. Cassens U, Barth IM, Baumann C, et al. Factors affecting the efficacy of peripheral blood progenitor cells collections by large-volume leukaphereses with standardized processing volumes. Transfusion 2004;44:1593-602.
59. Rick O, Beyer J, Kingreen D, et al. Successful autologous bone marrow rescue in patients who failed peripheral blood stem cell mobilization. Ann Hematol 2000;79:681-6.
60. Damiani D, Fanin R, Silvestri F, et al. Randomized trial of autologous filgrastim-primed bone marrow transplantation versus filgrastim-mobilized peripheral blood stem cell transplantation in lymphoma patients. Blood 1997;90:36-42.
61. Lemoli RM, de Vivo A, Damiani D, et al. Autologous transplantation of granulocyte colony-stimulating factor-primed bone marrow is effective in supporting myeloablative chemotherapy in patients with hematologic malignancies and poor peripheral blood stem cell mobilization. Blood 2003;102:1595-600.
62. Tarella C, Caracciolo D, Gavarotti P, et al. Circulating progenitors following high-dose sequential (HDS) chemotherapy with G-CSF: Short intervals between drug courses severely impair progenitor mobilization. Bone Marrow Transplant 1995;16:223-8.
63. Law P. Graft processing storage and infusion. In: Ball E, Lister J, Law P, eds. Hematopoietic stem cell therapy. Philadelphia: Churchill Livingstone, 2000:312-21.
64. Parkins MD, Bahlis N, Brown C, et al. Overnight storage of autologous stem cell apheresis products before cryopreservation does not adversely impact early or long-term engraftment following transplantation. Bone Marrow Transplant 2006;38:609-14.

65. Rowley SD. Hematopoietic stem cell cryopreservation: A review of current techniques. J Hematother 1992;1:233-50.
66. Sauer-Heilborn A, Kadidlo D, McCullough J. Patient care during infusion of hematopoietic progenitor cells. Transfusion 2004;44:907-16.
67. Syme R, Bewick M, Stewart D, et al. The role of depletion of dimethyl sulfoxide before autografting: On hematologic recovery, side effects, and toxicity. Biol Blood Marrow Transplant 2004;10:135-41.
68. Calmels B, Lemarie C, Esterni B, et al. Occurrence and severity of adverse events after autologous hematopoietic progenitor cell infusion are related to the amount of granulocytes in the apheresis product. Transfusion 2007;47:1268-75.
69. Milone G, Mercurio S, Strano A, et al. Adverse events after infusions of cryopreserved hematopoietic stem cells depend on non-mononuclear cells in the infused suspension and patient age. Cytotherapy 2007;9:348-55.
70. Davis JM, Rowley SD, Braine HG, et al. Clinical toxicity of cryopreserved bone marrow graft infusion. Blood 1990;75:781-6.
71. Zambelli A, Poggi G, Da Prada G, et al. Clinical toxicity of cryopreserved circulating progenitor cells infusion. Anticancer Res 1998;18:4705-8.
72. Alessandrino P, Bernasconi P, Caldera D, et al. Adverse events occurring during bone marrow or peripheral blood progenitor cell infusion: Analysis of 126 cases. Bone Marrow Transplant 1999;23:533-7.
73. Keung YK, Lau S, Elkayam U, et al. Cardiac arrhythmia after infusion of cryopreserved stem cells. Bone Marrow Transplant 1994;14:363-7.
74. Curcoy AI, Alcorta I, Estella J, et al. Cryopreservation of HPCs with high cell concentration in 5-percent DMSO for transplantation to children (letter). Transfusion 2002;42:962.
75. Okamoto Y, Takaue Y, Saito S, et al. Toxicities associated with cryopreserved and thawed peripheral blood stem cell autografts in children with active cancer. Transfusion 1993;33:578-81.
76. Kamble R, Pant S, Selby GB, et al. Microbial contamination of hematopoietic progenitor cell grafts—incidence, clinical outcome, and cost-effectiveness: An analysis of 735 grafts. Transfusion 2005;45:874-8.
77. Padley DJ, Dietz AB, Gastineau DA. Sterility testing of hematopoietic progenitor cell products: A single-institution series of culture-positive rates and successful infusion of culture-positive products. Transfusion 2007;47:636-43.
78. Bender JG, To LB, Williams S, Schwartzberg LS. Defining a therapeutic dose of peripheral blood stem cells. J Hematother 1992;1:329-41.
79. Tricot G, Jagannath S, Vesole D, et al. Peripheral blood stem cell transplants for multiple myeloma: Identification of favorable variables for rapid engraftment in 225 patients. Blood 1995;85:588-96.
80. Weaver CH, Hazelton B, Birch R, et al. An analysis of engraftment kinetics as a function of the CD34 content of peripheral blood progenitor cell collections in 692 patients after the administration of myeloablative chemotherapy. Blood 1995;86:3961-9.
81. Weaver CH, Potz J, Redmond J, et al. Engraftment and outcomes of patients receiving myeloablative therapy followed by autologous peripheral blood stem cells with a low CD34+ cell content. Bone Marrow Transplant 1997;19:1103-10.
82. Bensinger WI, Longin K, Appelbaum F, et al. Peripheral blood stem cells (PBSCs) collected after recombinant granulocyte colonystimulating factor (rhG-CSF): An analysis of factors correlating with the tempo of engraftment after transplantation. Br J Haematol 1994;87:825-31.
83. Dreger P, Klöss M, Petersen B, et al. Autologous progenitor cell transplantation: Prior exposure to stem cell-toxic drugs determines yield and engraftment of peripheral blood progenitor cell but not of bone marrow grafts. Blood 1995;86:3970-8.
84. Boiron JM, Dazey B, Cailliot C, et al. Large-scale expansion and transplantation of CD34+ hematopoietic cells: In vitro and in vivo confirmation of neutropenia abrogation related to the expansion process without impairment of the long-term engraftment capacity. Transfusion 2006;46:1934-42.
85. Keating S, Suciu S, de Witte T, et al. The stem cell mobilizing capacity of patients with acute myeloid leukemia in complete remission correlates with relapse risk: Results of the EORTC-GIMEMA AML-10 trial. Leukemia 2003;17:60-7.
86. Feller N, Schuurhuis GJ, van der Pol MA, et al. High percentage of CD34-positive cells in autologous AML peripheral blood stem cell products reflects inadequate in vivo purging and low chemotherapeutic toxicity in a sub-

group of patients with poor clinical outcome. Leukemia 2003;17:68-75.
87. Jacquy C, Soree A, Lambert F, et al. A quantitative study of peripheral blood stem cell contamination in diffuse large-cell non-Hodgkin's lymphoma: One-half of patients significantly mobilize malignant cells. Br J Haematol 2000; 110:631-7.
88. Deisseroth AB, Zu Z, Claxton D, et al. Genetic marking shows that Ph+ cells present in autologous transplants of chronic myelogenous leukemia (CML) contribute to relapse after autologous bone marrow in CML. Blood 1994;83: 3068-76.
89. Moss TJ, Ross AA. The risk of tumor cell contamination in peripheral blood stem cell collections. J Hematother 1992;1:225-32.
90. Linker C. The role of autologous transplantation for acute myeloid leukemia in first and second remission. Best Pract Res Clin Haematol 2007;20:77-84.
91. Attal M, Harousseau JL, Facon T, et al. Single versus double autologous stem-cell transplantation for multiple myeloma. N Engl J Med 2003;349:2495-502.
92. Gribben JG, Freedman AS, Neuberg D, et al. Immunologic purging of marrow assessed by PCR before autologous bone marrow transplantation for B-cell lymphoma. N Engl J Med 1991;325:1525-33.
93. Stewart AK, Vescio R, Schiller G, et al. Purging of autologous peripheral-blood stem cells using CD34 selection does not improve overall or progression-free survival after high-dose chemotherapy for multiple myeloma: Results of a multicenter randomized controlled trial. J Clin Oncol 2001;19:3771-9.
94. Brugger W. Improving outcomes in transplantation. Semin Oncol 2002;29:23-6.
95. Novella E, Madeo D, Albiero E, et al. Effect of DCEP mobilizing regimen in in vivo purging of PBSC harvests in multiple myeloma. Leuk Lymphoma 2004;45:1497-9.
96. Pavlovsky S, Fernandez I, Milone G, et al. Autologous peripheral blood progenitor cell transplantation mobilized with high-dose cytarabine in acute myeloid leukemia in first complete remission. Ann Oncol 1998;9:151-7.
97. van Heeckeren WJ, Vollweiler J, Fu P, et al. Randomised comparison of two B-cell purging protocols for patients with B-cell non-Hodgkin lymphoma: In vivo purging with rituximab versus ex vivo purging with CliniMACS CD34 cell enrichment device. Br J Haematol 2006; 132:42-55.
98. Heimfeld S. HLA-identical stem cell transplantation: Is there an optimal CD34 cell dose? Bone Marrow Transplant 2003;31:839-45.
99. Pulsipher MA, Chitphakdithai P, Logan BR, et al. Donor, recipient, and transplant characteristics as risk factors after unrelated donor PBSC transplantation: Beneficial effects of higher CD34+ cell dose. Blood 2009;114:2606-16.
100. Lee SH, Lee MH, Lee JH, et al. Infused CD34+ cell dose predicts long-term survival in acute myelogenous leukemia patients who received allogeneic bone marrow transplantation from matched sibling donors in first complete remission. Biol Blood Marrow Transplant 2005;11: 122-8.
101. Zaucha JM, Gooley T, Bensinger WI, et al. CD34 cell dose in granulocyte colony-stimulating factor-mobilized peripheral blood mononuclear cell grafts affects engraftment kinetics and development of extensive chronic graft-versus-host disease after human leukocyte antigen-identical sibling transplantation. Blood 2001;98:3221-7.
102. Eapen M, Horowitz MM, Klein JP, et al. Higher mortality after allogeneic peripheral-blood transplantation compared with bone marrow in children and adolescents: The Histocompatibility and Alternate Stem Cell Source Working Committee of the International Bone Marrow Transplant Registry. J Clin Oncol 2004; 22:4872-80.
103. Perez-Simon JA, Diez-Campelo M, Martino R, et al. Impact of CD34+ cell dose on the outcome of patients undergoing reduced-intensity-conditioning allogeneic peripheral blood stem cell transplantation. Blood 2003;102: 1108-13.
104. Collins NH, Gee AP, Durett AG, et al. The effect of the composition of unrelated donor bone marrow and peripheral blood progenitor cell grafts on transplantation outcomes. Biol Blood Marrow Transplant 2010;16:253-62.
105. Dreger P, Haferlach T, Eckstein V, et al. G-CSF-mobilized peripheral blood progenitor cells for allogeneic transplantation: Safety, kinetics of mobilization, and composition of the graft. Br J Haematol 1994;87:609-13.
106. Favre G, Beksac M, Bacigalupo A, et al. Differences between graft product and donor side effects following bone marrow or stem cell

donation. Bone Marrow Transplant 2003;32: 873-80.

107. Bredeson C, Leger C, Couban S, et al. An evaluation of the donor experience in the Canadian multicenter randomized trial of bone marrow versus peripheral blood allografting. Biol Blood Marrow Transplant 2004;10:405-14.
108. Visani G, Lemoli R, Tosi P, et al. Use of peripheral blood stem cells for autologous transplantation in acute myeloid leukemia patients allows faster engraftment and equivalent disease-free survival compared with bone marrow cells. Bone Marrow Transplant 1999;24: 467-72.
109. Talmadge JE, Reed E, Ino K, et al. Rapid immunologic reconstitution following transplantation with mobilized peripheral blood stem cells as compared to bone marrow. Bone Marrow Transplant 1997;19:161-72.
110. Kanteti R, Miller K, McCann J, et al. Randomized trial of peripheral blood progenitor cell vs bone marrow as hematopoietic support for high-dose chemotherapy in patients with non-Hodgkin's lymphoma and Hodgkin's disease: A clinical and molecular analysis. Bone Marrow Transplant 1999;24:473-81.
111. Perry AR, Peniket AJ, Watts MJ, et al. Peripheral blood stem cell versus autologous bone marrow transplantation for Hodgkin's disease: Equivalent survival outcome in a single-centre matched-pair analysis. Br J Haematol 1999; 105:280-7.
112. Bensinger WI, Martin PJ, Storer B, et al. Transplantation of bone marrow as compared with peripheral-blood cells from HLA-identical relatives in patients with hematologic cancers. N Engl J Med 2001;344:175-81.
113. Ringden O, Labopin M, Bacigalupo A, et al. Transplantation of peripheral blood stem cells as compared with bone marrow from HLA-identical siblings in adult patients with acute myeloid leukemia and acute lymphoblastic leukemia. J Clin Oncol 2002;20:4655-64.
114. Schulenburg A, Fischer M, Kalhs P, et al. Immune recovery after conventional and non-myeloablative allogeneic stem cell transplantation. Leuk Lymphoma 2005;46:1755-60.
115. Storek J, Dawson MA, Storer B, et al. Immune reconstitution after allogeneic marrow transplantation compared with blood stem cell transplantation. Blood 2001;97:3380-9.
116. Couban S, Simpson DR, Barnett MJ, et al. A randomized multicenter comparison of bone marrow and peripheral blood in recipients of matched sibling allogeneic transplants for myeloid malignancies. Blood 2002;100:1525-31.
117. Stem Cell Trialists' Collaborative Group. Allogeneic peripheral blood stem-cell compared with bone marrow transplantation in the management of hematologic malignancies: An individual patient data meta-analysis of nine randomized trials. J Clin Oncol 2005;23: 5074-87.
118. Elmaagacli AH, Basoglu S, Peceny R, et al. Improved disease-free-survival after transplantation of peripheral blood stem cells as compared with bone marrow from HLA-identical unrelated donors in patients with first chronic phase chronic myeloid leukemia. Blood 2002;99:1130-5.
119. Schmitz N, Beksac M, Bacigalupo A, et al. Filgrastim-mobilized peripheral blood progenitor cells versus bone marrow transplantation for treating leukemia: 3-year results from the EBMT randomized trial. Haematologica 2005;90:643-8.
120. Schrezenmeier H, Passweg JR, Marsh JCW, et al. Worse outcome and more chronic GVHD with peripheral blood progenitor cells than bone marrow in HLA-matched sibling donor transplants for young patients with severe acquired aplastic anemia: A report from the European Group for Blood and Marrow Transplantation and the Center for International Blood and Marrow Transplant Research. Blood 2007;110:1397-400.
121. Dey BR, Shaffer J, Yee AJ, et al. Comparison of outcomes after transplantation of peripheral blood stem cells versus bone marrow following an identical nonmyeloablative conditioning regimen. Bone Marrow Transplant 2007; 40:19-27.
122. Executive Committee, American Society for Blood and Marrow Transplantation. The role of cytotoxic therapy with hematopoietic stem cell transplantation in the therapy of acute myeloid leukemia in children. Biol Blood Marrow Transplant 2007;13:500-1.
123. Lane TA. Umbilical cord blood grafts for hematopoietic transplantation in adults: A cup half empty or half full? Transfusion 2005; 45:1027-34.
124. Laughlin MJ, Eapen M, Rubinstein P, et al. Outcomes after transplantation of cord blood or bone marrow from unrelated donors in adults with leukemia. N Engl J Med 2004;351:2265-75.

125. Rocha V, Labopin M, Sanz G, et al. Transplants of umbilical-cord blood or bone marrow from unrelated donors in adults with acute leukemia. N Engl J Med 2004;351:2276-85.

126. Eapen M, Rubinstein P, Zhang MJ, et al. Outcomes of transplantation of unrelated donor umbilical cord blood and bone marrow in children with acute leukaemia: A comparison study. Lancet 2007;369:1947-54.

Chapter 31

Umbilical Cord Blood

David H. McKenna, MD; Diane M. Kadidlo, MT(ASCP)SBB; Jeffrey McCullough, MD; and Donna M. Regan, MT(ASCP)SBB

THE CLINICAL APPLICATIONS of umbilical cord blood (UCB) have continued to grow since the publication of the 16th edition of the *Technical Manual*. Larger multi-institutional trials involving double-unit UCB transplants are ongoing. Technologies for UCB processing are expanding, and novel cellular therapies involving UCB are increasingly used in Phase I and II trials. In addition, a UCB licensure guidance document has been finalized by the Food and Drug Administration (FDA). This chapter not only includes the fundamentals of UCB banking but also emphasizes the latest developments in the field.

INTRODUCTION

Transplantation

Once considered biological waste, UCB has become the most recently identified source of hematopoietic stem cells (HSCs) for transplantation. In 1972, a report by Milton and Norman Ende described the use of several UCB units as a source of HSCs in a "minitransplant" setting for a 16-year-old boy with leukemia.[1] Early laboratory studies provided some initial support for the presence of hematopoietic progenitor cells (HPCs) or HSCs in human UCB,[2-4] with one study[2] suggesting that UCB "might be used as a source of hematopoietic stem cells for the restoration of bone marrow function in humans." Subsequent experiments further established that certain cells within UCB were capable of hematopoietic multilineage differentiation.[5,6] Following more extensive and clinically practical studies that confirmed in-vitro functionality after cryopreservation and thawing,[7] the first related-donor UCB transplant was performed in October 1988.[8] After receiving an HLA-matched sibling UCB unit for the treatment of Fanconi anemia, that patient continues to be healthy in complete hematologic and immunologic do-

David H. McKenna, MD, Scientific and Medical Director, Molecular and Cellular Therapeutics, and Associate Professor of Laboratory Medicine and Pathology, University of Minnesota; Diane M. Kadidlo, MT(ASCP)SBB, Director, Molecular and Cellular Therapeutics, University of Minnesota; Jeffrey McCullough, MD, Director, Institute for Engineering in Medicine, and Professor of Laboratory Medicine and Pathology, University of Minnesota, St. Paul/Minneapolis, Minnesota; and Donna M. Regan, MT(ASCP)SBB, Executive Director, St. Louis Cord Blood Bank and Cellular Therapy Laboratory at SSM Cardinal Glennon Children's Medical Center, St. Louis, Missouri

The authors have disclosed no conflicts of interest.

nor reconstitution over 20 years later.[9] Since this early success, the use of UCB for hematopoietic reconstitution has increased markedly in both the related and unrelated settings.[10-13] Studies have shown UCB to be an acceptable alternative to HLA-matched marrow for pediatric patients[14,15] and for adults lacking an HLA-matched adult donor.[16,17]

Beyond containing HSCs with higher proliferative and self-renewal capacity,[18-21] UCB has additional advantages over marrow and peripheral blood. Clinical trials have shown a decreased incidence of graft-vs-host disease (GVHD), particularly acute disease, despite the lower HLA-matching requirements of UCB.[16,17,22] In-vitro and in-vivo animal research suggests that these particular attributes of UCB transplantation result from the naive immune system of UCB.[23-25] Additionally, transplant candidates with rare HLA types are often successful in finding an acceptably matched UCB unit; search time, in general, is markedly decreased compared to that for other HSC sources, because UCB units are HLA typed at the time they are banked.[26]

Banking

The first UCB bank, established by Hal E. Broxmeyer, provided UCB for the historic 1988 UCB transplant procedure[8] as well as for the successive four HLA-matched sibling transplant procedures.[27] As UCB gained initial acceptance as an HSC source in the related setting, the possibilities for unrelated units became apparent, supporting a rationale for the establishment of unrelated UCB banks. The first unrelated UCB bank was established by Pablo Rubinstein at the New York Blood Center in 1992.[28] Banks in Dusseldorf and Milan were established shortly thereafter. Recent reports indicate there are greater than 450,000 unrelated units banked worldwide for potential clinical use, with well over 20,000 unrelated UCB transplants performed to date.[29] Several private banks have been established worldwide for family use as well; it is uncertain how many "private" units have been stored and transplanted.

As with any emerging technology over time, UCB banking has evolved to become a more established, standardized practice. This chapter provides a description of the current generally accepted practices for UCB banking (primarily from a public bank's perspective), including donor-related issues, collection and processing methods, and storage and shipment, as well as transplant-center-related activities such as thawing, washing, and infusion. The text continues with a brief discussion of standards and regulations, including an overview of the recently finalized FDA guidance, "Minimally Manipulated, Unrelated Allogeneic Placental/Umbilical Cord Blood Intended for Hematopoietic Reconstitution for Specified Indications," of October 2009; it finishes with a look at the future through novel UCB-derived cellular therapies.

DONOR-RELATED ISSUES

Recruitment

The case for recruiting women to donate UCB is based on the idea that UCB, normally discarded as medical waste, can be recovered and used to save the life of another individual. Most women wish to donate when they become aware of the possibility,[30] but participation may be limited by the availability of a UCB bank servicing the area where the mother delivers.

Recruitment typically begins with physician/midwife education and distribution of informational materials to obstetrics offices or to prenatal classes. This approach allows for enlistment of support for the program while providing information to obstetric staff, empowering them to introduce the idea of UCB donation to pregnant women and respond to their initial inquiries. More detailed questions can subsequently be referred to UCB bank personnel.

Distributed materials about UCB donation usually include basic information, such as the name of the bank, the nature of the bank (whether public or private), the cost or lack of cost associated with donation, a list of participating hospitals, the medical uses of UCB, and a brief description of UCB collection. Information should also include the risks of UCB donation to the mother and infant and whether the unit will be available for use by the donating family. Within an informational packet, a UCB bank might include the health history questionnaire, which is used to solicit information about the pregnancy, risk factors of the parents, and medical history of first-degree family members. The UCB bank will explain to potential donors the need for their written permission (informed consent) to collect and store the cord blood for later use in transplantation or research. Participating mothers need to understand that their blood will be drawn and tested for certain infections such as hepatitis and human immunodeficiency virus to reduce transmission of disease through the transplantation of their infant's UCB. The UCB bank will emphasize that all information and test results obtained during the process are held strictly confidential to protect the identity and privacy of donors and that the family will not be approached to donate more cells after the delivery process.

The role of the mother's physician is critical. During pregnancy, a woman trusts her physician to provide reliable care and advice. What helps a woman decide to donate or store her UCB can be as simple as the recommendation offered by her physician. It is also important that recruitment materials be designed to appeal to all ethnic groups so that mothers of various backgrounds can identify with the program and be motivated to donate, thus achieving ethnic diversity in the UCB bank.

In spite of broad awareness campaigns and recruitment efforts, some women may not be aware of UCB donation or may not have registered to participate when they arrive for delivery. Therefore, informational material should also be available in the labor and delivery area. The extent to which women not previously informed about UCB donation can be recruited at this stage (ie, delivery) varies depending on the specific situation. However, in most cases, women have been previously informed of UCB donation but have not registered or completed the necessary documentation.

Pregnant women may also be solicited for UCB donation by private banks. For a fee, these banks will arrange for UCB to be collected and held in long-term storage for use only by that family. These banks provide written or video information that is specific to their bank.

Engaging mothers and arranging donation in advance is critical in achieving best results. Early education allows for more complete medical screening, comprehensive donor protection, availability of adequate supplies, and acquisition of adequate informed consent.

Informed Consent

With the recent recognition of UCB as a valuable medical resource rather than waste, informed consent must be obtained for its collection, processing, testing, storage, and medical use.[31-38] Although the UCB actually belongs to the newborn, consent is obtained from the mother because of her availability (and the infant's inability to give consent) and because testing of her blood for transmissible diseases is required. Consent from the father is not necessary and does not add to the safety of the UCB.[39]

Although consent for collection must precede delivery, UCB banks use different approaches in obtaining consent for further manufacture, testing, and use. Some UCB banks may choose to obtain a single consent statement covering all activities. Presented in the prenatal period, a single consent process affords the mother adequate time to seek information and consider her options under relatively low-stress circumstances. Others may use a phased consent process, which permits collection and, if the resulting harvest meets criteria for banking, involves approaching the mother later for permission to screen, process, test, and store. This latter approach facilitates collection from mothers who have not previously been introduced to UCB banking because it does not require immediate comprehension of the full program. Criteria have been suggested that protect the woman's ability to make an informed decision,[32] and the Advisory Council on Blood Stem Cell Transplantation (of the US Department of Health and Human

Services) has recommended that each bank have a policy that considers the stage of labor and stress of the mother, the amount of precounseling that has occurred, and the amount of time available for an adequate discussion.[40] Final judgment regarding the woman's ability to give intralabor consent should rest with the obstetric staff. Whatever approach is favored should be presented to the institutional review board at the organization, which is formally designated to approve, monitor, and review the research to protect the rights and welfare of the participants in the UCB program.

Health History and Medical Evaluation

The UCB must be as safe as possible for the recipient and not harbor genetic or transmissible diseases. A donor eligibility determination, based on donor screening and testing for relevant communicable disease agents and diseases, is required for all donors of cells or tissue. A robust health history is an essential screening tool, designed to solicit exposure to infectious disease and history of symptoms indicating genetic disorders, to minimize the potential for transmission of these conditions through transplantation. Although the infant is the donor, the medical health history is obtained by interviewing the mother and reviewing her medical record. The father's medical history may be solicited to identify any issues that might affect the quality of the UCB, but it is not required. If not secured before delivery, the history must be obtained no later than 7 days after delivery.[36] The history may be self-administered, with follow-up by bank staff, or it can be obtained through direct interview by bank staff or hospital staff who are adequately trained and capable of answering the mother's questions.

The approach of screening and testing the mother is admittedly more conservative than applying these tools to the infant donor. It is the mother's circulation that nourishes the fetus during pregnancy, and because of this shared physiology, her infectious exposures are relevant to determining eligibility. Also associated with risk are maternal conditions at labor and delivery, such as fever, prolonged time after rupture of the membranes, or use of antibiotics—all of which suggest possible bacterial contamination that could be transmitted through the UCB.

Medical screening includes an extensive family genetic history because the infant has not had an opportunity to manifest many inherited diseases. First-degree relatives with history of malignancy or parents who have been treated with chemotherapy will preclude donation. UCB used to compensate for deficiencies in specific genetic disorders will be tested for presence of the targeted enzyme when available.

In most cases, infants are not retested or reexamined at 6 to 12 months of age for the purpose of donor eligibility because of difficulty in locating some families, concern for parental and infant privacy, necessary recordkeeping for family tracing, and cost. In spite of the difficulties in reconnecting with a donor family, some programs pursue follow-up at extended intervals after birth to ensure lack of disease and instill confidence in the suitability of the product.

Donor Testing

After the medical screening described above, the second step in determining donor eligibility is laboratory testing. The strategy for UCB donation adheres to a similar algorithm as whole blood donation except that the tests are performed on maternal blood. This approach is taken because it is assumed that infectious disease present in the UCB would have originated from the mother, and thus the best chance of detecting infectivity would be in a maternal blood sample. Because testing is performed on maternal blood, it is necessary to obtain the mother's informed consent for testing as well as for collection of the UCB.

The requirement for hemoglobin screening of newborns is issued at the state level of government. Results can be obtained from the state laboratory, or the UCB bank may perform or contract testing to rule out collections from donors with hemoglobinopathies. Some UCB banks store units that have sickle cell or alpha thalassemia trait because these units may have unique HLA types needed for transplantation in minority patients. Units displaying homozygous abnormal hemoglobin or compound abnormal hemoglobin heterozygotes are unsuitable for transplantation. UCB units selected for transplantation for a patient with an inherited disease are tested for that specific disease before being used for transplantation.[41]

Regardless of who obtains the medical history or who tests maternal or UCB samples, final donor eligibility determination is the responsibility of the UCB bank medical director.

COLLECTION

The methods of UCB collection are quite simple with several similarities to whole blood collection, starting with the collection bags. Although a variety of collection bags may be used, the authors' experience has been primarily with a 250-mL bag containing 35 mL of a citrate-phosphate-dextrose solution (CPD; eg, Fenwal Inc., Lake Zurich, IL). Acid-citrate-dextrose (ACD) and lyophilized heparin are also acceptable as anticoagulants for UCB collection. A smaller container such as the 150-mL collection bag with CPD (eg, Pall Corp., Port Washington, NY) may also be used, but the lower maximum volume limit does not accommodate the occasional larger collection. Recently available are sterile collection bags for use in vaginal or cesarean section births that are FDA approved through a new drug application (NDA) and CE marked specifically for collection of cord blood (Pall Corp.). With the larger 250-mL bag, 35 mL of CPD adequately prevents clotting. Anticoagulant should be added to the bag before the collection. For ease of use and diminished risk of contamination, most banks use bags that are prefilled with anticoagulant by the manufacturer.

After delivery, the umbilical cord is clamped, cut, and separated from the infant. The timing of clamping should not interfere with routine delivery practice. UCB can be collected before (in utero) or after (ex utero) the placenta has been delivered. There are advantages and disadvantages to each method, but neither seems to be better overall.[42] A brief discussion of the two methods is included below. Regardless of collection method (ie, in vivo vs ex vivo), the process is rather straightforward and essentially identical. As in whole blood collection, the venipuncture needle is attached to the bag. After an appropriate umbilical vein is identified, the site is cleansed before venipuncture. Typically this involves first wiping with isopropanol, then scrubbing with a broad-spectrum topical microbicide (eg, povidone iodine) for at least 30 seconds. Some banks have chosen to use a broad-spectrum antimicrobial formulation of 2% chlorhexidine gluconate/70% isopropyl alcohol in place of traditional iodophors. A hemostat is placed on the tubing a few inches from the needle. The hemostat is unclamped once the vein has been accessed, allowing blood to flow into the bag. Removal of the hemostat before entrance into the vein may allow air, a possible contaminant, to enter the tubing. While the UCB is being collected (a 3- to 5-minute process), it should be gently mixed with the anticoagulant to prevent clotting. The umbilical cord will appear collapsed when the collection is complete. Placing the bag on a laboratory scale during collection allows the collector to monitor the volume and provides an additional means for assessing completion of collection.

Once the collection is complete, the tubing is "stripped" forcing the blood within the tubing into the collection bag and allowing it to mix with the anticoagulant. This can be accomplished most easily with a specialized blood banking tool (ie, tube stripper), although newer bags include a filtered vent to eliminate the need for additional equipment. The UCB unit can then be packed for transport to the cell processing laboratory. See "Shipment" for a discussion on liquid UCB unit transport for processing.

In-Utero Collection

In-utero collections are generally performed by the obstetrician or nurse/midwife after the newborn has been delivered and assessed, and the umbilical cord has been clamped and cut. If the well-being of the newborn, mother, or both is in question, the collection is not attempted. If the decision to collect is made, care must be taken to maintain the sanitary field as a means to protect the mother and infant from risk of infection. Unless a sterile bag or extension set is used, the traditional supplies are not sterile, and inadvertent misplacement could contaminate the surgical field.

For logistical reasons, it is advisable to have preassembled collection kits for in-utero collections. An instructional packet may be included, containing, for example, the donor information form, a collection procedure, a list of collection kit contents, the maternal medical history form, the consent form(s), and packaging and shipping instructions. Collection kits should include the following items: one or two collection bags, antimicrobial supplies, tubing closures, appropriate sample tubes for infectious disease testing, sample tube labels, product labels, biohazard and any other appropriate stickers (eg, temporary storage temperature), and a secondary specimen and product bag. In some cases, the hospital's maternal label may be used to identify maternal tubes and UCB product, provided that two forms of identification are present and precautions are taken to protect confidentiality of the donor. Validated containers are used for shipping, which may contain a temperature monitor if transit takes place over a distance.

The primary advantage of in-utero collections is the substantially lower cost of collection. Because dedicated UCB bank collection personnel are not needed, the cost of collection is limited to collection and shipping supplies. Initial costs and efforts associated with education and training of the physician/midwife collectors should also be considered. However, once the obstetrics practice groups are trained, hands-on experience will improve the quality of collections; in-service and educational sessions can serve as a refresher course as well as a means to demonstrate appreciation of the clinicians' support. A bank with a robust training program, regular collection site visits, and established communication can support quality collections. In addition to the economic advantages, several studies have suggested that better collections can be obtained by in-utero methods. Along with higher volume, greater nucleated and CD34+ cell counts as well as a greater number of colony-forming units (CFUs) may be seen with units collected by in-utero methods.[43,44]

Ex-Utero Collection

Ex-utero collections are often performed by dedicated UCB collection staff. An obvious advantage of this approach is the standardization of methods with limited personnel and a more controlled environment. With ex-utero collections, the placenta can be removed from the delivery suite and transported to a nearby clean room for the collection. The cord should be clamped within 3 to 5 seconds of the infant's delivery, and the placenta taken immediately by bank staff to a suitable site where it may be suspended in a device to allow collection of blood by gravity. Figure 31-1 shows an example of a collection apparatus that holds a

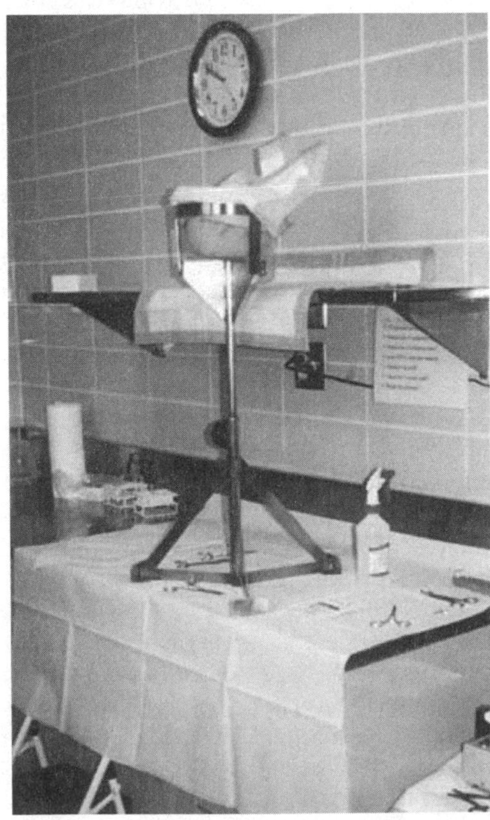

FIGURE 31-1. UCB collection apparatus.[45]

12-cup plastic bowl about 3 feet above the work surface. With this apparatus, the cord is passed through a 2-cm hole drilled through the base of the bowl. Collection proceeds as described above, after the surface of the cord has been prepared as described for the in-utero method. The placenta and cord are more accessible in the ex-utero setting, and therefore more manipulation, such as "milking" of the cord could increase collection volume so long as caution is used to prevent maternal contamination and lysis of cells. Speed is important in this process because the blood begins to clot and the volume and number of cells obtained will be inadequate if the collection is not performed quickly.

The cost of dedicated collection personnel may be substantial, depending upon the size and organization of the institution. The lack of availability of collectors on all shifts may limit the opportunity for participation. Perhaps secondary to the resulting standardization with dedicated collectors, benefits of ex-utero collections potentially include less clotting from inadequate mixing, less bacterial contamination, and fewer labeling errors.[42] Other investigators have questioned some of these findings.[46] Moreover, an earlier study by Wong et al hypothesized that a higher incidence of macroscopic clots with ex-utero collections consequently led to lower nucleated cell counts and CFUs.[47] Because data support both methods, either approach can lead to successful collection.[42]

PROCESSING

Methods

Most UCB products are cryopreserved in a laboratory that is dedicated to processing and preserving UCB and/or other HSCs and may be part of a hospital transfusion service or blood collection center. Methods of UCB cryopreservation have evolved significantly. In the early 1990s, UCB units were often stored in an unmanipulated state (ie, red cells and/or excess plasma were not removed before storage) in an effort to conserve the number of stem cells in the product.[28,48] Concern for infusion-related complications [associated with red cell incompatibility, free hemoglobin, and dimethylsulfoxide (DMSO)] and logistical issues surrounding limited storage capacity motivated an evaluation of processing methods designed to minimize red cell content and the size of the final UCB unit while limiting stem cell loss.

Today UCB processing laboratories use a variety of techniques for volume reduction, removal of red cells, or both. Most methods involve centrifugation, sedimentation, and/or filtration for reducing the red cell content, plasma volume, or both. Centrifugation for the removal of plasma is the simplest method in terms of cost and degree of manipulation, but it does not remove any of the red cells. The most common means of reducing red cell content has been the use of sedimenting agents such as hydroxyethyl starch (HES), gelatin, poligeline, and dextran. Such agents are effective and are used by many UCB banks.[49,50] Density separation by layering UCB cells over Percoll (Sigma-Aldrich, St. Louis, MO) or Ficoll Hypaque (Beckman Coulter Inc., Fullerton, CA) provides a mononuclear cell-enriched product essentially devoid of red cells.[51] More recently, leukocyte reduction filters and semiautomated methods have become commercially available, demonstrating in-vitro cell recoveries similar to the standard HES method.[49,52] Each of these methods has advantages and disadvantages in terms of cell recovery, red cell removal, processing time, and cost, and it is up to the individual laboratory to validate and determine which processing method is most appropriate for its situation. Factors such as process time, cost, maximization of storage, and production efficiency (number of UCB units processed per staff person per day) should be considered when deciding on an appropriate processing method. Cellular function, product integrity, and safety are considerations when developing a validation plan. Cell recovery (nucleated and CD34+), viability, clonogenic function (such as CFUs), and sterility testing (before and after cryopreservation) are typical validation performance measures.

One of the earliest methods for processing UCB was developed by Pablo Rubinstein[53]; modifications of this method are still commonly used today.[54] This process reduces red cell content using HES and depletes the units of plasma and anticoagulant to minimize the final product and cryoprotectant volumes. Figure 31-2 depicts a slightly modified version of the Rubinstein method.[45] Also, the reader is referred to Method 7-2 for a more detailed description.

The FDA has published final recommendations for the submission of a biologics license application (BLA) related to UCB products, providing guidance for UCB banks to demonstrate compliance with applicable regulatory requirements that ensure the safety, purity, potency, and effectiveness of UCB products (see "Regulations and Standards").[55] This document has compelled the industry to standardize manufacturing processes using reagents that have been approved for human use, and systems and supplies that have been cleared by the FDA. To date, the following systems have been FDA approved for processing UCB:

- Automation technology incorporated into the Sepax Cord Blood Processing System manufactured by Biosafe SA (Eysins, Switzerland), offers a closed and sterile process-

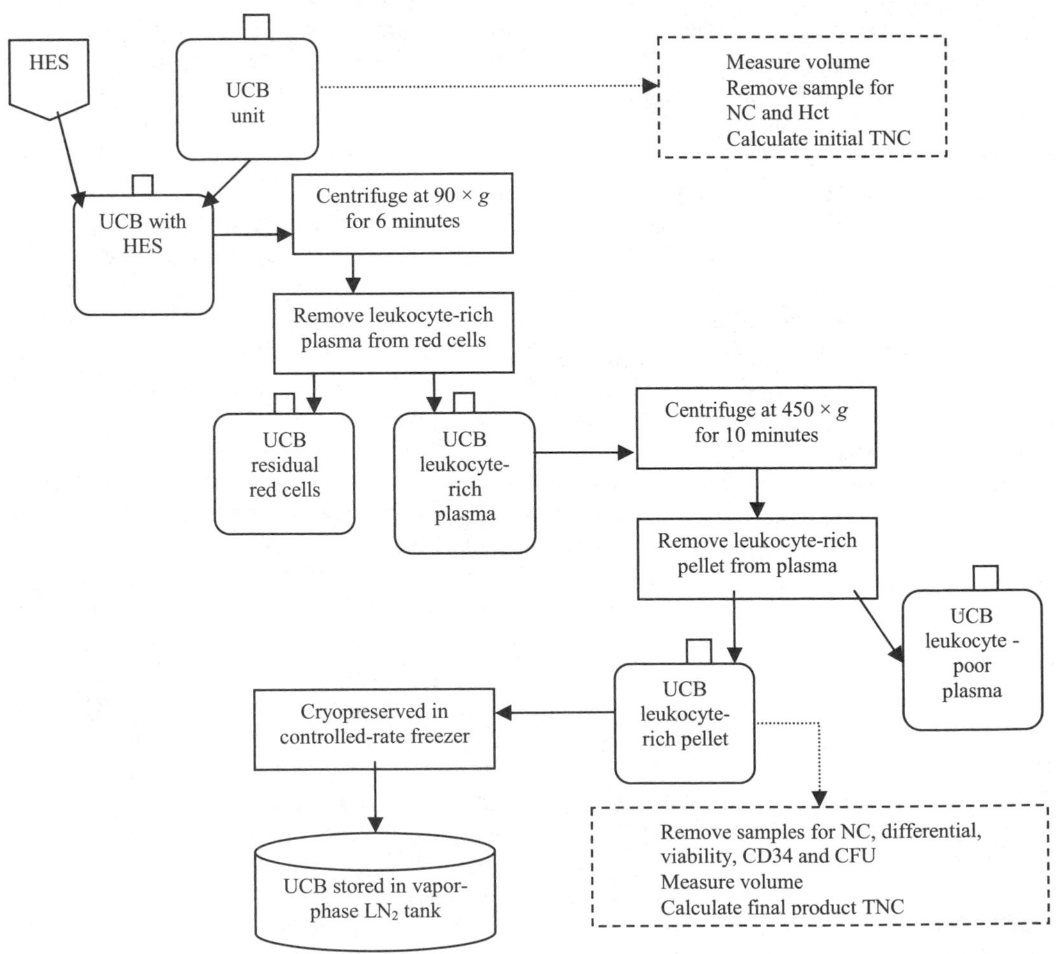

FIGURE 31-2. Umbilical cord blood (UCB) processing summary. Modified from Chrysler et al.[45]
CFU = colony-forming unit; Hct = hematocrit; HES = hydroxyethyl starch; LN_2 = liquid nitrogen; NC = nucleated cells; TNC = total nucleated cells.

ing system that efficiently harvests stem cells from UCB and is adaptable to a large-scale processing environment. The Sepax machine, essentially composed of a centrifuge with piston position sensors surrounding the entire chamber and pneumatic pump system, is operated by computer-controlled protocols to achieve component separation. Consumable kits consist of a large syringe-type barrel separation chamber with bags and tubing connected by a stopcock assembly. The Sepax system received FDA clearance in January 2007 and European CE mark approval in 2001.

- PrepaCyte-CB, a UCB processing system manufactured by BioE (St. Paul, MN), received FDA clearance in January 2009. PrepaCyte-CB is a sterile device composed of three integrally attached processing and storage bags containing the PrepaCyte-CB separation solution. While isolating total nucleated cells (TNC), PrepaCyte-CB removes virtually all red cells from the final processed UCB unit and requires only a standard laboratory centrifuge to concentrate desired cells after separation.

Quality Control Testing

Regardless of the method used for processing UCB, quality control (QC) testing to assess the adequacy of the product and process is essential. QC testing is generally performed upon receipt (before manipulation) and before cryopreservation. Typical QC assays include nucleated cell count, hematocrit, ABO/Rh typing, CD34+ cell enumeration, CFU assay, viability, sterility (aerobic, anaerobic, and fungal), and HLA typing. UCB products used for allogeneic transplantation must be typed for HLA Class I and Class II antigens, including *HLA-A*, *-B*, and *-DRB1* loci; HLA-C and -DQB typing is recommended.[34] Table 31-1 summarizes these basic QC tests. More details of QC testing of HSCs are provided in Chapter 29.

Cryopreservation and Long-Term Storage

Success for UCB banks hinges on the ability to preserve the integrity of UCB over substantial lengths of time. Freezing and storage methods must therefore be robust enough to ensure that the quality of the UCB unit is maintained for many years. The most common means of cryopreservation for UCB, as for marrow and peripheral blood, consists of freezing the cells in a cryogenic bag with a cryoprotectant solution of 10% DMSO.[56-58] One of the main advantages of using cryogenic bags rather than freezing vials is the ability to perform confirmatory HLA typing and QC testing from an integrally attached tubing segment. Not surprisingly, the Foundation for the Accreditation of Cellular Therapy (FACT) and the AABB have mandated the use of cryogenic bags with at-

TABLE 31-1. Summary of Quality Control Testing for UCB

Test	Method(s)
Cell counts	Hematology analyzer, manual differential
CD34+ cell enumeration	Flow cytometry (single or dual platform)
Viability assay	Dye exclusion (light microscopy), fluorescence microscopy, flow cytometry
Clonogenic assay	CFU (most common in clinical laboratories), LT-CICs
Sterility testing	Aerobic/anaerobic/fungal culture
HLA typing	Molecular
ABO/Rh typing	Serology
Hematocrit	Standard/routine

CFU = colony-forming unit; LT-CICs = long-term culture-initiating cells; UCB = umbilical cord blood.

tached segments for the freezing of UCB[34,36] until innovation provides an indisputable means of establishing identity and comparability.

It has been well established that slow cooling in a programmable controlled-rate freezing device at a rate of 1 C/minute will result in adequate recovery of HPCs.[57-59] Such instruments mitigate process variability and limit potential cell damage. As with all critical processes, the freezing process must be validated and procedures must be in place that address the use and operation of the controlled-rate freezer (or equivalent), expected cooling rates and freezing-curve parameters, endpoint freezing temperature, addition of cryoprotectant, final cell and cryoprotectant concentrations, and storage temperature.

Both the AABB and FACT have defined storage temperature limits for cryopreserved UCB to be ≤–150 C.[34,36] Once frozen, UCB units are typically transferred for long-term storage into a monitored liquid-nitrogen (LN_2) container, either immersed in liquid (at –196 C) or in vapor phase to minimize the potential for cross-contamination. Studies of the long-term effects of ultra-cold storage of UCB units have shown that retention of viabilities and/or proliferative function of UCB cells frozen in the liquid phase of LN_2 remains acceptable for greater than 23 years.[60,61]

To ensure the safety and stability of the stored UCB units, control measures should be established for product security and segregation, storage container monitoring, inventory control, and duration of storage. Storage containers should be located in a secure area to prevent unauthorized access. For units in which transmissible disease screening and testing is positive or incomplete, a designated quarantine storage area is necessary. To ensure that temperature and LN_2 levels are continuously maintained, a monitoring system should be in place with local and remote alarm capabilities. Alarm limits should be set to adequately allow for staff to respond to alarm notifications. All UCB product and reference sample storage locations should be cataloged using an inventory management system that allows for rapid retrieval. The duration of storage and product expiration dates should be defined in standard operating procedures, even when expiry dates have not been determined by the laboratory or bank.

Tests After Thawing and Stability Testing

The AABB requires that UCB products "shall have at least two integrally attached segments cryopreserved with the product."[36] These segments can be used for HLA confirmatory typing and product identity, ABO/Rh testing and product identity, viability, CD34+ cell analysis, progenitor assays, or others tests that may be useful in determining potency before releasing the UCB unit to a transplant facility.

SHIPMENT

With the vast number of commercial carriers available, UCB can be routinely transported to processing laboratories or transplant facilities within 24 hours. Ensuring that UCB units and products are properly packaged and shipped in order to prevent damage or deterioration during shipment is the responsibility of UCB collection facilities and processing laboratories. Validated packaging and shipping procedures should demonstrate that acceptable temperatures and the integrity of the unit are maintained.[36] Each institution defines its own shipping conditions (temperature, type of shipping container, packaging material, etc) for the transport of fresh and frozen UCB products. For newly collected UCB, the transit temperature requirements are not well defined, leaving each facility to determine transport temperature criteria and acceptable limits. Thus, fresh UCB units may be transported at room temperature, on ice, or with insulated precooled stabilizing packs. Wada et al observed a 1% decrease in viability for every 4-hour increase in transport time for newly collected UCB units that were shipped at ambient temperature.[62] A series of studies has shown that UCB can be preserved in CPD for up to 24 hours before processing and retain satisfactory cell recovery and progenitor content.[63-66] Storage at either room temperature or 1 to 4 C does not seem to make a large difference, but lower temperature may minimize growth of any contaminating bacteria.

Shipping methods must be well designed not only to preserve the quality and function of the UCB product but also to protect the safety of personnel involved in the shipping process.[34,45] The FDA, International Air Transport Association (IATA), US Department of Transportation (DOT), AABB, and FACT have established packaging and labeling requirements for shipping biologics.[34,36,67-69] The IATA requires that shipping containers withstand extreme external temperature variability and that the primary outer container be leakproof, constructed to resist breakage, and durable enough to withstand pressure changes and falls. Furthermore, an inner, secondary container such as a plastic resealable bag with enough absorbent material to contain the contents of the product in the event of a leak or break must also be used.[34,68]

Shipping Cryopreserved Units

Cryopreserved products are typically transported to transplant facilities in a portable LN_2 "dry" shipping container. Such shippers are insulated containers that allow for LN_2 to be absorbed into the vessel wall, creating an ultracold environment. FACT requires that LN_2 dry shippers be validated to maintain temperature of ≤–150 C for at least 48 hours past the time of delivery to the transplant facility.[34] For the portable LN_2 or "dry shipper" to be fully effective, it typically must be charged or filled with LN_2 24 hours before the estimated time of release from the processing laboratory. This allows for complete absorbance of the LN_2 into the wall of the shipping container. Improperly filled dry shippers present a risk of LN_2 leakage and, should a spill occur, may be subject to civil or criminal penalties as determined by the DOT.

Transport Labeling and Record Requirements

Both the AABB and FACT require continuous monitoring of the temperature during shipment[34,36] and require that the shipping container include the following: a listing of the name, address, and phone number of the shipping and receiving institution; the phrases "Medical Specimen," "Do Not Irradiate" (if applicable), and "Do Not X-Ray"; and biohazard labels (as appropriate).[34,36] Biological products must be packaged and shipped in compliance with all applicable government regulations. Transportation records that identify the shipping facility, date and time the unit was shipped and received, courier, and contents of each shipping container should be maintained.[34,36]

RECEIPT OF UCB FOR TRANSPLANTATION

UCB transplantation is a coordinated effort potentially involving the registry (in some cases), the UCB bank, and the cell processing laboratory and clinical team at the transplant center. UCB units typically are ordered by a program nurse coordinator, with selection based on institutional algorithms or guidelines. The coordinator may rely on the laboratory's medical or laboratory director for resolving questions related to a prospective UCB unit, including those associated with technical issues and donor medical history. It is advisable to involve the laboratory as early as possible in the unit selection process.[70]

The program nurse coordinator notifies the cell processing laboratory of the impending arrival of a UCB unit and any information relating to special handling (eg, size and dimensions of product canister, indications of risk factors requiring quarantine). When the unit is received at the laboratory, it is carefully unpacked and then examined before being placed into the LN_2 storage tank. The laboratory may have different thawing methods that are dependent on the bag or vessel in which the UCB is contained, so attention should be paid to this detail. The unit should be verified as frozen and intact. The dry shipper may be weighed to check for excessive LN_2 loss (in general, >10 lb). By examining the temperature-monitoring device included in the shipment, the technologist should confirm that the UCB remained within the acceptable range for shipment. Some continuous-recording devices allow for download and printout of temperature readings throughout shipment. If the temperature-monitoring device indicates a digital temperature, the temperature upon unpacking should be recorded. If the device has no temperature shown or the data cannot be downloaded upon receipt, the UCB bank should forward a copy of the data when it becomes available. If, for some reason, there is no temperature-monitoring device, a device from the transplant center should be inserted for several hours to ensure that the shipper can hold an acceptable temperature. The bank should be notified that no device was present in the shipment, and documentation of the bank's shipper validation should be requested.

The identity of the UCB unit should be verified at the time of inspection, before placement in storage. The product label should include the appropriate minimum partial label requirements—a unique product identifier (ie, unit number) and the proper product name. All other product information should be included on a tag attached to the product, the accompanying product paperwork, or both. The unit label or tag information should be checked against the accompanying UCB bank paperwork and the paperwork generated by the transplant program or coordinator. Any inconsistencies should be immediately and appropriately investigated.

The unit information, including donor medical history and infectious disease testing, should again be reviewed for completeness. If there are any comments not previously communicated to the receiving laboratory, particularly those related to the medical history, they should be referred to the medical director. The medical director should determine whether the information is significant and requires any further action, including notification of the transplant physician. If any infectious disease testing is found to be incomplete or positive at this time, the unit should be placed into quarantine storage, and the appropriate people (eg, laboratory supervisor, medical or laboratory director, nurse coordinator, transplant physician) should be notified. The product label or tag should be updated accordingly (eg, biohazard label), and a special medical release form may need to be completed.

Any further testing deemed necessary by the transplant center (eg, additional HLA testing, viability testing, CFU assays) should be performed as soon as possible on an attached segment, if one accompanies the unit. If the identity is in question and an attached segment is not available, a rapid (Class I serologic) HLA test is performed along with the standard product testing on the thawed product (ie, on the day of transplantation).[71]

THAWING AND WASHING OF UCB

Coordination of the transplantation requires consistent communication among all members of the clinical team. In the days before the planned transplant procedure, the coordinator should verify the correct infusion date with the clinical team, and both the coordinator and the laboratory should again review all records. The patient care unit should then be contacted at least one day before the day of transplantation to schedule an infusion time. Given the wide variety of types of products received from an increasing number of UCB banks, the most appropriate UCB thawing procedure must be determined based on the transplant center's validated method, the bank's recommendations, or whether the product was manufactured to reduce red cells and plasma (red cell reduced) or to deplete plasma only (red cell replete) before cryopreservation. These thawing procedures may not be identical and can be further complicated if the patient is enrolled in a clinical trial that requires a specific method.

Current practices for preparing UCB products for infusion include the traditional thaw-and-wash method, the thaw-and-dilution technique, or bedside thawing.[72,73] The rationale for preparing the product at the bedside is that potential cell loss from manipulation after thawing is eliminated, and the product is reconstituted in the recipient's circulation. However, this approach is not recommended because of the inability to rescue product if the bag integrity is compromised during thawing and because of the instability of cells exposed to DMSO after thawing should infusion be delayed. Furthermore, this method lacks the capacity for process control and product assessment.

The traditional washing method described in 1995[53] is recommended if exposure to DMSO, accumulation of free hemoglobin, and the volume of the product approach critical limits for recipients, particularly pediatric patients or those with underlying cardiac, pulmonary, or sensitizing conditions. More recently, because the majority of products are red cell reduced and because of concern for cell loss at the wash step, a dilution or simple reconstitution approach[74] has gained support. Both methods are initiated in similar fashion:

- The UCB product is carefully removed from the storage tank, and a thorough inspection is performed to evaluate the integrity of the container. Label verification of the product identity is conducted by two technologists.
- The unit is sealed within a clean or sterile transparent bag (eg, resealable zipper storage bags) and submerged in a 37 C waterbath containing clean or sterile water or saline. Gentle kneading of the UCB as it is thawing helps to accelerate the process, preventing recrystallization and consequential cell damage or death. Should a leak be discovered after initiating thawing, the site of the container break is determined and a hemostat is employed to prevent further escape of the product. The contents can then be aseptically transferred into another storage bag under a biological safety cabinet.[54]
- A thawing solution containing 10% dextran and a protein source, usually human serum albumin in final concentration of approximately 2.5% to 4.2%, is prepared in advance for diluting the product. The supplementation of a protein (albumin) solution has been proven to restore osmolarity and extend cell viability.[53] A volume of solution equaling (or exceeding) the volume of the UCB product is gradually added to the bag while gently mixing. The product and solutions are drained into a labeled transfer bag and left to equilibrate for 5 minutes. At this stage, if the product is to be reconstituted or diluted only, samples are removed for product testing.
- If the product is to be washed, the labeled transfer bag is then centrifuged at 400 × *g* for 15 minutes at 10 C. The supernatant is expressed, leaving behind a pellet of washed UCB cells. If it is the policy of the transplant laboratory to centrifuge the supernatant, the second labeled transfer bag is spun at 400 × *g* for 15 minutes at 10 C, the supernatant again expressed, and the two cell pellets combined into one labeled bag.
- The UCB cells are then resuspended in a volume of thawing solution appropriate for the weight of the patient and any concerns related to fluid overload.
- Some laboratories filter the resuspended product with a standard blood filter (170-260 microns).
- Samples are removed for QC tests, such as cell counts (TNC, CD34+, and CD3+), microbial culture (bacteria, fungi), confirmatory ABO/Rh typing, CFU assay, and viability testing (see "Evaluation and Quality Control of Hematopoietic Products" in Chapter 29). Final volume, dose, and recovery are determined, and following completion of paperwork and labeling, the unit can be released for infusion.[54]

It is anticipated that standardization of thawing procedures based on type of product will be forthcoming through the collaborative experience of the banking and transplant communities.

INFUSION OF UCB

At the time of infusion, the patient's understanding of the UCB transplant process from earlier discussions may have been limited as a result of emotional stress or other reasons. Hence, it is good practice to reiterate to the patient the general process, including graft selection, cell processing, infusion, potential side effects and adverse reactions, and plans for premedication. This explanation should take place on, or shortly before, the day of transplantation.

The general approach and potential adverse reactions are similar to those for other stem cell products.[75] A procedure for infusion is outlined below[45]:

- Once a cord blood unit has been thawed and washed, it is delivered to the patient care unit without delay.
- A form acknowledging receipt is signed by the nurse, who then notifies the patient's physician of the arrival of the UCB unit.
- Following physician approval for infusion and proper identification procedures, the unit is infused by intravenous (IV) drip or syringe push directly into a central line without a needle or pump. Some institutions use a standard blood filter at the bedside. If a filter is used in the laboratory after thawing and washing, a second standard blood filter at the bedside is not needed.
- The unit bag and IV tubing should be flushed with sterile saline after the unit bag empties to maximize cell dose. Sterile saline also may be added directly to the unit bag if the flow rate becomes unusually slow.

Because the final volume of a UCB unit is relatively low (roughly 60 to 100 mL with the thaw-wash methods detailed above), infusion is typically completed within 15 to 30 minutes of its receipt in the patient care unit.

The authors recommend that the thawed UCB be transfused as soon as possible, realizing that the administration of UCB may be delayed for a variety of reasons (eg, rapid serologic HLA typing, clinical necessity). Timely infusion is most likely to become an issue with UCB that has not been washed or diluted. Although Rowley and Anderson concluded that DMSO is not toxic to HSCs at clinically relevant concentrations (ie, 5%, 10%) at either 4 C or 37 C for up to 1 hour of incubation, they also noted that addition of 1% DMSO to culture dishes suppressed CFU assays.[76] It is important to note that these studies were performed on fresh cells.[76] Studies of the effects of DMSO on HSCs that have been previously cryopreserved are limited. However, some investigators have noted similar suppression of colony formation when thawed UCB samples are not washed and are immediately placed into CFU culture.[74,77] Thus, the possible functional defect caused by DMSO coupled with the not-infrequent need to hold clinical products before infusion raise the concern for cell injury with thawed UCB, again particularly when cells are not washed or diluted.

With regard to patient monitoring, it is recommended that vital signs be checked before infusion, immediately after infusion, and 1 hour after infusion at a minimum. Should an adverse reaction occur, more frequent monitoring would undoubtedly be required. The transplant physician and the medical director of the cellular therapy laboratory should be notified immediately of either an unexpected reaction or one that is moderate to severe. An investigation should be initiated and should include any appropriate laboratory testing (eg, direct antiglobulin test, Gram's stain, or culture). All of the monitoring information should be captured on the accompanying infusion form, which should be returned to the laboratory.

Reactions associated with HSC infusion may be very similar to those occasionally seen with blood transfusion (ie, allergic, hemolytic, and febrile reactions and those caused by microbial contamination). However, with combinations of the various processing methods for UCB (eg, red cell depletion, plasma reduction, postthaw washing step), some types of these reactions may be less likely to occur—that is, those attributed to red cell antigens and plasma proteins. Likewise, if red cell depletion and washing steps are included, renal compromise caused by infusion of red cells and free hemoglobin would not be expected as often as with other HSC sources. Reactions (ie, nausea, vomiting, cough, and headache) often attributed to DMSO would also be expected to be less common with washed UCB.[78,79] Bacterial contamination, which occurs with up to 5% of collections,[80-82] is usually not an issue with banked UCB units because banks would not routinely include these units in the useable inventory.

UCB infusions are generally very well tolerated; if reactions occur, they are typically mild and readily managed by the health-care team.[75] However, because a severe reaction is possible, aggressive IV hydration (eg, 2 to 6 hours before and 6 hours after infusion, with diuretics as needed) is recommended as a standard procedure. The general use of prophylactic antiemetics, antipyretics, and antihistamines is recommended as well.

REGULATIONS AND STANDARDS

FDA Regulations

In 1997, the FDA announced a novel risk-based tiered approach to the regulation of somatic cells and tissues.[83] The methodology outlined in the FDA "Proposed Approach to Regulation of Cellular and Tissue-Based Products" (February 27, 1997) was followed by the good tissue practice (GTP) regulations (2004),[67] requiring "that cells and tissues be handled according to procedures designed to prevent contamination and preserve [cell and] tissue function and integrity." This historic document has set the framework for cellular therapy laboratories to identify the agency's expectations for the prevention of disease transmission and laboratory process controls. Governed by three fundamentals, the GTP regulations are intended 1) to prevent unintentional use of contaminated tissue at risk for transmitting infectious disease, 2) to prevent improper processing of tissue that may cause damage or risk of contamination, and 3) to ensure the safety and efficacy of products that are more than minimally manipulated.[56,84-86] Based on these principles, all human cells, tissues, and cellular and tissue-based products (HCT/Ps) intended for unrelated use, regardless of degree of manipulation or potential risk, are required to comply with the requirements for donor testing and screening,[84] establishment registration,[87] and current GTP (cGTP).[67]

Since 2004, UCB banks have been required to register with the FDA as manufacturers of HCT/Ps and demonstrate compliance with cGTP regulations.[67] For UCB banks that manufacture or store more-than-minimally manipulated products (ie, UCB is activated, expanded, or genetically modified) or combine UCB with nontissue components, the FDA requires an investigational new drug (IND) application and adherence to licensure application requirements. Table 31-2 summarizes FDA regulations of HCT/Ps, including HPCs from UCB. [The official product name is HPC, Cord. The abbreviation HPC(C) used in this chapter is not intended to be used in the labeling process or on product labels.]

Minimally manipulated unrelated UCB has not been licensed; however, the FDA has long considered licensure as a way of improving the safety and quality of HPC(C) by instituting requirements that would be legally enforceable.[67] The FDA believed that compelling clinical safety and efficacy data existed for the development of product standards as an approach toward licensure. In 1998 the FDA issued the "Request for Proposed Standards for Unrelated Allogeneic Peripheral and Placental/Umbilical Cord Blood Hematopoietic Stem/Progenitor Cell Products; Request for Comments," asking the public to submit comments proposing establishment controls, process controls, and product standards for HPC(C) manufacturers.[88] Upon review of the submitted information, the FDA determined that sufficient data did exist to develop processing and product standards for granting licensure. Subsequently, the FDA released a guidance document for those UCB banks wishing to submit a BLA.[55] This document serves to assist HPC(C) manufacturers of unrelated, minimally manipulated UCB in their license application by identifying applicable regulatory requirements and manufacturing information to be submitted to the agency. It is the FDA's intent to grant licensure of products that are manufactured according to these recommendations. For establishments that manufacture HPC(C) products for autologous use or first- or second-degree blood relatives, the same manufacturing recommendations and regulations apply.[55]

The FDA recognizes that there will be circumstances in which the best available HPC(C) unit for a patient will not be a licensed unit. The unit 1) may be from UCB establish-

TABLE 31-2. Summary of FDA Regulations for HCT/Ps and HPCs, Cord[67,87,88]

Products Regulated	Specific Product
HCT/Ps that are or will be regulated as biological products	◆ All allogeneic, unrelated HCT/Ps derived from cord and peripheral blood ◆ HCT/Ps that are more than minimally manipulated (eg, expanded, activated, or genetically modified) ◆ HCT/Ps that are combined with a drug, device, or biological product ◆ HCT/Ps that are intended for nonhomologous use (eg, HCT/Ps intended for use in cardiac repair)
HPC(C) that are currently subject to biologics license application (BLA) requirements	◆ Allogeneic, unrelated, and minimally manipulated HPC(C) intended for hematopoietic reconstitution in patients with hematologic malignancies, certain lysosomal storage and peroxisomal enzyme deficiency disorders, primary immunodeficiency diseases, marrow failure, or beta thalassemias ◆ HPC(C) that are manufactured according to recommended establishment and process controls and that comply with all applicable regulatory requirements (licensure planned)
HPC(C) that are currently subject to investigational new drug (IND) requirements	◆ HPC(C) that are not FDA licensed and are: 1. Allogeneic, unrelated, and minimally manipulated 2. Intended for hematopoietic reconstitution in patients with hematologic malignancies, certain lysosomal storage and peroxisomal enzyme deficiency disorders, primary immunodeficiency diseases, marrow failure, or beta thalassemias 3. The only satisfactory treatment available ◆ HPC(C) manufactured in a US cord blood bank and intended to be used in the United States ◆ HPC(C) that were manufactured in a US cord blood bank before BLA approval and that do not meet licensing requirements ◆ HPC(C) prospectively manufactured in the United States and for which there is no satisfactory alternative

HCT/Ps = human cells, tissues, and cellular and tissue-based products; HPCs = hematopoietic progenitor cells; HPC(C) = HPCs, Cord.

ments in which a BLA is pending, 2) may not meet the licensing requirements, or 3) may be from a non-US UCB bank that has chosen not to apply for licensure. Under such circumstances, the FDA will require that an IND application be submitted. Recently the FDA released a draft guidance document to assist in the submission of that application.[89]

AABB and NetCord-FACT Standards

The AABB and NetCord-FACT have established professional standards for HPCs, including HPC(C).[34,36] The AABB has incorporated the requirements of HPC(C) processing facilities in its *Standards for Cellular Therapy Product Services*.[36] FACT and NetCord combined efforts to establish a unique set of standards specific for HPC(C) activities.[34] Both the AABB and NetCord-FACT have created standards that align with the FDA's good manufacturing practice (GMP) and GTP regulations and center on quality system essentials that include donor suitability, collection, processing control, document control, facility management, materials, records, storage, distribution, quality audits, quality plans, errors and deviations, labeling, personnel, equipment, validation, outcome review, and adverse event reporting.

NOVEL UCB-DERIVED CELLULAR THERAPIES

Cell Expansion

UCB continues to be a target of expansion studies, although historically, mobilized peripheral blood has been the primary starting material.[90] UCB is a logical focus for HSC expansion because UCB unit collection is a one-time event with a limited volume. Moreover, as discussed in the introductory paragraphs, HSCs derived from UCB have been shown to have a greater proliferative and self-renewal capacity[18-20]; hence, a higher likelihood of success with HSC expansion would be expected with UCB.

The majority of HSC expansion studies, including those with UCB, have involved enrichment for CD34+ or CD133+ cells and culture in media supplemented with a protein source (eg, human or fetal calf serum or albumin) and a cytokine cocktail (typically including stem cell factor, flt-3 ligand, and thrombopoietin).[90-92] Although success in clinical trials has been limited to date,[93,94] more recent research studies involving culture modifications have been promising.[95,96] Clinical trials incorporating these optimized methods and others are currently under way. Other means to improve the engraftment potential of UCB have been initiated as well. A few transplant centers have moved to the double-UCB-unit transplant strategy to overcome the limitation of cell counts.[97] Early success with this approach led to the subsequent initiation of two multicenter trials involving double-unit UCB transplantation. One study is a Phase II trial in adults with hematologic malignancy, sponsored by the Center for International Blood and Marrow Transplant Research; the other is a Phase III trial in children with high-risk leukemia and myelodysplasia sponsored by the National Heart, Lung, and Blood Institute. Both studies are ongoing with anticipated completion in the next several years. Studies involving coinfusion of mesenchymal stem or stromal cells (MSCs) with UCB have been encouraging as well,[98,99] and the initiation of clinical trials based on these studies can be expected.

Immunotherapy

There are a variety of immune cell types in UCB, several of which are being examined in basic and clinical research settings for potential clinical applications. Some of these prospective immunotherapies are discussed further below.

Natural Killer Cells

Natural killer (NK) cells are a subset of lymphocytes with critical roles in natural immunity and the regulation of hematopoiesis. NK cells represent about 10% to 20% of circulating lymphocytes, and they are easily isolated from adult peripheral blood by apheresis and immunomagnetic selection.[100] NK cells have been used successfully in the treatment of cancer,[101] and their use in this setting appears to be increasing. A recent report indicating the benefits of NK cells in the setting of mismatched HSC transplants[102] has encouraged the initiation of HSC-NK cell transplant strategies at several transplant centers.

UCB-derived NK cells have been characterized, and some investigators have shown encouraging results with potential therapeutic advantages over NK cells derived from marrow and peripheral blood.[103,104] Although the majority of nonclinical research on UCB-derived NK cells has used fresh UCB, NK cells can be isolated from thawed UCB units. Aside from the initial thaw, which includes addition of DNase, these methods are similar to those for apheresis mononuclear cell products [ie, immunomagnetic selection followed by incubation with interleukin 2 (IL-2)].

T Regulatory Cells

Naturally arising T regulatory cells are a discrete subpopulation of CD4+ T cells (approximately 5% to 10%) with an immunosuppressive function. They are characterized as CD4+/CD25+ cells that express FoxP3 protein, a transcription factor that controls expression of the IL-2 receptor α-chain (CD25) in natural CD4+/

CD25+ T regulatory cells but not in activated T cells in general.[105] Potential clinical applications of T regulatory cells include treatment of autoimmune disease and organ transplant (where enhancement of T regulatory function would be employed) as well as cancer and infectious disease (where reduction of T regulatory function would be sought).[105] UCB has been examined for the presence of T regulatory cells,[106] and these cells have been shown to have potent suppressor function.[107] In anticipation of trials in support of HSC transplantation, T regulatory cells have been shown to be resistant to GVHD immune-suppressive agents.[108] As with NK cells, production methods involve immunomagnetic selection and culture,[107] although optimal production methods have yet to be determined. Clinical trials have been initiated recently with promising results evident.[109]

Dendritic Cells

Dendritic cells (DCs) are a complex, diverse group of immune cells that serve a vital function in the immune response, being positioned at the interface between the innate and adaptive immune systems. DCs are often referred to as the "professional" antigen-presenting cells, possessing the ability to activate several types of immune effector cells such as B and T cells, NK-T cells, and NK cells.[110-112] To date, the primary sources of DCs for research and clinical trials have been CD34+ cells from blood or marrow (ie, immunomagnetic selection)[113] and blood-derived monocytes isolated by adherence technique[114] or other selection methods (eg, CD14+ cell selection[115] or counterflow centrifugal elutriation[116]). However, DCs have been successfully isolated and expanded from UCB, and clinical utility is apparent.[117,118]

DC culture systems have varied among researchers but typically include a protein-supplemented medium (eg, with human group AB or fetal calf serum), to which at least IL-4 and granulocyte-macrophage colony-stimulating factor are added to derive immature DCs. Following some days in culture, a DC maturing agent such as tumor necrosis factor alpha or poly-I:C and an antigen source are added.[112,114,115] The culture is continued for a few days (often 2-3), at which time mature DCs are harvested. The best method for the manufacture of clinically efficacious DCs has not been determined but is being actively pursued.[119]

Nonhematopoietic Stem Cells

There are other stem cells in UCB (ie, nonhematopoietic stem cells) that have only recently been discovered. The clinical value of these cells remains unknown; however, basic research with these cells has been promising. Two types of nonhematopoietic stem cells are briefly described below.

Mesenchymal Stem or Stromal Cells

The presence of MSCs in UCB was initially debated, with conflicting data in the literature.[120-122] However, UCB has since become an accepted source of MSCs, stem cells capable of differentiating into cells of connective tissue lineage.[123] Processing methods are similar to those described for marrow-derived MSCs, with an initial density centrifugation step followed by selection by adherence in culture.[124] More recently, methods of isolation and expansion of MSCs from Wharton's jelly have been described, indicating another use for the placenta and umbilical cord.[125] Again, as with most, if not all, of the UCB-derived novel cell therapies, optimal methods for production and clinical applicability have yet to be established.

Multipotent Stem Cells

Even more recently, UCB has been examined for the presence of cells capable of differentiating into cell types of all three embryonic layers (ie, endo-, ecto-, and mesoderm). Few groups have reported success in the literature.[126-128] The fact that such cells exist in UCB is an exciting prospect for the treatment of a variety of human diseases. Currently, however, these cells are limited to basic research, primarily being used as research tools to better understand human development and disease.

KEY POINTS

1. Umbilical cord blood (UCB) has evolved from being considered biological waste to acceptance as a viable source of hematopoietic stem cells (HSCs). Over 20,000 unrelated-donor UCB transplantations have been performed, and there are an estimated 450,000 unrelated UCB units banked worldwide.
2. Engaging mothers and arranging donation in advance is critical for achieving best results. Early education allows for more complete medical screening, comprehensive donor protection, availability of adequate supplies, and acquisition of adequate informed consent.
3. UCB can be collected before (in utero) or after (ex utero) the placenta has been delivered. There are advantages and disadvantages to each method, but neither seems to be better overall.
4. Coordination of the transplant event requires consistent communication among all members of the clinical team.
5. Given the wide variety of types of products from an increasing number of UCB banks, the most appropriate UCB thawing procedure must be determined based on the transplant center's validated method, the bank's recommendations, and/or how the product was manufactured.
6. Current practices for preparing UCB for infusion consist of the traditional thaw and wash method, the thaw and dilution technique, or bedside thawing.
7. UCB infusion reactions are similar, although typically less severe, when compared with those of other HSC sources. To avoid reactions, patients may be premedicated with antihistamines, antipyretics, and possibly antiemetics. Aggressive hydration may be warranted, depending on several factors, including the red cell volume of the unit(s) and patient-specific variables.
8. Several cell types within UCB (eg, mesenchymal stem cells, immune cells) are being investigated for clinical utility in the setting of various diseases.
9. In 2009 the Food and Drug Administration (FDA) released a guidance document for UCB banks wishing to submit a biologics license application (BLA). This guidance identifies applicable regulatory requirements and manufacturing information to be submitted to the FDA by manufacturers of unrelated, minimally manipulated UCB.
10. The FDA recognizes that some units may be needed that 1) are from UCB establishments in which a BLA is pending, 2) do not meet the licensing requirements, or 3) are from non-US UCB banks that have chosen not to apply for licensure. Under such circumstances, the FDA will require that an investigational new drug (IND) application be submitted.

REFERENCES

1. Ende M, Ende N. Hematopoietic transplantation by means of fetal (cord) blood: A new method. Va Med Mon 1972;99:276-80.
2. Knudtzon S. In vitro growth of granulocytic colonies from circulating cells in human cord blood. Blood 1974;43:357-61.
3. Vainchenker W, Guichard J, Breton-Gorius J. Growth of human megakaryocyte colonies in culture from fetal, neonatal, and adult peripheral blood cells: Ultrastructural analysis. Blood Cells 1979;5:25-42.
4. Hassan MW, Lutton JD, Levere RD, et al. In vitro culture of erythroid colonies from human fetal liver and umbilical cord blood. Br J Haematol 1979;41:477-84.
5. Nakahata T, Ogawa M. Hematopoietic colony-forming cells in umbilical cord blood with extensive capability to generate mono- and multipotential hematopoietic progenitors. J Clin Invest 1982;70:1324-8.
6. Leary AG, Ogawa M, Strauss LC, Civin CI. Single cell origin of multilineage colonies in culture. J Clin Invest 1984;74:2193-7.

7. Broxmeyer HE, Douglas GW, Hangoc G, et al. Human umbilical cord blood as a potential source of transplantable hematopoietic stem/progenitor cells. Proc Natl Acad Sci U S A 1989; 86:3828-32.
8. Gluckman E, Broxmeyer HE, Auerbach AD, et al. Hematopoietic reconstitution in a patient with Fanconi anemia by means of umbilical cord blood from an HLA-identical sibling. N Engl J Med 1989;321:1174-8.
9. Gluckman E, Rocha V. History of the clinical use of umbilical cord blood hematopoietic cells. Cytotherapy 2005;7:219-27.
10. Wagner JE, Kernan NA, Steinbuch M, et al. Allogeneic sibling cord blood transplantation in children with malignant and non-malignant disease. Lancet 1995;346:214-19.
11. Rubinstein P, Carrier C, Scaradavou A, et al. Outcomes among 562 recipients of placental-blood transplants from unrelated donors. N Engl J Med 1998;339:1565-77.
12. Laughlin MJ, Barker J, Bambach B, et al. Hematopoietic engraftment and survival in adult recipients of umbilical cord blood from unrelated donors. N Engl J Med 2001; 344: 1815-22.
13. Isoyama K, Ohnuma K, Kato K, et al. Cord blood transplantation from unrelated donors: A preliminary report from the Japanese Cord Blood Bank Network. Leuk Lymphoma 2003; 44:429-38.
14. Barker JW, Davies SM, DeFor T, et al. Survival after transplantation of unrelated donor umbilical cord blood is comparable to that of human leukocyte antigen-matched unrelated donor bone marrow: Results of a matched-pair analysis. Blood 2001;97:2957-61.
15. Rocha V, Cornish J, Sievers EL, et al. Comparison of outcomes of unrelated bone marrow and umbilical cord blood transplants in children with acute leukemia. Blood 2001;97: 2962-71.
16. Laughlin MJ, Eapen M, Rubinstein P, et al. Outcomes after transplantation of cord blood or bone marrow from unrelated donors in adults with leukemia. N Engl J Med 2004;351:2265-75.
17. Rocha V, Labopin M, Sanz G, et al. Transplants of umbilical cord blood or bone marrow from unrelated donors in adults with acute leukemia. N Engl J Med 2004;351:2276-85.
18. Broxmeyer HE, Hangoc G, Cooper S, et al. Growth characteristics and expansion of human umbilical cord blood and estimation of its potential for transplantation in adults. Proc Natl Acad Sci U S A 1992;89:4109-13.
19. Hows JM, Bradley BA, Marsh JCW, et al. Growth of human umbilical cord blood in long-term haemopoietic cultures. Lancet 1992;340:73-6.
20. Lansdorp PM, Dragowska W, Mayani H. Ontogeny-related changes in proliferative potential of human hematopoietic cells. J Exp Med 1993;178:787-91.
21. Vormoor J, Lapidot T, Pflumio F, et al. Immature human cord blood progenitors engraft and proliferate to high levels in severe combined immunodeficient mice. Blood 1994;83: 2489.
22. Rocha V, Wagner JE, Sobocinski K, et al. Comparison of graft-versus-host disease in children transplanted with HLA identical sibling umbilical cord blood versus HLA identical sibling bone marrow transplant. N Engl J Med 2000;342:1846-54.
23. Beck R, Lam-Po-Tang PR. Comparison of cord blood and adult blood lymphocyte normal ranges: A possible explanation for decreased severity of graft-versus-host disease after cord blood transplantation. Immunol Cell Biol 1994;72:440-4.
24. De La Selle V, Gluckman E, Bruley-Rosset M. Newborn blood can engraft adult mice without inducing graft-versus-host disease across non H-2 antigens. Blood 1996;87:3977-83.
25. D'Arena G, Musto P, Cascavilla N, et al. Flow cytometric characterization of human umbilical cord blood lymphocytes: Immunophenotypic features. Haematologica 1998;83:197-203.
26. Barker JN, Krepski TP, DeFor TE, et al. Searching for unrelated donor hematopoietic stem cells: Availability and speed of umbilical cord blood versus bone marrow. Biol Blood Marrow Transplant 2002;8:257-60.
27. Broxmeyer HE. Biology of cord blood cells and future prospects for enhanced clinical benefit. Cytotherapy 2005;7:209-18.
28. Rubinstein P, Rosenfield RE, Adamson JW, Stevens CE. Stored placental blood for unrelated bone marrow reconstitution. Blood 1993; 81:1679-90.
29. Rocha V, Gluckman E, on behalf of the Eurocord-Netcord Registry and European Blood and Marrow Transplant Group (2009). Improving outcomes of cord blood transplantation: HLA matching, cell dose, and other graft- and transplantation-related factors. Br J Haematol 2009;147:262-74.

30. Miller JP, Chrysler GR, Clay M, McCullough JJ. A survey of cord blood donors: Is intra-labor informed consent acceptable? (abstract) Transfusion 2001;41(Suppl 9S):24S-5S.
31. McCullough J, Clay M, Fautsch S, et al. Proposed policies and procedures for the establishment of a cord blood bank. Blood Cells 1994;20:609-26.
32. Vawter DE, Chrysler G, Clay M, et al. A phased consent policy for cord blood donation. Transfusion 2002;42:1268-74.
33. New York State Council on Human Blood and Transfusion Services. Guidelines for collection, processing and storage of cord blood stem cells. Albany, NY: New York State Department of Health, 1997.
34. NetCord, Foundation for the Accreditation of Cellular Therapy. International standards for cord blood collection, processing, and release for administration. 4th ed. Omaha, NE: FACT, 2010.
35. American Academy of Pediatrics. Cord blood banking for potential future transplantation: Subject review. Pediatrics 1999; 104:116-18.
36. Fontaine M, ed. Standards for cellular therapy product services. 5th ed. Bethesda, MD: AABB, 2011.
37. AMA Council on Ethical and Judicial Affairs. Code of Medical Ethics: E-2.165 Fetal umbilical cord blood. Current opinions with annotations. 1996-1997 ed. Chicago, IL: American Medical Association, 1997.
38. Committee on Obstetric Practice, Committee on Genetics. Routine storage of umbilical cord blood for potential future transplantation. Committee Opinion 183. Washington, DC: American College of Obstetricians and Gynecologists, 1997.
39. Askari SA, Miller J, Clay M, et al. The role of the paternal health history in cord blood banking. Transfusion 2002;42:1275-8.
40. Advisory Council on Blood Stem Cell Transplantation (ACBSCT) consensus recommendations to the Secretary of Health and Human Services (HHS). Full consensus recommendation 6. (September 21, 2009) Washington, DC: DHHS, 2009.
41. Wick M, Clay ME, Eastlund T, et al. Genetic testing of banked umbilical cord blood (letter). Cytotherapy 1999;1:275-8.
42. Lasky LC, Lane TA, Miller JP, et al. In utero or ex utero cord blood collection: Which is better? Transfusion 2002;42:1261-7.
43. Surbek DV, Schonfeld B, Tichelli A, et al. Optimizing cord blood mononuclear cell yield: A randomized comparison of collection before vs after placenta delivery. Bone Marrow Transplant 1998;22:311-12.
44. Solves P, Moraga R, Saucedo E, et al. Comparison between two strategies for umbilical cord blood collection. Bone Marrow Transplant 2003;31:269-73.
45. Chrysler G, McKenna D, Schierman T, et al. Umbilical cord blood banking. In: Broxmeyer HE, ed. Cord blood: Biology, immunology, banking, and clinical transplantation. Bethesda, MD: AABB Press, 2004:219-57.
46. Solves PS, Moraga R, Mirabet V, et al. In utero or ex utero cord blood collection: An unresolved question. Transfusion 2003;43:1174-5.
47. Wong A, Yuen PM, Li K, et al. Cord blood collection before and after placental delivery: Levels of nucleated cells, hematopoietic progenitor cells, leukocyte subpopulations and macroscopic clots. Bone Marrow Transplant 2001;27:133-8.
48. Kurtzberg J, Laughlin M, Graham M, et al. Placental blood is a source of hematopoietic stem cells for transplantation into unrelated recipients. N Engl J Med 1996;335:157-66.
49. Solves P, Mirabet V, Planelles D, et al. Red blood cell depletion with a semiautomated system or hydroxyethyl starch sedimentation for routine cord blood banking: A comparative study. Transfusion 2005;45:867-73.
50. Tsang KS, Li K, Huang DP, et al. Dextran sedimentation in a semi-closed system for cord blood banking of umbilical cord blood. Transfusion 2001;41:344-52.
51. Almici C, Carlo-Stella C, Wagner JE, Rizzoli V. Density separation and cryopreservation of umbilical cord blood cells: Evaluation of recovery in short-and long-term cultures. Acta Haematol 1996;95:171-5.
52. Takahashi TA, Rebulla P, Armitage S, et al. Multi-laboratory evaluation of procedures for reducing the volume of cord blood: Influence on cell recoveries. Cytotherapy 2006;8:254-64.
53. Rubinstein P, Dobrila L, Rosenfield RE, et al. Processing and cryopreservation of placental/umbilical cord blood for unrelated bone marrow reconstitution. Proc Natl Acad Sci U S A 1995;92:10119-22.
54. Alonso JM, Regan DM, Johnson CE, et al. A simple and reliable procedure for cord blood banking, processing, and freezing: St. Louis

and Ohio Cord Blood Bank experiences. Cytotherapy 2001;3:429-33.
55. Food and Drug Administration. Guidance for industry: Minimally manipulated, unrelated allogeneic placental/umbilical cord blood intended for hematopoietic reconstitution for specified indications. (October 2009) Rockville, MD: Office of Communication, Outreach, and Development, 2009.
56. Mayer EA, Hanna K, Gebbie K, eds. Institute of Medicine of the National Academies. Cord blood: Establishing a national hematopoietic stem cell bank program. Washington, DC: The National Academies Press, 2005.
57. Fraser JK, Cairo MS, Wagner E, et al. Cord blood transplantation study (COBLT): Cord blood bank standard operating procedures. J Hematother 1998;7:521-6.
58. Donaldson C, Armitage WJ, Denning-Kendall PA, et al. Optimal cryopreservation of human umbilical cord blood. Bone Marrow Transplant 1996;18:725-31.
59. Hunt CJ, Armitage SE, Pegg DE. Cryopreservation of umbilical cord blood II. Tolerance of CD34+ cells to multimolar dimethylsulfoxide and the effect of cooling rate on recovery after freezing and thawing. Cryobiology 2003;46:76-87.
60. Kobylka P, Ivanyi P, Breur-Vriesendorp BS. Preservation of immunological and colony forming capacities of long-term (15 years) cryopreserved cord blood cells. Transplantation 1998;65:1275-8.
61. Broxmeyer HE. Will iPS cells enhance therapeutic applicability of cord blood cells and banking? Cell Stem Cell 2010;6:21-4.
62. Wada R, Bradford A, Moogk M, et al. Cord blood units collected at a remote site: A collaborative endeavor to collect umbilical cord blood through the Hawaii Cord Blood Bank and store the units at the Puget Sound Blood Center. Transfusion 2004;44:111-18.
63. Hubel A, Carlquist D, Clay M, McCullough J. Short-term liquid storage of umbilical cord blood. Transfusion 2003;43:626-32.
64. Hubel A, Carlquist D, Clay M, McCullough J. Cryopreservation of cord blood after liquid storage. Cytotherapy 2003;5:370-6.
65. Hubel A, Carlquist D, Clay M, McCullough J. Liquid storage, shipment, and cryropreservation of cord blood. Transfusion 2004;44:518-25.
66. Solomon M, Wofford J, Johnson C, et al. Factors influencing cord blood viability assessment before cryopreservation. Transfusion 2010;50:820-30.
67. Food and Drug Administration. Current good tissue practice for human cell, tissue and cellular and tissue-based product establishments; inspection and enforcement; final rule. Docket No. 1997N-484P. Fed Regist 2004;69:68612-88.
68. International Air Transport Association. Dangerous goods regulations. 49th ed. Montreal, Canada: IATA, 2007.
69. Code of federal regulations. Hazardous materials regulations. Title 49, CFR Parts 171-180. Washington, DC: US Government Printing Office, 2010 (revised annually).
70. McCullough J, McKenna D, Kadidlo D, et al. Issues in the quality of umbilical cord blood stem cells for transplantation. Transfusion 2005;45:832-41.
71. McCullough J, McKenna D, Kadidlo D, et al. Mislabeled units of umbilical cord blood detected by a quality assurance program at the transplantation center. Blood 2009;114:1684-8.
72. Nagamura-Inoue T, Shioya M, Sugo M, et al. Wash-out of DMSO does not improve the speed of engraftment of cord blood transplantation: Follow-up of 46 adult patients with units shipped from a single cord blood bank. Transfusion 2003;43:1285-94.
73. Hahn T, Bunworasate U, George MC, et al. Use of nonvolume-reduced (unmanipulated after thawing) umbilical cord blood stem cells for allogeneic transplantation results in safe engraftment. Bone Marrow Transplant 2003;32:145-50.
74. Regan DM, Grunzinger Nelms LM, Wofford JD, et al. Comparison of cord blood product thawing methods on cell recovery and progenitor integrity (abstract). Cytotherapy 2005;7(Suppl 1):76.
75. McKenna D, Wagner J, McCullough J. Umbilical cord blood infusions are associated with mild reactions and are overall well-tolerated (abstract). Cytotherapy 2003;5:438.
76. Rowley SD, Anderson GL. Effect of DMSO exposure without cryopreservation on hematopoietic progenitor cells. Bone Marrow Transplant 1993;11:389-93.
77. Laroche V, McKenna D, Moroff G, et al. Cell loss and recovery in umbilical cord blood processing: A comparison of post-thaw and post-wash samples. Transfusion 2005;45:1909-16.

78. Davis JM, Rowley SD, Braine HG, et al. Clinical toxicity of cryopreserved bone marrow graft infusion. Blood 1990;75:781-6.
79. Stroncek DF, Fautsch SK, Lasky LC, et al. Adverse reactions in patients transfused with cryopreserved marrow. Transfusion 1991;31: 521-6.
80. Bornstein R, Flores AI, Montalban MA, et al. A modified cord blood collection method achieves sufficient cell levels for transplantation in most adult patients. Stem Cells 2005; 23:324-34.
81. M-Reboredo N, Diaz A, Castro A, Villaescusa RG. Collection, processing, and cryopreservation of umbilical cord blood for unrelated transplantation. Bone Marrow Transplant 2000;26:1263-70.
82. Lecchi L, Ratti I, Lazzari L, et al. Reasons for discard of umbilical cord blood units before cryopreservation. Transfusion 2000; 40:122-4.
83. Food and Drug Administration. Proposed approach to regulation of cellular and tissue-based products. Docket. No. 97N-0068. (February 27, 1997) Rockville, MD: Office of Communication, Outreach, and Development, 1997.
84. Food and Drug Administration. Eligibility determination for donors of human cells, tissues, and cellular and tissue-based products; final rule. Docket No. 1997N-0484S. Fed Regist 2004;69:29786-834.
85. Gee AP. Transplantation and the Food and Drug Administration: How will it affect your program? Cancer Res Ther Contr 1999;9:171-6.
86. Food and Drug Administration. FDA approach to the regulation of hematopoietic progenitor/stem cells derived from cord blood. Presentation by WJ Hartzler at the Workshop of the Institute of Medicine Committee for establishing a National Cord Blood Stem Cell Bank Program, Washington, DC, June 2, 2004.
87. Food and Drug Administration. Establishment registration and listing for manufacturers of human cellular and tissue-based products; final rule. Docket No. 97N-484R. Fed Regist 2001;66:5447-69.
88. Food and Drug Administration. Request for proposed standards for unrelated allogeneic peripheral and placental/umbilical cord blood hematopoietic stem/progenitor cell products; request for comments. Fed Regist 1998;63: 2985.
89. Food and Drug Administration. Draft guidance for industry and FDA staff: Investigational new drug applications (INDs) for minimally manipulated, unrelated allogeneic placental/umbilical cord blood intended for hematopoietic reconstitution for specified indications. (October 2009) Rockville, MD: Office of Communication, Outreach, and Development, 2009.
90. Devine SM, Lazarus HM, Emerson SG. Clinical application of hematopoietic progenitor cell expansion: Current status and future prospects. Bone Marrow Transplant 2003;31:241-52.
91. Lam AC, Li K, Zhang XB, et al. Preclinical ex vivo expansion of cord blood hematopoietic stem and progenitor cells: Duration of culture; the media, serum supplements, and growth factors used; and engraftment in NOD/SCID mice. Transfusion 2001;41:1567-76.
92. Madlambayan GJ, Rogers I, Purpura KA, et al. Clinically relevant expansion of hematopoietic stem cells with conserved function in a single-use, closed-system bioprocess. Biol Blood Marrow Transplant 2006;12:1020-30.
93. Pecora AL, Stiff P, Jennis A, et al. Prompt and durable engraftment in two older adult patients with high risk chronic myelogenous leukemia (CML) using ex vivo expanded and unmanipulated unrelated umbilical cord blood. Bone Marrow Transplant 2000;25:797-9.
94. Shpall EJ, Quinones R, Giller R, et al. Transplantation of ex vivo expanded cord blood. Biol Blood Marrow Transplant 2002;8:368-76.
95. Hofmeister CC, Zhang J, Knight KL, et al. Ex vivo expansion of umbilical cord blood stem cells for transplantation: Growing knowledge from the hematopoietic niche. Bone Marrow Transplant 2007;39:11-23.
96. Robinson SN, Ng J, Niu T, et al. Superior ex vivo cord blood expansion following co-culture with bone marrow-derived mesenchymal stem cells. Bone Marrow Transplant 2006;37: 359-66.
97. Barker JN, Weisdorf DJ, DeFor TE, et al. Transplantation of 2 partially HLA-matched umbilical cord blood units to enhance engraftment in adults with hematologic malignancy. Blood 2005;105:1343-7.
98. Kim DW, Chung YJ, Kim TJ, et al. Cotransplantation of third-party mesenchymal stromal cells can alleviate single-donor predominance and increase engraftment from double cord transplantation. Blood 2004;103:1941-8.

99. Nauta AJ, Kruisselbrink AB, Lurvink E, et al. Enhanced engraftment of umbilical cord blood-derived stem cells in NOD/SCID mice by cotransplantation of a second unrelated cord blood unit. Exp Hematol 2005;33:1249-56.
100. McKenna D, Sumstad D, Bostrom N, et al. GMP-production of natural killer cells for immunotherapy: A six year single institution experience. Transfusion 2007;47:520-8.
101. Miller JS, Soignier Y, Panoskaltsis-Mortari A, et al. Successful adoptive transfer and in vivo expansion of human haploidentical NK cells in cancer patients. Blood 2005;105:3051-7.
102. Ruggeri L, Capanni M, Urbani E, et al. Effectiveness of donor natural killer cell alloreactivity in mismatched hematopoietic transplants. Science 2002;295:2097-100.
103. Gardiner CM, O'Meara A, Reen DJ. Differential cytotoxicity of cord blood and bone marrow-derived natural killer cells. Blood 1998;91:207-13.
104. Dalle J-H, Menezes J, Wagner E, et al. Characterization of cord blood natural killer cells: Implications for transplantation and neonatal infections. Pediatr Res 2005;57:649-55.
105. Fehervari Z, Sakaguchi S. CD4+ T regs and immune control. J Clin Invest 2004;114:1209-17.
106. Takahata Y, Nomura A, Takada H, et al. CD25+CD4+ T cells in human cord blood: An immunoregulatory subset with naïve phenotype and specific expression of forkhead box p3 (Foxp3) gene. Exp Hematol 2004;32:622-9.
107. Godfrey WR, Spoden DJ, Ge YG, et al. Cord blood CD4+CD25+-derived T regulatory cell lines express FoxP3 protein and manifest potent suppressor function. Blood 2005;105:750-8.
108. Porter SB, Liu B, Rogosheske J, et al. Suppressor function of umbilical cord blood-derived CD4+CD25+ T regulatory cells exposed to graft-versus-host disease drugs. Transplantation 2006;82:23-9.
109. Brunstein C, Hippen KL, McKenna DH, et al. Adoptive transfer of umbilical cord blood (UCB)-derived regulatory T cells (Tregs) to recipients of nonmyeloablative unrelated double UCB transplantation (abstract). Blood 2009;114:513.
110. Banchereau J, Palucka AK. Dendritic cells as therapeutic vaccines against cancer. Nat Rev Immunol 2005;5:296-306.
111. Mohamadzadeh M, Luftig R. Dendritic cells: In the forefront of immunopathogenesis and vaccine development—a review. J Immune Based Ther Vaccines 2004;2:1.
112. Nestle FO, Farkas A, Conrad C. Dendritic-cell-based therapeutic vaccination against cancer. Curr Opin Immunol 2005;17:163-9.
113. Banchereau J, Palucka AK, Dhodapkar M, et al. Immune and clinical responses in patients with metastatic melanoma to CD34+ progenitor-derived dendritic cell vaccine. Cancer Res 2001;61:6451-8.
114. Moldenhauer A, Nociari MM, Dias S, et al. Optimized culture conditions for the generation of dendritic cells from peripheral blood monocytes. Vox Sang 2003;84:228-36.
115. Sorg RV, Ozcan Z, Brefort T, et al. Clinical-scale generation of dendritic cells in a closed system. J Immunother 2003;26:374-83.
116. Wong ECC, Maher VE, Hines K, et al. Development of a clinical-scale method for generation of dendritic cells from PBMC for use in cancer immunotherapy. Cytotherapy 2001;3:19-29.
117. Borras FE, Matthews NC, Patel R, Navarrete C. Dendritic cells can be successfully generated from CD34+ cord blood cells in the presence of autologous cord blood serum. Bone Marrow Transplant 2000;26: 371-6.
118. Hsu AKW, Kerr BM, Jones KL, et al. RNA loading of leukemic antigens into cord blood-derived dendritic cells for immunotherapy. Biol Blood Marrow Transplant 2006;12:855-67.
119. Kurlander RJ, Tawab A, Fan Y, et al. A functional comparison of mature human dendritic cells prepared in fluorinated ethylene-propylene bags or polystyrene flasks. Transfusion 2006;46:1494-504.
120. Erices A, Conget P, Minguell J. Mesenchymal progenitor cells in human umbilical cord blood. Br J Haematol 2000;109:235-42.
121. Goodwin H, Bicknese A, Chien S, et al. Multilineage differentiation activity by cells isolated from umbilical cord blood: Expression of bone, fat, and neural markers. Biol Blood Marrow Transplant 2001;7:581-8.
122. Mareschi K, Biasin E, Piacibello W, et al. Isolation of human mesenchymal stem cells: Bone marrow versus umbilical cord blood. Haematologica 2001;86:1099-100.
123. Bieback K, Kern S, Kluter H, Eichler H. Critical parameters for the isolation of mesenchymal stem cells from umbilical cord blood. Stem Cells 2004;22:625-34.
124. Pittenger MF, Mackay AM, Beck SC, et al. Multilineage potential of adult human mesenchymal stem cells. Science 1999;284:143-7.

125. Wang H-S, Hung S-H, Peng S-T, et al. Mesenchymal stem cells in the Wharton's jelly of the human umbilical cord. Stem Cells 2004;22:1330-7.

126. Lee OK, Kuo TK, Chen WM, et al. Isolation of multipotent mesenchymal stem cells from umbilical cord blood. Blood 2004;103:1669-75.

127. Kogler G, Sensken S, Airey J, et al. A new human somatic stem cell from placental cord blood with intrinsic pluripotent differentiation potential. J Exp Med 2004;200:123-35.

128. Berger MJ, Adams SD, Tigges BM, et al. Differentiation of umbilical cord blood-derived multilineage progenitor cells into respiratory epithelial cells. Cytotherapy 2006;8:480-7.

Chapter 32

◆32

Human Tissue Allografts and the Hospital Transfusion Service

◆

Lance D. Trainor, MD, and Rita A. Reik, MD

SURGICAL USE OF human tissue allografts (ie, allografts are tissues transferred between individuals of the same species) has grown dramatically in recent years. Every year, member organizations of the American Association of Tissue Banks (AATB) recover tissue from more than 30,000 donors and provide over 2 million tissue grafts for transplantation.[1] Many surgical specialties use human tissue, including orthopedics, plastic surgery, urology, neurosurgery, sports medicine, trauma, and reconstructive surgery. A growing number of increasingly sophisticated grafts are being produced by tissue suppliers to meet clinical needs. There is no regulatory requirement for the activities of a tissue-dispensing service to be managed in any particular department within the hospital or by any specific individual. However, because the tasks of ordering, receiving, storing, dispensing (issuing), tracking, tracing, investigating adverse events, and managing recalls are functions common to the transfusion service and the tissue-dispensing service, the AABB recommends a centralized model located within the transfusion service.[2]

TISSUE TRANSPLANTATION

Next to blood for transfusion, bone, tendons, and corneas are the most frequently used human tissues in the clinical setting. Numerous other tissues are selected for transplantation based on intrinsic qualities that meet the surgeon's functional requirements for the patient.[3] Cadaveric donors supply the vast majority of musculoskeletal, cardiovascular, ocular, and skin allografts. Tissues, including bones, tendons, cartilage, skin, corneas, veins, dura mater, fascia, and heart valves, are procured within 24 hours of death, after appropriate donor consent is obtained.[4] Aseptic surgical retrieval techniques minimize contamination with microorganisms from the donor and the surrounding environment.

Tissue retrieval agencies rely on multiple sources of information to determine donor eligibility, including social histories provided by next of kin, available medical records, autopsy reports, and physical assessment reports. These records, in addition to the circumstances of death, assist the tissue bank medical director in determining donor suitability. High-risk ac-

Lance D. Trainor, MD, Medical Director, Community Blood Centers of Florida, Lauderhill, Florida, and Rita A. Reik, MD, Medical Director, Transfusion Medicine Services, Memorial Healthcare System, Hollywood, Florida
The authors have disclosed no conflicts of interest.

tivities that may increase the chances of infectious disease transmission are evaluated and may lead to rejection of the donor. Allografts, similar to blood components, are released for transplantation only after testing for relevant communicable diseases is performed and determined to be acceptable (see Table 32-1).

Background and Definitions

Human tissue banking in the United States started nearly 60 years ago with the US Navy Tissue Bank. By the late 1990s, use of tissue allografts had become commonplace. From its original function of providing crude pieces of bone and soft tissues fashioned from cadaveric donors, the tissue banking industry has evolved into a highly innovative, continuously changing field. Collaboration between tissue bank scientists/engineers and end-user surgeons has resulted in a wide variety of tissue grafts that are lifesaving or life enhancing. Today's allografts may be processed to remove viable cells or preserved in such a way as to maintain cellular viability. They can be derived from a single tissue or multiple tissues acting as a functional unit. In some cases, processed human tissue may be combined with other biocompatible agents to achieve desired handling and functional characteristics. Bone allografts developed for spine surgery can be meticulously machined for compatibility with surgical instrumentation.

Autografts are tissues implanted into the same individual from whom they were removed. Bone surgically removed from a patient's ilium, shaped to desired dimensions, and immediately reimplanted into the vertebral disc space of the same patient is an example. The autograft bone is used to promote fusion of adjacent vertebrae, providing stability and relief from the pain of degenerative disc disease or trauma. Advantages of autografts are reduced disease transmission risks and ready availability of graft material. Disadvantages include morbidity associated with an additional surgical procedure for the patient, including pain and potential surgical-site infection. Additionally, the quality (eg, the strength) and quantity of the autologous tissue may not be adequate for the intended use, and removal of the patient's tissue may adversely affect function at the site from which it was removed.

Isografts, which are tissues transferred between genetically identical individuals such as identical twins, are uncommon. *Xenografts* are tissues that are transplanted from one species to another; a growing number of medical products are being developed from processed nonhuman animal tissues. Finally, *allografts,* as previously mentioned, are tissues transferred between individuals of the same species; the repertoire of such products distributed by tissue banks continues to expand.

Tissue Processing

Tissue processing is performed using aseptic technique in a bacteriologically controlled and climate-controlled environment.[5] After tissue

TABLE 32-1. Required Infectious Disease Testing for Tissue Grafts

Infectious Agent	Test Performed
Hepatitis B (HBV)	Hepatitis B surface antigen Hepatitis B core antibody (IgM and IgG)
Hepatitis C (HCV)	Hepatitis C antibody HCV nucleic acid testing
Human immunodeficiency virus (HIV)	HIV-1 and HIV-2 antibodies HIV-1 nucleic acid testing
Human T-cell lymphotropic virus (HTLV)	HTLV-I and HTLV-II antibodies*
Syphilis	Nontreponemal or treponemal-specific assay

*Required of tissues rich in viable leukocytes.

is procured from the deceased donor, grafts are debrided of extraneous soft tissue and cut to specification. In some cases more than 100 grafts can be produced from a single donor's gift. Increasingly popular precision bone grafts, including a growing array of spinal implants, are now crafted using sophisticated computer-aided cutting devices to meet exacting specifications required by modern surgical implantation instrumentation. These precisely milled allografts allow surgeons to operate quickly and efficiently. During the processing of the allograft, various solutions, including antibiotics, alcohols, and surfactants may be used to reduce the risk of bacterial contamination and to remove unnecessary lipids and extraneous biologic material. Depending on the type of graft, sterilization may or may not be possible; grafts containing viable cells cannot be subjected to sterilization processes without destroying cellular integrity. Ionizing radiation is the most frequently used sterilization technique; cobalt 60, electron beam, and X-ray are common sources of ionizing radiation. Ethylene oxide and various proprietary methods of tissue sterilization are also used by tissue processors.

Several methods of tissue preservation are available for long-term storage of human allografts, including freezing and freeze-drying (lyophilization). Both processes, similar to irradiation, are destructive to cell viability. The integrity of processed tissue can be enhanced through cryopreservation, a process in which tissues are frozen in a protective medium at a steady, controlled rate. Cryprotectants, such as glycerol or dimethylsulfoxide (DMSO), minimize cell damage caused by cell shrinkage and intracellular ice formation during the freezing process. Fresh, refrigerated grafts can be provided when cellular viability is particularly important, as with osteochondral allografts, where preservation of living chondrocytes is essential. These grafts in particular, which consist of an intact articular surface with associated soft tissue and bone, are being increasingly used for treating traumatic and degenerative joint conditions.

Clinical Use of Allografts

Allografts are used in a variety of surgical procedures.[6] Cadaveric human bone can be used to replace bone lost to degenerative disease, trauma, or malignancy. Although synthetic bone substitutes are available, allograft has specific advantages. Allogeneic bone is both osteoconductive and osteoinductive. In vivo, it can act as a scaffold that allows recipient capillary growth into the graft (osteoconductivity) and provides stimulation for the production of new bone (osteoinductivity) by exposing the patient's osteogenic progenitor cells to bone morphogeneic proteins (BMPs), a collection of growth factors found within bone that induce the formation of new bone. The intended result is creeping substitution, a process in which bone remodeling occurs through osteoclastic resorption of the implanted tissue and osteoblastic generation of new bone.

A variety of human tissues are used for transplantation.[7] Examples are listed in Table 32-2. Bone-tendon (Achilles tendon) or bone-tendon-bone (patellar-tibia tendon) grafts are commonly used for anterior cruciate ligament (ACL) repair. The allograft is implanted such that the tendon spans the joint space while the bone provides an anchor into the femur and/or tibia. Remodeling of the graft occurs over time with ingrowth of the recipient's own cells, resulting in restored joint stability.

Bone subjected to acid demineralization can be used alone or suspended in a biologically compatible carrier and applied to exposed bone surfaces. BMPs present in the demineralized bone product stimulate osteogenesis, fusion of adjacent bones, and healing. Newly formed bone provides structural support that can repair damage caused by osteoporosis, malignancy, or trauma.

The protective barrier of cadaveric skin can be used as a temporary wound dressing for severe burns to protect the underlying tissues from dehydration and environmental pathogens. Further, human skin can be processed to remove cellular elements, producing a collagen matrix sheet used in a variety of surgical settings, including hernia repair and soft tissue reconstruction. This acellular dermal

TABLE 32-2. Examples of Human Allograft Clinical Uses

Allograft Tissue	Surgical Use
Bone (cortical, corticocancellous, cancellous)	Skeletal reconstruction Spinal fusion Dental implant placement
Bone-tendon (Achilles tendon) Bone-tendon-bone (patellar tendon) Tendon (semitendinosus, gracilis, peroneus longus)	Anterior cruciate ligament repair Posterior cruciate ligament repair Rotator cuff restoration Biceps tendon rupture repair
Cardiac valves (aortic and pulmonary)	Valvular insufficiency correction Congenital cardiac defect repair
Cartilage (costal)	Facial reconstruction
Cornea	Keratoconus Traumatic scarring reversal Corneal ulcer excision
Decellularized skin	Hernia repair Soft tissue reconstruction Gingival restoration
Demineralized bone	Dental implant placement Spinal fusion
Dura mater	Dural defect/cerebrospinal leak repair
Fascia lata	Soft tissue reconstruction Pelvic floor support
Meniscus	Meniscus replacement
Osteoarticular/osteochondral graft (bone and joint cartilage)	Joint restoration
Pericardium	Dura patch Eyelid reconstruction Soft tissue reconstruction
Skin	Protection of underlying tissues after severe burns
Veins/arteries	Coronary artery bypass grafting Tissue revascularization Aneurysm repair Dialysis access shunts

matrix provides a scaffold for vascular ingrowth, cellular incorporation, and ultimately structural repair of the damaged tissue.

Cadaveric tissues are commonly used in ophthalmic surgery to treat a variety of ocular conditions. Thinning, scarring, or clouding of the cornea secondary to trauma, infection, or corneal diseases such as Fuchs dystrophy may necessitate a corneal transplant. In the most common procedure, penetrating keratoplasty, the ophthalmologist excises a circular section of the center of the cornea (called a button) and replaces it with donated cadaveric cornea. Scleral allografts have also been used in a variety of ophthalmic surgical procedures to treat glaucoma, scleral buckles, and traumatic deformities.

Although bone and soft tissue allografts can provoke an immune response in the recipient, such responses are generally not clinically significant, presumably because of a lack of residual cellular material in processed grafts.[8] As a result, it is not necessary to match most allografts to the recipient with respect to HLA or ABO type. Possible exceptions include veins, for which some clinicians request ABO compatibility, and frozen, unprocessed bone allografts containing marrow, red cells, or both. Published reports have documented the development of Rh(D), Fy(a), and Jk(b) antibodies in recipients following transplantation of unprocessed bone allografts.[9] Hospital transfusion services should be cognizant of these reports: if unprocessed bone is to be used for an Rh(D)-negative female of childbearing potential, future offspring may be at risk for developing hemolytic disease of the fetus and newborn, and Rh Immune Globulin prophylaxis should be considered if the Rh type of the allograft donor is positive or unknown.

Disease Transmission through Tissue Transplantation

Recipient safety is of paramount concern in tissue transplantation. Rare, sporadic transmission of infectious diseases, including, but not limited to, human immunodeficiency virus (HIV), hepatitis C virus, hepatitis B virus, and Creutzfeldt-Jakob disease (CJD) have been documented following tissue implantation.[10-13] In addition, bacterial and fungal infections from allografts have been associated with significant morbidity and death.[14-16] Possible sources of contaminants include donor flora as well as the recovery and processing environments and facilities. Fortunately, advances in screening, testing, and processing methodologies have led to improved safety profiles for current human tissue products.

REGULATIONS AND STANDARDS

In the United States, regulatory requirements exist for establishments that manufacture human tissues for transplantation such as tissue banks and tissue distribution intermediaries, which are establishments or persons engaged in the recovery, screening, testing, labeling, processing, storage, and/or distribution of human tissues for clinical use. These entities manufacture what the Food and Drug Administration (FDA) classifies as human cells, tissues, and cellular and tissue-based products (HCT/Ps), and they are the sources of tissue products for the transplanting surgeon. Exemptions from these regulatory requirements exist for tissue dispensing services, as described below.

Tissue Banks and Tissue Distribution Intermediaries

The FDA regulates the activities of tissue banks and tissue distribution intermediaries under the applicable sections of the *Code of Federal Regulations* (CFR): 21 CFR 1270 and 1271.[17] Tissue dispensing institutions such as hospitals, dental offices, or surgical centers that provide and use tissue within their own organizations are not subject to this oversight except under specific circumstances (ie, redistribution of allografts or autografts to affiliated institutions located at a different address, or sterilization of autografts). The three rules of 21 CFR 1271 concern 1) registration of tissue bank establishments, 2) donor eligibility, and 3) good tissue practice (GTP) related to handling HCT/Ps. Compliance with current GTP is required of tissue banks and tissue distribution intermediaries, as these practices promote optimum quality of the final tissue product.

Tissue Dispensing Services (Hospitals and Medical Facilities)

As mentioned above, 21 CFR 1270 and 1271 do not apply to facilities that only receive, store, and dispense tissue to a requesting surgeon in the same organization and engage in no further manufacturing or redistribution of the tissue product. However, voluntary accrediting organizations such as The Joint Commission, the AABB, the AATB, the College of American Pathologists (CAP) and the Association of peri-Operative Registered Nurses (AORN) all publish standards that apply to the practices of a tissue dispensing service.[5,18-22] Location within a hospital or medical facility and the scope of responsibilities of the tissue dispensing service will dictate applicable standards. Standards are updated regularly; therefore, periodic review of the most recent versions is required to ensure ongoing compliance.

The Joint Commission specifically requires that organizations assign oversight responsibility for a tissue program, use standardized procedures in tissue handling, maintain traceability of all tissues, and have a process for investigating and reporting adverse events. The AABB has provided guidance for handling tissue products that parallels that for blood, including standards relating to functions of a quality system, process control, and medical director oversight. CAP standards focus on centralization of tissue dispensing services, tracing tissue from donor to final disposition, and appropriate temperature storage. Qualifying suppliers (vendor qualification), tracking problems (adverse event investigation), and ensuring adherence to documented procedures are also obligatory. All three organizations have overlapping and similar standards that promote safety and quality of allograft transplantation.

Tissue Suppliers

The AATB and the Eye Bank Association of America (EBAA) are dedicated to ensuring that human tissues intended for transplantation are safe, of high quality, and available to the community. AATB's scope of standards includes all aspects of tissue banking, distribution, and dispensing services.[5] EBAA's scope encompasses all aspects of eye banking.[23] Membership is voluntary. Accreditation is based on verified compliance with established standards and periodic review. Both organizations serve as scientific and educational resources for professionals working in the field. Each offers certification for tissue or eye bank personnel through training and written examination. A tissue dispensing service may find AATB and EBAA accreditation of a supplier to be valuable information in performing a supplier qualification assessment.

HOSPITAL TISSUE SERVICES

The Blood Transfusion Service as a Tissue Dispensing Service

As previously mentioned, there is no requirement for a tissue dispensing service to be managed in any particular department or by any specific individual. The AABB recommends a centralized model within the transfusion service for the following reasons. More than any other department within the hospital, the transfusion service has expertise in providing an adequate supply of human-derived products that are perishable, potentially infectious, and sometimes in short supply and that require temperature-controlled storage. The tasks of ordering, receiving, storing, distributing (issuing), tracking, and tracing products as well as investigating adverse events, including complaints, recalls, and look-backs, are activities that are common to the transfusion service and tissue dispensing service.

RESPONSIBILITY FOR HOSPITAL-BASED TISSUE SERVICES

In the past, the handling of human allografts within US hospitals was unregulated, and responsibilities were not always clearly identified or delineated. Improvements have occurred in recent years as a result of increased oversight through requirements by standards-setting organizations. Since 2005, The Joint Commission has required hospitals under its purview to assign oversight responsibility for the acquisition, receipt, storage, and issuance of tissues. The Joint Commission allows an organization to have a centralized or decentralized process to manage these activities. In the centralized model, one department is responsible for all of the aforementioned tasks. In the decentralized model, multiple departments are responsible. In either model, designated oversight is required to coordinate tissue-related activities and ensure standardization of practices throughout the organization.

Written Standard Operating Procedures

Hospital tissue services must have written procedures (printed or electronic) for all functions pertaining to the acquisition, receipt, storage, issuance, and tracing of tissue grafts, as well as procedures for investigating adverse events and handling recalls.[20] Manufacturers' instructions should be incorporated into standard operating procedures (SOPs). Tissue services should also have a process for the development, validation, review, approval, and distribution of staff training and, certification of competency regarding new SOPs. Changes to existing procedures must follow the same process. When the blood bank or transfusion service is responsible for tissue, the AABB requires that the medical director approve medical and technical policies and procedures. In certain clinical situations, the handling of tissues may vary from SOP instructions. Such variances require justification, documentation, and approval by the medical director on a case-by-case basis.[20(p2)]

Tissue Supplier Qualification and Certification

In contrast to blood banks, tissue processors and distributors often specialize in providing particular types of products (grafts). As a result, a hospital tissue dispensing service may need to acquire human tissue products from numerous vendors, whereas the transfusion service generally obtains blood products from one or possibly two providers.

Tissue suppliers should be selected based on ability to reliably provide high-quality tissues that meet expectations for tissue availability, safety, and effectiveness. The hospital tissue service should establish certain minimal criteria for qualification of prospective suppliers. According to The Joint Commission, tissue supplier requirements must include evidence of FDA registration and state licensure, where state licensure is required. A written process for review and approval of suppliers is expected and should contain the elements listed in Table 32-3. A list of approved suppliers should be developed and maintained that includes documentation of each supplier's qualifications and certifications. Hospital tissue services should establish procedures to receive or monitor evidence of compliance or noncompliance, such as reviewing FDA warning letters and tissue allograft recalls or market withdrawals. Accreditation by AATB and/or EBAA may be desirable.

The qualification information for each supplier should be initially and annually reviewed and approved by the hospital tissue service director or medical director. At the review, the performance of suppliers in meeting the transplant facility's needs should be evaluated. Each year, it should be determined that the supplier remains registered with the FDA; AATB and/or EBAA accreditations may also be reconfirmed. FDA web postings should be viewed for information related to closures, recalls, or MedWatch reports. FDA inspection reports for tissue processors can be requested from the FDA through the Freedom of Information Act. Further use of a particular tissue supplier should depend in part on approval by the tissue service's director.

Additional requirements for tissue suppliers may be set in consultation with the hospital medical staff and transplanting surgeons. Complaints from surgeons concerning the supplier's tissue should be reviewed, along with any reports of infection possibly caused by transplanted allografts. Hospitals may consider using a medical staff committee to provide oversight in approving tissue suppliers.

Inspection of Incoming Tissue Grafts

Before being placed in storage, tissue allografts must be inspected upon receipt from a tissue supplier.[20(p8)] Incoming allografts must be inspected to ensure that the tissue container is

TABLE 32-3. Vendor Qualification Criteria for Human Allografts

Criterion	Documentation*/Performance
FDA registration†	Current Form FDA 3356
FDA inspection findings	Form FDA 483 findings, if any Warning letters and responses, if any
Voluntary accreditation, if available	Current AATB accreditation for tissues Current EBAA accreditation for ocular tissues
State license and registration if required by state law (varies from state to state)†	State license and registration (reviewed annually)
Reliable supply of needed tissues	Adequate notification of tissue shortages Ability to meet special requests Suitable length of time between receipt and expiration date
Transparency of the organization	Willingness to provide information regarding donor selection and tissue processing
Medical consultation	Accessibility of the tissue supplier's medical director
Quality assurance resources	Accessibility of the tissue supplier's quality assurance staff
New or trial tissue product support	Willingness to provide information on newly released tissue products
Professionalism of sales representatives	Representatives seek approval through designated channels before promoting or providing tissue within the hospital

*Copies acceptable.

†Required by The Joint Commission.

FDA = Food and Drug Administration; AATB = American Association of Tissue Banks; EBAA = Eye Bank Association of America.

intact and that the label is complete, appears accurate, and is adequately affixed and legible before acceptance into inventory. The Joint Commission requires that hospitals verify package integrity and ensure that the transport temperature was controlled and acceptable. Inspection of the shipping container for evidence of residual coolant (eg, wet ice for refrigerated grafts, dry ice for frozen grafts) may be useful to assess that the required tissue-specific storage environment was maintained during transportation. Many distributors use "validated" shipping containers that are tested to maintain required temperatures for a specified period of time. In this case, the receiver of the tissue simply needs to check that there is no damage to the container and that it has been received and opened within the specified time frame. Tissues requiring "ambient temperature" (defined as the temperature of the immediate environment) for storage and shipping, do not need to have the temperature verified upon receipt. However, tissues requiring "room temperature" storage should have temperatures verified and documented if the manufacturer has specified a temperature storage range in the package insert.[24] Regardless of the shipping and storage requirements, the incoming inspection results should be recorded along with the date, time, and name of the staff person conducting the inspection.

Tissue Allograft Storage

Like blood components, tissue grafts are stored under various conditions (see Table 32-4). Storage conditions depend on the nature of the tissue, method of preservation, and type of packaging. Hospital tissue services should store tissue allografts according to the processor's instructions in the allograft's package insert. Storage devices can include "ambient" and/or room-temperature cabinets, refrigerators, mechanical freezers, and liquid-nitrogen storage units. Continuous temperature monitoring of storage in refrigerators and freezers is required. Room-temperature storage equipment need only be monitored if required by the package insert for a particular allograft. Storage equipment should have functional alarms and emergency backup capability. Lyophilized (freeze-dried) tissues whose package insert instructions specify that they may be stored at "ambient temperature or colder" can tolerate a very broad range of temperatures and do not require monitoring.[25] Storage SOPs should address steps to be taken in case of temperature excursions from allowable limits or in the event of equipment or power failure. Emergency backup alternatives, including arrangements for temporary storage, should be detailed in written procedures, and staff should be appropriately trained.

Tissue Allograft Traceability and Record-Keeping

Proper management of human allografts requires that the hospital tissue service maintain comprehensive records of all steps of tissue handling, documented as they occur. Records should be accurate, legible, and indelible. They should identify the staff involved, the date, and the time when the tissue is accepted, prepared or processed. Records should be detailed and provide a clear history of actions performed while handling the tissue. Such records provide evidence that the SOPs were

TABLE 32-4. Storage Conditions for Commonly Transplanted Human Tissue[6]

Human Tissue	Storage Conditions	Temperature
Cardiovascular	Frozen, cryopreserved	–100 C or colder
Dura	Lyophilized	Ambient
Eye/cornea	Refrigerated	2-8 C
Sclera	Room temperature	Ambient
Musculoskeletal	Refrigerated	1-10 C
	Frozen, cryopreserved and non-cryopreserved (temporary storage less than 6 months)	–20 C to –40 C
	Frozen, cryopreserved and non-cryopreserved (long-term storage)	–40 C or colder
	Lyophilized	Ambient
Reproductive	Frozen, cryopreserved	LN_2 (liquid or vapor phase)
Skin	Refrigerated	1-10 C
	Frozen, cryopreserved	–40 C or colder
Soft tissue (eg, parathyroid)	Frozen, cryopreserved	Not established

followed and link the specific tissue allograft to the patient who received it. Tissue service records need to permit bidirectional traceability of all tissues from the donor and tissue supplier to the recipient(s) or other final disposition, including the occasional discard of tissue because of damage or other untoward effect on package integrity, opening of the tissue package in the operating room without use, or expiration. Records should be retained for 10 years after distribution, transplantation, discard, or expiration of tissue (whichever is latest).

Adequate record-keeping promotes transplantation safety by linking allograft and recipient. Documentation of tissue supplier, unique numeric or alphanumeric identifier(s), expiration date, and recipient name must be maintained for all tissue used.[20(p76)] The tissue supplier is responsible for ensuring traceability from donor to the hospital/consignee, and the hospital/consignee is responsible for ensuring traceability from receipt of the tissue to the recipient or other final disposition. If, for example, a tissue allograft is associated with infection in a recipient, other recipients receiving tissue grafts from the same donor can be evaluated for transplant-related infection only if traceability is maintained.

Tissue usage information cards supplied with the allograft by the tissue bank should be completed and returned. The information helps maintain traceability of the allograft and expedites tissue withdrawals or recalls if necessary.

Possible Tissue Allograft-Associated Adverse Events

Recognition and Reporting

Surgeons recognize that tissue allografts have risks that must be balanced with clinical benefits. Human allografts have been associated with bacterial, viral, fungal and prion transmissions. Additionally, allografts may have structural defects leading to unsuccessful outcomes sometimes as a result of donor selection or processing issues. Transplant surgeons play a critical role in the identification of allograft-associated adverse outcomes and need to immediately notify the hospital tissue service when such events are suspected. It should not be assumed that a tissue graft is free of microbial contamination because it is packaged in a sealed container or has been labeled as sterile. Viral infections can remain asymptomatic for weeks to months following surgery, and history of receipt of an allograft should be considered in the risk factor evaluation for patients that develop such infections. Prompt notification about the adverse event enables the hospital tissue service's staff and medical director to investigate cause, report the event to the tissue supplier, and institute corrective action. Early notification may prevent an untoward outcome for other recipients of an allograft from the same donor.

Investigation

Hospital tissue services are required to have procedures for the timely investigation of infections suspected to be caused by a tissue allograft. Since 2005, The Joint Commission has required that allograft-transmitted infections and other severe adverse events be reported by the hospital to the tissue supplier. Since May 25, 2005, the FDA has required tissue processors or tissue suppliers that recover, process, store, label, package, or distribute tissue to investigate and report adverse events to the FDA.[17]

Upon notification of an adverse event associated with a tissue allograft, the hospital tissue service should open an investigation. The tissue supplier should be promptly notified. Investigation of infections and other adverse events requires cooperation between the tissue dispensing service, clinicians, and the tissue supplier. Consultation with the hospital infection control department or an infectious disease specialist may be beneficial. Documents pertaining to the investigation and a final report identifying any corrective action, reviewed and approved by the tissue service's director, should be maintained in an adverse event file.

Although it is not mandatory for hospital tissue services to report tissue-related adverse events to the FDA, if there is reason to believe that a patient's infection was from a contaminated tissue allograft, hospitals can report this by using MedWatch, the FDA's voluntary reporting program. Similarly, the transplant surgeon can voluntarily report any infectious adverse event deemed to be associated with allograft use through the Medwatch system at http://www.fda.gov/medwatch or at http://www.hhs. gov/forms.

State departments of health have lists of communicable diseases that require reporting when the diseases are newly diagnosed. When there is a new diagnosis of HIV, hepatitis, or CJD in a tissue allograft recipient and the allograft is suspected to be a possible source, the state department of health should be notified by the patient's physician or by the director or medical director of the hospital tissue service. An epidemiologic investigation may be needed to establish whether the tissue allograft was a source of the recipient's infection. Because investigations can be very complex, early notification of the state department of health can result in timely assistance in the epidemiologic investigation, if needed.

Look-Back Investigations and Recalls

A tissue product "recall" or market withdrawal occurs when a tissue allograft is determined by the tissue processor to be compromised or potentially infectious. In such cases, other tissues derived from the same donor or tissue processing lot are also considered suspect. The tissue processor may recall all the tissues from that donor or processing lot, sequester any tissues in inventory, and notify any hospitals to which the allografts were shipped. The hospital may be instructed to quarantine any unused allografts in inventory, identify recipients, and/or notify the transplanting surgeon(s). Surgeons should evaluate recipients of these tissue grafts and may notify them of the rationale for the recall.

Look-back is performed when it is suspected or confirmed that a previously donated tissue was obtained from an infectious donor who had a false-negative blood test at the time of donation. The process is triggered when a donor who previously tested negative for infectious diseases is subsequently found to be infected with HIV; human T-cell lymphotropic virus, types I or II; viral hepatitis; or other infectious disease known to be transmitted by tissue. If the organization identifies recipients of tissues from deceased or living (eg, semen or femoral head) donors who are subsequently found to have positive test results for any of the diseases listed above, recipient notification is required. Because the vast majority of tissues used in hospitals are derived from deceased donors, look-back investigations are uncommon.

Tissue Autograft Collection, Storage, and Use

Surgical reconstruction using the patient's own tissues often has advantages over cadaveric tissue—for example, ready availability of donor tissue, rapid incorporation, appropriate dimensions, and relative safety from viral disease transmission. A bone flap removed during decompressive craniectomy surgery is a common example. In this procedure, a section of skull is removed by the neurosurgeon to reduce intracerebral pressure caused by brain swelling following trauma, stroke, or surgery. After removal, the fragment of skull is rinsed, packaged, frozen, and stored for future reimplantation during a procedure known as cranioplasty.[26]

There should be written procedures for aseptic collection of tissue autografts, microbial testing, packaging, storage, and subsequent issuance for use. Bacteria testing should be performed at the time of surgical removal and before packaging. Autografts should not be collected from patients who have bacteremia or who have bacterial or fungal infections within or adjacent to the tissue being removed for reimplantation at a later date. Tissue service procedures for incoming inspection, storage, and issuance should be similar to those procedures used for allografts. Autografts are usually stored within the hospital where they are collected, but they may be stored at an FDA-registered tissue bank off-site. Procedural recommendations have been published by AATB and AORN.

Occasionally, the patient has an autograft removed and stored at one hospital or off-site tissue bank but is subsequently transferred to a different hospital for reimplantation. If the autograft is requested from the original hospital or an off-site tissue bank for implantation, the receiving hospital tissue service needs to establish and document acceptability of the autograft. The hospital tissue service's medical director and/or staff should review applicable operative notes, bacterial cultures, and storage conditions. There needs to be assurance that appropriate procedures were followed and that the tissue is of satisfactory quality so that the patient is not placed at undue risk. Unexpected findings should be reviewed by the patient's surgeon and by the hospital tissue service's medical director.

Transfusion Service Support for Organ Transplantation

Organ transplantation is a complex undertaking that relies on the coordinated activities of the local organ procurement organization (OPO) and the hospital transplant team. Within the hospital, a successful transplant program requires an interdisciplinary team with well-defined policies, procedures, and communication pathways. The transfusion service is an integral component of the clinical transplantation program: appropriate blood testing and transfusion support before, during, and after transplantation contribute to optimal patient outcomes.

OPOs evaluate potential donors, obtain appropriate consent, and prepare organs for transportation. The United Network for Organ Sharing (UNOS) is a private, nonprofit organization that manages OPOs and the US organ transplant system under contract with the federal government. Guidelines for organ allocations are continually evolving and strive to achieve equitable distribution of life-enhancing and/or lifesaving organs. Factors such as severity of recipient illness, geographic proximity, and donor-recipient compatibility are considered. Human organs, unlike musculoskeletal allografts, are transported to the transplanting facility as soon as possible following procurement and undergo no additional "processing."

Unlike previously described musculoskeletal tissue implantation, ABO and HLA compatibility is an important consideration in organ transplantation. ABO antigens expressed on vascular endothelium of organs constitute strong histocompatibility barriers.[27] Major incompatibility between donor ABO antigens and recipient plasma can result in acute humoral rejection of the transplanted organ and concomitant thrombosis of graft vessels. As a result, UNOS requires ABO verification of donor and recipient before implantation as well as duplicate ABO typing of potential transplant recipients before listing on the Organ Procurement and Transplantation Network (OPTN) waiting list. However, ABO-incompatible kidney and other organ transplants have been successfully accomplished following a plasma exchange regimen.

The AABB publishes no standards related to organ transplantation. UNOS provides detailed policies and other information relevant to organ transplantation online (www.unos.org). Transfusion services that support organ transplantation should clearly understand the expectations of the transplant team. Blood bank services that may be required by a transplant program include provision of cytomegalovirus-reduced-risk components, blood irradiation, massive transfusion support, ABO subgroup typing, and immunohematology reference testing. Additionally, consultation for coagulopathy, often associated with end-stage liver disease and liver transplantation, may be desirable.

KEY POINTS

1. Surgical use of human allografts has grown dramatically in recent years, with over 1.5 million tissue grafts distributed annually by tissue banks in the United States. The majority of these grafts are obtained from deceased human donors who meet stringent infectious disease screening and testing requirements similar to those applied to blood donors.
2. Not all tissue allografts are sterile. Depending on the type of allograft, sterilization may not be possible, as it would jeopardize the viability of the cellular elements in the graft and adversely affect the graft's performance in vivo. Methods of sterilization include ionizing radiation, ethylene oxide, and some proprietary processes and techniques.
3. Human immunodeficiency virus, hepatitis C virus, hepatitis B virus, Creutzfeldt-Jakob disease, and bacterial and fungal transmission from allografts have been documented but are rare. Therefore, like blood components, allografts are released for use only after screening for infectious disease risk.
4. In general, bone and soft tissue allografts do not have to be matched for HLA or ABO type.
5. *Hospital-based tissue services* do not fall under regulatory oversight by the Food and Drug Administration (FDA) if their activities are limited to receiving, storing, and dispensing tissue to a requesting surgeon. However, The Joint Commission, the AABB, the American Association of Tissue Banks, the College of American Pathologists, and the Association of periOperative Registered Nurses publish standards that apply.
6. *Tissue banks* are organizations engaged in donor screening and testing and the recovery, packaging, labeling, processing, storage, and distribution of human tissues. Tissue banks are regulated by the FDA under the *Code of Federal Regulations* (21 CFR 1270 and 1271) as manufacturers of human cells, tissues, and cellular and tissue-based products.
7. There is no requirement by any regulatory or standards-setting organization for a hospital tissue dispensing service to be managed by a particular department or individual. However, the AABB favors a centralized model within the transfusion service.

REFERENCES

1. About AATB. McLean, VA: American Association of Tissue Banks, 2010. [Available at http://www.aatb.org (accessed February 20, 2011).]
2. Eastlund DT, Eisenbrey AB for the Tissue Committee. Guidelines for managing tissue allografts in hospitals. Bethesda, MD: AABB, 2006.
3. Trainor LD, Frizzo W. Human allografts and the transfusion service. ASCP Check Sample 2009:52:13-24.
4. Lavernia CJ, Malinin TI, Temple T, et al. Bone and tissue allograft use by orthopedic surgeons. J Arthroplasty 2004;19:430-5.
5. Pearson K, Dock N, Brubaker S, et al. Standards for tissue banking. 12th ed. McLean, VA: American Association of Tissue Banks, 2008.
6. Eisenbrey AB, Eastlund DT, Gottschall JL, eds. Hospital tissue management: A practitioner's handbook. 1st ed. Bethesda, MD: AABB, 2008.
7. Woll JE, Smith DM. Bone and connective tissue. Clin Lab Med 2005;25:499-518.
8. Malinin TI. Preparation and banking of bone and tendon allografts. In: Sherman OH, Minkoff J, eds. Arthroscopic surgery. Baltimore, MD: Williams and Wilkins, 1990:65-86.
9. Cheek RF, Harmon JV, Stowell CP. Red cell alloimmunization after a bone allograft. Transfusion 1995;35:507-9.
10. Eastlund T, Strong DM. Infectious disease transmission through tissue transplantation. In: Phillips GO, ed. Advances in tissue banking. Vol 7. Singapore: World Scientific Publishing, 2003:51-131.
11. Simonds RJ, Holmberg SD, Hurwitz RL, et al. Transmission of human immunodeficiency virus type 1 from a seronegative organ and tissue donor. N Engl J Med 1992;326:726-32.
12. Centers for Disease Control and Prevention. Hepatitis C virus transmission in an antibody-negative organ and tissue donor—United

States, 2000-2002. MMWR Morb Mortal Wkly Rep 2003;52:273-4, 276.

13. Centers for Disease Control and Prevention. Creutzfeldt-Jakob disease in patients who received a cadaveric dura mater graft—Spain, 1985-992. MMWR Morb Mortal Wkly Rep 1993; 42:560-3.
14. Schotveld JH, Raijmakers AJ, Henry Y, Zaal MJ. Donor-to-host transmitted Candida endophthalmitis after penetrating keratoplasty. Cornea 2005;24:887-9.
15. Eastlund T. Bacterial infection transmitted by human tissue allograft transplantation. Cell Tissue Bank 2006;7:147-66.
16. Centers for Disease Control and Prevention. Update: Allograft-associated bacterial infections—United States, 2002. MMWR Morb Mortal Wkly Rep 2002;51: 207-10.
17. Code of federal regulations. Human cells, tissues, and cellular and tissue-based products. Title 21, CFR Parts 1270 and 1271. Washington, DC: US Government Printing Office, 2010 (revised annually).
18. Transplant safety. In: Comprehensive accreditation manual for hospitals: The official handbook. Oakbrook Terrace, IL: The Joint Commission, 2009:TS-1-TS-8.
19. Standards for tissue storage and issuance. Accreditation manual for critical access hospitals. 2nd ed. Oakbrook Terrace, IL: The Joint Commission, 2003 (updated 2005).
20. Carson TH, ed. Standards for blood banks and transfusion services. 27th ed. Bethesda, MD: AABB, 2011.
21. Standards for laboratory accreditation. Northfield, IL: College of American Pathologists, 2000.
22. Recommended practices for surgical tissue banking. In: Perioperative standards and recommended practices. Denver, CO: AORN, 2008:599-612.
23. Medical standards. Washington, DC: Eye Bank Association of America, 2009.
24. Nether K, Sawchuk M, Brubaker S. Clarification of tissue storage requirements (letter). AORN J 2009;89:829-30.
25. Shrimp L. Heat resistance of allograft tissue. Cell Tissue Bank 2008;9:259-66.
26. Grossman N, Shemesh-Jan HS, Merkin V, et al. Deep-freeze preservation of cranial bones for future cranioplasty: Nine years of experience in Soroka University Medical Center. Cell Tissue Bank 2007;8:243-6.
27. Eastland T. The histo-blood group ABO system and tissue transplantation. Transfusion 1998; 38:975-88.

Methods

THE INCLUSION OF a method in this edition of the *Technical Manual* is a subjective decision of the authors and editors. Exclusion from the current edition does not necessarily indicate that its use is prohibited. However, some procedures were removed (beginning with the 16th edition) because the chemicals used in the procedures could present a safety risk or the methods are no longer needed or applicable. Readers are cautioned when referring to procedures in previous editions because they have not been reviewed for content and safety.

Methods given here are reliable, straightforward, and representative of current practice. Personnel should always consult the instructions from the manufacturer of a specific reagent and follow the directions provided.

Although the investigation of unusual problems often requires flexibility in thought and methodology, the adoption of uniform methods for routine procedures in the laboratory is imperative. In order for laboratory personnel to have reproducible and comparable results in a test procedure, it is essential that everyone in the laboratory perform the same procedure in the same manner.

General Laboratory Methods

INTRODUCTION

The methods outlined in the following sections are *examples* of acceptable procedures. Other acceptable procedures may be used by facilities if desired. To the greatest extent possible, the written procedures conform to the *Laboratory Documents: Development and Control; Approved Guideline* developed by the Clinical and Laboratory Standards Institute. As indicated in Title 21 of the *Code of Federal Regulations* (CFR), Part 606.65(e), the manufacturer's instructions (eg, product insert) for reagents and supplies licensed by the Food and Drug Administration (FDA) should be followed. Any deviation should be validated using appropriate controls and incorporated into a standard operating procedure before approval by the medical director. (Note: Deviations may also require concurrence from the FDA.) It is important to use Standard Precautions when appropriate.

Reagent Preparation

Many procedures include formulas for reagent preparation. Labels for reagents prepared inhouse must contain the following:

- Name of solution.
- Date of preparation.
- Expiration date (if known).
- Storage temperature and/or conditions.
- Mechanism to identify the person who prepared the solution.
- Universal hazardous substance label.

Temperatures

Whenever specific incubation or storage temperatures are given, the following ranges are considered satisfactory:

Stated Temperature	Acceptable Range
4 C	2-8 C
Room temperature	20-24 C
37 C	36-38 C
56 C	54-58 C

Centrifugation Variables

Centrifugation speeds (relative centrifugal force) and times should be standardized for each piece of equipment. (See Methods Section 8.)

Reference

1. Laboratory documents: Development and control; approved guideline. 5th ed. (CLSI Document GP02-A5, Vol. 26, No. 12.) Wayne, PA: Clinical and Laboratory Standards Institute, 2006.

METHOD 1-1. SHIPPING HAZARDOUS MATERIALS

Principle

It is the responsibility of the shipper of biologic or infectious material to properly classify, package, label, and document the substance being shipped.

For transport by mail of infectious materials, clinical specimens, or biologic products, the United States Postal Service (USPS) Dangerous Goods Regulations must be followed.[1,2] For interstate transport of infectious materials by ground or air, the United States Department of Transportation (DOT) regulations apply.[3] Most air carriers apply the International Air Transport Association (IATA)[4] regulations and the technical instructions of the International Civil Aviation Organization (ICAO).[5] These agencies adopt the recommendations of the United Nations (UN) Committee of Experts on the Transport of Dangerous Goods for the international transport of infectious substances and clinical specimens.

The Centers for Disease Control and Prevention (CDC)[6] and the IATA[7] provide packing and labeling requirements for shipments of infectious materials. Facilities should also consult their local carriers for additional requirements.

Procedure

1. *Classify the type of hazard:*
   If inadvertent exposure to human specimens occurs during shipment, the level of risk can be categorized.

- Category A substances contain infectious agents in a form that can cause permanent disability or life-threatening or fatal disease when otherwise healthy humans or animals are exposed to the substance. Examples include Ebola virus in any form, hepatitis B virus (HBV) in culture, and human immunodeficiency virus (HIV) in culture. AABB member facilities do not typically ship Category A substances.

  The proper shipping name and UN numbers are as follows:

  Infectious Substance, affecting humans, UN 2814; or
  Infectious Substance, affecting animals *only*, UN 2900.

- Category B substances contain or are suspected to contain infectious agents but do not meet the criteria for Category A. Examples include routine blood specimens from patients or donors who are known to be infected with HIV or HBV.

  The proper shipping name and UN number are as follows:

  Biological Substance, Category B, UN 3373.

- Exempt substances are those that do not contain infectious substances or are unlikely to cause disease in humans or animals. Patient samples that contain a Category B infectious substance and are transported for the purpose of research, diagnosis, investigational activities, or disease treatment or prevention are also considered exempt if they are transported by a private or contract carrier in a motor vehicle used exclusively to transport such materials. Examples of exempt substances include specimens from patients who are not suspected of having an infectious disease, blood products for transfusion, cellular therapy products for infusion, and reagents that have undergone pathogen inactivation.

  The shipping container is labeled as follows:

  Exempt human specimen, or
  Exempt animal specimen.

2. *Package and label according to the hazard category:*
   Both IATA and DOT provide detailed instruction on the amount of material that may be contained in one package, the types of packaging materials that may be used, and proper methods of packing for each hazard category. There are additional requirements for shipping specimens in dry ice or liquid nitrogen. It is up to the shipper to ensure that materials are packaged properly. The carrier will inspect the package for proper markings and labels, but they generally will not open the box to verify packaging. Packaging requirements apply to both air and land transportation.

Category A and B packages must bear the proper shipping name and UN label on the box.

If specimens are shipped in dry ice, the outer package must allow the release of carbon dioxide gas. Advance arrangements with the carrier are required when more than 2.3 kg of dry ice is contained in one package. The outer container must be marked with "Carbon dioxide, solid" or "Dry ice."

3. *Examples:*
Selected examples of specimen classification, applicable packaging, instructions, and labels are given in Table 1-1-1.

TABLE 1-1-1. Examples of Correct Packaging and Labeling of Specimens

If you are shipping:	Then classify as:	And use packing instruction:	And label:
◆ Known HIV virus in culture	UN 2814 Infectious Substance, affecting humans	IATA PI-602 or 49 CFR 173.196	INFECTIOUS SUBSTANCE 6
◆ Anti-HIV EIA-reactive blood specimen for HIV confirmatory Western blot testing	UN 3373 Biological Substance, Category B	IATA PI-650 or 49 CFR 173.199	UN3373
◆ Blood donor specimen for routine screening tests that include anti-HIV and HIV NAT	Exempt human specimen	See requirements below*	
◆ Lot-released blood component for transfusion	Not a hazardous material under DOT or IATA.	Not regulated by DOT or IATA.	
◆ Specimens on dry ice *(Use correct classification and packaging for the specimen, and additional instructions for dry ice.)*	Class 9, Miscellaneous	IATA PI-904 or 49 CFR 173.217	9

*Packaging requirements include the following:

- ◆ For exempt human or animal specimens:
  - A leak-proof primary receptacle(s).
  - A leak-proof secondary packaging.
  - An outer packaging of adequate strength for its capacity, mass, and intended use, with at least one surface having minimum dimensions of 100 mm × 100 mm.
- ◆ For liquids, absorbent material must be placed between the primary receptacle(s) and the secondary packaging. The amount of absorbent material must be able to absorb the entire contents so that during transport, any release or leak of a liquid substance will not reach the outer packaging and will not compromise the integrity of the cushioning material.
- ◆ If multiple, breakable, primary containers are placed in a single secondary packaging, they must be either individually wrapped or separated to prevent contact between them.
- ◆ The packaging must be marked "Exempt human specimen" or "Exempt animal specimen," as appropriate.

HIV = human immunodeficiency virus; UN = United Nations; IATA = International Air Transport Association; CFR = *Code of Federal Regulations*; EIA = enzyme immunoassay; NAT = nucleic acid testing; DOT = (US) Department of Transportation.

References

1. Code of federal regulations. Title 39 CFR. Washington, DC: US Government Printing Office, 2010 (revised annually). [Available at www.gpoaccess.gov/cfr (accessed January 9, 2011).]
2. Etiologic agent preparations, clinical specimens, and biological products. Domestic mail manual. Washington, DC: United States Postal Service, 2011 (revised annually). [Available at http://pe.usps.gov/text/dmm300/dmm300_landing.htm (accessed January 9, 2011).]
3. Code of federal regulations. Title 49, CFR Part 171-180. Washington, DC: US Government Printing Office, 2010 (revised annually). [Available at www.gpoaccess.gov/cfr (accessed January 9, 2011).]
4. Dangerous goods regulations. 52nd ed. Montreal, Canada: International Air Transport Association, 2011 (revised annually).
5. Technical instructions for the safe transport of dangerous goods by air. Documents 9284-AN/905. 2009-2010 ed. Montreal, Canada: International Civil Aviation Organization, 2009. [Available at http://www.icao.int/icaonet/dcs/9284/9284_2009_2010_add_02_corr_01_en.pdf (accessed January 9, 2011).]
6. Code of federal regulations. Title 42, CFR Part 72. Washington, DC: US Government Printing Office, 2010 (revised annually). [Available at www.gpoaccess.gov/cfr (accessed January 9, 2011).]
7. Dangerous Goods Panel, International Civil Aviation Organization. Guidance document: Infectious substances. Montreal, Canada: International Air Transport Association, 2010. [Available at http://www.iata.org/SiteCollectionDocuments/Documents/Guidance_Doc62DGR_51.pdf (accessed February 15, 2011).]

METHOD 1-1-1. MONITORING TEMPERATURE DURING SHIPMENT OF BLOOD

Principle

Some form of temperature indication or monitoring is desirable when shipping blood. The temperature of the contents of a shipping container used for whole blood or liquid-stored red cell components can be ascertained when the shipment is received, as follows:

Procedure

1. Open the shipping container and promptly place the sensing end of a calibrated liquid-in-glass or electronic thermometer between two bags of blood or components (labels facing out) and secure the "sandwich" with two rubber bands.
2. Close the shipping container.
3. After approximately 3 to 5 minutes, read the temperature.
4. If the temperature has exceeded the acceptable range, quarantine the units until their appropriate disposition can be determined.

Notes

Other suitable methods for monitoring shipments are as follows:

1. Use time/temperature indicators, one such indicator per shipping carton. These indicators will change color or show another visible indication if the temperature has exceeded the acceptable range.
2. Place a "high-low" thermometer in the shipping container. This simple, reusable thermometer measures and records the highest and lowest temperatures during any period.

METHOD 1-2. TREATING INCOMPLETELY CLOTTED SPECIMENS

Principle

Fibrin generation may continue in serum separated from incompletely clotted blood, especially during incubation at 37 C. The fibrin generation produces strands of protein that entrap red cells and that make it difficult to evaluate agglutination. Blood from patients who have recently received heparin may not clot at all, and blood from patients with excessive fibrinolytic activity may reliquefy or may contain protein fragments that interfere with examination for agglutination.

Materials

1. Thrombin: dry human/bovine thrombin or thrombin solution (50 units/mL in saline).
2. Glass beads.
3. Protamine sulfate: 10 mg/mL in saline.
4. Epsilon aminocaproic acid (EACA): 0.25 g/mL in saline.

Procedure

1. *To accelerate clotting*: Either of the following techniques may be used:
   a. Add to the specimen the amount of dry thrombin that adheres to the tip of an applicator stick or 1 drop of thrombin solution per mL of whole blood or serum. Allow 10 to 15 minutes for the clot to form. Use standard centrifugation to separate the clot and serum.
   b. Gently agitate the separated serum with small glass beads, at 37 C, for several minutes. Then, use low speed centrifugation to pellet the glass beads. Transfer the serum to another tube.
2. *To neutralize heparin:* Protamine sulfate can be added to the specimen to neutralize heparin; however, excess protamine promotes rouleaux formation and, in great excess, will inhibit clotting. Add 1 drop of protamine sulfate solution to 4 mL of whole blood, and wait 30 minutes to evaluate the effect on clotting. If clotting does not occur, add additional protamine sparingly. Note: protamine sulfate may work more rapidly when briefly incubated (5-10 minutes) at 37 C.
3. *To inhibit fibrinolytic activity:* Add 0.1 mL of EACA to 4 mL of whole blood.

Notes

1. The use of anticoagulated (eg, acid-citrate-dextrose or EDTA) collection tubes may help to avoid the problem of incompletely clotted specimens. The use of anticoagulated specimens must be validated in accordance with each standard operating procedure.
2. Because preparations of human thrombin may contain red cell antibodies, test results must be carefully observed for false-positive reactions. Quality control should be performed on thrombin reagents before or concurrent with their use to identify those with contaminating antibodies.

METHOD 1-3. SOLUTION PREPARATION PROCEDURE

Principle

The basic definitions, calculations, and instructions given below serve as a review of simple principles necessary for solution preparation.

1. Mole, gram-molecular weight: Weight, expressed in grams equal to the atomic or molecular weight of the substance.
2. Molar solution: A one molar (1 M) solution contains one mole of solute in a liter of solvent. The solvent is assumed to be distilled or deionized water unless otherwise indicated.
3. Gram-equivalent weight: Weight, in grams, of a substance that will produce or react with 1 mole of hydrogen ion.
4. Normal solution: A one normal (1 N) solution contains one gram-equivalent weight of solute in a liter of solution.
5. Percentage solutions: The percentage designation of a solution gives the weight or volume of solute present in 100 units of total solution. Percentage can be expressed as follows:
   a. Weight/weight (w/w), indicating grams of solute in 100 g of solution.
   b. Volume/volume (v/v), indicating milliliters of solute present in 100 mL of solution.
   c. Weight/volume (w/v), indicating grams of solute in 100 mL of solution. Unless otherwise specified, a solution expressed in percentage can be assumed to be w/v.

6. Water of crystallization, water of hydration: Molecules of water that form an integral part of the crystalline structure of a substance. A given substance may have several crystalline forms, with different numbers of water molecules intrinsic to the entire molecule. The weight of this water must be included in calculating molecular weight of the hydrated substance.
7. Anhydrous: The salt form of a substance with no water of crystallization.
8. Atomic weights (rounded to whole numbers): H, 1; O, 16; Na, 23; P, 31; S, 32; Cl, 35; K, 39.
9. Molecular weights:
   HCl: 1 + 35 = 36; NaCl: 23 + 35 = 58
   KCl: 39 + 35 = 74
   H_2O: (2 × 1) + 16 = 18
   NaH_2PO_4: 23 + (2 × 1) + 31 + (4 × 16) = 120
   $NaH_2PO_4 \bullet H_2O$: 23 + (2 × 1) + 31 + (4 × 16) + (2 × 1) + 16 = 138
   KH_2PO_4: 39 + (2 × 1) + 31 + (4 × 16) = 136
   H_2SO_4: (2 × 1) + 32 + (4 × 16) = 98

Examples

1. Molar solutions:
   1 M KH_2PO_4 = 136 g of solute made up to 1 L.
   0.15 M KH_2PO_4 = (136 × 0.15) = 20.4 g of solute made up to 1 L.
   0.5 M NaH_2PO_4 = (120 × 0.5) = 60 g of solute made up to 1 L.
2. Molar solution with hydrated salt:
   0.5 M $NaH_2PO_4 \bullet H_2O$ = (138 × 0.5) = 69 g of the monohydrate crystals made up to 1 L.
3. Normal solutions:
   1 N HCl = 36 g of solute made up to 1 L. One mole HCl dissociates into one mole H^+, so gram-equivalent weight and gram-molecular weight are the same.
   12 N HCl = (36 × 12) = 432 g of solute made up to 1 L.
   1 N H_2SO_4 = (98 ÷ 2) = 49 g of solute made up to 1 L. One mole H_2SO_4 dissociates to give two moles of H^+, so the gram-equivalent weight is half the gram-molecular weight.
4. Percentage solution:
   0.9% NaCl (w/v) = 0.9 g of solute made up to 100 mL of solution.

Notes

Accurate results require accurate preparation of reagents. It is important to carefully read and follow all instructions and labels.

1. Weigh only quantities appropriate for the accuracy of the equipment. The operator's manual should give these specifications.
2. Prepare the largest volume that is practical. There is greater accuracy in measuring larger volumes than smaller volumes. If a reagent balance is accurate to ± 0.01 g, the potential error in weighing 0.05 g (50 mg) will be 20%, whereas the potential error in weighing 0.25 g (250 mg) will be only 4%. If the solution retains its activity when stored appropriately, it is usually preferable to prepare a large volume. If the solution deteriorates rapidly, smaller volumes may be preferred to reduce waste.
3. Note whether a substance is in the hydrated or anhydrous form. If the instructions give solute weight for one form, and the available reagent is in another form, be sure to adjust the measurements appropriately. For example, if instructions for 0.5 M NaH_2PO_4 call for 60 g, and the reagent is $NaH_2PO_4 \bullet H_2O$, find the ratio between the weights of the two forms. The molecular weight of $NaH_2PO_4 \bullet H_2O$ is 138, and the molecular weight of NaH_2PO_4 is 120. Therefore, the ratio is 138 ÷ 120 = 1.15. Multiply the designated weight by the ratio (60 g × 1.15 = 69 g) to obtain the final weight needed.
4. Dissolve the solute completely before making the solution to the final volume. This is especially important for substances, such as phosphates, that dissolve slowly. For example, to make 500 mL of 0.15 M KH_2PO_4:

   a. Weigh 10.2 g of solute in a weighing boat or glass [(0.15 × 136) ÷ 2] because only 500 mL will be made.
   b. Place 350 mL of water in a 500-mL volumetric flask on a magnetic stirrer. Add the stirring bar and adjust it to a slow, steady stirring speed.
   c. Add 10.2 g of salt, then rinse the boat with several aliquots of water until no salt remains. Numerous small-volume rinses remove adherent material more effectively than a few larger volumes. Add the rinse water to the material in the flask and stir until the salt has completely dissolved.
   d. If pH measurement is unnecessary, add water to the 500-mL mark, adjusting the volume for the stirring bar, and mix thoroughly. For solutions needing pH adjustment, see the next step.
5. Adjust the pH of the solution before bringing it to its final volume so that the addition of water (or other solvent) does not markedly change the molarity. For example, to bring 500 mL of 0.1 M glycine to a pH of 3:
   a. Add 3.75 g of glycine (H_2NCH_2COOH: molecular weight, 75) to 400-475 mL of water in a beaker. Dissolve completely, using a magnetic stirrer.
   b. Add a few drops of concentrated (12 N) HCl and measure pH after acid is thoroughly mixed. Continue adding HCl until pH is 3.0.
   c. Transfer the solution to a 500-mL volumetric flask. Rinse beaker and stirring bar with aliquots of water, adding the rinse water to the flask. Use the rinses to contribute to the total 500-mL volume.
   d. Measure the pH of the solution at final volume.

References

1. Remson ST, Ackerman PG. Calculations for the medical laboratory. Boston, MA: Little, Brown & Co., 1977.
2. Henry JB, ed. Clinical diagnosis and management by laboratory methods. 18th ed. Philadelphia: WB Saunders, 1991.

METHOD 1-4. SERUM DILUTION PROCEDURE

Principle

Serum is sometimes diluted in saline or other diluents to determine its relative antibody concentration. It is customary to express the dilution as 1 part of serum *contained* in the total number of parts of the dilution. For example, to test the serum at one-tenth its original concentration, a dilution of 1 part in 10 may be made by mixing 1 mL of serum with 9 mL of saline. The *final volume is 10*, and the dilution is expressed as a 1-in-10 dilution. The diluted material contains one-tenth (1/10 or 0.1) of the unmodified serum. It is often customary to report the titer of an antibody as the reciprocal of the highest dilution that retains a 1+ agglutination. Therefore, serum that reacts at a dilution of 1/32 is considered to have a titer of 32. Note: A 1-in-10 dilution is 1 part in 9 parts, whereas a 1-to-10 or 1:10 is 1 part in 10 parts.

Procedure

1. To dilute an existing dilution:
   a. A new higher dilution can be prepared from diluted material by adding more diluent. The formula for calculating either the new higher final dilution or the amount of diluent to add to obtain a higher final dilution is as follows:

$$\frac{\text{reciprocal of present serum dilution}}{\text{volume of serum dilution used}} = \frac{\text{reciprocal of new final dilution}}{\text{total final volume}}$$

   b. *Example:* Serum dilution is 1 in 2, and volume of serum dilution is 1.0 mL. If 4.0 mL of saline is added, what will be the new final dilution?

$$\frac{2}{1} = \frac{X}{5}$$

$X = 10$, or a 1-in-10 dilution

2. To dilute a dilution to a specified volume:
   a. The formula for calculating the volume of diluent to add to a dilution to achieve a certain quantity of a new higher final dilution is as follows:

$$\frac{\text{reciprocal of present dilution}}{\text{volume of present dilution needed}}$$

$$= \frac{\text{reciprocal of final dilution}}{\text{total final volume required}}$$

   b. *Example:* Present serum dilution is 1 in 2, total final volume is 100 mL, and new final serum dilution is 1 in 10. How much serum (diluted 1 in 2) will have to be added to make up a final volume of 100 mL of a 1-in-10 dilution?

$$\frac{2}{X} = \frac{10}{100}$$

   X = 20, or 20 mL of serum (dilution of 1 in 2) must be added to 80 mL of diluent to obtain 100 mL of a 1-in-10 dilution.

METHOD 1-5. DILUTION OF PERCENTAGE SOLUTIONS PROCEDURE

Procedure

1. Dilutions can be prepared from more concentrated solutions by use of the following formula:

$$(\text{Volume}_1 \times \text{Concentration}_1) = (\text{Volume}_2 \times \text{Concentration}_2)$$
$$V_1 \times C_1 = V_2 \times C_2$$

   where V_1 and C_1 represent original volume and concentration, and V_2 and C_2 represent final desired volume and concentration.

2. *Example:* 30% albumin is available, but 2 mL of 6% albumin is needed. How should the albumin be diluted?

$$V_1 \times 30 = 2 \times 6$$
$$30V_1 = 12$$
$$V_1 = 12 \div 30 = 0.4$$

   Therefore, mix 0.4 mL of 30% albumin with 1.6 mL saline to obtain 2.0 mL of 6% albumin, or for small-volume use, mix 4 drops 30% albumin with 16 drops saline to obtain 20 drops of 6% albumin.

METHOD 1-6. PREPARING A 3% RED CELL SUSPENSION

Principle

A 3% red cell suspension is a common reagent in many serologic procedures. The suspension need not be exactly 3%; an approximation achieves the appropriate serum-to-cell ratio for most test procedures and for an adequate number of red cells so one can read and grade the reactions. The following steps are intended to help an individual gain confidence in approximating a 3% red cell suspension visually, both as a suspension of cells and in the appropriate size of the cell pellet achieved after centrifugation.

Materials

1. Whole blood sample.
2. Test tubes.
3. Disposable pipettes (1-mL and 10-mL serologic).
4. Saline.
5. Centrifuge (3000 rpm or equivalent).
6. Commercially prepared 3% reagent red cell suspension.

Procedure

To prepare 10 mL of a 3% red cell suspension:

1. Transfer at least 1 mL of whole blood to a 10-mL tube.
2. Wash the red cells in saline or phosphate-buffered saline (PBS), centrifuging for 5 minutes to pellet the cells. Repeat two or three times. The final supernate should be

clear and should be completely removed by aspiration.

3. Transfer 0.3 mL of the washed red cells to a tube with 9.7 mL of saline, PBS, or Alsever's solution.
4. Cap or cover the tube with parafilm. Thoroughly mix the red cells and saline by gently inverting the tube several times.
5. To compare the color and density of the suspension by eye, transfer a volume of the prepared suspension to a 10 × 75 mm tube. Also transfer a similar volume of a known 3% red cell suspension (eg, commercial reagent red cell suspension) to another 10 × 75 mm tube. Hold the two tubes in front of a light source to compare them.
6. To compare the size of the cell pellet expected from a 3% red cell suspension, transfer 1 drop of the prepared suspension to a 10 × 75 mm tube. Similarly, transfer 1 drop of a known 3% commercial reagent red cell suspension to another 10 × 75 mm tube. Centrifuge the tubes in a serologic centrifuge, using the spin time designated for "saline." The size of the two cell pellets should be similar.

Note

For best results use red cell suspensions on the day of preparation only unless stability for a longer time has been validated.

METHOD 1-7. PREPARING AND USING PHOSPHATE BUFFER

Principle

Mixtures of acids and bases can be prepared at specific pH values and used to buffer (render) other solutions to that pH. The following procedure includes a method for preparing phosphate-buffered saline (PBS), which can be used as a diluent in serologic tests.

Reagents

1. Prepare acidic stock solution (solution A) by dissolving 22.16 g of $NaH_2PO_4 \bullet H_2O$ in 1 L of distilled water. This 0.16 M solution of the monobasic phosphate salt (monohydrate) has a pH of 5.0.
2. Prepare alkaline stock solution (solution B) by dissolving 22.7 g of Na_2HPO_4 in 1 L of distilled water. This 0.16 M solution of the dibasic phosphate salt (anhydrous) has a pH of 9.0.

Procedure

1. Prepare working buffer solutions of the desired pH by mixing appropriate volumes of the two solutions. A few examples are as follows:

pH	Solution A	Solution B
5.5	94 mL	6 mL
7.3	16 mL	84 mL
7.7	7 mL	93 mL

2. Check the pH of the working solution before using it. If necessary, add small volumes of acid solution A or alkaline solution B to achieve the desired pH.
3. To prepare PBS of a desired pH, add one volume of phosphate buffer at that pH to nine volumes of normal saline.

References

1. Hendry EB. Osmolarity of human serum and of chemical solutions of biologic importance. Clin Chem 1961;7:156-64.
2. Dacie JV, Lewis SM. Practical haematology. 4th ed. London, England: J and A Churchill, 1968: 540-1.

METHOD 1-8. READING AND GRADING TUBE AGGLUTINATION

Principle

The purpose of grading reactions is to allow comparison of reaction strengths. This purpose is beneficial in detecting multiple antibody specificities or antibodies exhibiting dosage. For uniformity and reproducibility, the grading of agglutination reactions should be standardized among all members of the labo-

TABLE 1-8-1. Interpretation of Agglutination Reactions

Macroscopically Observed Findings	Designation	Score
One solid agglutinate	4+	12
Several large agglutinates	3+	10
Medium-size agglutinates, clear background	2+	8
Small agglutinates, turbid background	1+	5
Very small agglutinates, turbid background	$1+^{w}$	4
Barely visible agglutination, turbid background	w+ or +/–	2
No agglutination	0	0
Mixtures of agglutinated and unagglutinated red cells (mixed field)	mf	
Complete hemolysis	H	
Partial hemolysis, some red cells remain	PH	

ratory staff. Most laboratories define their own versions of a grading system, which is described in a written procedure available to all staff. Some systems use assigned numeric values (scores) for the observed reactions.

Materials

1. Centrifuged serologic tests for agglutination.
2. Agglutination viewer.

Procedure

1. Gently shake or tilt the tube to resuspend the red cell button in the tube. The tilt technique uses the solution meniscus to gently dislodge the red cell button from the wall of the tube.
2. Observe the way that cells are dispersed from the red cell button.
3. Record reactivity by comparing the agglutinates to the descriptions in Table 1-8-1. The reactivity should be assessed when the red cells have been completely resuspended from the button.

Interpretation

Refer to Table 1-8-1.

Red Cell Typing

METHOD 2-1. DETERMINING ABO GROUP OF RED CELLS—SLIDE TEST

Principle

See Chapter 12 for a discussion of the principles of testing for ABO groups.

Specimen

The reagent manufacturer's instructions must be consulted before slide tests are performed; some manufacturers recommend performing slide tests with whole blood, whereas others specify the use of red cell suspensions of lighter concentrations prepared in saline, serum, or plasma.

Reagents

1. Anti-A.
2. Anti-B.
3. Anti-A,B (optional).

All reagents must be used in accordance with the manufacturer's instructions.

Procedure

1. Place 1 drop of anti-A on a clean, labeled glass slide.
2. Place 1 drop of anti-B on a separate clean, labeled glass slide.
3. Place 1 drop of anti-A,B on a third slide—if parallel tests are to be performed with this reagent—or on a single, clean, labeled slide if this test is the only one performed.
4. Add to each drop of reagent on the slides 1 drop of well-mixed suspension (in saline, serum, or plasma) of the red cells to be tested. (Consult the reagent manufacturer's instructions to determine the correct cell concentration to be used.)
5. Mix the reagents and red cells thoroughly, using a clean applicator stick for each reagent. Spread the mixture over an area approximately 20 mm × 40 mm.
6. Gently tilt the slide from side to side continuously for up to 2 minutes. Do not place the slide over a heated surface, such as an Rh viewbox, during this period.
7. Read, interpret, and record the results of the reactions on all slides.

Interpretation

1. Strong agglutination of red cells in the presence of any ABO typing reagent constitutes a positive result.
2. A smooth suspension of red cells at the end of 2 minutes is a negative result.
3. Samples that give weak or doubtful reactions should be retested using Method 2-2.

Notes

1. Slide testing imposes a greater risk of exposure to infectious samples. Personnel should follow safety measures detailed in the facility's procedures manual.

2. Slide testing is not suitable for detection of ABO antibodies in serum or plasma.

METHOD 2-2. DETERMINING ABO GROUP OF RED CELLS AND SERUM—TUBE TEST

Principle

See Chapter 12 for a discussion of the principles of testing for ABO groups. The following procedure is an acceptable representative method, but the manufacturer's instructions for the specific reagents must be consulted.

Specimen

The reagent manufacturer's package insert must be consulted to determine specific specimen requirements. Generally, clotted or anticoagulated blood samples may be used for ABO testing. The red cells may be suspended in autologous serum, plasma, or saline, or they may be washed and resuspended in saline.

Reagents

1. Anti-A.
2. Anti-B.
3. Anti-A,B (optional).
4. 2% to 5% suspension of A_1, A_2, and B red cells. The red cells can be obtained commercially or prepared daily by the testing laboratory (Method 1-6). Note: The use of A_2 cells is optional.

All reagents must be used in accordance with the manufacturer's instructions.

Procedures

Testing Red Cells

1. Place 1 drop of anti-A in a clean, labeled test tube.
2. Place 1 drop of anti-B in a separate, clean, labeled tube.
3. Place 1 drop of anti-A,B in a third clean, labeled tube, if tests are to be performed with this reagent.
4. To each tube, add 1 drop of a 2% to 5% suspension (in saline, serum, or plasma) of the red cells to be tested. Alternatively, the equivalent amount of red cells can be transferred to each tube with clean applicator sticks.
5. Gently mix the contents of the tubes; then centrifuge for the calibrated spin time.
6. Gently resuspend the cell buttons, and examine them for agglutination.
7. Read, interpret, and record the test results. Compare the red cell test results with those obtained in the serum or plasma tests (see below).

Testing Serum or Plasma

1. Add 2 or 3 drops each of serum or plasma to two clean, labeled test tubes.
2. Add 1 drop of A_1 reagent red cells to the tube labeled A_1.
3. Add 1 drop of B reagent red cells to the tube labeled B.
4. Add A_2 red cells to a third appropriately labeled tube with 2 or 3 drops serum or plasma, if this optional test is being performed.
5. Gently mix the contents of the tubes; then centrifuge for the calibrated spin time.
6. Examine the serum overlying the red cell buttons for evidence of hemolysis. Gently resuspend the cell buttons, and examine them for agglutination.
7. Read, interpret, and record test results. Compare serum test results with those obtained in testing red cells (see above).

Interpretation

1. Agglutination of tested red cells and either hemolysis or agglutination in tests with serum or plasma constitute positive test results.
2. A smooth cell suspension after resuspension of the cell button is a negative test result.
3. Interpretation of serum or plasma and red cell tests for ABO is given in Table 12-1.

4. Any discrepancy between the results of the tests with serum or plasma and red cells should be resolved before an interpretation is recorded for the patient's or donor's ABO group (see Chapter 12).
5. Mixed-field agglutination should be investigated for possible cause.

Note

Positive reactions characteristically show 3+ to 4+ agglutination by reagent ABO antibodies; reactions between test serum and reagent red cells are often weaker. The serum tests may be incubated at room temperature for 5 to 15 minutes to enhance weak reactions. See Chapter 12 for a discussion of weakly reactive samples.

METHOD 2-3. DETERMINING ABO GROUP OF RED CELLS AND SERUM—MICROPLATE TEST

Principle

See Chapter 12 for a discussion of the principles of testing for ABO blood group. Microplate techniques can be used to test for antigens on red cells and for antibodies in serum. A microplate can be considered as a matrix of 96 "short" test tubes; the principles that apply to hemagglutination in tube tests also apply to tests in microplates.

Microplates may be rigid or flexible, with either U-shaped or V-shaped bottoms. U-shaped bottom plates are more widely used because results can be read either after centrifuging the plate and observing the characteristics of resuspended red cells or by observing the streaming pattern of the red cells when the plate is placed at an angle. Either reading technique permits estimation of the strength of agglutination.

Specimen

See Methods 2-1 and 2-2.

Equipment

1. Dispensers (optional): Semiautomated devices are available for dispensing equal volumes to a row of wells.
2. Microplate readers (optional): Automated photometric devices are available that read microplate results by the light absorbance in U-shaped bottom wells to differentiate between positive and negative test results. The microprocessor component of the reader interprets the reactions and prints the blood testing results. The manufacturer's instructions for the collection and preparation of serum or plasma and cell specimens must be followed.
3. Centrifuges: Special plate carriers can be purchased to fit common table-top centrifuges. Appropriate conditions must be established for each centrifuge. The following times and relative centrifugal forces, expressed as *g*, are suggested. Consult the manufacturer's directions for specific information.
   a. *For a flexible U-shaped bottom microplate:* 700 × *g* for 5 seconds for red cell testing and serum or plasma testing.
   b. *For a rigid U-shaped bottom microplate:* 400 × *g* for 30 seconds for red cell testing and serum or plasma testing.

Reagents

Many manufacturers supply ABO or Rh typing reagents that are licensed by the Food and Drug Administration for use as undiluted reagents in microplate tests.

1. Anti-A.
2. Anti-B.
3. Anti-A,B. Note: Use of this reagent is optional.
4. 2% to 5% suspension of group A_1, A_2, and B reagent red cells. The red cells can be obtained commercially or prepared daily by the testing laboratory (see Method 1-6). Note: The use of A_2 red cells is optional.

Procedure

Testing Red Cells

1. Place 1 drop of anti-A and 1 drop of anti-B in separate clean wells of a U-bottom microplate. If tests with anti-A,B are to be performed, add this reagent to a third clean well.
2. Add 1 drop of a 2% to 5% saline suspension of red cells to each well containing blood typing reagent.
3. Mix the contents of the wells by gently tapping the sides of the plate.
4. Centrifuge the plate at the appropriate conditions established for the centrifuge.
5. Resuspend the cell buttons by manually tapping the plate or with the aid of a mechanical shaker, or place the plate at an angle for the tilt-and-stream method.
6. Read, interpret, and record results. Compare red cell test results with those obtained in testing serum or plasma.

Testing Serum or Plasma

1. Add 1 drop of serum or plasma under test to each well.
2. Add 1 drop of a 2% to 5% suspension of A_1 and B reagent red cells to separate clean wells of a U-bottom microplate. If an optional test on A_2 red cells will be performed, add A_2 red cells to a third well.
3. Mix the contents of the wells by gently tapping the sides of the plate.
4. Centrifuge the plate at the appropriate conditions established for the centrifuge.
5. Resuspend the red cell buttons by manually tapping the plate or with aid of a mechanical shaker, or place the plate at an angle for the tilt-and-stream method.
6. Read, interpret, and record results. Compare test results on serum or plasma with those obtained in testing red cells.

Interpretation

1. Agglutination in any well of red cell tests or hemolysis or agglutination in any well of a serum test will constitute positive results.
2. A smooth suspension of red cells after resuspension of the cell button is a negative test result.
3. The interpretation of ABO tests is given in Table 12-1.
4. Any discrepancy between results on cell and serum or plasma tests should be resolved before an interpretation is recorded for the patient's or donor's ABO group (see Chapter 12).

Note

To enhance weak serum or plasma reactions, the plates may be incubated at room temperature for 5 to 10 minutes; then the centrifugation, reading, and recording steps may be repeated.

METHOD 2-4. INITIAL INVESTIGATION OF ABO GROUPING DISCREPANCIES PROCEDURE

Principle

To be considered valid, the results of red cell grouping and serum grouping should agree. This method describes a general approach to the initial investigation of an ABO grouping discrepancy caused by either missing reactions or unexpected positive reactions. (See Chapter 12 for a detailed discussion on ABO grouping.)

Procedure

1. Repeat ABO typing on the same sample. If initial tests were performed on red cells resuspended in serum or plasma, testing should be repeated after washing red cells several times with saline. This retest will eliminate many of the problems associated with plasma proteins or autoantibody.
2. Test a new sample. A new sample for testing should be requested when the ABO discrepancy reflects a disagreement

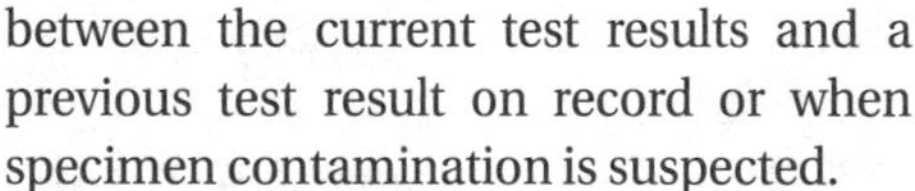

between the current test results and a previous test result on record or when specimen contamination is suspected.

3. Review the patient's medical history for medical conditions that could alter or interfere with ABO typing. This review can include the following:
   a. Medical diagnosis.
   b. Historical blood group.
   c. Transfusion history.
   d. Transplantation history.
   e. Current medications.
4. Review the results of plasma testing against autologous red cells and group O red cells in the antibody screen to evaluate potential interference by autoantibodies or alloantibodies. A direct antiglobulin test may be helpful. See Method 3-6.

METHOD 2-5. DETECTING WEAK A AND B ANTIGENS AND ANTIBODIES BY COLD TEMPERATURE ENHANCEMENT

Principle

Prolonged incubation at low temperatures can enhance antibody binding and detection of weak ABO antigens and antibodies. Because it is often unclear whether an ABO discrepancy is the consequence of weak antigens or of antibodies, testing both red cells and serum in parallel is recommended.

Specimen

1. Washed red cells to investigate missing red cell antigens.
2. Serum or plasma to investigate missing isoagglutinins.

Reagents

1. Monoclonal or polyclonal anti-A, anti-B, and anti-A,B.
2. A_1, A_2, B, and O reagent red cells (serum investigations).
3. 6% albumin.

Procedure

1. Set up tube test for red cell grouping as described in Method 2-2. (Note: When testing patients' red cells, it is recommended to also incubate cells with 6% albumin as a control to detect spontaneous or autoagglutination. During testing of patients' plasma, group O reagent red cells should be included to detect cold autoantibody or alloantibody.)
2. Incubate all tubes for 30 minutes at room temperature.
3. Centrifuge tubes according to reagent manufacturer's directions.
4. Gently resuspend cell buttons and examine for agglutination.
5. If no agglutination is observed, incubate tubes for 15 to 30 minutes at 4 C.
6. Centrifuge and examine for agglutination.

Interpretation

No interpretation can be made if the 6% albumin control for spontaneous agglutination is positive or if cold autoantibody or alloantibody is detected. See Chapter 12 for additional information on resolving ABO discrepancies.

Note

The manufacturer's directions for any reagent should be consulted regarding limitations of assay conditions for testing.

METHOD 2-6. CONFIRMING WEAK A AND B ANTIGENS USING ENZYME-TREATED RED CELLS

Principle

Enzyme treatment of red cells can enhance antigen-antibody reactions to ABO and other carbohydrate antigens.

Specimens

1. Washed, untreated autologous red cells.
2. Washed, enzyme-treated (ficin, papain, or bromelin) autologous red cells.

Reagents

1. Monoclonal or polyclonal anti-A, anti-B, and anti-A,B.
2. Reagents for enzyme treatment of red cells (see Methods 3-5-1 and 3-5-2).
3. Group O, enzyme-treated red cell control.

Procedure

1. Set up ABO tube test as described in Method 2-2. Red cell samples to be tested include untreated and enzyme-treated red cells.
2. Set up ABO tube test for enzyme-treated group O red cells as a control.
3. Incubate for 30 minutes at room temperature.
4. Centrifuge tubes according to reagent manufacturer's directions.
5. Gently resuspend red cell buttons and examine for agglutination.

Interpretation

Test results can be considered valid *only* if no reactivity is observed with the group O, enzyme-treated red cell control. Reactivity by anti-A, -B, or -A,B reagents with the enzyme-treated group O red cell control indicates excess enzyme treatment. No ABO interpretation can be made if the group O control is positive.

Notes

When no agglutination is observed after 30 minutes at room temperature, a modified procedure using enzyme-treated red cells and 15 to 30 minutes of incubation at 4 C may be used to further enhance detection of weak A and B expression.

METHOD 2-7. CONFIRMING WEAK A OR B SUBGROUP BY ADSORPTION AND ELUTION

Principle

Some weak ABO subgroups are too weak to be detected by direct agglutination, even after cold temperature and antibody enhancement. The presence of A antigens, B antigens, or both requires adsorbing anti-A or anti-B to red cells, followed by elution of bound antibody. The eluate is then evaluated for the presence of anti-A and anti-B by testing against A_1 and B reagent red cells.

Specimen

Red cells to be tested.

Reagents

1. Human anti-A and/or anti-B. Because some monoclonal ABO typing reagents are sensitive to changes in pH and osmolarity, the reagents may not be suitable for use in adsorption or elution tests.
2. Eluting agent: See Methods 4-3 and 4-4.
3. Group O red cell samples (three examples).
4. Group A_1 or B red cell samples as appropriate (three examples).

Procedure

1. Wash 1 mL of red cells to be tested at least three times with saline. Remove and discard supernatant saline after the last wash.
2. Add 1 mL of reagent anti-A (if weak A variant suspected) or 1 mL reagent anti-B (if weak B variant suspected) to washed red cells.
3. Mix red cells with antibody, and incubate at 4 C for 1 hour, mixing occasionally.
4. Centrifuge mixture to pack red cells. Remove all supernatant reagent.
5. Transfer red cells to a clean test tube.
6. Wash red cells at least eight times with large volumes (10 mL or more) of cold (4 C) saline. Save an aliquot of the final wash supernatant fluid, and test it in parallel with the eluate.
7. Use an elution method suitable for recovery of ABO antibodies [eg, heat (Method 4-3) or Lui freeze-thaw elution methods (Method 4-4)].

8. Test the eluate and the final wash solution (from step 6), in parallel, against three examples of group O red cells and three examples of red cells of the appropriate ABO type (A_1 or B cells). Add 2 drops of eluate or wash to 1 drop of red cells, and examine for agglutination after immediate centrifugation.
9. If no agglutination is observed after centrifugation, incubate for 15 to 30 minutes at room temperature and centrifuge.
10. If no agglutination is observed after room-temperature incubation, incubate at 37 C (15 minutes) and perform an indirect antiglobulin test.

Interpretation

1. The presence of anti-A or anti-B in the eluate indicates the presence of A or B antigen on test red cells. The results of the eluate are valid only if the following occur:
   a. The eluate reacts with all three antigen-positive cells, at any phase.
   b. The eluate is nonreactive with all three group O red cells.
   c. The final wash solution is nonreactive with all six cells tested.
2. Nonreaction of the eluate with antigen-positive red cells may indicate that the test red cells did not express A or B antigen. Alternatively, the lack of reaction could reflect failure to perform the eluate correctly.
3. Reactivity in the eluate with some or all of both antigen-positive and group O red cells indicates recovery of some other or additional antibody in the process.
4. If the wash solution reacts with antigen-positive red cells, the eluate results are invalid. The reaction can occur if unbound reagent antibody was not adequately removed by washing before the elution step or by dissociation of bound antibody during the wash process.
5. Adsorption and elution of A_1, B, or O red cells, or all three, can be performed and tested in parallel as positive and negative controls.

Reference

1. Beattie KM. Identifying the cause of weak or "missing" antigens in ABO grouping tests. In: The investigation of typing and compatibility problems caused by red blood cells. Washington, DC: AABB, 1975:15-37.

METHOD 2-8. TESTING SALIVA FOR A, B, H, Le^a, AND Le^b ANTIGENS

Principle

Approximately 78% of all individuals possess the Se gene that governs the secretion of water-soluble ABH antigens into all body fluids except cerebrospinal fluid. Such secreted antigens can be demonstrated in saliva by inhibition tests with ABH and Lewis antisera (see Chapter 12).

Specimen

1. Collect 5 to 10 mL of saliva in a small beaker or wide-mouth test tube. Most individuals can accumulate this amount in several minutes. To encourage salivation, the person may chew wax, paraffin, or a clean rubber band, but not gum or anything else that contains sugar or protein.
2. Centrifuge saliva at 900 to 1000 × *g* for 8 to 10 minutes.
3. Transfer the supernate to a clean test tube, and place it in a boiling waterbath for 8 to 10 minutes to inactivate salivary enzymes.
4. Recentrifuge at 900 to 1000 × *g* for 8 to 10 minutes, remove clear or slightly opalescent supernatant fluid, and discard the opaque or semisolid material. Dilute the supernatant fluid with an equal volume of saline.
5. Refrigerate, if testing is to be done within several hours. If testing will not be done on the day of collection, freeze the sample

and store it at –20 C. Frozen samples retain activity for several years.

Reagents

1. Human (polyclonal) anti-A and anti-B.
2. Anti-H lectin from *Ulex europaeus* obtained commercially or prepared by saline extraction of *U. europaeus* seeds.
3. Polyclonal (rabbit, goat, or human) anti-Le^a. There are no published data on the suitability of monoclonal Lewis antibodies.
4. A_1 and B red cells, as used in Method 2-2.
5. Group O, Le(a+b–) red cells.
6. Frozen or fresh saliva from persons known to be secretors or nonsecretors, to use as positive and negative controls. (See Notes.)

Procedure

Selection of Blood Grouping Reagent Dilution

1. Prepare doubling dilutions of the appropriate blood typing reagent: anti-A, anti-B, anti-H to determine ABH secretor status, or anti-Le^a to determine secretor status (see Method 3-7).
2. To 1 drop of each reagent dilution, add 1 drop of 2% to 5% saline suspension of red cells [A, B, O, or Le(a+) as appropriate].
3. Centrifuge each tube and examine macroscopically for agglutination.
4. Select the highest reagent dilution that gives 2+ agglutination.

Inhibition Test for Secretor Status

1. Add 1 drop of appropriately diluted blood grouping reagent to each of four tubes. For ABH studies, the tubes should be labeled "Secretor," "Nonsecretor," "Saline," and "Unknown." For Lewis studies, the labels will be "Lewis positive," "Lewis negative," "Saline," and "Unknown."
2. Add 1 drop of the appropriate saliva to each of the "Secretor," "Nonsecretor," and "Unknown" tubes, and 1 drop of saline to the tube marked "Saline."
3. Mix the contents of the tubes. Incubate the tubes for 8 to 10 minutes at room temperature.
4. Add 1 drop of 2% to 5% saline suspension of washed indicator red cells to each tube [A, B, O, or Le(a+), as appropriate].
5. Mix the contents of the tubes. Incubate the tubes for 30 to 60 minutes at room temperature.
6. Centrifuge each tube and inspect each red cell button macroscopically for agglutination.

Interpretation

1. Agglutination of indicator red cells by antibody in tubes containing saliva indicates that the saliva does not contain the corresponding antigen.
2. The failure of known antibody to agglutinate indicator red cells after incubation with saliva indicates that the saliva contains the corresponding antigen.
3. The failure of antibody in the saline control tube to agglutinate indicator red cells invalidates the results of saliva tests; the failure usually reflects use of reagents that are too dilute. Redetermine the appropriate reagent dilution, as described earlier, and repeat the testing.
4. For further interpretation, see Table 2-8-1.

Notes

1. For ABH status, use saliva from previously tested *Se* and *sese* persons. For Lewis testing, use saliva from a person whose red cells are Le(a+b–) or Le(a–b+) as the positive control; use saliva from a Le(a–b–) person as the negative control. Aliquots of saliva from persons of known secretor status may be frozen for later use.
2. This screening procedure can be adapted for the semiquantitation of blood group activity by testing serial saline dilutions of saliva. The higher the dilution needed to remove inhibitory activity, the more

TABLE 2-8-1. Interpretation of Saliva Testing

Testing with Anti-H				
Unknown Saliva	***Se* Saliva (H Substance Present)**	**Non-*Se* Saliva (H Substance Not Present)**	**Saline (Dilution Control)**	**Interpretation**
2+	0	2+	2+	Nonsecretor of H
0	0	2+	2+	Secretor of H
Testing with Anti-Le^a				
Unknown Saliva	**Le-Positive Saliva**	**Le-Negative Saliva**	**Saline (Dilution Control)**	**Interpretation**
2+	0	2+	2+	Lewis-negative
0	0	2+	2+	Lewis-positive*

*A Lewis-positive person shown to be a secretor of ABH can be assumed to have Le^b as well as Le^a in saliva. A Le(a+) person who is *sese* and does not secrete ABH substance will have only Le^a in saliva.

blood group substance is present in the saliva. Saliva should be diluted before it is incubated with antibody. To detect or to measure salivary A or B substance in addition to H substance, the same procedure can be used with diluted anti-A and anti-B reagents. The appropriate dilution of anti-A or anti B is obtained by titrating the reagent against A_1 or B red cells, respectively.

3. A Lewis-positive person shown to be a secretor of A, B, and H can be assumed to have Le^b as well as Le^a in his or her saliva. A Le(a+) person who does not secrete A, B, or H substances lacks the Se gene and will have only Le^a in his or her saliva.

METHOD 2-9. CONFIRMING ANTI-A_1 IN AN A_2 OR WEAK A SUBGROUP

Principle

A_2 and weak A subgroups can possess an anti-A_1 in serum or plasma, which will react with A_1 reagent cells during reverse or serum grouping. Anti-A_1 is a common cause of ABO discrepancies in A_2 and weak A subgroups.

Specimen

Red cells and serum or plasma to be evaluated.

Reagents

1. *Dolichos biflorus* lectin (anti-A1).
2. Group A_1, A_2, and O control red cells.

Procedure

Testing Red Cells

1. Add 1 drop of A_1 lectin to each test and control tube.
2. Add 1 drop of 2% to 5% saline suspension of red cells (Method 1-6) to the appropriate tubes.
3. Centrifuge 15 seconds.
4. Examine and record agglutination.

Testing Serum/Plasma (See Methods 2-2 and 2-3)

1. Serum should be tested against several examples (eg, two each) of A_1, A_2, and O red cells using established serum grouping methods.

Interpretation

1. The lectin should strongly agglutinate A_1 red cells (3+ to 4+) but should not agglutinate A_2 or O red cells. Group A red cells that fail to agglutinate with the lectin can be considered A_2 or another weak A subgroup.
2. Anti-A_1 in the patient's serum will agglutinate all A_1 samples. Anti-A_1 will not agglutinate autologous, A_2, or group O red cells. If the patient's serum agglutinates group A_2 or group O red cells, another cause for unexpected reactivity should be investigated.
3. If commercial lectin preparations are used, the manufacturer's directions should be followed for appropriate testing method and controls.

METHOD 2-10. RESOLVING ABO DISCREPANCIES CAUSED BY UNEXPECTED ALLOANTIBODIES

Principle

Some alloantibodies (eg, anti-P1 and anti-M) react at room temperature. Unexpected positive reactions resulting in an ABO discrepancy can occur if A_1 or B reagent red cells, or both, used for serum grouping are positive for the antigen.

Procedure

1. Test the patient's serum or plasma with antibody detection red cells at room temperature. If a cold-reactive alloantibody is identified, phenotype reagent A_1 and B red cells for the presence of the antigen if the information is not available from the manufacturer.
2. Test serum or plasma against A_1 and B red cells lacking the specific antigen of interest.
3. If the antibody detection test result is negative at room temperature, the patient may possess an alloantibody to a low-prevalence antigen present on A_1 or B reagent red cells. Retest the serum or plasma with other randomly selected A_1 and B red cell samples.

METHOD 2-11. DETERMINING SERUM GROUP WITHOUT CENTRIFUGATION

Principle

Strongly reactive cold autoantibodies, such as anti-I and anti-IH, can agglutinate adult red cells, including reagent red cells, at room temperature. With few exceptions, agglutination by these cold agglutinins is weaker than that caused by anti-A and anti-B. One method to identify anti-A and anti-B in the presence of cold antibodies is by using a "settled reading."

Specimen

Serum or plasma to be evaluated.

Reagents

A_1, B, and O reagent red cells.

Procedure

1. Warm serum and reagent red cells to 37 C.
2. Add 2 to 3 drops serum to prelabeled (A_1, B, O) clean test tubes.
3. Add 1 drop of the appropriate reagent red cells to each of the labeled tubes.
4. Mix contents and incubate at 37 C for 1 hour.
5. Remove and examine for agglutination. Do not centrifuge samples (settled reading).

Notes

1. Weak examples of anti-A and anti-B may not be detected by this method.
2. If the group O red cell control shows agglutination, no valid conclusion can be made regarding ABO type.

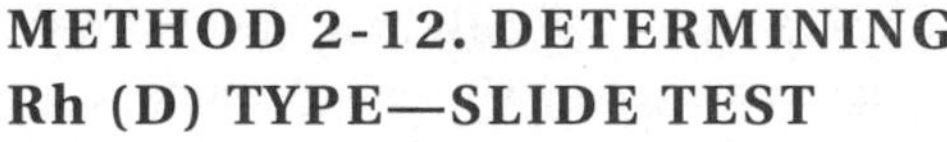

METHOD 2-12. DETERMINING Rh (D) TYPE—SLIDE TEST

Principle

For a discussion of Rh (D) typing principles, see Chapter 13.

Specimen

Red cells from clotted or anticoagulated blood samples may be used. The red cells may be suspended in autologous serum, plasma, or saline or may be washed and resuspended in saline. Slide tests produce optimal results with a higher concentration of red cells than required for tube tests.

Reagents

The reagent anti-D must specifically indicate that it is suitable for slide tests. The manufacturer's instructions will indicate the type of reagent control to use.

Cautions

Slide testing imposes a much greater risk of biohazard exposure. Personnel should follow safety measures detailed in the facility's procedures manual. Evaporation of the reaction mixture can cause the red cells to aggregate and be misinterpreted as agglutination. Tests for weak D expression cannot be performed by slide testing.

Procedure

1. Prewarm the glass slides on an Rh viewbox to 40 to 50 C before testing.
2. Place 1 drop of anti-D onto a clean, labeled slide.
3. Place 1 drop of the appropriate control reagent, if needed, onto a second labeled slide. Follow the manufacturer's instructions for the reagent control. For tests using a low-protein anti-D, a negative result on slide testing with anti-A or anti-B serves as the control reaction.
4. To each slide, add 2 drops of a well-mixed 40% to 50% suspension of red cells in serum or plasma.
5. Use a clean applicator stick to thoroughly mix the cell suspension and reagent over an area approximately 20 mm × 40 mm.
6. Place the slide(s) on the viewbox and tilt it gently while continuously observing for agglutination. Inspect for macroscopic agglutination and read within 2 minutes. Do not mistake drying of the reaction mixture or rouleaux for agglutination.
7. Interpret and record the results.

Interpretation

1. Agglutination with anti-D and no agglutination on the control slide constitute a positive test result and indicate that the red cells are D positive.
2. No agglutination with either anti-D or the control suggests the red cells are D negative. Testing by an indirect antiglobulin procedure (IAT; see Method 2-15) will detect weak expression of D not detected on slide testing.
3. If agglutination is observed on the control slide, results of anti-D testing must not be interpreted as positive without further testing.
4. Drying around the edges of the mixture must not be confused with agglutination.

METHOD 2-13. DETERMINING RH (D) TYPE—TUBE TEST

Specimen

Red cells from clotted or anticoagulated blood samples may be used. The red cells may be suspended in autologous serum, plasma, or saline or may be washed and resuspended in saline.

Reagents

Suitable reagents include low-protein monoclonal reagents and high-protein polyclonal reagents. The manufacturer's instructions will indicate the type of reagent control to use.

Procedure

1. Place 1 drop of anti-D into a clean, labeled test tube. Note: The addition of the reagent to the tube *before* the addition of the red cell suspension acts as a visual check for the presence of the anti-D to eliminate false-negative reactions caused by failure to add the reagent.
2. Place 1 drop of the appropriate control reagent to a second labeled tube.
3. Add 1 drop of a 2% to 5% suspension of the red cells in saline, serum, or plasma. Alternatively, an equivalent amount of red cells to be tested can be transferred to each tube with a clean applicator stick.
4. Mix gently and centrifuge for the time, and at the speed, specified by the manufacturer.
5. Gently resuspend the red cell button and examine for agglutination. If red cells were added by transfer with an applicator stick, addition of 1 drop of saline will aid resuspension of the cell button.
6. Grade reactions and record the test and control results.

Interpretation

1. Agglutination in the anti-D tube, combined with a smooth suspension in the control tube, indicates that the red cells are D positive.
2. No agglutination of the red cells in both the anti-D and the control tubes is a negative test result. A sample from a patient may be designated as D negative at this point. AABB *Standards for Blood Banks and Transfusion Services* requires donor blood and infants of mothers being evaluated for Rh Immune Globulin to be tested further for the presence of weak D antigen.
3. A negative tube test result with anti-A and/or anti-B is a valid negative control if a low-protein anti-D reagent is used for testing.
4. Agglutination in the control tube invalidates the test. Methods for removal of IgM or IgG antibody from the red cells may be required. See Methods 2-17 through 2-21.

Reference

1. Carson TH, ed. Standards for blood banks and transfusion services. 27th ed. Bethesda, MD: AABB, 2011.

METHOD 2-14. DETERMINING RH (D) TYPE—MICROPLATE TEST

Specimen

Follow the manufacturer's instructions. Automated methods may require the use of samples drawn into a specific anticoagulant.

Reagents

Use only anti-D reagents approved for use in microplate tests. Consult the manufacturer's instructions for specific reagents, equipment, and proper controls.

Procedure

1. Place 1 drop of anti-D reagent into a clean well of the microplate. If the reagent requires use of an Rh control, add 1 drop of the control to a second well.
2. Add 1 drop of a 2% to 5% saline suspension of red cells to each well.
3. Mix the contents by gently tapping the sides of the plate.
4. Centrifuge the plate at the appropriate conditions according to the manufacturer's instructions.
5. Resuspend the cell buttons by manually tapping the plate or with the aid of a microplate shaker, or place the plate at an angle for the tilt-and-stream method.
6. Examine for agglutination, read, interpret, and record the results.
7. To enhance weak reactions, incubate tests with negative results at 37 C for 15 to 30 minutes and repeat steps 4 to 6.

Interpretation

1. Agglutination in the anti-D well, combined with a smooth suspension in the control well, indicates that the red cells are D positive.
2. No agglutination of the red cells in both the anti-D and the control wells is a negative test result. A sample from a patient may be designated as D negative at this point. AABB *Standards for Blood Banks and Transfusion Services* requires donor blood and infants of mothers being evaluated for Rh Immune Globulin to be tested further for the presence of weak D antigen.
3. A negative test result with anti-A and/or anti-B is a valid negative control if a low-protein anti-D reagent is used for testing.

Reference

1. Carson TH, ed. Standards for blood banks and transfusion services. 27th ed. Bethesda, MD: AABB, 2011.

METHOD 2-15. TESTING FOR WEAK D

Principle

Some weak D antigens are recognized only by an indirect antiglobulin (IAT) procedure. AABB *Standards for Blood Banks and Transfusion Services* requires detection of weak D when typing donor units, but this is not required for pretransfusion testing of patients' samples.

Specimen

Follow the manufacturer's instructions.

Reagents

Not every anti-D reagent is suitable for the weak D test. Consult the manufacturer's package insert for test procedures and appropriate controls.

1. Antihuman globulin reagent, either polyspecific or anti-IgG.
2. IgG-coated control cells.

Procedure

1. If a tube test was performed for the direct anti-D test, the same tube may be used for the weak D test if an appropriate reagent was used. Go to step 5.
2. Place 1 drop of anti-D in a clean, labeled test tube.
3. Place 1 drop of the appropriate control reagent in a second, labeled test tube.
4. To each tube, add 1 drop of 2% to 5% saline-suspended red cells.
5. Mix and incubate the test and control tubes according to the reagent manufacturer's directions. This is typically 15 to 30 minutes at 37 C.
6. If desired, centrifuge and read after incubation by gently resuspending the red cell button, and examine for agglutination.
7. Wash the red cells at least three times with saline.
8. Add antiglobulin reagent according to the manufacturer's directions.
9. Mix gently and centrifuge according to the calibrated spin time for the centrifuge.
10. Gently resuspend and examine for agglutination, grade, and record.
11. Add IgG-coated control cells to confirm the validity of negative antiglobulin test results.

Interpretation

1. Agglutination in the anti-D tube, combined with a smooth suspension in the control tube, indicates that the red cells are D positive. It is incorrect to report the results as "D^u positive" or "D negative, D^u positive."
2. No agglutination of the red cells in both the anti-D and the control tubes is a negative test result.

3. It is permissible to use a direct antiglobulin test on the test cells as a control, but an IAT procedure with an Rh or albumin control reagent is preferable because this ensures that all reagent components that might cause a false-positive result are represented.
4. Agglutination at any phase in the control tube invalidates the test, and no interpretation can be made. IgG removal from the red cells may be helpful (see Methods 2-20 and 2-21).

Reference

1. Carson TH, ed. Standards for blood banks and transfusion services. 27th ed. Bethesda, MD: AABB, 2011.

METHOD 2-16. PREPARING AND USING LECTINS

Principle

Saline extracts of seeds react with specific carbohydrates on red cell membranes and make useful typing reagents that are highly specific at appropriate dilutions. Diluted extract of *Dolichos biflorus* agglutinates A_1 red cells but not A_2. *Ulex europaeus* extract reacts with the H determinant; it agglutinates in a manner proportional to the amount of H present ($O>>A_2>>B>>A_1>>A_1B$ red cells). Other lectins useful for special purposes include *Arachis hypogaea* (anti-T), *Glycine max* (anti-T, -Tn), *Vicia graminea* (anti-N), and the *Salvia* lectins (*S. horminum*, anti-Tn/Cad; *S. sclarea*, anti-Tn). To investigate red cell polyagglutination, prepare and test the red cells with *Arachis, Glycine, Salvia,* and *Dolichos* lectins. The anticipated reactions with various types of polyagglutinable red cells are shown in Table 2-16-1. If commercially made lectins are used, follow the manufacturer's instructions.

Reagents

Seeds may be obtained from health-food stores, pharmacies, or commercial seed companies. The seeds should be raw.

Procedure

1. Grind the seeds in a food processor or blender until the particles look like coarse sand. A mortar and pestle may be used, or seeds can be used whole.
2. In a large test tube or small beaker, place ground seeds and three to four times their volume of saline. (Seeds vary in the quantity of saline they absorb.)
3. Incubate at room temperature for 4 to 12 hours, stirring or inverting occasionally.
4. Transfer supernatant fluid to a centrifuge tube, and centrifuge for 5 minutes to obtain a clear supernatant. Collect and filter the supernatant fluid, and discard the seed residue.

TABLE 2-16-1. Reactions between Lectins and Polyagglutinable Red Cells

	T	Th	Tk	Tn	Cad
*Arachis hypogaea**	+	+	+	0	0
Dolichos biflorus†	0	0	0	+	+
Glycine max (soja)	+	0	0	+	+
Salvia sclarea	0	0	0	+	0
Salvia horminum	0	0	0	+	+

*T and Th cells give weaker reactions with *Arachis* after protease treatment; Tk reactivity is enhanced after protease treatment.

†A and AB cells may react because of anti-A reactivity of *Dolichos* lectin.

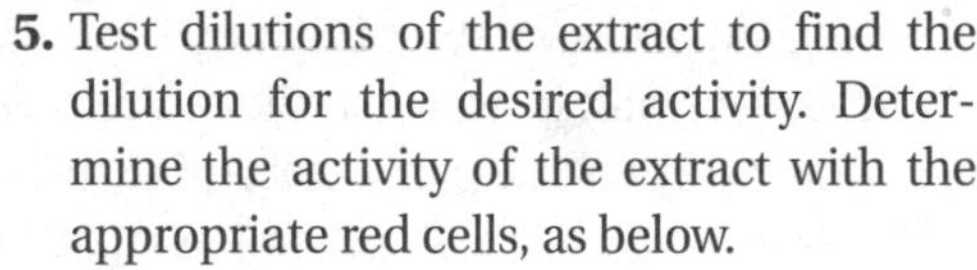

5. Test dilutions of the extract to find the dilution for the desired activity. Determine the activity of the extract with the appropriate red cells, as below.

For Dolichos biflorus:

- **a.** Add 1 drop of 2% to 5% saline suspension of known A_1, A_2, A_1B, A_2B, B, and O red cells to appropriately labeled tubes.
- **b.** Add 1 drop of the extract to each tube.
- **c.** Centrifuge for calibrated time.
- **d.** Inspect for agglutination and record results.
- **e.** The lectin should agglutinate A_1 and A_1B red cells but not A_2, A_2B, B, or O red cells. The native extract often agglutinates all the red cells tested. To make the product useful for reagent purposes, add enough saline to the extract so that there is 3+ or 4+ agglutination of A_1 and A_1B red cells, but not of A_2, A_2B, B, or O red cells.

For Ulex europaeus:

- **a.** Add 1 drop of 2% to 5% saline suspension of known A_1, A_2, A_1B, B, and O red cells to appropriately labeled tubes.
- **b.** Add 1 drop of extract to each tube.
- **c.** Centrifuge for the calibrated time.
- **d.** Inspect for agglutination and record results.
- **e.** The strength of the agglutination should be in the order of O>>A_2>>B>>A_1>>A_1B.
- **f.** Dilute extract with saline, if necessary, to a point that O red cells show 3+ or 4+ agglutination, A_2 and B red cells show 1+ to 2+ agglutination, and A_1 or A_1B red cells are not agglutinated.

Notes

1. To facilitate grinding hard seeds, one should cover the seeds with saline and soak them for several hours before grinding. The container used for soaking should not be tightly closed because some beans release gas during the soaking process, which could cause the container to explode.
2. The saline extracts may be stored in the refrigerator for several days; they may be stored indefinitely if frozen.
3. Tests should include a positive and negative control.

METHOD 2-17. REMOVING AUTOANTIBODY BY WARM SALINE WASHES

Principle

Red cells heavily coated with autoantibodies can spontaneously agglutinate or autoagglutinate and lead to false-positive reactions with anti-A, -B, and -D. Washing red cells with warm saline will often remove sufficient autoantibody to allow determination of ABO and Rh type.

Specimen

Red cells with spontaneous agglutination or autoagglutination interfering with red cell antigen typing.

Reagents

1. Warm isotonic saline.
2. Monoclonal or polyclonal anti-A and anti-B.
3. Control reagent such as 6% albumin.

Procedure

1. Warm red cell suspension to 37 C for 15 minutes to 1 hour.
2. Wash cells with warm (37 C) saline several times to remove autoantibody.
3. Type washed red cells with anti-A, anti-B, and anti-D and 6% albumin as described in earlier methods (Methods 2-1 to 2-3). If the control is still positive, see Methods 2-18 through 2-21.

METHOD 2-18. USING SULFHYDRYL REAGENTS TO DISPERSE AUTOAGGLUTINATION

Principle

Red cells heavily coated with IgM autoantibodies can spontaneously agglutinate during centrifugation, leading to false-positive reactions in red cell typing and direct antiglobulin (DAT) tests. Dithiothreitol (DTT) or 2-mercaptoethanol (2-ME) can reduce the disulfide bonds of IgM molecules, decreasing their polyvalency and ability to directly agglutinate red cells.

Specimen

Red cells with IgM autoagglutination interfering with red cell antigen typing.

Reagents

1. 0.01 M DTT: 0.154 g of DTT dissolved in 100 mL of phosphate-buffered saline (PBS) at pH 7.3; store at 4 C.
2. 0.1 M stock 2-ME: 0.7 mL of a 14 M stock solution of 2-ME diluted in 100 mL of PBS at pH 7.3; 2-ME should be stored in a dark glass container at 4 C.
3. PBS at pH 7.3.
4. Antigen-positive control red cells for antigen typing to be treated in parallel.
5. Red cell typing antisera.
6. 6% albumin (control reagent).

Procedure

1. Wash red cells three times with saline, and dilute to a 50% concentration in PBS.
2. Add an equal volume of 0.01 M DTT in PBS or 0.1 M 2-ME in PBS to the red cell suspension.
3. Incubate at 37 C for 15 minutes (DTT) or 10 minutes (2-ME).
4. Wash red cells three times in saline, and dilute to 2% to 5% suspension in saline.
5. Test the treated cells with 6% albumin (immediate-spin test) to make sure the cells do not spontaneously agglutinate. If the test result is negative, the red cells are now ready for use in red cell typing tests.

Notes

1. Treated red cells should not agglutinate in 6% albumin.
2. Antigen-positive control red cells should react equally strongly with typing reagent before and after treatment.
3. This procedure is normally used only for ABO forward typing, Rh determination, and the DAT.
4. Kell system antigens may be weakened or destroyed by DTT and 2-ME treatment. Js^a and Js^b may be more sensitive than other Kell antigens to this concentration of DTT.

Reference

1. Judd WJ, Johnson S, Storry JR. Judd's methods in immunohematology. 3rd ed. Bethesda, MD: AABB Press, 2008.

METHOD 2-19. USING GENTLE HEAT ELUTION TO TEST RED CELLS WITH A POSITIVE DAT

Principle

Red cells that are heavily coated with IgG may spontaneously agglutinate in high-protein reagents and will cause false-positive antihuman globulin (AHG) test results. If one is to perform red cell antigen typing, it may be necessary to dissociate antibody from the cells by elution without damaging membrane integrity or altering antigen expression. The gentle heat elution procedure used to prepare immunoglobulin-free red cells differs from procedures that are intended to recover active antibody.

Specimen

Test red cells with a positive direct antiglobulin test (DAT) result.

Reagent

AHG.

Procedure

1. Place one volume of washed antibody-coated red cells and three volumes of normal saline in a test tube of appropriate size. In another tube, place the same volumes of saline and washed red cells positive for the antigen under test. This step will provide a check that the elution technique does not destroy the antigen reactivity.
2. Incubate the contents of both tubes at approximately 45 C for 10 to 15 minutes. The tubes should be agitated frequently. The time of incubation should be roughly proportional to the degree of antibody coating, as indicated by the strength of antiglobulin reactivity.
3. Centrifuge the tubes and discard the supernatant saline.
4. Test the red cells for the degree of antibody removal by comparing a DAT on the treated red cells with the DAT on untreated red cells. If the antibody coating is reduced but still present, steps 1 through 3 can be repeated; the control red cells should be subjected to a similar second treatment.
5. Test the treated red cells for the desired antigen.

Notes

1. This procedure may be unnecessary if IgM monoclonal reagents are available; such reagents cause direct agglutination and are not usually affected by bound immunoglobulin.
2. As with untreated patients' red cells, results of antigen testing in recently transfused patients should be interpreted with caution because of the potential presence of donor red cells.

METHOD 2-20. DISSOCIATING IgG BY CHLOROQUINE FOR ANTIGEN TESTING OF RED CELLS WITH A POSITIVE DAT

Principle

Red cells giving a positive direct antiglobulin test (DAT) result cannot be tested accurately with blood typing reagents that require an indirect antiglobulin technique. Under controlled conditions, chloroquine diphosphate dissociates IgG from the red cell membrane with little or no damage to its integrity. Use of this procedure permits complete phenotyping of red cells coated with warm-reactive autoantibody, including tests with reagents solely reactive by indirect antiglobulin techniques.

Specimen

Red cells with a positive DAT resulting from IgG coating.

Reagents

1. Chloroquine diphosphate solution prepared by dissolving 20 g of chloroquine diphosphate in 100 mL of saline. Adjust to pH 5.1 with 1 N NaOH, and store at 2 to 8 C.
2. Control red cells carrying a single-dose expression of antigens for which the test samples are to be phenotyped.
3. Anti-IgG antiglobulin reagent.

Procedure

1. To 0.2 mL of washed IgG-coated cells, add 0.8 mL of chloroquine diphosphate solution. Similarly treat the control sample.
2. Mix and incubate at room temperature for 30 minutes.
3. Remove a small aliquot (eg, 1 drop) of the treated test cells and wash them four times with saline.
4. Test the washed cells with anti-IgG.
5. If this treatment has rendered the cells nonreactive with anti-IgG, wash the total

volume of treated test cells and control cells three times in saline and make a 2% to 5% suspension in saline to use in subsequent blood typing tests.

6. If the treated red cells react with anti-IgG after 30 minutes of incubation with chloroquine diphosphate, steps 3 and 4 should be repeated at 30-minute intervals (for a maximum incubation period of 2 hours), until the sample tested is nonreactive with anti-IgG. Then proceed as described in step 5.

Notes

1. Chloroquine diphosphate does not dissociate complement proteins from the cell membrane. If red cells are coated with both IgG and C3, only anti-IgG should be used in tests performed after chloroquine treatment.
2. Incubation with chloroquine diphosphate should not extend beyond 2 hours. Prolonged incubation at room temperature or incubation at 37 C may cause hemolysis and loss of red cell antigens.
3. Some denaturation of Rh antigens may occur.
4. Many serologists run chloroquine-treated control cells for each antigen tested. Select control cells that are positive for the antigen corresponding to the antisera that will be used to type the patient's cells.
5. Chloroquine diphosphate may not completely remove antibody from sensitized red cells. DAT results on red cells from some persons, particularly those with a strongly positive initial test result, may only be diminished in strength.
6. In addition to its use for removal of autoantibodies, this method can be used for removal of Bg (HLA)-related antigens from red cells. Appropriate Bg controls should be used.
7. If a commercial kit is used, manufacturer's instructions should be followed for testing and controls.

References

1. Edwards JM, Moulds JJ, Judd WJ. Chloroquine dissociation of antigen-antibody complexes: A new technique for phenotyping red blood cells with a positive direct antiglobulin test. Transfusion 1982;22:59-61.
2. Swanson JL, Sastamoinen R. Chloroquine stripping of HLA-A,B antigens from red cells (letter). Transfusion 1985;25:439-40.

METHOD 2-21. USING ACID GLYCINE/EDTA TO REMOVE ANTIBODIES FROM RED CELLS

Principle

Acid glycine/EDTA can be used to dissociate antibody molecules from red cell membranes. The procedure is routinely used for blood typing tests or adsorption procedures. All common red cell antigens can be detected after treatment with acid glycine/EDTA except antigens of the Kell system, Bg antigens, and Er antigens. Thus, red cells treated in this manner cannot be used to determine these phenotypes.

Specimen

Red cells giving a positive direct antiglobulin test (DAT) result.

Reagents

1. 10% EDTA prepared by dissolving 2 g of disodium ethylenediamine tetraacetic acid (Na_2EDTA) in 20 mL of distilled or deionized water.
2. 0.1 M glycine-HCl buffer (pH 1.5) prepared by diluting 0.75 g of glycine to 100 mL with isotonic (unbuffered) saline. Adjust the pH to 1.5 using concentrated HCl.
3. 1.0 M TRIS-NaCl prepared by dissolving 12.1 g of Tris(hydroxymethyl) aminomethane (TRIS) and 5.25 g of sodium chloride (NaCl) to 100 mL with distilled or deionized water.

Procedure

1. Wash the red cells to be treated six times with isotonic saline.
2. In a test tube, mix together 20 volumes of 0.1 M acid glycine-HCl (pH 1.5) with five volumes of 10% EDTA. This mixture is the acid glycine/EDTA reagent.
3. Place 10 volumes of washed red cells in a clean tube.
4. Add 20 volumes of acid glycine/EDTA.
5. Mix the contents of the tube thoroughly.
6. Incubate the mixture at room temperature for no more than 2 to 3 minutes.
7. Add one volume of 1.0 M TRIS-NaCl, and mix the contents of the tube.
8. Centrifuge at 900 to 1000 × *g* for 1 to 2 minutes; then aspirate and discard the supernatant fluid.
9. Wash the red cells four times with saline.
10. Test the washed red cells with anti-IgG. If nonreactive with anti-IgG, the cells are ready for use in blood typing or adsorption procedures. If the DAT is still positive, one additional treatment can be performed.

Notes

1. Overincubation of red cells with acid glycine/EDTA causes irreversible damage to red cell membranes.
2. Include a parallel control reagent, such as 6% bovine albumin or inert plasma, when typing treated red cells.
3. Use anti-IgG, not a polyspecific antiglobulin reagent, in step 10.
4. Many serologists run acid glycine/EDTA-treated control red cells for each antigen tested. Select control red cells that are positive for the antigen corresponding to the antisera that will be used to type the patient's cells.
5. If a commercial kit is used, manufacturer's instructions should be followed for testing and controls.

References

1. Louie JE, Jiang AF, Zaroulis CG. Preparation of intact antibody-free red cells in autoimmune hemolytic anemia (abstract). Transfusion 1986;26:550.
2. Champagne K, Spruell P, Chen J, et al. EDTA/glycine-acid vs. chloroquine diphosphate treatment for stripping Bg antigens from red blood cells (abstract). Transfusion 1996;36(Suppl):21S.
3. Reid ME, Lomas-Francis C. The blood group antigen factsbook. 2nd ed. London, UK: Elsevier Academic Press, 2004.

METHOD 2-22. SEPARATING TRANSFUSED FROM AUTOLOGOUS RED CELLS BY SIMPLE CENTRIFUGATION

Principle

Newly formed autologous red cells generally have a lower specific gravity than transfused red cells and will therefore concentrate at the top of the column of red cells when blood is centrifuged in a microhematocrit tube. This provides a simple method for recovering autologous red cells in a blood sample from recently transfused patients. Note: Red cells from patients with hemoglobin S or spherocytic disorders are not effectively separated by this method (see Method 2-23 for an alternative procedure).

Specimen

Red cells from whole blood collected into EDTA.

Materials

1. Microhematocrit centrifuge.
2. Plain (not heparinized) glass or plastic hematocrit tubes.
3. Sealant.

Procedure

1. Wash the red cells three times in saline. For the last wash, centrifuge them at 900 to 1000 × *g* for 5 to 15 minutes. Remove as much of the supernatant fluid as possible without disturbing the buffy coat. Mix thoroughly.

2. Fill 10 microhematocrit tubes to the 60-mm mark with well-mixed washed red cells.
3. Seal the ends of the tubes by heat or with sealant.
4. Centrifuge all tubes in a microhematocrit centrifuge for 15 minutes.
5. Cut the microhematocrit tubes 5 mm below the top of the column of red cells. This 5-mm segment contains the least dense, hence youngest, circulating red cells.
6. Place the cut microhematocrit tubes into larger test tubes (10 or 12 × 75 mm), add saline, and mix well to flush the red cells from the microhematocrit tubes. Then, either 1) centrifuge them at 1000 × *g* for 1 minute and remove the empty hematocrit tubes or 2) transfer the saline-suspended red cells to a clean test tube.
7. Wash the separated red cells three times in saline before resuspending them to 2% to 5% in saline for testing.

Notes

1. Separation is better if the sample is obtained 3 or more days after transfusion rather than shortly after transfusion.
2. The red cells should be mixed continuously while the microhematocrit tubes are being filled.
3. Separation techniques are effective only if the patient is producing normal or above-normal numbers of reticulocytes. This method will be ineffective in patients with inadequate reticulocyte production.
4. Some red cell antigens may not be as strongly expressed on reticulocytes as on older cells. Particular attention should be given to determinations of the E, e, c, Fy[a], Jk[a], and Ge antigens.

References

1. Reid ME, Toy P. Simplified method for recovery of autologous red blood cells from transfused patients. Am J Clin Pathol 1983;79:364-6.
2. Vengelen-Tyler V, Gonzales B. Reticulocyte rich RBCs will give weak reactions with many blood typing antisera (abstract). Transfusion 1985;25:476.

METHOD 2-23. SEPARATING TRANSFUSED FROM AUTOLOGOUS RED CELLS IN PATIENTS WITH HEMOGLOBIN S DISEASE

Principle

Red cells from patients with sickle cell disease, either hemoglobin SS or SC, are resistant to lysis by hypotonic saline, in contrast to red cells from normal persons and those with hemoglobin S trait. This procedure permits isolation of autologous red cells from patients with hemoglobin SS or SC disease who have recently been transfused.

Specimen

Red cells to be evaluated.

Reagents

1. Hypotonic saline (0.3% w/v NaCl): NaCl, 3 g; distilled water to 1 L.
2. Normal saline (0.9% w/v NaCl): NaCl, 9 g; distilled water to 1 L.

Procedure

1. Place 4 or 5 drops of red cells into a 10 or 12 × 75-mm test tube.
2. Wash the cells six times with 0.3% NaCl, or until the supernatant fluid no longer contains grossly visible hemoglobin. For each wash, centrifuge at 1000 × *g* for 1 minute.
3. Wash the cells twice with 0.9% NaCl to restore tonicity. For each wash, centrifuge at 200 × *g* for 2 minutes to facilitate removal of residual stroma.
4. Resuspend the remaining intact red cells to a 2% to 5% concentration for phenotyping.

Notes

1. Larger volumes, for use in adsorption studies, can be processed in a 16 × 100-mm test tube.

2. When using the hypotonic saline technique, one must be careful to remove the stroma from the lysed cells because stroma can adsorb typing serum and produce false-negative typing results.

Reference

1. Brown D. A rapid method for harvesting autologous red cells from patients with hemoglobin S disease. Transfusion 1988;28:21-3.

Antibody Detection, Identification, and Compatibility Testing

◆

METHOD 3-1. USING IMMEDIATE-SPIN COMPATIBILITY TESTING TO DEMONSTRATE ABO INCOMPATIBILITY

Principle

See Chapter 15 for a discussion of the principles of compatibility testing.

Specimen

Patient serum or plasma may be used. The age of the specimen must comply with the pretransfusion specimen requirements in AABB *Standards for Blood Banks and Transfusion Services.*[1]

Reagents

1. Normal saline.
2. Donor red cells.

Procedure

1. Prepare a 2% to 5% suspension of donor red cells in normal saline or EDTA saline. Some serologists using serum for testing prefer to suspend the donor red cells in EDTA saline because high-titer anti-A or anti-B can initiate complement coating, which can cause steric hindrance of agglutination.[2] The use of a patient's sample collected in EDTA is an alternative approach to prevent this phenomenon.
2. Label a tube for each donor red cell suspension being tested with the patient's serum.
3. Add 2 drops of the patient's serum or plasma to each tube.
4. Add 1 drop of the suspension of donor red cells to the appropriate test tube.
5. Mix the contents of the tube(s) and centrifuge according to the calibration of the centrifuge.
6. Examine the tube(s) for hemolysis, gently resuspend the red cell button(s), and examine for agglutination.
7. Read, interpret, and record test results.

Interpretation

1. Agglutination or hemolysis constitutes a positive (incompatible) test result.
2. A smooth suspension of red cells after resuspension of the red cell button constitutes a negative result and indicates a compatible immediate-spin crossmatch.

References

1. Carson TH, ed. Standards for blood banks and transfusion services. 27th ed. Bethesda, MD: AABB, 2011.
2. Judd WJ, Steiner EA, O'Donnell DB, Oberman HA. Discrepancies in ABO typing due to prozone: How safe is the immediate-spin crossmatch? Transfusion 1988;28:334-8.

METHOD 3-2. DETECTING ANTIBODIES TO RED CELL ANTIGENS—INDIRECT ANTIGLOBULIN TESTS

Principle

For a discussion of the principles of saline testing, albumin testing, low-ionic-strength saline (LISS) testing, and polyethylene glycol (PEG) indirect antiglobulin testing, see Chapter 15.

Specimen

Serum or plasma may be used. The age of the specimen must comply with pretransfusion specimen requirements in AABB *Standards for Blood Banks and Transfusion Services.*

Reagents

1. Normal saline.
2. Bovine albumin (22%).
3. LISS, made as follows:
   a. Add 1.75 g of NaCl and 18 g of glycine to a 1-liter volumetric flask.
   b. Add 20 mL of phosphate buffer prepared by combining 11.3 mL of 0.15 M KH_2PO_4 and 8.7 mL of 0.15 M Na_2HPO_4.
   c. Add distilled water to the 1-liter mark.
   d. Adjust the pH to 6.7 ± 0.1 with NaOH.
   e. Add 0.5 g of sodium azide as a preservative.
4. PEG, 20% w/v: To 20 g of 3350 MW PEG, add phosphate-buffered saline (PBS) pH 7.3 (see Method 1-7) to 100 mL. PEG is also available commercially.
5. Antihuman globulin (AHG) reagent. Polyspecific or anti-IgG may be used unless otherwise indicated.
6. Group O antibody detection cells. Pooled group O antibody-detection cells may be used only for donor testing. Testing of patient samples must be performed with unpooled cells.
7. A 2% to 5% suspension of donor red cells in saline.
8. IgG-coated red cells.

Note

LISS may be used as an additive (see Method 3-2-2) or for the suspension of test red cells (see Method 3-2-3). LISS preparations are also available commercially.

Reference

1. Carson TH, ed. Standards for blood banks and transfusion services. 27th ed. Bethesda, MD: AABB, 2011.

METHOD 3-2-1. SALINE INDIRECT ANTIGLOBULIN TEST PROCEDURE

Procedure

1. Add 2 drops of serum or plasma to properly labeled tubes.
2. Add 1 drop of 2% to 5% saline-suspended reagent group O red cells or donor red cells to each tube and mix.
3. Centrifuge and observe for hemolysis and agglutination. Grade and record the results.
4. Incubate at 37 C for 30 to 60 minutes.
5. Centrifuge and observe for hemolysis and agglutination. Grade and record the results.
6. Wash the red cells three or four times with saline, and completely decant the final wash.
7. Add AHG to the dry red cell button according to the manufacturer's directions. Mix well.
8. Centrifuge and observe for agglutination. Grade and record the results.
9. Confirm the validity of negative results by adding IgG-coated red cells.

METHOD 3-2-2. ALBUMIN OR LISS-ADDITIVE INDIRECT ANTIGLOBULIN TEST PROCEDURE

Procedure

1. Add 2 drops of serum or plasma to properly labeled tubes.
2. Add an equivalent volume of 22% bovine albumin or LISS additive (unless the manufacturer's directions state otherwise).
3. Add 1 drop of a 2% to 5% saline-suspended reagent or donor red cells to each tube and mix.
4. For albumin, incubate at 37 C for 15 to 30 minutes. For LISS, incubate for 10 to 15 minutes or follow the manufacturer's directions.
5. Centrifuge and observe for hemolysis and agglutination. Grade and record the results.
6. Perform the indirect antiglobulin test (IAT) described in Method 3-2-1, steps 6 through 9.

METHOD 3-2-3. LISS INDIRECT ANTIGLOBULIN TEST PROCEDURE

Procedure

1. Wash reagent or donor red cells three times in normal saline, and completely decant the saline.
2. Resuspend the cells to a 2% to 3% suspension in LISS.
3. Add 2 drops of serum to a properly labeled tube.
4. Add 2 drops of LISS-suspended red cells, mix, and incubate at 37 C for 10 to 15 minutes or follow the manufacturer's directions.
5. Centrifuge and observe for hemolysis and agglutination by gently resuspending the red cell button. Grade and record results.
6. Perform the IAT described in Method 3-2-1, steps 6 through 9.

METHOD 3-2-4. PEG INDIRECT ANTIGLOBULIN TEST PROCEDURE

Procedure

1. For each red cell sample to be tested, mix 2 drops of test serum, 4 drops of 20% PEG in PBS, and 1 drop of a 2% to 5% suspension of red cells.
2. Incubate at 37 C for 15 minutes.
3. DO NOT CENTRIFUGE.
4. Wash the red cells four times with saline, and completely decant the final wash.
5. Perform the IAT described in Method 3-2-1, steps 7 through 9, using anti-IgG.
   Note: The manufacturer's instructions should be followed for the proper use of commercial PEG solutions.

Interpretation (for Antiglobulin Tests, Methods 3-2-1 through 3-2-4)

1. The presence of agglutination/hemolysis after incubation at 37 C constitutes a positive test result.
2. The presence of agglutination after addition of AHG constitutes a positive test result.
3. Antiglobulin test results are negative when no agglutination is observed after initial centrifugation followed by agglutination with the addition of IgG-coated red cells and centrifugation. If the IgG-coated red cells are not agglutinated, the negative result is invalid and the test must be repeated.

Controls

The procedure used for the detection of unexpected antibodies in pretransfusion testing should be checked daily with weak examples of antibody. Control sera can be prepared from reagent grade typing sera diluted with 6% bovine albumin to give 2+ reactions by an IAT. Human sources of IgG antibodies are also acceptable.

Notes

1. The incubation times and the volume and concentration of red cells indicated are those given in the literature. Individual laboratories may choose to standardize techniques with somewhat different values. See Chapter 15 for other limitations when modifying procedures. In all cases, the manufacturer's package insert should be consulted before modifying a procedure.
2. For the saline procedure (Method 3-2-1), step 3 may be omitted to avoid the detection of antibodies reactive at room temperature.
3. For the PEG procedure, omit centrifugation after 37 C incubation because red cells will not resuspend readily. Use anti-IgG rather than polyspecific AHG to avoid unwanted positive reactions caused by C3-binding autoantibodies. Precipitation of serum proteins when PEG is added appears to be related to elevated serum globulin levels. The problem becomes apparent when the IgG-coated red cells are nonreactive or unexplained weak reactions are detected.[2] At least four washes of the red cells at AHG phase, with agitation, will fully resuspend the red cells and usually prevent the problem from occurring. Alternatively, the test may have to be repeated using a method that does not use PEG.
4. Steps 6 through 9 of the IAT (Method 3-2-1) should be performed without interruption.

References

1. Carson TH, ed. Standards for blood banks and transfusion services. 27th ed. Bethesda, MD: AABB, 2011.
2. Hoffer J, Koslosky WP, Gloster ES, et al. Precipitation of serum proteins by polyethylene glycol (PEG) in pretransfusion testing. Immunohematology 1999;15:105-7.

METHOD 3-3. PREWARMING PROCEDURE

Principle

Prewarming may be useful in the detection and identification of red cell antibodies that bind to antigen only at 37 C. The test is particularly useful for testing sera of patients with cold-reactive autoantibody activity that may mask the presence of clinically significant antibodies. However, use of the prewarming technique for this application has become controversial.[1,2] It has been shown to result in decreased reactivity of some potentially significant antibodies, and weak antibodies can be missed.[3] The technique should be used with caution and not used to eliminate unidentified reactivity.

Strong cold-reactive autoantibodies may react in prewarmed tests; other techniques such as cold allo- or autoadsorption or dithiothreitol treatment of plasma may be required to detect underlying clinically significant antibodies.

Specimen

Serum or plasma may be used. The age of the specimen must comply with pretransfusion specimen requirements in AABB *Standards for Blood Banks and Transfusion Services.*[4]

Reagents

1. Normal saline.
2. Anti-IgG.
3. Commercially available group O antibody detection red cells. Pooled group O antibody detection red cells may be used only for donor testing. Testing of patient samples must be performed with unpooled red cell samples.
4. IgG-coated red cells.

Procedure

1. Prewarm a container of saline to 37 C.
2. Label one tube for each reagent or donor sample to be tested.

3. Add 1 drop of 2% to 5% saline-suspended red cells to each tube.
4. Place the tubes containing red cells and a tube containing a small volume of the patient's serum and a pipette at 37 C; incubate for 5 to 10 minutes.
5. Using the prewarmed pipette, transfer 2 drops of prewarmed serum to each tube containing prewarmed red cells. Mix without removing tubes from the incubator.
6. Incubate at 37 C for 30 to 60 minutes.
7. Without removing the tubes from the incubator, fill each tube with prewarmed (37 C) saline. Centrifuge and wash three or four times with 37 C saline.
8. Add anti-IgG according to the manufacturer's directions.
9. Centrifuge and observe for reaction. Grade and record the results.
10. Confirm the validity of negative results by adding IgG-coated red cells.

Notes

1. The prewarming procedure described earlier will not detect alloantibodies that agglutinate at 37 C or lower and are not reactive in the antiglobulin phase. If detection of these antibodies is desired, testing and centrifugation at 37 C are required. If time permits, a tube containing a prewarmed mixture of serum and cells can be incubated at 37 C for 60 to 120 minutes, and the settled red cells can be examined for agglutination by resuspending the button without centrifugation.
2. Cold-reactive antibodies may not be detectable when room temperature saline instead of 37 C saline is used in the wash step.[2] The use of room temperature saline may avoid the elution of clinically significant antibody(ies) from reagent red cells that can occur with the use of 37 C saline. Some strong cold-reactive autoantibodies, however, may still react and therefore require the use of 37 C saline to avoid their detection.

References

1. Judd WJ. Controversies in transfusion medicine. Prewarmed tests: Con. Transfusion 1995;35:271-5.
2. Mallory D. Controversies in transfusion medicine. Prewarmed tests: Pro—why, when, and how—not if. Transfusion 1995;35:268-70.
3. Leger RM, Garratty G. Weakening or loss of antibody reactivity after prewarm technique. Transfusion 2003;43: 1611-14.
4. Carson TH, ed. Standards for blood banks and transfusion services. 27th ed. Bethesda, MD: AABB, 2011.

METHOD 3-4. DETECTING ANTIBODIES IN THE PRESENCE OF ROULEAUX—SALINE REPLACEMENT

Principle

Patient samples with abnormal concentrations of serum proteins, altered serum-protein ratios, or high-molecular-weight volume expanders can aggregate reagent red cells and can mimic agglutination. Rouleaux are red cell aggregates that adhere along their flat surfaces, giving a "stacked coin" appearance microscopically.

Specimen

Serum or plasma to be evaluated.

Reagents

1. Saline.
2. A_1, B, and O reagent red cells.

Procedure

After routine incubation and resuspension, proceed with the following steps if the appearance of the resuspended red cells suggests rouleaux formation. The saline replacement technique is best performed by the test tube method.

1. Recentrifuge the serum (or plasma) or cell mixture.

2. Remove the serum, leaving the red cell button.
3. Replace the serum with an equal volume of saline (2 drops).
4. Resuspend the red cell button gently, and observe for agglutination. Rouleaux will disperse when suspended in saline. True agglutination is stable in the presence of saline.

Notes

1. In some instances, simple dilution of serum 1:3 with saline is sufficient to prevent rouleaux and to detect ABO isoagglutinins.
2. Review of the patient's recent medical history and other laboratory results may be helpful (eg, history of multiple myeloma).

Reference

1. Issitt PD, Anstee DJ. Applied blood group serology. 4th ed. Durham, NC: Montgomery Scientific Publications, 1998:1135.

METHOD 3-5. ENZYME PROCEDURES

For a discussion of the principles of enzyme testing, see Chapter 16.

METHOD 3-5-1. PREPARING FICIN ENZYME STOCK, 1% W/V

Principle

The ficin preparations used in blood banking differ from lot to lot. Each time a stock enzyme solution is prepared, its reactivity should be tested, and incubation periods should be standardized for optimal effectiveness (see Method 3-5-3).

Reagents

1. Dry ficin powder, 1 g.
2. Phosphate-buffered saline (PBS), pH 7.3 (see Method 1-7).
3. Phosphate buffer, pH 5.4.

Procedure

1. Place 1 g of powdered ficin in a 100-mL volumetric flask. Handle the ficin carefully; it is harmful if it gets in the eyes or is inhaled. It is desirable to wear gloves, mask, and apron, or to work under a hood.
2. Add PBS, pH 7.3, to 100 mL to dissolve the ficin. Agitate vigorously by inversion, rotate for 15 minutes, or mix with a magnetic stirrer until mostly dissolved. The powder will not dissolve completely.
3. Collect clear fluid, either by filtration or centrifugation, and prepare small aliquots. Store the aliquots at –20 C or colder. Do not refreeze a thawed solution.

METHOD 3-5-2. PREPARING PAPAIN ENZYME STOCK, 1% W/V

Principle

The papain preparations used in blood banking differ from lot to lot. Each time a stock enzyme solution is prepared, its reactivity should be tested, and incubation periods should be standardized for optimal effectiveness (see Method 3-5-3).

Reagents

1. L-cysteine hydrochloride (0.5 M), 0.88 g in 10 mL distilled water.
2. Dry papain powder, 2 g.
3. Phosphate buffer (0.067 M at pH 5.4), prepared by combining 3.5 mL of Na_2HPO_4 and 96.5 mL of KH_2PO_4.

Procedure

1. Add 2 g of powdered papain to 100 mL of phosphate buffer (pH 5.4). Handle papain carefully; it is harmful to mucous membranes. Use appropriate protective equipment.
2. Agitate enzyme solution for 15 minutes at room temperature.

3. Collect clear fluid by filtration or centrifugation.
4. Add L-cysteine hydrochloride, and incubate solution at 37 C for 1 hour.
5. Add phosphate buffer (pH 5.4) to final volume of 200 mL. Store aliquots at –20 C or colder. Do not refreeze aliquots.

METHOD 3-5-3. STANDARDIZING ENZYME PROCEDURES

Principle

For a two-stage enzyme procedure, the optimal treatment time must be determined for each new lot of stock solution. The following technique for ficin can be modified for use with other enzymes.

Reagents

1. 1% stock solution of ficin in PBS, pH 7.3.
2. Several sera known to lack unexpected antibodies.
3. Anti-D that agglutinates only enzyme-treated D+ red cells and does not agglutinate untreated D+ red cells.
4. Anti-Fy^a of moderate or strong reactivity.
5. D+ and Fy(a+b–) red cell samples.
6. Antihuman globulin (AHG) reagent. Polyspecific or anti-IgG may be used unless otherwise indicated.
7. IgG-coated red cells.

Procedure

1. Prepare 0.1% ficin by diluting one volume of stock ficin solution with nine volumes of PBS, pH 7.3.
2. Label three tubes: 5 minutes, 10 minutes, and 15 minutes.
3. Add equal volumes of washed red cells and 0.1% ficin to each tube.
4. Mix and incubate at 37 C for the time designated. Incubation times are easily controlled if the 15-minute tube is prepared first, followed by the 10- and 5-minute tubes at 5-minute intervals. Incubation will be complete for all three tubes at the same time.
5. Immediately wash the red cells three times with large volumes of saline.
6. Resuspend treated red cells to 2% to 5% in saline.
7. Label four tubes for each serum to be tested: untreated, 5 minutes, 10 minutes, and 15 minutes.
8. Add 2 drops of the appropriate serum to each of the four tubes.
9. Add 1 drop of the appropriate red cell suspension to each of the labeled tubes.
10. Mix and incubate at 37 C for 15 minutes.
11. Centrifuge and examine for agglutination by gently resuspending the red cell button.
12. Proceed with the IAT test described in Method 3-2-1, steps 6 through 9.

Interpretation

Table 3-5-3-1 shows possible results with D+, Fy(a+b–) cells and the sera indicated. In this case, the optimal incubation time would be 10 minutes. Incubation for only 5 minutes does not completely abolish Fy^a activity or maximally enhance anti-D reactivity. Incubation for 15 minutes causes false-positive AHG reactivity with inert serum.

If incubation for 5 minutes overtreats the red cells, it is preferable to use a more dilute working solution of enzyme than to reduce incubation time, because it is difficult to accurately monitor very short incubation times. Additional tests can evaluate a single dilution at different incubation times, or a single incubation time can be used for different enzyme dilutions.

METHOD 3-5-4. EVALUATING ENZYME-TREATED RED CELLS

Principle

After optimal incubation conditions have been determined for a lot of enzyme solution, treated red cells should be evaluated before use to demonstrate that they are adequately, but not excessively, modified. Satisfactory enzyme treatment should produce red cells that are directly agglutinated by an antibody

TABLE 3-5-3-1. Hypothetical Results with D+, Fy(a+b–) Red Cells

Cells and Enzyme		Inert Serum	Anti-D	Anti-Fy[a]
Untreated	37 C incubation	0	0	0
	Antihuman globulin (AHG) test	0	1+	3+
5 minutes	37 C incubation	0	1+	0
	AHG test	0	2+	1+
10 minutes	37 C incubation	0	2+	0
	AHG test	0	2+	0
15 minutes	37 C incubation	0	2+	0
	AHG test	W+	2+	W+

that reacts only by IAT with untreated cells; however, enzyme-treated red cells should not be agglutinated or aggregated by inert serum.

Specimen

Enzyme-treated red cells.

Reagents

1. Sera known to contain antibody that will agglutinate enzyme-treated red cells.
2. Sera free of any unexpected antibodies.
3. Antihuman globulin (AHG) reagent. Polyspecific or anti-IgG may be used unless otherwise indicated.
4. IgG-coated red cells.

Procedure

1. Select an antibody that agglutinates enzyme-treated red cells positive for the antigen but gives only AHG reactions with unmodified red cells. Many examples of human-source anti-D behave in this way.
2. Add 2 drops of the selected antibody-containing serum to a tube labeled "positive."
3. Add 2 drops of a serum free of unexpected antibodies to a tube labeled "negative."
4. Add 1 drop of 2% to 5% suspension of enzyme-treated red cells to each tube.
5. Mix and incubate 15 minutes at 37 C.
6. Centrifuge and resuspend the red cells by gentle shaking.
7. Examine macroscopically for the presence of agglutination.
8. Perform the IAT described in Method 3-2-1, steps 6 through 9, on the tube labeled "negative."

Interpretation

There should be agglutination in the "positive" tube and no agglutination in the "negative" tube. If agglutination occurs in the "negative" tube, the red cells have been overtreated; if agglutination does not occur in the "positive" tube, treatment has been inadequate.

METHOD 3-5-5. ONE-STAGE ENZYME PROCEDURE

Specimen

Serum or plasma to be tested.

Reagent

1. Reagent red cells.
2. Antihuman globulin (AHG) reagent. Polyspecific or anti-IgG may be used unless otherwise indicated.
3. IgG-coated red cells.

Procedure

1. Add 2 drops of serum to an appropriately labeled tube.

2. Add 2 drops of a 2% to 5% saline suspension of reagent red cells.
3. Add 2 drops of 0.1% papain solution and mix well.
4. Incubate at 37 C for 15 minutes.
5. Centrifuge; gently resuspend the red cells and observe them for agglutination. Grade and record the results.
6. Proceed with the IAT described in Method 3-2-1, steps 6 through 9.

METHOD 3-5-6. TWO-STAGE ENZYME PROCEDURE

Specimen

Serum or plasma to be tested.

Reagents

1. Reagent red cells.
2. Antihuman globulin (AHG) reagent. Polyspecific or anti-IgG may be used unless otherwise indicated.
3. IgG-coated red cells.

Procedure

1. Prepare a diluted enzyme solution (papain or ficin) by adding 9 mL of PBS, pH 7.3, to 1 mL of stock enzyme.
2. Add one volume of diluted enzyme to one volume of packed, washed reagent red cells.
3. Incubate at 37 C for the time determined to be optimal for that enzyme solution.
4. Wash treated red cells at least three times with large volumes of saline, and resuspend the red cells to a 2% to 5% concentration in saline.
5. Add 2 drops of serum or plasma to be tested to an appropriately labeled tube.
6. Add 1 drop of 2% to 5% suspension of enzyme-treated red cells.
7. Mix and incubate for 15 minutes at 37 C.
8. Centrifuge; gently resuspend the red cells and observe for agglutination. Grade and record the results.
9. Proceed with the IAT described in Method 3-2-1, steps 6 through 9.

Notes

1. An alternative method for steps 4 and 5 (Method 3-5-5) or steps 7 and 8 (Method 3-5-6) is to incubate the serum and enzyme-treated cells at 37 C for 60 minutes and to examine the settled cells for agglutination without centrifugation. This examination can be useful for serum with strong cold-reactive agglutinins and can sometimes prevent false-positive results.
2. Microscopic examination is not recommended for routine use and is particularly inappropriate with enzyme-enhanced tests; false-positive reactions will often be detected.
3. Either papain or ficin may be used in a two-stage procedure.
4. Enzyme preparations are available commercially. The manufacturer's directions should be followed for appropriate use and quality control.

References

1. Issitt PD, Anstee DJ. Applied blood group serology. 4th ed. Durham, NC: Montgomery Scientific Publications, 1998.
2. Judd WJ, Johnson S, Storry J. Judd's methods in immunohematology. 3rd ed. Bethesda, MD: AABB Press, 2008.

METHOD 3-6. PERFORMING A DIRECT ANTIGLOBULIN TEST

Principle

See Chapter 17 for a discussion of the principles of direct antiglobulin testing.

Specimen

Red cells from an EDTA-anticoagulated blood sample.

Reagents

1. Antihuman globulin (AHG) reagent: polyspecific antiglobulin reagent, anti-IgG, anti- complement antisera.

2. A control reagent (eg, saline or 6% albumin) is required when all antisera tested give a positive result.
3. IgG-coated red cells.
4. Complement-coated red cells, if instructed by the manufacturer.

Procedure

1. Dispense 1 drop of a 2% to 5% suspension of red cells into each tube.
2. Wash each tube three or four times with saline. Completely decant the final wash.
3. Immediately add antisera and mix. For the amount of antisera required, refer to the manufacturer's directions.
4. Centrifuge according to the manufacturer's directions. For anticomplement, the manufacturer may indicate a delay before centrifugation.
5. Examine the cells for agglutination. Grade and record the reaction.
6. If using polyspecific AHG or anticomplement, incubate nonreactive tests at room temperature if indicated by the manufacturer; then centrifuge and read again.
7. Confirm the validity of negative results as indicated by the manufacturer (eg, add IgG-coated red cells to tests containing anti-IgG).
8. Centrifuge according to the manufacturer's directions.
9. Examine the cells for agglutination and record the reaction.

Interpretation

1. The direct antiglobulin test (DAT) is positive when agglutination is observed either after immediate centrifugation or after the centrifugation that followed room-temperature incubation. IgG-coated red cells usually give immediate reactions, whereas complement coating may be more easily demonstrable after incubation.[1,2] Monospecific AHG reagents are needed to confirm which globulins are present.
2. The DAT is negative when no agglutination is observed at either test phase and the IgG-coated cells added in step 7 are agglutinated. If the IgG-coated cells are not agglutinated, the negative DAT result is considered invalid, and the test must be repeated. A negative DAT does not necessarily mean that the red cells have no attached globulin molecules. Polyspecific and anti-IgG reagents detect 150 to 500 molecules of IgG per cell, but patients may still experience autoimmune hemolytic anemia when IgG coating is below this level.[2]
3. No interpretation can be made if the control reagent is reactive. This may indicate the presence of a strong cold autoagglutinin or spontaneous agglutination due to warm-reactive IgM or IgG antibodies. Warming the red cells to 37 C and/or washing with warm (37 C) saline should resolve reactivity due to cold autoagglutinins. Spontaneous agglutination requires treatment of the red cells with dithiothreitol or 2-aminoethylisothiouronium bromide (see Method 3-10).

Notes

1. Steps 2 through 5 should be performed without interruption.
2. Initial testing may be performed with polyspecific reagent only. If the DAT is negative with polyspecific reagent, no further testing is necessary. If the DAT is positive with polyspecific reagent, perform the DAT with monospecific reagents, anti-IgG, and anticomplement, to determine which globulins are present.
3. Additional washes may be needed when testing cord samples contaminated with Wharton's jelly.

References

1. Klein HG, Anstee DJ. Mollison's blood transfusion in clinical medicine. 11th ed. Oxford, England: Blackwell Publishing, 2005.
2. Petz LD, Garratty G. Immune hemolytic anemia. Philadelphia: Churchill-Livingstone, 2004.

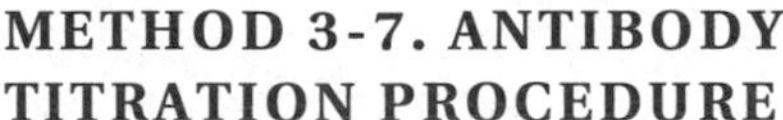

METHOD 3-7. ANTIBODY TITRATION PROCEDURE

Principle

Titration is a semiquantitative method used to determine the concentration of antibody in a serum sample or to compare the strength of antigen expression on different red cell samples. The usual applications of titration studies are as follows: 1) estimating antibody activity in alloimmunized pregnant women to determine whether and when to perform more complex invasive investigation of the fetal condition (see Chapter 22); 2) elucidating autoantibody specificity (see Chapter 17); 3) characterizing antibodies as having high titer and low avidity, traits common in antibodies to antigens of the Knops and Chido/Rodgers systems, Cs^a, and JMH (see Chapter 16); and 4) observing the effect of sulfhydryl reagents on antibody behavior, to determine immunoglobulin class (IgG or IgM; see Method 3-8).

Specimen

Serum or plasma antibody to be titrated.

Reagents

1. Red cells that express the antigen(s) corresponding to the antibody specificity(ies), in a 2% to 5% saline suspension. Uniformity of red cell suspensions is very important to ensure comparability of results.
2. Saline. (Note: Dilutions may be made with albumin if desired.)

Procedure

The master dilution technique for titration studies is as follows:

1. Label 10 test tubes according to the serum dilution (eg, 1 in 1, 1 in 2, etc). A 1-in-1 dilution means one volume of serum undiluted; a 1-in-2 dilution means one volume of serum in a final volume of two, or a 50% solution of serum in the diluent.
2. Deliver one volume of saline to all test tubes except the first (undiluted, 1 in 1) tube.
3. Add an equal volume of serum to each of the first two tubes (undiluted and 1 in 2).
4. Using a clean pipette, mix the contents of the 1-in-2 dilution several times, and transfer one volume into the next tube (the 1-in-4 dilution).
5. Continue the same process for all dilutions, using a clean pipette to mix and transfer each dilution. Remove one volume of diluted serum from the final tube, and save it for use if further dilutions are required.
6. Label 10 tubes for the appropriate dilutions.
7. Using separate pipettes for each dilution, transfer 2 drops of each diluted serum into the appropriately labeled tubes, and add 2 drops of a 2% red cell suspension. Alternatively, for convenience, add 1 drop of a 3% to 4% suspension of red cells as supplied by the reagent manufacturer, although this method is less precise.
8. Mix well and test by a serologic technique appropriate to the antibody (see Chapter 16).
9. Examine test results macroscopically; grade and record the reactions. The prozone phenomenon (see Chapter 10) may cause reactions to be weaker in the more concentrated serum preparations than in higher dilutions. If one is to avoid misinterpretation of results, it may be preferable to examine first the tube containing the most dilute serum and then to proceed through the more concentrated samples to the undiluted specimen.

Interpretation

1. Observe the highest dilution that produces 1+ macroscopic agglutination. The titer is reported as the reciprocal of the dilution level (eg, 32—*not* 1 in 32 or 1:32). (See Table 3-7-1.) If there is agglutination in the tube containing the most dilute serum, the endpoint has not been

TABLE 3-7-1. Examples of Antibody Titers, Endpoints, and Scores

		Reciprocal of Serum Dilution											
		1	**2**	**4**	**8**	**16**	**32**	**64**	**128**	**256**	**512**	**Titer***	**Score**
Sample #1	Strength	3+	3+	3+	2+	2+	2+	1+	±	±	0	64(256)	
	Score	10	10	10	8	8	8	5	3	2	0		64
Sample #2	Strength	4+	4+	4+	3+	3+	2+	2+	1+	±	0	128(256)	
	Score	12	12	12	10	10	8	8	5	3	0		80
Sample #3	Strength	1+	1+	1+	1+	±	±	±	±	±	0	8(256)	
	Score	5	5	5	5	3	3	3	2	2	0		33

*The titer is often determined from the highest dilution of serum that gives a reaction 1+ (score 5). This reaction may differ significantly from the titration endpoint (shown in parentheses), as with the reactions of an antibody with high-titer, low-avidity characteristics, manifested by Sample #3.

reached, and additional dilutions should be prepared and tested.

2. In comparative studies, a significant difference in titer is three or more dilutions. Variations in technique and inherent biologic variability can cause duplicate tests to give results that differ by one dilution in either direction. Serum containing antibody at a true titer of 32 may show, on replicate tests, the endpoint in the 1-in-32 tube, the 1-in-64 tube, or the 1-in-16 tube.
3. Titer values alone can be misleading if the strength of agglutination is not also evaluated. The observed strength of agglutination can be assigned a number, and the sum of these numbers for all tubes in a titration study represents the score, another semiquantitative measurement of antibody reactivity. The arbitrarily assigned threshold for significance in comparing scores is a difference of 10 or more between different test samples (see Table 3-7-1).
4. Antibodies with high-titer and low-avidity characteristics generally have a titer greater than 64, with most tubes showing consistently weak reactivity.
5. Table 3-7-1 shows the results obtained with three sera, each of which shows no more agglutination after 1:256 dilution. The differences in score, however, indicate considerable variation in strength of reactivity.

Notes

Titration is a semiquantitative technique. Technical variables greatly affect the results, and care should be taken to achieve the most uniform practices possible.

1. Measurements are more accurate with large volumes than with small volumes; a master dilution technique (see earlier) gives more reliable results than individual dilutions for a single set of tests. The volume needed for all planned tests should be calculated, and an adequate quantity of each dilution should be prepared.
2. Careful pipetting is essential. Pipettes with disposable tips that can be changed after each dilution are recommended.
3. The age, phenotype, and concentration of the test red cells will influence the results.
4. The optimal time and temperature of incubation, and the time and force of centrifugation, should be used consistently.
5. When the titers of several antibody-containing sera are to be compared, all of them should be tested against red cells (preferably freshly collected) from the same donor. If this is not possible, the tests should use a pool of reagent red cells from donors of the same phenotype. Comparisons are valid only when specimens are tested concurrently.
6. When a single serum is to be tested against different red cell samples, all red cell samples should be collected and preserved in the same manner and diluted to the same concentration before use. Material from the master dilution should be used for all the tests. Comparisons are valid only when specimens are tested concurrently.
7. When performing a titration for anti-D for hemolytic disease of the fetus and newborn, see Method 5-3.
8. Other titration methods have been described that may show less variation.[1]

Reference

1. AuBuchon JP, de Wildt-Eggen J, Dumont LJ, et al. Reducing the variation in performance of antibody titrations. Arch Pathol Lab Med 2008;132:1194-201.

METHOD 3-8. USING SULFHYDRYL REAGENTS TO DISTINGUISH IgM FROM IgG ANTIBODIES

Principle

Treating IgM antibodies with sulfhydryl reagents abolishes both agglutinating and complement-binding activities. Observations of antibody activity before and after sulfhydryl treatment are useful in determining immunoglobulin class. Sulfhydryl treatment can also be used to abolish IgM antibody activity to permit detection of coexisting IgG antibodies. For a discussion of IgM and IgG structures, see Chapter 10.

Specimen

2 mL of serum or plasma to be treated.

Reagents

1. Phosphate-buffered saline (PBS) at pH 7.3.
2. 0.01 M dithiothreitol (DTT) prepared by dissolving 0.154 g of DTT in 100 mL of pH 7.3 PBS. Store at –18 C or lower.

Procedure

1. Dispense 1 mL of serum or plasma into each of two test tubes.
2. To one tube (labeled dilution control), add 1 mL of pH 7.3 PBS.
3. To the other tube (labeled test), add 1 mL of 0.01 M DTT.
4. Mix and incubate at 37 C for 30 to 60 minutes.
5. Use the DTT-treated and dilution control samples in standard procedures.

Interpretation

1. Reactivity in the dilution control serum and no reactivity in the DTT-treated serum indicate an IgM antibody.
2. Reactivity in the dilution control serum and in the DTT-treated serum indicates an IgG antibody or an IgG and IgM mixture. Titration studies may be necessary to distinguish between them (see Table 3-8-1).
3. No reactivity in the dilution control serum indicates dilution of weak antibody reactivity and an invalid test.

Control

A serum or plasma sample known to contain an IgM antibody should be treated and tested in parallel.

Notes

1. 2-mercaptoethanol can also be used for this purpose (see Method 2-18 for preparation).
2. Sulfhydryl reagents used at low concentration may weaken antigens of the Kell system. For investigation of antibodies in the Kell system, it may be necessary to use other methods.

TABLE 3-8-1. Effect of Dithiothreitol on Blood Group Antibodies

	Reciprocal of Serum Dilution					
Test Sample	**2**	**4**	**8**	**16**	**32**	**Interpretation**
Serum + DTT	3+	2+	2+	1+	0	IgG
Serum + PBS	3+	2+	2+	1+	0	
Serum + DTT	0	0	0	0	0	IgM
Serum + PBS	3+	2+	2+	1+	0	
Serum + DTT	2+	1+	0	0	0	IgG + IgM*
Serum + PBS	3+	2+	2+	1+	0	

*May also indicate only partial inactivation of IgM.
Note: DTT = dithiothreitol; IgG = immunoglobulin, gamma class; IgM = immunoglobulin M; PBS = phosphate-buffered saline.

3. Gelling of a serum or plasma sample may be observed during treatment with DTT. This gelling can occur if the DTT has been prepared incorrectly and has a concentration above 0.01 M. Gelling may also occur if serum and DTT are incubated too long. An aliquot of the sample undergoing treatment can be tested after 30 minutes of incubation; if the activity thought to be caused by IgM has disappeared, there is no need to incubate further. Gelled samples cannot be tested for antibody activity because overtreatment with DTT causes the denaturation of all serum proteins.

Reference

1. Klein HG, Anstee D. Blood transfusion in clinical medicine. 11th ed. Oxford, England: Blackwell Scientific, 2005.

METHOD 3-9. USING PLASMA INHIBITION TO DISTINGUISH ANTI-CH AND -RG FROM OTHER ANTIBODIES WITH SIMILAR CHARACTERISTICS

Principle

For a discussion of the principles of plasma inhibition of anti-Ch and -Rg, see Chapters 14 and 16.

Specimen

Serum or plasma to be tested.

Reagents

1. Reactive red cell samples.
2. A pool of six or more normal plasma samples.
3. 6% bovine albumin (see Method 1-5).
4. Anti-IgG.
5. IgG-coated red cells.

Procedure

1. Prepare serial twofold dilutions of test serum in saline. The dilution range should be from 1 in 2 to 1 in 512, or to one tube beyond the known titer (Method 3-7). The volume prepared should be not less than 0.3 mL for each red cell sample to be tested.
2. For each red cell sample to be tested, place 2 drops of each serum dilution into each of two sets of appropriately labeled 10 or 12 × 75-mm test tubes.
3. To one set, add 2 drops of pooled plasma to each tube.
4. To the other set, add 2 drops of 6% albumin to each tube.
5. Gently agitate the contents of each tube and incubate the tubes at room temperature for at least 30 minutes.
6. Add 1 drop of a 2% to 5% suspension of red cells to each tube.
7. Gently agitate the contents of each tube and incubate the tubes at 37 C for 1 hour.
8. Wash the cells four times in saline, add anti-IgG, and centrifuge according to the manufacturer's directions.
9. Resuspend the cell buttons and examine for agglutination; confirm all nonreactive tests microscopically. Grade and record the results.
10. Confirm the validity of negative results by adding IgG-coated red cells.

Interpretation

1. Inhibition of antibody activity in the tubes to which plasma has been added suggests anti-Ch or anti-Rg specificity; this inhibition is often complete.
2. The presence of partial inhibition suggests the possibility of additional alloantibodies. This can be tested by preparing a large volume of inhibited serum and testing it against a reagent red cell panel to see if the nonneutralizable activity displays antigenic specificity.
3. Lack of reactivity in the control (6% albumin) indicates dilution of weakly reactive antibody and an invalid test.

Notes

1. Antibodies to other plasma antigens may also be partially inhibited by plasma.[1]
2. Adsorption with C4-coated red cells is an alternative procedure that may be used for identifying anti-Ch or anti-Rg and for detecting underlying alloantibodies.[2]

References

1. Reid ME, Lomas-Francis C. The blood group antigen factsbook. 2nd ed. San Diego: Academic Press, 2004.
2. Ellisor SS, Shoemaker MM, Reid ME. Adsorption of anti-Chido from serum using autologous red blood cells coated with homologous C4. Transfusion 1982;22: 243-5.

METHOD 3-10. TREATING RED CELLS USING DTT OR AET

Principle

Dithiothreitol (DTT) and 2-aminoethylisothiouronium bromide (AET) are efficient reducing agents that can disrupt the tertiary structure of proteins by irreversibly reducing disulfide bonds to free sulfhydryl groups. Without tertiary structure, protein-containing antigens can no longer bind antibodies that are specific for them. Red cells treated with DTT or AET will not react with antibodies in the Kell blood group system, most antibodies in the Knops system, or most examples of anti-LW^a, -Yt^a, -Yt^b, -Do^a, -Do^b, -Gy^a, -Hy, and -Jo^a. These inhibition techniques may be helpful in identifying some of these antibodies or in determining if a serum contains additional underlying alloantibodies.

Specimen

Red cells to be tested.

Reagents

1. Prepare 0.2 M DTT by dissolving 1 g of DTT powder in 32 mL of phosphate-buffered saline (PBS), pH 8.0. Divide it into 1-mL volumes, and freeze aliquots at –18 C or colder.
2. PBS at pH 7.3 (see Method 1-7).
3. Prepare 6% AET by dissolving 0.6 g of AET in 10 mL distilled water, and bring the pH to 8 by slowly adding 5 N NaOH.
4. Red cells known to be positive for the antigen in question and, as a control, red cells known to be positive for K, which is consistently disrupted by DTT or AET.
5. Anti-K, either in reagent form or strongly reactive in a serum specimen.

Procedure—DTT

1. Wash one volume of the test cells and the control cells with PBS. After decanting, add four volumes of 0.2 M DTT, pH 8.0.
2. Incubate at 37 C for 30 to 45 minutes.
3. Wash four times with PBS. Slight hemolysis may occur; if hemolysis is excessive, repeat the procedure using fresh red cells and a smaller volume of DTT (eg, two or three volumes).
4. Resuspend the cells to a 2% to 5% suspension in PBS.
5. Test DTT-treated cells with serum containing the antibody in question. Test K+ red cells with anti-K.

Procedure—AET

1. Combine four volumes of the prepared AET solution with one volume of washed, packed red cells to be treated.
2. Incubate for 20 minutes at 37 C, mixing every 5 minutes.
3. Wash treated cells with PBS five to seven times or until the supernatant is clear.
4. Resuspend the cells to a 2% to 5% suspension in PBS.
5. Test AET-treated cells with serum containing the antibody in question. Test K+ red cells with anti-K.

Interpretation

1. The control K+ red cells should give negative reactions when tested with anti-K; if

not, the DTT or AET treatment has been inadequate. Other antigens in the Kell system can also serve as the control.
2. If reactivity of the test serum is eliminated, the suspected antibody specificity may be confirmed. Enough red cell samples should be tested to exclude most other clinically significant alloantibodies.

Note

Treatment of red cells with 0.2 M DTT or 6% AET will denature or weaken all antigens of the Kell, Cartwright, LW, Dombrock, and Knops systems. Lower concentrations of DTT may selectively denature particular blood group antigens (ie, 0.002 M DTT will denature only Js^a and Js^b antigens, while other Kell antigens will not be affected). This property may aid in certain antibody investigations.

References

1. Advani H, Zamor J, Judd WJ, et al. Inactivation of Kell blood group antigens by 2-aminoethylisothiouronium bromide. Br J Haematol 1982; 51:107-15.
2. Branch DR, Muensch HA, Sy Siok Hian S, Petz LD. Disulfide bonds are a requirement for Kell and Cartwright (Yt^a) blood group antigen integrity. Br J Haematol 1983;54: 573-8.

METHOD 3-11. NEUTRALIZING ANTI-Sd^a WITH URINE

Principle

For a discussion of anti-Sd^a neutralization by urine, see Chapter 16.

Specimen

Serum or plasma suspected of containing anti-Sd^a.

Reagents

1. Urine from a known Sd(a+) individual, or from a pool of at least six individuals of unknown Sd^a type, and prepared as follows: Collect urine and immediately boil it for 10 minutes. Cool. Using 10-mm-interior-diameter cellulose membrane tubing (12,400 MW cut off), dialyze it against phosphate-buffered saline (PBS), pH 7.3, at 4 C for 48 hours. Change PBS several times. Centrifuge. Dispense supernatant into aliquots, which can be stored at –20 C until thawed for use.
2. PBS, pH 7.3 (see Method 1-7).

Procedure

1. Mix equal volumes of thawed urine and test serum.
2. Prepare a dilution control tube containing equal volumes of serum and PBS.
3. Prepare a urine control tube by mixing equal volumes of thawed urine and PBS.
4. Incubate all tubes at room temperature for 30 minutes.
5. Mix 1 drop of each test red cell sample with 4 drops from each of the tubes: neutralized serum, serum with PBS, and urine with PBS. Test each one using standard procedures.

Interpretation

1. Persistent agglutination in the serum sample incubated with urine means either that partial or no neutralization was achieved or that underlying antibodies are present. Microscopic examination may be helpful; agglutination caused by anti-Sd^a has a refractile, mixed-field appearance on microscopic examination.
2. No agglutination in the neutralized tube with persistent agglutination in the dilution control tube and absence of hemolysis and agglutination in the urine control tube indicate that the antibody has been neutralized and is quite probably anti-Sd^a.
3. The absence of agglutination in the dilution control tube means that the dilution in the neutralization step was too great for the antibody present, and the results of the test are invalid.

4. The urine control tube provides assurance that no substances in the urine are agglutinating or damaging the red cells.

Note

Urine may also contain ABO and Lewis blood group substances, depending upon the ABO, Lewis, and secretor status of the donor.

Reference

1. Judd WJ, Johnson S, Storry J. Judd's methods in immunohematology. 3rd ed. Bethesda, MD: AABB Press, 2008.

METHOD 3-12. ADSORPTION PROCEDURE

Principle

See Chapter 16.

Specimen

Serum or plasma containing antibody to be adsorbed.

Reagents

Red cells (eg, autologous or allogeneic) that carry the antigen corresponding to the antibody specificity to be adsorbed.

Procedure

1. Wash the selected red cells at least three times with saline.
2. After the last wash, centrifuge the red cells at 800 to 1000 × *g* for at least 5 minutes, and remove as much of the supernatant saline as possible. Additional saline may be removed by touching the red cell mass with a narrow piece of filter paper.
3. Mix appropriate volumes of the packed red cells and serum, and incubate at the desired temperature for 30 to 60 minutes.
4. Mix the serum or cell mixture periodically throughout the incubation phase.
5. Centrifuge the red cells at 800 to 1000 × *g* for 5 minutes to pack cells tightly. Centrifuge at the incubation temperature, if possible, to avoid dissociation of antibody from the red cell membranes.
6. Transfer the supernatant fluid, which is the adsorbed serum, to a clean test tube. If an eluate is to be prepared, save the red cells.
7. Test an aliquot of the adsorbed serum, preferably against a reserved unused aliquot of the red cells used for adsorption, to see if all antibody has been removed.

Interpretation

If reactivity remains, the antibody has not been completely removed. No reactivity signifies that antibody has been completely adsorbed.

Notes

1. Adsorption is more effective if the area of contact between the red cells and serum is large. Use of a large-bore test tube (13 mm or larger) is recommended.
2. Multiple adsorptions may be necessary to remove an antibody completely; however, each successive adsorption increases the likelihood that the serum will be diluted and unadsorbed antibodies weakened.
3. Repeat adsorptions should use a fresh aliquot of red cells and not the red cells from the earlier adsorption.
4. Enzyme pretreatment of adsorbing red cells can be performed to increase antibody uptake for enzyme-resistant antigens.

Reference

1. Judd WJ, Johnson S, Storry J. Judd's methods in immunohematology. 3rd ed. Bethesda, MD: AABB Press, 2008.

METHOD 3-13. USING THE AMERICAN RARE DONOR PROGRAM

Principle

The American Rare Donor Program (ARDP) helps to locate blood products for patients requiring rare or unusual blood. The ARDP maintains a database of rare donors submitted by immunohematology reference laboratories (IRLs) that are accredited by the AABB or the American Red Cross (ARC). Donors are considered rare because of the absence of a high-prevalence antigen, the absence of multiple common antigens, or IgA deficiency.

All requests to the ARDP must originate from an AABB- or ARC-accredited IRL to ensure that the patient in question has been accurately evaluated and reported. All shipping and rare-unit fees are established by the shipping institution.

Procedure

1. A hospital blood bank, transfusion service, or blood center identifies a patient who needs rare blood.
2. The institution contacts the nearest AABB- or ARC-accredited IRL to supply the needed blood.
3. If the IRL cannot supply the blood, it contacts the ARDP. *All* requests to the ARDP *must* come from an AABB- or ARC-accredited IRL (or another rare donor program). Requests received directly from a nonaccredited facility will be referred to the nearest accredited institution.
4. The institution contacting the ARDP (requesting institution) *must* confirm the identity of the antibody(ies) by serologic investigation or by examining the serologic work performed by another institution.
5. ARDP staff search their database for centers that have identified donors with the needed phenotype and contact the centers for availability of units. The ARDP staff give the name(s) of the shipping center(s) to the requesting institution.
6. The requesting and shipping institutions should discuss and agree on charges and testing requirements before units are shipped.
7. If an initial search does not result in a sufficient number of units, the following mechanisms can be used by the ARDP staff to obtain needed units: 1) communicating with all ARDP participating centers, alerting them to search their inventories and/or recruit donors matching the needed phenotype, or 2) contacting other rare donor files such as those administered by the World Health Organization, Japanese Red Cross, or similar organizations.

Investigation of a Positive DAT

◆

ELUATES

After an eluate is prepared, it should be tested by an appropriate technique for the type of antibody being investigated. Eluates prepared for the detection of IgG antibodies should be incubated at 37 C and converted to the antiglobulin test. Heat eluates prepared for detection of IgM antibodies may first be incubated at room temperature for 15 to 30 minutes and, if nonreactive, then incubated at 37 C, centrifuged, read for agglutination, and subsequently converted to the antiglobulin phase. IgM agglutinins may not be detectable at the antiglobulin phase.

Supernatant fluid from the final wash of the red cells to be eluted should be tested in parallel with the eluate and found to be nonreactive to ensure that antibody detected in the eluate is only red-cell-bound antibody and not free antibody from the plasma. Also, transferring the red cells to a clean tube before the elution step eliminates the possibility of dissociating any plasma antibody that may have nonspecifically bound to the test tube during preparation.

METHOD 4-1. COLD-ACID ELUTION PROCEDURE

Principle

Elution of antibodies at low pH is probably the result of disruption of the electrostatic bonds in proteins and changes to the tertiary structure. This method is suitable for recovery of warm-reactive auto- and alloantibodies.

Specimens

1. Red cells washed four to six times with large volumes of saline.
2. Supernatant saline from the final wash of the red cells to be eluted.

Reagents

1. Glycine-HCl (0.1 M, pH 3.0), prepared by dissolving 3.75 g of glycine and 2.922 g of sodium chloride in 500 mL of deionized or distilled water. Adjust the pH to 3.0 with 12 N HCl. Store at 4 C. Use chilled.
2. Phosphate buffer (0.8 M, pH 8.2), prepared by dissolving 109.6 g of Na_2HPO_4 and 3.8 g of KH_2PO_4 in approximately 600 mL of deionized or distilled water and adjusting the final volume to 1 L. Adjust the pH, if necessary, with either 1 N NaOH or 1 N HCl. Store at 4 C (see Note 1).
3. NaCl, 0.9%, at 4 C. Use chilled.

Procedure

1. Place the glycine-HCl and the saline in an ice waterbath.
2. Place 1 mL of red cells in a 13 × 100-mm test tube and chill in an ice waterbath for 5 minutes before adding the glycine-HCl.
3. Add 1 mL of chilled saline and 2 mL of chilled glycine-HCl to the red cells.
4. Mix and incubate the tube in an ice waterbath (0 C) for 1 minute.
5. Quickly centrifuge the tube at 900 to 1000 × *g* for 2 to 3 minutes.

6. Transfer the supernatant eluate into a clean test tube, and add 0.1 mL of pH 8.2 phosphate buffer for each 1 mL of eluate.
7. Mix and centrifuge at 900 to 1000 × *g* for 2 to 3 minutes.
8. Transfer the supernatant eluate into a clean test tube, and test it in parallel with the supernatant saline from the final wash.

Notes

1. Phosphate buffer will crystallize during storage at 4 C. Redissolve it at 37 C before use.
2. Acidity may cause hemolysis of the reagent red cells used in testing the eluate. Addition of 22% bovine albumin (one part to four parts of eluate) may reduce such hemolysis.

References

1. Judd WJ, Johnson ST, Storry J. Judd's methods in immunohematology. 3rd ed. Bethesda, MD: AABB Press, 2008.
2. Rekvig OP, Hannestad K. Acid elution of blood group antibodies from intact erythrocytes. Vox Sang 1977;33:280-5.

METHOD 4-2. GLYCINE-HCL/EDTA ELUTION PROCEDURE

Principle

Dissociation of antibodies from red cells enables the identification of auto- or alloantibodies. Elution methods used in conjunction with adsorption techniques are also useful in detecting weak antigen expression on the adsorbing red cells, as well as in separating mixtures of antibodies against red cell antigens.

Specimen

Red cells positive by the direct antiglobulin test (DAT) washed six times with large volumes of saline (saving the last wash).

Reagents

1. Disodium EDTA (10% w/v): Na_2EDTA, 10 g; add distilled water to 100 mL.
2. Glycine-HCl (0.1 M at pH 1.5): 0.75 g glycine diluted to 100 mL with 0.9% NaCl; adjust to pH 1.5 with 12 N HCl.
3. TRIS-NaCl (1 M): Tris(hydroxymethyl) aminomethane (TRIS) or TRIZMA BASE, 12.1 g; NaCl, 5.25 g; distilled water to 100 mL.
4. Supernatant saline from the final wash of the red cells to be tested.

Procedure

1. In a test tube, mix together 20 volumes (eg, drops) of 0.1 M glycine-HCl buffer and five volumes of 10% EDTA. This mixture is the eluting solution.
2. In a 12 × 75-mm tube, place 10 volumes of packed red cells.
3. Add 20 volumes of the eluting solution to the red cells, mix well, and incubate at room temperature for 2 minutes. Do not overincubate.
4. Add 1 volume of TRIS-NaCl, mix, and immediately centrifuge the tube at 900 to 1000 × *g* for 60 seconds.
5. Transfer the supernatant eluate into a clean test tube, and carefully adjust it dropwise to pH 7.0 to 7.4 with 1 M TRIS-NaCl. The pH can be checked with pH paper.
6. Centrifuge at 900 to 1000 × *g* for 2 to 3 minutes to remove the precipitate.
7. Transfer the supernatant eluate into a clean test tube and test it in parallel with the supernatant saline from the final wash.

Notes

1. Once the red cells have been rendered DAT negative, they may be tested for the presence of blood group antigens, except those in the Kell system and Er^a, as those antigens are denatured by glycine-HCl/

EDTA. Wash the red cells at least three times in saline before use.
2. Red cells modified with glycine-HCl/EDTA may be treated with a protease and used in autologous adsorption studies.
3. Overincubation with the eluting solution (step 3) will irreversibly damage the red cells.
4. TRIS-NaCl is very alkaline, and only a few drops should be required to attain the desired pH (step 5).
5. Aliquots of the reagents can be stored frozen, and one tube of each can be thawed just before use. The 10% EDTA may precipitate when stored at 2 to 8 C.
6. Stored eluate (4 C or frozen) may be more stable if albumin is added (3 volumes of 22% bovine albumin for every 10 volumes of eluate). If albumin is added to the eluate, the albumin also should be added to the last wash.

Reference

1. Byrne PC. Use of a modified acid/EDTA elution technique. Immunohematology 1991;7:46-7.

METHOD 4-3. HEAT ELUTION PROCEDURE

Principle

Heat elution uses an increase in temperature to dissociate antibodies from red cells. This method is best suited for the investigation of ABO hemolytic disease of the fetus and newborn and for the elution of IgM antibodies from red cells. It should not be used routinely for the investigation of IgG auto- or alloantibodies.

Specimens

1. Red cells positive by the direct antiglobulin test (DAT), washed four to six times with large volumes of saline (see Note).
2. Supernatant saline from the final wash of the red cells to be eluted.

Reagent

6% bovine albumin (see Method 1-5).

Procedure

1. Mix equal volumes of washed packed cells and 6% bovine albumin in a 13 × 100-mm test tube.
2. Place the tube at 56 C for 10 minutes. Agitate the tube periodically during this time.
3. Centrifuge the tube at 900 to 1000 × *g* for 2 to 3 minutes.
4. Immediately transfer the supernatant eluate into a clean test tube, and test in parallel with the supernatant saline from the final wash.

Note

For optimal recovery of cold-reactive antibodies, the red cells should be washed in ice-cold saline to prevent dissociation of bound antibody before elution.

References

1. Judd WJ, Johnson ST, Storry JR. Judd's methods in immunohematology. 3rd ed. Bethesda, MD: AABB Press, 2008.
2. Landsteiner K, Miller CP Jr. Serological studies on the blood of primates. II. The blood groups in anthropoid apes. J Exp Med 1925;42:853-62.

METHOD 4-4. LUI FREEZE-THAW ELUTION PROCEDURE

Principle

As red cells freeze, extracellular ice crystals form that attract water from their surroundings. This increases the osmolarity of the remaining extracellular fluid, which then extracts water from the red cells. The red cells shrink, resulting in lysis. As the membranes are disrupted, antibody is dissociated. This method is used primarily for the investigation of ABO hemolytic disease of the fetus and newborn.

Specimens

1. Red cells washed four to six times with large volumes of saline.
2. Supernatant saline from the final wash of the red cells to be eluted.

Procedure

1. Mix 0.5 mL of the red cells to be tested with 3 drops of saline in a test tube.
2. Cap the tube, then rotate the tube to coat the tube wall with cells.
3. Place the tube in a horizontal position in a freezer at –6 C to –70 C for 10 minutes.
4. Remove the tube from the freezer and thaw it quickly with warm, running tap water.
5. Centrifuge for 2 minutes at 900 to 1000 × *g*.
6. Transfer the supernatant eluate to a clean test tube, and test it in parallel with the supernatant saline from the final wash.

References

1. Judd WJ, Johnson ST, Storry JR. Judd's methods in immunohematology. 3rd ed. Bethesda, MD: AABB Press, 2008.
2. Feng CS, Kirkley KC, Eicher CA, et al. The Lui elution technique: A simple and efficient method for eluting ABO antibodies. Transfusion 1985;25:433-4.

IMMUNE HEMOLYTIC ANEMIA SERUM/PLASMA METHODS

Included in this section are methods used to remove warm or cold autoantibody reactivity (eg, adsorptions) so that alloantibody detection tests and diagnostic tests for differentiating the immune hemolytic anemias can be performed. See Chapter 17 for a discussion of the immune hemolytic anemias.

METHOD 4-5. COLD AUTOADSORPTION PROCEDURE

Principle

Although most cold autoantibodies do not cause a problem in serologic tests, some potent cold-reactive autoantibodies may mask the concomitant presence of clinically significant alloantibodies. In these cases, adsorbing the serum in the cold with autologous red cells can remove the autoantibody, permitting detection of underlying alloantibodies. In the case of most nonpathologic cold autoantibodies, a simple quick adsorption of the patient's serum with enzyme-treated autologous red cells will remove most cold antibody. Washing the red cells with warm (37 C) saline before treatment will help to dissociate cold autoantibody from the red cells. Performing autoadsorption with red cells treated with ZZAP, a combination of proteolytic enzyme and dithiothreitol (DTT), is more efficient. Complement is removed in addition to IgM and IgG,[1] and the red cells are simultaneously enzyme-treated, thereby enhancing the uptake of free autoantibody from the serum.

Specimens

1. 1 mL of serum or plasma to be adsorbed.
2. One or more 1-mL aliquots of autologous red cells. See Note 1 to determine number of aliquots.

Reagents

1. 1% cysteine-activated papain or 1% ficin (see Methods 3-5-1 and 3-5-2).
2. Phosphate-buffered saline (PBS), pH 7.3 (see Method 1-7).
3. 0.2 M DTT prepared by dissolving 1 g of DTT in 32.4 mL of pH 7.3 PBS. Dispense into 3-mL aliquots and store at –18 C or colder.

Procedure

1. Prepare ZZAP reagent[2] by mixing 0.5 mL of 1% cysteine-activated papain with 2.5 mL of 0.2 M DTT and 2 mL of pH 7.3 PBS. Alternatively, use 1 mL of 1% ficin, 2.5 mL of 0.2 M DTT, and 1.5 mL of pH 7.3 PBS.
2. Add 2 mL of ZZAP reagent to 1 mL of autologous red cells. There is no need to

wash the red cells before treatment. Mix and incubate at 37 C for 30 minutes.

3. Wash the cells three times in saline. Centrifuge the last wash for at least 5 minutes at 900 to 1000 × *g* and remove as much of the supernatant saline as possible.
4. To the tube of ZZAP-treated red cells, add 1 mL of the autologous serum. Mix and incubate at 4 C for 30 minutes.
5. Centrifuge at 900 to 1000 × *g* for 4 to 5 minutes and transfer the serum into a clean tube.
6. Steps 2 through 5 may be repeated if the first autoadsorption does not satisfactorily remove the autoantibody activity. See Note 1.
7. After the final adsorption, test the serum with reagent red cells for alloantibody activity.

Notes

1. Sufficient cold autoantibody can usually be removed in one or two adsorptions.
2. If the reactivity of the autoantibody is not diminished, the target autoantigen may have been destroyed by either the enzyme or the DTT. The adsorption should be repeated against untreated autologous red cells washed several times in warm saline.

References

1. Branch DR. Blood transfusion in autoimmune hemolytic anemias. Lab Med 1984; 15:402-8.
2. Branch DR, Petz LD. A new reagent (ZZAP) having multiple applications in immunohematology. Am J Clin Pathol 1982;78:161-7.

METHOD 4-6. DETERMINING THE SPECIFICITY OF COLD-REACTIVE AUTOAGGLUTININS

Principle

For a discussion of specificity of cold-reacting autoantibodies, see Chapter 17.

Specimens

1. Serum or plasma, separated at 37 C from a blood sample maintained and/or allowed to clot at 37 C, or plasma, separated from an anticoagulated sample after periodic inversion at 37 C for approximately 15 minutes.
2. Autologous red cells.

Reagents

Test red cells of the following phenotypes:

1. A pool of two or more examples of adult group O I adult red cells; these can be the reagent cells routinely used for alloantibody detection.
2. Group O i cord red cells.
3. The patient's own (autologous) red cells, washed at least three times with 37 C saline.
4. Red cells of the same ABO group as the patient, if the patient is not group O. If the patient is group A or AB, use both A_1 and A_2 cells.
5. Saline or phosphate-buffered saline (PBS), pH 7.3 (see Method 1-7).

Procedure

1. Prepare serial twofold dilutions of the serum or plasma in saline or PBS. The dilution range should be from 1 in 2 to 1 in 4096 (12 tubes), and the volumes prepared should be more than the total volume needed to test all of the desired red cells. For example, diluting 0.4 mL of serum with 0.4 mL of saline would be sufficient to test three red cell examples. See Notes 1 and 2. See Method 3-7.
2. Label a set of 12 tubes with the dilution (eg, 2, 4, 8, etc) for each kind of red cells to be tested (eg, adult, cord, autologous).
3. Dispense 2 drops of each dilution into the appropriate tubes.
4. Add 1 drop of a 3% to 5% saline suspension of each red cell sample to the appropriate set of tubes.

5. Mix and incubate at room temperature for 30 to 60 minutes.
6. Centrifuge for 15 to 20 seconds at 900 to 1000 × *g*. Examine the tubes one by one macroscopically for agglutination, starting with the set of tubes at the highest dilution for each cell tested (ie, read all the tubes for each dilution as a set). Grade and record the results.
7. Incubate the tubes at 4 C for 1 to 2 hours.
8. Centrifuge for 15 to 20 seconds at 900 to 1000 × *g*. Immediately place the tubes in a rack in an ice waterbath. Examine the tubes as in step 6. Grade and record the results.

Interpretation

Table 4-6-1 summarizes the reactions of the commonly encountered cold-reactive autoantibodies. In cold agglutinin syndrome, anti-I is seen most frequently, but anti-i may also be encountered. When cord cells react stronger than adult cells, the specificity may be anti-i, but adult i red cells need to be tested to confirm that these reactions are due to anti-i and not anti-I^T. Some examples of anti-I react more strongly with red cells that have a strong expression of H antigen (eg, O and A_2 cells); such antibodies are called anti-IH. Rarely, the specificity may be anti-Pr, which should be suspected if all the cells tested react equally. Anti-Pr can be confirmed by testing enzyme-treated cells; anti-Pr does not react with enzyme-treated cells, whereas anti-I and anti-i react better with enzyme-treated cells. Anti-Pr reacts equally with untreated red cells of I or i phenotypes.

Notes

1. It is important to use separate pipettes or pipette tips for each tube when preparing serum dilutions because the serum carried from one tube to the next when a single pipette is used throughout may cause falsely high titration endpoints. The difference can convert a true titer of 4000 to an apparent titer of 100,000 when the use of separate pipettes is compared with the use of a single pipette.
2. Serum dilutions can be prepared more accurately with large volumes (eg, 0.5 mL) than with small volumes.
3. Potent examples of cold-reactive autoantibodies generally do not show apparent specificity until titration studies are performed; this specificity may not even be apparent with dilutions at room temperature or 4 C. In such circumstances, tests can be incubated at 30 to 37 C. Differential reactivity may be more apparent if incubation times are prolonged and agglutination is evaluated after settling, without centrifugation. Settled readings

TABLE 4-6-1. Typical Relative Reactivity Patterns of Cold Autoantibodies

	Antibody Specificity				
Red Cells	**Anti-I**	**Anti-i**	**Anti-I^T**	**Anti-IH**	**Anti-Pr**
O I adult	+	0/↓	0/↓	+	+
O i cord	0/↓	+	+	↓	+
O i adult	0/↓	+	0/↓	↓	+
A_1 I adult	+	0/↓	0/↓	↓	+
Autologous	+	0/↓	0/↓	↓	+
O I enzyme-treated	↑	↑	↑	↑	0

+ = reactive; 0 = nonreactive; ↓ = weaker reaction; ↑ = stronger reaction.

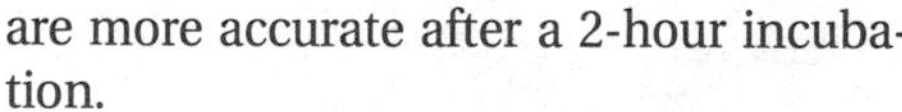

are more accurate after a 2-hour incubation.

4. This procedure can be used to determine both the titer and the specificity. If incubations are started at 37 C (set up prewarmed, ie, all reactants at 37 C before combining) and readings are taken sequentially after incubation at each temperature (eg, 37 C, 30 C, room temperature, 4 C), the specificity, titer, and thermal amplitude of the autoantibody can be determined with a single set of serum dilutions.
5. If testing will also be performed at 30 C and 37 C, include in parallel a test of the neat (undiluted) serum.

Reference

1. Petz LD, Garratty G. Immune hemolytic anemias. 2nd ed. Philadelphia: Churchill Livingstone, 2004.

METHOD 4-7. COLD AGGLUTININ TITER PROCEDURE

Principle

Cold-reactive autoantibodies, if present at very high titers, may suggest a pathologic cold agglutinin disease. This may result in overt hemolysis and systemic symptoms and may indicate underlying B-cell hematologic neoplasia.

Specimen

Serum or plasma, separated at 37 C from a sample maintained and/or allowed to clot at 37 C, or plasma, separated from an anticoagulated sample after periodic inversion at 37 C for approximately 15 minutes.

Reagents

1. A pool of two or more examples of washed group O I adult red cells (eg, antibody detection cells).
2. Phosphate-buffered saline (PBS), pH 7.3 (see Method 1-7).

Procedure

1. Prepare serial twofold dilutions of the patient's serum or plasma in PBS. The dilution range should be from 1 in 2 to 1 in 4096 (12 tubes). See Notes 1 and 2. See Method 3-7.
2. Mix 2 drops of each dilution with 1 drop of a 3% to 5% suspension of red cells.
3. Mix and incubate at 4 C for 1 to 2 hours.
4. Centrifuge the tubes for 15 to 20 seconds at 900 to 1000 × g, then place the tubes in a rack in an ice waterbath. Examine the tubes one by one macroscopically for agglutination, starting with the tube at the highest dilution. Grade and record the results.

Interpretation

The titer is the reciprocal of the highest serum dilution at which macroscopic agglutination is observed. Titers above 64 are considered elevated, but hemolytic anemia resulting from cold-reactive autoagglutinins rarely occurs unless the titer is ≥1000. Titers below 1000 may be obtained when the autoantibody has a different specificity (eg, anti-i) or if the cold agglutinin is of the less-common low-titer, high-thermal-amplitude type. If the patient has a positive direct antiglobulin test (DAT) because of complement only and has clinical signs of hemolytic anemia, specificity and thermal amplitude studies should be performed (see Method 4-6).

Notes

1. It is important to use separate pipettes for each tube when preparing serum dilutions because the serum carried from one tube to the next when a single pipette is used throughout may cause falsely high titration endpoints.
2. Serum dilutions can be prepared more accurately with large volumes (eg, 0.5 mL) than with small volumes.

Reference

1. Petz LD, Garratty G. Immune hemolytic anemias. 2nd ed. Philadelphia: Churchill Livingstone, 2004.

METHOD 4-8. ADSORBING WARM-REACTIVE AUTOANTIBODIES USING AUTOLOGOUS RED CELLS

Principle

Warm-reactive autoantibodies in serum may mask the concomitant presence of clinically significant alloantibodies. Adsorption of the serum with autologous red cells can remove autoantibody from the serum, permitting detection of underlying alloantibodies. However, autologous red cells in the circulation are coated with autoantibody. Autologous adsorption of warm-reactive autoantibodies can be facilitated by dissociating autoantibody from the red cell membrane, thereby uncovering antigen sites that can bind free autoantibody to remove it from the serum. Some autoantibody can be dissociated by a gentle heat elution for 3 to 5 minutes at 56 C. Subsequent treatment of the cells with enzymes enhances the adsorption process by removing membrane structures that otherwise hinder the association between antigen and antibody. The most effective procedure involves the use of ZZAP reagent,[1] a mixture of a proteolytic enzyme and the sulfhydryl reagent dithiothreitol (DTT). ZZAP removes immunoglobulins and complement from the red cells and enhances the adsorption process. Red cells from patients transfused within the last 3 months should not be used for autoadsorption because transfused red cells present in the circulation are likely to adsorb the alloantibodies that are being sought. See Chapter 17.

Specimens

1. 1 mL of serum or plasma (or eluate) to be adsorbed.
2. One or more 1-mL aliquots of autologous red cells. See Note 3.

Reagents

1. 1% cysteine-activated papain or 1% ficin (see Methods 3-5-1 and 3-5-2).
2. Phosphate-buffered saline (PBS), pH 7.3 (see Method 1-7).
3. 0.2 M DTT prepared by dissolving 1 g of DTT in 32.4 mL of pH 7.3 PBS. Dispense into 3-mL aliquots and store at –18 C or colder.

Procedure

1. Prepare ZZAP reagent by mixing 0.5 mL of 1% cysteine-activated papain with 2.5 mL of 0.2 M DTT and 2 mL of pH 7.3 PBS. Alternatively, use 1 mL of 1% ficin, 2.5 mL of 0.2 M DTT, and 1.5 mL of pH 7.3 PBS.
2. Add 2 mL of ZZAP reagent to each of two tubes containing 1 mL of packed red cells. There is no need to wash the red cells before treatment. Mix and incubate at 37 C for 30 minutes with periodic mixing.
3. Wash the red cells three times in saline. Centrifuge the last wash for at least 5 minutes at 900 to 1000 × *g* and remove as much supernatant saline as possible.
4. Add serum to an equal volume of ZZAP-treated red cells, mix, and incubate at 37 C for approximately 30 to 45 minutes.
5. Centrifuge and carefully remove serum.
6. If the original serum reactivity was only 1+, proceed to step 7; otherwise, repeat steps 4 and 5 once more using the once-adsorbed patient's serum and a second aliquot of ZZAP-treated cells. See Note 3.
7. Test the adsorbed serum against group O reagent cells. If reactivity persists, repeat steps 4 and 5.

Interpretation

One or two adsorptions ordinarily remove sufficient autoantibody so that alloantibody reactivity, if present, is readily apparent. If the twice-autoadsorbed serum reacts with defined specificity, as shown by testing against a small antibody identification panel, then the defined specificity of the antibody is probably an alloantibody. If the serum reacts with all cells on the panel, 1) additional autoadsorptions are necessary, 2) the serum contains antibody to a high-prevalence antigen, or 3) the serum contains an autoantibody (eg, anti-Kp^b) that does not react with ZZAP-treated cells and thus will not be adsorbed by this procedure. To check this latter possibility, test the reactive autoadsorbed serum against reagent cells that have been pretreated with the ZZAP reagent.

Notes

1. ZZAP treatment destroys all Kell system antigens and all other antigens that are destroyed by proteases (eg, M, N, Fy^a, and Fy^b), as well as the antigens of the LW, Cartwright, Dombrock, and Knops systems. If the autoantibody is suspected to have specificity to a high-prevalence antigen in any of these blood groups, an alternative procedure is to perform autoadsorption with untreated autologous cells or autologous cells treated only with 1% ficin or 1% cysteine-activated papain.
2. Cold autoantibodies reactive at room temperature can also be present in the serum of about 35% of patients with warm-reactive autoantibodies. Removal of these cold antibodies can be facilitated by placing the serum and cell mixture at 4 C for about 15 minutes after incubation at 37 C.
3. As a guide, when the original serum reactivity is 1+ in the low-ionic-strength saline indirect antiglobulin test (LISS-IAT), usually only one adsorption is required. Antibodies with 2+ to 3+ reactivity will generally be removed in two to three adsorptions. Performing greater than four adsorptions increases the risk of diluting alloantibody reactivity.

Reference

1. Branch DR, Petz LD. A new reagent (ZZAP) having multiple applications in immunohematology. Am J Clin Pathol 1982;78:161-7.

METHOD 4-9. ADSORBING WARM-REACTIVE AUTOANTIBODIES USING ALLOGENEIC RED CELLS

Principle

Adsorption of serum with selected red cells of known phenotypes will remove autoantibody and leave alloantibodies to most common blood group antigens. The specificity of the antibodies that remain after adsorption can be confirmed by testing against a panel of reagent red cells. This procedure can be used to detect underlying alloantibodies if the patient has been recently transfused, or if insufficient autologous red cells are available. Treating the adsorbing cells with enzyme or ZZAP typically enhances the adsorption process. In addition, the treated red cells will lack the antigens destroyed by dithiothreitol (DTT) and/or enzymes (see Chapter 16).

Specimen

Serum/plasma containing warm-reactive autoantibodies or eluate from direct antiglobulin test (DAT)-positive cells.

Reagents

1. 1% cysteine-activated papain or 1% ficin (see Methods 3-5-1 and 3-5-2).
2. ZZAP reagent (papain or ficin plus 0.2 M DTT). See Method 4-8.
3. Phosphate-buffered saline (PBS), pH 7.3 (see Method 1-7).
4. Adsorbing red cells *when the patient's phenotype is unknown:* Group O red cells of the phenotypes R_1R_1, R_2R_2, and rr; one of these cells should be Jk(a–), and one should be Jk(b–). Additionally, if the red cells are to be enzyme-treated only, at least one of the samples should also be K–; the cells can be treated with enzyme or ZZAP to denature other antigens (see Table 17-5 and Note 1).

   Adsorbing red cells *when the patient's phenotype is known:* The red cells can be selected to match the patient's phenotype, or at least they should have the same Rh and Kidd phenotypes if the cells can be treated with enzyme or ZZAP to denature other antigens.

The red cells can be reagent cells or from any blood specimen that will yield a sufficient volume of red cells. See Note 2. Reserve a sample of these red cells to test for completeness of adsorption (step 7).

Procedure

1. Wash 1 mL of each red cell specimen once in a large volume of saline, centrifuge to pack the cells, and remove the supernatant saline. There is no need to wash packed red cells before treatment with ZZAP.
2. To each volume of washed packed cells, add one volume of 1% enzyme solution or two volumes of working ZZAP reagent. Mix the cells by inverting several times.
3. Incubate at 37 C: 15 minutes for enzyme or 30 minutes for ZZAP. Mix periodically throughout incubation.
4. Wash the red cells three times with large volumes of saline. Centrifuge at 900 to 1000 × *g* for at least 5 minutes and remove the last wash as completely as possible to prevent dilution of the serum.
5. For each of the red cell specimens, mix one volume of treated cells with an equal volume of the patient's serum and incubate at 37 C for 30 minutes, mixing occasionally.
6. Centrifuge at 900 to 1000 × *g* for approximately 5 minutes and harvest the supernatant serum.
7. Test the sample(s) of adsorbed serum against the cells (untreated) used for adsorption, respectively, for completeness of adsorption. If reactivity is present, repeat steps 5 through 7 until no reactivity remains. Consider the phenotype of the adsorbing red cells when evaluating completeness of adsorption; reactivity may persist if it is directed to an antigen destroyed by enzyme or DTT treatment; for example, anti-Fy[a] in the adsorbed serum will react with untreated Fy(a+) adsorbing red cells if they were treated for adsorption. The three samples of adsorbed serum can then be tested against antibody detection/panel cells and the results compared for demonstration of persisting and removed antibody activity. See Chapter 17.

Notes

1. The s antigen may not be denatured by a particular enzyme or ZZAP solution. The s antigen status of the adsorbing red cells may need to be considered.
2. If the autoantibody is very strong, three or more aliquots of adsorbing cells should be prepared. As a guide, when the original serum reactivity is 1+ in the low-ionic-strength saline indirect antiglobulin test (LISS-IAT), usually only one adsorption is required. Antibodies with 2+ to 3+ reactivity will generally be removed in two to three adsorptions. Performing greater than four adsorptions increases the risk of diluting alloantibody reactivity. The use of a higher proportion of cells to serum/eluate may enhance adsorption effectiveness.
3. A visible clue to the effectiveness of adsorption is clumping of the enzyme- or ZZAP-treated cells when they are mixed with the serum, especially when strong antibodies are present.
4. Because the treated red cells will lack the antigens destroyed by DTT and/or enzymes, adsorption with untreated red cells may be tried if the autoantibody is not removed with treated red cells.

References

1. Branch DR, Petz LD. A new reagent (ZZAP) having multiple applications in immunohematology. Am J Clin Pathol 1982;78:161-7.
2. Judd WJ, Johnson ST, Storry JR. Judd's methods in immunohematology. 3rd ed. Bethesda, MD: AABB Press, 2008.

METHOD 4-10. POLYETHYLENE GLYCOL ADSORPTION PROCEDURE

Principle

Polyethylene glycol (PEG) enhances the adsorption of antibody by untreated red cells. Testing the adsorbed aliquot against a panel of red cells can identify the specificity of antibodies that remain after adsorption. This method can be used for both autologous and allogeneic adsorption.

Specimen

Serum or plasma to be tested.

Reagents

1. PEG, 20% (20 g PEG, 3350 MW, in 100 mL of PBS, pH 7.3) or commercial PEG enhancement reagent.
2. Autologous red cells or ABO-compatible allogeneic red cells of known phenotype (see Table 17-5). Reserve a sample of these red cells to test for completeness of adsorption (step 5).

Procedure

1. Wash aliquots of red cells in large volumes of saline three times and centrifuge for 5 to 10 minutes at 1000 × *g*. Remove all residual saline.
2. To 1 volume (eg, 1 mL) of red cells, add 1 volume of serum and 1 volume of PEG. Mix well and incubate at 37 C for 15 minutes.
3. Centrifuge the serum/PEG/cell mixture for 5 minutes and harvest the adsorbed serum/PEG mixture.
4. To test the adsorbed serum, add 4 drops of the serum/PEG mixture to 1 drop of test red cells, incubate for 15 minutes at 37 C, and proceed to the antiglobulin test with anti-IgG. The larger volume of serum tested (4 drops) is required to account for the dilution of the serum by the PEG. See Notes 3 and 4.
5. To check for completeness of adsorption, test the adsorbed serum against the red cells used for the adsorption. If positive, repeat the adsorption by adding the adsorbed serum to a fresh aliquot of red cells but do not add additional PEG. If the test result was negative, test the adsorbed serum with a panel of cells.

Notes

1. Red cells for adsorption may be chemically modified (eg, with enzymes or ZZAP) before adsorption if denaturation of antigens is desired.
2. Although many laboratories successfully use the PEG adsorption method, some serologists have reported a weakening or loss of antibody reactivity in some samples when compared with results obtained using a different technique. To accommodate this potential weakening of antibody reactivity, some serologists test 6 drops of the PEG-adsorbed serum.
3. Test the adsorbed serum on the day it was adsorbed. Weak antibody reactivity may be lost upon storage of PEG-adsorbed sera, possibly as a result of precipitation of the protein noticeable after 4 C storage.
4. Agglutination of the adsorbing red cells does not occur when PEG is used; therefore, there is no visible clue to the efficiency of the adsorption process. As a guide, when the original serum reactivity is 1+ in the low-ionic-strength saline indirect antiglobulin test (LISS-IAT), usually only one adsorption is required. Antibodies with 2+ to 3+ reactivity will generally be removed in two adsorptions.

References

1. Leger RM, Garratty G. Evaluation of methods for detecting alloantibodies underlying warm autoantibodies. Transfusion 1999;39:11-16.
2. Leger RM, Ciesielski D, Garratty G. Effect of storage on antibody reactivity after adsorption in the presence of polyethylene glycol. Transfusion 1999;39:1272-3.

METHOD 4-11. PERFORMING THE DONATH-LANDSTEINER TEST

Principle

IgG autoantibodies that cause paroxysmal cold hemoglobinuria (PCH) act as biphasic hemolysins in vitro. The IgG autoantibodies bind to the red cells at cold temperatures, and as the test is warmed to 37 C, complement is activated and lysis of the red cells occurs. The patient for whom this procedure should be considered is one with a positive direct antiglobulin test (DAT) result due to C3; demonstrable hemoglobinemia, hemoglobinuria, or both; and no evidence of autoantibody activity in the serum or the eluate made from the DAT-positive cells. For a discussion of PCH, see Chapter 17.

Specimen

Serum separated from a freshly collected blood sample maintained at 37 C. See Note 1.

Reagents

1. Freshly collected pooled normal sera known to lack unexpected antibodies, to use as a source of complement.
2. 50% suspension of washed group O red cells that express the P antigen (eg, antibody detection cells).

Procedure

1. Label three sets of three 10 × 75-mm test tubes as follows: A1-A2-A3; B1-B2-B3; C1-C2-C3.
2. To tubes 1 and 2 of each set, add 10 volumes (eg, drops) of the patient's serum.
3. To tubes 2 and 3 of each set, add 10 volumes of fresh normal serum.
4. To all tubes, add one volume of the 50% suspension of washed P-positive red cells and mix well.
5. Place the three "A" tubes in a bath of melting ice for 30 minutes and then at 37 C for 1 hour.
6. Place the three "B" tubes in a bath of melting ice and keep them in melting ice for 90 minutes.
7. Place the three "C" tubes at 37 C and keep them at 37 C for 90 minutes.
8. Gently mix and centrifuge all tubes. Examine the supernatant fluid for hemolysis.

Interpretation

The Donath-Landsteiner test is considered positive when the patient's serum, with or without added complement, causes hemolysis in the tubes that were incubated first in melting ice and then at 37 C (ie, tubes A1 and A2) and there is no hemolysis in any of the tubes maintained throughout at 37 C (ie, tubes C1, C2) or in melting ice (ie, tubes B1, B2). The A3, B3, and C3 tubes serve as controls of the normal sera complement source and should not manifest hemolysis.

Notes

1. To avoid loss of antibody by autoadsorption before testing, the patient's blood should be allowed to clot at 37 C, and the serum separated from the clot at this temperature.
2. Active complement is essential for demonstration of the antibody. Because patients with PCH may have low levels of serum complement, fresh normal serum should be included in the reaction medium as a source of complement.
3. If a limited amount of blood is available (eg, from young children), set up tubes A-1, A-2, A-3, C-1, and C-2; if there is only enough serum for two tests (ie, 20 drops), set up tubes A-2, A-3, and C-2.
4. To demonstrate the P specificity of the Donath-Landsteiner antibody, ABO-compatible p red cells should be tested in a second set of tubes A-1, A-2, and A-3. No lysis should develop in these tubes, confirming the P specificity of the antibody.

References

1. Judd WJ, Johnson ST, Storry JR. Judd's methods in immunohematology. 3rd ed. Bethesda, MD: AABB Press, 2008.
2. Dacie JV, Lewis SM. Practical hematology. 7th ed. New York: Churchill Livingstone, 1991:500-1.

METHOD 4-12. DETECTING DRUG ANTIBODIES BY TESTING DRUG-TREATED RED CELLS

Principle

Some drugs, principally penicillin and many cephalosporins, can induce an IgG immune response that can be detected by testing red cells treated with the drug. The preparation of the drug used should, to the extent possible, be the same as what was given to the patient. Antibodies to either penicillin or cephalothin may cross-react with cells treated with the other drug (ie, penicillin antibodies may attach to cephalothin-treated cells and vice versa). Antibodies to other cephalosporins may react with cephalothin-treated cells.

For drugs other than penicillin and the cephalosporins, refer to published reports for the method used to treat the red cells. Normal sera may contain weak antibodies to penicillin or cephalosporins, presumably as a result of environmental exposure. Results definitive for a penicillin-induced positive DAT are reactivity of the eluate against the penicillin-treated red cells and no reactivity of the eluate against the uncoated red cells.

Specimen

Serum or plasma *and* eluate (and last wash) to be studied.

Reagents

1. 0.1 M sodium barbital buffer (BB) at pH 9.6 to 9.8, prepared by dissolving 2.06 g of sodium barbital in 80 mL of distilled or deionized water. Adjust the pH to between 9.6 and 9.8 with 0.1 N HCl. Bring total volume to 100 mL. Store at 2 to 8 C.
2. Phosphate-buffered saline (PBS), pH 7.3 (see Method 1-7).
3. Drug (eg, penicillin, cephalosporin).
4. Washed, packed, group O red cells.
5. Normal sera/plasma (antibody free) as a negative control.
6. Positive control serum/plasma, if available.
7. Antihuman globulin or anti-IgG.
8. IgG-coated red cells.

Procedure

1. Prepare drug solutions just before use. See Notes 1 and 2.
   a. For penicillin-treated cells, dissolve 600 mg of penicillin in 15 mL of BB. This high pH is optimal, but if the buffer is unavailable, PBS, pH 7.3, can be used. Add 1 mL of red cells. In a separate tube, prepare control cells by adding 1 mL of untreated red cells (without the drug) to 15 mL of the same buffer. Incubate both tubes for 1 hour at room temperature with occasional mixing. Wash three times and prepare a 5% suspension in PBS.
   b. For cephalosporin-treated cells, dissolve 400 mg of the drug in 10 mL of PBS, pH 7.3. Add 1 mL of red cells. In a separate tube, prepare control cells by adding 1 mL of untreated red cells (without the drug) to 10 mL of PBS. Incubate both tubes for 1 hour at 37 C with occasional mixing. Wash three times and prepare a 5% suspension in PBS.
2. Label two sets of tubes (drug-treated and untreated) for each sample to be tested: serum, eluate, last wash, PBS, negative control sera/plasma, and positive control. If the drug is known to cause nonimmunologic protein adsorption, also test a 1-in-20 dilution of the patient's serum and the controls (negative and positive).
3. Add 2 or 3 drops of each sample to the appropriate tube.
4. Add 1 drop of a 5% saline suspension of drug-treated red cells to one set of tubes. Add 1 drop of a 5% saline suspension of

untreated red cells to the second set of tubes.

5. Incubate the tubes at 37 C for 60 minutes. Centrifuge and examine for hemolysis and agglutination. Record the results.
6. Wash the cells four times in saline, and test by an indirect antiglobulin technique using polyspecific antihuman globulin or anti-IgG reagent. Centrifuge and examine for agglutination. Record the results.
7. Confirm the validity of negative test results by adding IgG-coated red cells.

Interpretation

Reactivity (hemolysis, agglutination, and/or positive indirect antiglobulin test result) with drug-treated cells, but not with untreated cells, indicates that drug antibodies are present (see Note 4). No hemolysis will be seen in tests with plasma or the eluate.

Negative results without a positive control can be interpreted to mean only that drug antibodies were not detected. The drug may or may not be bound to the test red cells.

Notes

1. The volume of drug-treated red cells can be scaled down as long as the ratio of the 40 mg/mL drug solution to red cells is constant (eg, 120 mg penicillin in 3 mL BB plus 0.2 mL red cells, or 100 mg cephalosporin in 2.5 mL PBS plus 0.25 mL red cells).
2. Drug-treated red cells may be kept in PBS at 4 C for up to 1 week; however, there may be some weakening of drug coating upon storage. Drug-treated and untreated red cells may also be stored frozen.
3. Cephalosporins do not require a high pH for optimal coating of red cells. In fact, a lower pH (ie, pH 6 to 7) decreases nonspecific protein adsorption seen when a high pH buffer is used. The least amount of nonspecific protein adsorption by drug-treated red cells will occur if a pH 6.0 buffer is used, but this leads to a slight decrease in coating by the drug.
4. To control for nonspecific protein adsorption of normal sera observed with some cephalosporins (eg, cephalothin), test the control sera and the test serum at a 1-in-20 dilution in PBS. Normal sera diluted 1 in 20 generally do not react nonspecifically. Thus, reactivity of the diluted serum with the drug-treated cells but not with the untreated cells indicates that drug antibody is present.
5. When antibodies are not detected with drug-treated red cells, test for drug antibodies in the presence of the drug (see Method 4-13). Antibodies to some third-generation cephalosporins (eg, ceftriaxone) do not react with drug-treated red cells.

Reference

1. Petz LD, Garratty G. Immune hemolytic anemias. 2nd ed. Philadelphia: Churchill Livingstone, 2004.

METHOD 4-13. DETECTING DRUG ANTIBODIES BY TESTING IN THE PRESENCE OF DRUG

Principle

Some drug antibodies are demonstrable when the patient's serum is tested in the presence of soluble drug (or metabolite) against untreated or enzyme-treated red cells. In the past, this has been referred to as the "immune complex" method, although the actual mechanism has not been proven.[1]

Specimen

The patient's serum.

Reagents

1. The drug under investigation, in the same form (powder, tablet, capsules) that the patient is receiving.
2. Phosphate-buffered saline (PBS) at pH 7.0 to 7.4.

3. Fresh, normal serum known to lack unexpected antibodies, as a source of complement.
4. Pooled group O reagent red cells, 5% suspension: one aliquot treated with a proteolytic enzyme, and one untreated.
5. Polyspecific antihuman globulin reagent.
6. IgG-coated red cells.

Procedure

1. Prepare a 1-mg/mL solution of the drug in PBS. Centrifuge to remove any particulate matter, and adjust the pH of the supernatant fluid to approximately 7 with either 1 N NaOH or 1 N HCl, as required, if the pH is below 5 or above 8.
2. Label two sets of three tubes (untreated and enzyme-treated) for the following test mixtures:
   a. Patient's serum + drug.
   b. Patient's serum + PBS.
   c. Patient's serum + complement (normal serum) + drug.
   d. Patient's serum + complement (normal serum) + PBS.
   e. Normal serum + drug.
   f. Normal serum + PBS.
3. Add two volumes (eg, 2 drops) of each component to the appropriate tubes (eg, 2 drops of serum + 2 drops of drug).
4. Add 1 drop of a 5% saline suspension of untreated group O reagent red cells to one set of tubes. Add 1 drop of a 5% saline suspension of enzyme-treated group O reagent red cells to the second set of tubes.
5. Mix and incubate at 37 C for 1 to 2 hours, with periodic gentle mixing.
6. Centrifuge, examine for hemolysis and agglutination, and record the results.
7. Wash the cells four times in saline, and test with a polyspecific antiglobulin reagent.
8. Centrifuge, examine for agglutination, and record the results.
9. Confirm the validity of negative test results by adding IgG-coated red cells.

Interpretation

Hemolysis, direct agglutination, or positive indirect antiglobulin tests can occur together or separately. Reactivity in any of the tests containing the patient's serum to which the drug was added, and absence of reactivity in the corresponding control tests containing PBS instead of the drug, indicate that antibody to the drug is present. See Note 4.

Notes

1. The drug may be more easily dissolved by incubation at 37 C and vigorous shaking of the solution. If the drug is in tablet form, crush it with a mortar and pestle and remove any visible outer tablet coating material before adding PBS.
2. Not all drugs will dissolve completely in PBS. Consult the manufacturer or a reference such as the Merck Index for the solubility of the drug in question. A previous report of drug-induced immune hemolytic anemia resulting from the drug in question may provide information on the drug solution preparation.
3. When available, a serum or plasma known to contain antibody with the drug specificity being evaluated should be included as a positive control.
4. Tests without the drug added may be positive if autoantibodies or circulating drug-antibody immune complexes are present in the patient's sample. Autoantibody reactivity would be persistent over time, whereas circulating immune complexes are transient.
5. Testing with enzyme-treated red cells and the addition of fresh normal serum as a source of complement may increase the sensitivity of the test.
6. If testing in the presence of the drug and tests with drug-treated red cells (Method 4-12) are noninformative, consider testing with a metabolite of the drug.[2]

References

1. Petz LD, Garratty G. Immune hemolytic anemias. 2nd ed. Philadelphia: Churchill Livingstone, 2004.
2. Johnson ST, Fueger JT, Gottschall JL. One center's experience: The serology and drugs associated with drug-induced immune hemolytic anemia—a new paradigm. Transfusion 2007; 47:697-702.

Hemolytic Disease of the Fetus and Newborn

METHOD 5-1. TESTING FOR FETOMATERNAL HEMORRHAGE—THE ROSETTE TEST

Principle

This test detects D+ red cells in the blood of a D– woman whose fetus or recently delivered infant is D+. When reagent anti-D is added to maternal blood containing D+ fetal cells, fetal red cells become coated with anti-D. When D+ reagent cells are subsequently added, easily visible rosettes are formed, with several red cells clustered around each antibody-coated D+ red cell.

Although the number of rosettes is roughly proportional to the number of D+ red cells present in the original mixture, this test provides only qualitative information about fetal-maternal admixture. Specimens giving a positive result should be subjected to further testing to quantify the number of fetal cells. The acid-elution procedure given below and flow cytometry are acceptable choices. If a commercial test is available, the directions in the package insert should be followed.

Specimen

A 2% to 5% saline suspension of washed red cells from a maternal blood sample.

Reagents

Prepared reagents are commercially available. The steps below can be used for in-house preparation.

1. Negative control: a 2% to 5% saline suspension of washed red cells known to be D–.
2. Positive control: a 2% to 5% saline suspension of a mixture containing approximately 0.6% D+ red cells and 99.4% D– red cells. The positive control can be prepared by adding 1 drop of a 2% to 5% suspension of D+ control cells to 15 drops of a 2% to 5% suspension of washed D– control cells. Mix well, then add 1 drop of this cell suspension to 9 drops of the 2% to 5% suspension of D– red cells. Mix well.
3. Indicator red cells: a 2% to 5% saline suspension of group O, R_2R_2 red cells. Either enzyme-treated or untreated cells in an enhancing medium can be used.
4. High-protein reagent anti-D serum. Some monoclonal/polyclonal blended reagents are unsuitable for use in this method. The antisera selected for use should be evaluated for suitability before incorporation into the test procedure.

Procedure

1. To each of three test tubes, add 1 drop (or the volume specified in the manufacturer's instructions) of reagent anti-D.
2. Add 1 drop of maternal cells, negative control cells, and positive control cells to the appropriately labeled tubes.
3. Incubate at 37 C for 15 to 30 minutes, or as specified by the manufacturer's instructions.

4. Wash cell suspensions at least four times with large volumes of saline, to remove all unbound reagent anti-D. Decant saline completely after last wash.
5. To the dry cell button, add 1 drop of indicator cells and mix thoroughly to resuspend them.
6. Centrifuge the tubes for 15 seconds at 900 to 1000 × *g*.
7. Resuspend the cell button and examine the red cell suspension microscopically at 100× to 150× magnification.
8. Examine at least 10 fields and count the number of red cell rosettes in each field.

Interpretation

The absence of rosettes is a negative result. With enzyme-treated indicator cells, up to one rosette per three fields may occur in a negative specimen. With untreated indicator cells and an enhancing medium, there may be up to six rosettes per five fields in a negative test. The presence of more rosettes than these allowable maxima constitutes a positive result, and the specimen should be examined using a test that quantifies the amount of fetal blood present.

The presence of rosettes or agglutination in the negative control tube indicates inadequate washing after incubation, allowing residual anti-D to agglutinate the D+ indicator cells. A strongly positive result is seen with red cells from a woman whose Rh phenotype is weak D rather than D–; massive fetomaternal hemorrhage may produce an appearance difficult to distinguish from that caused by a weak D phenotype, and a quantitative test for fetal cells should be performed. If the infant's cells are shown to be weak D, a negative result on the mother's specimen should be interpreted with caution. In this situation, a quantitative test that does not rely on D antigen expression should be performed.

Reference

1. Sebring ES, Polesky HF. Detection of fetal maternal hemorrhage in Rh immune globulin candidates. Transfusion 1982;22:468-71.

METHOD 5-2. TESTING FOR FETOMATERNAL HEMORRHAGE—MODIFIED KLEIHAUER-BETKE TEST

Principle

Fetal hemoglobin resists elution from red cells under acid conditions, whereas adult hemoglobin is eluted. When a thin blood smear is exposed to an acid buffer, hemoglobin from adult red cells is leached into the buffer so that only the stroma remains; fetal cells retain their hemoglobin and can be identified by a positive staining pattern. The approximate volume of fetomaternal hemorrhage can be calculated from the percentage of fetal red cells in the maternal blood film.

Specimen

Maternal anticoagulated whole blood sample.

Reagents

Prepared reagents are commercially available in kits. The directions below can be used for in-house preparations.

1. Stock solution A (0.1 M of citric acid): $C_6H_8O_7 \bullet H_2O$, 21.0 g, diluted to 1 liter with distilled water. Keep refrigerated.
2. Stock solution B (0.2 M of sodium phosphate): $Na_2HPO_4 \bullet 7H_2O$, 53.6 g, diluted to 1 liter with distilled water. Keep refrigerated.
3. McIlvaine's buffer, pH 3.2: Add 75 mL of stock solution A to 21 mL of stock solution B. Prepare fresh mixture for each test. This buffer mixture should be brought to room temperature or used at 37 C.
4. Erythrosin B, 0.5% in water.
5. Harris hematoxylin (filtered).
6. 80% ethyl alcohol.
7. Positive control specimen: Ten parts of anticoagulated adult blood, mixed with one part of anticoagulated ABO-compatible cord blood.
8. Negative control specimen: Anticoagulated adult blood.

Procedure

1. Prepare very thin blood smears, diluting blood with an equal volume of saline. Air dry.
2. Fix the smears in 80% ethyl alcohol for 5 minutes.
3. Wash the smears with distilled water.
4. Immerse the smears in McIlvaine's buffer, pH 3.2, for 11 minutes at room temperature or 5 minutes at 37 C. This reaction is temperature sensitive.
5. Wash the smears in distilled water.
6. Immerse the smears in erythrosin B for 5 minutes.
7. Wash the smears completely in distilled water.
8. Immerse the smears in Harris hematoxylin for 5 minutes.
9. Wash the smears in running tap water for 1 minute.
10. Examine the smears dry using 40× magnification, count a total of 2000 red cells, and record the number of fetal cells observed.
11. Calculate the percentage of fetal red cells in the total counted.

Interpretation

1. Fetal cells are bright pink and refractile; normal adult red cells appear as very pale "ghosts."
2. The conversion factor used to indicate the volume (as mL of whole blood) of fetomaternal hemorrhage is the percentage of fetal red cells observed times 50.

Note

The accuracy and precision of this procedure are poor, and decisions regarding Rh Immune Globulin (RhIG) dosage in massive fetomaternal hemorrhage should be made accordingly. If there is a question regarding the need for additional RhIG, it is preferable to administer another dose to prevent the risks of undertreatment. (See Table 22-1 for dosage.)

Reference

1. Sebring ES. Fetomaternal hemorrhage—incidence and methods of detection and quantitation. In: Garratty G, ed. Hemolytic disease of the newborn. Arlington, VA: AABB, 1984:87-118.

METHOD 5-3. USING ANTIBODY TITRATION STUDIES TO ASSIST IN EARLY DETECTION OF HEMOLYTIC DISEASE OF THE FETUS AND NEWBORN

Principle

Antibody titration is a semiquantitative method of determining antibody concentration. Serial twofold dilutions of serum are prepared and tested for antibody activity. The reciprocal of the highest dilution of plasma or serum that gives a 1+ reaction is referred to as the titer (ie, 1 in 128 dilution; titer = 128).

In pregnancy, antibody titration is performed to identify women with significant levels of antibodies that may lead to hemolytic disease of the fetus and newborn (HDFN) and, for low-titer antibodies, to establish a baseline for comparison with titers found later in pregnancy. Titration of non-Rh antibodies should be undertaken only after discussion with the obstetrician about how the data will be used in the clinical management of the pregnancy. The significance of titers has been sufficiently established only for anti-D (using a saline technique).

Specimen

Serum for titration (containing potentially significant unexpected antibodies to red cell antigens), 1 mL. If possible, test the current sample in parallel with the most recent previously submitted (preceding) sample from the current pregnancy.

Materials

1. Antihuman IgG: need not be heavy chain specific.
2. Isotonic saline.

3. Volumetric pipettes, or equivalent: 0.1- to 0.5-mL delivery, with disposable tips.
4. Red cells: group O reagent red cells, 2% suspension. (See note 1 regarding the selection of red cells for testing.) Avoid using Bg+ red cells because they may result in falsely high values, especially with sera from multiparous women.
5. IgG-coated red cells.

Quality Control

1. Test the preceding sample in parallel with the most recent sample.
2. Prepare the dilutions using a separate pipette for each tube. Failure to do so will result in falsely high titers because of carryover.
3. Confirm all negative reactions with IgG-coated red cells (see step 9 below).

Procedure

1. Using 0.5-mL volumes, prepare serial twofold dilutions of serum in saline. The initial tube should contain undiluted serum and the doubling dilution range should be from 1 in 2 to 1 in 2048 (total of 12 tubes). (See Method 3-7.)
2. Place 0.1 mL of each dilution into appropriately labeled test tubes.
3. Add 0.1 mL of the 2% suspension of red cells to each dilution. Alternatively, for convenience, add 1 drop of a solution of a 3% to 4% suspension of red cells as supplied by the reagent manufacturer, although this method is less precise.
4. Gently agitate the contents of each tube; incubate at 37 C for 1 hour.
5. Wash the red cells four times with saline; completely decant the final wash supernatant.
6. To the dry red cell buttons thus obtained, add anti-IgG according to the manufacturer's directions.
7. Centrifuge as for hemagglutination tests.
8. Examine the red cells macroscopically; grade and record the reactions.
9. Add IgG-coated red cells to all negative tests; recentrifuge and examine the tests for macroscopic agglutination; repeat the testing if the tests with IgG-coated red cells are nonreactive.

Interpretation

The titer is reported as the reciprocal of the highest dilution of serum at which 1+ agglutination is observed. A titer ≥16 (this value may vary according to the laboratory) is considered significant and may warrant further monitoring for HDFN.

Notes

1. The selection of the most suitable phenotype of red cells to use when performing titration studies for HDFN is controversial. Some workers select red cells that have the strongest expression of antigen, such as R_2R_2 for anti-D. Others select red cells with the phenotype that would be expected in fetal circulation—ie, red cells that express a single dose of the antigen, such as R_1r for testing for anti-D. Whichever viewpoint is followed, it is important that the laboratory be consistent and use red cells of the same phenotype for future titrations to test the same patient's serum.
2. Titration studies should be performed upon initial detection of the antibody; save an appropriately labeled aliquot of the serum (frozen at –20 C or colder) for comparative studies with the next submitted sample.
3. When the titer (eg, >16) and the antibody specificity have been associated with HDFN, it is recommended that repeat titration studies be performed every 2 to 4 weeks, beginning at 18 weeks' gestation; save an aliquot of the serum (frozen at –20 C or colder) for comparative studies with the next submitted sample.
4. When invasive procedures (eg, amniocentesis) have demonstrated fetal compromise and are being used to monitor the pregnancy, use the optimal method for follow-up of fetal well-being. However,

if initial studies do not show fetal compromise or the Liley curve result is borderline, additional titrations may be helpful as a means of following the pregnancy in a less invasive manner.

5. Each institution should develop a policy to ensure a degree of uniformity in reporting and interpreting antibody titers.

6. For antibodies to low-prevalence antigens, consider using putative paternal red cells, having established that they express the antigen in question.

7. Do not use enhancement techniques [albumin, polyethylene glycol, low-ionic-strength saline (LISS)] or enzyme-treated red cells because falsely elevated titers may be obtained. Gel testing is not recommended.

8. LISS should not be used as a diluent in titration studies; nonspecific uptake of globulins may occur in serum-LISS dilutions.

9. Failure to obtain the correct results may be caused by 1) incorrect technique, notably failure to use separate pipette tips for each dilution, or 2) failure to adequately mix thawed frozen serum.

10. Other titration methods have been described that may show less variation.[6]

References

1. Issitt PD, Anstee DJ. Applied blood group serology. 4th ed. Durham, NC: Montgomery Scientific Publications, 1998:1067-9.
2. Judd WJ, Luban NLC, Ness PM, et al. Prenatal and perinatal immunohematology: Recommendations for serologic management of the fetus, newborn infant, and obstetric patient. Transfusion 1990;30:175-83.
3. Judd WJ, Johnson ST, Storry J. Judd's methods in immunohematology. 3rd ed. Bethesda, MD: AABB Press, 2008.
4. Judd WJ. Practice guidelines for prenatal and perinatal immunhematology, revisited. Transfusion 2001;41:1445-52.
5. Judd WJ for the Scientific Section Coordinating Committee. Guidelines for prenatal and perinatal immunohematology. Bethesda, MD: AABB, 2005.
6. AuBuchon JP, de, Dumont LJ, et al. Reducing the variation in performance of antibody titrations. Arch Pathol Lab Med 2008; 132:1194-201.

Blood Collection, Component Preparation, and Storage

◆

METHOD 6-1. SCREENING DONORS FOR ANEMIA—COPPER SULFATE METHOD

Principle

This method estimates the hemoglobin content of blood from its specific gravity. A drop of blood in contact with copper sulfate solution of specific gravity 1.053 becomes encased in a sac of copper proteinate, which prevents dispersion of the fluid or any change in specific gravity for about 15 seconds. If the specific gravity of the blood is higher than that of the solution, the drop will sink within 15 seconds; if not, the drop will hesitate and remain suspended or rise to the top of the solution. A specific gravity of 1.053 corresponds to a hemoglobin concentration of 12.5 g/dL.

This is not a quantitative test; it shows only whether the prospective donor's hemoglobin is below or above the acceptable level of 12.5 g/dL. False-positive reactions are rare; donors whose drop of blood sinks nearly always have an acceptable hemoglobin level. False-negative reactions occur fairly commonly and can cause inappropriate deferral.[1,2] Measuring hemoglobin by another method or determining hematocrit sometimes reveals that the prospective donor is acceptable.

Reagents and Materials

1. Copper sulfate solution at specific gravity 1.053, available commercially. Store in tightly capped containers to prevent evaporation. Keep solution at room temperature or bring to room temperature before use.
2. Sterile gauze, antiseptic wipes, and sterile lancets.
3. Containers for the disposal of sharps and other biohazardous materials.
4. Capillary tubes and dropper bulbs or a device to collect capillary blood without contact.

Procedure

1. Into a labeled, clean, dry tube or bottle, dispense a sufficient amount (at least 30 mL) of copper sulfate solution to allow the drop to fall approximately 3 inches. Change the solution daily or after 25 tests. Be sure that the solution is adequately mixed before beginning each day's determinations.
2. Clean the site of the skin puncture thoroughly with antiseptic solution and wipe it dry with sterile gauze.
3. Puncture the finger firmly, near the end but slightly to the side, with a sterile, disposable lancet or springloaded, disposable needle system. A good free flow of blood is important. Do not squeeze the puncture site repeatedly because this may dilute the drop of blood with tissue fluid and lower the specific gravity.
4. Collect the blood in a capillary tube without allowing air to enter the tube.

5. Let one drop of blood fall gently from the tube at a height about 1 cm above the surface of the copper sulfate solution.
6. Observe for 15 seconds.
7. Dispose of lancets and capillary tubes in appropriate biohazard containers. Dispose of gauze appropriately; gauze contaminated with droplets of blood that subsequently dry such that the item is stained but not soaked or caked may be considered nonhazardous.

Interpretation

1. If the drop of blood sinks, the donor's hemoglobin is at an acceptable level for blood donation.
2. If the drop of blood does not sink, the donor's hemoglobin may not be at an acceptable level for blood donation. If time and equipment permit, it is desirable to perform a quantitative measurement of hemoglobin or hematocrit.

Notes

1. A certificate of analysis from the manufacturer should be obtained with each new lot of copper sulfate solution.
2. Used solution should be disposed of as biohazardous or chemical material because of the blood in the container. Refer to local and state laws regarding disposal.
3. Use care to prevent blood from contaminating work surfaces, the donor's clothing, or other persons or equipment.
4. Cover the container between uses to prevent evaporation.

References

1. Lloyd H, Collins A, Walker W, et al. Volunteer blood donors who fail the copper sulfate screening test: What does failure mean, and what should be done? Transfusion 1988;28:467-9.
2. Morris MW, Davey FR. Basic examination of blood. In: Henry JB, ed. Clinical diagnosis and management by laboratory methods. 20th ed. Philadelphia: WB Saunders, 2001:479-519.

METHOD 6-2. PREPARING THE DONOR'S ARM FOR BLOOD COLLECTION

Detailed instructions are specific to each manufacturer and should be followed as indicated. The following procedure is written in general terms as an example.

Principle

Iodophor compounds, or other sterilizing compounds, are used to sterilize the venipuncture site before blood collection.

Materials

1. Scrub solution: Disposable povidone-iodine scrub 0.75% or disposable povidone-iodine swab stick 10%; available in prepackaged single-use form.
2. Preparation solution: 10% povidone-iodine; available in prepackaged single-use form.
3. Sterile gauze.

Procedure

1. Apply tourniquet or blood pressure cuff; identify venipuncture site; then release tourniquet or cuff.
2. Scrub area at least 4 cm (1.5 inches) in all directions from the intended site of venipuncture (ie, 8 cm or 3 inches in diameter) for a minimum of 30 seconds with 0.7% aqueous solution of iodophor compound. Excess foam may be removed, but the arm need not be dry before the next step.
3. Starting at the intended site of venipuncture and moving outward in a concentric spiral, apply "prep" solution; let stand for 30 seconds or as indicated by manufacturer.
4. Cover the area with dry, sterile gauze until the time of venipuncture. After the skin has been prepared, it must not be touched again. Do not repalpate the vein at the intended venipuncture site.

Notes

1. For donors sensitive to iodine (tincture or povidone preparations), another method (eg, ChloraPrep 2% chlorhexidine and 70% isopropyl alcohol) should be designated by the blood bank physician. Green soap should not be used.
2. For donors sensitive to both iodine and chlorhexidine, a method using only isopropyl alcohol could be considered. The preferred procedure is the use of a 30-second up-and-down scrub, followed by enough time for the skin to dry. A second scrub is then applied. This method may require a variance from the Food and Drug Administration.

Reference

1. Goldman M, Roy G, Fréchette N, et al. Evaluation of donor skin disinfection methods. Transfusion 1997;37:309-12.

METHOD 6-3. COLLECTING BLOOD AND SAMPLES FOR PROCESSING AND COMPATIBILITY TESTS

Principle

Blood for transfusion and accompanying samples is obtained from prominent veins on the donor's arm, usually in the area of the antecubital fossa.

Materials

1. Sterile collection bag containing anticoagulant, with integrally attached tubing and needle.
2. Metal clips and hand sealers.
3. Balance system to monitor volume of blood drawn.
4. Sterile gauze and instruments (scissors, hemostats, forceps).
5. Test tubes for sample collection.
6. Device for stripping blood in the tubing.
7. Dielectric sealer (optional).

Procedure

1. Ask donor to confirm his or her identification.
2. Ensure that all labeling on blood container, processing tubes, retention segment, and donor records is correct.
3. Prepare the donor's arm as described in Method 6-2 for arm preparation for blood collection.
4. Inspect bag for any defects and discoloration. The anticoagulant and additive solutions should be inspected for particulate contaminants.
5. Position bag below the level of the donor's arm.
   a. If a balance system is used, be sure the counterbalance is level and adjusted for the amount of blood to be drawn. Unless metal clips and a hand sealer are used, make a very loose overhand knot in the tubing. Hang the bag, and route the tubing through the pinch clamp. To prevent air from entering the line, a hemostat should be applied to the tubing before the needle is uncapped.
   b. If a balance system is not used, be sure to monitor the volume of blood drawn.
6. Reapply tourniquet, or inflate blood pressure cuff. Ask the donor to open and close his or her hand until the previously selected vein is again prominent.
7. Uncover sterile needle, and perform the venipuncture immediately. A clean, skillful venipuncture is essential for collection of a full, clot-free unit. Once the bevel has penetrated the skin, palpation of the skin above the needle stem may be performed with a gloved finger, provided the needle is not touched. When the needle position is acceptable, tape the tubing to the donor's arm to hold the needle in place, and cover the site with sterile gauze.
8. Release the hemostat. Open the temporary closure between the interior of the bag and the tubing.
9. Ask the donor to open and close his or her hand slowly every 10 to 12 seconds during collection.

10. Keep the donor under observation throughout the donation process. The donor should never be left unattended during or immediately after the donation.
11. Mix blood and anticoagulant gently and periodically (approximately every 45 seconds) during collection. Mixing may be done by hand or by continuous mechanical mixing.
12. Be sure blood flow remains fairly brisk so that coagulation activity is not triggered. If there is continuous, adequate blood flow and constant agitation, rigid time limits are not necessary. However, units requiring more than 15 minutes to draw may not be suitable for preparation of platelets, Fresh Frozen Plasma (FFP), or Cryoprecipitated AHF. The time required for collection can be monitored by indicating the time of phlebotomy or the maximal allowable time (start time plus 15 minutes) on the donor's record.
13. Monitor volume of blood being drawn. If a balance is used, the device will interrupt blood flow after the proper amount has been collected. Generally, devices that are designed to mix the blood during collection also permit interruption of the flow when the preset amount is collected. One mL of blood weighs at least 1.053 g, indicated by the minimum allowable specific gravity for donors. A convenient figure to use is 1.06 g/mL; a unit containing 405 to 550 mL should weigh 429 to 583 g plus the weight of the container and anticoagulant. A 500-mL bag collection should weigh 565 to 671 g plus the weight of the container and anticoagulant.
14. Clamp the tubing near the venipuncture using a hemostat, metal clip, or other temporary clamp. Release the blood pressure cuff or tourniquet to 20 mm Hg or less, and fill the tube(s) for blood processing sample(s) by a method that prevents contamination of the contents of the bag. This process can be done in several ways.
    a. If the blood collection bag contains an in-line needle, make an additional seal with a hemostat, metal clip, hand sealer, or tight knot made from a previously prepared loose knot just distal to the in-line needle. Open the connector by separating the needles. Insert the proximal needle into a processing test tube, remove the hemostat, allow the tube to fill, and reclamp the tubing. The donor needle is now ready for removal.
    b. If the blood collection bag contains an in-line processing tube, be certain that the processing tube or pouch is full when the collection is complete and that the original clamp is placed near the donor needle. The entire assembly may now be removed from the donor.
    c. If a straight-tubing assembly set is used, the following procedure should be followed. Place a hemostat on the tubing, allowing about four segments between the hemostat and the needle. Pull tight the loose overhand knot made in step 5a. Release the hemostat, and strip a segment of the tubing free of blood between the knot and the needle (about 1 inch in length). Reapply the hemostat, and cut the tubing in the stripped area between the knot and the hemostat. Fill the required tube(s) by releasing the hemostat, and then reclamp the tubing with the hemostat. Because this system is open, Biosafety Level 2 precautions should be followed.
    d. If a blood collection set that includes a sample diversion pouch is used, the following procedure should be followed. A hemostat is applied above the Y-junction before phlebotomy. Immediately after the phlebotomy, the hemostat is released to allow the blood to flow to the pouch. The sample pouch should be positioned below the donor's arm. Ensure that blood is not flowing into the tubing leading to the collection bag. Fill the pouch with 30 to 35 mL of blood or as recommended by the manufacturer. Once the pouch is filled, apply a hemostat or Robert's clamp to the tubing

between the donor needle and the pouch. Break the in-line cannula in the tubing that leads from the donor needle to the collection bag to allow the blood to flow into the collection bag.

Sample tubes are collected from the pouch as follows. Sample tubes must be collected within 4 minutes or as recommended by the manufacturer from the time the hemostat is applied to stop the flow into the pouch. The manufacturer-supplied access device is inserted into the sampling site of the pouch by clockwise rotation. A sample tube is allowed to slide into the access device with a straight motion, and the tube is allowed to fill until the blood flow spontaneously stops. These steps are repeated for all sample tubes.

15. Deflate the cuff and remove the tourniquet. Remove the needle from the donor's arm, if not already removed. Apply pressure over the gauze, and ask the donor to raise his or her arm (elbow straight) and to hold the gauze firmly over the phlebotomy site with the other hand.

16. Discard the needle assembly into a biohazard container designed to prevent the accidental injury to, and contamination of, personnel.

17. Strip donor tubing as completely as possible into the bag, starting at the seal. To prevent the blood from clotting in the tubing, work quickly. Invert the bag several times to mix the contents thoroughly; then allow the tubing to refill with anticoagulated blood from the bag. Repeat this procedure a second time.

18. Seal the tubing attached to the collection bag into segments, leaving a segment number clearly and completely readable. Attach a unit identification number to one segment to be stored as a retention segment. Knots, metal clips, or a dielectric sealer may be used to make segments suitable for compatibility testing. It must be possible to separate segments from the unit without breaking sterility of the bag. If a dielectric sealer is used, the knot or clip should be removed from the distal end of the tubing after creating a hermetic seal.

19. Reinspect the container for defects.

20. Recheck numbers on the container, processing tubes, donation record, and retention segment.

21. Place blood at appropriate temperature. Whole blood from which platelet concentrate will not be prepared should be placed at 1 to 6 C after collection unless it must be transported from the collection site to the processing laboratory. In that case, the blood must be placed in a temporary storage area having sufficient coolant capacity to cool the blood continuously toward a range between 1 and 10 C until the blood arrives at the processing laboratory. If platelets are to be prepared, blood should not be chilled but should be stored in a manner intended to reach a temperature of 20 to 24 C until platelets are separated. Platelets must be separated within 8 hours after collection of the unit of Whole Blood or within the time frame specified in the directions for use of the blood collecting, processing, and storage system. Time within which platelets must be separated may exceed 8 hours in Europe.

Notes

1. If the needle is withdrawn and venipuncture is attempted again, preparation of the site must be repeated as in the method for arm preparation for blood collection, and blood is drawn into a new collection set.
2. In addition to routine blood donor phlebotomy, this procedure may be adapted for use in therapeutic phlebotomy.
3. AABB *Standards for Blood Banks and Transfusion Services* requires that a diversion pouch be used for any blood collection from which platelets will be prepared.

References

1. Carson TH, ed. Standards for blood banks and transfusion services. 27th ed. Bethesda, MD: AABB, 2011:21.
2. Smith LG. Blood collection. In: Green TS, Steckler D, eds. Donor room policies and procedures. Arlington, VA: AABB, 1985:25-45.
3. Huh YO, Lightiger B, Giacco GG, et al. Effect of donation time on platelet concentrates and fresh frozen plasma. Vox Sang 1989;56:21-4.
4. Sataro P. Blood collection. In: Kasprisin CA, Laird-Fryer B, eds. Blood donor collection practices. Bethesda, MD: AABB, 1993:89-103.

METHOD 6-4. PREPARING RED BLOOD CELLS FROM WHOLE BLOOD

Principle

Red Blood Cells (RBCs) are obtained by removal of supernatant plasma from centrifuged whole blood. The volume of plasma removed determines the hematocrit of the component. When RBCs are preserved in citrate-phosphate-dextrose-adenine-1 (CPDA-1), maximal viability during storage requires an appropriate ratio of cells to preservative. A hematocrit of 80% or lower in CPDA-1 RBC units ensures the presence of adequate glucose for red cell metabolism for up to 35 days of storage.

Materials

1. Freshly collected whole blood, obtained by phlebotomy as described in Method 6-3. Collect blood in a collection unit with integrally attached transfer container(s).
2. Plasma extractor.
3. Metal clips and hand sealer.
4. Instruments (scissors, hemostats).
5. Dielectric sealer (optional).
6. Refrigerated centrifuge.
7. Scale.

Procedure

1. If platelet-rich plasma will not be prepared, centrifuge whole blood using a "heavy" spin, with a temperature setting of 4 C. Heavy spin using 5000 × *g* for 5 minutes or 5000 × *g* for 7 minutes (plus deceleration time) should generally be sufficient. Each individual laboratory must establish its own parameters. If one is to calculate relative centrifugal force (RCF) in *g*, the formula in Fig 6-4-1 should be used. Centrifuge whole blood using a "light" spin if platelet-rich plasma is to be harvested. Light spin consisting of 2000 × *g* for 3 minutes (plus deceleration time) should generally be sufficient. Each individual laboratory must establish its own parameters for light spin.
2. Place the primary bag containing centrifuged blood on a plasma expressor, and release the spring, allowing the plate of the expressor to contact the bag.
3. Temporarily clamp the tubing between the primary and satellite bags with a hemostat; if a mechanical sealer will not be used, make a loose overhand knot in the tubing.
4. If two or more satellite bags are attached, apply the hemostat to allow plasma to flow into only one of the satellite bags. Penetrate the closure of the primary bag. A scale, such as a dietary scale, may be used to measure the expressed plasma. Remove the appropriate amount of plasma to obtain the desired hematocrit. An automated expressor may also be used for this purpose.
5. Reapply the hemostat when the desired amount of supernatant plasma has entered the satellite bag. Seal the tubing between the primary bag and the satellite bag in two places.
6. Check that the satellite bag has the same donor number as that on the primary bag, and cut the tubing between the two seals.

Notes

1. If blood was collected in a single bag, modify the above directions as follows: Before centrifugation, attach a transfer bag to the Whole Blood unit using a sterile connection device. Alternatively, after

placing the bag on the expressor, apply a hemostat to the tubing of a sterile transfer bag, aseptically insert the cannula of the transfer bag into the outlet port of the bag of blood, release the hemostat, and continue as outlined above. However, the expiration date will change as a result of the open system.

2. For 450 mL of whole blood collection, the removal of 230 to 256 g (225 to 250 mL) of plasma and preservation of the red cells in the anticoagulant-preservative solution will generally result in a red cell component with a hematocrit between 70% and 80%. Correspondingly, for 500 mL of whole blood collection, the removal of 256 to 281 g (250 to 275 mL) of plasma and the preservation of the red cells in the anticoagulant-preservative solution will generally result in a red cell component with a hematocrit between 70% and 80%.
3. The use of an additive solution allows removal of a greater volume of plasma in step 4. After the plasma has been removed, the additive solution is allowed to flow from the attached satellite bag into the red cells. This process will result in a hematocrit of 55% to 65%. Be sure that an appropriate label and dating period are used.

METHOD 6-5. PREPARING PRESTORAGE RED BLOOD CELLS LEUKOCYTES REDUCED FROM WHOLE BLOOD

Principle

The general principle and materials of preparation of RBCs apply, except that the red cells are filtered using a special leukocyte reduction filter. All red cell leukocyte reduction filters licensed in the United States remove platelets to some degree. Anticoagulated whole blood may be filtered, from which only platelet-poor plasma (leukocyte reduced) and red cells may be made. However, the Food and Drug Administration (FDA) has approved a platelet-sparing, whole blood leukocyte reduction filter. Alternatively, the red cells may be filtered in additive solution, potentially allowing the preparation of platelets, plasma, and red cells. Non-leukocyte-reduced red cells may also undergo leukocyte reduction after preparation by attaching a leukocyte reduction filter connected to a storage container using a sterile connecting device.

Procedure

1. Before centrifugation, the anticoagulated whole blood may be filtered by hanging the container upside down and allowing the blood to flow through an in-line filter by gravity into a secondary container. The steps in Method 6-4 for the preparation of RBCs are then followed [see note 3 in that method, for addition of additive solution (AS)].
2. The anticoagulated whole blood may be centrifuged with the in-line filter attached. After centrifugation, the plasma is expressed. The AS is added, and the red cells in the AS are filtered by gravity, as in step 1 above.
3. A red cell component prepared using a red cell preparation method either in residual anticoagulated plasma or in additive solution (AS-1, AS-3, AS-5) may have a secondary container with an in-line filter attached using a sterile connecting device. Filtration can proceed according to the manufacturer's directions using gravity, as in step 1. The tim-

$$\text{RCF} = 28.38 \times \text{R} \times (\text{RPM}/1000)^2 \text{ or}$$

$$\text{RPM} = \sqrt{[RCF/(28.38 \times R)]} \times 1000$$

where:

RCF = relative centrifugal force ($\times g$)
R = radius in inches
RPM = revolutions per minute

FIGURE 6-4-1. Formula for calculating relative centrifugal force. From Naval Blood Research Laboratory. [Available at http://www.nbrl.org/SOP/ACP215/collection.html (accessed January 24, 2011).]

ing of this filtration is often within 24 hours of collection but can be up to 5 days or as directed by the manufacturer of the filter.

4. Red cells that are leukocyte reduced are labeled "Red Blood Cells Leukocytes Reduced." There is no specific label for prestorage leukocyte reduction.

Notes

1. If the collection system does not include an in-line filter, a sterile connecting device can be used to attach a leukocyte reduction filter to the collection system. The filter should be used according to the manufacturer's directions.
2. Generally, whole-blood-derived platelets can be manufactured only before leukocyte reduction. However, an FDA-approved, platelet-sparing, whole blood leukocyte reduction filter has recently become available.

METHOD 6-6. REJUVENATING RED BLOOD CELLS[1]

Principle

Rejuvenation is a process to restore depleted metabolites and to improve the function and posttransfusion survival of stored red cells. The rejuvenating solution is not intended for intravenous administration; after warm incubation with the solution, the Red Blood Cell (RBC) units either are glycerolized for frozen storage or are washed and kept at 1 to 6 C for transfusion within 24 hours.

The rejuvenating solution approved by the Food and Drug Administration (FDA) contains pyruvate, inosine, phosphate, and adenine. The solution's use is permitted only with RBCs prepared from whole blood collected into citrate-phosphate-dextrose (CPD), citrate-phosphate-dextrose-dextrose (CP2D), or citrate-phosphate-dextrose-adenine-1 (CPDA-1). The solution may be added at any time between 3 days after collection of the blood and 3 days after the expiration of the unit. However, the use of the rejuvenation solution with RBC units before 14 days of storage is not routinely performed because the treated cells may develop supranormal levels of 2,3-diphosphoglycerate, which impairs oxygen uptake.

Reagents and Materials

1. RBCs stored at 1 to 6 C and prepared from whole blood collected in CPD, CP2D, or CPDA-1. After collection, RBCs suspended in CPD from day 3 to day 24 (or in CPDA-1, from day 3 to day 38) may be used. RBCs stored in additive solution 1 (AS-1) can be rejuvenated, but they can be stored frozen for only 3 years. The rejuvenation solution is not approved by the FDA for red cells preserved in CP2D, AS-3, and AS-5. However, satisfactory postrejuvenation survival of red cells preserved in CP2D AS-3, CPD AS-3, and CPD AS-5 has been described in the literature.
2. Red Blood Cell Processing Solution, in 50-mL sterile vial (Rejuvesol, Cytosol Laboratories, Braintree, MA), which is also called rejuvenating solution. (See note 1.)
3. Waterproof plastic bag.
4. Metal clips and hand sealer.
5. Sterile airway.

Procedure

1. Connect the container of rejuvenating solution to the RBCs using a transfer set and aseptic technique.
2. Allow 50 mL of rejuvenating solution to flow by gravity into the container of red cells. Gently agitate the cell/solution mixture during this addition. Note that a sterile airway is required if the solution is in a bottle.
3. Seal the tubing near the blood bag, and incubate the mixture for 1 hour at 37 C. Either a dry incubator or circulating waterbath can be used. If placed in a waterbath, the container should be completely immersed; use of a waterproof overwrap is essential to prevent contamination.

4. For use within 24 hours, wash the rejuvenated cells with saline [2 L unbuffered 0.9% sodium chloride (NaCl)] by the use of an approved protocol. Storage of the washed cells from the start of the wash procedure should be at 1 to 6 C for no longer than 24 hours.
5. If the rejuvenated cells are to be cryopreserved, the standard glycerolization protocol adequately removes the rejuvenation solution from the processed cells. Expiration date remains 10 years from the date of collection.
6. Be sure that units are appropriately labeled and that all applicable records are complete.

Notes

1. At the time of publication, rejuvenation solution was not available from the manufacturer.
2. RBCs prepared from 500 mL whole blood collected in CPD, stored in AS-1 for 48 days, and subsequently rejuvenated have been successfully glycerolized and deglycerolized.[2] In this procedure, 50 mL of Rejuvesol solution was used for each unit of outdated AS-1 RBCs.

References

1. Valeri CR, Zaroules CG. Rejuvenation and freezing of outdated stored human red cells. N Engl J Med 1972;287:1307-13.
2. Valeri CR, Ragno G, Houten PV, et al. Automation of the glycerolization of red blood cells with the high-separation bowl in the Haemonetics ACP 215 instrument. Transfusion 2005;45:1621-7.

METHOD 6-7. USING HIGH-CONCENTRATION GLYCEROL TO CRYOPRESERVE RED CELLS—MERYMAN METHOD[1]

Principle

Cryoprotective agents make possible the long-term (10 or more years) preservation of red cells in the frozen state. High-concentration glycerol is particularly suitable for this purpose. A practical method for Red Blood Cells (RBCs) collected in a 450-mL bag is described below.

Materials

1. Donor blood, collected into citrate-phosphate-dextrose (CPD), citrate-phosphate-dextrose-dextrose (CP2D), citrate-phosphate-dextrose-adenine-1 (CPDA-1), or an additive solution (AS).
   a. Complete all blood processing on units intended for freezing.
   b. RBCs preserved in CPD, CP2D, or CPDA-1 may be stored at 1 to 6 C for up to 6 days before freezing.
   c. RBCs preserved in AS-1 and AS-3 may be stored at 1 to 6 C for up to 42 days before freezing.
   d. RBCs that have undergone rejuvenation (see Method 6-6) may be processed for freezing up to 3 days after their original expiration date.
   e. RBCs that are in any preservative solution and that have been entered for processing must be frozen within 24 hours of puncturing the seal.
2. Storage containers, either polyvinyl chloride (PVC) or polyolefin bags.
3. 6.2 M of glycerol lactate solution (400 mL).
4. Cardboard or metal canisters for freezing.
5. Hypertonic (12%) NaCl solution.
6. 1.6% NaCl, 1 liter for batch wash.
7. Isotonic (0.9%) NaCl with 0.2% dextrose solution.
8. 37 C waterbath or 37 C dry warmer.
9. Equipment for batch or continuous-flow washing, to deglycerolize cells frozen in high-concentration glycerol.
10. Freezer tape.
11. Freezer (–65 C or colder).

Procedure

Preparing RBCs for Glycerolization

1. Prepare RBCs from Whole Blood units by removal of supernatant anticoagulant-

preservative or additive solution. Weigh the RBC unit to be frozen, and obtain the net weight of the red cells. The combined weight of the cells and the collection bag should be between 260 g and 400 g.

2. Underweight units can be adjusted to approximately 300 g either by the addition of 0.9% NaCl or by the removal of less plasma than usual. Record the weight; if applicable, document the amount of NaCl added.
3. Record the Whole Blood number, the ABO group and Rh type, the anticoagulant, the date of collection, the date frozen, the expiration time, and the identity of the person performing the procedure. If applicable, document the lot number of the transfer bag.
4. Warm the red cells and the glycerol to at least 25 C by placing them in a dry warming chamber for 10 to 15 minutes or by allowing them to remain at room temperature for 1 to 2 hours. The temperature must not exceed 42 C.
5. Apply a "Frozen Red Blood Cells" label to the freezing bag in which the unit will be frozen. The label must include the name of the facility freezing the unit, Whole Blood number, ABO group and Rh type, and the expiration date. The label must also include tracking for the date collected, the date frozen, and the cryoprotective agent used.

Glycerolization

1. Document the lot numbers of the glycerol; the freezing bags; and, if used, the 0.9% NaCl.
2. Place the container of red cells on a shaker, and add approximately 100 mL of glycerol as the red cells are gently agitated.
3. Turn off the shaker and allow the cells to equilibrate, without agitation, for 5 to 30 minutes.
4. Allow the partially glycerolized cells to flow by gravity into the freezing bag.
5. Add the remaining 300 mL of glycerol slowly in a stepwise fashion, with gentle mixing. Add smaller volumes of glycerol for smaller volumes of red cells. The final glycerol concentration is 40% w/v. Remove any air from the bag.
6. Allow some glycerolized cells to flow back into the tubing so that segments can be prepared. Preferably, two segments should be prepared so that the unit may be crossmatched and/or phenotyped before a decision to thaw.
7. Maintain the glycerolized cells at temperatures between 25 and 32 C until freezing. The recommended interval between removing the RBC unit from refrigeration and placing the glycerolized cells in the freezer should not exceed *4 hours.*

Freezing and Storage

1. Place the glycerolized unit in a cardboard or metal canister, and place it flat in a freezer at –65 C or colder.
2. Label the top edge of the canister with freezer tape marked with the Whole Blood number, the ABO group and Rh type, and the expiration date.
3. Do not bump or handle the frozen cells roughly.
4. The freezing rate should be less than 10 C/minute.
5. Store the frozen RBCs at –65 C or colder for up to 10 years. For blood of rare phenotypes, a facility's medical director may wish to extend the storage period. The unusual nature of such units and the reason for retaining them past the routine 10-year storage period must be documented.

Thawing and Deglycerolizing

1. Put an overwrap on the protective canister containing the frozen cells, and place it in either a 37 C waterbath or 37 C dry warmer.
2. Agitate it gently to speed thawing. The thawing process takes at least 10 minutes. The temperature of the thawed cells should be 37 C.

3. After the cells have thawed, use a commercial instrument for batch or continuous-flow washing to deglycerolize cells. Follow the manufacturer's instructions.
4. Record the lot numbers and manufacturer of all the solutions and software used. Apply a "Deglycerolized Red Blood Cells" label to the transfer pack; be sure that the label includes identification of the collecting facility, the facility preparing the deglycerolized cells, the ABO group and Rh type of the cells, the Whole Blood number, and the expiration date and time.
5. Dilute the unit with a quantity of hypertonic (12%) NaCl solution appropriate for the size of the unit. Allow it to equilibrate for approximately 5 minutes.
6. Wash the cells with 1.6% NaCl until deglycerolization is complete. Approximately 2 liters of wash solution are required. To check for residual glycerol, see Method 6-9.
7. Suspend the deglycerolized cells in isotonic (0.9%) NaCl with 0.2% dextrose.
8. Fill the integrally attached tubing with an aliquot of cells sealed in such a manner that it will be available for subsequent compatibility testing.
9. Deglycerolized RBCs must be stored at 1 to 6 C for no longer than 24 hours. (A closed system has been licensed that allows storage of deglycerolized RBCs at 1 to 6 C for 2 weeks. The closed system deglycerolization requires that the glycerolization step also be performed by a closed system in accordance with the manufacturer's instructions).

Notes

1. An aliquot of the donor's serum or plasma should be frozen and stored at –65 C or colder for possible future use if new donor screening tests are implemented.
2. When new donor screening tests have been implemented and stored units do not have aliquots available for testing, the units may have to be issued with a label stating that the test has not been performed. The reason for distributing an untested component should be documented. If a specimen from the donor is obtained and tested after the unit was stored, the date of testing should be noted on the unit when it is issued.
3. Glycerolization and deglycerolization of leukocyte-reduced RBCs obtained from 500-mL Whole Blood units and stored in AS-1 and AS-3 have been successful.[2] In-vivo recoveries were greater than 80%, and chromium-51 tagged $t_{1/2}$ value was greater than 40 days for the two additive solutions. The amount of glycerol added to red cells may be adjusted to achieve 40% w/v concentration. For this calculation, the assumption is made that each 100 mL of glycerol contains 57 g of glycerol.

References

1. Meryman HT, Hornblower M. A method for freezing and washing RBCs using a high glycerol concentration. Transfusion 1972;12:145-56.
2. Bandarenko N, Hay SN, Holmberg J, et al. Extended storage of AS-1 and AS-3 leukoreduced red blood cells for 15 days after deglycerolization and resuspension in AS-3 using an automated closed system. Transfusion 2004; 44:1656-62.

METHOD 6-8. USING HIGH-CONCENTRATION GLYCEROL TO CRYOPRESERVE RED CELLS—VALERI METHOD[1]

Principle

Red Blood Cells (RBCs) collected in an 800-mL primary collection bag in citrate-phosphate-dextrose-adenine (CPDA-1) and stored at 1 to 6 C for 3 to 38 days can be biochemically rejuvenated and frozen with 40% w/v glycerol in the 800-mL primary container. See the method for rejuvenation of RBCs for additional information (Method 6-6).

Materials

1. Quadruple plastic bag collection system with 800-mL primary bag.
2. Hand sealer clips.
3. Empty, 600-mL polyethylene cryogenic vials [eg, Corning 25702 (Corning Incorporated Life Sciences, Lowell, MA) or Fisher 033746 (Thermo Fisher Scientific, Waltham, MA)].
4. Sterile connection device with wafers.
5. Freezer tape.
6. 600-mL transfer bag.
7. 50 mL of Red Blood Cell Processing Solution (Rejuvesol, Cytosol Laboratories, Braintree, MA). (Note: At the time of publication, rejuvenation solution was not available from the manufacturer.)
8. Heat-sealable 8" × 12" plastic bags.
9. Rejuvenation harness [Fenwal 4C1921 (Fenwal Inc., Lake Zurich, IL) or Cutter 98052 (Cutter Biological, Berkeley, CA)].
10. Sterile filtered airway needle [eg, BD Nokor (Becton Dickinson, Franklin Lakes, NJ)] for Fenwal rejuvenation harness only.
11. 500 mL of glycerolyte 57 solution (Fenwal 4A7833) or 500 mL of 6.2 M glycerolization solution (Cytosol PN5500).
12. Labels—Red Blood Cells Frozen Rejuvenated.
13. Corrugated cardboard storage box (7" × 5.5" × 2" outside dimensions).
14. Heat sealing device.
15. Plastic bag for overwrapping.

Procedure

Preparation of RBCs for Glycerolization

1. Collect 450 mL of whole blood in the primary bag. Invert the bag, fold it about 2 inches from the base, secure the fold with tape, and place the bag upright in a centrifuge. Centrifuge and remove all visible supernatant plasma. The hematocrit of the RBC unit must be 75% ± 5%.
2. Store RBCs at 1 to 6 C in the 800-mL primary bag, along with the adapter port on the tubing that connects the primary bag and transfer pack.
3. Centrifuge the stored cells to remove all visible plasma before undertaking rejuvenation. The gross weight and net weight of the red cells should not exceed 352 g and 280 g, respectively.
4. Transfer the plasma to the integrally connected transfer pack, fold the integral tubing, and replace the hand sealer clip (not crimped).
5. Using a sterile connection device, attach an empty 600-mL transfer pack to the integral tubing of the primary collection bag.
6. If desired, transfer 1 mL of plasma to each of three cryogenic vials to be used for future testing.

Biochemical Modification of the Cells[2]

1. For the Fenwal rejuvenation harness: Aseptically insert the needle of the Y-type Fenwal harness into the rubber stopper of a 50-mL Red Blood Cell Processing Solution bottle, and insert the coupler of the set into the adapter port of the primary collection bag. Insert the filtered airway needle into the rubber stopper of the Red Blood Cell Processing Solution bottle.
2. For the Cutter rejuvenation harness: Aseptically insert the vented white spike with the drip chamber into the rubber stopper of the Red Blood Cell Processing Solution bottle, and insert the nonvented spike into the special adapter port on the primary collection bag.
3. With gentle manual agitation, allow 50 mL of Red Blood Cell Processing Solution to flow directly into the red cells.
4. Heat-seal the tubing of the harness set that connects the Red Blood Cell Processing Solution to the adapter port. The second tubing of the harness Y-set is used to add glycerol (see below).
5. Completely overwrap the 800-mL primary bag, the integrally connected empty transfer pack, and the coupler of the Y-type harness; incubate them in a 37 C waterbath for 1 hour.

Glycerolization

1. Remove the numbered crossmatch segments, leaving the initial segment and number attached to the collection bag. Weigh the unit.
2. Using the values shown in Table 6-8-1, determine the amount of glycerol to be added, on the basis of the gross or net weight of the unit.
3. Aseptically insert the coupler of the rejuvenation harness into the outlet port of the rubber stopper on the glycerol solution bottle. For the Fenwal harness only, insert a filtered airway needle into the vent portion of the glycerol bottle stopper.
4. Place the bag on a shaker. Add the amount of glycerol shown in Table 6-8-1 for the first volume while the bag is shaking at low speed (180 oscillations/minute).
5. Equilibrate the mixture for 5 minutes without shaking, and add the second volume. Equilibrate it for 2 minutes. Add the third volume of glycerol, using vigorous manual shaking.
6. Heat-seal the tubing between the empty bottle of glycerol and the tubing proximal to the adapter port. Ensure that the transfer pack remains integrally attached to the primary collection bag.
7. Centrifuge the mixture of red cells and glycerol, and transfer all visible supernatant glycerol to the transfer pack, resuspend, and mix. Note that this step differs from the one in Method 6-7.
8. Seal the tubing 4 inches from the primary collection bag, detach the transfer pack containing the supernatant fluid, and discard it.
9. Affix an overlay blood component label, the facility label, and an ABO/Rh label. Record the expiration date on the label.
10. Weigh the unit just before freezing, and record the weight.
11. Fold over the top portion of the primary bag (approximately 2 inches). Place the primary bag into a plastic bag overwrap, and heat-seal the outer bag across the top so that there is as little air as possible between the bags.
12. Place one vial of plasma and the plastic bag containing the glycerolized red cells in the cardboard box. Store the other two vials, suitably identified, at –65 C or colder for future testing, if needed.
13. Affix a "Frozen Rejuvenated Red Blood Cells" label, an ABO/Rh label, a facility label, and the original unit number on the outside of the box. Record separately or affix on the cardboard box the collection, freezing, and expiration dates.
14. Freeze the unit in a –80 C freezer. No more than 4 hours should be allowed to elapse between the time the unit was removed from the 4 C refrigerator and the time the cells are placed in the –80 C freezer.

Thawing and Deglycerolization

See Method 6-7. Note, however, that the supernatant glycerol is removed before freezing. Therefore, only two salt solutions (the hypertonic 12% saline and the 0.9% saline-0.2% dextrose solution) are used in the deglycerolization process.

Note

Glycerolization and deglycerolization of leukocyte-reduced RBCs obtained from 500-mL Whole Blood units and stored in AS-1 and AS-3 have been successful.[2] In-vivo recoveries were greater than 80%, and chromium-51 tagged $t_{1/2}$ value was greater than 40 days for the two additive solutions.[3] The amount of glycerol added to red cells may be adjusted to achieve 40% w/v concentration. For this calculation, the assumption is made that each 100 mL of glycerol contains 57 g of glycerol.

References

1. Valeri CR, Ragno G, Pivacek LE, et al. A multicenter study of in vitro and in vivo values in human RBCs frozen with 40% (wt/vol) glycerol and stored after deglycerolization for 15 days at 4 C in AS-3: Assessment of RBC processing in the ACP 215. Transfusion 2001;41:933-9.
2. Rejuvesol package insert. Braintree, MA: Cytosol Laboratories, 2002.

3. Bandarenko N, Hay SN, Holmberg J, et al. Extended storage of AS-1 and AS-3 leukoreduced red blood cells for 15 days after deglycerolization and resuspension in AS-3 using an automated closed system. Transfusion 2004; 44:1656-62.

METHOD 6-9. CHECKING THE ADEQUACY OF DEGLYCEROLIZATION OF RED BLOOD CELLS

Principle

Glycerolization of red cells for frozen storage creates a hyperosmolar intracellular fluid, which must be restored to physiologically compatible levels before the cells are transfused. Inadequately deglycerolized red cells will be hemolyzed by contact with normal saline, or with serum or plasma if subjected to crossmatching. During deglycerolization, the last solution in contact with the cells is normal saline that contains low concentration of dextrose. The easiest way to determine adequacy of glycerol removal is to determine the level of free hemoglobin (mg/dL) in the final wash. An adequate estimate of hemolysis can be achieved by comparing the color of the final wash fluid with the blocks in a commercially available color comparator. Alternatively, normal saline can be added to an aliquot of deglycerolized cells, and the color of the supernatant fluid can be evaluated against the color comparator.

Materials and Equipment

1. Semiautomated instrument for deglycerolizing cryopreserved Red Blood Cells (RBCs).
2. Transparent tubing, as part of disposable material used to deglycerolize individual unit.
3. Color comparator, available commercially.

Procedure

Final Wash Method

1. Interrupt the last wash cycle at a point when wash fluid is visible in the tubing leading to the disposal bag.
2. Hold the comparator block next to an accessible segment of tubing and against a well-lighted white background.
3. Note coloration of the wash fluid, which should be no stronger than the block, indicating 3% hemolysis (ie, 3% of the red cells are hemolyzed).
4. If the level of hemolysis is excessive, continue the wash process until the color is within acceptable limits.
5. Record observation for the individual unit and for the quality assurance program.
6. If unacceptable hemolysis occurs repeatedly, document the corrective action.

Other Methods for Quality Control of Deglycerolized RBCs

1. Hand-held refractometer: A hand-held refractometer [eg, TS meter, Model 10400A (Cambridge Scientific Instruments, Cambridge, UK)] may be used according to the manufacturer's instructions. A small amount of supernatant is transferred to the measuring prism, and the instrument is held against a light source. The refraction value should be less than 30 to ensure that the glycerol level is less than 1 g%.
2. Osmolality: Osmometer [Fiske Model 2400 (American Instrument Exchange, Haverhill, MA)] can be used to measure osmolality according to the manufacturer's instructions. A small amount of supernatant is transferred to an osmometer cuvette, and osmolality of the sample is measured. The value should not exceed 400 mOsm/kg H_20 to ensure that the residual glycerol concentration is less than 1 g%.

References

1. Quality control of deglycerolized red blood cells. Boston, MA: Naval Blood Research Laboratories, 2007. [Available at http://www.nbrl.org/SOP/115/qualitycontrol.html (accessed January 24, 2011).]
2. Umlas J, O'Neill TP. Use of refractive index to measure the adequacy of glycerol removal from previously frozen erythrocytes. Transfusion 1980;20:720-4.

METHOD 6-10. PREPARING FRESH FROZEN PLASMA FROM WHOLE BLOOD

Principle

Plasma is separated from cellular blood elements and is frozen to preserve the activity of labile coagulation factors. Plasma must be placed in the freezer within 8 hours or the time frame specified in the directions for use of the blood collecting, processing, and storage system.

Materials

1. Freshly collected whole blood, ob-tained by phlebotomy as described in Method 6-3, in a collection unit with integrally attached transfer container(s).
2. Metal clips and hand sealer.
3. Instruments (scissors, hemostats).
4. Dielectric sealer (optional).
5. Plasma extractor.
6. Freezing apparatus.
7. Refrigerated centrifuge.
8. Scale.

Procedure

1. Centrifuge blood soon after collection, using a "heavy" spin (see Method 6-4 for preparation of RBCs). Use a refrigerated centrifuge at 1 to 6 C unless also preparing platelets (see Method 6-13 for preparation of platelets from whole blood).
2. Place the primary bag containing centrifuged blood on a plasma extractor, and place the attached satellite bag on a scale adjusted to zero. Express the plasma into the satellite bag, and weigh the plasma.
3. Seal the transfer tubing with a dielectric sealer or metal clips but do not obliterate the segment numbers of the tubing. Place another seal nearer the transfer bag.
4. Label the transfer bag with the unit number before it is separated from the original container. Affix a Fresh Frozen Plasma (FFP) component label and record the volume of plasma on the label.
5. Cut the tubing between the two seals. The tubing may be coiled and taped against the plasma container, leaving the segments available for any testing desired.
6. Store the plasma at –18 C or colder within 8 hours of phlebotomy.

METHOD 6-11. PREPARING CRYOPRECIPITATED AHF FROM WHOLE BLOOD

Principle

Coagulation Factor VIII (antihemophilic factor, or AHF) can be concentrated from freshly collected plasma by cryoprecipitation. Cryoprecipitation is accomplished by slow thawing of Fresh Frozen Plasma (FFP) at 1 to 6 C.

Materials

1. FFP (≥200 mL) prepared as described in Method 6-10 with at least one integrally attached transfer container.
2. Metal clips and hand sealer.
3. Clean instruments (scissors, hemostats).
4. Dielectric sealer (optional).
5. Plasma extractor.
6. Refrigerated centrifuge.
7. Freezing apparatus: Suitable freezing devices include 1) blast freezers or mechanical freezers capable of maintaining temperatures of –18 C or colder, 2) dry ice, or 3) an ethanol dry ice bath. In a bath of 95% ethanol and chipped dry ice, freezing will be complete in about 15 minutes.

8. 1 to 6 C circulating waterbath or refrigerator.
9. Scale.

Procedure

1. Allow FFP to thaw at 1 to 6 C by placing the bag in a 1 to 6 C circulating waterbath or in a refrigerator. If thawed in a waterbath, use a plastic overwrap (or other means) to keep container ports dry.
2. When the plasma has a slushy consistency, separate liquid plasma from the cryoprecipitate by one of the procedures below:
   a. Centrifuge the plasma at 1 to 6 C using a "heavy" spin. (See Method 6-4 for preparation of Red Blood Cells.) Hang the bag in an inverted position, and allow the separated plasma to flow rapidly into the transfer bag, leaving the cryoprecipitate adhering to the sides of the primary bag. To prevent the cryoprecipitate from dissolving and flowing out of the bag, separate the cryoprecipitate from the plasma promptly. Ten to 15 mL of supernatant plasma may be left in the bag for resuspension of the cryoprecipitate after thawing. Refreeze the cryoprecipitate immediately.
   b. Place the thawing plasma in a plasma expressor when approximately one-tenth of the contents are still frozen. With the bag in an upright position, allow the supernatant plasma to flow slowly into the transfer bag, using the ice crystals at the top as a filter. The cryoprecipitate paste will adhere to the sides of the bag or to the ice. Seal the bag when ~90% of cryoprecipitate-reduced plasma has been removed. Refreeze the cryoprecipitate immediately.
3. The cryoprecipitate should be refrozen within 1 hour of thawing. Store at –18 C or colder, preferably at –30 C or colder, for up to 12 months from collection.

Note

Cryoprecipitated AHF may be prepared from FFP at any time within 12 months of collection. The expiration date of Cryoprecipitated AHF is 12 months from the date of phlebotomy, not from the date it was prepared.

METHOD 6-12. THAWING AND POOLING CRYOPRECIPITATED AHF

Principle

Cryoprecipitated AHF should be rapidly thawed at 30 to 37 C but should not remain at this temperature once thawing is complete. The following method permits rapid thawing and pooling of this component.

Materials

1. Circulating waterbath at 37 C (waterbaths designed for thawing plasma are available commercially, as are specially designed dry heat devices).
2. Medication injection ports.
3. Sterile 0.9% NaCl for injection.
4. Syringes and needles.

Procedure

1. Cover the container with a plastic overwrap to prevent contamination of the ports with unsterile water, or use a device to keep the containers upright with the ports above water. Place container in 37 C waterbath.
2. Resuspend the thawed precipitate carefully and completely, either by kneading it into the residual 10 to 15 mL of plasma or by adding approximately 10 mL of 0.9% NaCl and gently resuspending.
3. Pool by inserting a medication injection site into a port of each bag. Aspirate contents of one bag into a syringe, and then inject into the next bag. Use the ever-increasing volume to flush each subsequent bag of as much dissolved cryopre-

cipitate as possible until all contents are in the final bag.

Notes

1. Thawed Cryoprecipitated AHF prepared for transfusion must be stored at room temperature. If pooled for immediate transfusion, it must be administered within 4 hours. Thawed single units, if not entered, must be administered within 6 hours of thawing if intended for replacement of Factor VIII. Pools of thawed individual units may not be refrozen.
2. Prepooled Cryoprecipitated AHF may be prepared by pooling 4 to 10 units at the time of initial preparation and will have an expiration date of 1 year. No diluent can be added to the product before freezing. Pooling is generally performed with the use of a sterile connection device but may use an "open" system. Prestorage pooled Cryoprecipitated AHF has an expiration time of 4 hours when an "open" system is used, or 6 hours oncc thawed if prepared using a sterile connection device. Pooled Cryoprecipitated AHF should be frozen within 2 hours of preparation and may be stored for 1 year from the date of collection. In accordance with AABB *Standards for Blood Banks and Transfusion Services*,[3] the pool must con tain a minimum of 150 mg of fibrinogen and 80 IU of coagulation Factor VIII times the number of components in the pool. The pool must be labeled with ABO/Rh. If 1 unit in a pool is Rh positive, then the pool must be labeled Rh positive. Thawed pools may not be refrozen.

References

1. Joint UKBTS/NIBSC Professional Advisory Committee. Cryoprecipitate pooled, leucocyte depleted. In: Guidelines for the blood transfusion service in the United Kingdom. 7th ed. Sheffield, UK: National Blood Service, 2005. [Available at http://www.transfusionguidelines.org.uk/index.asp?Publication=RB&Section=25&pageid=969 (accessed January 24, 2011).]
2. Smith KJ, Hodges PA. Preparation of pooled cryoprecipitate for treatment of hemophilia A in a home care program. Transfusion 1984;24:520-3.
3. Carson TH, ed. Standards for blood banks and transfusion services. 27th ed. Bethesda, MD: AABB, 2011:27.
4. Code of federal regulations. Title 21, CFR Part 640.54. Washington, DC: US Government Printing Office, 2010 (revised annually).

METHOD 6-13. PREPARING PLATELETS FROM WHOLE BLOOD

Principle

Platelets can be prepared by the platelet-rich plasma (PRP) method or by the buffy-coat method. In the PRP method, PRP is separated from whole blood by "light-spin" centrifugation, the platelets are concentrated by "heavy-spin" centrifugation, and the supernatant plasma is subsequently removed. In the buffy-coat method, whole blood is centrifuged at "high speed" with subsequent collection of the buffy coat. The buffy coat is then centrifuged at "low speed" to concentrate platelets and to remove red cells and white cells. Both methods are described below.

Materials

1. Freshly collected whole blood, obtained by phlebotomy as described in Method 6-3, in a collection unit with two integrally attached transfer containers. The final container must bc made of a plastic approved for platelet storage. Keep blood at room temperature (20 to 24 C) before separating PRP from the red cells. This separation must take place within 8 hours of phlebotomy or within the time frame specified in the directions for use of the blood collecting, processing, and storage system.
2. In-line filter (if preparing prestorage leukocyte-reduced components).
3. Metal clips and hand sealer.
4. Instruments (scissors, hemostats).
5. Plasma extractor.
6. Dielectric sealer (optional).

7. Centrifuge, calibrated as in Method 8-4.
8. Scale.
9. Rotator.

Procedure

For Preparation of PRP Platelets

1. Do not chill the blood at any time before or during platelet separation. If the temperature of the centrifuge is 1 to 6 C, set the temperature control of the refrigerated centrifuge at 20 C, and allow the temperature to rise to approximately 20 C. Centrifuge the blood using a "light" spin (see Method 6-4).
2. Express the PRP into the transfer bag intended for platelet storage. Seal the tubing twice between the primary bag and Y connector of the two satellite bags and cut between the two seals. Place the red cells at 1 to 6 C.
3. Centrifuge the PRP at 20 C using a "heavy" spin (see Method 6-4 for preparation of Red Blood Cells).
4. Express the platelet-poor plasma into the second transfer bag, and seal the tubing. Some plasma should remain on the platelet button for storage, but no exact volume can be designated. AABB *Standards for Blood Banks and Transfusion Services*[1] requires that sufficient plasma remain with the platelet concentrate to maintain the pH at 6.2 or higher for the entire storage period. This pH level usually requires a minimum of 35 mL of plasma when storage is at 20 to 24 C, but 50 to 70 mL is preferable.
5. The platelet concentrate container should be left stationary, with the label side down, at room temperature for approximately 1 hour.
6. Resuspend the platelets in either of the following ways:
   a. Manipulate the platelet container gently by hand to achieve uniform resuspension.
   b. Place the container on a rotator at room temperature. The slow, gentle agitation should achieve uniform resuspension within 2 hours.
7. Maintain the platelet suspension at 20 to 24 C with continuous gentle agitation.
8. Platelets should be inspected before issue to ensure that no platelet aggregates are visible.

For Preparation of Buffy-Coat Platelets[2]

1. Whole blood should be stored at 20 to 24 C before centrifugation.
2. Centrifuge whole blood at "high" speed [eg, 2800 × *g* for 11.5 minutes using Beckman J6ME centrifuge (Tritech Inc., Edgewater, MD).]
3. Remove supernatant plasma from the top of the container, and red cells from the bottom of the container of a specially designed collection set manually or by using an automated instrument. Approximately 50 mL of buffy coat remains in the bag.
4. Pool buffy coats from 4 to 6 units and centrifuge at "low" speed (eg, 700 × *g* for 5 minutes using Beckman J6ME centrifuge). Transfer supernatant PRP manually or by an automated instrument into platelet storage bag. Filter platelets to remove leukocytes during the transfer.

For Preparation of Prestorage Leukocyte-Reduced Platelets

Prestorage leukocyte-reduced (LR) platelets may be prepared from whole blood using in-line filtration of the PRP. The resulting intermediate product is a filtered PRP, from which LR platelet concentrate and LR plasma may be manufactured.

Note

The supernatant plasma may be frozen promptly and stored as Fresh Frozen Plasma (FFP) if the separation and freezing are completed within the time frame specified in the directions for use of the blood collecting, processing, and storage system. The volume of FFP prepared after platelet preparation will be substantially less than that prepared directly from whole blood.

References

1. Carson TH, ed. Standards for blood banks and transfusion services. 27th ed. Bethesda, MD: AABB, 2011:28.
2. Turner CP, Sutherland J, Wadhwa M, et al. In vitro function of platelet concentrates prepared after filtration of whole blood or buffy coat pools. Vox Sang 2005;88:164-71.
3. Sweeney JD, Holme S, Heaton WAL, Nelson E. Leukodepleted platelet concentrates prepared by in-line filtration of platelet rich plasma. Transfusion 1995;35:131-6.
4. Sweeney JD, Kouttab N, Penn LC, et al. A comparison of prestorage leukoreduced whole blood derived platelets with bedside filtered whole blood derived platelets in autologous stem cell transplant. Transfusion 2000;40:794-800.

METHOD 6-14. REMOVING PLASMA FROM PLATELETS (VOLUME REDUCTION)

Principle

Although optimal storage of platelets requires an adequate volume of plasma, a few patients may not tolerate large-volume infusion. Stored platelets may be centrifuged and much of the plasma removed shortly before transfusion, but appropriate resuspension is essential. The platelets must remain at room temperature, without agitation, for 20 to 60 minutes before resuspension into the remaining plasma. Transfusion must take place within 4 hours of the time the platelet bag was entered. Volume reduction can be performed on individual or pooled units.

No consensus exists regarding the optimal centrifugation rate. One study[1] found 35% to 55% platelet loss in several units centrifuged at 500 × *g* for 6 minutes, compared with 5% to 20% loss in units centrifuged at 5000 × *g* for 6 minutes or 2000 × *g* for 10 minutes. The authors recommend 2000 × *g* for 10 minutes, to avoid any risk that a higher centrifugal force might inflict on the plastic container. A study by Moroff et al[2] found mean platelet loss to be less than 15% in 42 units centrifuged at 580 × *g* for 20 minutes. High *g* forces are of theoretical concern because they may damage the platelets when they are forced against the wall of the container and also increase the possibility of container breakage.

Materials

1. Apheresis Platelets or Platelets prepared from whole blood as described in Method 6-13.
2. Metal clips and hand sealer.
3. Scissors, hemostats.
4. Dielectric sealer (optional).
5. Centrifuge, calibrated as in Method 8-4.
6. Plasma extractor.

Procedure

1. Pool platelets, if desired, into a transfer pack, using standard technique. Single platelet concentrates may need volume reduction for pediatric recipients. Apheresis components may be processed directly.
2. Centrifuge at 20 to 24 C, using one of the following protocols:
   a. 580 × *g* for 20 minutes.
   b. 2000 × *g* for 10 minutes.
   c. 5000 × *g* for 6 minutes.
3. Without disturbing the contents, transfer the bag to a plasma extractor. Remove all but 10 to 15 mL plasma from single units, or somewhat more volume, proportionately, from a pool or from a component prepared by apheresis.
4. Mark expiration time on bag as 4 hours after the time the unit was entered or units were pooled.
5. Leave bag at 20 to 24 C without agitation for 20 minutes if centrifuged at 580 × *g*, or for 1 hour if centrifuged at 2000 or 5000 × *g*.
6. Resuspend platelets as described in Method 6-13.

Notes

1. If a sterile connection device is used for removing plasma from a hemapheresis component or individual platelet concentrate, the unit can be considered sterile and it is not necessary to impose the 4-hour expiration interval required for entered platelets. However, no data exist to support storage of reduced-volume platelet concentrates; therefore, it is preferable to transfuse them as soon as possible.
2. Reduced-volume platelet concentrates may not be distributed as a licensed product.
3. Platelets that have been pooled must be used within 4 hours of entering the units, whether or not they have been volume reduced. Pooled platelets may not be distributed as a licensed product.

References

1. Simon TL, Sierra ER. Concentration of platelet units into small volumes. Transfusion 1984; 24:173-5.
2. Moroff G, Friedman A, Robkin-Kline L, et al. Reduction of the volume of stored platelet concentrates for use in neonatal patients. Transfusion 1984;24:144-6.

Transplantation of Cells and Tissue

METHOD 7-1. INFUSING CRYOPRESERVED HEMATOPOIETIC CELLS

Principle

The purpose of this procedure is to outline the steps to be performed before the infusion of cryopreserved hematopoietic progenitor cells (HPCs) can be started, as well as the steps necessary to infuse the cells. The method presented below should be considered a representative example of methods in current use.

Materials and Equipment

1. Standard IV setup.
2. Bags of $NaHCO_3$ and KCl combined at a 50:20 ratio mEq/L.
3. Urine output toilet insert.
4. pH sticks.
5. 650 mg acetaminophen.
6. 1 mg/kg diphenhydramine—limit = 50 mg.
7. Antiemetics.
8. Thawed HPCs (see laboratory procedure for thawing details).
9. Standard infusion set (blood administration set may be used).
10. Patient infusion record.
11. *Circular of Information for the Use of Cellular Therapy Products.*

Procedure

1. If the product volume is greater than 300 mL, hydration should be initiated with 0.25% normal saline and $NaHCO_3$ at least 3 hours before infusion. The $NaHCO_3$ is added to ensure alkaline urine. The goal is to achieve a urine output of 2 to 3 mL/kg/hour and a urine pH of 7.0.
2. At 15 to 30 minutes before HPC infusion, medicate with the following:
   a. Diphenhydramine, 1 mg/kg (maximum = 50 mg).
   b. Antiemetics, as necessary.
3. Repeat medications if additional cells are to be infused after a break of more than 4 hours.
4. Infuse thawed HPC aliquots rapidly (50 mL over 5-10 minutes) to minimize clumping.
5. Maintain an infusion record with vital signs and adverse events, as appropriate.

Notes

1. Infusion protocols should be defined in the appropriate (nursing and/or laboratory) procedures manual. Medical staff administering the product need to be familiar with adverse signs of blood transfusion: fever, chills, dyspnea, bronchospasm, hypotension, cyanosis, rash or hives, chest or back pain, and any other change in condition. Dimethylsulfoxide (DMSO) toxicity is the most common complication of cryopreserved HPC product administration. Symptoms result from histamine release and include flushing, rash, chest tightness, nausea and vomiting, and cardiovascular instability. The *Circular of Information for the Use of Cellular Therapy Products* contains

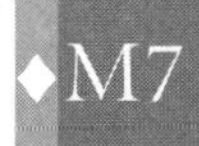

detailed descriptions of the side effects and hazards related to the infusion of HPC products.[1] HPCs should not be infused through leukocyte-reduction filters. However, depending on the protocol, cells may be filtered through a standard blood administration set—for example, a 170-micron filter.

2. Adverse reactions to the infusion of HPC products are documented on a "Report of Adverse Reaction Form." A copy should be kept in the laboratory. These forms are completed by nursing and laboratory staff. Certain adverse reactions related to HPC administration are required to be reported to the Center for Biologics Evaluation and Research (CBER) of the Food and Drug Administration (FDA). The definitions of reportable adverse reactions and the requirements for reporting them are specified in the *Code of Federal Regulations* (21 CFR 1271.350).[2] Updated information about CBER reporting requirements may be found on the FDA website.[3]
3. If the total infusion volume contains greater than 1 g/kg of DMSO, it is recommended that the product be infused over 2 days. For reference, 100 mL of cryopreserved cells in a 10%-DMSO-based cryoprotectant contains 10 g of DMSO. Consult the cellular therapy laboratory medical director if the product exceeds this limit.

References

1. AABB, America's Blood Centers, American Association of Tissue Banks, American Red Cross, American Society for Apheresis, American Society for Blood and Marrow Transplantation, College of American Pathologists, Foundation for the Accreditation of Cellular Therapy, ICCBBA, International Society for Cellular Therapy Joint Accreditation Committee, National Marrow Donor Program, Netcord. Circular of information for the use of cellular therapy products. Bethesda, MD: AABB, 2009. [Available at http://www.aabb.org/resources/bct/Documents//coi_ct 1109.pdf (accessed February 17, 2011).]
2. Code of federal regulations. Title 21, CFR Part 1271.350. Washington, DC: US Government Printing Office, 2010 (revised annually).
3. Food and Drug Administration. Biological product deviations: Includes human tissue and cellular and tissue-based product (HCT/P) deviation reporting. Rockville, MD: CBER Office of Communication, Outreach, and Development, 2010. [Available at http://www.fda.gov/BiologicsBloodVaccines/SafetyAvailability/ReportaProblem/BiologicalProductDeviations/default.htm (accessed February 17, 2011).]

METHOD 7-2. PROCESSING UMBILICAL CORD BLOOD

Principle

The method below, representative of several methods in current use, reduces red cell content and concentrates leukocyte content in cord blood units. It minimizes the final product volume (optimizing storage space) and cryoprotectant volumes (decreasing potential infusion-related complications).

Materials and Equipment

1. Collected umbilical cord blood.
2. Hydroxyethyl starch (HES; 6% w/v).
3. Blood component centrifuge.
4. Plasma expressor.
5. Transfer bags.
6. Sterile dimethylsulfoxide (DMSO).
7. Controlled-rate freezer.
8. Liquid-nitrogen freezer.
9. Automated hematology analyzer.
10. Flow cytometry facilities.

Procedure

1. Combine the cord blood product (5 parts) in a bag with HES (1 part).
2. Centrifuge the mixture at 90 × *g* for 6 minutes with no brake.
3. Express the leukocyte-rich plasma into a secondary bag.
4. Centrifuge the leukocyte-rich plasma at 450 × *g* for 10 minutes.

5. Express the leukocyte-poor plasma into a third bag.
6. Cryopreserve the remaining leukocyte pellet (approximate volume, 20-23 mL) using a controlled-rate freezer (final product concentration, 10% DMSO and 1% dextran 40).
7. Store the product in a vapor-phase liquid-nitrogen storage container (<–135 C).
8. Quality control parameters that should be measured include nucleated cell count and hematocrit of the starting umbilical cord unit, and nucleated cell count, leukocyte differential, viability, and CD34 count on an aliquot from the frozen product.

Note

See Fig 31-2 in Chapter 31 for a summary diagram of this procedure.

References

1. Chrysler G, McKenna D, Schierman T, et al. Umbilical cord blood banking. In: Broxmeyer HE, ed. Cord blood: Biology, immunology, banking, and clinical transplantation. Bethesda, MD: AABB Press, 2004:219-57.
2. Rubenstein P, Dobrilla L, Rosenfield RE, et al. Processing and cryopreservation of placental/umbilical cord blood for unrelated bone marrow reconstitution. Proc Natl Acad Sci U S A 1995;92:10119-22.

METHOD 7-3. INVESTIGATING ADVERSE EVENTS AND INFECTIONS FOLLOWING TISSUE ALLOGRAFT USE

Principle

Transplanting surgeons are responsible for reporting to the hospital tissue service any recipient infection where there is a likelihood or suspicion that the infection originated from a contaminated tissue allograft.

Early reporting allows actions to take place to determine the source of contamination, to develop corrective actions, and to limit further spread of infection. Early reporting also facilitates the identification and evaluation of other patients who may have received contaminated tissue from the same donor and who may have experienced a similar infection.

Hospital tissue services are responsible for investigating adverse events and infections and for reporting those occurrences to the tissue processor and supplier.

Materials

Adverse event file.

Procedures

Quarantine, Record-Keeping, and Notification

1. Immediately sequester, quarantine, and cease further distribution of any existing, unused tissue allografts from the same donor, if any are known to be in the hospital tissue service's inventory. Tissue allografts from the same donor or processing lot can be identified by a donor-specific numerical identifier that can be obtained from the tissue supplier. Unused tissue from the same donor may be needed to test for contamination and should be quarantined but not destroyed until all investigations are complete.
2. If quarantined tissue allografts from the same donor are later cleared of possible contamination, there should be a documented quality assurance review and approval by the tissue service's medical director before they are removed from quarantine and placed in releasable inventory.
3. Initiate an investigation and open an adverse event file. The adverse event file should contain a record of all investigative actions and the final report after it has been reviewed and approved by the hospital tissue service's medical director.
4. Notify the hospital tissue service's medical director as soon as possible. Immediate actions by the medical director should include a review of the patient's illness and a discussion with the transplant sur-

geon to confirm the type of infection and possible contributing factors and to confirm that the allograft is suspected to be involved with causing the infection.

5. Notify the tissue processor (name is in package insert) and tissue supplier (if not the same) promptly so appropriate actions, such as quarantining tissues from the same donor, can take place and the tissue supplier (tissue bank, tissue processor, tissue distribution intermediaries) can conduct its own investigation as to the possible origin of the contaminant from an infected donor or from acquisition during tissue recovery, tissue processing, or storage.
6. Notify hospital risk management, especially if the infection is likely to be from the allograft.
7. If a serious infection is determined to have been caused by the allograft, notify The Joint Commission.
8. If the recipient is seriously or fatally ill from an allograft, the hospital tissue service should consider voluntary notification of the Food and Drug Administration (FDA) through MedWatch (notification is mandatory for tissue processors and suppliers).

Hospital Investigation

1. Cooperate with the ongoing investigation by the tissue processor.
2. With the aid of the hospital tissue service's medical director and hospital infection control, investigate whether patient or hospital factors could have contributed to the infection.
3. If the infection is viral (eg, human immunodeficiency virus, hepatitis C virus, hepatitis B virus), consider the presence of behavioral risk factors in the tissue allograft recipient (eg, hemophiliac receiving coagulation factors, injecting drug user, prostitute, male who had sex with another male, transfusion recipient, etc).
4. Investigate whether the patient's infection could have been hospital-acquired. This is particularly important when the infection is bacterial or fungal. In collaboration with the hospital's infection control or epidemiology service, the hospital tissue service needs to determine whether the infection could have been acquired from the hospital environment, supplies, equipment, or staff. Determine whether there have been recent outbreaks of infections by the same organism. An investigation and assessment by the hospital infection control service, a clinical infectious disease specialist, or both may be needed. The state department of health can also be involved if needed.
5. Request a report of the tissue supplier's investigation. If the tissue supplier discovers contamination of the tissue and its source, the investigation in the hospital can be brief.
6. If the infection may be allograft associated, conduct a sentinel event investigation. If the source of the infection is uncertain or is determined to be hospital acquired rather than allograft acquired, the hospital should conduct a root cause analysis, look for contributing factors, and implement corrective and preventive actions, as needed.

Confidentiality

1. During the investigation of an adverse event, pertinent confidential patient medical information may be shared with the investigative teams of the hospital, the public health department, and the tissue supplier (in accordance with the Health Insurance Portability and Accountability Act).
2. The tissue supplier is required to investigate adverse events reported to the supplier and report those activities to the FDA.

Review of Supplier Certification

1. If the tissue allograft is determined to be the probable or confirmed cause of the

recipient infection, review the qualifications of the tissue supplier. Obtain and review information to determine whether tissues from that supplier are less safe or less effective than others. Information can be obtained by consulting the FDA (eg, MedWatch reports, FDA inspection findings), by interviewing the tissue supplier quality assurance officer or medical director, and by determining whether there have been infections in other patients who received tissues from the same tissue bank.

2. If the tissue supplier or tissue processor refuses to provide needed information, quarantine all other tissue allografts in the hospital inventory previously obtained from the supplier. Suspend that supplier's certification and approvals and obtain tissue from other suppliers.

Final Assessment

1. After the investigation is complete, prepare a written final report identifying the cause of the patient's infection and determining whether the tissue allograft was unlikely, likely, probably, or confirmed to be the cause of the infection. The investigation documents, conclusion, final report, and any corrective actions should be reviewed and approved in writing by the hospital tissue service's medical director. Place the final report in the adverse event file.
2. If corrective actions were taken, an evaluation should be made at a later date to document that actions are in place and are effective.

Final Reports to Others

1. A report of the investigation written by, or reviewed and approved by, the tissue service's medical director should be provided to the following entities:
   - **a.** The transplant surgeon who originally reported the infection.
   - **b.** The tissue processor and supplier.
   - **c.** The hospital tissue services committee.
2. If the hospital tissue service determines that either 1) the recipient infection was caused by the allograft or 2) the organism was hospital acquired, and that 3) the infection is fatal, life-threatening, or has resulted in permanent impairment of a body function or permanent damage to a body structure, then notify The Joint Commission and conduct a sentinel event investigation.
3. If a transmitted contagious infection is diagnosed in the recipient and is reportable according to state law, notify the state department of health in writing.
4. It is not mandatory for the hospital to report adverse events to the FDA. However, if the hospital tissue service determines that the adverse event caused by the tissue 1) involves a communicable disease; 2) is fatal, life-threatening, or results in permanent impairment of a body function or permanent damage to a body structure; or 3) necessitates medical or surgical intervention, then the hospital can voluntarily notify the FDA by MedWatch (21 CFR 1271.350). MedWatch reports are accepted online (see http://www.fda.gov/Safety/MedWatch/HowToReport/ucm085568.htm); by telephone at 1-800-FDA-1088; by FAX at 1-800-FDA-0178; or by mail to MedWatch, Food and Drug Administration, HF-2, 5600 Fishers Lane, Rockville, MD 20857.

Methods Section 8

Quality Control

METHOD 8-1. VALIDATING COPPER SULFATE SOLUTION

Principle

Copper sulfate solution can be checked for suitability in donor screening by observing the behavior (sinking or floating) of drops of blood of known hemoglobin concentration.

Materials

1. Copper sulfate—specific gravity 1.053.
2. Capillary tubes.
3. Worksheet for recording results.

Procedure

1. Obtain several (three to six, if possible) blood samples with known hemoglobin levels. Samples should include hemoglobin levels slightly above and below 12.5 g/dL.
2. Gently place a drop of each blood sample into a vial of copper sulfate solution of stated specific gravity of 1.053.
3. Drops of all blood samples with hemoglobin at or above 12.5 g/dL must sink and those with hemoglobin levels below 12.5 g/dL must float.
4. Record the date of testing; the manufacturer, lot number, and expiration date of the copper sulfate; sample identity; the results; and the identity of the person performing the test.
5. Document the corrective action taken if the results are outside acceptable limits.

Reference

1. Philips RA, Van Slyke DD, Hamilton PB, et al. Measurement of specific gravities of whole blood and plasma by standard copper sulfate solutions. J Biol Chem 1950;183:305-30.

METHOD 8-2. STANDARDIZING AND CALIBRATING THERMOMETERS

Principle

Thermometers used during laboratory testing and in the collection (donor suitability), processing, and storage of blood components and reagents should be calibrated and standardized to ensure accurate indication of temperatures. Calibration should be performed at temperatures close to the temperature at which the thermometers will be used. Over time, liquid-in-glass thermometers may give a different reading at a given temperature because of permanent changes in the volume of the bulb related to relaxation of the glass.[1] Each thermometer should be calibrated before initial use and periodically thereafter, as well as any time there is reason to suspect change or damage. Calibration must be verified for all electronic thermometers, even those described as "self-calibrating."

Materials

1. National Institute of Standards and Technology (NIST)-certified thermometer or thermometer with NIST-traceable calibration certificate.

2. Thermometer to be calibrated.
3. Suitable container (eg, 250-500 mL beaker).
4. Water.
5. Crushed ice.
6. 37 C waterbath.
7. Worksheet for recording results.

METHOD 8-2-1. CHECKING LIQUID-IN-GLASS LABORATORY THERMOMETERS

Procedure

1. Before choosing a thermometer for a particular application, consider all the governing factors; be sure that the thermometer will be used at its proper immersion; and follow the manufacturer's instructions for its proper use. When using a certified thermometer, read and follow the applicable notes. Be sure to include any correction factors noted on the certificate for the NIST-traceable thermometer and apply them in calculations.
2. Categorize the thermometers by key factors, such as immersion, increments, and temperature of intended use. Test them in groups, comparing similar thermometers. Do not attempt to compare dissimilar thermometers in a single procedure.
3. Number each thermometer being tested (eg, place a numbered piece of tape around the top of each thermometer or use the manufacturer's serial number).
4. Perform calibration with water at a temperature close to that which the thermometer will monitor.
5. To calibrate at 37 C, place the thermometers to be tested and the NIST thermometer at a uniform depth in a standard 37 C waterbath, making sure that the tips of all devices are at the same level in the liquid.[1]
6. To calibrate at 1 to 6 C, fill a suitable container with water. Add crushed ice until the approximate desired temperature is reached. Place the thermometers to be tested and the NIST thermometer at a uniform depth in the water/ice mixture, making sure that the tips of all devices are at the same level and are in the liquid, not the upper ice.
7. Stir constantly in a random motion until the temperature equilibrates, approximately 3 to 5 minutes.
8. Observe temperatures. Record each thermometer's identification and results. Acceptance criteria depend on the level of precision required, but for most blood banking applications, agreement within 1 C between the two thermometers may be considered acceptable. If the reading varies by more than one degree from the standard, the thermometer may be returned to the distributor (if newly purchased), labeled with the correction factor (degrees different from the NIST thermometer) that must be applied to each reading, or discarded.
9. Complete the calibration record with the date of testing and identity of the person who performed the test.

Notes

1. If a thermometer is to be used for temperatures over a range greater than a few degrees (eg, 10 degrees), a three-point calibration should be performed. Use water of appropriate temperature. Test at temperatures just below, just above, and at the midway point of intended use. All results should be within 1 C of the NIST thermometer to be considered acceptable.
2. Thermometers should be observed routinely for any split in the column because this will cause inaccurate readings. The methods for reuniting the separation can be found in CLSI Standard I2-A2.[2] When this occurs, document corrective action and recalibrate the thermometer.

References

1. Wise JA. A procedure for the effective recalibration of liquid-in-glass thermometers. NIST special publication 819. Gaithersburg, MD: National Institute of Standards and Technology, 1991.

2. Temperature calibration of water baths, instruments, and temperature sensors. 2nd ed; approved standard I2-A2 Vol. 10 No. 3. Wayne, PA: National Committee for Clinical Laboratory Standards (now CLSI), 1990.

METHOD 8-2-2. CHECKING ELECTRONIC ORAL THERMOMETERS

Procedure

1. Use any of the following methods to verify calibration:
   a. Follow manufacturer's instructions for verifying calibration.
   b. Use a commercially available calibration device by following the instructions provided by the device's manufacturer.
   c. Calibrate the thermometer by inserting the probe in a waterbath that has a temperature in the range to be tested using a NIST-certified thermometer.
2. A result is acceptable if the readings agree within acceptable tolerances. If not, document and remove from use.
3. Record the date of testing, thermometer identification numbers, temperature readings, and the identity of the person performing the test.

METHOD 8-3. TESTING BLOOD STORAGE EQUIPMENT ALARMS

Blood storage refrigerators and freezers must be equipped with a system for continuous temperature monitoring and an audible alarm. If a storage unit goes into alarm, it is essential that personnel know the appropriate actions to take. Directions for such events should be available in a conspicuous location, and personnel should be trained to initiate these actions if the temperature cannot be corrected rapidly. The alarm on each storage unit should be checked periodically for proper functioning. Monthly checks are appropriate until consistent behavior of a particular storage unit has been demonstrated. Thereafter, alarms should be tested regularly and frequently enough to detect malfunctions as well as to achieve and maintain personnel competency. For equipment in good condition, quarterly checks are usually sufficient. Because alarms may be disconnected or silenced during repairs, it is also prudent to verify alarm functioning after repairs.

The high and low temperatures of activation must be checked and the results recorded. AABB *Standards for Blood Banks and Transfusion Services*[1] requires that the alarm be set to activate at a temperature that will allow appropriate intervention before blood or components reach unacceptable conditions. Because of the diversity of equipment available, it is not possible to give specific instructions for all applicable alarm systems. If the equipment user's manual does not provide suitable directions for testing the alarm, consult the manufacturer or other equipment storage expert. The facility procedures manual must include a detailed description of the method(s) in local use. (See Appendix 1-4 in Chapter 1 for quality control testing intervals.)

METHOD 8-3-1. TESTING REFRIGERATOR ALARMS

Principle

Refrigerator temperatures may increase above acceptable limits for several reasons, including the following:

1. Improperly closed door.
2. Insufficient refrigerant.
3. Compressor failure.
4. Dirty or blocked heat exchanger.
5. Loss of electrical power.

Materials

1. Calibrated thermometer.
2. Pan large enough to hold the thermocouple container.
3. Water.
4. Crushed ice.
5. Table salt.
6. Worksheet for recording results.

Procedure

1. Verify that the alarm circuits are operating, the alarm is switched on, and the starting temperature is 1 to 6 C. Immerse an easy-to-read calibrated thermometer in the container with the alarm thermocouple.
   For low activation:
2. Place the container with the thermocouple and thermometer in a pan containing an ice and water slush at a temperature of –4 C or colder. To achieve this temperature, add several spoonfuls of table salt to the slush.
3. Close the refrigerator door to avoid changing the temperature of the storage compartment. Keep the container in the pan of cold slush, and gently agitate it periodically until the alarm sounds.
4. Record this temperature as the low-activation temperature.
   For high activation:
5. Place the container with thermocouple and thermometer in a pan containing cool water (eg, 12 to 15 C).
6. Close the refrigerator door. Allow the fluid in the container to warm slowly, with occasional agitation.
7. Record the temperature at which the alarm sounds as the high-activation temperature.
8. Record the date of testing, the refrigerator identification, the thermometer identification, and the identity of the person performing the test.
9. If temperatures of activation are too low or too high, take appropriate corrective actions such as those suggested by the manufacturer, record the nature of the corrections, and repeat the alarm check to document that the corrections were effective.

Notes

1. The thermocouple for the alarm should be easily accessible and equipped with a cord long enough so that it can be manipulated easily.
2. The thermocouple for the continuous temperature monitor need not be in the same container as that of the alarm. If it is in the same container, a notation should be made in the records that explains any out-of-range temperature registered as a result of the alarm check.
3. When the temperatures of alarm activation are checked, the temperature change should occur slowly enough so that the measurements and recording are accurate. Too rapid a change in temperature may give the false impression that the alarm does not sound until an inappropriate temperature is registered.
4. The low temperature of activation should be greater than 1 C (eg, 1.5 C); the high temperature of activation should be less than 6 C (eg, 5.5 C).
5. Alarms should sound simultaneously at the site of the refrigerator and at the location of remote alarms, when employed. If remote alarms are used, the alarm check should include a verification that the alarm sounded at the remote location.
6. The amount of fluid in which the thermocouple is immersed must be no larger than the volume of the smallest component stored in that refrigerator. The thermocouple may be immersed in a smaller volume, but this means that the alarm will go off with smaller temperature changes than those registered in a larger volume of fluid. Excessive sensitivity may create a nuisance.
7. With the one-time assistance of a qualified electrician, the required refrigerator alarm checks of units with virtually inaccessible temperature probes can be performed with an electrical modification cited by Wenz and Owens.[2]

References

1. Carson TH, ed. Standards for blood banks and transfusion services. 27th ed. Bethesda, MD: AABB, 2011:5.

2. Wenz B, Owens RT. A simplified method for monitoring and calibrating refrigerator alarm systems. Transfusion 1980;20:75-8.

METHOD 8-3-2. TESTING FREEZER ALARMS

Principle

Freezer temperatures may rise to unacceptable levels for a variety of reasons. Common causes of rising temperatures include the following:

1. Improperly closed freezer door or lid.
2. Low level of refrigerant.
3. Compressor failure.
4. Dirty or blocked heat exchanger.
5. Loss of electrical power.

Materials

1. Protection for the freezer contents (eg, a blanket).
2. Calibrated thermometer or thermocouple independent from that built into the system.
3. Warm water or an oven mitt.
4. Worksheet for recording results.

Procedure

1. Protect frozen components from exposure to elevated temperatures during the test.
2. Use a thermometer or thermocouple, independent from that built into the system that will accurately indicate the temperature of alarm activation. Compare these readings with the temperatures registered on the recorder.
3. Warm the alarm probe and thermometer slowly (eg, in warm water, by an oven-mitt-covered hand, exposure to air). The specific temperature of activation cannot be determined accurately during rapid warming, and the apparent temperature of activation will be too high.
4. Record the temperature at which the alarm sounds, the date of testing, the identity of the person performing the test, the identity of the freezer and calibrating instrument, and any observations that might suggest impaired activity.
5. Return the freezer and the alarm system to their normal conditions.
6. If the alarm sounds at too high a temperature, take appropriate corrective actions such as those suggested by the manufacturer, record the nature of the correction, and repeat the alarm check to document that the corrections were effective.

Notes

1. Alarms should sound simultaneously at the site of the freezer and at the location of the remote alarms, when employed. If remote alarms are used, the alarm check should include a verification that the alarm sounded at the remote location.
2. Test battery function, electrical circuits, and power-off alarms more frequently than the activation temperature. Record function, freezer identification, date, and identity of person performing the testing.
3. For units with the sensor installed in the wall or in air, apply local warmth to the site or allow the temperature of the entire compartment to rise to the point at which the alarm sounds. Remove the frozen contents or protect them with insulation while the temperature rises.
4. For units with the thermocouple located in antifreeze solution, pull the container and the cables outside the freezer chest for testing, leaving the door shut and the contents protected.
5. For units with a tracking alarm that sounds whenever the temperature reaches a constant interval above the setting on the temperature controller, set the controller to a warmer setting and note the temperature interval at which the alarm sounds.
6. Liquid-nitrogen freezers must have alarm systems that activate at an unsafe level of contained liquid nitrogen.

METHOD 8-4. CALIBRATING CENTRIFUGES FOR PLATELET SEPARATION

Principle

Successful preparation of platelet concentrates requires adequate but not excessive centrifugation; the equipment used must perform in a consistent and dependable manner. Each centrifuge used to prepare platelets should be calibrated upon receipt and after adjustment or repair. Functional calibration of the centrifuge for both the preparation of platelet-rich plasma (PRP) from whole blood and the subsequent preparation of platelet concentrates from PRP can be performed during the same procedure.

Materials

1. Freshly collected whole blood, obtained by phlebotomy into a bag with two integrally attached transfer containers.
2. A specimen of blood from the donor, anticoagulated with EDTA and collected in addition to the specimens drawn for routine processing.
3. Metal clips and hand sealer or dielectric sealer.
4. Clean instruments (scissors, hemostats, tubing stripper).
5. Plasma extractor.
6. Centrifuge suitable for preparation of platelet concentrates.
7. Worksheet for recording results.

Procedure

For Preparation of PRP

1. Perform a platelet count on the anticoagulated specimen.
2. Calculate and record the number of platelets in the Whole Blood unit: platelets/µL × 1000 × mL of whole blood = number of platelets in whole blood.
3. Prepare PRP at a selected speed and time. (See Method 6-4 for preparation of Red Blood Cells (RBCs) or see guidance provided by the centrifuge manufacturer.)
4. Place a temporary clamp on the tubing so that one satellite bag is closed off. Express the PRP into the other satellite bag. Seal the tubing close to the primary bag, leaving a long section of tubing, or the "tail." Disconnect the two satellite bags from the primary bag. Do not remove the temporary clamp between the satellite bags until the platelets are prepared (see next section).
5. Strip the tubing and "tail" several times so that they contain a representative sample of PRP.
6. Seal off a segment of the "tail" and disconnect it so that the bag of PRP remains sterile.
7. Perform a platelet count on the sample of PRP in the sealed segment. Calculate and record the number of platelets in the bag of PRP: platelets/µL × 1000 × mL of PRP = number of platelets in PRP.
8. Calculate and record the percentage of yield: (number of platelets in PRP × 100) divided by (number of platelets in whole blood) = % yield.
9. Repeat the above process three or four times with different donors, using different speeds and times of centrifugation; compare the yields achieved under each set of test conditions.
10. Select the shortest time and lowest speed combination that results in the highest percentage of platelet yield without unacceptable levels of red cell content in the PRP.
11. Record the centrifuge identification, the calibration settings selected, the date, and the identity of the person performing the calibration.

For Preparation of Platelets

1. Centrifuge the PRP (as prepared above) at a selected time and speed to prepare platelets. (See Method 6-4 for preparation of RBCs, or see the guidance provided by the centrifuge manufacturer.)

2. Remove the temporary clamp between the two satellite bags, and express the supernatant plasma into the second attached satellite bag, leaving approximately 55 to 60 mL volume in the platelet bag. Seal the tubing, leaving a long section of tubing attached to the platelet bag.
3. Allow the platelets to rest for approximately 1 hour.
4. Place the platelets on an agitator for at least 1 hour to ensure that they are evenly resuspended. Platelet counts performed immediately after centrifugation will not be accurate.
5. Strip the tubing several times, mixing tubing contents well with the contents of the platelet bag. Seal off a segment of the tubing and disconnect it, so that the platelet bag remains sterile.
6. Perform a platelet count on the contents of the segment.
7. Calculate and record the number of platelets in the concentrate: platelets/μL × 1000 × mL of platelets = number of platelets in platelet concentrate.
8. Calculate and record the percentage of yield.
9. Repeat the above process with PRP from different donors, using different speeds and times of centrifugation; compare the yields achieved under each set of test conditions.
10. Select the shortest time and lowest speed combination that results in the highest percentage of platelet yield in the platelet concentrate.
11. Record the centrifuge identification, the calibration settings selected, the date performed, and the identity of the person performing the calibration.

Notes

1. It is not necessary to perform functional recalibration of a centrifuge unless the instrument has undergone adjustments or repairs, or unless component quality control indicates that platelet counts have fallen below acceptable levels. However, timer, speed, and temperature calibrations of the centrifuge should occur on a regularly scheduled basis (see Appendix 1-4 in Chapter 1 for suggested quality control performance intervals).
2. Each centrifuge used for preparing platelets must be calibrated individually. Use the conditions determined to be optimal for each instrument.
3. When counting platelet samples on an instrument intended for whole blood, it may be necessary to use a correction factor to obtain accurate results.
4. When determining the appropriate time and speed of centrifugation, one should consider other products that will be prepared from the whole blood. Final size and hematocrit of red cell and plasma volume made available for further processing are important factors to consider.
5. In one study,[1] the average number of platelets in a typical Whole Blood unit was 1.14×10^{11}. This figure was based on an average 238,000/μL platelet count of blood donors and an average 478 mL of whole blood collected per unit. PRP from such units contained 8.3×10^{10} platelets, and the platelet concentrates contained 7.9×10^{10} platelets.[1] Average yield in a platelet concentrate was 69%.[1]
6. In one study,[2] platelet concentrate samples collected in dry K_2EDTA (1.5 mg/mL) and then counted in a flow cell cytometer gave higher platelet counts than the samples collected without the EDTA—probably the result of microaggregates in samples without EDTA.

References

1. Kahn R, Cossette I, Friedman L. Optimum centrifugation conditions for the preparation of platelet and plasma products. Transfusion 1976;16:162-5.
2. McShine R, Das P, Smit Sibinga C, Brozovic B. Effect of EDTA on platelet parameters in blood and blood components collected with CPDA-1. Vox Sang 1991; 61:84-9.

METHOD 8-5. CALIBRATING A SEROLOGIC CENTRIFUGE

Principle

Each centrifuge should be calibrated upon receipt, after adjustments or repairs, and periodically. Calibration evaluates the behavior of red cells in solutions of different viscosities, not the reactivity of different antibodies.

For Immediate Agglutination

Materials

1. Test tubes, 10 × 75 mm or 12 × 75 mm (whichever size is routinely used in the laboratory).
2. Worksheet for recording results.
3. For saline-active antibodies:
    - Serum from a group A person (anti-B) diluted with 6% albumin to give 1+ macroscopic agglutination (3 mL of 22% bovine albumin + 8 mL of normal saline = 6% bovine albumin). See Method 1-5.
    - *Positive control:* Group B red cells in a 2% to 5% saline suspension.
    - *Negative control:* Group A red cells in a 2% to 5% saline suspension.
4. For high-protein antibodies:
    - Anti-D diluted with 22% albumin to give 1+ macroscopic agglutination.
    - *Positive control:* D+ red cells in a 2% to 5% saline suspension.
    - *Negative control:* D– red cells in a 2% to 5% saline suspension.

Procedure

1. For each set of tests (saline and high-protein antibodies), label five test tubes for positive reactions and five for negative reactions.
2. In quantities that correspond to routine use, add diluted anti-B to each of 10 tubes for the saline test and add diluted anti-D to each of 10 tubes for the high-protein test. Add serum and reagents in quantities that correspond to routine use.
3. Add the appropriate control cell suspension to one set of tubes (one positive and one negative tube for the saline test, and one positive and one negative tube for the high-protein antibody test). Centrifuge immediately for the desired time interval (eg, 10 seconds).
4. Observe each tube for agglutination and record observations. (See example in Table 8-5-1.)
5. Repeat steps 2 and 3 for each time interval (eg, 15, 20, 30, and 45 seconds). Do not allow cells and sera to incubate before centrifugation.
6. Select the optimal time of centrifugation, which is the shortest time required to fulfill the following criteria:
    a. The supernatant fluid is clear.

TABLE 8-5-1. Example of Serologic Centrifuge Test Results*

	Time in Seconds				
Criteria	**10**	**15**	**20**	**30**	**45**
Supernatant fluid is clear	No	No	Yes	Yes	Yes
Cell button is clearly delineated	No	No	No	Yes	Yes
Cells are easily resuspended	Yes	Yes	Yes	Yes	Yes
Agglutination is observed	±	±	1+	1+	1+
Negative tube is negative	Yes	Yes	Yes	Yes	Resuspends roughly

*The optimal time for centrifugation in this example is 30 seconds.

b. The cell button is clearly delineated and the periphery is sharply defined, not fuzzy.
c. The cell button is easily resuspended.
d. Agglutination in the positive tubes is as strong as determined in preparing reagents.
e. There is no agglutination or ambiguity in the negative tubes.

In the example shown in Table 8-5-1, these criteria are met by the 30-second and the 45-second spins; the optimal time for these tests in this centrifuge is 30 seconds.

7. Record centrifuge identification, the times selected, the date, and the identity of the person performing the calibration.

For Washing and Antiglobulin Testing

Tests in which antihuman globulin (AHG) serum is added to red cells may require centrifugation conditions different from those for immediate agglutination. Centrifugation conditions appropriate for both washing and AHG reactions can be determined in one procedure. Note that this procedure does not monitor the completeness of washing; use of IgG-coated cells to control negative AHG reactions provides this check. The following procedure addresses only the mechanics of centrifugation.

Materials

1. AHG reagent, unmodified.
2. Saline, large volumes.
3. Test tubes, 10 × 75 mm or 12 × 75 mm (whichever size is routinely used in the laboratory).
4. Worksheet for recording results.
5. *Positive control:* a 2% to 5% saline suspension of D+ red cells incubated for 15 minutes at 37 C with anti-D diluted to give 1+ macroscopic agglutination after addition of AHG.
6. *Negative control:* a 2% to 5% suspension of D+ red cells incubated for 15 minutes at 37 C with 6% albumin. (Note: D– red cells incubated with diluted anti-D may also be used as a negative control.)

Procedure

1. Prepare five test tubes containing 1 drop of positive cells and five tubes containing 1 drop of negative control cells.
2. Fill tubes with saline and centrifuge them in pairs, one positive and one negative, for different times (eg, 30, 45, 60, 90, and 120 seconds). The red cells should form a clearly delineated button, with minimal cells trailing up the side of the tube. After the saline has been decanted, the cell button should be easily resuspended in the residual fluid. The optimal time for washing is the shortest time that accomplishes these goals.
3. Repeat washing process on all pairs three more times, using time determined to be optimal.
4. Decant supernatant saline thoroughly.
5. Add AHG to one positive control test tube and one negative control test tube. Centrifuge immediately for the desired interval (eg, 10 seconds).
6. Observe each tube for agglutination and record observations.
7. Repeat steps 5 and 6 for each interval (eg, 15, 20, 30, and 45 seconds). Do not allow cells and AHG to incubate before centrifugation.
8. Select optimal time as in immediate agglutination procedure.
9. Record centrifuge identification, the times selected, the date, and the identity of the person performing the calibration.

Note

Periodic recalibration is performed to verify that the timing in use continues to be the optimal timing. This may be accomplished by using a shortened version of the procedures outlined above. For example, use the current timing for a particular centrifuge and each medium and those times just above and just below the current timing.

METHOD 8-6. TESTING AUTOMATIC CELL WASHERS

Principle

Antihuman globulin (AHG) is inactivated readily by unbound immunoglobulin. The red cells to which AHG will be added must be washed free of all proteins and suspended in a protein-free medium. A properly functioning cell washer must add large volumes of saline to each tube, resuspend the cells, centrifuge them adequately to avoid excessive red cell loss, and decant the saline to leave a dry cell button.

Materials

1. Test tubes routinely used in the laboratory, 10 × 75 mm or 12 × 75 mm.
2. Additive routinely used to potentiate antigen-antibody reactions.
3. Human serum, from patient or donor.
4. IgG-coated red cells known to give a 1 to 2+ reaction in antiglobulin testing.
5. Normal saline.
6. AHG reagent, anti-IgG or polyspecific.
7. Worksheet for recording results.

Procedure

1. To each of 12 tubes, add potentiator and human serum in quantities that correspond to routine use, and 1 drop of IgG-coated red cells.
2. Place the tubes in a centrifuge carrier, seat the carrier in the cell washer, and start the wash cycle.
3. After addition of saline in the second cycle, stop the cell washer. Inspect the contents of all tubes. There should be an approximately equal volume of saline in all tubes; some variation is acceptable. Tubes should be approximately 80% full, to avoid splashing and cross-contamination. (Refer to manufacturer's instructions for specific requirements.) Record observations.
4. Observe all tubes to see that the red cells have been completely resuspended. Record observations.
5. Continue the washing cycle.
6. After addition of saline in the third cycle, stop the cell washer and inspect tubes as above. Record observations.
7. Complete the wash cycle.
8. At the end of the wash cycle, inspect all tubes to see that saline has been completely decanted and that each tube contains a dry cell button. Record observations.
9. Add AHG according to the manufacturer's directions, centrifuge, and examine all tubes for agglutination. If the cell washer is functioning properly, the size of the cell button should be the same in all tubes. All tubes should show the same degree of agglutination. Record observations.
10. Record identity of centrifuge, the date of testing, and the identity of the person performing the testing.

Notes

1. Further investigation is needed if:
   a. The amount of saline varies significantly from tube to tube or cycle to cycle.
   b. The cell button is not resuspended completely after being filled with saline.
   c. Any tube has weak or absent agglutination in the antiglobulin phase.
   d. Any tube has a significant decrease in the size of the cell button.
2. Cell washers that automatically add AHG should also be checked for uniform addition of AHG. In step 9 above, AHG would be added automatically, and failure of addition would be apparent by absence of agglutination. The volume of AHG should be inspected and found to be equal in all tubes. The volume of AHG delivered automatically by cell washers should be checked monthly to ensure that it is as specified in the manufacturer's directions and that delivery is uniform in all tubes.

3. Some manufacturers market AHG colored with green dye for use in automated cell washers so that it will be immediately obvious if no reagent has been added.

METHOD 8-7. MONITORING CELL COUNTS OF APHERESIS COMPONENTS

Principle

When cellular components are prepared by apheresis, it is essential to determine cell yields without compromising the sterility of the component.

Materials

1. Component collected by apheresis.
2. Metal clips and hand sealer or dielectric sealer.
3. Tubing stripper.
4. Clean instruments (scissors, hemostats).
5. Test tubes.
6. Cell-counting equipment.
7. Worksheet for recording results.

Procedure

1. Ensure that the contents of the apheresis component bag are well mixed.
2. Strip the attached tubing at least four times, mixing the contents of the tubing with the contents of the bag, to ensure that the contents of the tubing accurately represent the entire contents of the bag.
3. Seal a 5- to 8-cm (2- to 3-inch) segment distal to the collection bag. There should be approximately 2 mL of fluid in the segment. Double-seal the end of the tubing next to the component bag and detach the segment.
4. Empty the contents of the segment into a suitably labeled tube.
5. Determine and record cell counts in cells/mL.
   a. For results reported as cells/μL, change values to cells/mL by multiplying by 1000 (or 10^3).
   b. For results reported as cells/L, change values to cells/mL by dividing by 1000 (or 10^3).
6. Multiply cells/mL by the volume of the component, in mL, to obtain total cell count in the component.
7. Record component's identity, the date, and the identity of the person performing the testing.

Note

Refer to manufacturer's directions for any additional requirements.

METHOD 8-8. COUNTING RESIDUAL WHITE CELLS IN LEUKOCYTE-REDUCED BLOOD AND COMPONENTS—MANUAL METHOD

Principle

The residual white cell content of leukocyte-reduced (LR) whole blood and components can be determined using a large-volume hemocytometer. For red-cell-containing components, the red cells in the aliquot to be counted are first lysed. 0.01% Turk's solution is used to stain the leukocyte nuclei. The Nageotte counting chamber has a volume 56 times that of the standard hemocytometer. Accuracy of counting is improved by examining a larger volume of minimally diluted specimen, compared with standard counting techniques.

Materials

1. Hemocytometer chamber with 50-μL counting volume (eg, Nageotte Brite Line Chamber, Biotrans GmbH, Dreieich, Germany).
2. 0.01% Turk's solution.
3. Red cell lysing agent (eg, Zapoglobin, Coulter Electronics, Brea, CA), for red-cell-containing components only.
4. Pipettor (40 μL and 100 μL) with disposable pipette tips.

5. Talc-free gloves, clean plastic test tubes, plastic petri dish, and filter paper.
6. Light microscope with 10× ocular lens and 20× objective.
7. Worksheet for recording results.

Procedure

1. Dilute and stain LR blood and component samples as follows:
   a. For red-cell-containing components:
      1. Pipette 40 µL of lysing agent into a clean test tube.
      2. Place a representative sample of the component to be tested in a clean test tube. The hematocrit of the sample to be tested should not exceed 60%.
      3. Pipette 100 µL of the sample into the tube containing 40 µL of lysing agent. Rinse the pipette several times to mix the two fluids, until the pipette tip is no longer coated with intact red cells.
      4. Pipette 360 µL of 0.01% Turk's solution into the mixture, and mix fluids by pipetting up and down several times. The final volume is now 500 µL.
   b. For platelets:
      1. Place a representative sample of the platelet in a clean test tube.
      2. Pipette 100 µL of the platelet sample into a clean test tube.
      3. Pipette 400 µL of 0.01% of Turk's solution into the 100 µL of platelets, and mix fluids by pipetting up and down several times. The final volume is now 500 µL.
2. Fit the hemocytometer with a cover slip; using a pipette, load the mixture until the counting area is completely covered but not overflowing.
3. Cover the hemocytometer with a moist lid to prevent evaporation (a plastic petri dish into which a piece of damp filter paper has been placed works well), and let it rest undisturbed for 10 to 15 minutes to allow the white cells to settle in the counting area of the chamber.
4. Remove the moist lid, place the hemocytometer on the microscope and—using a 20× objective—count the white cells present in the entire 50-µL volume of the counting chamber. White cells appear as intact cells that are refractile with a blue gray color.
5. Calculate and record results.
   a. White cell concentration:
      leukocytes/µL = (cells counted/50 µL) × 5
      where 50 µL is the volume counted and 5 is the dilution factor resulting from the addition of lysing agent and Turk's solution.
   b. Total white cell content of the LR component:
      leukocytes/component = leukocytes/µL × 1000 µL/mL × volume in mL of the component.
6. Record the component's identity, the date obtained, and the identity of the person performing the testing.

Notes

1. White cells deteriorate during refrigerated storage; counts on stored blood or red cell components may give inaccurate results.
2. Use of talc-free gloves is recommended because talc particles that contaminate the counting chamber can be misread as white cells.
3. Filtration of the Turk's solution (0.22 micron) is recommended if the counting chamber demonstrates a large amount of particulates.
4. The accuracy of the counting method can be validated from a reference sample with a high white cell content that has been quantified by another means. This reference sample can be used for serial dilutions in blood or a component that has been rendered extremely leukocyte reduced by two passages through a leukocyte-reduction filter. Counts obtained on the serially diluted samples can be com-

pared with the expected concentration derived by calculation.

5. This counting technique is not known to be accurate at concentrations lower than 1 white cell/μL.

References

1. Lutz P, Dzik WH. Large-volume hemocytometer chamber for accurate counting of white cells (WBCs) in WBC-reduced platelets; validation and application for quality control of WBC-reduced platelets prepared by apheresis and filtration. Transfusion 1993;33:409-12.
2. Dzik WH, Szuflad P. Method for counting white cells in white cell-reduced red cell concentrates (letter). Transfusion 1993;33: 272.

Appendices

APPENDIX 1. Normal Values in Adults

Determination	SI Units	Conventional Units
Alanine aminotransferase	4-36 U/L at 37 C	4-36 U/L at 37 C
Bilirubin, total	2-21 μmol/L	0.1-1.2 mg/dL
Haptoglobin	0.6-2.7 g/L	60-270 mg/dL
Hematocrit		
Males	0.40-0.54	40-54%
Females	0.38-0.47	38-47%
Hemoglobin (Hb)		
Males	135-180 g/L	13.5-18.0 g/dL
Females	120-160 g/L	12.0-16.0 g/dL
Hemoglobin A_2	0.015-0.035 total Hb	1.5-3.5% total Hb
Hemoglobin F	0-0.01 total Hb	<1% total Hb
Hemoglobin (plasma)	5-50 mg/L	0.5-5.0 mg/dL
Immunoglobulins		
IgG	8.0-18.0 g/L	800-1801 mg/dL
IgA	1.1-5.6 g/L	113-563 mg/dL
IgM	0.5-2.2 g/L	54-222 mg/dL
IgD	5.0-30 mg/L	0.5-3.0 mg/dL
IgE	0.1-0.4 mg/L	0.01-0.04 mg/dL
Methemoglobin	<0.01 total Hb	<1% total Hb
Platelet count	$150\text{-}450 \times 10^9$/L	$150\text{-}450 \times 10^3$/μL
Red cells		
Males	$4.6\text{-}6.2 \times 10^{12}$/L	$4.6\text{-}6.2 \times 10^6$/μL
Females	$4.2\text{-}5.4 \times 10^{12}$/L	$4.2\text{-}5.4 \times 10^6$/μL
Reticulocyte count	$25\text{-}75 \times 10^9$/L	$25\text{-}75 \times 10^3$/μL
Viscosity, relative	1.4-1.8 × water	1.4-1.8 × water
White cells	$4.5\text{-}11.0 \times 10^9$/L	$4.5\text{-}11.0 \times 10^3$/μL

APPENDIX 2. Selected Normal Values in Children

Age		Bilirubin (total)	
		SI Units	Conventional Units
Cord	Preterm	<30 mmol/L	<1.8 mg/dL
	Term	<30 mmol/L	<1.8 mg/dL
0-1 day	Preterm	<137 mmol/L	<8 mg/dL
	Term	<103 mmol/L	<6 mg/dL
1-2 days	Preterm	<205 mmol/L	<12 mg/dL
	Term	<137 mmol/L	<8 mg/dL
3-7 days	Preterm	<274 mmol/L	<16 mg/dL
	Term	<205 mmol/L	<12 mg/dL
7-30 days	Preterm	<205 mmol/L	<12 mg/dL
	Term	<120 mmol/L	<7 mg/dL
Thereafter	Preterm	<34 mmol/L	<2 mg/dL
	Term	<17 mmol/L	<1 mg/dL

Age	Hemoglobin	WBC	Platelets
26-30 weeks' gestation	11.0-15.8 g/dL	1.7-7.1 $\times 10^9$/L	180,000-327,000/μL
Term	13.5-19.5 g/dL	9-30 $\times 10^9$/L	150,000-450,000/μL
1-3 days	14.5-22.5 g/dL	9.4-34 $\times 10^9$/L	213,000/μL (mean)
2 weeks	13.4-19.8 g/dL	5-20 $\times 10^9$/L	170,000-500,000/μL
1 month	10.7-17.1 g/dL	4-19.5 $\times 10^9$/L	343,000/μL (mean)
2 months	9.4-13.0 g/dL	5-15 $\times 10^9$/L	210,000-650,000/μL
6 months	11.1-14.1 g/dL	6-17.5 $\times 10^9$/L	210,000-560,000/μL
6 months-2 years	10.5-13.5 g/dL	6-17 $\times 10^9$/L	200,000-550,000/μL
2-6 years	11.5-13.5 g/dL	5-15.5 $\times 10^9$/L	210,000-490,000/μL
6-12 years	11.5-15.5 g/dL	4.5-13.5 $\times 10^9$/L	170,000-450,000/μL
12-18 years			
Male	13.0-16.9 g/dL	4.5-13.5 $\times 10^9$/L	180,000-430,000/μL
Female	12.0-16.0 g/dL	4.5-13.5 $\times 10^9$/L	180,000-430,000/μL

APPENDIX 2. Selected Normal Values in Children (Continued)

Age	IgG	IgM	IgA
Newborn	831-1231 mg/dL	6-16 mg/dL	<3 mg/dL
1-3 months	312-549 mg/dL	19-41 mg/dL	8-34 mg/dL
4-6 months	241-613 mg/dL	26-60 mg/dL	10-46 mg/dL
7-12 months	442-880 mg/dL	31-77 mg/dL	19-55 mg/dL
13-24 months	553-971 mg/dL	35-81 mg/dL	26-74 mg/dL
25-36 months	709-1075 mg/dL	42-80 mg/dL	34-108 mg/dL
3-5 years	701-1157 mg/dL	38-74 mg/dL	66-120 mg/dL
6-8 years	667-1179 mg/dL	40-80 mg/dL	79-169 mg/dL
9-11 years	889-1359 mg/dL	46-112 mg/dL	71-191 mg/dL
12-16 years	822-1070 mg/dL	39-79 mg/dL	85-211 mg/dL

Activated Partial Thromboplastin Time	
Preterm	70 seconds
Full-term	45-65 seconds

Prothrombin Time	
Preterm	12-21 seconds
Full-term	13-20 seconds

Reprinted with permission from The Harriet Lane Handbook. 15th ed. St. Louis, MO: Mosby, 2000.

APPENDIX 3. Typical Normal Values in Tests of Hemostasis and Coagulation (Adults)

Test	Normal Value
Activated partial thromboplastin time	25-35 seconds
Bleeding time	2-8 minutes
Coagulation factors	500-1500 U/L
Fibrin degradation products	<10 mg/L
Fibrinogen	2.0-4.0 g/L
Plasma D-dimers	<200 mg/L
Protein C	70-1400 U/L
Protein S (total)	70-1400 U/L
Prothrombin time	10-13 seconds
Thrombin time	17-25 seconds

Reprinted with permission from Henry JB. Clinical diagnosis and management by laboratory methods. 20th ed. Philadelphia: WB Saunders, 2001.

APPENDIX 4. Coagulation Factor Values in Platelet Concentrates

Factor/Protein	Normal Range	Day 0	Day 1	Day 2	Day 3	Day 4	Day 5
II %	78-122	104	91-96	96	85-94	90	90
V %	47-153	78-98	69-78	50	36-47	28	24-35
VII %	51-168	108	93-117	88	80-103	75	72
VIII %	48-152	68-126	85-99	76	68-76	75	39-70
IX %	62-138	72-105	100-106	95	91-98	93	63-97
X %	58-142	66-101	93-94	92	85-88	84	60-83
XI %	52-148	91-111	106-108	103	96-98	101	86-110
XII %	46-126	117	107-112	116	106-123	123	131
C %	57-128	106	102	101	98	99	100
S %	83-167	95	75	61	40	32	31
Antithrombin %	88-126	103	99	101	102	103	97
Plasminogen %	60-140	140	133	126	122	124	117
Fibrinogen mg/dL	198-434	217-308	278-313	310	265-323	302	221-299
Ristocetin cofactor %	50-150	106	124	125	133	116	127

Note: Coagulation factor % = 100 × coagulation factor units/mL.

Reproduced with permission from Brecher ME, ed. Collected questions and answers. 6th ed. Bethesda, MD: AABB, 2000.

APPENDIX 5. Approximate Normal Values for Red Cell, Plasma, and Blood Volumes

	Infant[1]		Adult[2]	
	Premature	Term Birth at 72 hours	Male	Female
Red Cell Volume mL/kg	50	40	26	24
Plasma Volume mL/kg	58	47	40	36
Blood Volume mL/kg	108	87	66	60

The adult values should be modified to correct for:

1. Below age 18: increase values by 10%.
2. Weight loss:
   a. Marked loss within 6 months—calculations made at original weight.
   b. Gradual loss over a longer time—calculations made at present weight and raised 10% to 15%.
3. Obese and short: values are reduced by 10%.
4. Elderly: values are reduced by 10%.
5. Pregnancy[3]:

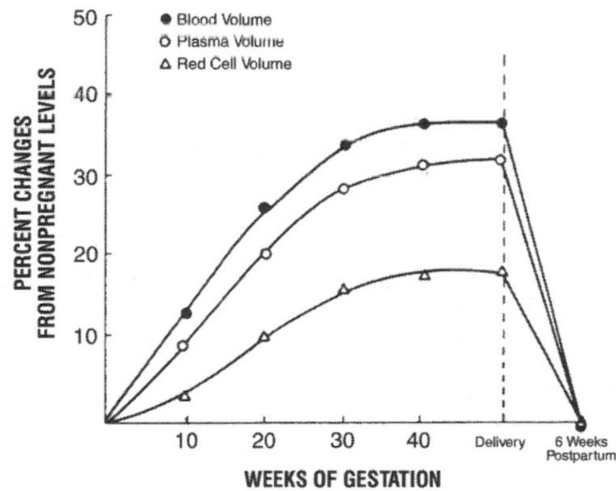

Estimation of Body Surface Area[4]:

$$BSA(m^2) = \sqrt{\frac{Ht(cm) \times Wt(kg)}{3600}} \text{ or } \sqrt{\frac{Ht(in) \times Wt(lb)}{3131}}$$

Blood Volume (BV)[5]:

$BV = 2740\ mL/m^2$—males

$BV = 2370\ mL/m^2$—females

Hematocrit[6]:

Venous hematocrit = H_V (blood obtained by vein or finger puncture)

Whole-body hematocrit = H_B

$H_B = (Hv) \times (0.91)$

References

1. Miller D. Normal values and examination of the blood: Perinatal period, infancy, childhood and adolescence. In: Miller DR, Baehner RL, McMillan CW, Miller LP, eds. Blood diseases of infancy and childhood. St. Louis: C V Mosby, 1984:21,22.
2. Albert SN. Blood volume. Springfield, IL. Charles C. Thomas, 1963:26.
3. Peck TM, Arias F. Hematologic changes associated with pregnancy. Clin Obstet Gynecol 1979; 22:788.
4. Mosteller RD. Simplfied calculation of body-surface area. N Engl J Med 1987;317:1098.
5. Shoemaker WC. Fluids and electrolytes in the acutely ill adult. In: Shoemaker WC, Ayres S, Grenvik A, et al, eds. Textbook of critical care. 2nd ed. Philadelphia: WB Saunders Co., 1989: 1130.
6. Klein HG, Anstee D. Mollison's blood transfusion in clinical medicine. 11th ed. Oxford: Blackwell Publishing, 2005:849.

APPENDIX 6. Blood Group Antigens Assigned to Systems

In 1980, the International Society of Blood Transfusion (ISBT) formed a Working Party on Terminology for Red Cell Surface Antigens. The task of this group was to devise a uniform nomenclature that would be both eye- and machine-readable. The numeric system proposed by this group was not intended to replace traditional terminology but, instead, to enable communication using computer systems where numbers are necessary. It also provides a genetical classification for blood groups. ISBT terminology uses uppercase letters and Arabic numbers for system and antigen codes. Each system, collection, or series of antigens is given a number (eg, ABO system = 001), and each antigen within the system is given a number (eg, A = 001, B = 002). Sinistral zeros may be omitted. Thus, in ISBT terminology, the A antigen would be written using computer code as 001001, or using the system symbol, as ABO1.

Periodically, the Working Party meets to update assignment of antigens to systems, collections, and series. The table below lists the blood group systems and the antigens assigned to those systems. Other red cell antigens are assigned to collections and to series of high- and low-incidence antigens. Although all terms in the table are acceptable, the *Technical Manual* and *TRANSFUSION* choose to use traditional terminology in most cases. Further information on blood group terminology, which antigens are assigned to the collections, and the series of high- and low-incidence antigens can be found in the references.

Symbol/(Number)	Antigen (ISBT Number)			
ABO (ABO/001)	A(ABO1)			
	B (ABO2)			
	A,B (ABO3)			
	A1 (ABO4)			
MNS	M (MNS1)	M^{e} (MNS13)	Dantu (MNS25)	ERIK (MNS37)
(MNS/002)	N (MNS2)	Mt^{a} (MNS14)	Hop (MNS26)	Os^{a} (MNS38)
	S (MNS3)	St^{a} (MNS15)	Nob (MNS27)	ENEP (MNS39)
	s (MNS4)	Ri^{a} (MNS16)	En^{a} (MNS28)	ENEH (MNS40)
	U (MNS5)	Cl^{a} (MNS17)	En^{a}KT (MNS29)	HAG (MNS41)
	He (MNS6)	Ny^{a} (MNS18)	'N' (MNS30)	ENAV (MNS42)
	Mi^{a} (MNS7)	Hut (MNS19)	Or (MNS31)	MARS (MNS43)
	M^{c} (MNS8)	Hil (MNS20)	DANE (MNS32)	ENDA (MNS44)
	Vw (MNS9)	M^{v} (MNS21)	TSEN (MNS33)	ENEV (MNS45)
	Mur (MNS10)	Far (MNS22)	MINY (MNS34)	MNTD (MNS46)
	M^{g} (MNS11)	s^{D} (MNS23)	MUT (MNS35)	
	Vr (MNS12)	Mit (MNS24)	SAT (MNS36)	

APPENDIX 6. Blood Group Antigens Assigned to Systems (Continued)

Symbol/(Number)	Antigen (ISBT Number)			
P (P/003)	P1 (P1)			
Rh (RH/004)	D (RH1)	Hr (RH18)	Rh33 (RH33)	CELO (RH58)
	C (RH2)	hr^S (RH19)	Hr^B (RH34)	Dav (RH47)
	E (RH3)	VS (RH20)	Rh35 (RH35)	JAL (RH48)
	c (RH4)	C^G (RH21)	Be^a (RH36)	STEM (RH49)
	e (RH5)	CE (RH22)	Evans (RH37)	FPTT (RH50)
	f (RH6)	D^W (RH23)	Rh39 (RH39)	MAR (RH51)
	Ce (RH7)	c-like (RH26)	Tar (RH40)	BARC (RH52)
	C^W (RH8)	cE (RH27)	Rh41 (RH41)	JAHK (RH53)
	C^X (RH9)	hr^H (RH28)	Rh42 (RH42)	DAK (RH54)
	V (RH10)	Rh29 (RH29)	Crawford (RH43)	LOCR (RH55)
	E^W (RH11)	Go^a (RH30)	Nou (RH44)	CENR (RH56)
	G (RH12)	hr^B (RH31)	Riv (RH45)	CEST (RH57)
	Hr_o (RH17)	Rh32 (RH32)	Sec (RH46)	
Lutheran (LU/005)	Lu^a (LU1)	Lu6 (LU6)	Lu12 (LU12)	Au^a (LU18)
	Lu^b (LU2)	Lu7 (LU7)	Lu13 (LU13)	Au^b (LU19)
	Lu3 (LU3)	Lu8 (LU8)	Lu14 (LU14)	Lu20 (LU20)
	Lu4 (LU4)	Lu9 (LU9)	Lu16 (LU16)	Lu21 (LU21)
	Lu5 (LU5)	Lu11 (LU11)	Lu17 (LU17)	
Kell (KEL/006)	K (KEL1)	K11 (KEL11)	Km (KEL20)	KUCI (KEL32)
	k (KEL2)	K12 (KEL12)	Kp^c (KEL21)	KANT (KEL33)
	Kp^a (KEL3)	K13 (KEL13)	K22 (KEL22)	KASH (KEL34)
	Kp^b (KEL4)	K14 (KEL14)	K23 (KEL23)	VONG (KEL28)
	Ku (KEL5)	K16 (KEL16)	K24 (KEL24)	KALT (KEL29)
	Js^a (KEL6)	K17 (KEL17)	VLAN (KEL25)	KTIM (KEL30)
	Js^b (KEL7)	K18 (KEL18)	TOU (KEL26)	KYO (KEL31)
	Ul^a (KEL10)	K19 (KEL19)	RAZ (KEL27)	

(Continued)

APPENDIX 6. Blood Group Antigens Assigned to Systems (Continued)

Symbol/(Number)		Antigen (ISBT Number)		
Lewis (LE/007)	Le^a (LE1)	Le^{bH} (LE4)		
	Le^b (LE2)	ALe^b (LE5)		
	Le^{ab} (LE3)	BLe^b (LE6)		
Duffy (FY/008)	Fy^a (FY1)	Fy4 (FY4)		
	Fy^b (FY2)	Fy5 (FY5)		
	Fy3 (FY3)	Fy6 (FY6)		
Kidd (JK/009)	Jk^a (JK1)			
	Jk^b (JK2)			
	Jk3 (JK3)			
Diego (DI/010)	Di^a (DI1)	WARR (DI7)	Vg^a (DI13)	Fr^a (DI20)
	Di^b (DI2)	ELO (DI8)	Sw^a (DI14)	SW1 (DI21)
	Wr^a (DI3)	Wu (DI9)	BOW (DI15)	
	Wr^b (DI4)	Bp^a (DI10)	NFLD (DI16)	
	Wd^a (DI5)	Mo^a (DI11)	Jn^a (DI17)	
	Rb^a (DI6)	Hg^a (DI12)	KREP (DI18)	
			Tr^a (DI19)*	
Yt (YT/011)	Yt^a (YT1)			
	Yt^b (YT2)			
Xg (XG/012)	Xg^a (XG1)	CD99 (XG2)		
Scianna (SC/013)	Sc1 (SC1)	Rd (SC4)	SCAN (SC7)	
	Sc2 (SC2)	STAR (SC5)		
	Sc3 (SC3)	SCER (SC6)		

APPENDIX 6. Blood Group Antigens Assigned to Systems (Continued)

Symbol/(Number)	Antigen (ISBT Number)		
Dombrock (DO/014)	Do^a (DO1)		
	Do^b (DO2)		
	Gy^a (DO3)		
	Hy (DO4)		
	Jo^a (DO5)		
	DOYA (DO6)		
Colton (CO/015)	Co^a (CO1)		
	Co^b (CO2)		
	Co3 (CO3)		
Landsteiner-Wiener (LW/016)	LW^a (LW5)		
	LW^{ab} (LW6)		
	LW^b (LW7)		
Chido/Rodgers (CH/RG /017)	Ch1 (CH/RG1)	Rg1 (CH/RG11)	
	Ch2 (CH/RG2)	Rg2 (CH/RG12)	
	Ch3 (CH/RG3)		
	Ch4 (CH/RG4)		
	Ch5 (CH/RG5)		
	Ch6 (CH/RG6)		
	WH (CH/RG7)		
H (H/018)	H (H1)		
Kx (XK/019)	Kx (XK1)		
Gerbich (GE/020)	Ge2 (GE2)	Wb (GE5)	Dh^a (GE8)
	Ge3 (GE3)	Ls^a (GE6)	GEIS (GE9)
	Ge4 (GE4)	An^a (GE7)	

(Continued)

APPENDIX 6. Blood Group Antigens Assigned to Systems (Continued)

Symbol/(Number)	Antigen (ISBT Number)			
Cromer (CROM/021)	Cr^a (CROM1)	Dr^a (CROM5)	WES^b (CROM9)	ZENA (CROM13)
	Tc^a (CROM2)	Es^a (CROM6)	UMC (CROM10)	CROV (CROM14)
	Tc^b (CROM3)	IFC (CROM7)	GUTI (CROM11)	CRAM (CROM15)
	Tc^c (CROM4)	WES^a (CROM8)	SERF (CROM12)	
Knops (KN/022)	Kn^a (KN1)	McC^a (KN3)	Yk^a (KN5)	Sl2 (KN7)
	Kn^b (KN2)	Sl1 (KN4)	McC^b (KN6)	Sl3 (KN8)*
				KCAM (KN9)
Indian (IN/023)	In^a (IN1)	INFI (IN3)		
	In^b (IN2)	INJA (IN4)		
Ok (OK/024)	Ok^a (OK1)			
Raph (RAPH/025)	MER2 (RAPH1)			
John Milton Hagen (JMH/026)	JMH (JMH1)	JMHL (JMH3)	JMHM (JMH5)	
	JMHK (JMH2)	JMHG (JMH4)		
I (I/027)	I (I1)			
Globoside (GLOB/028)	P (GLOB1)			
Gill (GIL/029)	GIL (GIL1)			
RHAG (RHAG/030)	Duclos (RHAG1)	Ol^a (RHAG2)	Duclos-like (RHAG3)	

*Provisional.

Daniels GL, Fletcher A, Garratty G, et al. Blood group terminology 2004. From the ISBT committee on terminology for Red Cell Surface Antigens. Vox Sang 2004;87:304-16.

Daniels G, Flegel WH, Fletcher A, et al. International Society of Blood Transfusion Committee on Terminology for Red Cell Surface Antigens: Cape Town report. Vox Sang 2007;92:250-3.

Garratty G, Dzik W, Issitt PD, et al. Terminology for blood group antigens and genes—historical origins and guidelines in the new millennium. Transfusion 2000;40:477-89.

Daniels G. Human blood groups. 2nd ed. Oxford: Blackwell Science, 2002.

APPENDIX 7. Examples of Gene, Antigen, and Phenotype Symbols in Conventional and International Society of Blood Transfusion Terminology

System	Genes*	Antigens	Phenotypes
ABO	$A\ A^1\ A^2\ B$	A A1 B	A A_1 A_2 B A_1B
Rh	*D C c E e* *RH*1 RH*2*	D C c E e RH1 RH2	D+ C+ c+ E− e+ RH:1,2,3,−4,5
MNS	*M N S s* *MNS*1 MNS*4*	M N S s MNS1 MNS4	M+ N+ S− s+ MNS:1,2,−3,4
Lewis	*Le le*	Le^a Le^b LE1 LE2	Le(a+) Le(a−b+) LE:−1,2
Kell	$K\ k\ Kp^a\ Kp^b$ *KEL*1 KEL*3*	K k Kp^a Kp^b KEL1 KEL3	K− k+ Kp(a+) Js(a−) KEL:−1,2,3,−6
Kidd	$Jk^a\ Jk^b$ *JK*1 JK*2*	Jk^a Jk^b Jk3 JK1 JK2 JK3	Jk(a+b−) Jk:3 JK:1,−2,3

*Serologically defined alleles.

Daniels GL, Fletcher A, Garratty G, et al. Blood group terminology 2004. From the ISBT Committee on Terminology for Red Cell Surface Antigens. Vox Sang 2004;87:304-16. [Available at http://blood.co.uk/ibgrl > ISBT Terminology and Workshops > ISBT Committee on Terminology for Red Cell Surface Antigens.]

APPENDIX 8. Examples of Correct and Incorrect Terminology*

Term Description	Correct Terminology	Incorrect Terminology
Phenotype	Fy(a+)	Fy^{a+}, $Fy^{(a+)}$, $Fya^{(+)}$, Fya(+), $Duffy^a$+, $Duffy^a$-positive
Phenotype	Fy(a+b−)	Fy^{a+b-}, $Fy^{(a+b-)}$, $Fy^a(+)^b(-)$, $Fy^{a(+)b(-)}$
Antibody	Anti-Fy^a	Anti Fy^a, Anti-Duffy
Antigen	K	Kell (name of system), K1
Antibody	Anti-k	Anti-Cellano, anti-K2
Phenotype	KEL:1, KEL:−2	KEL1+, K1+, KEL(1), K(1), KEL1−, KEL1-negative, K1-negative
Phenotype	A Rh+, B Rh−	A+ (means positive for A antigen) B− (means negative for B antigen)
Phenotype	M+ N−	M(+), MM (implies unproven genotype)
Phenotype	RH:−1,−2,−3,4,5	RH:−1,−2,−3,+4,+5 RH:−1,−2,−3, 4+,5+

*Modified from Issitt L. Blood group nomenclature. In: Blood groups: Refresher and updates (syllabus). Bethesda, MD: AABB, 1995.

Note: The examples shown may not represent the only correct terminologies. In the Rh system, for example, use of CDE terminology is also acceptable and is more commonly used.

APPENDIX 9. Distribution of ABO/Rh Phenotypes by Race or Ethnicity*

Race or Ethnicity	Number	Phenotype Distribution (%)†							
		O Rh+	O Rh–	A Rh+	A Rh–	B Rh+	B Rh–	AB Rh+	AB Rh–
White non-Hispanic	2,215,623	37.2	8.0	33.0	6.8	9.1	1.8	3.4	0.7
Hispanic‡	259,233	52.6	3.9	28.7	2.4	9.2	0.7	2.3	0.2
Black non-Hispanic	236,050	46.6	3.6	24.0	1.9	18.4	1.3	4.0	0.3
Asian§	126,780	39.0	0.7	27.3	0.5	25.0	0.4	7.0	0.1
North American Indian	19,664	50.0	4.7	31.3	3.8	7.0	0.9	2.2	0.3
All donors	3,086,215	39.8	6.9	31.5	5.6	10.6	1.6	3.5	0.6

*Used with permission from Garratty G, Glynn SA, McEntire R, et al for the Retrovirus Epidemiology Donor Study. ABO and Rh(D) phenotype frequencies of different racial/ethnic groups in the United States. Transfusion 2004;44:703-6.

†Percentages may not add up to 100.0% because of rounding.

‡Hispanic includes Mexican (68.8%), Puerto Rican (5.0%), Cuban (1.6%), and other Hispanic donors (24.6%).

§Asian includes Chinese (29.8%), Filipino (24.1%), Indian (13.8%), Japanese (12.7%), Korean (12.5%), and Vietnamese (7.1%) donors.

APPENDIX 10. Example of a Maximum Surgical Blood Order Schedule

Procedure	Units*	Procedure	Units*
General Surgery		*Orthopedics*	
Breast biopsy	T/S	Arthroscopy	T/S
Colon resection	2	Laminectomy	T/S
Exploratory laparotomy	T/S	Spinal fusion	3
Gastrectomy	2	Total hip replacement	3
Laryngectomy	2	Total knee replacement	T/S
Mastectomy, radical	T/S	*Obstetrics/Gynecology*	
Pancreatectomy	4	Abdomino-perineal repair	T/S
Splenectomy	2	Cesarean section	T/S
Thyroidectomy	T/S	Dilation and curettage	T/S
Cardiac-Thoracic		Hysterectomy, abdominal	T/S
Aneurism resection	6	Hysterectomy, laparoscopic	T/S
Redo coronary artery bypass graft	4	Hysterectomy, radical	2
Primary coronary artery bypass graft	2	*Urology*	
Lobectomy	T/S	Bladder, transurethral resection	T/S
Lung biopsy	T/S	Nephrectomy, radical	3
Vascular		Prostatectomy, transurethral	T/S
Aortic bypass with graft	4	Radical prostatectomy, perineal	2
Endarterectomy	T/S	Renal transplant	2
Femoral-popliteal bypass with graft	2		

*Numbers may vary with institutional practice.
T/S = type and screen.

APPENDIX 11. Directory of Organizations

AABB
8101 Glenbrook Road
Bethesda, MD 20814-2749
(301) 907-6977
Fax: (301) 907-6895
http://www.aabb.org

American Association of Tissue Banks (AATB)
1320 Old Chain Bridge Road, Suite 450
McLean, VA 22101
(703) 827-9582
Fax: (703) 356-2198
http://www.aatb.org

American Medical Association (AMA)
515 N. State Street
Chicago, IL 60654
(800) 621-8335
http://www.ama-assn.org

American Red Cross (ARC)
National Headquarters
2025 E Street, NW
Washington, DC 20006
(800) 733-2767
http://www.redcross.org

American Society for Apheresis (ASFA)
375 West 5th Avenue, Suite 201
Vancouver, BC, V5Y 1J6, Canada
(604) 484-2851
Fax: (604) 874-4378
http://www.apheresis.org

American Society for Clinical Pathology (ASCP)
35 West Monroe Street, Suite 1600
Chicago, IL 60603
(800) 267-2727
Fax: (312) 541-4998
http://www.ascp.org

American Society for Histocompatibility and Immunogenetics (ASHI)
15000 Commerce Parkway, Suite C
Mount Laurel, NJ 08054
(856) 638-0428
Fax: (856) 439-0525
http://www.ashi-hla.org

American Society of Anesthesiologists (ASA)
520 N. Northwest Highway
Park Ridge, IL 60068-2573
(847) 825-5586
Fax: (847) 825-1692
www.asahq.org

American Society of Hematology (ASH)
2021 L Street, NW, Suite 900
Washington, DC 20036
(202) 776-0544
Fax: (202) 776-0545
http://www.hematology.org

American Society of Pediatric Hematology/Oncology
4700 W. Lake Avenue
Glenview, IL 60025
(847) 375-4716
http://www.aspho.org

America's Blood Centers (ABC)
725 15th Street, NW, Suite 700
Washington, DC 20005
(202) 393-5725
Fax: (202) 393-1282
http://www.americasblood.org

Armed Services Blood Program Office (ASBPO)
5109 Leesburg Pike, Suite 698
Falls Church, VA 22041-3258
(703) 681-8024
Fax: (703) 681-7541
http://www.militaryblood.dod.mil

Association of Donor Recruitment Professionals (ADRP)
P.O. Box 150790
Austin, TX 78715
(512) 658-9414
Fax: (866) 498-6527
http://www.adrp.org

APPENDIX 11. Directory of Organizations (Continued)

College of American Pathologists (CAP)
325 Waukegan Road
Northfield, IL 60093-2750
(800) 323-4040
Fax: (847) 832-8000
http://www.cap.org

Foundation for the Accreditation of Cellular Therapy (FACT)
c/o University of Nebraska Medical Center
986065 Nebraska Medical Center
Omaha, NE 68198-6065
(402) 559-1950
Fax: (402) 559-1951
http://www.factwebsite.org

ICCBBA, Inc.
P.O. Box 11309
San Bernardino, CA 92423-1309
(909) 793-6516
Fax: (909) 793-6214
http://www.iccbba.org

International Society for Cellular Therapy (ISCT)
375 West 5th Avenue, Suite 201
Vancouver, BC, V5Y 1J6, Canada
(604) 874-4366
Fax: (604) 874-4378
http://www.celltherapysociety.org

International Society of Blood Transfusion (ISBT)
Jan van Goyenkade 11
1075 HP Amsterdam
The Netherlands
+ 31 (0) 20 570 9636
Fax: + 31 (0) 20 673 7306
http://www.isbt-web.org

The Joint Commission (TJC)
1 Renaissance Boulevard
Oakbrook Terrace, IL 60181
(630) 792-5000
Fax: (630) 792-5005
http://www.jointcommission.org

National Heart, Lung, and Blood Institute
Bldg. 31,Room 5A52
31 Center Drive, MSC 2486
Bethesda, MD 20892
(301) 592-8573
Fax: (240) 629-3246
http://www.nhlbi.nih.gov

National Hemophilia Foundation (NHF)
116 West 32nd Street, 11th Floor
New York, NY 10001
(212) 328-3700
Fax: (212) 328-3777
http://www.hemophilia.org

National Marrow Donor Program (NMDP)
3001 Broadway Street NE, Suite 100
Minneapolis, MN 55413-1753
(800) 627-7692; (612) 627-5800
http://www.marrow.org

Plasma Protein Therapeutics Association (PPTA)
147 Old Solomons Island Road, Suite 100
Annapolis, MD 21401
(202) 789-3100
Fax: (410) 263-2298
http://www.pptaglobal.org

Society for the Advancement of Blood Management
350 Engle Street
Englewood, NJ 07631
(602) 343-7458; (480) 699-6763
Fax: (602) 343-2301
http://www.sabm.org

United Network for Organ Sharing (UNOS)
P.O. Box 2484
Richmond, VA 23218
(804) 782-4800
Fax: (804) 782-4817
http://www.unos.org

APPENDIX 12. Resources for Safety Information

Centers for Disease Control and Prevention (CDC)
Office of Health and Safety, Biosafety Branch
Mail Stop F-05
1600 Clifton Road
Atlanta, GA 30333
(800) 232-4636
Fax: (770) 488-4760
http://www.cdc.gov/od/ohs

Clinical and Laboratory Standards Institute (CLSI)
940 West Valley Road, Suite 1400
Wayne, PA 19087-1898
(610) 688-0100
Fax: (610) 688-0700
http://www.clsi.org

Department of Transportation (DOT)
Office of Hazardous Materials Standards
1200 New Jersey Ave. S.E. (East Bldg., 2nd Floor)
Washington, DC 20590
(202) 366-4433
Fax: (202) 366-3666
DOT Hazardous Materials Information Center: (800) 467-4922
http://hazmat.dot.gov

Environmental Protection Agency (EPA)
Office of Emergency Management (5104A)
1200 Pennsylvania Avenue, NW
Washington, DC 20460
(202)564-8600
http://www.epa.gov/emergencies

Environmental Protection Agency (EPA)
Office of Solid Waste (5305P)
1200 Pennsylvania Avenue, NW
Washington, DC 20460
(800) 424-9346
http://www.epa.gov/waste

Food and Drug Administration (FDA)
Center for Biologics Evaluation and Research
Division of Blood Applications, HFM-370
1401 Rockville Pike
Rockville, MD 20852-1448
(301) 827-1800
FAX: (301) 827-3535
http://www.fda.gov/cber

International Air Transport Association (IATA)
800 Place Victoria, P.O. Box 113
Montreal, QC, H4Z 1M1, Canada
(514) 874-0202
Fax: (514) 874-9632
http://www.iata.org

International Civil Aviation Organization (ICAO)
999 University Street
Montreal, QC, H3C 5H7, Canada
(514) 954-8219
Fax: (514) 954-6077
http://www.icao.int

National Fire Protection Association (NFPA)
1 Batterymarch Park
Quincy, MA 02169-7471
(617) 770-3000
Fax: (617) 770-0700
http://www.nfpa.org

National Institute for Occupational Safety and Health (NIOSH)
Education and Information Division
4676 Columbia Parkway
Cincinnati, OH 45226-1998
(800) 232-4636; (513) 533-8328
Fax: (513) 533-8347
Clinicians' Postexposure Prophylaxis Hotline: (888) 448-4911
http://www.cdc.gov/niosh

National Institutes of Health (NIH)
Division of Occupational Health and Safety
13 South Drive, MSC 5760
(Bldg. 13, Room 3K04)
Bethesda, MD 20892-0003
(301) 496-2960
Fax: (301) 402-0313
http://dohs.ors.od.nih.gov

Nuclear Regulatory Commission (NRC)
11555 Rockville Pike
Rockville, MD 20852-2738
(800) 368-5642; (301) 415-7000
Fax: (301) 415-8200
For Safety and Security Concerns: (800) 695-7403
http://www.nrc.gov

APPENDIX 12. Resources for Safety Information (Continued)

Occupational Safety and Health Administration (OSHA)
200 Constitution Avenue, NW
Washington, DC 20210
(800) 321-6742
http://www.osha.gov

US Postal Service (USPS)
475 L'Enfant Plaza, SW
Washington, DC 20260
(800) 275-8777
http://www.usps.com

Index

Page numbers in italics refer to figures or tables

B

C

E

G

H

I

J

K

L

M

N

S

T

U

V

W

X

Y-Z